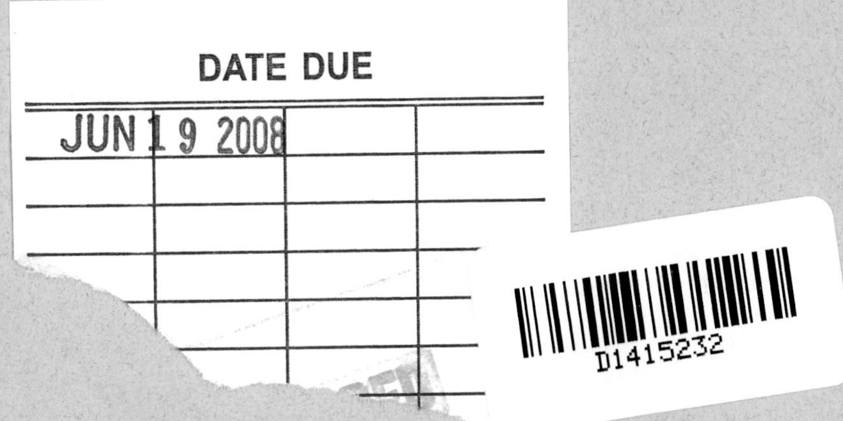

Pediatric Orthopaedics and Sports Medicine

THE REQUISITES IN PEDIATRICS

SERIES EDITOR **Louis M. Bell,** M.D.
Patrick S. Pasquariello, Jr. Professor of Pediatrics
University of Pennsylvania School of Medicine
Chief, Division of General Pediatrics
The Children's Hospital of Philadelphia
Philadelphia, Pennsylvania

COMING SOON IN
THE REQUISITES IN PEDIATRICS SERIES

Endocrinology

Nephrology and Urology

Toxicology

Pulmonology

Cardiology

Infectious Diseases

Pediatric Orthopaedics and Sports Medicine

THE REQUISITES IN PEDIATRICS

John P. Dormans, M.D.
Professor of Orthopaedic Surgery
University of Pennsylvania School of Medicine
Chief of Orthopaedic Surgery
The Children's Hospital of Philadelphia
Philadelphia, Pennsylvania

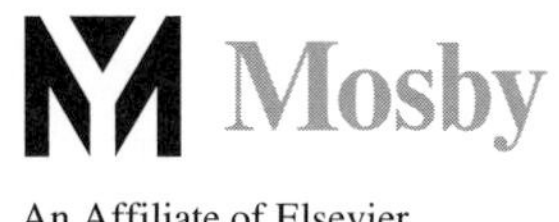

An Affiliate of Elsevier

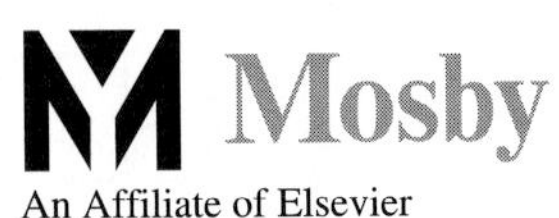

An Affiliate of Elsevier

11830 Westline Industrial Drive
St. Louis, Missouri 63146

THE REQUISITES
THE REQUISITES
THE REQUISITES
THE REQUISITES
THE REQUISITES
™

Acquisitions Editor: Judith Fletcher
Developmental Editor: Kimberley Cox
Project Manager: Jeff Gunning

PEDIATRIC ORTHOPAEDICS AND SPORTS MEDICINE: THE REQUISITES IN PEDIATRICS
ISBN 0-323-01826-2

Notice

Pediatrics is an ever-changing field. Standard safety precautions must be followed, but as new research and clinical experience broaden our knowledge, changes in treatment and drug therapy may become necessary or appropriate. Readers are advised to check the most current product information provided by the manufacturer of each drug to be administered to verify the recommended dose, the method and duration of administration, and contraindications. It is the responsibility of the treating physician, relying on experience and knowledge of the patient, to determine dosages and the best treatment for each individual patient. Neither the Publisher nor the editor assumes any liability for any injury and/or damage to persons or property arising from this publication.

The Publisher

First Edition 2004.

Library of Congress Cataloging-in-Publication Data

Pediatric orthopaedics and sports medicine: the requisites in pediatrics / edited by John P. Dormans.
p. cm.
ISBN 0-323-01826-2
1. Pediatric orthopedics. 2. Pediatric sports medicine. I. Dormans, John P.
[DNLM: 1. Bone Diseases—Child. 2. Bone and Bones—injuries—Child. 3. Orthopedics—methods—Child. 4. Sports Medicine—methods—Child. WE 225 P371 2004]
RD732.3.C48P433 2004
618.92′7—dc22 2003044272

Printed in the United States of America.

Last digit is the print number: 9 8 7 6 5 4 3 2 1

About the Editor

John P. Dormans, M.D., is Chief of Orthopaedic Surgery at The Children's Hospital of Philadelphia (CHOP) and Professor of Orthopaedic Surgery at the University of Pennsylvania School of Medicine. He holds The Children's Hospital of Philadelphia Endowed Chair in Pediatric Orthopaedic Surgery and is a Research Associate at the Stokes Research Institute at CHOP. He also is Co-director of the Pediatric Orthopaedic Fellowship at CHOP.

Dr. Dormans completed a pediatric orthopaedic fellowship at the Hospital for Sick Children in Toronto, Ontario, Canada. Dr. Dormans has been at CHOP and the University of Pennsylvania School of Medicine since 1990 and has been the recipient of both the Jesse T. Nicholson Award for Excellence in Clinical Teaching (awarded by the senior Orthopaedic Residency Class of 1993) and also the Dean's Award for Excellence in Clinical Teaching from the University of Pennsylvania School of Medicine (in 1995). He was a Sashawegi Suzuki traveling fellow to Japan in 1996 and completed both the Program for Chiefs of Clinical Services and the Advanced Program for Chiefs of Clinical Services at the Harvard School of Public Health Department of Health Policy and Management. He has served as President of the Medical Staff at CHOP and twice as President of Children's Surgical Associates, the multispecialty surgical group at CHOP. His practice focuses on children with spinal deformity and musculoskeletal tumors.

Dr. Dormans has published more than 150 articles, has authored more than 65 chapters in various books, and has edited or coedited 4 medical textbooks. He is an Associate Editor for the *Journal of Bone and Joint Surgery*, is an Advisory Editor for *Clinical Orthopaedics and Related Research*, and is on the editorial board of the *Journal of Pediatric Orthopaedics*. He serves on the board of directors of the Pediatric Orthopaedic Society of North America and the Scoliosis Research Society.

Dr. Dormans has a strong interest in orthopaedic care of children in developing countries. He serves on the International Affairs Committee of the American Academy of Orthopaedic Surgeons. He has worked in various countries, including Ethiopia, Bulgaria, Uganda, and Indonesia, and currently serves as Chairman of the Board of Directors for Orthopaedics Overseas. Dr. Dormans lives in Gladwyne, Pennsylvania, with his wife and four children.

Contributors

Benjamin Chang, M.D. Assistant Professor, Department of Surgery, Division of Plastic Surgery, University of Pennsylvania School of Medicine; Assistant Surgeon, The Children's Hospital of Philadelphia, Philadelphia, Pennsylvania

Lawson A. B. Copley, M.D. Clinical Assistant Professor, University of Texas Southwestern; Staff Orthopaedic Surgeon, Children's Medical Center of Dallas and Texas Scottish Rite Hospital for Children, Dallas, Texas

Randy Q. Cron, M.D., Ph.D. Assistant Professor of Pediatrics, University of Pennsylvania School of Medicine; Attending Physician, Division of Rheumatology, The Children's Hospital of Philadelphia, Philadelphia, Pennsylvania

Richard S. Davidson, M.D. Associate Professor, Department of Pediatrics, University of Pennsylvania School of Medicine; Staff Physician, The Children's Hospital of Philadelphia and Shriners Hospital of Philadelphia, Philadelphia, Pennsylvania

John P. Dormans, M.D. Chief of Orthopaedic Surgery, The Children's Hospital of Philadelphia, Professor of Orthopaedic Surgery, University of Pennsylvania School of Medicine; Philadelphia, Pennsylvania

Denis S. Drummond, M.D. Professor of Orthopaedic Surgery, University of Pennsylvania School of Medicine; Emeritus Director, Orthopaedic Surgery, The Children's Hospital of Philadelphia, Philadelphia, Pennsylvania

Bulent Erol, M.D. Research Fellow, The Children's Hospital of Philadelphia, Philadelphia, Pennsylvania

Richard S. Finkel, M.D. Clinical Associate Professor in Neurology and Pediatrics, University of Pennsylvania School of Medicine; Director, Neuromuscular Program, The Children's Hospital of Philadelphia, Philadelphia, Pennsylvania

John M. Flynn, M.D. Assistant Orthopaedic Surgeon, The Children's Hospital of Philadelphia; Assistant Professor of Orthopaedic Surgery, University of Pennsylvania School of Medicine, Philadelphia, Pennsylvania

Theodore J. Ganley, M.D. Assistant Professor of Orthopaedic Surgery, University of Pennsylvania School of Medicine; Orthopaedic Director of Sports Medicine, The Children's Hospital of Philadelphia, Philadelphia, Pennsylvania

John R. Gregg, M.D. Clinical Associate Professor of Surgery, University of Pennsylvania School of Medicine; Senior Surgeon, The Children's Hospital of Philadelphia, Philadelphia, Pennsylvania

B. David Horn, M.D. Assistant Professor of Orthopaedic Surgery, University of Pennsylvania School of Medicine; Attending Pediatric Orthopaedic Surgeon, The Children's Hospital of Philadelphia, Philadelphia, Pennsylvania

Frederick S. Kaplan, M.D. Isaac & Rose Nassau Professor of Orthopaedic Molecular Medicine, Chief, Division of Metabolic Bone Diseases and Molecular Medicine, Department of Orthopaedic Surgery, Hospital of the University of Pennsylvania, Philadelphia, Pennsylvania

Bong S. Lee, M.D. Clinical Associate Professor of Orthopedic Surgery, University of Pennsylvania School of Medicine; Director of Pediatric Hand Surgery, The Children's Hospital of Philadelphia, Philadelphia, Pennsylvania

Julia E. Lou, B.A. Research Coordinator, The Children's Hospital of Philadelphia, Philadelphia, Pennsylvania

Sameer Nagda, M.D. Clinical Instructor, Department of Orthopaedic Surgery, University of Pennsylvania School of Medicine, Philadelphia, Pennsylvania

Bruce R. Pawel, M.D. Assistant Professor, Department of Pathology and Laboratory Medicine, University of Pennsylvania School of Medicine; Pathologist, The Children's Hospital of Philadelphia, Philadelphia, Pennsylvania

Kristan A. Pierz, M.D. Assistant Professor of Orthopaedics, University of Connecticut School of Medicine; Orthopaedic Surgeon, Connecticut Children's Medical Center, Hartford, Connecticut

Kristen Pryor, M.S.N. Certified Registered Nurse Practitioner, The Children's Hospital of Philadelphia, Philadelphia, Pennsylvania

Benjamin D. Roye, M.D., M.P.H. Attending Physician, Beth Israel Hospital, New York, New York

Lisabeth V. Scalzi, M.D. Assistant Professor of Internal Medicine and Pediatrics, Case Western Reserve University School of Medicine; Attending, Division of Rheumatology, Rainbow Babies & Children's Hospital, Cleveland, Ohio

Lee S. Segal, M.D. Associate Professor, Department of Orthopaedics, and Rehabilitation, Pennsylvania State University College of Medicine; Chief, Division of Pediatric Orthopaedics, Milton S. Hershey Medical Center, Hershey, Pennsylvania

David A. Spiegel, M.D. Adjunct Associate Professor, Department of Surgery, University of Minnesota Medical School; Acting Assistant Chief of Staff, Shriners Hospitals for Children/Twin Cities, Minneapolis, Minnesota

Lisa States, M.D. Thomas Jefferson University Medical School; Chief of Nuclear Medicine, Alfred I. duPont Hospital for Children, Wilmington, Delaware; Attending, Thomas Jefferson University Hospital, Philadelphia, Pennsylvania

Junichi Tamai, M.D. Assistant Professor of Orthopaedic Surgery, University of Cincinnati College of Medicine; Staff, Cincinnati Children's Hospital Medical Center, Cincinnati, Ohio

David M. Wallach, M.D. Assistant Professor of Orthopaedics, Pennsylvania State University College of Medicine; Staff Physician, Milton S. Hershey Medical Center, Hershey, Pennsylvania

Lawrence Wells, M.D. Assistant Professor of Orthopaedic Surgery, University of Pennsylvania School of Medicine; Staff Physician, The Children's Hospital of Philadelphia, Philadelphia, Pennsylvania

Foreword

Pediatrics has a depth and richness that is unique among medical specialties because it deals with the growth and development of infants, children, and adolescents. Physicians caring for children must enlist family members or care providers to help in carrying out preventive health measures or in treating disease.

With this in mind, the concept for the **Requisites in Pediatrics** series was formed. This entailed the following steps: Gather a group of pediatric subspecialists willing to edit a series of books that, in total, represent the requisite knowledge in pediatrics. Ask the physician editors to include the essential fund of pediatric knowledge, to choose topics that could be considered suitable for a "curriculum" or "refresher course" in pediatrics for students, nurse practitioners, resident physicians, and primary care providers. Encourage the authors to leave the discussion of those esoteric diseases that often appear at the bottom of the differential diagnosis list for the exhaustive subspecialty textbooks; rather, to include the common pediatric conditions—conditions that physicians caring for children and adolescents need to know about and understand. Furthermore, ask the editors to include practical information about when to refer to a specialist; what laboratory testing should be performed to assist the subspecialist in his or her search for the difficult diagnosis; and the "major points" to remember for each disease or condition discussed; and so on.

This lofty ideal has its beginning in *Pediatric Orthopaedics and Sports Medicine: The Requisites in Pediatrics*, edited by John Dormans. This is the first in a series of ten books exploring the pediatric subspecialties of Pulmonology, Endocrinology, Infectious Diseases, Toxicology, Cardiology, Nephrology and Urology, Adolescent Medicine, and Gastroenterology.

Dr. Dormans has edited an outstanding book that fulfills our hopes and philosophy for the first installment of **Requisites in Pediatrics.** The book is an up-to-date text for understanding those common orthopaedic conditions that we face as primary care providers.

The book is organized into four topic areas. Trauma and Injury to the spine and pelvis, upper extremities, and lower extremities are discussed in the first three chapters. Disorders of the Bone, including infections, metabolic disorders, and spine, hip, upper extremity, and lower extremity disorders are discussed in Chapters 4 through 9. An excellent and practical discussion of Sports Medicine is found in Chapter 10. The final 5 chapters are dedicated to Conditions of Special Significance in Pediatric Orthopaedics. These include the often difficult-to-diagnose musculoskeletal tumors in Chapter 11; synovial disorders (arthritis and spondyloarthropathies) in Chapter 12; the complex disorder of cerebral palsy in Chapter 13; spina bifida in Chapter 14; and, finally, the inherited and acquired diseases of muscle in Chapter 15, "Muscular Dystrophy and Arthrogryposis." These chapters include practical information and illustrations that demonstrate the techniques of performing the proper physical examination—explaining, for example, the components of a normal gait and comparing that with the gait in children with cerebral palsy.

As a general pediatrician and educator, I extend my appreciation to the authors of this book. As I read through the chapters, I am impressed with the organization of the topics and the practical nature of the clinical information provided. We hope you enjoy this first volume in the **Requisites in Pediatrics** series.

Louis M. Bell, M.D.

Preface

The **Requisites in Pediatrics** series is an attempt to concisely summarize a "requisite" knowledge of pediatrics for a broad group of medical specialists. This series has its beginning in *Pediatric Orthopaedics and Sports Medicine: Requisites in Pediatrics.* This book is the first in a planned series of ten textbooks exploring the pediatric subspecialties of Pulmonology, Endocrinology, Infectious Diseases, Toxicology, Cardiology, Nephrology and Urology, Hematology and Oncology, and Gastroenterology.

Pediatric Orthopaedics and Sports Medicine: Requisites in Pediatrics is an up-to-date text for understanding the common orthopaedic conditions faced by primary care providers. My fellow authors and I have attempted to assemble an essential fund of pediatric orthopaedic knowledge, and we have chosen topics that could be considered suitable subjects for curriculum or "refresher courses" for students, nurse practitioners, resident physicians, primary care providers, and other specialists. We have included the most common pediatric orthopaedic conditions—conditions that physicians and surgeons caring for infants, children, and adolescents need to know and understand. The book includes practical information and illustrations demonstrating the technique of appropriate physical examination, major points for each condition, imaging "Pearls," and indications for referral to a specialist. The book is organized into four sections: Trauma and Injury, Disorders of Bone, Sports Medicine, and Conditions of Special Significance in Pediatric Orthopaedics.

We intended to have fun writing this book and to make it enjoyable to read. At the same time, we strove to cover the material well enough that this would be the only book you would need for a thorough introduction to pediatric orthopaedic surgery . . . the "requisites." We believe that if you have the perseverance to read this book from cover to cover, you will have the foundation for being better able to care for children with orthopaedic problems who present to you for evaluation. You will find the material rewarding in your practice, be it primary care, pediatrics, radiology, surgery, orthopaedic surgery, pediatric orthopaedic surgery, or other specialty. We hope you enjoy and benefit from *Pediatric Orthopaedics and Sports Medicine: Requisites in Pediatrics.*

John P. Dormans, M.D.
Chief of Orthopaedic Surgery
The Children's Hospital of Philadelphia
Professor of Orthopaedic Surgery
University of Pennsylvania School of Medicine
Philadelphia, Pennsylvania

Acknowledgments

A lot of people must be acknowledged whenever you embark on as grandiose a project as creating a new book. Many people deserve credit for this book. These special people can be grouped into six categories: chapter authors, reviewers, Elsevier staff, colleagues, mentors, and last but not least, my support system (i.e., family).

Chapter authors: I am indebted to the many friends and colleagues who took time away from their busy lives to contribute to this book. I know this project took valuable time away from other projects and your families; I appreciate the time and effort. Many of the chapter authors are past fellows or trainees at The Children's Hospital of Philadelphia (CHOP) or the University of Pennsylvania School of Medicine. It is very rewarding to see you doing so well in your academic careers.

Reviewers: Leslie Moroz has been a valuable organizer and helper with this project and has kept my research, academic affairs, and the papers moving forward while I was preoccupied with the book. Additional thanks to Bea Chestnut, Catherine O'Shea, and Jennifer Millman in CHOP Orthopaedics.

Elsevier staff: To Kim Cox, Managing Editor; Jeffrey Gunning, Project Manager; and many others at Elsevier: thank you. You have been a terrific team to work with.

Colleagues: My colleagues in pediatric orthopaedic surgery at CHOP and Penn also deserve credit. These are colleagues who put up with my preoccupation with "The Book" and other projects: Richard Davidson, John Gregg, Bong Lee, Malcolm Ecker, Jack Flynn, Ted Ganley, David Horn, Larry Wells, Angela Smith, Ben Chang, and Roger Cornwall. They are in my opinion the greatest group of pediatric orthopaedic surgeons ever assembled in one division. It is not hard to be successful with a great supporting clinical staff in the Division of Orthopaedic Surgery. Thanks also to Kenro Kusumi, our Director of Pediatric Orthopaedic Basic Science Research at CHOP, who altered the course of my research interests and is an important friend. Thanks also to our Division Manager at CHOP, Nancy Collins, for holding it all together. And finally, thanks to all my current and past fellows, who have provided me with endless educational experiences and who created the vitality necessary for learning. *You* make *us* better surgeons. Each of you is very special to me (but unfortunately the royalties are fairly low so don't expect a free book). I am biased, but I believe that there is no better place than CHOP to practice the art and science of pediatric orthopaedic surgery.

Mentors: On a professional level, I thank Denis Drummond, who gave me a great opportunity and has been a true friend, supporter, and mentor; he also is an outstanding pediatric orthopaedic surgeon. Denis provided me with a chance to work at two legendary institutions—CHOP and Penn—with people who love their trade/art/profession. I also thank my mentors during my fellowship at the Hospital for Sick Children in Toronto: Peter Armstrong, Ivan Krajbich, Robert Salter, and especially the late Mercer Rang, who had a major impact on my career and view of academic life.

Support system: Nan, my wife, who has put up with an incredible amount, is truly an awesome person. What a clever move on my part—marrying someone who is supportive, beautiful, and a great mother and wife. For her:

> . . . Love is not love
> Which alters when it alteration finds,
> Or bends with the remover to remove:
> O, no! It is an ever-fixed mark,
> That looks on tempests and is never shaken . . . .
>
> William Shakespeare

To our children, Nicholas, Andrea, Laura, and Katie, products of this hybrid vigor: you are sensational children/friends. For you, I wish the best.

In closing, one of my favorite quotes:

> Nothing that is worth doing can be achieved in our lifetime; therefore we must be saved by hope. Nothing which is true or beautiful or good makes complete sense in any immediate context of history; therefore we must be saved by faith. Nothing we do, however virtuous, can be accomplished alone; therefore we must be saved by love.
>
> Reinhold Niebuhr

The greatest of these is love.

Thanks to all!

Happy trails.

John P. Dormans, M.D.
Chief of Orthopaedic Surgery
The Children's Hospital of Philadelphia
Professor of Orthopaedic Surgery
University of Pennsylvania School of Medicine
Philadelphia, Pennsylvania

Contents

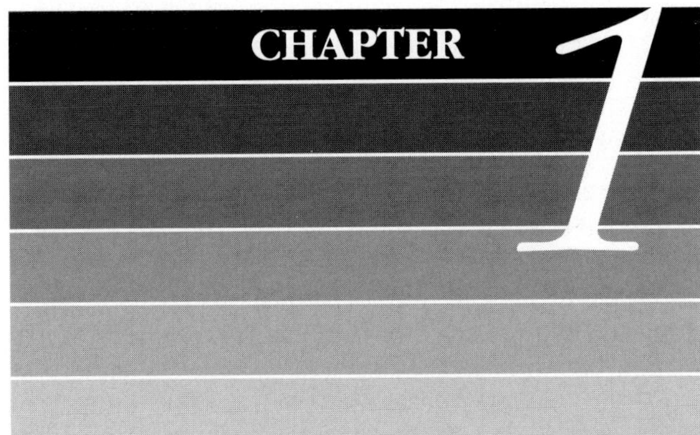

Spine and Pelvis Trauma

LEE S. SEGAL

Trauma remains the leading cause of death and disability in children older than 1 year despite all our attempts at injury prevention.[1] The long-term morbidity from traumatic injuries in children is directly related to the severity of the associated head and musculoskeletal injuries. Ten percent of pediatric trauma admissions are due to multiple injuries, with motor vehicle–related accidents the most common cause of injury.[1] After multiple trauma, the patterns and responses to injury in children are different from those in adults. Anatomic, biomechanical, and physiologic differences in children contribute to these different responses to injury.

Fractures of the spine and pelvis in children are uncommon injuries, most often occurring after high-energy trauma such as pedestrian–motor vehicle accidents. These traumatic injuries to the axial skeleton are quite different in children and adults, and the often-quoted saying "Children are not small adults" applies. The unique features of the child's spine and pelvis lead to different patterns of injuries, and treatment considerations must take into account the dynamic elements of growth and remodeling. This chapter focuses on the clinical and radiographic evaluation of these injuries as well as the management of specific traumatic spine and pelvis injuries in skeletally immature patients.

TRAUMATIC INJURIES OF THE SPINE

Traumatic injuries to the spine occur infrequently in children, accounting for only 5% of all injuries to both the spinal cord and the vertebral column.[2] An understanding of the unique features of the pediatric spine is critical to making a proper diagnosis and providing the appropriate treatment for these potentially catastrophic injuries. The anatomic, physiologic, and biomechanical differences in the spines of children and adults contribute to the different mechanisms of injury, fracture patterns, and levels of injury seen in the two age groups. The dynamic element of growth in children may affect the outcome in pediatric spine trauma. Vertebral body height can be restored after compression fractures, with subsequent growth secondary to remodeling. Further growth of the spinal column in a child with a spinal cord injury, however, may contribute to a progressive spinal deformity such as scoliosis.

Unique Characteristics of the Pediatric Spine

The anatomic and physiologic characteristics of the pediatric cervical spine evolve over time, developing more adult-like features after the child reaches age 8 to 10 years. Children younger than 8 years demonstrate greater range of motion than adults. This difference is due in part to the relative ligamentous laxity, muscle weakness, incomplete ossification of the cervical spine, and horizontal orientation of the facet joints in younger children.[3] McGrory and colleagues[4] have identified two distinct groups of cervical spine injuries on the basis of age, with different patterns and mechanisms of injury. In children younger than 11 years, injury to the upper cervical spine (occiput to C3) predominates. These children have relatively horizontal facet joints that offer little resistance to shear forces from trauma. The fulcrum of motion in the sagittal plane is more proximal in this age group at the C3-C4 level. With the disproportionately larger head size and ligamentous laxity of such children, traumatic injuries to the upper cervical spine are common. The injuries tend to occur more often from falls, and the mortality rate is higher. In children 11 to 15 years, the anatomy of the cervical spine develops more adult-like characteristics, and the injuries are similar to those in adults. The subaxial or lower cervical spine (C3-C7) has a greater rate of involvement, with injuries often occurring with sports or recreational activities, and carries a higher risk of permanent spinal cord injury.

During transport or immobilization on an adult backboard, the disproportionate head size in a young child forces the neck into an undesirable position: flexion and anterior translation of the upper cervical spine. Modifications to the backboard so as to stabilize the cervical spine in a relative neutral position have been recommended for use in a child younger than 6 years. The modifications include lowering the child's head with an occipital recess and raising the chest on a mattress pad so that the occiput is 1 to 2 inches below the level of the back.[5]

The thoracolumbar spine in the skeletally immature patient possesses several unique features that alter its response to traumatic injuries. The presence of the ring apophysis contributes to the developing contour and width of the vertebral body during growth. Under certain single or repetitive axial loads, the apophysis can slip or separate into the spinal canal, giving rise to clinical findings that mimick those of a herniated intervertebral disk.[6] Because the intervertebral disks are well hydrated in children, the high energy of spinal trauma can be dissipated over several levels of the spine, resulting in injuries to several contiguous and noncontiguous levels.[7]

The greater elasticity of the ligamentous complex of the spinal column in response to high-energy trauma may lead to traumatic spinal cord injury without radiographic abnormality (SCIWORA). This situation occurs when a force applied to the flexible spine exceeds the tensile limits of the relatively inelastic spinal cord. Stretching of the spinal cord occurs under these conditions and leads to distraction or ischemic injury to the spinal cord. No obvious fracture is identified on radiographs or computed tomography (CT) scans. SCIWORA is associated with complete and incomplete lesions, is more common in younger children, and may be associated with delayed presentation.[8]

Mechanisms of Pediatric Spine Injury

Different mechanisms of injury predispose children to spinal trauma according to their age at the time of injury. Infants and toddlers are prone to spinal trauma after falls and motor vehicle accidents (MVAs). Adolescents sustain traumatic spinal injuries after participation in sports and recreational activities such as diving.[4] The specific causes of spinal trauma unique to children are child abuse, birth trauma, and the use of passive seat-belt restraint systems.

Several reports in the literature have increased our awareness that spinal trauma can occur as part of the spectrum of injuries in the battered child syndrome. Three percent of all spine fractures in children are the direct result of child abuse.[9] In one reported series, the average age of a child with a spine fracture due to child abuse was 22 months.[10] Many spine injuries related to child abuse are not recognized initially because of the lack of neurologic involvement and the absence of gross deformity. The majority of such injuries occur at the thoracolumbar junction, and the demonstration of multiple spinous process fractures or multiple compression fractures on radiographs should raise the index of suspicion for child abuse. In suspected cases, a lateral radiograph of the thoracolumbar spine should be part of the routine skeletal survey.

Trauma to the spine or spinal cord should be suspected in neonates after a difficult or traumatic delivery and unexplained hypotonia or delay in development. In the evaluation of the "floppy infant," one should consider magnetic resonance imaging (MRI) or somatosensory evoked potentials (SSEPs).[11] Injury to the upper cervical spine may occur with cephalic presentations, and injury to the lower cervical spine and thoracic spine during breech deliveries.[7]

The mandatory use of seat-belt restraint systems has increased the incidence of flexion-distraction or Chance fracture of the lumbar spine in children. The unique characteristics of the small pelvis, the higher center of gravity, and the typical slouched posture of a child prevent the normal or intended positioning of the lap belt across the pelvis.[12] At the time of frontal impact, the properly positioned lap belt is intended to dissipate the deceleration forces through the pelvis and the hips. Children tend to "submarine under" the seat belt, allowing the lap belt to improperly ride up to the level of the midlumbar spine. The lap belt then acts as an anterior fulcrum that generates the flexion-distraction mechanism of injury (Fig. 1-1). In addition to the spinal injury, there may be associated injury to the spinal cord, resulting in paraplegia and life-threatening visceral injury.[12,13]

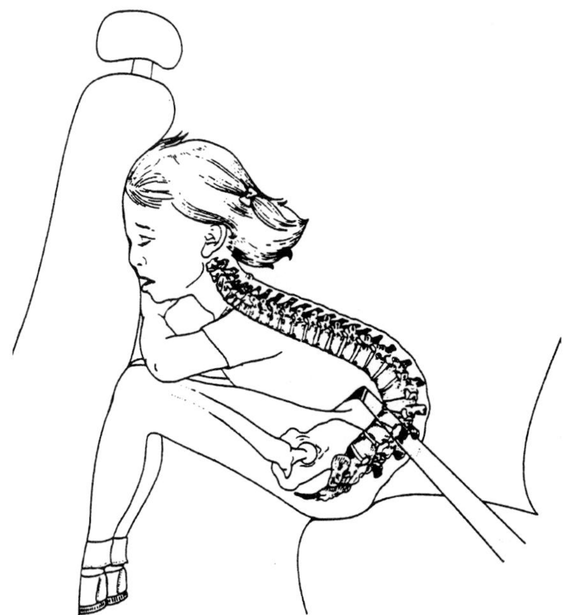

Figure 1-1 Lap belt injury in a child at the time of impact. The lap belt rides up over iliac crests to create a bending moment at the midlumbar region and generate a flexion-distraction injury. (From Johnson DL, Falci S: The diagnosis and treatment of pediatric lumbar spine injuries caused by rear seat lap belts. Neurosurgery 26:434-441, 1990.)

Hoy and Cole[14] described the pediatric cervical seat belt syndrome in seven children wearing either three-point or four-point restraint systems. They noted a wide range of injuries in these children, including fractures and fracture-dislocations of the upper and lower cervical spine, spinal cord injuries, head injuries, and laryngeal fractures. These investigators proposed the following mechanisms of injury for this syndrome: in three-point restraint systems, flexion of the neck over the poorly fitting sash, which has moved up across the neck, and in properly fitting four-point systems, hyperflexion injuries produced by the deceleration forces on the child's disproportionately large head.

Evaluation

Infants or children with suspected spine injuries should be properly immobilized to prevent motion that could cause injury to the spinal cord or other injuries. Children with a history of high-energy trauma, such as a motor vehicle–related injury or a fall, with loss of consciousness or altered mental status, with complaints of neck pain or guarding, or with associated head or facial trauma should be immobilized in a rigid cervical collar with sandbags on either side. Careful logrolling and other spinal precautions should be maintained by health care personnel until appropriate screening radiographs can be obtained.

The clinical examination of a child with a suspected spine injury can be extremely difficult. Often the child is quite young, frightened, and unable to communicate the location of the pain. The physical examination must closely evaluate the upper cervical spine in a young child because of the higher risk of injury to this area. With any signs of facial or head trauma, the upper cervical spine should be carefully evaluated as well. There may be muscle spasm about the paraspinal or sternocleidomastoid muscles. Torticollis may be a presenting physical sign of C1-C2 rotary instability. There may be tenderness about the posterior neck along the interspinous process ligaments or along the thoracolumbar spine. Evaluation of the skin for any cutaneous signs, such as abrasions and bruising, is important. The presence of a bandlike pattern of ecchymosis around the abdomen or iliac crest, described as the "lap belt sign," may indicate an underlying lumbar spine fracture and associated visceral injuries (Fig. 1-2). A thorough neurological examination should be performed to assess motor strength, sensation, reflexes, and proprioception. Rectal examination to evaluate for the bulbocavernosus reflex should be performed in children with suspected acute spinal cord injury to detect when the period of spinal shock is over.

Imaging

After appropriate immobilization of the cervical spine, radiographs of the cervical spine are obtained as part of the trauma series in the pediatric trauma patient. Other radiographs, including those of the thoracolumbar spine, should be obtained as clinically indicated. Anteroposterior (AP) and lateral views of the cervical spine and an open-mouth view of the odontoid constitute the trauma series. The C7-T1 junction should be visible on the lateral radiograph. If the cervicothoracic

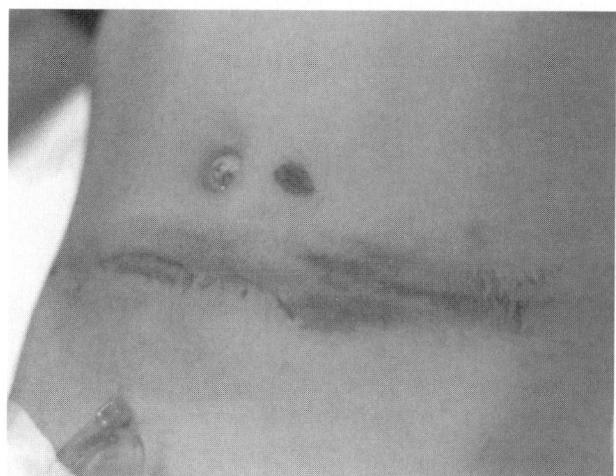

Figure 1-2 Lap belt sign in a child sustaining a Chance fracture of the lumbar spine. A transverse band of contusion and ecchymosis was caused by the lap belt.

junction cannot be seen, additional views, such as a swimmer's view, or a CT scan should be acquired.

Like the physical examination, the radiographic assessment of a child's spine can be difficult. Plain radiographs alone can miss up to 50% of cervical spine injuries.[7] Incomplete ossification as well as the greater motion of the pediatric spine contribute to the variability of radiographic findings that can easily be mistaken for traumatic injuries (Box 1-1).[15] In the skeletally immature patient, the vertebral bodies of the cervical spine may appear wedge-shaped and can be confused with compression fractures. The odontoid process may be anteriorly angulated in 4% of normal children. The synchondrosis at the base of the odontoid, the secondary centers of ossification of the spinous processes, and the apical tip of the odontoid are examples of areas of incomplete ossification that can be incorrectly interpreted as fractures.

Pseudosubluxation of the cervical spine at the C2-C3 and C3-C4 articulations is a normal radiographic variant in children. It is a reflection of the greater mobility and incomplete ossification of this area in young children. Pseudosubluxation is present in up to 20% of children younger than 7 years.[16] The spinolaminar line drawn along the posterior arch from the first to the third cervical vertebra on a radiograph, is useful in differentiating pseudosubluxation from true injury. The lack of normal cervical lordosis is seen in up to 14% of children. In both of these conditions, extension of the neck corrects the radiographic findings. Overriding of the anterior arch of C1 on the odontoid can be seen in up to 20% of children, reflecting incomplete ossification of both the anterior arch of C1 and the odontoid.[15] All of these normal radiographic variables must be interpreted in conjunction with the physical findings. Rapid resolution of symptoms with return of a full range of motion in a child suggests a normal variant. On the other hand, continuous muscle spasm, limited range of motion, or tenderness in a child warrants further investigation with other imaging studies.[15]

Evaluation of lateral radiographs should initially focus on the four lines that correspond to the anterior and posterior vertebral bodies, the spinolaminar line, and the tips of the spinous processes from the C1 through C7 vertebral bodies.[15] Each of these four lines should have a smooth contour (Fig. 1-3). Because of the importance of the upper cervical spine in young children, greater attention should be focused on the C1-C2 level. In children younger than 8 years, the atlantodens interval (ADI), which is the space between the anterior arch of C1 and the anterior border of the odontoid, should not be greater than 4 to 4.5 mm. If these lateral views are normal, flexion-extension radiographs should be obtained under physician guidance if the child is alert and cooperative. Soft tissue swelling should be evaluated on the lateral radiograph as well. Caution must be exercised in the interpretation of these studies in a crying child.

Box 1-1 Unique Characteristics of the Pediatric Cervical Spine

- Anterior angulation of the odontoid process (4%)
- Overriding anterior arch of C1 on the odontoid (20%)
- C1-C2 atlanto-dens interval can be up to 4-4.5 mm in normal children
- Decreased cervical lordosis (14%)
- C2-C3 and C3-C4 pseudosubluxation can be misinterpreted for instability (20% in children up to 7 years old)
- Basilar synchondrosis of C2 can be mistaken for an odontoid fracture
- Tip of odontoid (ossiculum terminale) can be confused with a fracture
- Neurocentral synchondroses and multiple ossification centers of C1 can mimic fracture appearance
- Rounding of anterior vertebral bodies can mimic compression fractures
- Secondary centers of spinous processes can be mistaken for avulsion fractures
- Spinal cord injury without radiographic abnormality (SCIWORA) (at both cervical and thoracolumbar levels)

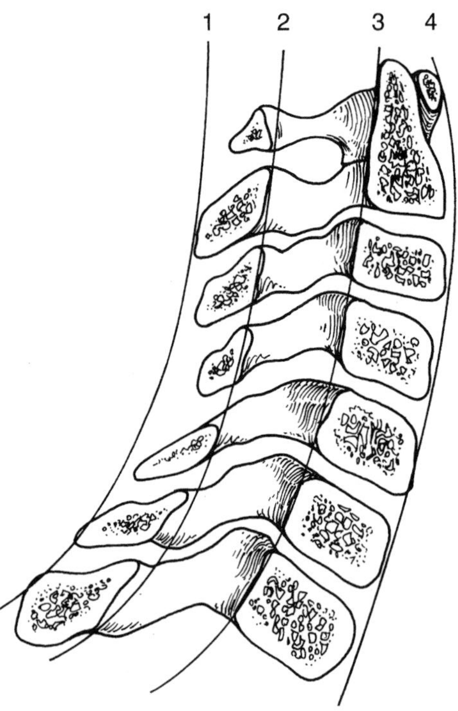

Figure 1-3 Four lines of the normal lateral cervical spine: 1, spinous processes; 2, spinolaminar line; 3, posterior vertebral body line; 4, anterior vertebral body line. (From Copley LA, Dormans JP: Cervical spine disorders in infants and children. J Am Acad Orthop Surg 6:207, 1998.)

The retropharyngeal space should be less than 7 mm, and the retrotracheal space should be less than 14 mm in children[15]; and both spaces may be increased in a crying child without injury.

Other imaging studies should be obtained in children for whom radiographic findings are equivocal and in whom the mechanism of injury and physical findings are highly suspicious for an underlying spine or spinal cord injury. An uncooperative child or an unconscious, intubated child in whom absence of cervical spine injury ("clearance") would also warrant other studies, such as computed tomography (CT) or magnetic resonance imaging (MRI).[15] CT scans can be quite helpful in delineating injuries such as fractures that are not well visualized on plain radiographs and may be confused with normal variants of the pediatric spine. One must be aware that a CT scan may miss a fracture if the orientation of the scan is in the same plane as the fracture. Three-dimensional CT scan reconstruction images have improved our ability to evaluate difficult injuries of the pediatric cervical spine. Dynamic CT scans should be considered in the child who presents with a painful torticollis and suspected atlantoaxial rotary instability.[17] CT scans are essential in the assessment of thoracolumbar spine fractures to assess the extent of osseous injury such as canal compromise in burst fractures, to check for an unrecognized posterior lamina or facet fracture, and to evaluate the relative stability of a fracture pattern that may influence treatment decisions.

MRI is the imaging study of choice in the child presenting with a spine fracture and an associated neurologic deficit. It is also warranted in the child with suspected SCIWORA to determine the location and evaluate the extent of spinal cord injury. Advancements in the techniques of MRI have refined the evaluation of injuries to the spinal cord, ligaments, and other soft tissues, the intervertebral disks, and the cartilaginous or unossified pediatric spine. Most level I pediatric trauma centers routinely use MRI for evaluation of the cervical spine in the intubated, unconscious child. MRI also has an important role in accurately determining fracture pattern and stability as well as the degree of acute spinal cord injury, if present, in thoracolumbar fractures.

Cervical Spine Injuries

The type and level of traumatic injuries to the pediatric cervical spine depend on the age of the child at the time of injury. In children younger than 10 years, injuries tend to be located in the upper cervical spine, and a higher percentage are subluxations and dislocations without associated fractures. Older children have more adult-like fracture patterns in the lower or subaxial cervical spine.[4] A complete review of all injuries to the pediatric cervical spine is beyond the scope of this chapter, which instead addresses the management of injuries unique to the younger child.

Occiput-C1 dislocation is a rare injury, frequently associated with severe head trauma and other injuries. The dislocation is often fatal, but some children are now surviving this catastrophic injury as a result of rapid response and resuscitation in the field. Many of these children are quadriplegic and require ventilator support, having complete spinal cord injuries below the level of the brainstem. Radiographs may miss this injury if the dislocation spontaneously reduces, but several radiographic parameters can be used to evaluate for it. One is the Powers ratio; a ratio greater than 1 is suggestive of possible occiput-C1 dislocation.[15] MRI and CT are beneficial in confirming the injury. Early treatment by halo immobilization, either alone or with posterior spine fusion and internal fixation, is recommended to mobilize the child into an upright position and promote pulmonary care.

Atlas fractures, rare injuries in children, are caused by axial loads, and the specific pattern of injury depends on the position of the head at the time of impact. Disruptions of both the anterior and posterior rings of the atlas occur as the occipital condyles are forced into the lateral masses of C1. The presence of a persistent synchondrosis may result in only a single break in the ring in children. Rates of spinal cord injury and nonunion of atlas fractures are extremely low. Rupture of the transverse atlantal ligament can be associated with this fracture pattern as the lateral masses are driven apart, subsequently resulting in atlantoaxial instability. CT scans best define the specific fracture patterns of the atlas (Fig. 1-4). The recommended treatment for atlas

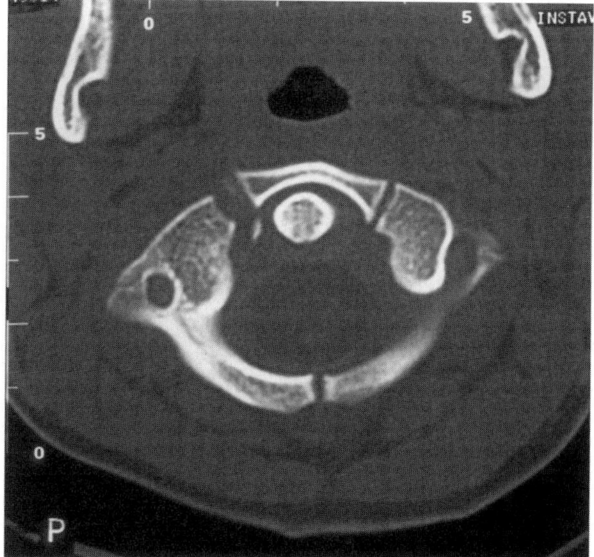

Figure 1-4 Computed tomography scan of an atlas fracture in a 5-year-old child. Note the "single break" in the ring of C1 with the synchondrosis still present.

fractures is immobilization in either Minerva cast or halo and vest.

Fractures of the ring of C2 are believed to result from hyperextension injuries. Also known as hangman's fractures, they tend to be minimally displaced and heal with cast or halo-vest immobilization (Fig. 1-5).

Odontoid fractures in children most often occur at the base within the body of the C2 vertebra and below the level of the facet joints. Normal variants of the cervical spine, as previously discussed, can be mistaken for fractures of the odontoid process. These injuries are usually Salter-Harris type I physeal fractures through the synchondrosis. In a series of odontoid fractures in children reported in 1999 by Odent and colleagues,[18] the mean age at the time of fracture was 30 months. The majority of injuries had occurred in MVAs. Eight of the children had been riding in forward-facing car seats, and four had been restrained in rear-facing car seats. The risk of neurologic injury is thought to be low with this injury. Displaced fractures are easily reduced in extension and posterior translation, then immobilized with Minerva cast or halo and vest. An intact periosteal hinge at the base of the odontoid gives stability to the fracture and facilitates reduction.[7] Because odontoid fractures are located within the body of C2 and are physeal type fractures, they typically heal rapidly, within 6 to 8 weeks, and have a low rate of non-union. There is controversy about whether the etiology of this entity is developmental or traumatic. Failure to identify and properly immobilize an odontoid fracture in a child may be responsible for the development of an os odontoideum, in which the fracture line is usually proximal to the body of C2.

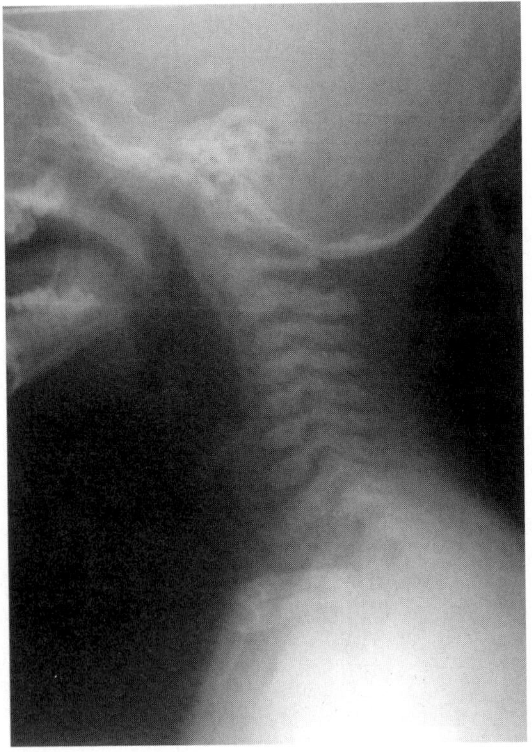

Figure 1-5 C2 fracture (hangman's fracture) in a 2-year-old child.

Atlantoaxial instability may occur after a traumatic event, although it is more commonly seen in chronic progressive conditions such as Down syndrome. In children for whom a history of trauma is obtained, radiographic demonstration of an ADI greater than 5 mm is suggestive of C1-C2 instability. The ADI is measured from the anterior cortex of the dens to the posterior cortex of the anterior ring of C1. Atlantoaxial instability may occur after atlas fractures with disruption of the transverse atlantal ligament or with odontoid fractures. Initial treatment is conservative, consisting of a trial of immobilization for 2 to 3 months. Posterior arthrodesis is indicated at the C1-C2 level for continued instability after the initial immobilization.[7]

Atlantoaxial rotary instability in children manifests as torticollis, pain, and limited range of motion of the neck. Although this condition can occur after trauma, it is more commonly seen after upper respiratory infection, otorhinolaryngologic surgery, and other inflammatory conditions. There is often a delay in diagnosis. Four types of subluxation of increasing severities have been described, depending on the degree and direction of displacement and reflecting the integrity of the C1-C2 ligaments.[19] The diagnosis is made from radiographs and dynamic CT scans that demonstrate the fixed nature of the subluxation.[17] Treatment with head halter traction and cervical collar immobilization is often effective if duration of symptoms is less than 1 month. Symptoms of longer duration may require posterior arthrodesis from C1 to C2. The indications for surgery include neurologic involvement, failure to achieve and maintain correction of a deformity present for longer than 3 months, and recurrence of the deformity after 6 to 8 weeks of nonoperative care.[17]

Injuries of the lower cervical spine are more common in older children and adolescents, and the fracture patterns have more adult-like characteristics. Such fractures include wedge- or compression-type fractures, facet dislocations, and fracture-dislocations. Ligamentous injury with instability may also occur in children. Pennecot and associates[20] reported on 16 children with ligamentous disruption, 11 of whom had injuries at or below the C3 level. The patients presented with stiff neck and loss of lordosis, representing protective muscle spasm of the cervical spine. Radiographs showed widening of the interspinous process space, kyphosis at the disk space, and loss of parallelism of the facet joints. Surgery was indicated in patients who had persistent pain and progressive deformity.[20]

The majority of pediatric cervical spine fractures can be treated in a closed fashion with cervical collar or halo immobilization. Compression fractures are thought to be the most common fracture type, occurring after flexion–axial load injuries. They are stable fractures that can be associated with spinous process, laminar, and anterior teardrop fractures off the vertebral body. Flexion-extension radiographs should be obtained after 4 to 6 weeks of immobilization to assess stability of the posterior ligaments.

Facet dislocations in the pediatric spine may be unilateral or bilateral and may be associated with fracture of the facet (Fig. 1-6). Prereduction MRI should be performed to evaluate the status of the spinal cord and the intervertebral disks. Bilateral facet dislocations tend to be unstable and are associated with a greater risk of neurologic involvement. Closed reduction of the facet dislocation should initially be attempted with gentle, guided traction. If the dislocations do not reduce easily, open reduction and posterior fusion are indicated. Fracture-dislocations of the cervical spine are often the results of high-energy trauma and strongly associated spinal cord injuries. The goals of treatment for these fractures are early reduction and surgical stabilization.

Physeal fracture through the vertebral end plates is a cervical spine injury unique to children. The inferior end plate is more commonly involved. Identification of this fracture on radiographs can be difficult, because spontaneous reduction and normal realignment may occur. MRI may be used to identify this injury as well as SCIWORA in a child with neurologic deficits. These fractures are typically unstable and may require surgical stabilization.

Thoracolumbar Spine Injuries

The management of pediatric thoracolumbar fractures requires thoughtful consideration of the stability of the fracture pattern, coronal or sagittal plane deformities, neurologic deficit if present, and other associated injuries. The integrity or stability of the spinal column can be determined with a number of different methods. The three-column concept of the spine, which divides the thoracolumbar spine into anterior, middle, and posterior columns, can be applied to pediatric spine fractures.[21] The spinal injury is thought to be unstable if two or more columns of the spine are involved, particularly when there is ligamentous disruption. The mechanism of injury and the direction of forces applied to the spine at the time of injury contribute to the specific fracture patterns identified on the radiographs and other imaging studies. In general, the majority of these injuries are stable, the risk of spinal cord injury is low compared with the risk in adults, and most cases can be treated conservatively.

Compression fractures of the spine occur primarily in the thoracic spine and most often are due to a flexion

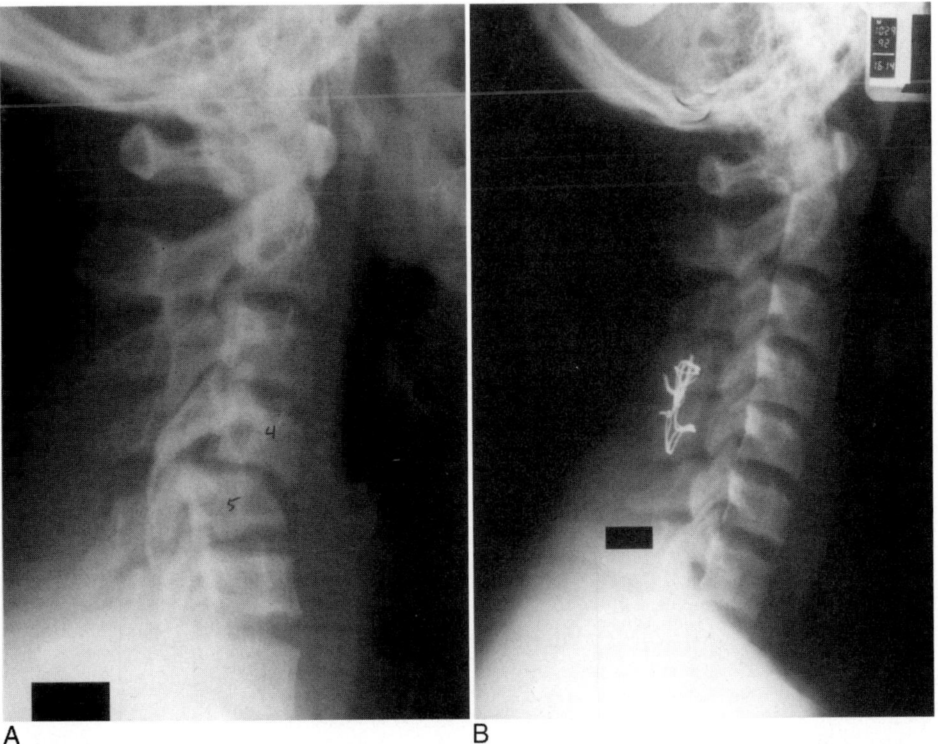

Figure 1-6 A-B C4-C5 unilateral facet fracture-dislocation with incomplete neurologic deficit sustained by a 15-year-old boy while playing football. The patient underwent open reduction and posterior arthrodesis with wire fixation and had full neurologic recovery.

mechanism of injury. These fractures tend to be stable, involving only the anterior column of the spine. The thoracic rib cage gives inherent stability to these injuries. Wedging of the anterior vertebral bodies with less than 50% loss of anterior vertebral height is often noted. Multiple contiguous compression fractures can be found; they result from the greater flexibility of the spine and hydration of the intervertebral disks, which enable the forces to be dissipated over several levels. The increased elasticity of the posterior ligamentous complex in the child is thought to contribute to the higher incidence of multiple compression fractures noted at the thoracolumbar junction and lumbar spine after lap belt injuries. Despite the flexion-distraction mode of injury, only the anterior column fails in flexion in skeletally immature persons.[13,22] The ability of the skeletally immature spine to spread out the traumatic forces over several vertebral levels minimizes the incidence of neurologic injury. The majority of these stable fractures can be treated nonoperatively, but the extent of kyphosis and wedging may influence treatment decisions. In younger children, reconstitution of anterior vertebral body height predictably occurs. Child abuse and pathologic causes must be considered when multiple compression fractures of the spine are seen in children.

The management of flexion-distraction injuries of the thoracolumbar spine should address both the fracture itself and the potential for associated intra-abdominal injuries. Approximately two-thirds of patients with these injuries also have intra-abdominal injuries that may be life threatening (Fig. 1-7); the most common are tears or perforations of the small and large bowel, disruptions of the mesentery, and abdominal vascular structures.[12,13] It is common for diagnosis of such injuries to be delayed because their clinical signs often overlap with those of the spinal fracture.[13] As noted earlier, the incidence of neurologic injury is low in children because of the flexibility of the spine. Specific management of this spinal injury depends on the extent of deformity, the stability of the fracture, the associated injuries, and the presence of a neurologic deficit.

Four types of flexion-distraction injuries have been described; they define the distraction plane of injury through the ligaments, bone, or the intervertebral end plates.[13] Disruption of the posterior ligamentous complex usually results in an unstable fracture that will not heal on its own. The fracture is thought to be stable when it extends through bone in only the posterior column of the spine (pedicles) and when it can potentially heal without operative intervention. Hyperextension casting or bracing is indicated in neurologically intact patients with stable fracture patterns. Surgery is indicated for patients with unstable fractures, significant kyphotic deformity, or neurologic injury (Fig. 1-8). Patients may also benefit from operative stabilization of such a fracture if they have associated abdominal injuries

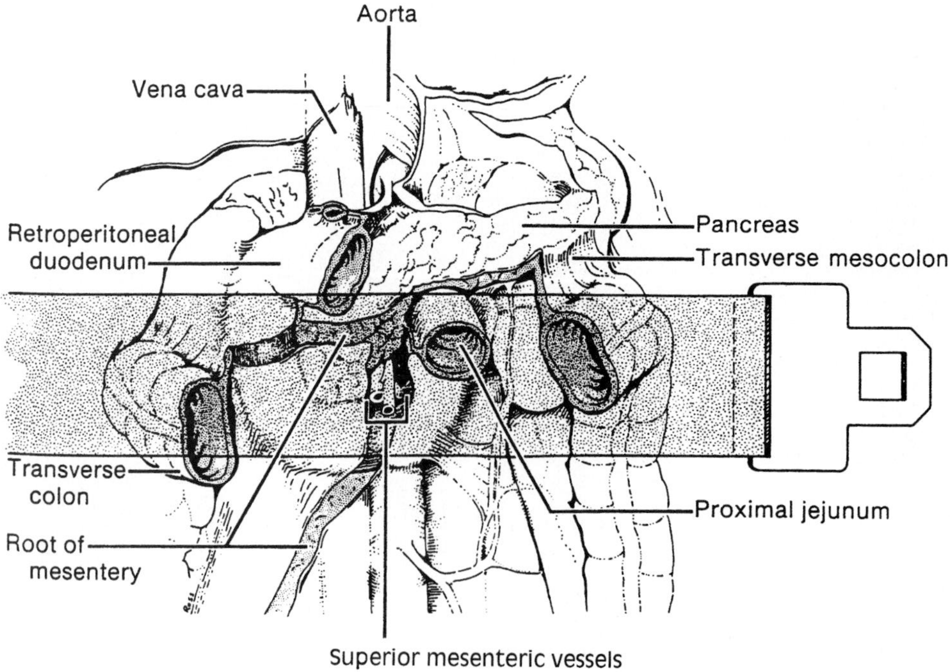

Figure 1-7 Intra-abdominal structures attached in the retroperitoneum at the midlumbar region vulnerable to injury in a lap belt injury. (From Johnson DL, Falci S: The diagnosis and treatment of pediatric lumbar spine injuries caused by rear seat lap belts. Neurosurgery 26:434-441, 1990.)

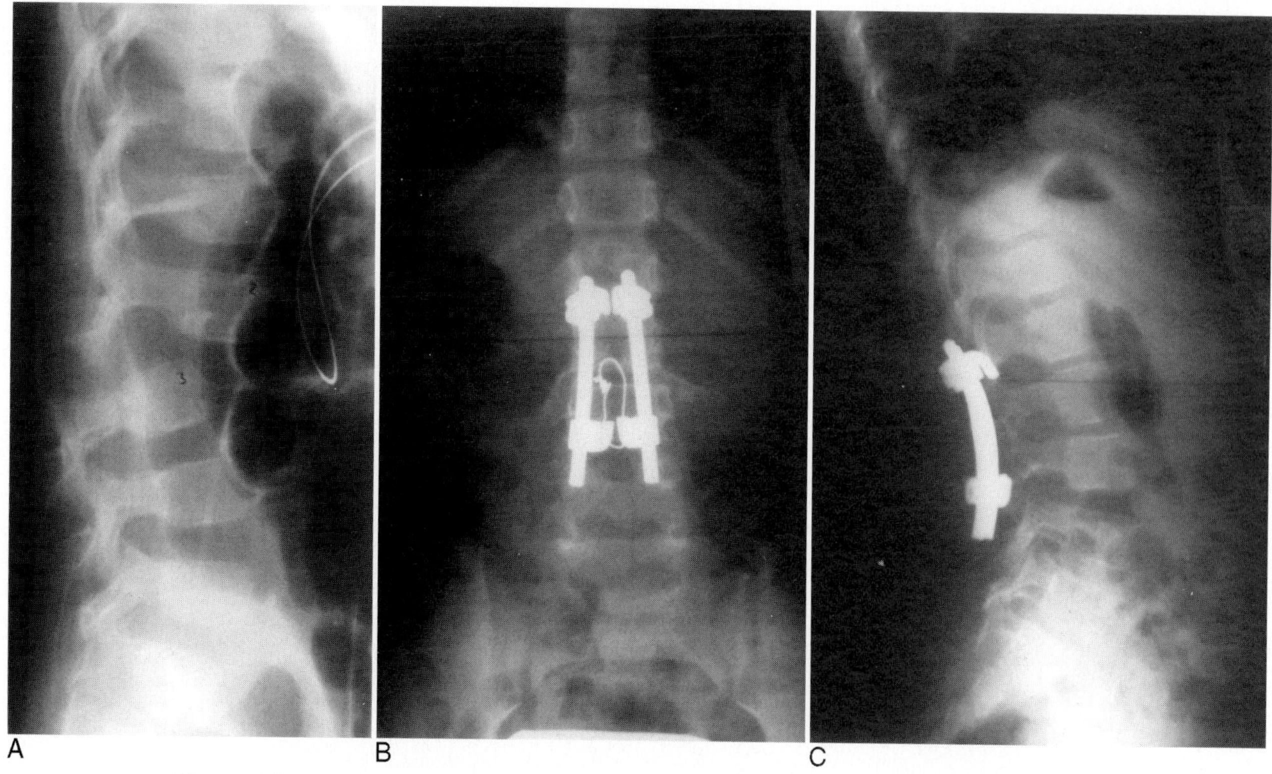

Figure 1-8 **A** to **C**, Flexion-distraction injury in a 4-year-old child restrained with a lap belt. Despite the near dislocation of the spine at the L2-L3 level, the child had normal neurologic function. Open reduction and posterior fusion with compression instrumentation were performed to stabilize the injury.

that require surgery, because hyperextension casting may not be possible, and internal fixation of the fracture would promote early mobilization.

Burst fractures account for only 10% of all pediatric thoracolumbar fractures and are more common in older children approaching skeletal maturity. In a study reported by Lalonde and coworkers,[23] the mean age of children sustaining burst fractures was 14.4 years. The greater flexibility of the skeletally immature spinal column in younger children is able to dissipate the concentrated compressive forces that result in burst fractures. Such fractures result from axial load and flexion forces applied to the spine. Failure of the middle column occurs as the vertebral end plate fails and the intervertebral disk is forced into the vertebral body, leading to retropulsion of bone into the spinal canal. The spinal canal is larger relative to the spinal cord and cauda equina in children than in adults, and a greater degree of canal compromise is tolerated without impingement of the cord or cauda equina.[23] Burst fractures occurring distal to the L1 level tend also to have a lower incidence of permanent neurologic injury, because the cauda equina is more tolerant of compression than the spinal cord. Hyperextension casting or bracing can be considered in the child (typically an adolescent) who is neurologically intact, has a stable fracture pattern, and has minimal kyphotic deformity. The severity of spinal canal compromise is usually not a factor in decision-making for treatment of burst fractures. In addition to the larger relative canal dimensions in children, resorption of the retropulsed bone fragments predictably occurs with remodeling. Operative decompression and stabilization with internal fixation are indicated for unstable burst fractures in patients with significant kyphotic deformity (often > 20 degrees) or neurologic deficits (Fig. 1-9). The individual fracture pattern and surgeon's preference often determine whether an anterior or posterior approach is used.

Spinal Cord Injury Without Radiographic Abnormality

Children may have a complete or incomplete spinal cord injury after a traumatic event even when radiographic and CT findings are normal. SCIWORA is unique to the pediatric population. It is a consequence of a stretch or distraction injury to the relatively flexible spinal column that exceeds the tensile limits of the underlying spinal cord in a skeletally immature individual. Numerous theories have been proposed to explain the spinal cord injury, including stretch or traction injury,

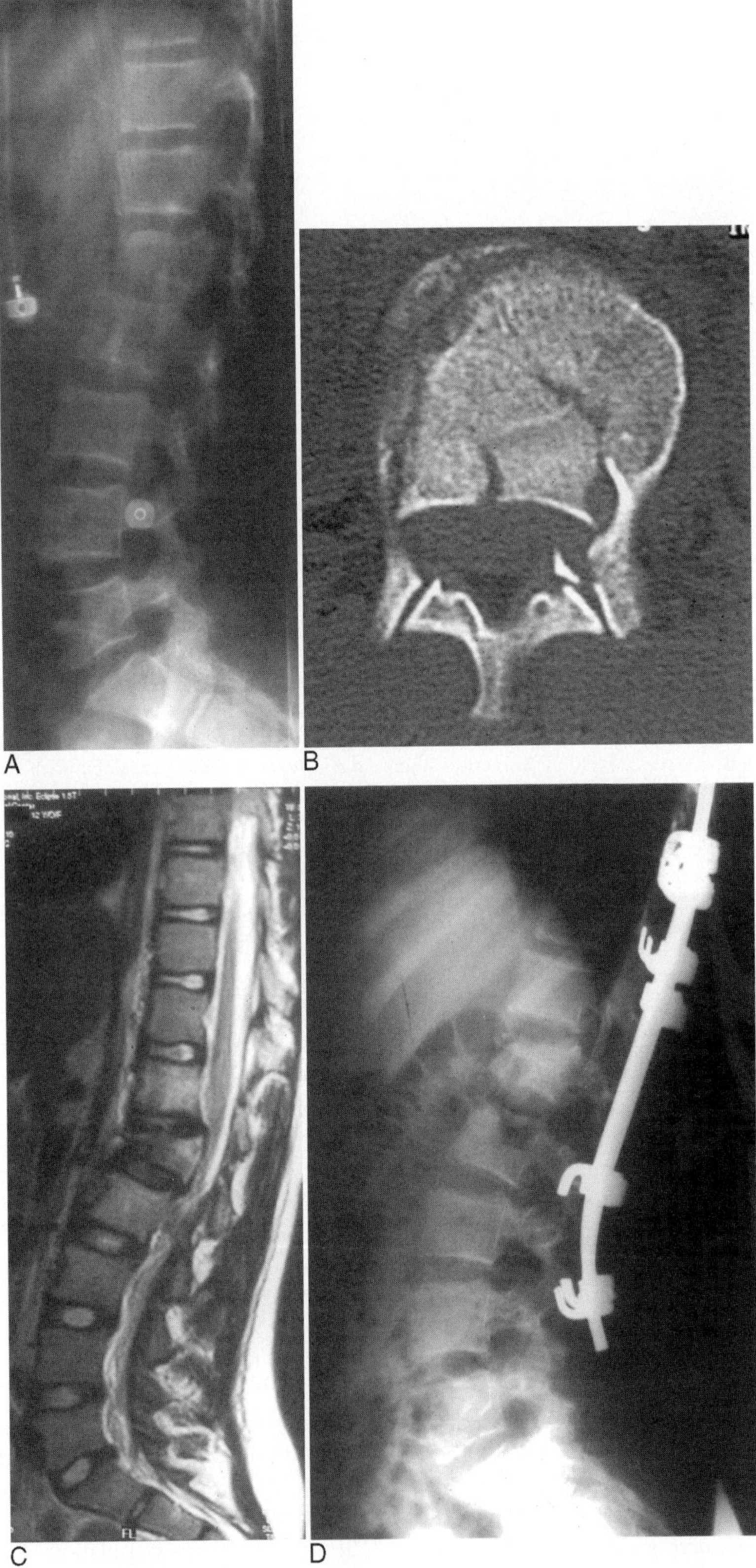

Figure 1-9 **A,** L1 burst fracture in a 12-year-old girl after a motor vehicle accident. Neurologic function was intact. **B,** Computed tomography scan shows failure of the middle column with retropulsion of bone fragments into the spinal canal. **C,** Magnetic resonance image demonstrates impingement of the spinal cord at the level of the conus. **D,** Lateral radiograph obtained after posterior arthrodesis and instrumentation from T10 to L3.

vascular compromise or ischemic injury, and transient disk herniation or end plate separation. The injury often occurs after a high-energy traumatic event such as a pedestrian–motor vehicle accident or a fall from a significant height. The neurologic deficit must be thoroughly assessed, and the child evaluated for the associated injuries that frequently occur with SCIWORA. This unique injury is often noted in children 8 years or younger, commonly occurs at the cervicothoracic junction, and is more likely to be a complete spinal cord injury in these young patients.[8]

Children with incomplete spinal cord injuries should be treated with the expectation of neurologic improvement. MRI best defines the location and extent of injury to the cord, ligaments, and unossified cartilage (Fig. 1-10). Management is guided by the stability of the spinal column injury and the severity of injury to the spinal cord. The role of steroids in the management of progressive neurologic deficits has not been defined. Fusion of the spine is indicated in children with unstable spine injuries or progressive neurologic deficits. Otherwise, patients with SCIWORA should be immobilized with an orthosis for 6 to 8 weeks, at which point the stability of the spine should be reevaluated with physician-guided radiographs. For all patients with complete or incomplete SCIWORA, a spinal cord rehabilitative program should be started when other acute injuries allow. Because children with spinal cord injuries are at risk for development of progressive spinal deformities such as scoliosis, follow-up should be maintained until they reach skeletal maturity.

TRAUMATIC INJURIES OF THE PELVIS

Fractures of the pelvis are uncommon in children. The incidence of these fractures as seen at major pediatric trauma centers ranges from 2% to 5%,[24-26] and the majority are stable injuries not requiring intervention. Watts[27] stated that only ten fractures involving the pelvic ring should be expected at a children's hospital each year. Despite the relatively rare occurrence, the presence of a pelvic fracture in the trauma setting is often an indication of other potentially life-threatening injuries that take precedence over the skeletal injury.

The mechanisms of injury for pediatric pelvic fractures are different in children and adults. In the majority of cases, pelvic fracture is the result of trauma sustained in pedestrian–motor vehicle accidents, often occurring as a child runs into the street and is struck by an oncoming car. Most studies report this mode of injury to occur in 60% of pelvic fractures.[28] In 30% of pelvic fractures, the child or adolescent is either the passenger or the driver involved in an MVA; in contrast, this is the most common mode of injury in adults. Falls and other miscellaneous injuries account for the remaining 10% of injuries causing pelvic fractures in children.

Anatomy

The evaluation and management of traumatic injuries to the pelvis in pediatric patients must take into account several unique features. The skeletally immature pelvis is quite flexible and plastic as a result of the high percentage of cartilage and the porous nature of the cortical bone. The greater elasticity of the posterior sacroiliac joints and the anterior symphysis pubis enables the pediatric pelvis to absorb significant amounts of energy and allows for large amounts of displacement before a fracture occurs.[3,27-29] The pelvis can easily "bend but not break" when subjected to the significant forces of high-energy trauma. Unlike in adults, single breaks or fractures in the pelvic ring are seen in children, and the majority of pelvic fractures are stable. The presence of cartilage within the pelvis can delay radiographic diagnosis of fractures involving the cartilage, resulting in growth disturbances.

The presence of primary and secondary centers of ossification in the developing pelvis can easily be confused with fractures. The child's pelvis consists of three primary ossification centers (the ilium, ischium, and the pubis) that meet at the triradiate cartilage and fuse around the age of 16 to 18 years (Fig. 1-11). The growth of the acetabulum involves the complex interaction of interstitial growth within the triradiate cartilage complex, appositional growth at the periphery of the cartilage, and periosteal new bone formation at the acetabular margins,[30] The concavity of the acetabulum forms from the direct mechanical response to a reduced spherical femoral head. The triradiate cartilage within the chondro-osseous complex of the acetabulum can prematurely close if injured, most often after a crush type injury, resulting in a possible limb length discrepancy, progressive acetabular dysplasia, and possible hip subluxation.[31] The secondary centers of ossification are the anterior superior and inferior spines, the iliac crest, and the ischial tuberosity. The age of appearance and fusion for each of these apophyses is different, and they can be pulled or avulsed off the pelvis by forceful muscle contractions.[32]

Evaluation

Children who sustain pelvic fractures often have multiple injuries that can be life threatening and require initial resuscitative measures in the field and the emergency room as established by the Advanced Trauma Life Support (ATLS) protocol. A history of the accident and the mechanism of injury should be obtained, if possible. The primary survey centers on the evaluation and

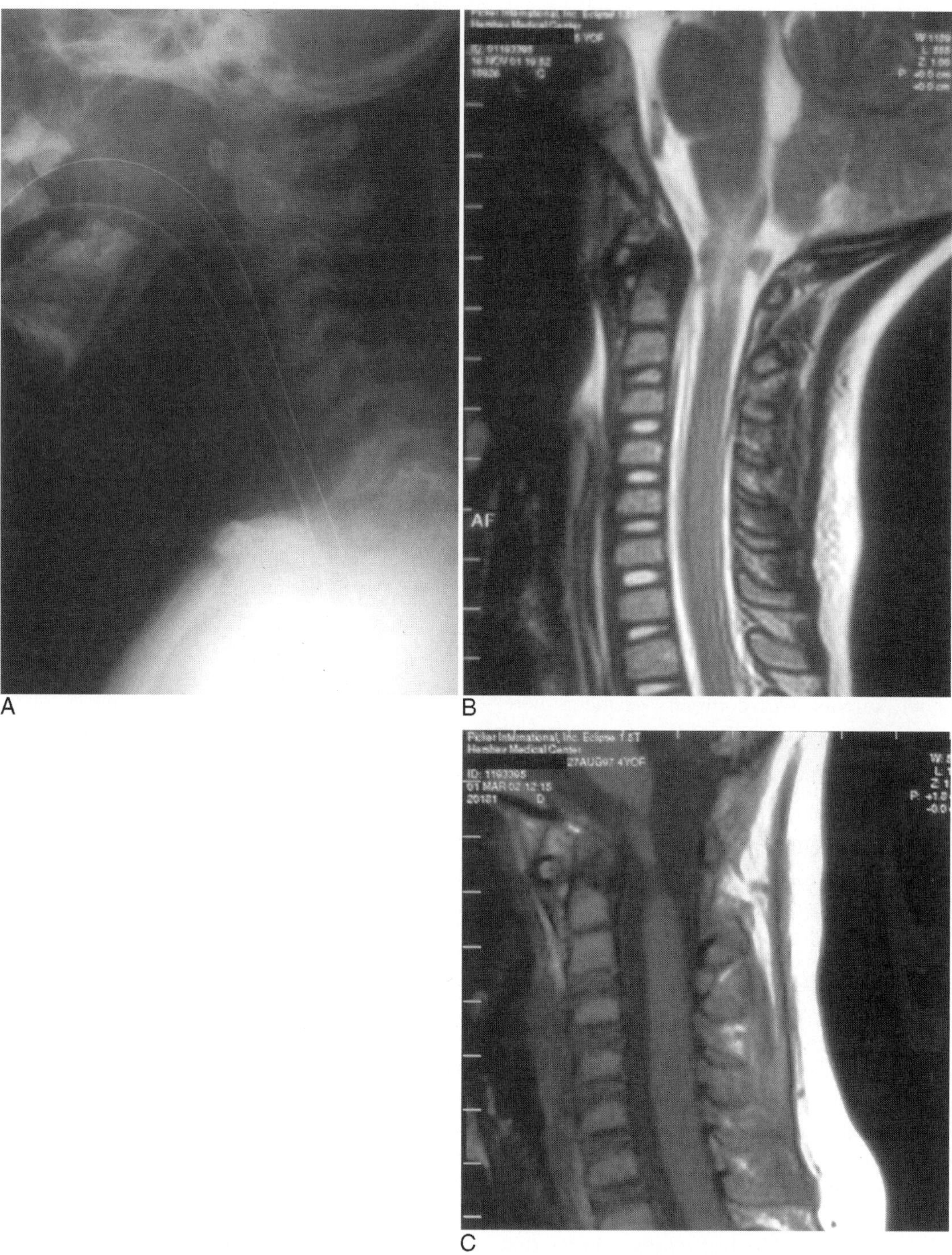

Figure 1-10 Four-year-old child with spinal cord injury without radiographic abnormality (SCIWORA) after a motor vehicle accident. **A,** Lateral radiograph of the cervical spine obtained on admission. No obvious fracture or dislocation was noted. **B,** Magnetic resonance image reveals contusion at the level of the brainstem and upper cervical spinal cord. **C,** Magnetic resonance image obtained 4 months after injury shows marked atrophy of the spinal cord at the craniocervical junction.

treatment of these potentially life-threatening injuries and includes the ABCs (airway assessment, breathing or ventilation, and circulatory status). A brief neurologic examination and exposure of the child are needed to complete the primary survey.

Detailed examination of the pelvis begins with inspection of the skin for any signs of contusion, ecchymosis, abrasions, or lacerations about the pelvis and perineum. The location of these cutaneous signs may often help define the pattern of injury to the pelvis, such as a lateral

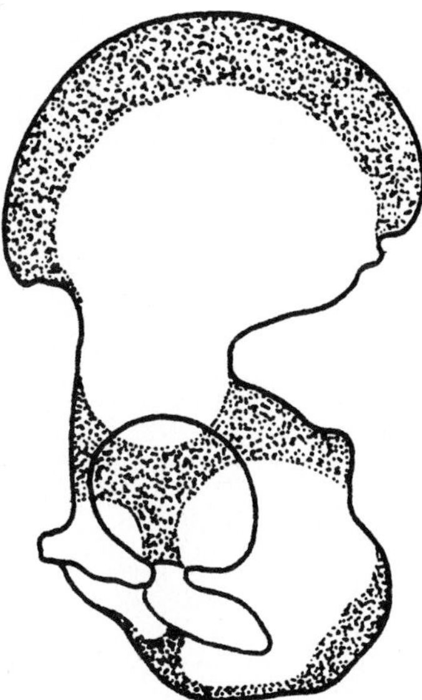

Figure 1-11 Confluence of the triradiate cartilage at the junction of the three pelvic bones and within the acetabulum. (From Bucholz RW, Ezaki M, Ogden JA: Injury to the acetabular triradiate physeal cartilage. J Bone Joint Surg Am 64:600-609, 1982.)

compression injury. Any laceration of the skin suggests an open pelvic fracture and should be probed or explored to define the depth of the laceration and determine whether it communicates with a spike of bone from a pelvic fracture. The landmarks of the pelvis should be palpated for tenderness, symmetry, and abnormal motion. Lateral compression at the iliac crests and AP compression at the symphysis pubis help identify instability or pain from a pelvic fracture. An apparent limb length discrepancy may represent an unstable pelvic fracture with a vertical shear component. Milch identified the following three signs as representative of pelvic fractures: (1) Destot sign, a superficial hematoma below the inguinal ligament or in the scrotum; (2) Roux sign, decreased distance between the greater trochanter on the involved side and the pubic spine; and (3) Earle sign, a bony prominence or hematoma detected on rectal examination.[33] Lacerations within the rectum strongly indicate an open pelvic fracture.

Thorough neurologic and vascular assessments of the lower extremities should also be performed in the trauma bay. Traumatic injuries involving the sacroiliac joint can result in stretching or disruption of the lumbosacral plexus. A detailed evaluation of sensation and muscle strength in the legs determines whether a neurologic deficit is present.

Imaging

A screening AP radiograph of the pelvis, without use of a gonadal shield, is routinely performed during the secondary survey of a pediatric trauma patient. Additional radiographs, including inlet and outlet views, are obtained to evaluate specific injuries to the pelvic ring after the child is stabilized. The inlet view, directed at an angle of 30 to 45 degrees caudad, helps define disruptions of the posterior pelvic ring such as at the sacroiliac joints. The tangential view, directed 40 to 45 degrees cephalad, is used to evaluate anterior pelvic ring injuries. When fractures of the acetabulum are suspected from the screening radiographs, the 45-degree oblique views (iliac and obturator oblique) described by Judet are obtained to better define the fracture.[33]

CT scans are being used with growing frequency when a pelvic fracture is noted or suspected from a screening radiograph. CT scans of the pelvis can be readily obtained at the same time other CT studies are requested for pediatric trauma patients, such as abdominal and head scans. The pelvis can be scanned with the use of 2- to 3-mm cuts extending from the L5 vertebra to the lower end of the pelvis. The use of soft tissue windows in addition to bone windows is helpful in defining the extent of pelvic hematoma. CT scans are important in determining the severity of injury to the posterior sacroiliac joints, occult posterior pelvic ring fractures of the ilium and the sacrum, posterior wall fractures of the acetabulum after fracture-dislocations of the hip, and intra-articular fragments within the hip joint after reduction of a hip dislocation (Fig. 1-12).

Technetium (^{99m}Tc) bone scans can also be obtained to detect occult or nondisplaced fractures of the pelvis. Injuries to the lower urinary tract should be investigated in pelvic fractures that result in wide displacement of the anterior pelvic ring. Retrograde urethrograms are obtained to delineate traumatic bladder injuries before insertion of Foley catheters, and intravenous pyelograms help define renal or urethral anatomy and function.

Associated Injuries

> The pelvis is like a suit of armor: when it is damaged there is much more concern about its contents than about the structure itself.
>
> *Mercer Rang*[34]

The presence of a pediatric pelvic fracture should alert the clinician that the child has experienced a significant high-energy trauma and may have other potentially life-threatening injuries. The incidence of associated injuries in children with a pelvic fracture is high. They may be intra-abdominal injuries, neurovascular and other intrapelvic injuries, genitourinary injuries, and closed-head injuries. Evaluation and treatment of these injuries take priority over the obvious pelvic fracture seen on the screening radiograph obtained as part of the trauma survey. Long-term morbidity in children with fractures of

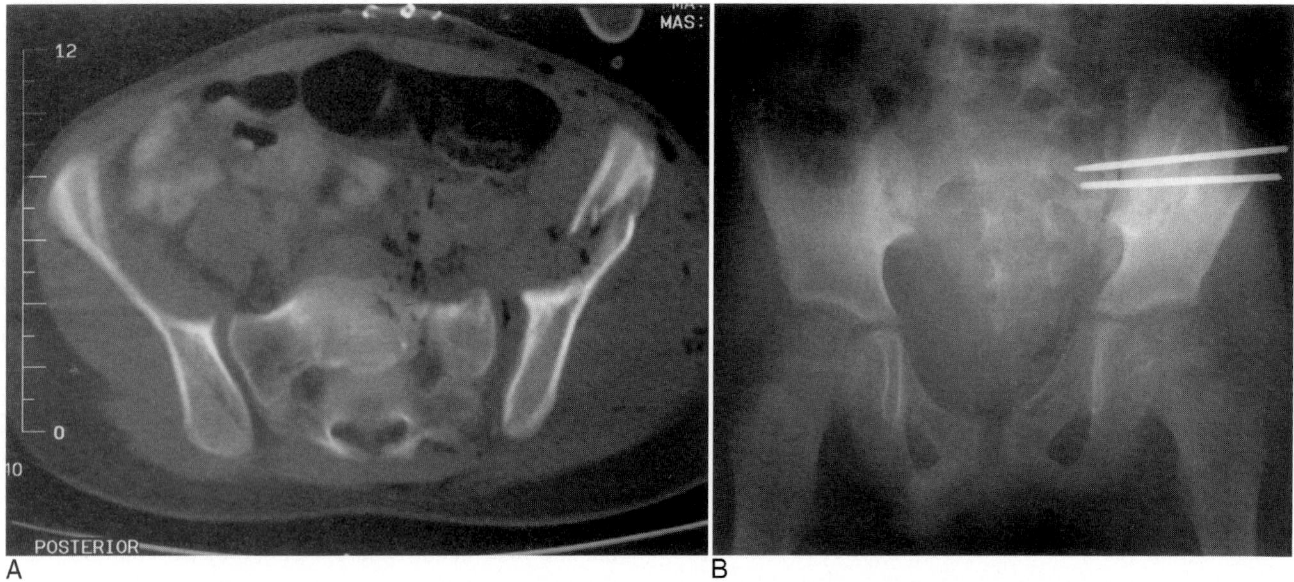

Figure 1-12 **A,** Computed tomography scan of a 10-year-child demonstrating widening of the left sacroiliac joint with associated iliac wing fracture. **B,** Postoperative radiograph showing fixation of the left sacroiliac joint with pin fixation.

the pelvis is more often the result of the associated injuries than of the skeletal injury itself.[3]

Numerous studies have evaluated the predictive risks of associated injuries that occur with pediatric pelvic fractures. These injuries may be difficult to diagnose in a child in the trauma setting. A child's age, noncompliance, or unconsciousness may limit his or her ability to communicate. Bond and associates[24] noted a 60% risk of concomitant abdominal injuries when multiple pelvic fractures were present. McIntyre and colleagues[26] found that unstable pelvic ring disruptions involving both the anterior and posterior parts of the pelvis were the only variables associated with life-threatening hemorrhage and higher blood transfusion requirements. Vazquez and Garcia[35] reported that the presence of a pelvic fracture and another skeletal fracture was associated with a significantly higher incidence of head and abdominal injuries. A study by Silber and colleagues[28] showed that 54% of children with pelvic fractures have associated nonpelvic fractures.

Concomitant abdominal or visceral injuries occur along with fractures of the pelvis in 20% of cases, often involving the spleen, liver, pancreas, or bowel.[24,26,28] The high costal margin of the rib cage and the poorly developed abdominal wall musculature contribute to the high incidence of these injuries in children. Chest traumas, such as pulmonary contusion and pneumothorax, also occur concurrently in 12% to 20% of pelvic fractures in children, in part due to the greater compliance of the chest wall.[26,28] Children may be at lower risk for injuries to the bladder and urethra than adults, primarily because of the decreased incidence of "straddle" fractures (bilateral fractures of the superior and inferior pubic rami) in children.[28] Closed-head injuries occur frequently with pelvic fractures in children, ranging from 21% to 61%, and are the most common cause of death in children with pelvic fractures.[28,34]

The overall mortality rate for children with pelvic fractures ranges from 2% to 12%.[29,35-37] The mortality rate is higher in adults (17%), for whom fatal exsanguination from the pelvic fracture itself is one of the leading causes of death. The lower rate of life-threatening hemorrhage after pelvic fractures in children may have several contributing factors. As noted previously, pelvic fractures in children most commonly occur after pedestrian-motor vehicle accidents, and a lateral compression fracture pattern results. The mechanism of injury is different in adults, usually the result of an anteroposterior force leading to an "open-book" fracture pattern that can increase pelvic volume and the potential for fatal bleeding. Lateral compression fractures of the pelvis in children do not increase pelvic volume, accounting for a lower risk of life-threatening hemorrhage.[28] The thick periosteal sleeve of the pediatric pelvis may also limit the amount of displacement in a fracture, contributing to a more stable fracture pattern and minimizing the potential for bleeding. In addition, children's blood vessels are thought to be more vasoreactive, a feature that may also limit the amount of bleeding from these smaller vessels.[24]

Classification

The use of classification schemes for fractures in general are important to define the severity of the fracture and other associated injuries, determine treatment, and allow assessment of outcomes. Factors critical in the analysis of pelvic fractures are stability, anatomic location, and mechanism of injury. Many different classification systems have evolved to describe both pediatric and adult pelvic fractures. Quimby[36] classified pediatric pelvic fractures as corresponding to the severity of the associated injuries, such as visceral injuries requiring operative exploration and those with significant hemorrhage. This classification represents a logical approach because the associated injuries can be life threatening and take precedence over the majority of pelvic fractures in initial evaluation and management. The major disadvantage of this system is the lack of defining the skeletal injury.

The Torode and Zieg classification scheme is frequently used for pediatric pelvic fractures.[3,28,37] This scheme predicts the potential associated injuries and expected outcomes with four types of pelvic fracture patterns of increasing severity, taking into account the anatomic and physiologic differences of the response of a child's pelvis to high-energy trauma (Fig. 1-13).[37] Type I fractures are avulsion fractures of the pelvis that commonly occur through the cartilaginous apophyseal growth plates. Type II pelvic fractures involve the iliac wing and are more common as isolated injuries in children than in adults. A laterally directed force against the pelvis in a pedestrian–motor vehicle accident is the most common mechanism of injury. Type III fractures are defined as simple ring fractures. They can be fractures of the pubic rami or disruptions of the pubic symphysis (diastasis) that are stable injuries. Because of the plasticity of the pelvis and the elasticity of the joints in a child, the posterior sacroiliac joint ligaments remain intact. Type III fractures tend to be stable, even with displaced fracture fragments. They can occur from AP compression, lateral compression, or vertical shear mechanisms of injury. Type IV fractures are unstable pelvic fractures; they include bilateral pubic rami or straddle fractures, fractures of the left or the right pubic rami (or the equivalent injury involving the pubic symphysis), disruption of the sacroiliac joint or fracture adjacent to it, and acetabular fractures. Type IV fractures represent the most severe injuries with the highest incidence of associated injuries to other organ systems. In their series, Torode and Zieg[37] found the greatest risk for growth disturbances, long-term disability and mortality, in type IV fractures.

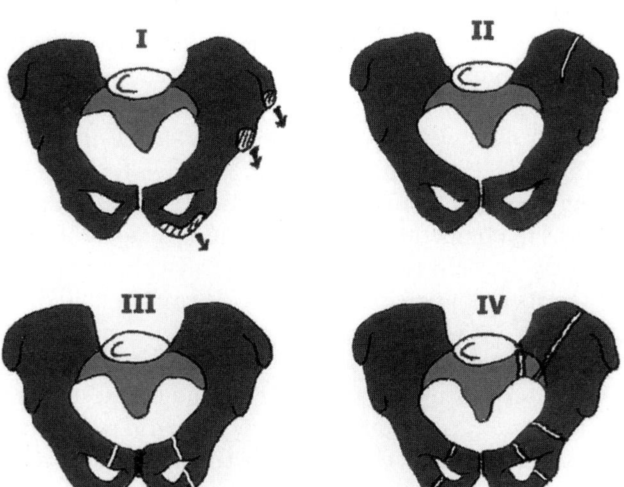

Figure 1-13 Torode and Zieg classification of pediatric pelvic fractures. (From Torode I, Zieg D: Pelvic fractures in children. J Pediatr Orthop 5:77-79, 1985.)

The presence of an open triradiate cartilage defining a skeletally immature pelvis has been proposed as an important radiographic marker that differentiates pediatric pelvic fractures from the adult-like pelvic fracture patterns and outcomes observed in older children and adolescents before skeletal maturity.[27] The incidence of unstable pelvic disruptions, such as diastasis of the pubic symphysis or the sacroiliac joints, is lower in the skeletally immature patient. The greater elasticity of the sacroiliac joints and the pubic symphysis, as well as the plasticity of the pelvis itself in the skeletally immature patient, accounts for these differences.

Management of Pelvic Fractures

The majority of pediatric pelvic fractures are stable injuries that need little more than 4 to 6 weeks of recumbency or no weight-bearing to allow for predictable healing. The thick periosteal sleeve of the pediatric pelvis gives inherent stability to most pelvic fractures. Even with mild fracture displacement, both healing and remodeling readily occur, and long-term morbidity is rare with stable pelvic fractures.[38] Progressive weight-bearing is permitted when patients are comfortable with activities such as transfers, and as much as the associated injuries allow. Pain from motion at the fracture site diminishes with early fracture healing and decreased motion of the fracture fragments. Patients are then rapidly encouraged to move, initially with crutches or a walker (partial weight-bearing), then with full and independent weight-bearing. Some children may benefit from a hip spica cast to obtain pain control, painless mobility, and an earlier discharge from the hospital.

A more aggressive approach is needed for unstable pelvic fractures such as the type IV fractures described by Torode and Zieg.[37] These fractures, often involving both the anterior and posterior pelvic ring, have the highest risk of long-term deformity and disability. Patients with these unstable fracture patterns also have the highest risk of associated abdominal or closed-head injuries, and rarely, can be hemodynamically unstable. The goals of treatment for these severe fractures, which are often both rotationally and vertically unstable, are to prevent deformity, restore joint congruity, minimize growth disturbances, and obtain hemodynamic stability.[38] Reduction of such fractures can be achieved by either closed or open methods.

Older methods of closed reduction consist of the use of a pelvic sling for open-book injuries with separation of the pubic symphysis of more than 3 cm, and the use of distal femoral skeletal traction for vertical shear injuries. External fixation of pelvic fractures is still widely used, particularly with open-book fractures and disruption of the anterior sacroiliac joint ligaments (Fig. 1-14). In the hemodynamically unstable child or adolescent, the application of an external fixation frame can rapidly close the pelvis and decrease pelvic volume, effectively exerting a tamponade effect and minimizing further hemorrhage from the fracture. On rare occasions, angiographic embolization is required to control life-threatening bleeding in a child.

There are several indications for open reduction and internal fixation of pelvic fractures. For some fractures, these methods are performed in combination with external fixation of the anterior pelvic ring (Fig. 1-15); indications include open displaced pelvic fractures, displaced and rotationally unstable pelvic fractures that cannot be reduced by closed methods, displaced vertical shear fractures (with disruption of the posterior sacroiliac joint complex), and open-book type fractures with more than 3 cm of separation of the symphysis pubis that are associated with hemorrhage or requiring exploratory laparotomy. Open reduction and internal fixation are thought to facilitate the care of the child with multiple injuries.

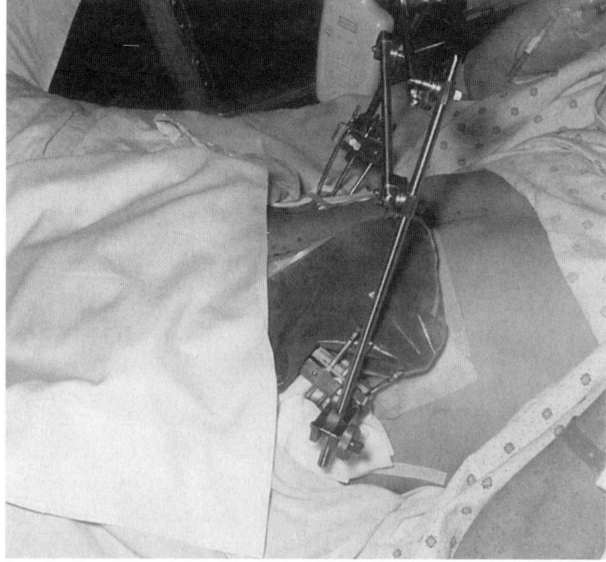

Figure 1-14 External fixation of the pelvis in a 14-year-old child after an open pelvic fracture. Note the diverting colostomy.

Avulsion Fractures

The presence of apophyses about the pelvic ring in children often results in avulsion fractures, which most often occur in adolescents after competitive athletic events. The apophyses or secondary centers of ossification are located at the iliac crest, anterior superior iliac spine (ASIS), anterior inferior iliac spine (AIIS), and the ischium (Fig. 1-16). The apophyses tend to appear and fuse later than the epiphyseal centers of long bones. Forceful concentric or eccentric contractures of large muscle groups can generate sufficient tension across an open pelvic apophysis to cause an avulsion fracture. Displacement of the avulsed fragment of bone depends on the specific avulsion fracture and can be limited by additional soft tissue attachments to the apophysis.[32]

The majority of these injuries can be treated nonoperatively. Early recognition of the injury, which often has a classic presentation, is important. Patients are often between 13 and 17 years old, present with a sudden onset of pain about the pelvis, and commonly describe having felt a "pop" in the thigh or hip region. Palpation about the pelvis for areas of tenderness and resistance testing of specific muscle groups should localize the site of injury. Tenderness about the ischium and pain with knee extension due to the pull of the hamstrings on the ischial apophysis are suggestive of an avulsion injury to the ischial tuberosity. Radiographs of the pelvis demonstrate and confirm the avulsion fracture, often diagnosed from the history and clinical examination. The radiographs may also disclose avulsion injuries of the greater or lesser trochanter. When patients present without a clear traumatic episode, infectious or neoplastic processes such as osteomyelitis or Ewing sarcoma may be evident on plain radiographs.

The majority of avulsion fractures of the pelvis can be treated conservatively with a graduated rehabilitative program of partial or foot-flat weight-bearing on crutches for 6 weeks or until there is evidence of healing of the avulsion fracture is present; a progressive strengthening program should be initiated before the patient returns to competitive sports activities.[32] If avulsion fractures are properly treated, operative reattachment or excision because of persistent disability is rarely required.

Acetabular Fractures

Fractures of the acetabulum in children are uncommon injuries, accounting for 12% of pediatric pelvic fractures.[31] The presence of an open triradiate cartilage in the pelvis in children makes the pattern of injuries, prognosis, and complications of acetabular fracture different from those seen in adults. The chondro-osseous complex involving the triradiate cartilage is formed by the

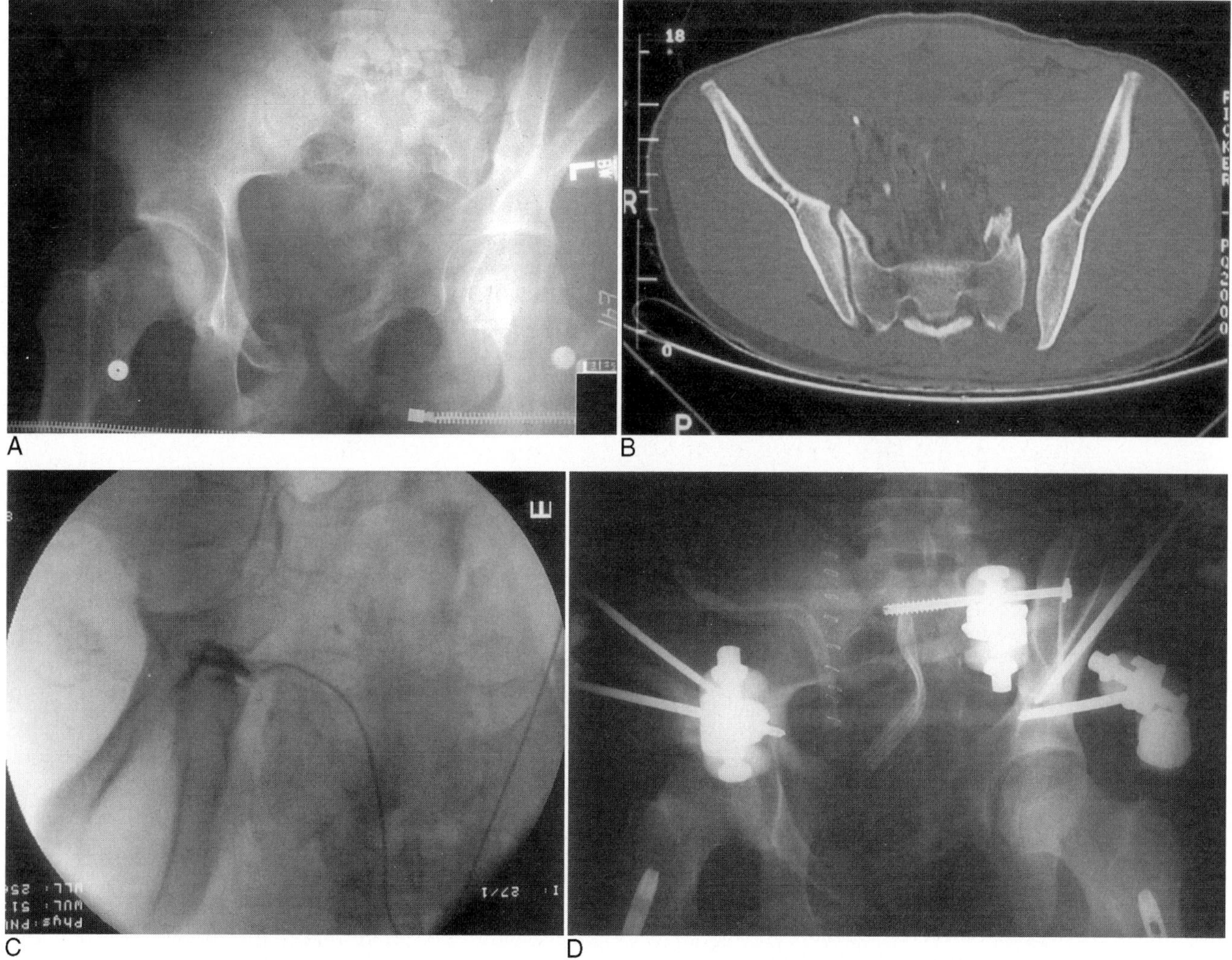

Figure 1-15 Torode and Zieg type IV pelvic fracture in a 16-year-old boy after a motor vehicle accident. The boy also sustained severe head and intra-abdominal injuries. **A,** Anteroposterior radiograph of the pelvis shows a straddle fracture of the anterior ring and disruption of the left sacroiliac (SI) joint. The patient was hemodynamically unstable upon admission. **B,** Computed tomography scan of the pelvis showing the left SI joint injury and an associated sacral fracture. **C,** Angiographic embolization was performed to control life-threatening hemorrhage. **D,** Stabilization of the anterior ring with external fixation and internal fixation of the posterior ring with a left SI joint screw.

confluence of the ischium, innominate, and pubic bones. Normal growth and development of the pediatric acetabulum occur by interstitial and appositional growth.[30] Injuries to the acetabulum can occur from a shearing force, resulting in a Salter-Harris type I or II injury, or from a crush-type injury, leading to a Salter-Harris type V injury (Fig. 1-17). Crush injury has a poorer prognosis, which may lead to premature closure of the triradiate cartilage and subsequent growth disturbance. Crush injuries are often missed on initial radiographs. In addition to the chondro-osseous injury, disruption of the blood supply to the germinal zone of the physis or growth plate of the triradiate cartilage may contribute to a growth disturbance of the acetabulum.[31]

Prognosis depends on the age of the child at the time of injury as well as the extent of the chondro-osseous injury.[31,39] Premature closure of the triradiate cartilage in a young child leads to a progressively shallow or dysplastic acetabulum. Over time, the growing femoral head is displaced superiorly and laterally, eventually resulting in hip subluxation. Because progressive acetabular dysplasia may not be noted for several years after a fracture, patients with suspected injury to the triradiate cartilage must be monitored until they reach skeletal maturity.[31,37,39]

Evaluation of pediatric patients with acetabular fractures requires the three standard radiographic views of the pelvis—AP, internal oblique, and external oblique

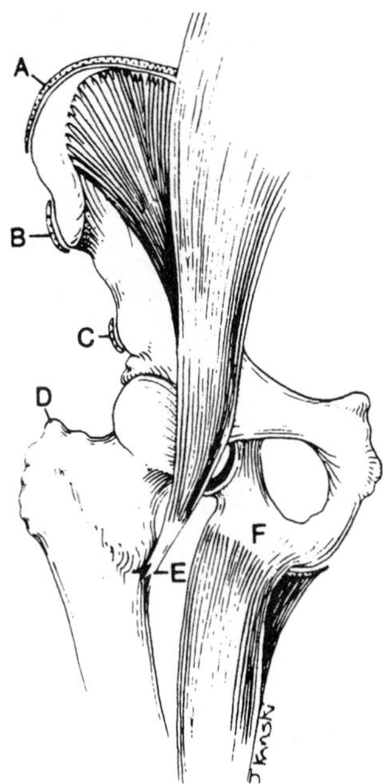

Figure 1-16 Sites of apophyseal avulsion fractures off the pediatric pelvis. A, iliac crest; B, anterior superior iliac spine; C, anterior inferior iliac spine; D, greater trochanter; E, lesser trochanter; F, ischial tuberosity. (From Fernbach SK, Wilkinson RH: Avulsion injuries of the pelvis and proximal femur. AJR Am J Roentgenol 137:581-584, 1981.)

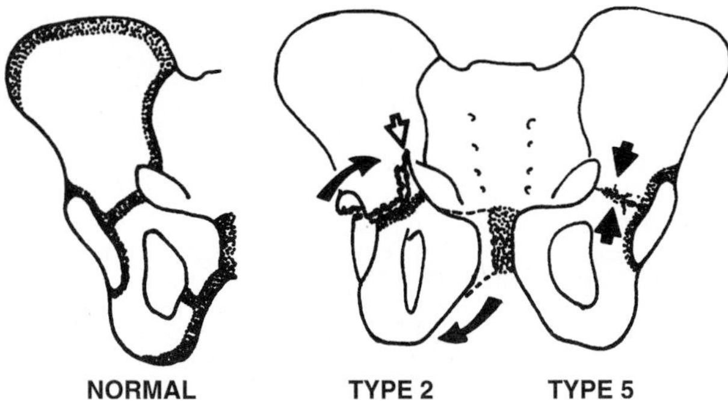

Figure 1-17 Salter-Harris type II and type V physeal fractures of the pediatric acetabulum. (From Bucholz RW, Ezaki M, Ogden JA: Injury to the acetabular triradiate physeal cartilage. J Bone Joint Surg Am 64:600-609, 1982.)

images (Judet views). These views help define the extent and pattern of the fracture. Dislocations of the femoral head frequently occur with acetabular fractures, and urgent reduction of the dislocation is critical to reduce the risk of avascular necrosis of the femoral head. CT scans are mandatory in the postreduction assessment of fracture-dislocations of the acetabulum to evaluate for joint space widening or joint incongruity. Loose cartilage fragments causing joint incongruity are easily missed on plain radiographs. CT scanning can be performed at the time of the initial trauma evaluation so as to identify other injuries to the pelvic ring and define the extent of the injury. The management of acetabular fractures depends on the extent and severity of the injury. Options for treatment include bed rest, no weight-bearing, skeletal traction, percutaneous internal fixation, and open reduction with internal fixation (Figs. 1-18 and 1-19). The indications for the surgical procedure are fractures that involve the major weight-bearing surface of the acetabulum with more than 2 mm of displacement and unstable fracture-dislocations of the posterior wall.[33]

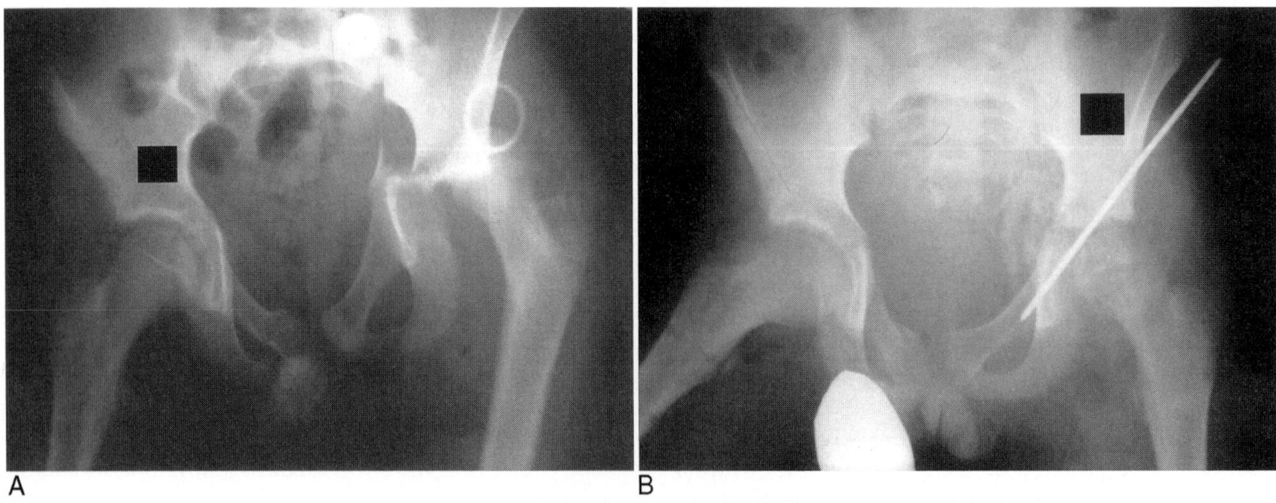

Figure 1-18 Left acetabular fracture-dislocation in an 11-year-old boy after a motor vehicle accident. He sustained multiple injuries, including a closed-head injury, a right forearm fracture, and a right femur fracture. **A,** Anteroposterior radiograph demonstrating the left Salter-Harris type II acetabular fracture and dislocation of the femoral head. **B,** Open reduction with pin fixation of the left acetabular fracture.

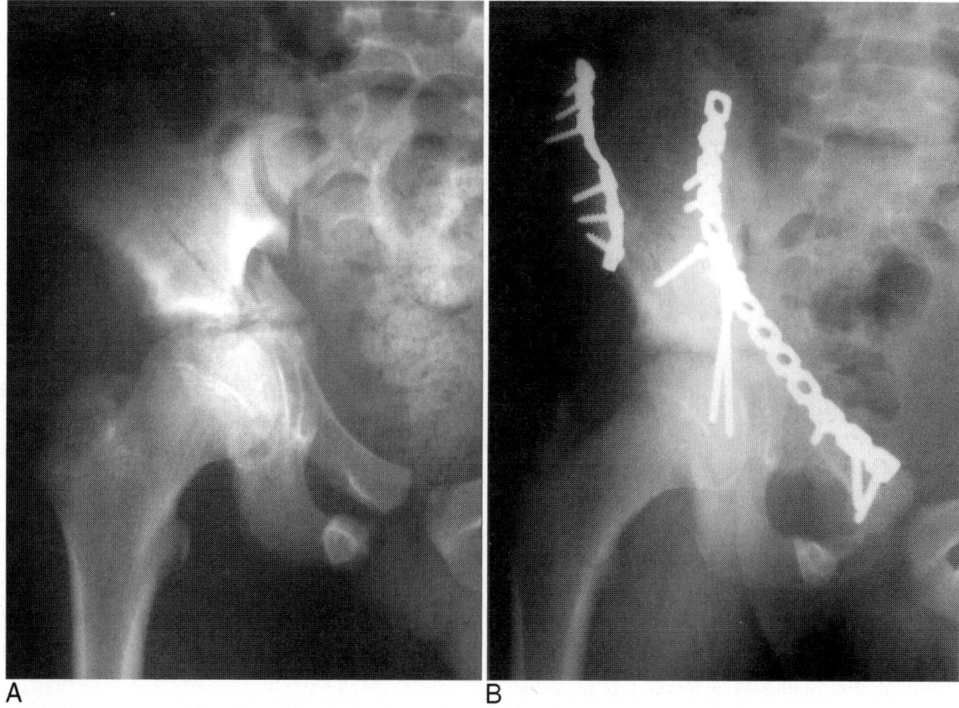

Figure 1-19 Right Salter-Harris type II fracture of the acetabulum and associated iliac wing fracture in a 14-year-old child after a motor vehicle accident. **A,** Anteroposterior radiograph of the right acetabular fracture. **B,** Open reduction and internal fixation of the right acetabular and iliac wing fractures.

MAJOR POINTS

Pediatric spinal and pelvic fractures are uncommon injuries, often occurring after high-energy traumatic events.

The unique mechanisms of injury and the anatomic differences characteristic of the pediatric spine contribute to the different fracture patterns and responses to injuries seen in children.

A thorough understanding of the normal developmental anatomy of the pediatric cervical spine and its normal variants is critical to the evaluation of cervical spine injuries in children.

The presence of the lap belt sign may indicate a flexion-distraction mechanism of injury to the lumbar spine and the potential for associated intra-abdominal injuries.

Radiographic demonstration of pelvic fracture is highly suggestive of high-energy trauma, and the physician must be aware of the high risk of associated life-threatening injuries.

The greater flexibility and plasticity of the skeletally immature pelvis contribute to the differences in fracture patterns and responses to injury from those seen in adults.

The majority of pelvic fractures in children is stable and can be managed conservatively. The risk of life-threatening hemorrhage and death from pelvic fractures is lower in children than in adults.

REFERENCES

1. Cramer KE:The pediatric polytrauma patient. Clin Orthop 318125-135, 1995.
2. Hadley MN, Zabramski JM, Browner CM, et al: Pediatric spinal trauma: Review of 122 cases of spinal cord and vertebral column injuries. J Neurosurg 68:18-24, 1988.
3. Garvin K, McCarthy R, Barnes C, et al: Pediatric pelvic ring fractures. J Pediatr Orthop 10:577-582, 1990.
4. McGrory BJ, Klassen RA, Chao EY, et al: Acute fractures and dislocations of the cervical spine in children and adolescents. J Bone Joint Surg Am 75:988-995, 1993.
5. Herzenberg JE, Hensinger RN, Dedrick DK, et al: Emergency transport and positioning of young children who have an injury of the cervical spine: The standard backboard may be hazardous. J Bone Joint Surg Am 71:5-22, 1989.
6. Sovio OM, Ball HM, Beauchamp RD, Tredwell SJ: Fracture of the lumbar vertebral apophysis. J Pediatr Orthop 5:550-552, 1985.
7. Flynn JM, Dormans JP: Spine trauma in children. Semin Spine Surg 10:7-16, 1998.
8. Yngve DA, Harris WP, Herndon WA, et al: Spinal cord injury without osseous spine fracture. J Pediatr Orthop 8:153-159, 1988
9. King J, Diefendorfer D, Apthorp J, et al: Analysis of 429 fractures in 189 battered children. J Pediatr Orthop 8:585-589, 1988.
10. Kleinman PK, Marks SC: Vertebral body fractures in child abuse: Radiologic-histopathologic correlates. Invest Radiol 27:715-722, 1992.

11. Bell HJ, Dykstra DD: Somatosensory evoked potentials as an adjunct to diagnosis of neonatal spinal cord injury. J Pediatr 106:298-301, 1985.

12. Johnson DL, Falci S: The diagnosis and treatment of pediatric lumbar spine injuries caused by rear seat lap belts. Neurosurgery 26:434-441, 1990.

13. Rumball K, Jarvis J: Seat-belt injuries of the spine in young children. J Bone Joint Surg Br 74:571-574, 1992.

14. Hoy GA, Cole WG: The pediatric cervical seat belt syndrome. Injury 24:297-299, 1993.

15. Dormans JP: Evaluation of children with suspected cervical spine injury. J Bone Joint Surg Am 84:124-132, 2002.

16. Swischuk LE: Anterior displacement of C2 in children: Physiologic or pathologic? Radiology 122:759-763, 1977.

17. Philips WA, Hensinger RN: The management of atlanto-axial subluxation in children. J Bone Joint Surg Am 71:664-668, 1989.

18. Odent T, Langlais J, Glorion C, et al: Fractures of the odontoid process: A report of 15 cases in children younger than 6 years. J Pediatr Orthop 19:51-54, 1999.

19. Fielding JW, Hawkins RJ: Atlanto-axial rotary fixation (fixed rotary subluxation of the atlanto-axial joint). J Bone Joint Surg Am 59:37-44, 1977.

20. Pennecot GF, Leonard P, Peyrot Des Gachons S: Traumatic ligamentous instability of the cervical spine. J Pediatr Orthop 4:346-352, 1984.

21. Denis F: The three column spine and its significance in the classification of acute thoracolumbar spinal injuries. Spine 8:817-831, 1983.

22. Sturm PF, Glass RB, Sivit CJ, et al: Lumbar compression fractures secondary to lap-belt use in children. J Pediatr Orthop 15:521-523, 1995.

23. Lalonde F, Letts M, Yang JP, Thomas K: An analysis of burst fractures of the spine in adolescents. Am J Orthop 30:115-120, 2001.

24. Bond S, Gotshall C, Eichelberger M: Predictors of abdominal injury in children with pelvic fractures. J Trauma 31:1169-1173, 1991.

25. Ismail N, Bellemore J, Moll HD, et al: Death from pelvic fractures: Children are different. J Pediatr Surg 31:82-85, 1996.

26. McIntyre RC, Bensard DD, Moore EE, et al: Pelvic fracture geometry predicts risk of life-threatening hemorrhage in children. J Trauma 35:423-429, 1993.

27. Watts HG: Fractures of the pelvis in children. Orthop Clin North Am 7:615-624, 1976.

28. Silber JS, Flynn JM, Koffler KM, et al: Analysis of the cause, classification, and associated injuries of 166 consecutive pelvic fractures. J Pediatr Orthop 21:446-450, 2001.

29. Silber JS, Flynn JM: Changing patterns of pediatric pelvic fractures with skeletal maturation: Implications for classification and management. J Pediatr Orthop 22:22-26, 2002.

30. Ponseti IV: Growth and development of the acetabulum in the normal child: Anatomical, histological, and roentgenographical studies. J Bone Joint Surg Am 60:575-585, 1978.

31. Bucholz R, Ezaki M, Ogden J: Injury to the acetabular triradiate physeal cartilage. J Bone J Surg Am 64:600-609, 1982.

32. Metzmaker JN, Pappas A: Avulsion fractures of the pelvis. Am J Sports Med 13:349-358, 1985.

33. Canale ST, Beaty JH: Pelvic and hip fractures. In Rockwood CA Jr, Wilkins KE, Beaty JH (eds): Fractures in Children, 4th ed. Philadelphia, Lippincott-Raven, 1996, pp 1109-1147.

34. Rang M: Children's Fractures, 2nd ed. Philadelphia, JB Lippincott, 1983, pp 233-241.

35. Vazquez WD, Garcia VF: Pediatric pelvic fractures combined with an additional skeletal injury is an indicator of significant injury. Surg Gynecol Obstet 177:486-492, 1993.

36. Quimby WC: Fractures of the pelvis and associated injuries in children. J Pediatr Surg 1:353-364, 1966.

37. Torode I, Zieg D: Pelvic fractures in children. J Pediatr Orthop 5:76, 1985..

38. Blasier RD, McAfee J, White J, et al: Disruption of the pelvic ring in pediatric patients. Clin Orthop 376:87-95, 2000.

39. Heeg M, Klassen H, Visser J: Acetabular fractures in children and adolescents. J Bone Joint Surg Br 71:418-421, 1989.

CHAPTER 2

Upper Extremity Injuries

JOHN M. FLYNN
SAMEER NAGDA

Injuries to the hand, forearm, arm, and shoulder are the most common musculoskeletal injuries sustained by children.[17] Though most can be successfully treated and can heal uneventfully, careful attention to certain principles of diagnosis and management are crucial to a consistently good outcome. Many skeletal injuries in children involve the growth plate. These injuries are commonly classified into five types, known as Salter-Harris types I through V (Fig. 2-1).

HAND INJURIES

General Principles

The pediatric hand is a very common site for injury. Children are constantly exploring their surroundings, so their hands are continuously exposed to potential accidents. The incidence of hand fractures increases sharply after age 8 years, peaks in boys at age 13 years, when they are often participating in contact sports. Physeal injuries represent between 10% and 40% of hand fractures.[1] The most common physeal fracture is the Salter-Harris type (SH) II variant. The thumb and the little finger are the most commonly injured digits.

The immature hand has epiphyses at both the proximal end and the distal end of all tubular bones. However, secondary ossification centers develop only in the proximal end of the thumb metacarpal and distal ends of the other four metacarpals. As a child reaches skeletal maturity, the irregularity of the physeal zones increases,[2] and a fracture through the physis can be transmitted through several zones. This development may account for the

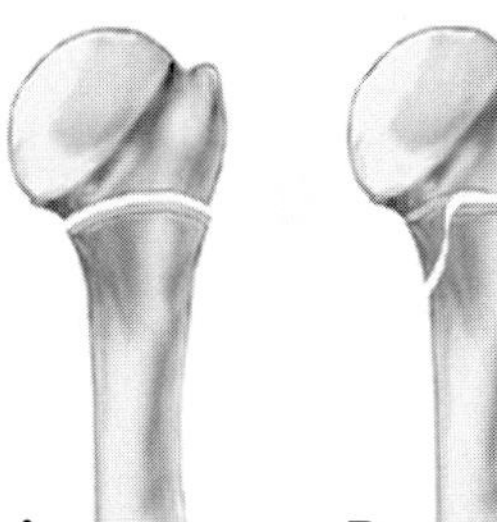

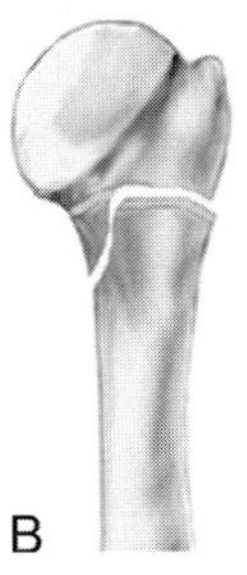

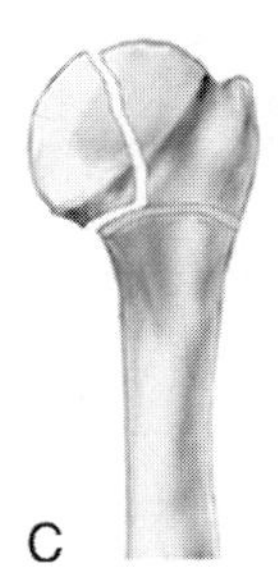

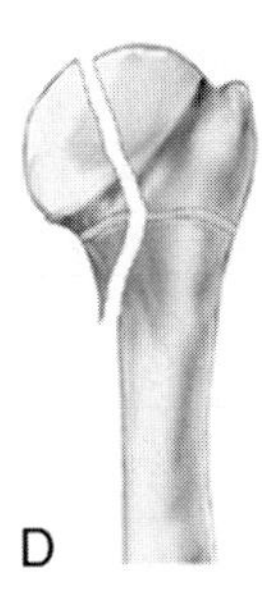

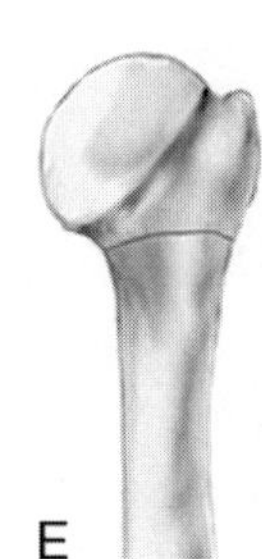

Figure 2-1 Salter-Harris Classification of Physeal Fractures. A, Type I: fracture through the physis. **B,** Type II: fracture through physis extending through metaphysis. **C,** Type III: fracture through physis extending through epiphysis. **D,** Type IV: fracture through the metaphysis and epiphysis. **E,** Type V: compression-type fracture.

partial growth arrest seen after some physeal fractures. SH I and SH II fractures occur more often in younger patients, whereas SH III and SH IV fractures are seen more commonly in children approaching skeletal maturity.[3]

The ligaments of the child are stronger than the physeal and epiphyseal bone. For that reason, tendon and ligamentous injuries are uncommon. Extensor tendons insert onto the epiphyses of the terminal phalanges. The flexor digitorum profundus inserts onto the distal phalanx, and the flexor digitorum superficialis onto the middle phalanx. All interphalangeal joints have collateral ligaments that insert onto the metaphysis and epiphysis of the respective bones. The ligaments also insert onto the volar plate. The volar plate is a soft tissue structure that functions to stabilize the joint against hyperextension forces.

Nail bed injuries are very common in children. An awareness and understanding of nail bed anatomy are essential for anyone treating these injuries. Figure 2-2 diagrams the anatomy of the distal phalanx in a child. The nail bed is composed of a germinal matrix and a sterile matrix. The germinal matrix produces the cells that make up the overlying nail.

Evaluation of the pediatric hand can be a challenge. Injured children are usually very apprehensive about allowing anyone to come near them. Even a parent can be an obstacle to a complete evaluation. Calming both parties before any examination is critical. Examining other, uninvolved areas first can give the child some comfort and allow the examiner to ease into the examination. The first thing to assess for is an open injury. Palpation of the hand provides an indication of injured areas, although bony landmarks are often difficult to feel. Tenderness at the insertion site of a ligament or tendon can provide clues to soft tissue injuries. Range of motion, both passive and active, should be measured at every joint, and the stability of all joints against varus and valgus forces

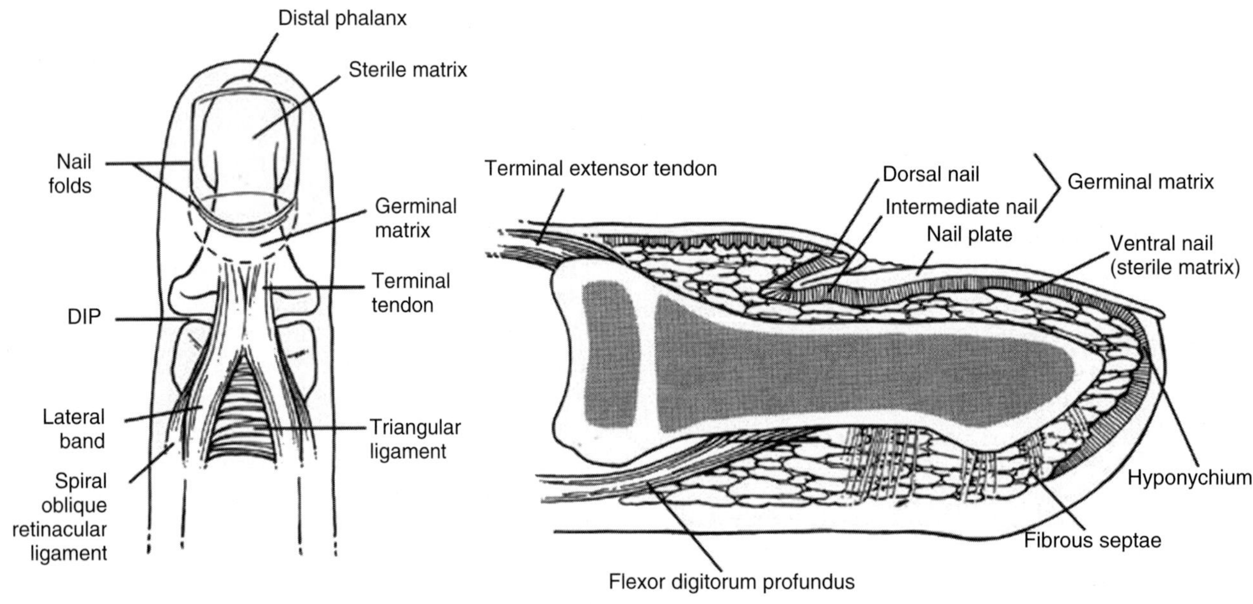

Figure 2-2 Anatomy about the distal phalanx. A, The skin, nail, and extensor apparatus share a close relation with the bone of the distal phalanx. Specific anatomical structures at the terminal aspect of the digit are labeled. **B,** This lateral view of the nail demonstrates the tendon insertions and the specific anatomy of the specialized nail tissues. (From Rockwood CA Jr, Wilkins KE, Beaty JH: Fractures in Children, 4th ed. Philadelphia, Lippincott-Raven, 1996.)

should be checked. Volar plate integrity should also be assessed with gentle hyperextension testing.

Neurologic examination can be very difficult in children. One clue to possible nerve injury is excessive bleeding from a wound around the area of the digital nerve, because laceration of the digital artery is often associated with an injury to the digital nerve. One helpful way to assess nerve injury is the "wrinkle test," which is performed as follows: The digit is immersed in warm water for 5 minutes. In denervated digits, there will be wrinkling of the volar skin.

Radiographic evaluation should include anteroposterior (AP), lateral, and oblique views. Oblique views are helpful for assessing intra-articular injuries.

Treatment of any hand injury begins with proper pain control. Conscious sedation is used when manipulation of a fracture is required. Digital blocks are very effective for phalangeal and nail bed injuries. Lidocaine is effective, but epinephrine should never be used. Lidocaine should be injected from the dorsal surface of the hand on both sides of the metacarpophalangeal (MCP) joint. The physician should insert the needle almost to the volar surface and retract the needle as the anesthetic is injected. Injection should never be made in a circle around the circumference of digit, because the circulation to the digit could be compromised.

An orthopaedic surgeon should be consulted for manipulation of a fracture. Repeated attempts to reduce physeal fractures will increase the chances of premature growth arrest. Early reduction before swelling occurs makes the reduction easier and can help prevent increased swelling. Immobilization should be achieved immediately after the reduction.

SPECIFIC FRACTURES OF THE HAND

Phalangeal Fractures

Fractures of the distal phalanx are very common. They can range from closed avulsion fractures to high-energy crush injuries.

The orthopaedist should be consulted for crush injuries of the distal phalanx. They can manifest as severe comminution of the underlying bone, disruption of the nail bed, and significant soft tissue injury. One must be careful to preserve all possible tissue during evaluation and treatment. The nail is removed if not already off. The nail bed injury often manifests as a stellate laceration. The wound is irrigated because this is an open fracture. Antibiotics and tetanus prophylaxis are given. The nail bed should be loosely approximated with 6-0 or smaller absorbable suture. The healing potential in children is excellent, and loose approximation will allow healing. Treatment of the nail bed injury often acts as a splint to bring the underlying fracture together (Fig. 2-3).

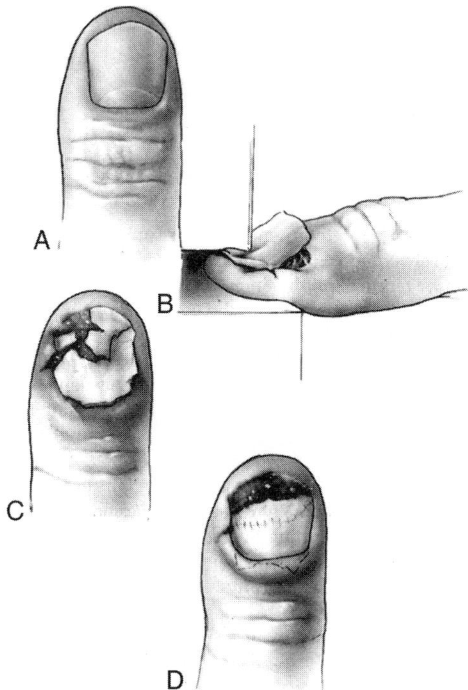

Figure 2-3 **A** and **B,** The normal nail with the most common mechanism of trauma. **C,** The resulting stellate laceration of the nail bed often accompanied with distal phalanx fracture. **D,** The resulting repair of a nail bed with the nail replaced as a stent. (From Lovell W, Winter R: In Morrissy RT, Weistein SL [eds]: Pediatric Orthopaedics. Philadelphia, Lippincott-Raven, 1996.)

After repair of the nail bed, the nail is replaced onto the bed with the end of it inserted under the nail fold. It should also be sutured in place. A nail substitute can be fashioned from the sterile suture packaging. Using the contralateral nail as a guide, one can cut a piece off the wrapping and use it in place of a destroyed or missing nail. These injuries often involve significant tissue destruction.

Hand surgery consultation should be obtained if there is any question regarding management. Regardless of how confident one is with management of hand injuries, the patient should always be referred to a hand surgeon for follow-up.

Mallet Finger

A mallet finger deformity is a common presentation of distal phalanx injuries. The child complains of pain and inability to extend the distal portion of the digit after a hyperextension injury. It is similar to the mallet finger injury in adults, but the underlying pathology is different. In adults, the cause is a disruption of the tendon, but in children, it is an avulsion fracture. Children younger than 5 years have a SH I or SH II injury, with the flexor tendon still attached to the distal piece and pulling it in a volar direction. Children closer to adolescence usually have an SH III injury. Common physeal injuries are shown in Figure 2-4.

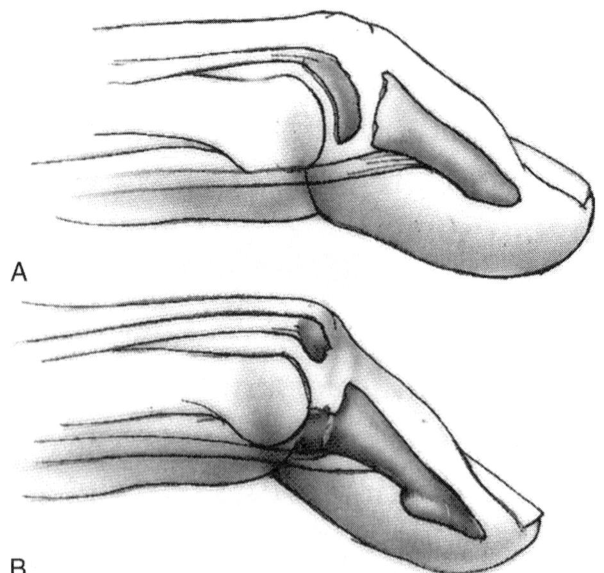

Figure 2-4 In the child and the adolescent, mallet finger fractures are very different. A, A Salter type I fracture seen in a child. **B,** A Salter type III fracture seen in an adult patient nearing skeletal maturity. (From Lovell W, Winter R: In Morrissy RT, Weistein SL [eds]: Pediatric Orthopaedics. Philadelphia, Lippincott-Raven, 1996.)

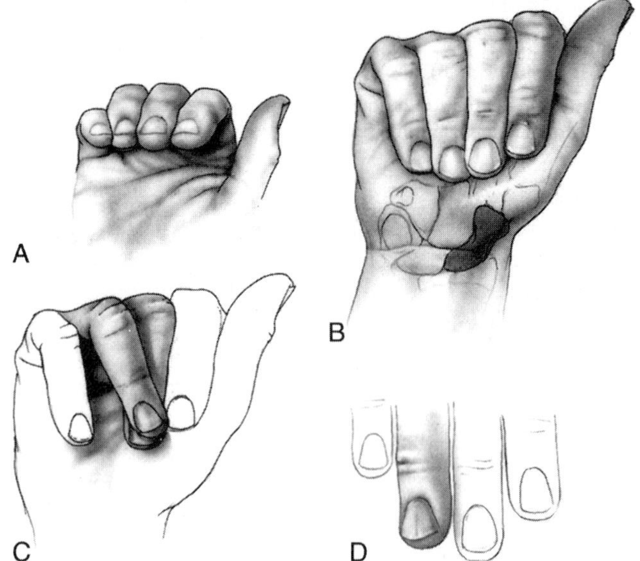

Figure 2-5 In the uninjured hand, all nail beds are parallel **(A)** and, with flexion, all fingertips point to the scaphoid tubercle **(B).** In malrotation, all fingertips do not point to the scaphoid tubercle **(C),** and the nail beds are not parallel **(D).** (From Lovell W, Winter R: In Morrissy RT, Weistein SL [eds]: Pediatric Orthopaedics. Philadelphia, Lippincott-Raven, 1996.)

Regardless of the obvious nature of the diagnosis, plain radiographs should be obtained to assess the displacement of the fracture. The patient should be splinted with the digit in extension for 3 to 4 weeks. Hand surgery consultation should be arranged to ensure close follow-up. Some patients closer to skeletal maturity may need operative fixation for severely displaced fractures.

Another easily overlooked injury is the "jersey finger" injury. This injury is essentially the opposite of the mallet finger and usually occurs in adolescents near skeletal maturity. It is most often the result of a true flexor tendon avulsion and is classically seen in a football player whose finger gets caught in an opposing player's jersey. The patient has a history of a forced extension of a flexed digit. Inability to flex the digit at the distal interphalangeal (DIP) joint is pathognomonic. Plain radiographs should be performed, and a hand surgery consultation should be arranged immediately. Surgical intervention is usually required to reattach the tendon and should be performed within 7 to 10 days of the injury.

Fractures of the proximal and middle phalanges can be classified into the following four groups: physeal, shaft, neck, and intra-articular (condylar). Careful examination with observation, palpation, and range-of-motion testing should reveal any associated soft tissue injuries or rotational deformities. It is essential to assess the level of rotational deformity can. Often a significant deformity is present even though initial finding is subtle finding (Fig. 2-5).

Plain radiographs are essential in the diagnosis and pretreatment planning. Oblique views may show intra-articular extension better than AP or lateral views. Lateral views offer details of any sagittal plane deformity. An orthopaedic surgeon should be consulted for a displaced or intra-articular fracture. The orthopaedist may use a pencil as a fulcrum over which angulation can be reduced (Fig. 2-6). SH II fractures are extremely common and can be managed with immobilization alone if there is no significant displacement. Overall, most proximal and middle phalangeal fractures can be treated with nonoperative management

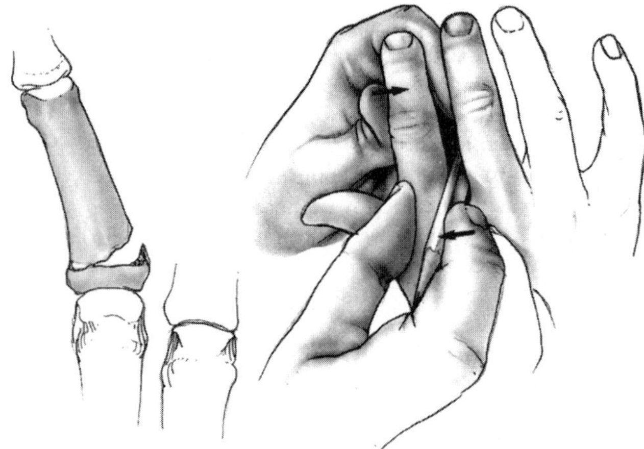

Figure 2-6 The "extra octave" fracture is hard to reduce and hold in place. The pencil technique is a way to manipulate this fracture, although some physicians believe that the pencil is distal to the apex of the fracture, hindering a satisfactory reduction. (From Lovell W, Winter R: In Morrissy RT, Weistein SL [eds]: Pediatric Orthopaedics. Philadelphia, Lippincott-Raven, 1996.)

consisting of closed reduction and casting for 3 to 4 weeks. Outcomes are usually excellent, as healing and remodeling in children are significant.

Fingertip Amputations

Distal fingertip amputations and avulsions can be gruesome injuries, and both patients and parents may be hysterical at presentation. The history is often similar to that for a crush injury, but the force causes an avulsion rather than a true crush. The orthopaedist must evaluate for the extent of tissue deficit, the amount of visible bone, and the presence of vessel or nerve injury. The avulsed part may be missing or too damaged to salvage. If the piece is brought in by the parents, its quality must be assessed. Even if the tissue is not viable, it may still serve as a biologic dressing to cover any visible bone in the short term. The piece should be irrigated and placed in a damp, saline-soaked gauze until after the finger has been cleaned. Motor and sensory examinations should be performed on the proximal portion before any digital nerve block is performed. Excessive bleeding signals a digital vessel injury, and direct pressure should be applied until the bleeding stops. Antibiotic and tetanus prophylaxis should be administered. A hand surgeon should be consulted immediately because operative management is often indicated.

The wound should be irrigated after a good digital nerve block has been obtained. One can reassess the wound after irrigating and débride any nonviable tissue. Significant tissue deficit should be evaluated and managed by an experienced hand surgeon. If the distal piece is intact, it can be placed on the proximal piece and approximated with 5-0 or 6-0 absorbable sutures. If the amputation traverses through the nail bed, a meticulous repair should be performed, and the nail fold should be splinted with the technique described for crush injuries. Once the repair is complete, the wound should be dressed with sterile gauze and copious amounts of padding. Close follow-up by a hand surgeon is critical to monitor for any signs of infection or necrosis of the distal piece. Outcomes vary for fingertip amputations and avulsions and are usually better for extremely young children.

Nail Bed Injuries

Nail bed injuries are common injuries in children and can easily be missed. Often the only clue on physical examination is a subungual hematoma. A hematoma larger than 25% of the nail bed should raise suspicion of bed injury and prompt a direct visual evaluation of the nail bed. Plain radiographs should be obtained to assess for a concomitant fracture. A hand surgeon should be consulted immediately. A digital nerve block is established by injection of 1% plain lidocaine around the radial and ulnar digital nerve at the proximal end of the digit to be treated. After this block is performed, the nail should be elevated with a blunt instrument such as a Freer elevator. If a laceration is identified, it should be repaired meticulously; 6-0 absorbable suture can be used to approximate the edges. The nail should be used as a splint. This repair can be performed in an emergency department setting. Close follow-up with a hand surgeon should be arranged. Outcomes of nail bed injuries are good overall. Meticulous repair of the laceration improves the chances of a good outcome.

Fractures of the Metacarpals

The metacarpals, unlike the phalanges, are relatively protected by their position within the hand. The relative mobility of the metacarpals varies, with the second and third metacarpals having less mobility. Fractures can occur at the head, neck, shaft, or base. The neck is the most common site of fracture. Fracture patterns of the metacarpal shaft are similar to those of the phalangeal shaft. Fractures of the second and third metacarpals tend to have less displacement because of the surrounding soft tissue. The injury can occur from a direct blow, a rotational force, or an axial load.

Fractures of the metacarpal head are seen most commonly as SH II fractures of the fifth digit in adolescents. Physeal injuries of the other metacarpals are rarely seen.[4] Radiographic evaluation of the hand usually shows the fracture. A hand radiograph is taken with the dorsum of the hand against the cassette and the MCP joint flexed 65 degrees. The beam is angled 15 degrees to the ulnar side of the hand. There is a risk of avascular necrosis of the head in such a fracture. It is postulated that the risk is greater with a hematoma collection at the fracture site.[5] Therefore, some orthopaedists advocate aspiration of the hematoma. Metacarpal head fractures can be treated by the orthopaedist with closed reduction and splinting in the safe position. Fractures that are reduced but remain unstable, however, require pin fixation. Displaced fractures of the metacarpal head often require open reduction and internal fixation. It is recommended that a hand surgeon be consulted for these fractures.

Fractures of the metacarpal neck are the most common metacarpal (MC) fractures in children.[6] These fractures are analogous to the boxer's fracture in adults. Examination of the hand shows significant swelling over the area. An obvious bump may be visible over the fracture site. Routine radiographs show the fracture. Radiographic evaluation of the degree of angulation of the fracture can often be difficult because of superimposed digits on the lateral view. Oblique views can often aid in delineating the digits. Neck fractures are usually treated with closed methods. The Jahss reduction maneuver is performed by flexion of the MCP to 90 degrees, is followed by the application of pressure on the dorsal aspect of the metacarpal proximal to the fracture. Pressure on the volar side of the distal fragment can aid the reduction. The hand should then be placed in the safe position with the wrist in 10 to 15 degrees of extension, the MCP joint in flexion, and the proximal interphalangeal (PIP) joint in extension. Postreduction radiographs should always be obtained. In some patients near skeletal maturity, unstable fractures of the metacarpal neck may require pin fixation. Such patients should be seen by a hand surgeon as soon as possible.

Fractures of the metacarpal shaft can be transverse, oblique, or spiral. Usually the result of direct trauma, these fractures must be evaluated for rotational deformity, as follows: The patient is asked to make a fist. All the fingers should point to the scaphoid, and all the nail beds should be parallel. Routine radiographs show this fracture. Angular and rotational deformity must be corrected by the orthopaedic surgeon before splinting or casting. The surgeon usually performs the correction with closed reduction by exaggerating the injury and then reducing the fracture in one motion. After reduction is obtained, the hand should be splinted in the safe position. Unstable fractures with residual rotational malalignment may need pin fixation, and a hand surgery should be consulted. A rotational deformity of even 10 degrees can be enough to cause overlapping of the fingers.

Fractures of the base of the metacarpal are uncommon in children. They are usually the result of high-energy trauma. They can occur from an axial load resulting in a stable compression fracture. High-energy trauma usually leads to a fracture-dislocation at the carpometacarpal (CMC) level. Radiographic evaluation should include a 30-degree pronated or supinated oblique view, which aids assessment of any joint dislocation or subluxation. Significant fracture-dislocations should alert one to search for associated soft tissue injury. Reduction of the dislocation or fracture should be followed by a thorough examination to assess stability of the joint. Splinting in the safe position is an option. However, some orthopaedists leave the PIP joint free to move.

Fractures of the head and shaft of the thumb metacarpal are treated just as those of the other digits. Fractures of the base of the thumb metacarpal can manifest as simple transverse fractures or intra-articular fractures. SH III and SH IV fractures of the base in children most closely resemble the Bennett fracture in adults. Examination of the thumb shows swelling similar to that in other metacarpal fractures. Malrotation can be assessed by checking for the perpendicular relationship of the thumb's nail plate with the other nail plates. Fractures of the base of the thumb without intra-articular extension can be treated with closed reduction and immobilization. Angulation of up to 20 degrees can be accepted. Unstable fractures should be stabilized with pin fixation in the operating room. Displaced intra-articular fractures also need operative intervention, and a hand surgeon should be consulted. The outcomes are usually excellent. The immobilization period is usually 4 to 6 weeks.

Ulnar collateral ligament (UCL) injury of the thumb (also known as gamekeeper's thumb) is commonly encountered in adolescent patients. Usually the result of an abduction force applied to the thumb, the injury can range from a sprain of the UCL to an avulsion fracture from the proximal phalanx. The patient presents with pain over the ulnar side of the thumb. Examination should include stressing the MCP joint of the thumb in extension and flexion. Lack of a distinct endpoint or opening up of the joint more than 45 degrees farther than in the other thumb is indicative of a tear in the UCL. Routine radiographs will differentiate between an avulsion fracture and a tear. Stress radiographs may be needed to visualize the fracture. Immobilization in a cast for 3 to 4 weeks is usually all that is needed for fractures and incomplete tears. A complete tear requires operative repair, and a hand surgeon should be consulted.

Metacarpal fractures are usually immobilized for 3 to 4 weeks. This period should be followed by an examination to assess tenderness at the fracture site. Correlation of tenderness at the fracture site with radiographic evidence of non-union should prompt one to consider immobilization for longer than 4 weeks. Outcomes for metacarpal fractures are excellent if rotational malalignment or angular deformity is assessed at the time of primary treatment.

Fractures of the Carpal Bones

Fractures of the carpal bones in children are exceedingly rare. Most occur in the adolescent patient from a fall on an outstretched hand. The patient complains of pain over the dorsum of the hand. The physical findings are consistent with pain over the affected bone. The most commonly fractured bone is the scaphoid. Pain is typically located in the anatomic snuffbox. Good-quality radiographs (AP, lateral, and scaphoid views) should be obtained. Radiographic findings are normal in about 10% of scaphoid fractures. It is essential that this fracture not be missed, because most complications result from late presentations or missed diagnosis. Any patient with pain in the anatomic snuffbox should be treated by the orthopaedic surgeon with use of a thumb spica cast for 10 to 14 days even if radiographs are normal. The patient should be examined after this time with a second set of radiographs. Continued pain with normal radiographic findings should prompt one to obtain a bone scan or magnetic resonance imaging (MRI). Treatment consists of use of a thumb spica cast for 4 to 6 weeks. Occasionally, surgical fixation may be necessary for displaced fractures of the carpal bones. Outcomes are usually good, non-union and avascular necrosis being the major complications.

Dislocations of the Hand

Dislocations of the hand in children are relatively uncommon. The collateral ligaments and volar plate are stronger than the physeal bone. Any force strong enough to produce a dislocation usually causes a fracture. Occasionally a patient presents with an acute dislocation. Physical examination usually shows an apparent deformity and inability to move a certain joint. An inspection to evaluate for open dislocation is obviously important. Prereduction neurovascular examination is also important. The blood supply distal to the dislocation can be compromised, and the nerve placed in excessive traction. Radiographs are equally important to assess for any fractures.

Reduction can be attempted after a digital nerve block or with conscious sedation. Slight traction followed by reduction of the joint is usually all that is required. Occasionally, the physician encounters an irreducible dislocation of a joint, for which a hand surgeon should be consulted. It is likely that an interposed ligament or volar plate is hindering the reduction. Operative reduction may be necessary. Also, postreduction stressing of the joint is important to evaluate for ligamentous and volar plate injury. Immobilization of the joint with buddy taping for a few weeks is usually sufficient. Follow-up with a hand surgeon is indicated.

A "jammed finger" is a common injury that is actually not a dislocation. Patients usually complain of tenderness at a joint and have a history of a longitudinal force applied to the finger. Physical examination reveals tenderness and swelling over a joint. Motion is painful. The diagnosis is one of exclusion. All possible bone and soft tissue injuries should be ruled out. The cause of this common entity is unknown. However, it may be due to a sprain of one of the collateral ligaments. Patients and parents should be warned that discomfort may last up to 9 months after the injury. Swelling about the joint may remain as a residual thickening around the joint. Treatment is symptomatic, consisting of warm compresses and the use of buddy taping during activities.

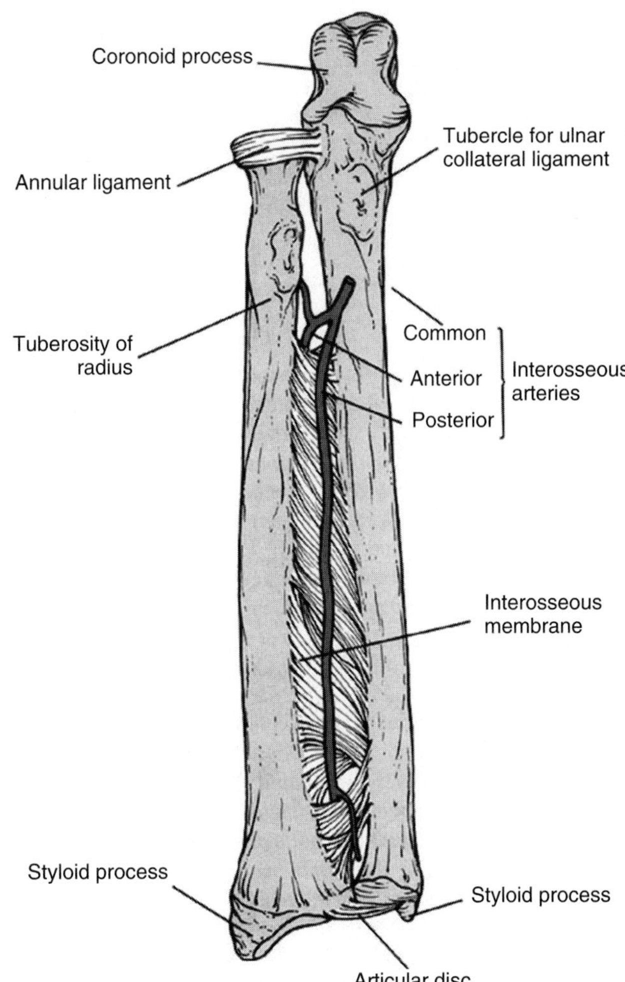

Figure 2-7 The interosseous membrane, ligaments, and bony landmarks. (From Green NE: Skeletal Trauma in Children, 2nd ed., Philadelphia, WB Saunders, 1998.)

FRACTURES OF THE RADIUS AND ULNA

Fractures of the Distal Radius and Ulna

General Considerations

Fractures of the wrist and forearm are very common in children, accounting for nearly half of all fractures seen in the skeletally immature. The most common mechanism of injury is a fall on the outstretched hand. About 80% of forearm fractures are injuries to the distal third of the radius and ulna, 15% involve the middle third, and the rest are rare fractures of the proximal third of the radius or ulnar shaft. The majority of forearm fractures, especially in younger children, are greenstick or buckle fractures.

Several important anatomic features should be considered by anyone managing these injuries (Fig. 2-7). The ulna is a straight, triangular bone. The radius, however, is rectangular distally, triangular in the middle third, and cylindrical in the proximal third. The radius has a gentle bow throughout the extent of its shaft, which is critical in enabling it to rotate around the ulna during pronation and supination (Fig. 2-8). The interosseous membrane attaches along the lateral border of the ulna and the medial border of the radius. The radius has a tuberosity just below its proximal neck that is the site of insertion of the biceps tendon. This tuberosity is located directly opposite (180 degrees from) the radial styloid. Understanding of this relationship can be valuable to determining rotational alignment after fracture reduction.

Fracture management is also greatly aided by an understanding of the connection between the radius and ulna. With articulations proximally and distally and an interosseous membrane in the middle, the radius and ulna act as a two-bone complex. Managing injuries to the complex requires an understanding of this relationship,

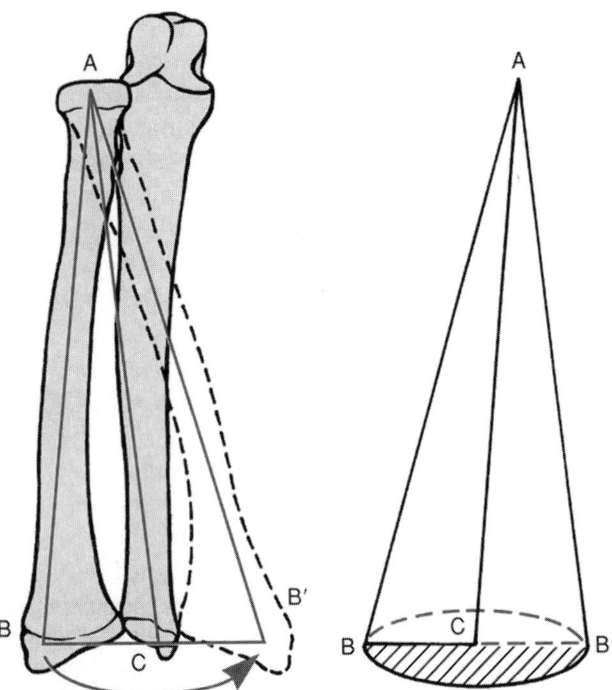

Figure 2-8 The rotation of the radius on the ulna has a mechanical axis from the center of the radial head to the ulnar styloid. (From Green NE: Skeletal Trauma in Children, 2nd ed. Philadelphia, WB Saunders, 1998.)

because a significantly displaced injury to one bone is often associated with an injury to the other. Detecting the second, subtle injury (e.g., a radial head dislocation with a greenstick ulnar fracture) requires an appreciation of the radioulnar relationship. The interosseous membrane is stretched to its full length when the forearm is in neutral to 30 degrees of supination.[7] As the forearm is pronated, the radius rotates around the ulna, and the interosseous membrane relaxes. Thus, the treating surgeon usually immobilizes the arm in neutral to 30 degrees of supination so that after healing, the interosseous membrane is not contracted and forearm motion has been regained.

Distally, the triangular fibrocartilage complex (TFCC) consists of an articular disk and a number of fibers that connect the ulna to the carpus and to the distal radius. The ulnar styloid, which is sometimes fractured in wrist injuries, is a key source of attachment of these ligaments. Fortunately, unlike adults, children rarely sustain injuries to the TFCC that require treatment. Proximally, the radius articulates with the capitellum and is connected to the ulna by a complex of tissues including the annular ligament.

A few developmental features of the forearm are also worth discussion. The distal radial physis, a common location of injury, closes very late in development. Typically closure occurs around 17 years in girls and 18 years in boys. The distal ulnar physis closes about a year earlier. Separate ossification centers at the radial styloid can be confused for a fracture in children between 1 and 2 years of age. At the elbow, the proximal ulnar ossification center appears around age 10. This also can have a bipartite ossification center that is commonly mistaken for an avulsion fracture.

The treating physician must have knowledge of the muscles attached to the radius and ulna and the forces they exert in order to understand typical patterns of fracture displacement and the deforming forces on the bones after reduction (Fig. 2-9). Distally, the pronator quadratus, some extensors and adductors, and the wrist extensors tend to pronate and extend a distal radius fracture fragment. The stronger force, however, is the brachioradialis, which inserts laterally above the radial styloid. More proximally, the pronator quadratus inserts

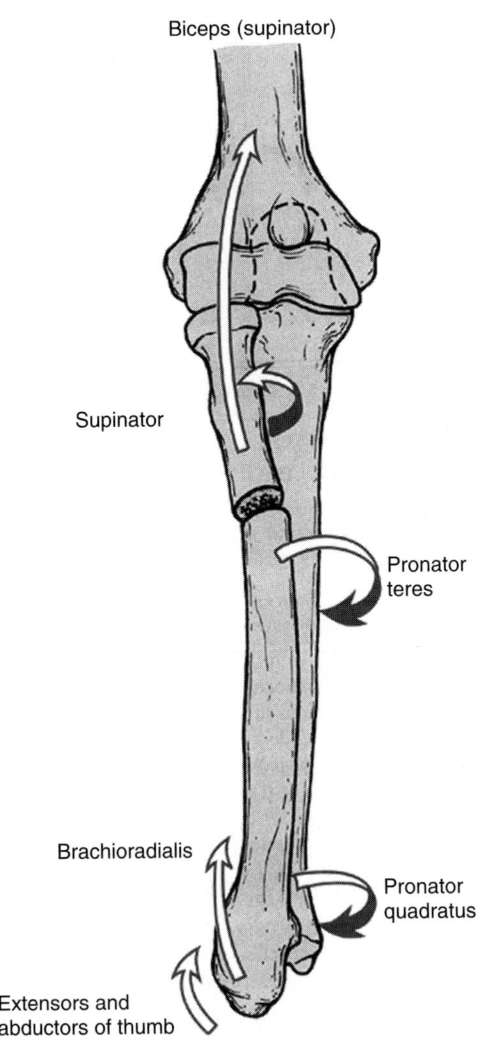

Figure 2-9 Main deforming muscular forces of the forearm. (From Green NE: Skeletal Trauma in Children, 2nd ed. Philadelphia, WB Saunders, 1998.)

in the middle third of the radius; this muscle will pronate the shaft in all fractures proximal to its insertion. In the proximal third of the radius, there is a strong supination force from the supinator and the biceps. The biceps will also serve to flex the proximal radius. Understanding these forces, most surgeons treat proximal fractures with forearm supination, and middle or distal third fractures with neutral forearm position or slight forearm pronation.

Finally, in addition to understanding mechanism of injury, anatomy, development, and mechanics of the forearm, the treating physician must appreciate the tremendous remodeling potential of the forearm in children. This remodeling potential is the single most important reason that most forearm fractures in children can be treated with cast immobilization, whereas many similar fractures in adults require operative reduction and internal fixation. Remodeling is greatest in young children, in fractures near a rapidly growing physis, in fractures that are in the plane of motion of the adjacent joint, and in fractures with greater angulation. Thus, the typical apex-volar angulation of the distal radius fracture in a 5-year-old child has tremendous remodeling potential—adjacent to the distal radius physis, it is in the plane motion of the wrist joint, and nearly 12 years of physeal growth remain to drive the remodeling. Typically, about 10 degrees of angulation per year can be corrected with remodeling. Radialward angulation of the distal radius, caused by the pull of the brachioradialis muscle, corrects more slowly. Bayonet apposition corrects reliably in younger children. Rotational malalignment does not remodel, although shoulder abduction can functionally compensate for loss of pronation.

Physeal Injuries to the Distal Radius and Ulna

Distal radial physeal fractures are the most common growth plate injury in children. The vast majority occur after age 10 (younger children are more likely to sustain a metaphyseal buckle fracture). The majority of distal radial physeal fractures are the SH II type. SH I fractures are much less common. Although many fractures are called type I, careful inspection of radiographs often shows a small Thurston-Holland metaphyseal fragment. Most distal radial and ulnar physeal fractures occur from a fall on an outstretched hand. Many such fractures in teenagers are high-energy injuries, sustained during roller-blading, skateboarding, or falls in sports.

On physical examination, displaced forearm physeal fractures show deformity, tenderness, and swelling at the fracture site. Because the fracture is usually displaced dorsally, the volar periosteum is often disrupted. It is critical that the initial evaluation include a careful inspection of the skin around the forearm, as very subtle, pinpoint openings in the skin represent an open fracture caused by the sharp volar metaphyseal fragment. Careful neurologic evaluation is also important. Higher-energy injuries may cause a neuropraxia of the median nerve or an acute carpal tunnel syndrome. Physical examination should also include palpation of the hand below and the elbow above the fracture to search for associated injuries. In fractures without significant swelling and deformity, diagnosis of a nondisplaced distal radius fracture is confirmed by the presence of specific tenderness over the distal radial physis.

Radiographs should include good-quality AP and lateral views centered at the wrist. In addition, radiographs of the whole forearm, including the elbow, are valuable to rule out associated injuries. In an occult or nondisplaced fractures, the pronator fat pad sign may alert the physician to the presence of an injury.

Nondisplaced SH I fracture at the distal radius, ulna, or both can be splinted and referred to the orthopaedist for evaluation and management within a few days. A simple, well-padded volar splint extending from the metacarpal heads to the proximal forearm gives sufficient comfort and safety to the injured child. If an elastic bandage wrap is used, it should be applied with no tension as to avoid finger swelling, which is commonly seen a few days later if the wrap is stretched during splint application.

Displaced fractures should be reduced by the orthopaedist with the use of conscious sedation or general anesthesia. Most fractures are dorsally displaced, with disruption of the volar periosteum (Fig. 2-10). The reduction maneuver involves volarward pressure on the distal fragments with slight traction. A long-arm splint or cast is used to hold reduction. A three-point mold, with dorsal pressure distal and proximal to the fracture and volar pressure at the fracture, works with the intact periosteum to maintain reduction during the 4 weeks of cast immobilization. In children in whom more than 1 or 2 years of growth remain, up to 50% displacement is acceptable. Second attempts at reduction performed more than 3 days after injury are thought to risk physeal arrest. Irreducible fractures may result from interposed tissue, especially on the volar side. The tissue may include the median nerve or radial artery, so careful examination is important. Open or closed reduction with Kirschner wire (K-wire) fixation is used for irreducible fractures, fractures associated with acute carpal tunnel syndrome, and after irrigation and débridement of open fractures.

Long-term outcome after distal radial and ulnar physeal fractures is usually excellent. Dorsal angulation of up to 30 to 40 degrees remodels satisfactorily in a child in whom significant growth remains. Physeal arrest after distal radius fractures is quite rare, occurring in less than 10% of these common injuries. Most orthopaedists monitor patients with displaced distal radial physeal fractures for up to a year to be certain that there is no growth arrest. Because remodeling is excellent and intra-articular fractures and TFCC injuries are rare in children, late deformity and disability are rarely encountered after these fractures.

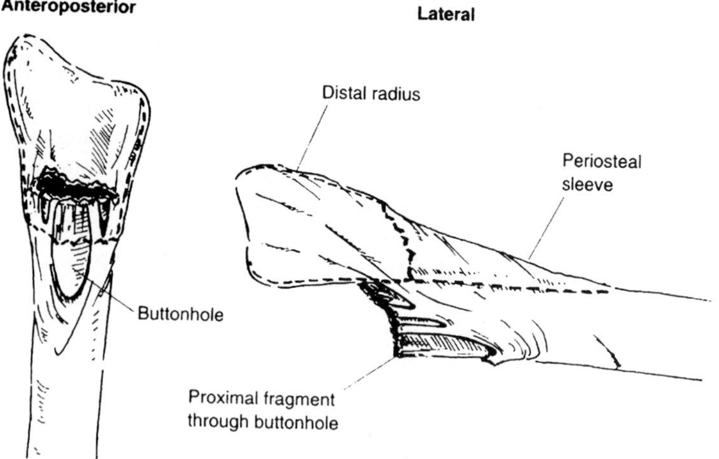

Figure 2-10 In completely displaced pediatric forearm fractures, the periosteum is torn and elevated. In cases of reversed fracture obliquity, it becomes difficult to reduce the bone end to end with longitudinal traction, because the periosteum tightens around the buttonholed proximal end. However, the elevated periosteum does provide a framework for rapid cortical remodeling as bone and callus form along the elevated margin. (From Noonan KJ, Price CT: Forearm and distal radius fractures in children. J Am Acad Orthop Surg 6:146-156, 1998.)

Metaphyseal Fractures of the Distal Radius and Ulna

Metaphyseal fractures to the arm occur during early childhood as well as during the adolescent growth spurt, when the trabecular bone of the metaphysis is thought to weaken temporarily during rapid growth. Most fractures are caused by a fall on an outstretched hand, usually with some pronation of the wrist. The vast majority displace dorsally.

Nondisplaced buckle fractures (Fig. 2-11) either can be splinted by the physician or in the emergency department, and the patient is then sent to the orthopaedist for later casting or can be casted by the orthopaedist at the time of injury. Three weeks in a short-arm cast allows healing of most buckle fractures. Greenstick fractures, which involve a break on the tension (usually volar) cortex, are treated similarly with slightly longer protection. After 4 weeks in a short-arm or long-arm cast, most fractures are healed, and the patients have no tenderness at the fracture site. The orthopaedist can place a short-arm cast first, then test pronation and supination in the cast. If the child is comfortable, there is no need to extend the cast above the elbow.

Complete fractures (Fig. 2-12) require closed reduction by the orthopedic surgeon. Once adequate conscious sedation is obtained, the fracture is reduced by recreation of the deformity (extreme volar angulation) and reduction with a volarward pressure. A carefully prepared cast, with three-point molding (Fig. 2-13), is applied. Neutral or slight pronation of the forearm is preferred. A long-arm cast is used for completely displaced fractures. An initial follow-up visit with radiographs is arranged for 5 to 10 days after injury. If the angulation is unacceptable at this time, a second reduction can be performed. In children younger than 10 years, up to 30 degrees of dorsal angulation or 20 degrees of radial angulation yield a good result. In older children, less than half of this displacement should be accepted.

Galeazzi Fracture

Galeazzi fracture, a distal radius fracture with disruption (or its equivalent) of the TFCC, is a relatively rare injury in children. In adults, Galeazzi fracture is more common than Monteggia lesions. This incidence pattern is reversed in children. Galeazzi fractures are thought to occur from a fall on the outstretched hand with extreme hand or wrist pronation. The equivalent fractures in children include a radius fracture with a distal ulnar physeal injury. Generally, these injuries can be successfully treated by closed reduction and immobilization in a long-arm cast for 6 weeks. The forearm should be casted in

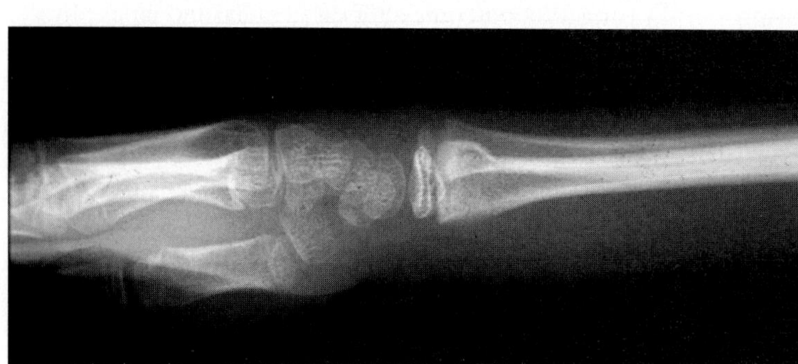

Figure 2-11 Radial fracture buckle.

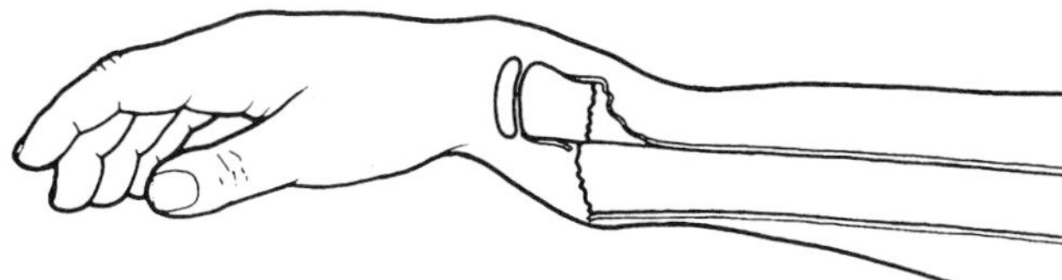

Figure 2-12 Usually, the periosteum is intact on the dorsal side and disrupted on the volar side in metaphyseal forearm fractures. (From Rockwood CA Jr, Wilkins KE, Beaty JH: Fractures in Children, 4th ed. Philadelphia, Lippincott-Raven, 1996.)

slight pronation. Open reduction and pin fixation of Galeazzi fracture are rarely necessary in children.

Injuries to the Shafts of the Radius and Ulna

Diaphyseal Fractures of the Radius and Ulna

Radial and ulnar diaphyseal fracture can be more difficult to treat because the limits of acceptable reduction are much more stringent than for distal radial fractures. A significant malunion of a forearm diaphyseal fracture can lead to a permanent loss of pronation and supination and, sometimes, an unsightly curvature or prominence in the forearm. Fortunately, diaphyseal fractures are four times less common than distal radius fractures and are seen more frequently in younger children, in whom remodeling potential is better. Like most other fractures in the upper extremity, these injuries are caused by a fall on an outstretched arm, usually with a significant rotational component. An understanding this rotational component is quite valuable to the reduction, especially in greenstick fractures.

The physician should note the rotation of the arm, the neurovascular status, the location of the deformity, and the status of the compartment pressures. Although upper extremity compartment syndrome is rare, the most common cause is a severe radial and ulnar diaphyseal fracture. Radiographs should include two views at right angles to one another that show the entire extent of the forearm on the same film. The wrist and the elbow should be clearly visualized. The fracture location and pattern should be noted. In fractures with a dorsal angulation, the distal fragment is pronated; in fractures with a volar angulation, the distal fragment is supinated. The key to reduction of these greenstick fractures is reversal of this rotation. In complete fractures, the widths of the diaphyseal fragments at the fracture site should be studied. A significant discrepancy in the width of the bone ends adjacent to the fracture suggests a rotational deformity (Fig. 2-14). Additionally, the relationship of the bicipital tuberosity to the radial styloid should be noticed—in anatomic alignment, the bicipital tuberosity should be opposite the radial styloid.

An orthopaedist should be consulted for every angulated or displaced radial and ulnar diaphyseal fracture, which requires manipulative closed reduction under conscious sedation or general anesthesia (Fig. 2-15). Once the child is comfortably sedated, the fracture can be reduced by rotation of the palm toward the angulation (Fig. 2-16) (e.g., supination of the hand to correct the pronation deformity of a dorsally angulated fracture). Acceptable reduction is 10 to 20 degrees of angulation in children younger than 10 years but no more than

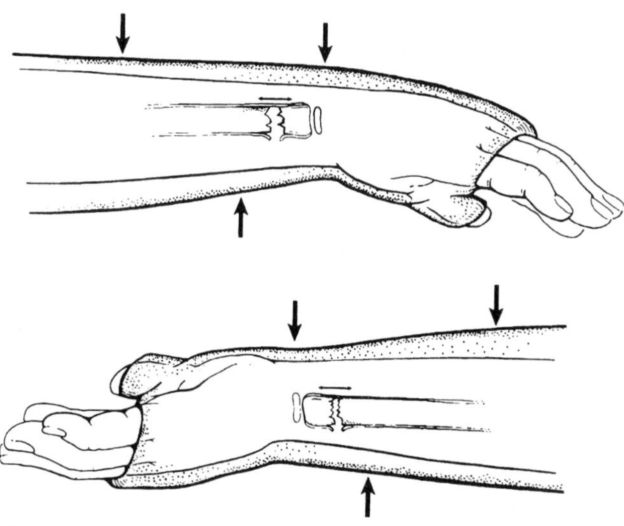

Figure 2-13 Three-point molding of a forearm cast. (From Rockwood CA Jr, Wilkins KE, Beaty JH: Fractures in Children, 4th ed. Philadelphia, Lippincott-Raven, 1996.)

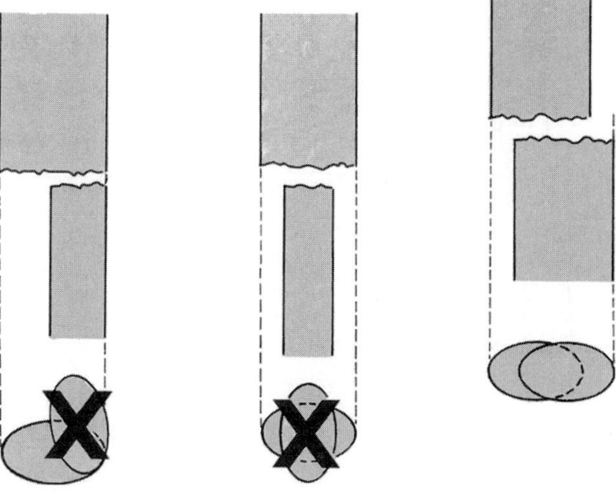

Figure 2-14 Matching of the width and shape of the fracture fragments on radiographs is essential to ensure correct rotational alignment. (From Green NE: Skeletal Trauma in Children, 2nd ed. Philadelphia, WB Saunders, 1998.)

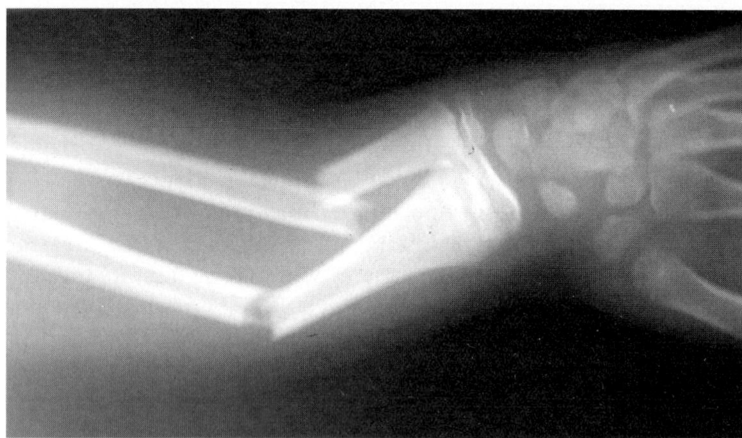

Figure 2-15 Radius and ulna fracture.

10 degrees of angulation in older children and adolescents. Bayonet apposition is acceptable at union, but correction to near-anatomic alignment should be sought at the time of injury. Because diaphyseal fractures heal much more slowly than distal metaphyseal fractures, clinical and radiographic evaluation should be performed at 1 week and 2 weeks after injury. Loss of reduction is common. If loss of reduction causes an unacceptable alignment, a second manipulation or even limited internal fixation with wires or plates can be used even several weeks after injury. Cast immobilization should be continued for at least 6 weeks. Sometimes, in high-energy fractures, open fractures, or fractures in adolescents, up to 8 weeks of cast immobilization may be required. The arm should be immobilized in a well-molded long-arm cast with a flat ulnar border and a good interosseous mold (Fig. 2-17). Some orthopaedists prefer to include the thumb, although this is not our practice. The major causes of treatment failure in these fractures are a lack of understanding of the rotational component of the fracture and poor technical skills in making the cast.

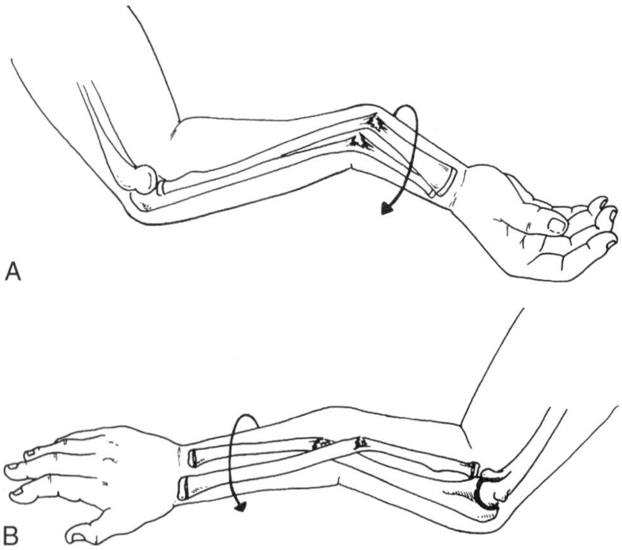

Figure 2-16 The angulation in greenstick forearm fractures results from rotation, which must be corrected for reduction. (From Rockwood CA Jr, Wilkins KE, Beaty JH: Fractures in Children, 4th ed. Philadelphia, Lippincott-Raven, 1996.)

Plastic Deformation of the Radius, Ulna, or Both

In young children, especially those younger than 7 years, the radius and ulnar shafts can deform plastically rather than fracture completely. Deformation occurs when the injury force exceeds the yield point—but not the failure point—of the bone.[8] In young children in whom there is no cosmetic deformity and who have full range of motion, casting without reduction is acceptable. However, if the arm appears bowed or motion is lost, reduction should be attempted in the operating room. A great amount of force is applied at a very slow rate over a long period to correct the plastic deformation. The arm is then immobilized in a long-arm cast for 4-6 weeks.

Monteggia Fractures

Monteggia fractures describes a group of injuries that involve radial humeral dislocation and ulnar fracture. Although these injuries represent less than 1% of all pediatric forearm fractures, they receive great attention because their recognition and treatment can be challenging. Most Monteggia fractures occur in children

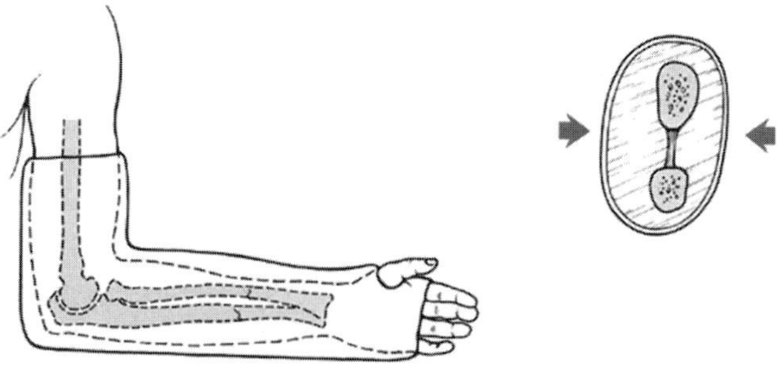

Figure 2-17 Ideal shape for a long-arm cast. (From Green NE: Skeletal Trauma in Children, 2nd ed. Philadelphia, WB Saunders, 1998.)

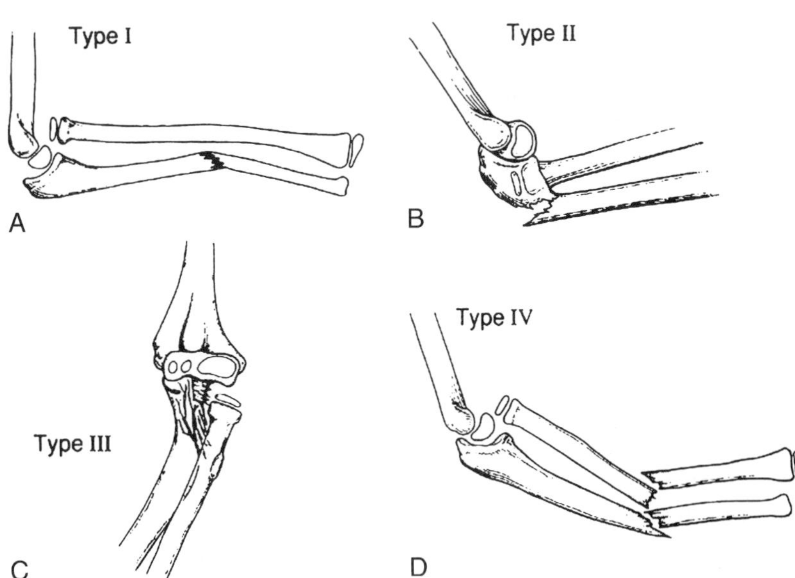

Figure 2-18 Bado's Classification of Monteggia Fractures. **A,** Type I (anterior dislocation): The radial head is dislocated anteriorly; the ulna has a short oblique or greenstick fracture in the diaphyseal or proximal metaphyseal area. **B,** Type II (posterior dislocation): The radial head is dislocated posteriorly and posterolaterally; the ulna is usually fractured in the metaphysis in children. **C,** Type III (lateral dislocation): There is lateral dislocation of the radial head with a greenstick metaphyseal fracture of the ulna. **D,** Type IV (anterior dislocation with radius shaft fracture): The pattern of injury is the same as with a type I injury, with the addition of a radius shaft fracture below the level of the ulna fracture. (From Rockwood CA Jr, Wilkins KE, Beaty JH: Fractures in Children, 4th ed. Philadelphia, Lippincott-Raven, 1996.)

younger than 10 years. Many isolated radial head dislocations discovered late are probably missed traumatic lesions rather than congenital dislocations.

Bado[9] developed what is now a commonly accepted classification of Monteggia fractures (Fig. 2-18). Type I fractures involve anterior dislocation of the radial head, type II fractures posterior dislocation of the radial head, type III fractures lateral dislocation of the radial head, and type IV fractures a segmental radius fracture with dislocation of the radial head. In each case, the ulna angulates in the direction of the radial head dislocation. There are also a large number of Monteggia equivalents, which involve various fracture combinations of the proximal ulna, radial neck, and physis. Most fractures occur through a fall on an outstretched hand with extreme pronation of the forearm caused by the weight of the body over the planted hand; the extreme pronation dislodges the radial head anteriorly (type I). With the same trauma and severe supination, a type II lesion is produced. Type III lesions may be caused by a fall with a varus force, fracturing the ulna and dislodging the radial head laterally. Type IV fractures are usually due to pronation at the time of the fall on the outstretched hand.

High-quality radiographs are mandatory for successful management of Monteggia fractures. Views of the whole forearm as well as isolated elbow radiographs should be obtained. The radial head should point toward the center of the capitellum on all views (Fig. 2-19). The treating physician should persist until a true lateral radiograph of the elbow is achieved. Without such a view, it is easy to miss subtle anterior subluxation of the radial head.

A careful neurologic examination is essential, because up to 20% of Monteggia fractures manifest as a nerve palsy.[9,10] The most common finding is a posterior interosseous nerve palsy associated with type III lesions.

Treatment involves an initial attempt at closed reduction with conscious sedation or general anesthesia. The reduction maneuver varies with the fracture type. Type I fractures are reduced with forearm supination and complete elbow flexion. The observant orthopaedist detects a "clunking" sensation when the radial head relocates. A well-molded long-arm cast is then applied for 4 to 6 weeks. Type II fractures, more commonly seen in older

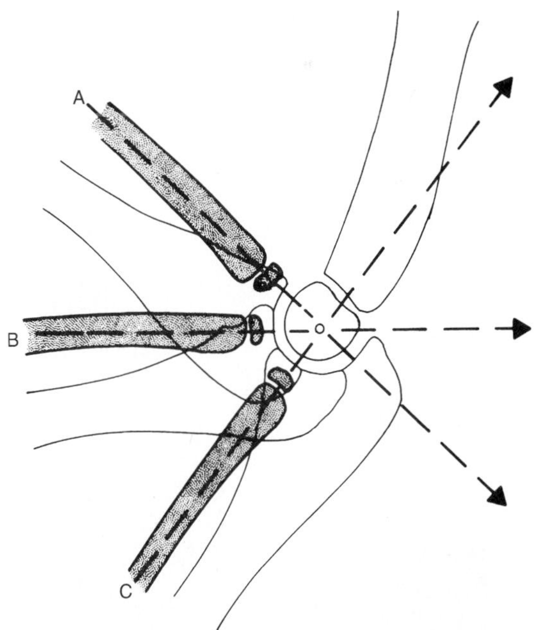

Figure 2-19 Composite drawing with the elbow in various degrees of flexion. A line drawn down the long axis of the radius bisects the capitellum of the humerus, regardless of the degree of flexion or extension of the elbow. (From Rockwood CA Jr, Wilkins KE, Beaty JH: Fractures in Children, 4th ed. Philadelphia, Lippincott-Raven, 1996)

children and adolescents, are reduced with forearm extension. Maintaining a reduction may be difficult in a long-arm cast with the elbow flexed; if this is the case, K-wire fixation of the ulna is a relatively simple way to maintain reduction in a long-arm cast. Type III fractures require correction of the varus angulation for reduction of the radial head (Fig. 2-20). This maneuver can be challenging, because the orthopaedist must fight the deforming force of a greenstick proximal ulna fracture in order to keep the radial head reduced. As with type II fractures, failure of simple closed techniques can be addressed with K-wire fixation of the proximal ulna in the operating room after reduction under fluoroscopic guidance. Type IV fractures are very difficult to treat with a simple closed reduction; often the radial shaft fracture must be internally fixed with either a plate or wires to successfully reduce the radial head.

The treating orthopaedic surgeon must be vigilant about monitoring a Monteggia fracture after reduction. Follow-up examinations and radiography once or twice in the first 3 weeks should be performed to ensure that the radial head remains reduced. If there is any question about the reduction, the surgeon should remove the cast and repeat the radiographs until the issue is clarified. It is better to have to reperform a reduction lost because of cast removal than to discover weeks later that the radial head has redislocated while the ulnar fracture has healed.

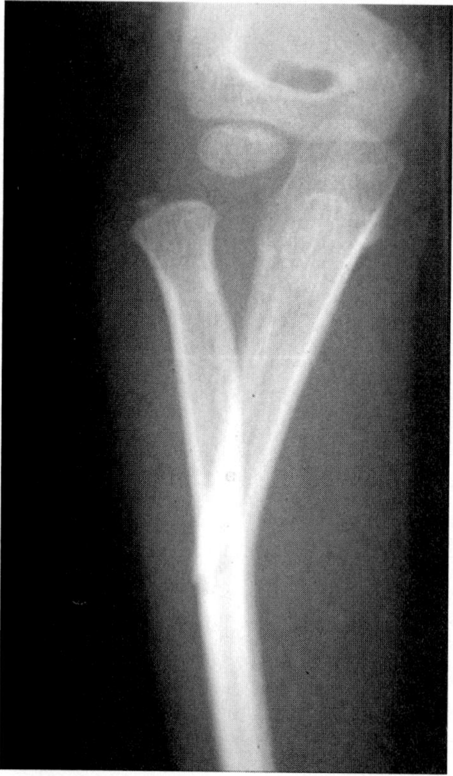

Figure 2-20 Type III Monteggia lesion.

Complications of Monteggia fractures include failure of recognition, failure of reduction, loss of reduction, nerve injury, late stiffness, avascular necrosis of the radial head, and radioulnar synostosis. If a Monteggia fracture is missed, late reconstruction involves restoration of ulnar length and alignment and an open reduction of the radial head, often with reconstruction of the annular ligament.

Fractures of the Proximal Radius and Ulna

Fractures of the Proximal Radius

The so-called radial head fracture is a fairly common childhood injury. Many such fractures are minimally displaced. In children, a displaced intra-articular fracture is rare. Because the radial head's relationship with the capitellum is critical in maintaining forearm rotation, optimal reduction of angulation—and more important, translation—offers the best chance of a good functional result (Fig. 2-21). Evaluation at the time of injury should include a search for associated injuries and radiographs that show the forearm and wrist as well as the elbow anatomy. The neurovascular examination should focus on the radial nerve.

An attempt should be made to reduce all displaced proximal radial fractures with conscious sedation or general anesthesia. This attempt can be aided by injection of a local anesthetic into the radiocapitellar joint and evacuation of the hematoma before reduction. After an attempt at closed reduction, up to 30 degrees of angulation but minimal translation can be accepted. If there is more than 30 degrees of angulation, reduction should be attempted again. If reduction under conscious sedation fails, further attempts should be made under fluoroscopic guidance in the operating room.

Several different maneuvers can be helpful in reducing a radial head fracture. With the elbow extended, a valgus force can be placed directly over the radial head to achieve a reduction. If this fails, the flexion-pronation technique is very valuable. With pressure over the radial head, the elbow extended, and the forearm in supination, the orthopaedist pronates the forearm while fully flexing the elbow (Fig. 2-22). Even 100% radial head dislocations can be reduced with this maneuver. When all closed measures fail, a small K-wire or awl introduced through a small lateral incision to push the fractured fragment back into position.[11]

Complications after radial head fracture are more common than is generally appreciated. Loss of motion is the most common. For this reason, immobilization should last for no more than 3 or 4 weeks in children. Avascular necrosis of the radial head and heterotopic ossification have also been described.

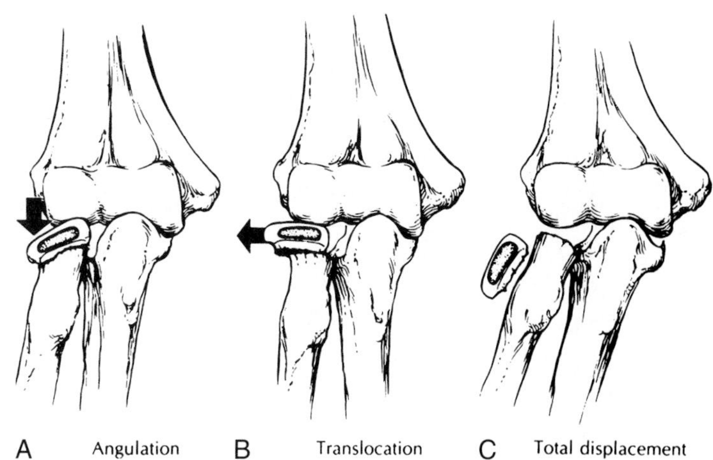

Figure 2-21 Displacement patterns in proximal radius fracture. The radial head can be angulated **(A)**, translocated **(B)**, or completely displaced **(C)**. (From Rockwood CA Jr, Wilkins KE, Beaty JH: Fractures in Children, 4th ed. Philadelphia, Lippincott-Raven, 1996)

Fractures of the Proximal Ulna

Olecranon fractures are uncommon in children. They may occur from a fall on an outstretched hand or a direct blow to the elbow. Most are minimally displaced metaphyseal fractures. Avulsion fractures have also been described in children with osteogenesis imperfecta.[12,13] Displaced intra-articular fractures of the proximal ulna are managed with open reduction and internal fixation with either a tension band technique or compression fixation with an interfragmentary screw.

FRACTURES OF THE ELBOW

General Principles

Although elbow fractures are less common than forearm and wrist fractures, many pediatric elbow fractures receive more attention because more aggressive management is needed to achieve a good result. Improper management of elbow injuries remains a common source of disability and malpractice litigation. Many elbow injuries are intra-articular, involve the physeal cartilage, or may result in rare pediatric malunion or nonunion with permanent functional loss.

As the distal humerus develops, a series of ossification centers appear (Fig. 2-23); these ossification centers can be mistaken for fractures by the inexperienced physician. The capitellar ossification center appears first, between the ages of 6 months and 2 years, followed by those in the medial epicondyle, the trochlea, and then the lateral epicondyle. The medial epicondyle is the last to fuse to the distal humerus, usually in the mid-teenage years. The vascular supply around the elbow is very good (Fig. 2-24). This explains the rapid healing of metaphyseal fractures and the rich collateral network that allows profusion of the hand even when the distal brachial artery is occluded at the time of a severe supracondylar humerus fracture.

Careful radiographic evaluation is an essential part of diagnosing and managing pediatric elbow injuries. The elbow has anterior and posterior fat pads (Fig. 2-25). The entire distal humerus is intra-articular. A distal humeral fracture causes a hemarthrosis and elevates the fat pads. The posterior fat pad sign is the most important

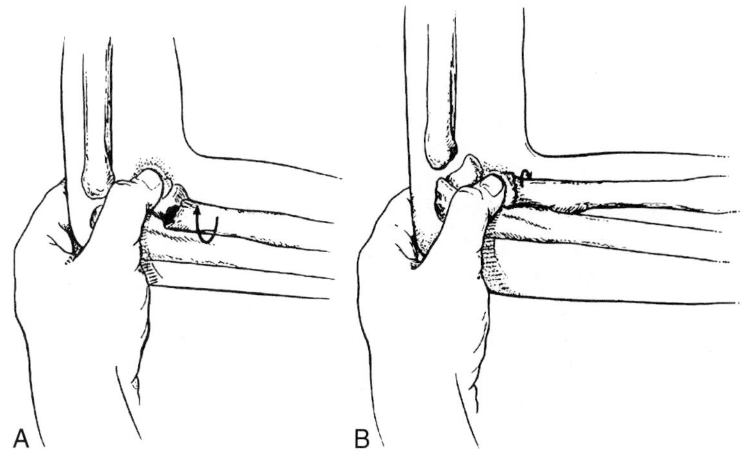

Figure 2-22 Flexion-pronation, Israeli technique. (From Rockwood CA Jr, Wilkins KE, Beaty JH: Fractures in Children, 4th ed. Philadelphia, Lippincott-Raven, 1996.)

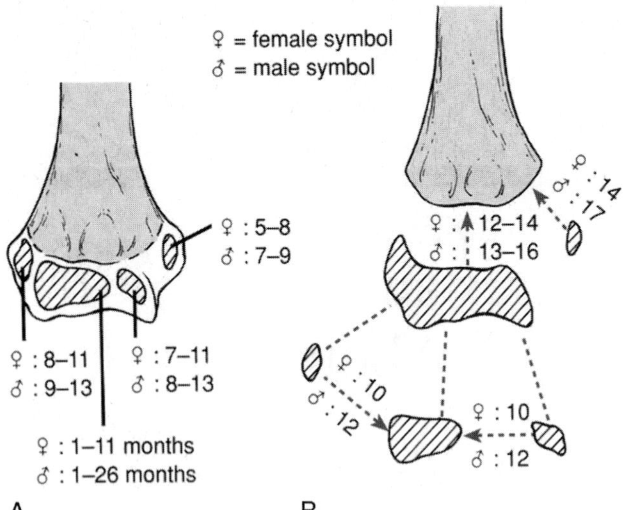

Figure 2-23 Ossification and fusion of the growth centers of the distal end of the humerus. A, Appearance of the ossification centers. **B,** Fusion of the ossification centers. (From Green NE: Skeletal Trauma in Children, 2nd ed. Philadelphia, WB Saunders, 1998.)

sign of an occult fracture. When it is present, there is a 70% chance of a fracture.[14]

Several lines or radiographic relationships are important in evaluating elbow injuries in children. On the AP view, the Baumann angle (Fig. 2-26) is measured from the intersection of a line drawn down the center of the humeral shaft and a second line drawn through the capitellar physis. The angle in the injured arm should be within a few degrees of the angle in the uninjured arm. On a lateral view, a line drawn along the anterior humerus is valuable in assessing the amount of extension of a supracondylar fracture. Generally, the anterior humeral line should bisect the capitellum (Fig. 2-27). An anterior humeral line that passes anterior to the entire capitellum confirms significant extension of the distal humeral fracture fragment.

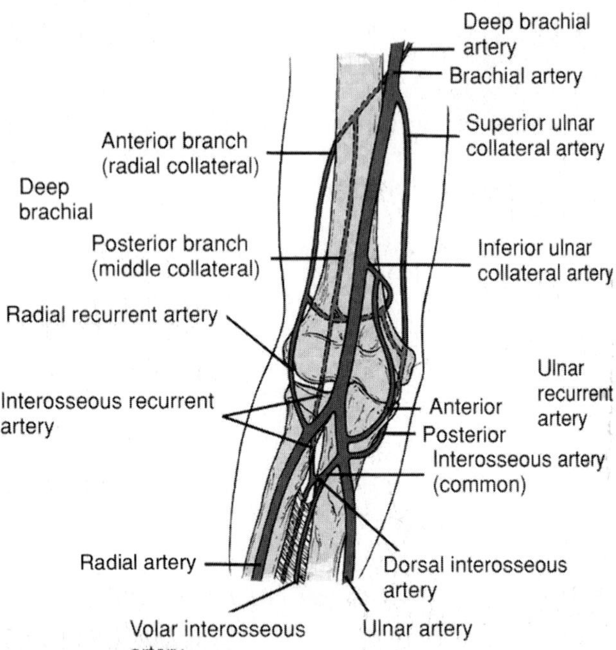

Figure 2-24 The vascular supply about the elbow is rich, with excellent collateral circulation. The collateral circulation is usually sufficient to maintain viability of the extremity in the event of occlusion of the brachial artery. (From Green NE: Skeletal Trauma in Children, 2nd ed. Philadelphia, WB Saunders, 1998.)

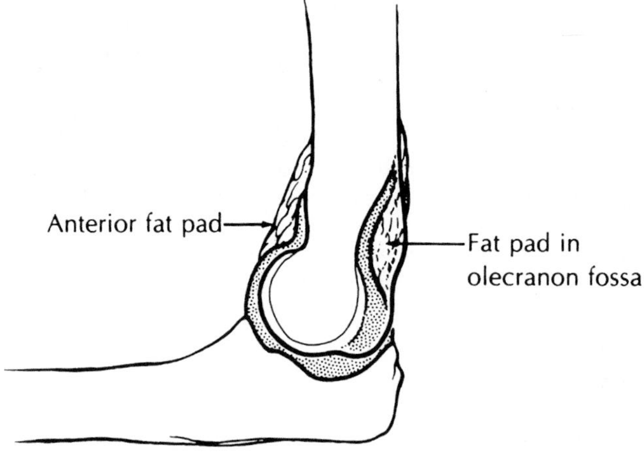

Figure 2-25 The elbow fat pads. Some of the coronoid fat pad lies anterior to the shallow coronoid fossa. The olecranon fat pad lies totally within the deeper olecranon fossa. (From Rockwood CA Jr, Wilkins KE, Beaty JH: Fractures in Children, 4th ed. Philadelphia, Lippincott-Raven, 1996.)

Supracondylar Fractures of the Humerus

Supracondylar fractures of the humerus occur most frequently in children younger than 8 years. Many young children with lax ligaments can hyperextend their

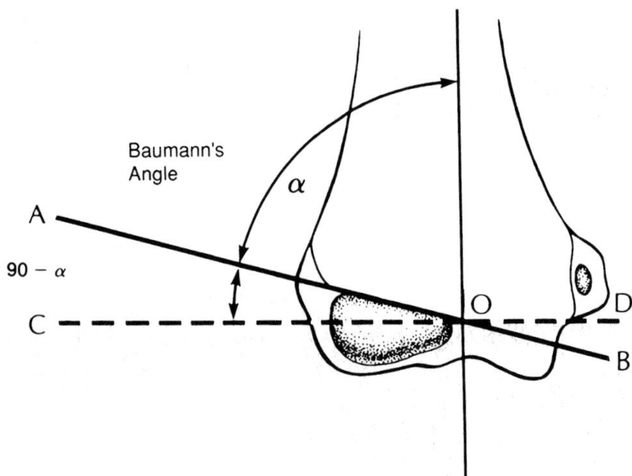

Figure 2-26 Bauman's angle (α). (From Rockwood CA Jr, Wilkins KE, Beaty JH: Fractures in Children, 4th ed. Philadelphia, Lippincott-Raven, 1996.)

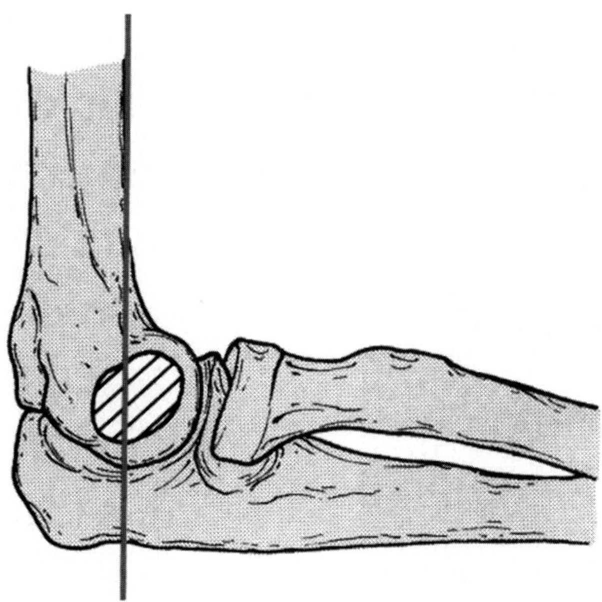

Figure 2-27 The anterior humeral line is drawn down the outer edge of the anterior cortex of the distal humerus. As the line is drawn distally through the capitellum, it should pass through the middle of the capitellum. (From Rockwood CA Jr, Wilkins KE, Beaty JH: Fractures in Children, 4th ed. Philadelphia, Lippincott-Raven, 1996.)

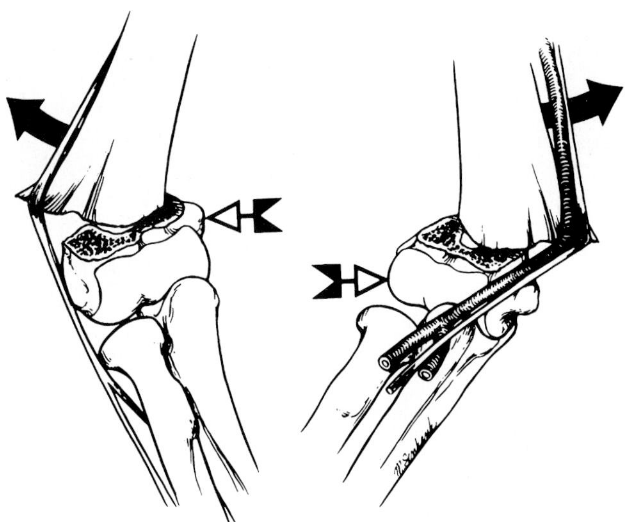

Figure 2-28 In a supracondylar fracture, there is risk of injury to the radial nerve, brachial artery, and median nerve. (From Rockwood CA Jr, Wilkins KE, Beaty JH: Fractures in Children, 4th ed. Philadelphia, Lippincott-Raven, 1996.)

elbows. When such a child falls on an outstretched hand, this elbow hyperextension allows the olecranon to act as a wedge in the olecranon fossa, placing a tension force across the anterior humerus. If this force is sufficient, the anterior cortex is disrupted, and a type I supracondylar fracture (see later) is produced. With further force, the fracture can become partially or completely displaced, resulting in a more significant injury. The distal humerus is a narrow area of rapidly remodeling bone in the young child, making this region particularly vulnerable to injury. The very narrow width of the distal humerus also limits the bony stability necessary to hold a closed reduction of a displaced injury. Thus, before pinning was popularized, the completely displaced supracondylar humerus fracture treated in a cast would often rotate and angulate into varus, creating the so-called gunstock deformity.

Many supracondylar humerus fractures are severe injuries in children and require careful evaluation and operative management. At the time of the evaluation, the integrity of the skin should be confirmed, and the neurovascular status should be checked carefully. Nerve injuries occur in 10% to 15% of all supracondylar fractures (Fig. 2-28). The most common nerve injury is of the anterior interosseous nerve;[15] it can be checked for by evaluation of flexion of the thumb and the distal phalanx of the index finger. The radial nerve is most commonly injured when the distal fragment is displaced in a posterior-medial direction. Ulnar nerve injury is less common than median and radial nerve injuries. The ulnar nerve should nevertheless be assessed carefully, because pinning sometimes affects the ulnar nerve, and documentation of the nerve's preoperative status is valuable in managing this potential complication.

Extension-type supracondylar humerus fractures are the most common source of fracture-associated vascular injury in children. In an emergency room setting, the physician should assess the color and viability of the hand and the presence or absence of a radial pulse. The compartments of the forearm should be assessed carefully, especially with the possibility of a vascular injury.

Traditionally, the Gartland classification has been used to describe supracondylar humerus fractures in children. A type I fracture is nondisplaced, a type II fracture involves angulation with an intact posterior cortex, and a type III fracture is complete displacement of the distal humeral fragment. Often in type III fractures, the humeral metaphysis tears through the brachialis muscle and can be palpated directly beneath the skin (Fig. 2-29). The presence of ecchymosis and a puckering of the skin at the fracture site indicate a very severe injury. Although the Gartland classification is valuable as a radiographic description, it may be easier to think of two types of supracondylar fractures, those that can be casted and those that need closed reduction and pinning. Fractures in which the anterior humeral line intersects the capitellum and the medial column has not collapsed can be treated with a cast for 3 weeks. All other fractures are currently treated with closed reduction and pinning.

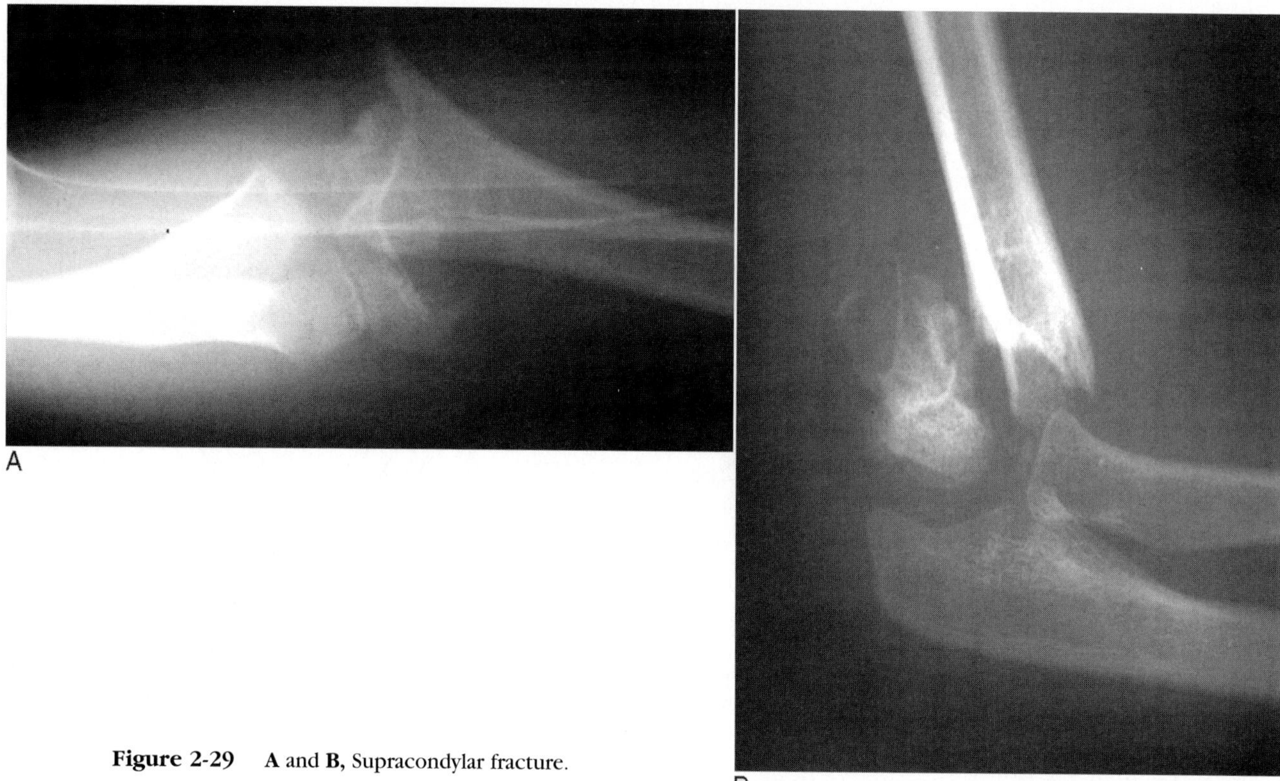

Figure 2-29 **A** and **B,** Supracondylar fracture.

In fractures with either unacceptable extension or medial collapse, simple evaluation and splinting should be performed in the emergency room. No reduction should be attempted. In more severe fractures, closed reduction and pinning are generally performed within the first 24 hours after injury. With the child asleep and the elbow prepared for surgery, the orthopaedic surgeon reduces the fracture by correcting varus and valgus and then flexing the elbow fully, using the posterior periosteum to hold the distal humerus in position as pins are placed. The commonly used fixation strategies involve two lateral pins, crossed medial and lateral pins, and two lateral pins and a medial pin. If, after pinning, the hand is well perfused even though a radial pulse cannot be felt, it is safe to observe the child closely rather than explore the artery.

Complications after supracondylar humerus fractures in children include loss of motion, cubitus varus, persistent neurologic deficit, and avascular necrosis of the trochlea. Cubitus varus can be avoided by confirmation of a satisfactory Baumann angle after stable fixation is applied. Volkman ischemic contracture, fairly common in the past, when closed reduction alone was used, has been virtually eliminated by the use of pinning. After pinning, the elbow can be immobilized in only 70 to 80 degrees of flexion, avoiding the forearm ischemia caused in the past when the elbow was flexed to more than 90° degrees and the brachial artery was occluded because of arm position and swelling. The most common nerve injury associated with supracondylar fracture is neuropraxia, which resolves without surgical intervention.

Flexion supracondylar fractures are 50 times less common than the extension type. They generally occur when a child falls directly onto the elbow. Most displaced flexion supracondylar humerus fractures require internal fixation with pins. The ulnar nerve is the nerve most commonly injured with flexion supracondylar fractures.

A rare fracture is the distal humeral epiphyseal separation. It generally occurs in children younger than 5 years who fall on an outstretched hand and sustain an extension injury to the elbow. Reduction and treatment are similar to those for displaced supracondylar fractures, with one exception: Reduction after 3 to 5 days is not recommended because it risks causing a growth arrest of the distal humeral physis.

Lateral Condyle Fractures

Fractures of the lateral condyle of the distal humerus are the second most common elbow fractures in children. They can be caused by avulsion, when a varus force is transmitted to the distal humerus during a fall on the outstretched hand, or by a direct blow to the capitellum by the humeral head through a fall on the outstretched hand.

The Milch classification is most commonly used to describe lateral condyle fractures (Fig. 2-30). The Milch type I fracture is an SH IV fracture that passes from the metaphysis through the capitellar ossification center into the joint. The elbow is usually stable in these injuries. In a Milch type II fracture, the fracture line passes medial to the capitellum into the trochlear grove of the distal humerus; this is an SH II fracture. The Milch type II fracture is much more common than the Milch type I and can be associated with elbow subluxation.

A second classification that is more valuable to surgeons describes the stages of displacement (Fig. 2-31). A type I fracture is nondisplaced, with an intact cartilaginous epiphyseal hinge. A type II fracture is complete but not rotated. A type III fracture is completely displaced with the capitellum rotated out of the radiohumeral joint. Some type I fractures (according to this classification) can be treated with a cast, but the other types must be treated with either closed or open reduction and pinning.

Evaluation at the time of injury involves a careful examination for other injuries and AP and lateral radiographs of the elbow. An oblique radiograph of the elbow often shows the greatest displacement of the fracture.

Most lateral condyle fractures are treated surgically. A lateral condyle fracture with less than 2 mm of displacement can be treated in a long-arm cast for 4 to 6 weeks. Radiographs should be obtained 1 week and 2 weeks after injury to ensure that late displacement has not occurred. Fractures with more than 2 mm of displacement are evaluated fluoroscopically in the operating room. Most require open reduction and internal fixation. Two K-wires are used to secure fixation after anatomic reduction. Occasionally, a fresh, minimally displaced lateral condyle fracture can be treated satisfactorily with closed reduction and percutaneous pinning.

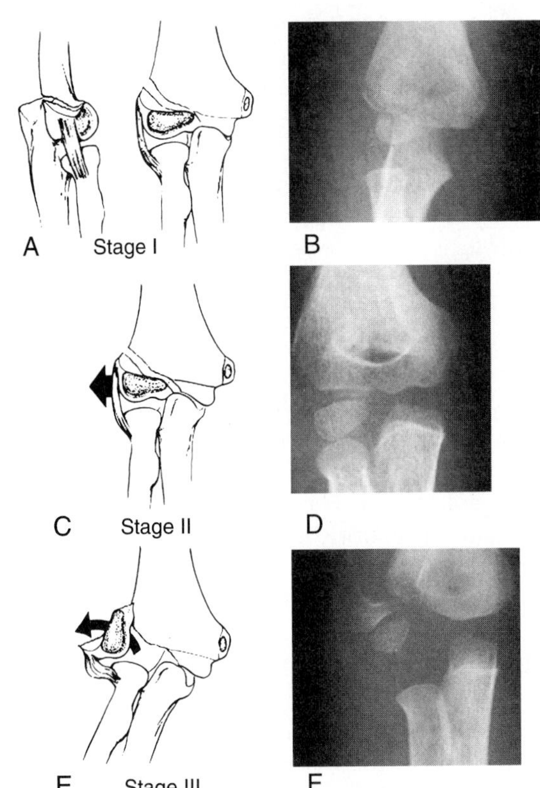

Figure 2-31 Stages of displacement of lateral condyle fractures. (From Rockwood CA Jr, Wilkins KE, Beaty JH: Fractures in Children, 4th ed. Philadelphia, Lippincott-Raven, 1996.)

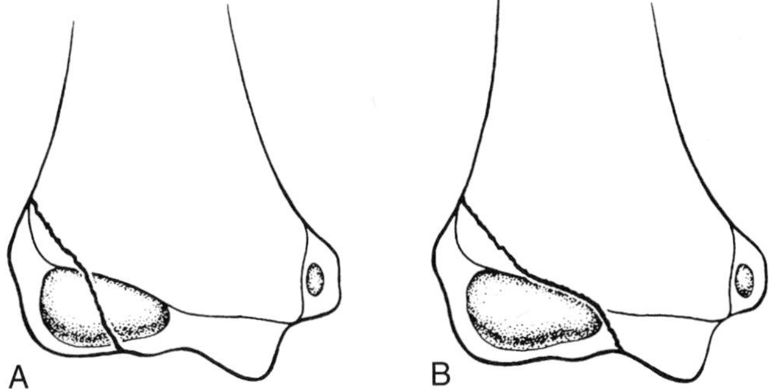

Figure 2-30 Physeal fractures of the lateral condyle. **A,** Salter-Harris type IV physeal injury (Milch type I). **B,** Salter-Harris type II physeal injury (Milch type II). (From Rockwood CA Jr, Wilkins KE, Beaty JH: Fractures in Children, 4th ed. Philadelphia, Lippincott-Raven, 1996.)

One must keep in mind several important complications when treating lateral condyle fractures. These injuries are one of the rare pediatric fractures that can proceed to non-union. Because the fracture fragment is bathed in synovial fluid, is largely cartilage, and has a relatively tenuous blood supply, non-union occurs in a displaced, neglected fracture. Late treatment of a neglected non-union involves observation or open reduction, stable compression fixation, and bone grafting. Cubitus valgus may occur with non-union and may be associated with a tardy ulnar nerve palsy.

Medial Epicondyle Fractures

Most medial epicondyle fractures occur in adolescent boys. The injury is thought to be due to a valgus force combined with contraction of the forearm flexors-supinator complex. The same combination of forces also causes an elbow dislocation. Therefore, the evaluating physician should never forget the association of medial epicondyle fractures with elbow dislocations. These injuries occur together in nearly 50% of cases of elbow dislocations. The neurovascular status, particularly the ulnar nerve, should be evaluated, and other associated injuries should be ruled out. The physician should study the AP and lateral radiographs of the elbow to determine the extent of displacement of the medial epicondyle. These injuries can be particularly subtle in younger children, in whom the medial epicondyle is barely ossified. One must remember that the medial epicondyle is a fairly posterior structure that may be difficult to appreciate on a lateral radiograph.

The treatment of nondisplaced medial epicondyle fractures involves cast immobilization for 3 weeks followed by range-of-motion exercises. Shorter immobilization may be wise in the child with an elbow dislocation, which may be associated with greater stiffness after casting. The treatment of displaced medial epicondyle fractures is controversial. For a fracture displaced only 2 to 5 mm, most pediatric orthopaedists recommend cast immobilization for 3 weeks. In fractures with more than 5 mm of displacement, internal fixation is standard for most specialists, especially in the dominant arm of an athlete. Although several studies have documented high levels of function with nonoperative treatment of widely displaced medial epicondyle fractures, most surgeons currently fix such injuries. Families are generally not satisfied with the fibrous non-union that would be expected without treatment, even if it would eventually become asymptomatic.

The major complication of medial epicondyle fractures is a loss of terminal elbow extension. This development is particularly common if the fracture is associated with elbow dislocation or immobilization lasted for an extended period.

Elbow Dislocations

Although elbow dislocation is a very rare injury in the young child, it is seen with some frequency in the adolescent. The mechanism that produces supracondylar fracture in a 5- or 6-year-old child causes elbow dislocation in a teenager. Elbow dislocations result when the proximal radius and ulna are driven posteriorly by a force directed through the forearm, usually after a fall on the outstretched hand. The dislocation may occur with either flexion or extension of the elbow. If there is a valgus component to the force, avulsion of the medial epicondyle may occur. Because the medial epicondyle may become incarcerated in the joint (Fig. 2-32) or may be too subtle to recognize, the physician must remember the relationship between elbow dislocation and the medial epicondyle when evaluating such injuries.

In a child with a suspected elbow dislocation, the initial evaluation should consist of a careful neurovascular examination, palpation of the upper extremity for other injuries, and an assessment of skin integrity. AP and lateral radiographs of the elbow and forearm should be evaluated for determination of the direction and extent of the dislocation as well as for incarcerated medial epicondyle fracture and other associated injuries.

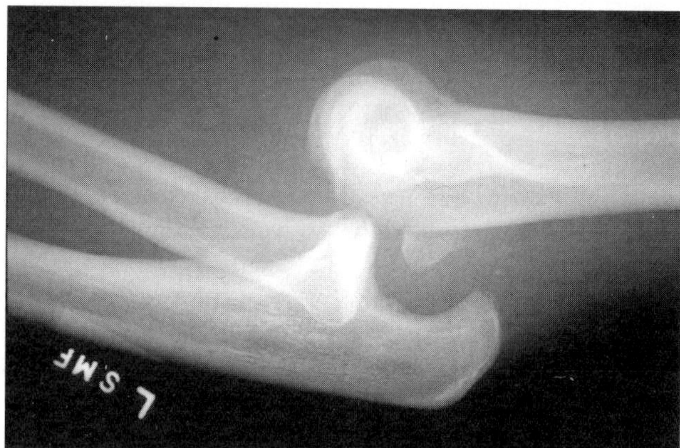

Figure 2-32 Elbow dislocation with entrapped medial epicondyle.

The treatment of an elbow dislocation in children involves prompt reduction of the dislocation with the use of conscious sedation. The reduction is generally quite easy, so general anesthesia is rarely required. The orthopaedist achieves reduction either through a traction maneuver or by pushing posteriorly over the olecranon (Fig. 2-33) to reduce the displacement of the ulnar and radius onto the humerus. When there is lateral displacement in addition to the posterior displacement, correcting the lateral displacement first avoids entrapment of the median nerve within the joint during reduction.[16] The reduction should be performed with the forearm supinated. A satisfying "clunk" is usually felt at reduction. The elbow should then be taken through a gentle range of motion to assess stability.

Postreduction radiographs are essential. The AP and lateral radiographs of the elbow should be assessed for the congruency of the radial and ulnar articulations with the humerus and for incarceration of the medial epicondyle within the joint. The most common cause of an incongruent joint relationship is interposed tissue at the time of reduction. The tissue is usually the medial ligament and muscle attached medial epicondyle. If tissue interposition is noted, an open reduction to remove the interposed soft tissue is generally best. The postreduction assessment should also include an evaluation of nerve function. There are several alarming reports of an entrapped median nerve at the time of elbow reduction.

Significant soft tissue disruption occurs at the time of an elbow dislocation. However, the greatest risk after these injuries is of elbow stiffness rather than recurrent dislocation. For this reason, immobilization should last for only 2 to 3 weeks, followed by a supervised return to motion. In general, full terminal extension is avoided until 4 to 6 weeks after injury (depending on stability).

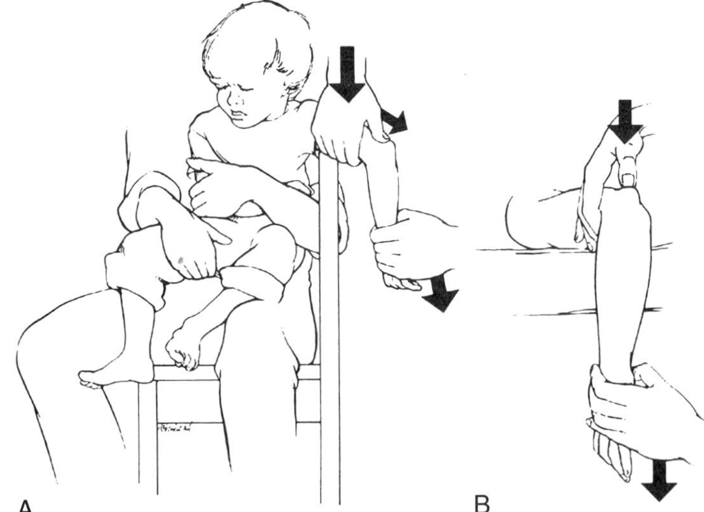

Figure 2-33 **A** and **B,** Reduction of elbow dislocation by "pusher" techniques. (From Rockwood CA Jr, Wilkins KE, Beaty JH: Fractures in Children, 4th ed. Philadelphia, Lippincott-Raven, 1996.)

We generally prefer a cast for immobilization, because splints and elastic wraps are more likely to cause skin problems and become malpositioned during recovery.

Complications of elbow dislocation include loss of motion, neurovascular injury, and recurrent dislocation. A careful assessment of stability and a return to early range of motion are the best ways to prevent elbow stiffness. The family should be counseled that terminal elbow extension may be slow to return. Ulnar and median nerve injuries have been reported in several series of elbow dislocations. Some injuries occur at the time of injury, but the median nerve can be injured by entrapment at reduction. As mentioned previously, recurrent dislocation is a rare problem after this elbow injury in children. If recurrent dislocation does not respond to immobilization, surgical reattachment or reconstruction of the elbow-stabilizing ligaments may be required.

Nursemaid's Elbow

Nursemaid's elbow represents the single most common upper extremity injury of childhood that is definitively treated by the primary care physician. These injuries are most common in the young child, usually younger than 4 years, but are seen in early school-age children as well. Recurrence after the initial injury is quite common. The pediatrician may encounter a worried parent who notes several "elbow dislocations" in a preschool child over the course of a year.

It is important to understand the pathophysiology of this injury. Nursemaid's elbow is not a dislocation of the radial head, but entrapment of a portion of the annular ligament between the radial head and the capitellum (Fig. 2-34). After the initial injury, there is a small tear in this annular ligament, which is also stretched, explaining the frequency of the recurrent injury. The mechanism of injury is generally pronation of the forearm with traction. Typically this mechanism occurs when an adult is holding the child's hand or forearm and the child pulls away. It can also occur when the child falls with pronation of the forearm.

Initial assessment after injury should focus on localization of the area of tenderness, a search for other injuries along the upper extremity, and a standard neurovascular examination. Good-quality AP and lateral

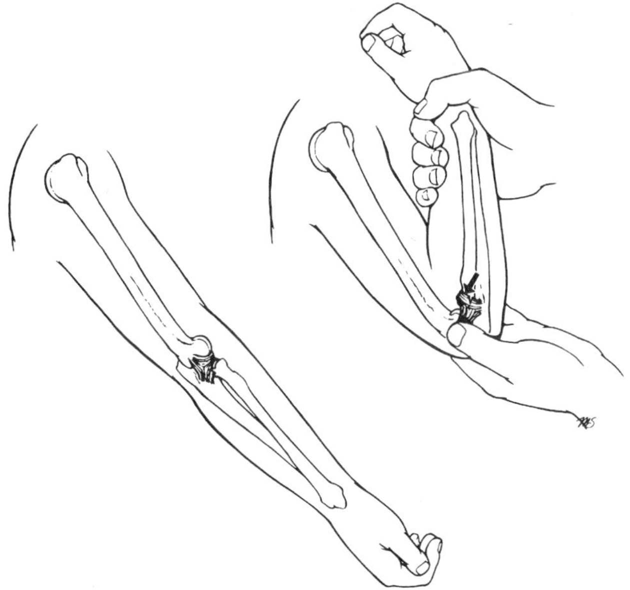

Figure 2-34 **Reduction technique of nursemaid's elbow.** *Left,* The forearm is first supinated. *Right,* The elbow is then hyperflexed. The surgeon's thumb is placed laterally over the radial head so as to feel the characteristic snapping as the ligament is reduced. (From Rockwood CA Jr, Wilkins KE, Beaty JH: Fractures in Children, 4th ed. Philadelphia, Lippincott-Raven, 1996.)

radiographs of the elbow should be studied carefully to ensure that other injuries are not present. In children with recurrent nursemaid's elbows in whom the diagnosis is confirmed by history and examination, reduction may be performed by the parent or physician without another series of radiographs.

Reduction of nursemaid's elbow involves full supination of the forearm and maximal flexion of the elbow. The child's supinated hand should come to be opposed to the anterior surface of the shoulder with maximal flexion. The most common reason for orthopaedic consultation after an unsuccessful nursemaid's reduction is failure to maximally flex the elbow at the time of the initial reduction.

Once the reduction has been performed, the child should be observed for a few minutes to ascertain full use of the injured arm. With reduction performed soon after injury, the child will rapidly adopt full use of the arm and show no signs of residual symptoms. In cases of missed nursemaid's elbow or multiple attempts at reduction over several days, inflammation of the annular ligament may cause symptoms for a day or so after the reduction. In longer-standing cases or cases in which a complete reduction cannot be ascertained in an anxious child who is difficult to examine, elbow ultrasonography can reassure the parents and the physician that there is no longer any interposed tissue and that there are no other occult injuries masquerading as nursemaid's elbow.

Complications after nursemaid's elbow are rare. The most common problem is recurrence. Recurrence generally ceases to be a problem as the child is older than 6 or 7 years and the annular ligament thickens and strengthens, thus resisting injury.

Rare Injuries of the Elbow

A few very rare pediatric elbow injuries are worthy of mention without detailed description or treatment guidelines. T-condylar distal humerus fractures are seen occasionally in older children and teenagers. They result from a fall with a direct blow on the elbow. The ulna is driven up into the distal humerus, splitting the humerus longitudinally in addition to causing a transverse or spiral fracture more proximally. The vast majority of these injuries are displaced and require operative reduction and fixation. For widely displaced fractures in older children, a combination of plates and screws is used to obtain stable fixation and allow early motion of the injured elbow.

Articular fractures of the capitellum and trochlea are very rare in children. Generally, the biomechanics of the condylar epiphysis dictate that force applied in this region causes a lateral condyle or supracondylar fracture rather than the cartilaginous shear fractures of the capitellum or trochlea. Articular fractures generally require open reduction and fixation or débridement with drilling. Medial condyle fractures are extremely rare injuries. In a major children's hospital treating thousands of fractures per year, physicians may observe a medial condyle fracture once every 1 or 2 years. Treatment of displaced medial condyle fractures involves open or closed reduction and pinning. A lateral epicondyle fracture is also quite rare. It generally involves an avulsion of the lateral epicondyle and attached soft tissues. A short period of cast immobilization is usually a satisfactory treatment.

FRACTURES OF THE HUMERUS AND SHOULDER REGION

Fractures of the Humeral Shaft

Fractures of the humeral shaft account for about 2% to 5% of all fractures in children.[18] The incidence is highest in children younger than 3 years and older that 12 years. Transverse or short oblique fracture patterns usually result from direct blunt. Spiral fracture patterns, however, can occur from a twisting mechanism and may suggest child abuse. A transverse fracture pattern does not rule out child abuse.

Assessment of a patient with trauma to the arm should begin with an inspection to look for open fractures and should be followed by a thorough neurovascular examination. The radial nerve is especially vulnerable to injury with humeral shaft fractures. Nerve injuries with humeral shaft fractures are usually a result of traction, and most resolve within 3 to 6 months. The brachial artery should also be evaluated through assessment of distal pulses. The shoulder and the elbow should be included in the radiographic examination of the humerus.

A child's humerus has a great deal of remodeling potential, allowing for a wide range of acceptable deformity. Children younger than 5 years can tolerate 70 degrees of angulation and total displacement, children 5 to 12 years old 40 to 70 degrees of angulation, and children older than 12 years old 40 degrees of angulation and 50% apposition.[18] Shortening of 1 to 2 cm is acceptable because bony overgrowth will occur. A thorough neurologic examination is especially important if reduction of the fracture is undertaken to appose the fracture fragments. A nerve that was previously intact, but is compromised after the reduction is an indication for surgical exploration. Immobilization with a coaptation splint (Fig. 2-35) or a functional brace (often referred to as a Sarmiento brace) is valuable to maintain alignment of the fracture fragments. Humeral shaft fracture in a newborn can be managed by splinting of the arm to the chest wall, which can often be achieved by placing a safety pin to connect the sleeve to the front of the child's shirt.

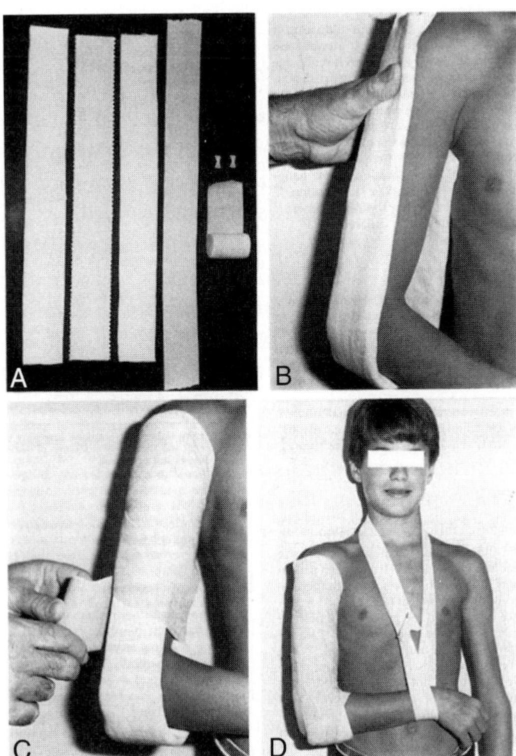

Figure 2-35 Coaptation splints with collar and cuff. (From Rockwood CA Jr, Wilkins KE, Beaty JH: Fractures in Children, 4th ed. Philadelphia, Lippincott-Raven, 1996.)

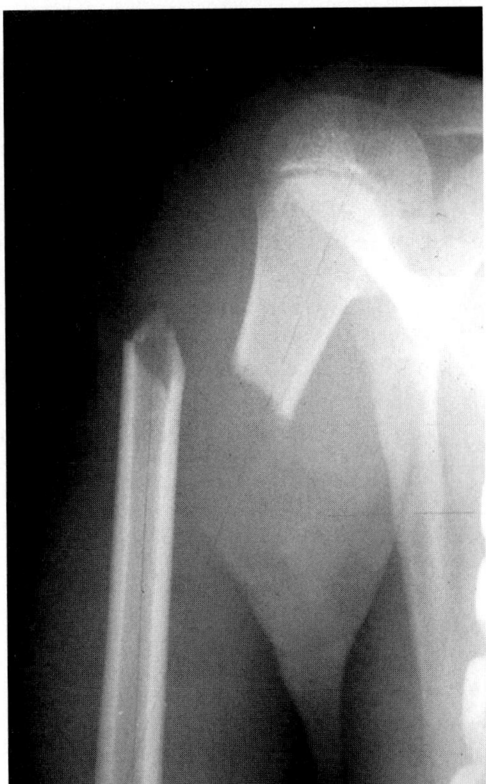

Figure 2-36 Proximal humerus fracture.

Children with humeral shaft fractures usually do very well with nonoperative treatment. Complications after humeral shaft fractures include the previously mentioned nerve palsies. Vascular injuries can be devastating, and a high index of suspicion and prompt treatment are vital in preventing complications. Malunion and nonunion of a humeral shaft fracture are uncommon problems in children. Compartment syndrome is a rare complication, but it has been reported.[19] A small discrepancy in limb length is common but is usually less than 1 cm, and patients tolerate it well.

Fractures of the Proximal Humerus

Fractures of the proximal humerus are relatively uncommon injuries, accounting for less than 5% of all fractures in children.[6] The mechanism is usually a fall on an outstretched arm. Proximal humeral fracture can occur during birth and manifest as a pseudoparalysis; it is usually a result of an excessive hyperextension and external rotation force during delivery.

Fracture patterns tend to vary according to the age group. Neonates and children younger than 5 years usually sustain SH I fractures (Fig. 2-36). Children between 5 and 10 years often present with metaphyseal fractures; these are usually transverse or short oblique fractures. Children older than 11 years usually have SH II fractures.[20] Examination of the involved extremity should involve a thorough neurologic examination, including evaluation of the axillary nerve. Good-quality plain radiographs should include an axillary view to rule out associated dislocation.

SH I fractures in children require no reduction. The patients have excellent remodeling potential, and immobilization in a sling and swathe for 2 to 3 weeks is usually sufficient for healing. Metaphyseal fractures in patients 5 to 10 years old also usually need no reduction. If the fracture is angulated more than 50 degrees, closed reduction by the orthopaedist is recommended to improve the alignment. SH II fractures with less than 20 to 30 degrees of angulation and less than 50% displacement can be managed in a sling without reduction. Reduction is usually accomplished by external rotation, abduction, and forward flexion of the arm; such a reduction often requires operative fixation to secure the fragments.

The fractures usually are healed by 4 to 6 weeks, at which time some light activity can be permitted. Patients with severe angulation may lose some range of motion but are still very functional. Limb length inequalities are usually minimal, and nerve injuries usually resolve with 3 to 6 months.

Glenohumeral Joint Subluxation and Dislocation

The shoulder joint is a ball-and-socket articulation. Although the glenoid functions as the socket, its relatively flat surface allows for greater range of motion at the expense of stability. The shoulder capsule and rotator cuff muscles are the main sources of stability at this joint. Fortunately, shoulder dislocations in children are rare. Most occur in adolescents near skeletal maturity. In one series of 500 dislocations, only 8 had occurred in children younger than 10 years.[21]

The majority of traumatic dislocations are anterior. The mechanism of injury is a force that abducts and externally rotates the outstretched arm. Posterior dislocations are rare and usually occur as a result of seizures. Atraumatic dislocations can occur from inherent ligamentous laxity, such as in patients with Ehlers-Danlos syndrome. This syndrome should be suspected in a shoulder dislocation for which there is no clear-cut traumatic event.

Physical examination should include a thorough neurovascular evaluation with special interest on axillary nerve function. Radiographic evaluation is important even when the diagnosis is obvious. A complete shoulder series should be obtained, the axillary view being the most important for diagnosis. Prereduction radiographs are important to document associated fractures before reduction is undertaken. Postreduction films should also be obtained.

Prompt closed reduction of a traumatic shoulder dislocation should be undertaken by the orthopaedist using one of the many accepted techniques. The key to any reduction is conscious sedation with, possibly, muscle relaxation. The traction-countertraction method utilizes a sheet placed in the affected axilla and around the patient for countertraction. The affected extremity is then gently distracted in line with the deformity until the muscles are fatigued and the humeral head relocates. Improper technique can result in iatrogenic fractures of the glenoid or humeral head. Postreduction radiographs should be taken to document proper location of the head. The arm and shoulder should be immobilized in a sling for 2 to 3 weeks before activity is resumed.

The most common complication is recurrent dislocation, which is seen in 50% to 100% of cases and is more common in younger patients. Recurrent shoulder dislocations may require surgical reconstruction. Axillary nerve injuries can also occur; most are neuropraxic injuries that resolve with time. Most patients with atraumatic dislocations do very well with vigorous rehabilitation and strengthening of the musculature around the joint.

Fractures of the Clavicle Shaft

The clavicle is an S-shaped bone that articulates with the thorax medially and the shoulder joint laterally. It is the most commonly fractured bone in neonates and children.[22] Neonatal fractures occur from direct trauma during birth, most often as result of a tight birth canal. They can often be missed initially, manifesting as pseudoparalysis of the affected extremity or a bump over the fracture 7 to 10 days after the injury. Childhood fractures are usually the result of a fall on the affected shoulder or direct trauma to the clavicle during sports. The child often holds the affected arm with the other arm and tilts the head toward the fracture. Tenderness over the clavicle makes the diagnosis fairly easy. As always, a thorough neurovascular examination is important to diagnose brachial plexus injuries.

Radiographic evaluation is useful and is usually all that is required. In neonates, ultrasonography can sometimes be used. Radiographic evaluation can help differentiate fracture from congenital pseudarthrosis of the clavicle, a rare disorder that is usually right-sided.[23] Evaluation of the radiograph by an experienced observer may be necessary to differentiate the two entities.

Most midshaft clavicle fractures, even with significant displacement, can be treated in a figure-of-eight splint. A sling is an acceptable option either with or without the figure-of-eight splint. Bot open fractures and significant tenting of the skin from a fracture fragment (Fig. 2-37) necessitate an immediate orthopaedic consultation for surgical management. Clavicle fractures of birth can be treated with a safety pin attaching the sleeve to the baby's clothing as a sling. Most fractures in neonates heal well without complications, and some may heal before they are ever diagnosed. In most children, deformity remodels over time. In older children, a resid-

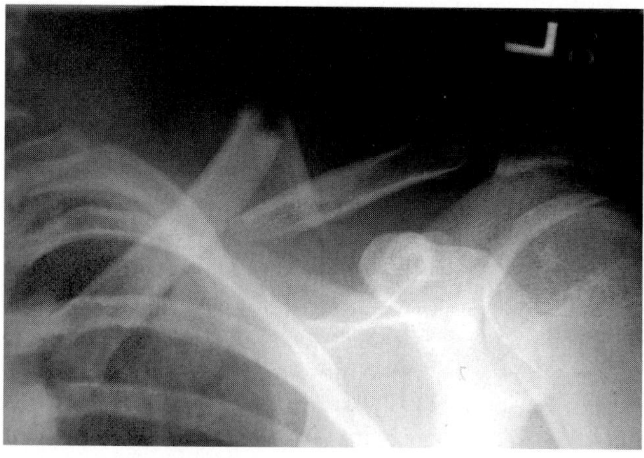

Figure 2-37 Segmental clavicle fracture.

ual deformity manifesting as a bump may remain but rarely affects function. Complications of clavicle shaft fracture include malunion, brachial plexus injury, and vascular injury.

Injuries around the Acromioclavicular Joint

Injuries to the lateral end of the clavicle account for 10% to 12% of all clavicular fractures.[6] Unlike in adults, these injuries are less likely to be acromioclavicular dislocations and more likely to be pseudodislocations represented by distal clavicular fractures. The immature clavicle has a thick periosteum, to which the coracoclavicular and acromioclavicular ligaments attach. Injury is usually fracture of the bone, which tends to slip out of this periosteum. Adolescent patients nearing skeletal maturity are more likely to suffer true acromioclavicular joint dislocations.

Injuries to the acromioclavicular joint are usually from a direct blow to the lateral end of the clavicle or from a fall in which the child lands on the affected shoulder. The patient commonly presents with pain and swelling over the joint. More severe injuries may show a deformity over the area. The child usually supports the affected arm with the other arm. The examination should include palpation of the rest of the clavicle and shoulder as well as the entire upper extremity.

Radiographic evaluation with shoulder films may be sufficient. However, radiographs centered over the acromioclavicular joint are often needed for proper evaluation. Views of the other acromioclavicular joint may also be helpful. A Stryker notch projection is helpful in demonstrating fracture of the coracoid (Fig. 2-38).

Distal clavicular injuries are classified according to the severity. Less severe injuries are managed nonoperatively. Open fractures or significantly displaced fractures with tenting of the skin require immediate orthopaedic consultation. Most fractures in children younger than 16 years are likely to heal well with nonoperative management in a sling, because of the thick periosteum that is still intact and attached to the ligaments. True acromioclavicular joint dislocations in older children should be managed like those in adults. Outcomes are excellent, with healing usually complete by 4 to 6 weeks.

Rare Injuries about the Shoulder

Injuries to the medial end of the clavicle and sternoclavicular joint are rare in children, representing only about 5% of clavicular fractures.[24] The mechanism is usually a lateral force applied to the shoulder. As with distal clavicular injuries, the lateral force produces a physeal injury rather than a pure dislocation of the sternoclavicular joint. Occasionally, the injury results from a direct blow to the sternoclavicular joint, in which case the displacement is posterior.

Posterior displacement should be evaluated promptly and carefully to assess for neurovascular damage and injury to important mediastinal structures. Any complaints by the patient of trouble breathing or swallowing should be taken seriously. Pulses in the affected extremity should be carefully measured and compared with those on the other side. Diminution or absence of pulses suggests vascular injury.

The patient usually holds the affected arm across the chest and has pain with palpation over the sternoclavicular joint. A chest x-ray may suffice for evaluation of the injury. Signs of mediastinal injury should be excluded. CT scanning of the chest can provide an accurate assessment of injury and displacement.

Fractures of the medial end of the clavicle have excellent healing and remodeling potential in children. Reduction is indicated only for posterior displacement. It should be performed by an orthopaedic consultant, and may have to be an emergency procedure. Surgical treatment is rarely indicated and outcomes are excellent.

Fractures of the scapula (Fig. 2-39) are extremely rare, accounting for less than 1% of all fractures in children.[6] Fractures of the scapular spine and body are usually the result of a direct high-energy blow and often have associated injuries. Trauma and orthopaedic specialists should be consulted for diagnosis and treatment of the associated injuries. Scapular fractures are usually minimally displaced because the musculature surrounding the fragments often keeps them in place. Conservative treatment is usually indicated.

Scapular neck fractures can be either isolated or associated with clavicular fractures. Isolated injuries are usually stable and need only conservative treatment. Scapular fractures in combination with clavicular fractures are unstable and require orthopaedic consultation.

Glenoid fractures are commonly associated with shoulder dislocations and should be ruled out in any patient with a dislocation. They can range from small avulsion fractures to large intra-articular fragments that cause severe disability and shoulder instability. Orthopaedic consultation should be obtained when this fracture is suspected. CT scanning may delineate the fracture pattern better than plain radiographs.

Scapular fractures, by themselves, usually have good outcomes. However, the patient may have many other significant injuries with serious sequelae. Most scapular fractures are treated nonoperatively, with immobilization in a sling. However, orthopaedic and trauma specialists should be consulted immediately when this injury is diagnosed.

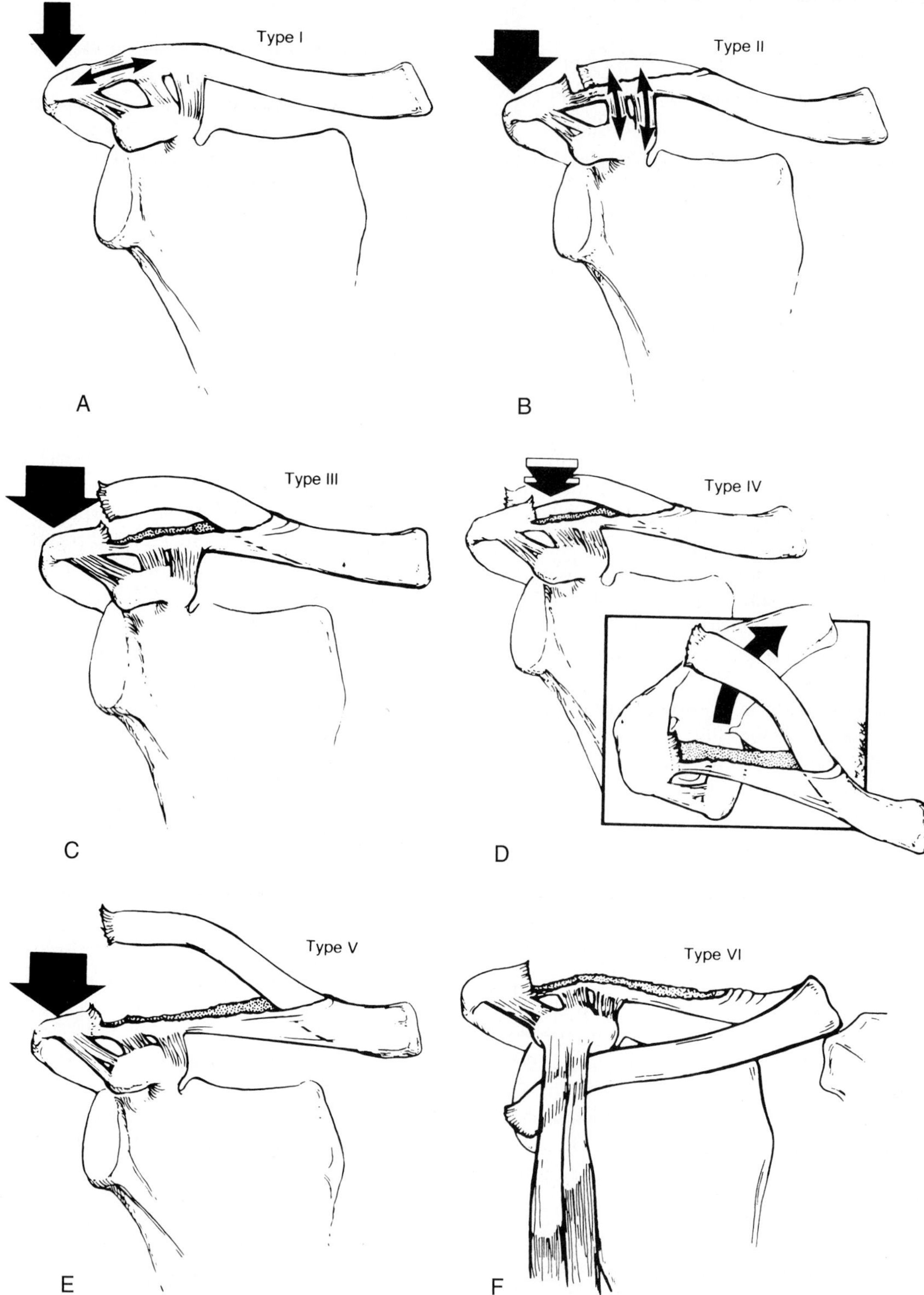

Figure 2-38 Rockwood's classification of clavicular-acromioclavicular joint injuries in children. (From Rockwood CA Jr, Wilkins KE, Beaty JH: Fractures in Children, 4th ed. Philadelphia, Lippincott-Raven, 1996.)

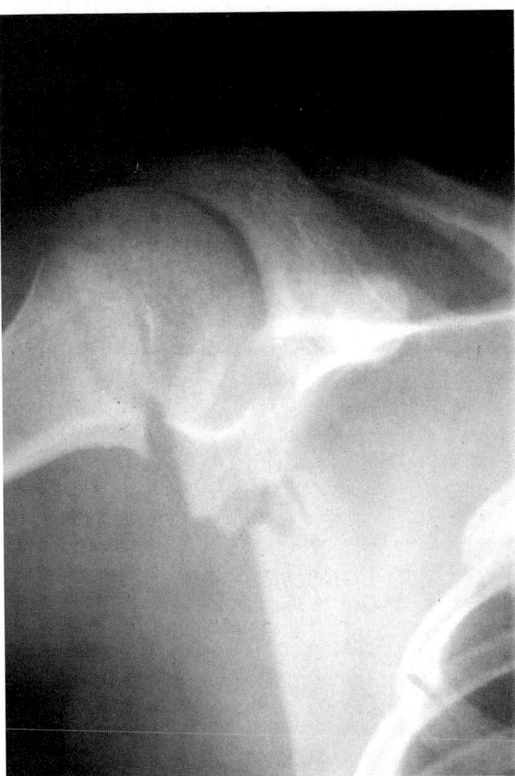

Figure 2-39 Scapula fracture.

SUMMARY

Upper extremity injuries are very common in children. Most can be treated with a cast or reduction and pinning if cast treatment does not confer satisfactory stability to the injured bone or joint. Careful history and physical examination, followed by proper imaging, provide the key starting points for successful management.

MAJOR POINTS

The pediatric hand is a very common site for injury. The incidence of hand fractures increases sharply after age 8 years and the peak in boys is at 13 years, when they often participate in contact sports.

A mallet finger deformity is a common presentation of distal phalanx injuries. Children younger than 5 years have a Salter-Harris type (SH) I or SH II injury with the flexor tendon still attached to the distal piece, pulling it in a volar direction. Children closer to adolescence usually have an SH III injury.

A hematoma greater than 25% of the nail bed should raise suspicion of nail bed injury and prompt a direct visual evaluation of the nail bed.

Fractures of the metacarpal shaft must be evaluated for rotational deformity. The patient is asked to make a fist. All fingers should point to the scaphoid and all the nail beds should be parallel.

Fracture management is also greatly aided by an understanding of the connection between the radius and ulna. With articulations proximally and distally and an interosseous membrane in the middle, the radius and ulna act as a two-bone complex. Managing injuries to this complex requires an understanding of this relationship, because a significantly displaced injury to one bone is often associated with an injury to the other.

Most surgeons treat proximal fractures with forearm supination, and middle or distal third fractures with a neutral forearm position or slight forearm pronation.

Long-term outcome after distal radius and ulnar physeal fracture is usually excellent. Dorsal angulation up to 30 or 40 degrees remodels satisfactorily in a child in whom significant growth remains.

Radial and ulnar diaphyseal fracture can be more difficult to treat because the limits of acceptable reduction are much more stringent than for distal radial fractures. A significant malunion of a forearm diaphyseal fracture can lead to a permanent loss of pronation and supination and, sometimes, an unsightly curvature or prominence in the forearm.

Acceptable reduction of diaphyseal forearm fractures is 10 to 20 degrees of angulation in children younger than 10 years but no more than 10 degrees of angulation in older children and adolescents.

High-quality radiographs are mandatory for successful management of Monteggia fractures.

Although elbow fractures are less common than forearm and wrist fractures, many pediatric elbow fractures receive more attention because they need more aggressive management for a good result. Improper management of elbow injuries remains a common source of disability and malpractice litigation.

The posterior fat pad sign is the most important indication of an occult fracture of the distal humerus. When the posterior fat pad sign is seen, there is a 70% chance of a fracture.

Nerve injuries occur in 10% to 15% of all supracondylar fractures of the humerus. The most common nerve injury is of the anterior interosseous nerve.

Most lateral condyle humerus fractures are treated surgically. Lateral condyle fractures with less than 2 mm of displacement can be treated in a long-arm cast for 4 to 6 weeks. Radiographs should be obtained 1 week and 2 weeks after injury to ensure that late displacement has not occurred. Fractures with more than 2 mm of displacement are evaluated fluoroscopically in the operating room.

The evaluating physician should never forget the association of medial epicondyle fractures with elbow dislocations. These injuries occur together in nearly 50% of cases of elbow dislocations.

(Continued)

MAJOR POINTS—cont'd

Nursemaid's elbow is not a dislocation of the radial head. Instead, it involves the entrapment of a portion of the annular ligament between the radial head and the capitellum. After the initial injury, there is a small tear in this annular ligament and it is stretched, explaining the frequency of recurrence of this injury.

Reduction of nursemaid's elbow involves full supination of the forearm and maximal flexion of the elbow. The child's supinated hand should come to be opposed to the anterior surface of the shoulder with maximal flexion.

A child's humerus has a great deal of remodeling potential, allowing for a wide range of acceptable deformity. Children younger than 5 years can tolerate 70 degrees of angulation and total displacement; children 5 to 12 years 40 to 70 degrees of angulation, and children older than 12 years 40 degrees of angulation and 50% apposition.

Shoulder dislocations in children are rare. Most occur in the adolescent near skeletal maturity. In one series of 500 dislocations, only 8 had occurred in children younger than 10 years.

Clavicle fractures of birth can be treated with a safety pin placed to attach the sleeve to the baby's clothing as a sling. Most fractures in neonates heal well without complications, and some may heal before they are ever diagnosed.

REFERENCES

1. Hastings H 2nd, Simmons BP: Hand fractures in children: A statistical analysis. Clin Orthop 188:120-130, 1984.
2. Brighton CT: Clinical problems in epiphyseal plate growth and development. Instruct Course Lect XXIII: 105-122, 1974.
3. Green DP: Hand injuries in children. Pediatr Clin North Am 24:903-918, 1977.
4. Beatty E, Light TR, Belsole RJ, Ogden JA: Wrist and hand skeletal injuries in children. Hand Clin 6:723-738, 1990.
5. Crock HV, Chari PR, Crock MC: The blood supply of the wrist and hand bones in man. In Tubiana R (ed): The Hand, vol. 1. Philadelphia, WB Saunders, 1981, pp 335-349.
6. Rockwood CA Jr, Wilkins KE, Beaty JH: Fractures in Children, 4th ed. Philadelphia, Lippincott-Raven, 1996.
7. Christensen JB: A study of the interosseous distance between the radius and ulna during rotation of the forearm J Bone Joint Surg 46B:778-779, 1964.
8. Mabrey JD, Fitch RD: Plastic deformation in pediatric fractures: Mechanism and treatment. J Pediatr Orthop 9:310-314, 1989.
9. Bado JL:The Monteggia lesion. Clin Orthop 50:71-86, 1967.
10. Olney BW, Menelasu MB: Monteggia and equivalent lesions in childhood. J Pediatr Orthop 9:219-223, 1989.
11. Dormans JP: Arthrographically assisted percutaneous manipulation of displaced and angulated radial neck fractures in children: Description of a technique for reduction and a new radiograhic sign. J Orthop Tech 2:77-81, 1994.
12. Di Cesare PE, Sew-Hoy A, Krom W: bilateral isolated olecranon fractures in an infant as presentation of osteogenesis imperfecta. Orthopaedics 15:741-743, 1992.
13. Mudgal CS: Olecranon fractures in osteogenesis imperfecta: A case report. Acta Orthop Belg 58:453-456, 1992.
14. Skaggs DL, Mirzayan R: The posterior fat pad sign in association with occult fracture of the elbow in children. J Bone Joint Surg Am 81:1429-433, 1999.
15. Dormans JP, Squillante R: Nerve injuries associated with supracondylar fractures of the distal humerus in children. J Hand Surg 20A:1-4, 1995.
16. Magnuson PB: Fractures. Philadelphia, JB Lippincott, 1933, pp 58-99.
17. Cheng JC, Shen WY: Limb fracture pattern in different pediatric age groups: A study of 3,350 children. J Orthop Trauma 7:15-22, 1993.
18. Beaty JH: Fractures of the proximal humerus and shaft in children. Instruct Course Lect 41:369-372, 1992.
19. Mubarak SJ, Carroll NC: Volkmann's contracture in children: Aetiology and prevention. J Bone Joint Surg Br 61:285-293, 1979.
20. Dameron TB Jr, Reibel DB: Fractures involving the proximal humeral epiphyseal plate. J Bone Joint Surg Am 51:289-297, 1969.
21. Rowe CR: Prognosis in dislocations of the shoulder. J Bone Joint Surg 38A:957-977, 1956.
22. Stanley D, Trowbridge EA, Norris SH: The mechanism of clavicular fractures: A clinical and biomechanical analysis. J Bone Joint Surg 70B:461-464, 1988.
23. Kite JH: Congenital pseudarthrosis of the clavicle. South. Med. J 61:703-710, 1968.
24. Browner BD, Jupiter JB: Skeletal Trauma: Fractures, Dislocations, Ligamentous Injuries, 2nd ed. Philadelphia, WB Saunders, 1992.

CHAPTER 3

Lower Extremity Fractures

B. DAVID HORN
LAWRENCE WELLS
JUNICHI TAMAI

Lower extremity fractures in children are common, and although it is commonly believed that these fractures heal without serious problems, complications are encountered during their treatment. Furthermore, many of these complications do not correct with growth and development. A review of malpractice claims filed against orthopaedic surgeons published in the American Academy of Orthopaedic Surgeons' *Bulletin* found that "closed treatment of children's fractures resulted in the most frequent and expensive complications."[1] An important key to the successful treatment of pediatric lower extremity fractures is a thorough understanding of the unique anatomy and physiology of the skeletally immature musculoskeletal system. Children are not small adults; they sustain unique injuries not seen in adults, and treatment of a child's fracture must take into consideration the unique physiology, psychology, and development of the child.

MECHANISMS OF FRACTURE UNIQUE TO CHILDREN

Most lower extremity fractures in children have a straightforward mechanism of injury, similar to those resulting in adult fractures. Some fractures, however, occur from mechanisms unique to children and adolescents. These include birth injuries, child abuse, and pathologic fractures (Box 3-1).

Birth Injuries

Birth injuries can occur during either a vaginal or caesarean delivery (although much more common in vaginal deliveries) and may result in lower extremity fractures. Lower extremity fractures that occur during birth may be associated with neuromuscular disorders or skeletal dysplasias. Risk factors for birth fractures are breech presentation, prolonged labor, high birth weight, and the use of obstetrical maneuvers during delivery. Neonates with fractures typically present with limb

Box 3-1 Mechanisms of Injury for Lower Extremity Injuries in Children

- Birth injuries
- Child abuse
- Pathologic fractures

swelling, pseudoparalysis, pain, and crepitus. Femur fractures and proximal femoral epiphyseal separations (type I hip fractures or Salter-Harris type I fractures of the proximal femoral physis—see later) may occur as birth fractures. Treatment of femur fractures in the neonate and young infant is discussed later in this chapter. Proximal femoral epiphyseal separations may be difficult to diagnose with plain radiographs because the femoral head does not ossify until a child is 4 to 6 months old. Additional imaging modalities, such as hip arthrography, ultrasonography, and bone scanning or magnetic resonance imaging (MRI) may be needed to confirm the diagnosis. Treatment of these injuries is discussed later in the chapter.

Child Abuse

Child abuse should be suspected in nonambulatory children with lower extremity long bone fractures.[2] No fracture patterns or types are pathognomonic for child abuse; any type of fracture may result from nonaccidental trauma. Lower extremity fractures that are suggestive of intentional injury, however, include femur fractures in nonambulatory children and distal femoral metaphyseal corner fractures. Other findings suggestive of child abuse are a described mechanism of injury that is inconsistent with the physical findings, an unexplained delay in seeking treatment after injury, a history of similar injuries, and the presence of multiple fractures or soft tissue injuries in different stages of healing. State laws mandate that cases of suspected child abuse be reported to social welfare agencies. Many hospitals now have multidisciplinary teams to further evaluate and treat patients who are suspected victims of child abuse. From an orthopaedic perspective, lower extremity fractures resulting from abuse should be treated in accordance with standard principles and techniques.

Pathologic Fractures

Pathologic fractures can also occur in lower extremities. A pathologic fracture occurs when normal, physiologic stresses occur through areas of abnormal, weakened bone (Fig. 3-1). The abnormal bone may be secondary to a malignant neoplasm, such as Ewing sarcoma, a benign condition, such as unicameral bone cyst, or a metabolic condition such as a skeletal dysplasia. Treatment of a pathologic fracture involves treatment of the fracture as well as an evaluation of the process underlying it. This may require further imaging studies, laboratory tests, or a biopsy of the lesion.

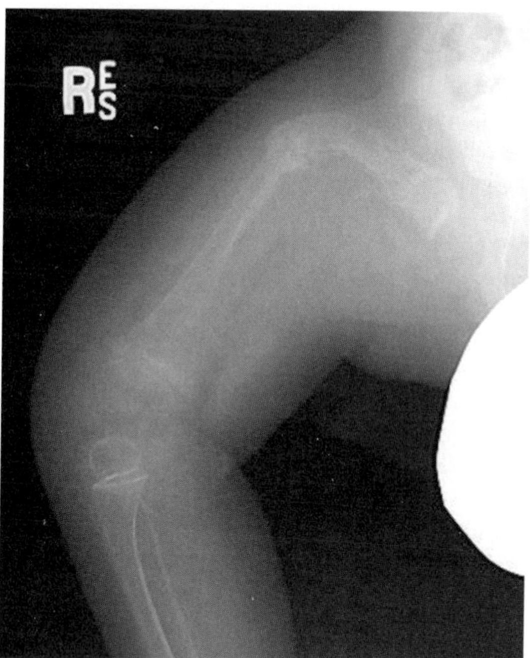

Figure 3-1 Pathologic femur fracture in a 4-year-old child with osteogenesis imperfecta.

PELVIC FRACTURES

Pelvic fractures in children encompass a wide spectrum of injuries, from sports-related avulsion fractures to life-threatening unstable pelvic ring fractures. The wide variety of pelvic fractures makes it difficult to apply a simple, comprehensive classification system in the analysis of children's pelvic fractures. A simple classification system formulated by Watts[3] describes three general types of pelvic fractures: avulsion fractures, pelvic ring fractures, and acetabular fractures (Box 3-2).

Avulsion Fractures

Avulsion fractures typically occur secondary to athletic injuries that involve running and jumping. The most common mechanism of injury is an eccentric contraction of a muscle, which causes a traction injury to a cartilaginous apophysis.[4] The location of muscle origins about the pelvis determines the sites of these injuries: The sartorius originates from the anterior superior iliac spine (ASIS), the direct head of the rectus femoris arises from the anterior inferior iliac spine, and the hamstring and adductor muscles originate from the ischial tuberosity.

Box 3-2 Watts Classification of Pelvic Fractures[42]

- Avulsion fractures
- Pelvic ring fractures
- Acetabular fractures

Violent contraction of the sartorius muscle, particularly when the muscle is elongated (such as when the hip is extended and the knee flexed) can lead to ASIS avulsion fractures. Eccentric hamstring contractions can lead to ischial avulsion fractures, whereas tension injuries of the rectus femoris muscle can lead to avulsion fractures of the ASIS.

Evaluation

Patients with avulsion fractures frequently describe a "pop" coupled with a sudden onset of pain and difficulty bearing weight. Physical examination reveals point tenderness over the affected region, and the diagnosis may be confirmed with radiographs or computed tomography (CT) (Fig. 3-2).

Management

For fractures with less than 2 cm of displacement, treatment is expectant, consisting of relief of weight-bearing and physical therapy. Fractures with more than 2 cm of displacement are best treated with open reduction and internal fixation.[4]

Pelvic Ring Fractures

Pelvic ring fractures in children account for between 2.4% and 7.5% of pediatric hospital admissions for blunt trauma. These are high-energy injuries, and 75% of children with pelvic ring fractures have significant associated injuries to intra-abdominal, genitourinary, or central nervous system structures.[5] The mortality rate from pediatric pelvic fractures is about 3.5%, with most fatalities occurring from injuries associated with the pelvic fracture (such as traumatic brain injury) rather than from the bleeding and hypovolemic shock seen in adult pelvic fractures.

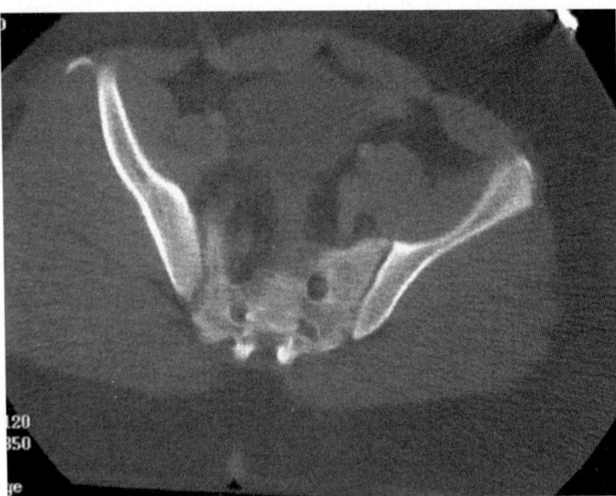

Figure 3-2 Computed tomography scan of an avulsion fracture of the anterior superior iliac spine.

There are several significant anatomic and mechanical differences accounting for this difference. A child's pelvis is more malleable than an adult's because the bones of the child's pelvis are less dense and more porous. A skeletally immature pelvis also contains more cartilage than a mature one, also making the skeletally immature pelvis relatively pliable and allowing for elastic deformation before failure. A thick, stout periosteum overlies the bones of children. This periosteum imparts fracture stability, limits fracture displacement, and helps contain bleeding after a fracture. Finally, ossification anomalies and synchondroses, particularly the synchondrosis between the inferior pubic ramus and the ischium, can have the radiographic appearance of a fracture, and their presence may be confused with a fracture (Fig. 3-3).

For these reasons, children with pelvic fractures are less likely than adults to have significant bleeding, and are more likely to have only a single break in the pelvic ring as well as a stable injury. These differences also help explain why long-term complications associated with pediatric pelvic fractures are usually secondary to either the associated injuries or a pelvic growth disturbance.

Fracture Pattern

Pelvic ring fractures in children occur in two general patterns, depending on the skeletal maturity of the individual.[6] The first pattern occurs in children who are skeletally immature—defined by the presence of an open triradiate cartilage. Fractures in skeletally immature patients are marked by failure of the bone before disruption of the ligament. Injuries in this pattern are

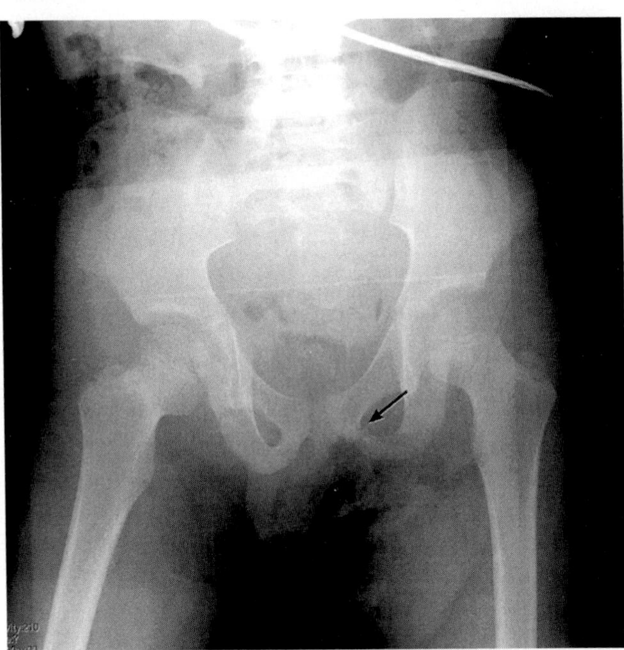

Figure 3-3 Anteroposterior radiograph of the pelvis of an 8-year-old boy. The *arrow* indicates the synchondrosis, which may be mistaken for a fracture.

frequently stable and can usually be treated by nonoperative means.

Skeletally mature patients—in whom the triradiate cartilage is closed—tend to have injuries similar to those seen in adults. They are more likely to have unstable injuries, including sacroiliac joint disruption, diastasis of the symphysis pubis, and associated acetabular fractures. For both skeletally mature and immature patients, the AO/ASIF system, a classification system based on mechanism of injury, can be used to categorize these injuries (Table 3-1). AO/ASIF type A fractures are stable injuries; they include isolated rami fractures and iliac wing fractures. Type B fractures are rotationally unstable but vertically stable; they include "open book" fractures that typically result from anterior compressive forces. Type C fractures are rotationally and vertically unstable (see Fig. 3-4A).

Management

Treatment of pelvic ring fractures initially requires a thorough and comprehensive assessment of the patient. Children with these fractures often have multiple injuries, such as concomitant neurologic, gastrointestinal, and genitourinary injuries. Appropriate imaging studies, including inlet and outlet radiographs of the pelvis, are needed. Judet views (oblique radiographs) of the pelvis may be useful to search for associated acetabular fractures. CT is sensitive in evaluating pelvic fractures and is the imaging modality of choice in the evaluation of complex injuries to the pelvis.

Stable pelvic (AO/ASIF type A) fracture or fractures involving a single break in the pelvic ring can be treated symptomatically with protected weight-bearing, followed by rehabilitation. Patients with diastasis of the pubic symphysis, or those with an "open book" fracture (type B), can be treated either nonoperatively or operatively with anterior fixation alone. Small amounts of diastasis (3 cm) can be treated nonoperatively with a pelvic sling or cast. The rare fracture with more than 3 cm of displacement should be considered for operative stabilization through use of either internal or external fixation. Unstable pelvic fractures with significant posterior disruption (unstable type B and type C fractures) can be treated with posterior stabilization.[5] This can be accomplished through percutaneous placement of screws across the sacroiliac joint or with sacral bars (see Fig. 3-4B). Posterior stabilization can be supplemented with anterior fixation of the pubic symphysis by internal or external fixation.

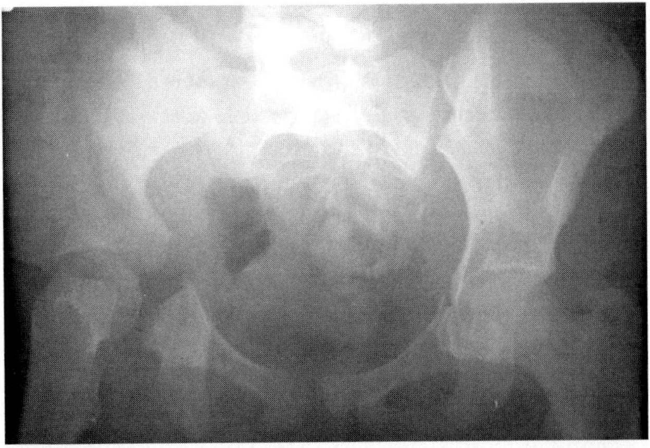

A

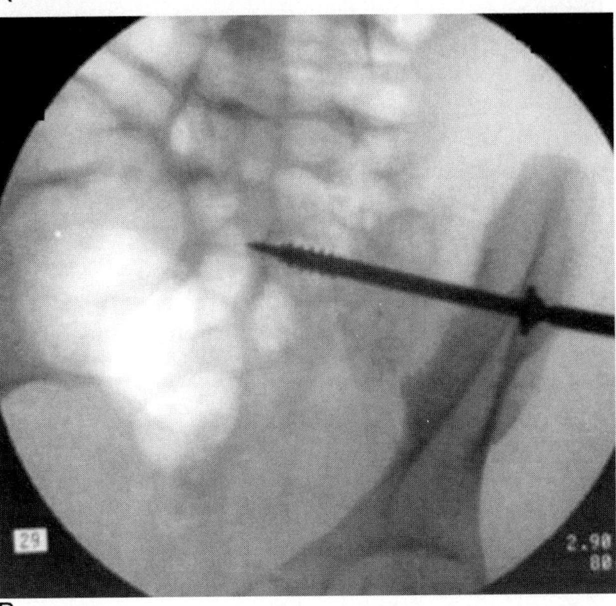

B

Figure 3-4 **A,** Anteroposterior radiograph of the pelvis showing a vertically unstable pelvic fracture. **B,** Percutaneous screw fixation of the sacroiliac joint was performed to provide posterior stabilization of the fracture.

Table 3-1 AO/ASIF Classification of Pelvic Ring Fractures

Type A	Stable
	Include:
	  Isolated rami fractures
	  Iliac wing fractures

Type B	Rotationally unstable Vertically stable Mechanism—anterior compressive forces Include open book fractures
Type C	Rotationally and vertically unstable

Complications

Although complications are common in pediatric pelvic fractures, the outcomes are better in children than in adults. Complications of pelvic fractures in children include heterotopic ossification, limb length discrepancy, and pelvic growth disturbance. Because of the last possibility, the pediatric patient with a pelvic fracture should be monitored for at least 1 year after injury.[3,5]

Acetabular Fractures

In younger children with an open triradiate cartilage, fractures of the acetabulum can be categorized according to the Salter-Harris classification (Fig. 3-5). Most fractures are Salter-Harris type I, II, or V injuries (Fig. 3-6). In older children and adolescents, in whom the triradiate cartilage is closed, the classification system devised by Letournel and Judet can be used (Fig. 3-7). Children with suspected acetabular fractures should be evaluated with plain radiographs (including Judet views) as well as CT.

Management

Stable fractures with less than 2 mm of intra-articular displacement can be treated nonoperatively with no weight-bearing until fracture healing. Fractures that involve more than 2 mm of displacement or are unstable should be treated with open or closed reduction and internal fixation. A central fracture-dislocation requires prompt reduction with skeletal traction, followed by open reduction and internal fixation.

Complications

Complications of acetabular fractures in younger children primarily occur from premature closure of the triradiate cartilage. This development produces a shallow, dysplastic acetabulum and may lead to hip subluxation. Post-traumatic arthrosis of the hip may develop in acetabular fractures that heal with an articular incongruity, whereas avascular necrosis (AVN) of the femoral head may occur after fracture of the hip accompanied by hip dislocation.

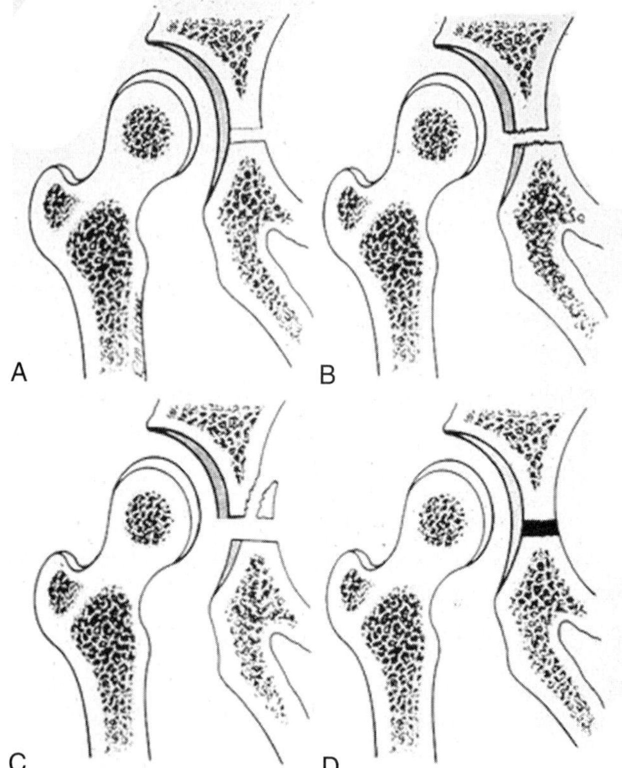

Figure 3-5 Salter-Harris classification of acetabular fractures. A, Normal configuration of the triradiate cartilage; **B,** Salter-Harris type I fracture; **C,** Salter-Harris type II fracture; **D,** Salter-Harris type V injury to the triradiate cartilage.

HIP DISLOCATIONS

Hip dislocation may also occur in children without an associated acetabular or femoral fracture. The majority of dislocations are posterior, and in 75% of cases, hip dislocations occur secondary to high-energy injuries (Fig. 3-8A).[7] In children younger than 10 years, however, ligamentous laxity often leads to hip dislocations from low-energy trauma.

Management

Reduction of a hip dislocation within 6 hours of injury is recommended to minimize AVN of the femoral head. Adequate relaxation is required in reduction of a dislocated hip to prevent physeal damage and fracture during reduction. Hip dislocations in younger children can generally be reduced in the emergency department with the use of conscious sedation, whereas reductions in older children should be performed with the use of general anesthesia. After reduction, plain radiographs or a CT scan should be carefully evaluated for any hip joint incongruity (see Fig. 3-8B), which may indicate incarceration of soft tissue within the hip joint. After a satisfactory closed reduction, a period of spica casting, use of hip abduction pillow, or no weight-bearing should be instituted to allow for soft tissue healing. Open reduction should be performed for a dislocation that is irreducible by closed methods, a late-presenting dislocation, and interposition soft tissue in the hip joint preventing a congruous reduction.

Complications

Complications of hip dislocations in children include AVN (8%), myositis ossificans, redislocation, neurovascular injury, and post-traumatic arthrosis of the hip.[7]

HIP FRACTURES

Hip fractures in children account for less than 1% of all children's fractures.[8,9] These injuries result from high-energy trauma and are frequently associated with injury to the chest, head, or abdomen. Treatment of hip fractures in children is associated with a complication rate of up to 60%, with an overall AVN rate of 50%, and a malunion rate of up to 30%.[8] The unique blood supply to the

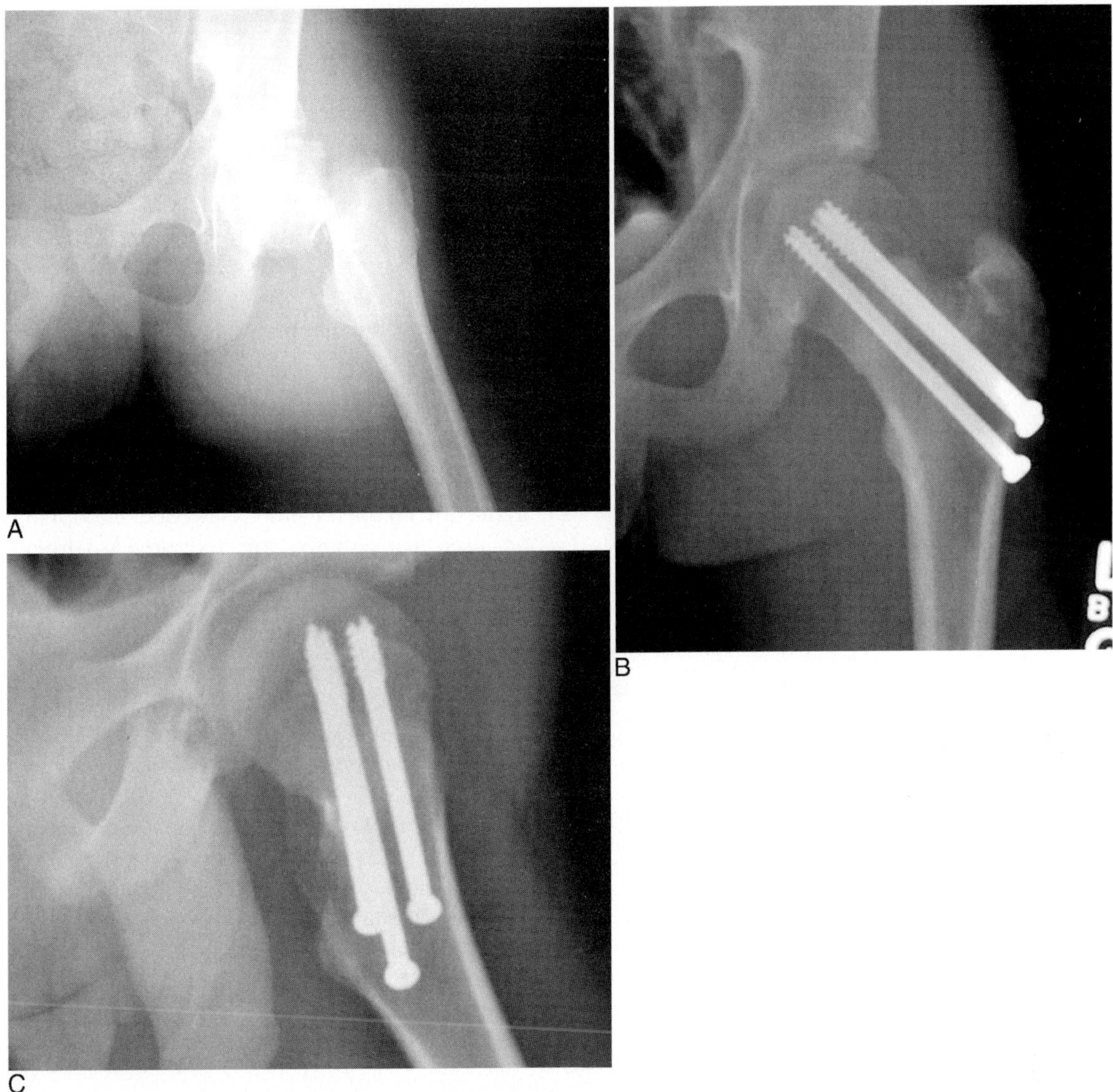

Figure 3-6 **A,** Type II femoral neck fracture in a 12-year-old boy. **B** and **C,** Fracture after open reduction and internal fixation with three cannulated screws.

femoral head accounts for the high rate of AVN seen with this injury. In infancy, the femoral head derives blood supply from metaphyseal vessels originating from the medial and lateral femoral circumflex arteries. These vessels transverse the proximal femoral physis and vascularize the proximal femoral epiphysis.[10] By 2 years of age, however, with normal growth and development of the proximal femoral physis, these vessels involute, and the cartilaginous physis of the proximal femur becomes a barrier to blood flow to the femoral head. At this point, the blood supply to the proximal femoral epiphysis derives from the lateral epiphyseal vessels, which are the terminal vessels arising from the medial femoral circumflex artery. These posterosuperior and posteroinferior retinacular vessels lie on the femoral neck and are vulnerable to injury during fracture of the hip.[10] It is believed that damage to these vessels at the time of injury leads to AVN of the femoral head. This belief is underscored by the finding that the rate of AVN in pediatric hip fractures is generally related to the extent of fracture displacement present as well as to fracture location.

Classification

Pediatric hip fractures are classified according to the system of Delbet.[11] This system classifies hip fractures into four types according to their location. Type I fractures are transphyseal separations; type II fractures occur in the femoral neck and are also known as transcervical fractures; type III fractures are cervicotrochanteric (which are similar to adult basocervical fractures); and type IV fractures are intertrochanteric.

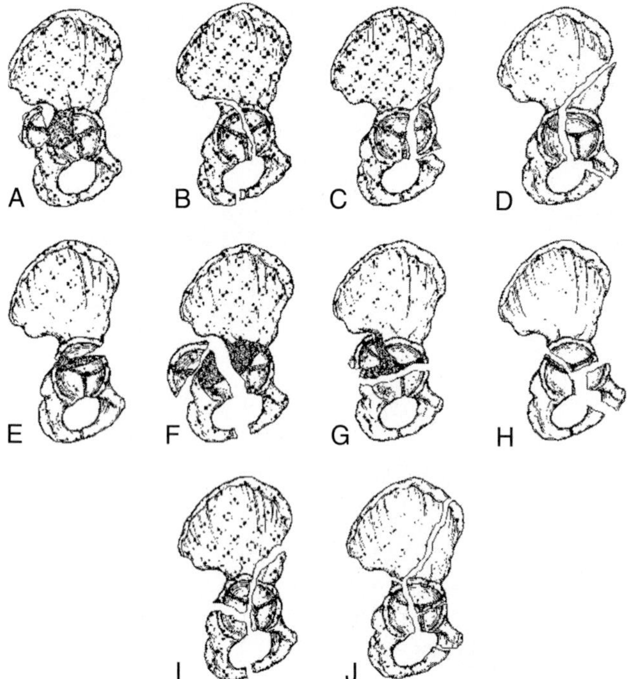

Figure 3-7 Letournel and Judet classification of acetabular fracture. **A,** Posterior wall fracture, often associated with impaction on the intact side of the fracture margin. **B,** Posterior column fracture. **C,** Anterior wall fracture. **D,** Anterior column fracture. **E,** Transverse fracture pattern. **F,** Associated posterior column and posterior wall fractures. **G,** Associated transverse and posterior wall fractures. **H,** T-shaped fracture. **I,** Associated anterior column and posterior hemitransverse fractures. **J,** Both-column fracture. (From Swiontkowski MF: Fractures and dislocations about the hips and pelvis. In Green NE, Swiontkowski MF [eds]: Skeletal Trauma in Children, vol 3, 3rd ed. Philadelphia, WB Saunders, 2003, p 376.)

Management

In general, treatment principles for pediatric hip fractures consist of urgent treatment, achievement of an anatomic reduction (either open or closed), stable internal fixation (avoiding the physis if possible), and spica casting.[9] A capsulotomy to decompress the hip joint is also recommended to minimize tamponade of the retinacular blood vessels by the fracture hematoma. Type I fractures are uncommon, representing only about 8% of hip fractures. They usually occur in infants and young children; type I fractures in infants can be secondary to birth trauma. In about 50% of type I fractures, there is an associated dislocation of the proximal femoral epiphysis.[11] Type I fractures require urgent reduction and, frequently, an open method is needed. Smooth pins should be used to stabilize the fracture, as threaded pins should not be used across a physis, and the pin fixation should be supplemented with a spica cast. Type I fractures in children older than 2 years have an 80% rate of AVN. In younger children, particularly those with fractures secondary to birth trauma, the AVN rate is lower, most likely because these are low-energy injuries.

Type II fractures are the most common hip fracture in children, accounting for many of the complications.[9,11] They should be treated with anatomic reduction (open if necessary) followed by screw or pin fixation. Screw threads should avoid the physis if possible, so smooth transphyseal pins may have to be used for fixation in younger children. The AVN rate for type II fractures is 50%.

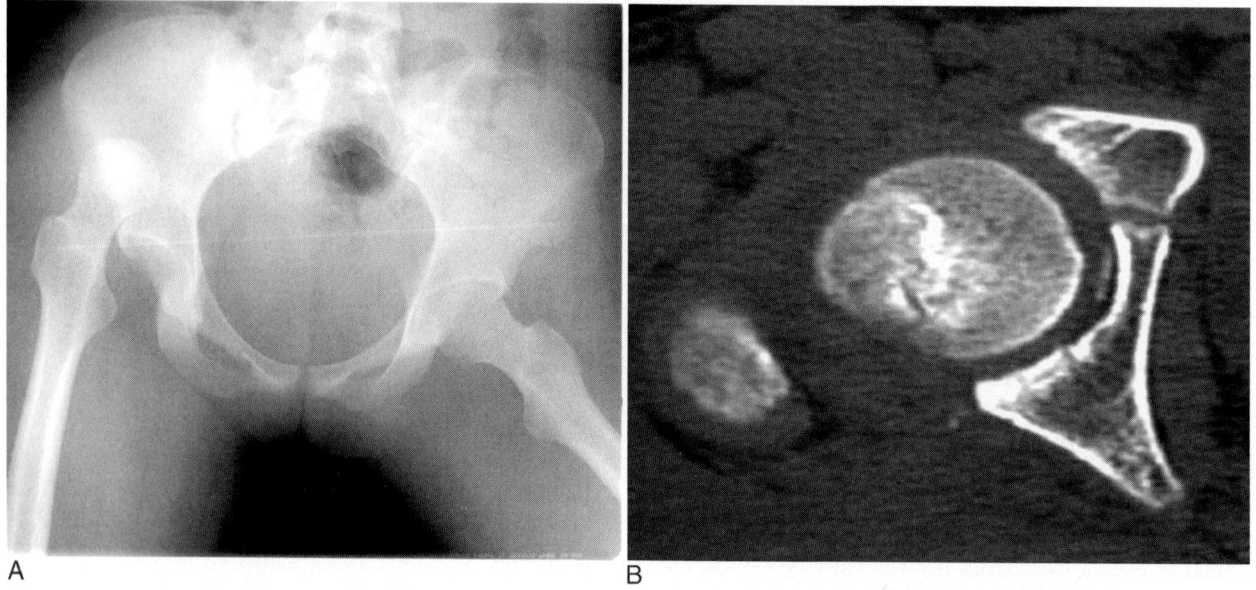

Figure 3-8 **A,** Traumatic hip dislocation in an 11-year-old girl who was struck by a car. **B,** Postreduction computed tomography scan showing a bony fragment trapped in the hip joint, which required an arthrotomy for treatment.

Type III fractures, or cervicotrochanteric fractures, occur at the base of the femoral neck. They are the second most common type of hip fracture in children and are analogous to adult basocervical hip fractures. Like Type II fractures, cervicotrochanteric hip fractures should be treated with urgent, anatomic reduction, stable internal fixation using smooth pins or screws (crossing the physis if necessary), and a spica cast (see Fig. 3-6A, B and C). For type III hip fractures that are displaced, the AVN rate is 25%.[11] Type IV, or intertrochanteric, hip fractures have the best prognosis. These are commonly stable, and in children 8 years or older, type IV fractures can be treated with a hip spica cast alone. Displaced fractures in children older than 8 years are best treated with open reduction and internal fixation. Type IV fractures have an AVN rate of less than 10%.[11]

Complications

Complications of hip fractures in children include malunion, non-union, and AVN. Studies have suggested that these complications can be minimized with early anatomic reduction, internal fixation, and spica cast immobilization.[9] Malunion usually results in a coxa vara and is secondary to a poor quality reduction; open reduction should be performed if an adequate closed reduction cannot be obtained. Small degrees of coxa vara will remodel, but correction of larger malunions may require femoral osteotomy. Non-unions typically result from a combination of a malreduction and inadequate fracture stabilization. Varus malunion results in shear forces across the fracture site, contributing to the nonunion. Treatment should consist of a valgus femoral subtrochanteric osteotomy (to convert the shear forces across the fracture site to compression), bone grafting, internal fixation, and spica casting.

The rates of non-union and malunion seem to be decreasing with the use of anatomic reduction and internal fixation of these injuries. AVN is related to both fracture location and displacement. There is no simple, reliable treatment for postfracture AVN of the femoral head. Children younger than 8 to 10 years can be treated with abduction bracing (similar to treatment for Legg-Calvé-Perthes disease), whereas early vascularized fibula strut grafting may be of value in older children to promote healing of the avascular bone and to prevent femoral head collapse.

FEMUR FRACTURES

Fractures of the femur in children occur commonly. All age groups, from early childhood to adolescence, can be affected. The mechanisms of injury vary from low-energy twisting-type injuries (seen in falls from playground equipment) to high-velocity injuries (seen in motor vehicle accidents in which the femur fracture is one of several injuries) (Table 3-2).[12] Additional trauma includes life-threatening head, chest, and abdominal injuries that often take priority over the management of the femur fracture.

As shown in Table 3-2 fracture patterns and epidemiology in femur fractures can be categorized according to age group. For each age group, a particular subset of issues must be addressed as management and treatment plans are formulated. Treatment algorithms based on age, fracture pattern, associated injuries, socio-economic factors, and family dynamics are the guiding principles by which fractures are managed today, and they continue to evolve with new technology.

Mechanism of Injury

The vast majority of femur fractures occurs as a result of low-energy events, such as falls from playground equipment, mishaps on roller blades or skateboards, and in contact sports such as football. These low-energy injuries occur primarily in children 5 to 10 years old (see Table 3-2).

Femur fractures in children younger than 2 years raise the concern for child abuse. In the absence of an underlying metabolic or neurologic disease process such as myelomeningocele (MM), muscular dystrophy (MD), osteogenesis imperfecta (OI), or cerebral palsy (CP), child abuse or endangerment should be considered. Additional "red flags" for possible child abuse include a delay in seeking prompt medical attention and a history that is not compatible with the injury (Box 3-3). In a study by Thomas and colleagues,[13] 22% of children younger than 5 years and 39% of children younger than 1 year at the time of fracture had been victims of child abuse. Injury patterns are not specific. Fractures can vary in location from proximal to midshaft or distal with or without metaphyseal corner involvement, and can be transverse from a direct blow or spiral or oblique from a twisting mechanism (Fig. 3-9). By obtaining a thorough history, conducting a complete physical examination and

Table 3-2 Injury Mechanism and Fracture Pattern in Femur Fractures

Injury Mechanism	Fracture Pattern
Torsion	Spiral pattern
Direct blow	Transverse
High energy	Comminuted/compound/open

From Staheli LT: Fractures of the shaft of the femur. In Rockwood C, Wilkins K, King R (eds): Fractures in Children. Philadelphia, JB Lippincott, 1984.

Box 3-3 "Red Flag" Findings in Possible Child Abuse

- Femur fracture in a child younger than walking age
- Delay in seeking prompt medical attention
- Metaphyseal corner fractures
- Rib fractures and/or multiple injuries in different stages of healing

Data from Scherl SA, Miller L, Lively N, et al: Accidental and nonaccidental femur fractures in children. Clin Orthop 376:96-105, 2000; and Thomas SA, Rosenfield NS, Leventhal JM, et al: Long-bone fractures in young children: Distinguishing accidental injuries from child abuse. Pediatrics 88:471-476, 1991.

skeletal survey, and obtaining a social services evaluation, one can recognize the pattern of abuse and minimize the risk of repeat events that can often result in fatalities.

Playground or sports-related fractures are usually isolated injuries with a specific history and timely recruitment of medical attention. Mechanism of injury can be varied, but it is usually consistent with a fall during sports. Although underlying primary bone disease (MM, MD, OI, CP), weakened bones due to osteopenia (Fig. 3-10), or pathologic fracture (Fig. 3-11) secondary to tumor should be ruled out, the usual scenario is that the bone quality is normal.

High-energy fracture usually occurs as a result of a motor vehicle accident, in which the patient was either an occupant of the vehicle or a pedestrian struck by a motor vehicle. For example, the Waddell triad describes (Fig. 3-12) a femur fracture resulting from a car bumper striking the thigh, a chest or thoracic injury from impact of the hood, and a head injury as a result of being thrown by the initial impact. All-terrain vehicles and motorcycle injuries also contribute to high-energy trauma, particularly in adolescents.

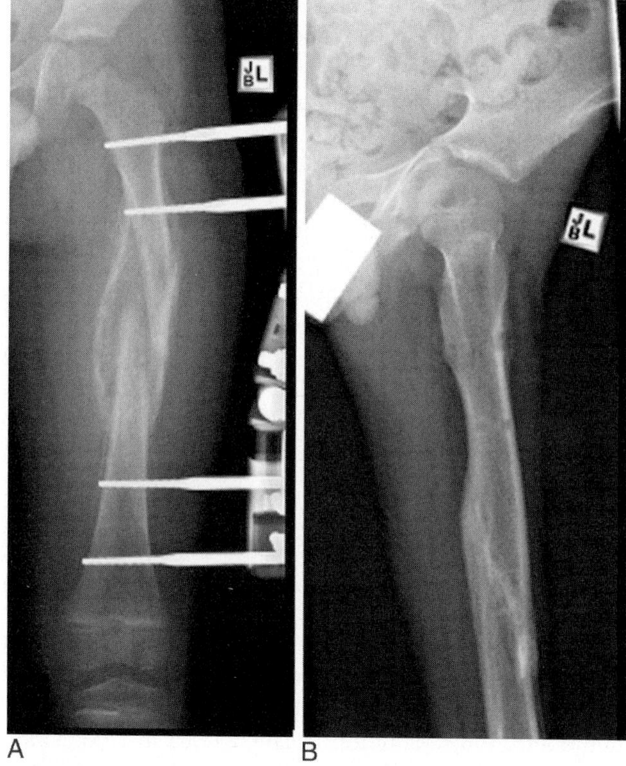

Figure 3-9 Spiral oblique femur fracture, interval healing **(A)** and healed **(B)**.

Fractures can vary by location—subtrochanteric, diaphyseal, or supracondylar (Fig. 3-13)—or may involve the growth plate. The mechanism of injury (i.e., direct blow or twisting) can be inferred from the fracture pattern (Tables 3-2 and 3-3). Special consideration must be given

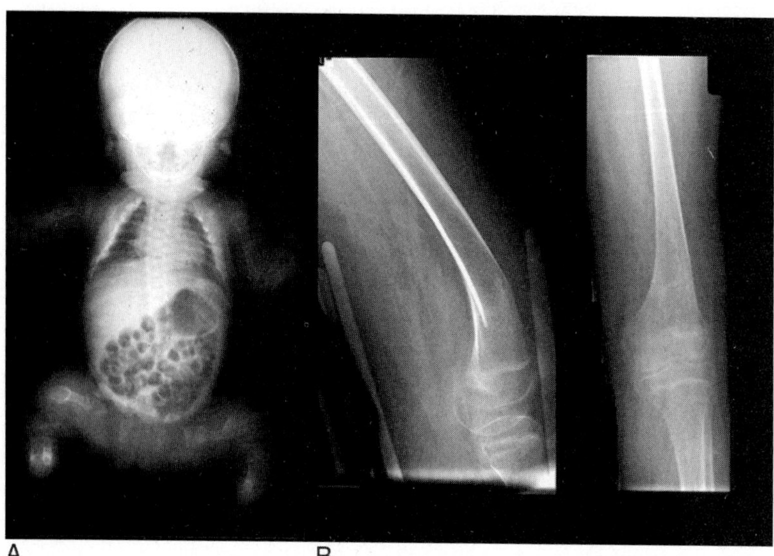

Figure 3-10 Distal femur fractures due to osteogenesis imperfecta **(A)** and muscular dystrophy **(B)**.

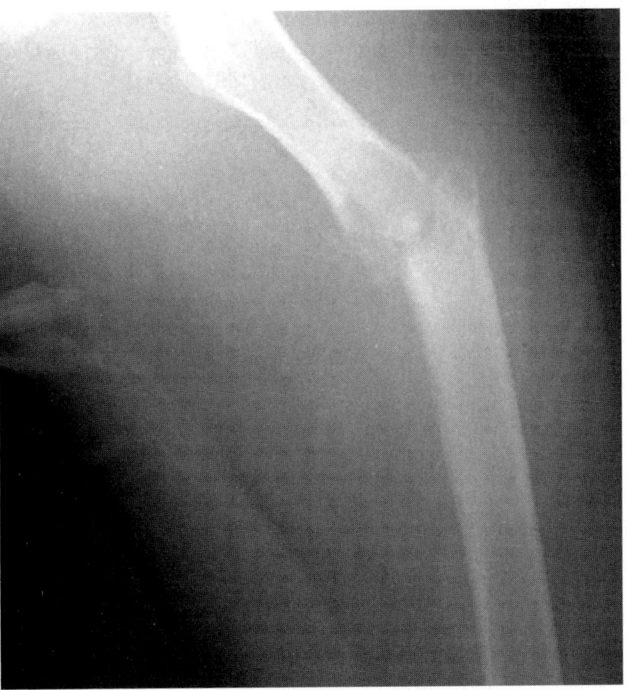

Figure 3-11 Cystic lesion leading to pathologic femur fracture.

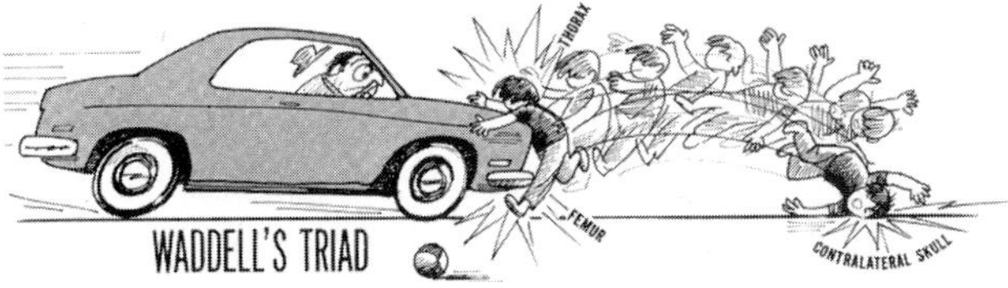

Figure 3-12 Waddell's triad of femur, chest, and head injuries. (From Rang M [ed]: Children's Fractures, 2nd ed. Philadelphia, Lippincott Williams & Wilkins, 1983, p 63.)

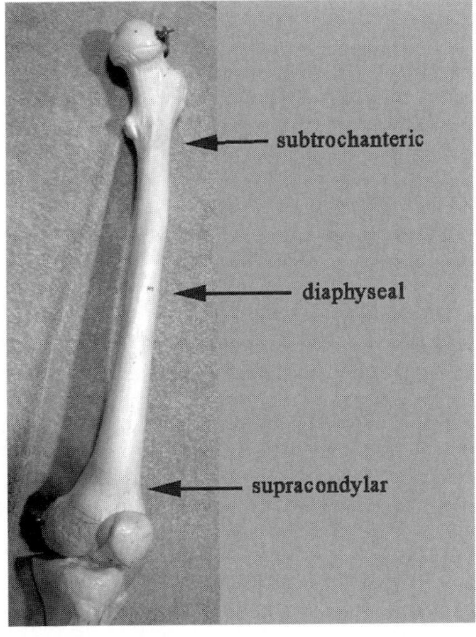

Figure 3-13 Anatomy of the femur.

Table 3-3 Common Locations of Injury in Femur Fractures

Location	Prevalence (%)
Middle third	66
Proximal third	17
Distal third	12
Subtrochanteric region	5

From Tachdjian MO: Fractures and dislocations. In Pediatric Orthopaedics, 2nd ed. Philadelphia, WB Saunders, 1990.

to injuries that involve the growth plate. Depending on the severity of injury, the long-term outcome can be affected by partial or complete growth arrest and subsequent angular deformity or limb length discrepancy in up to 30% of patients.

Fracture Pattern

Growth Plate Fractures

Sixty-six percent of the longitudinal growth of the leg occurs from the contribution of growth plates about the knee, that is, the distal femoral and proximal tibial growth plates (Table 3-4).

Although a variety of classification schemes has been developed for growth plate fractures, the system most commonly used is the Salter-Harris classification (Fig. 3-14). It describes various injury patterns to the physis and can identify the injuries at greatest risk for long-term growth disturbance. The Salter-Harris type II fracture is the most common pattern seen.

Principles of treatment are achievement of an "anatomic" reduction (Fig. 3-15A) and stabilization until healing has occurred. Anatomic reduction often requires operative treatment to maintain a perfect reduction (see Fig. 3-15B).

Table 3-4 Relative Contributions of Lower Limb Physes to Longitudinal Growth

Location of Physis	Contribution (%)
Proximal femur	18
Distal femur	39
Proximal tibia	27
Distal tibia	16

From Tachdjian MO: Limb length discrepancy. In Pediatric Orthopaedics, 2nd ed. Philadelphia, WB Saunders, 1990.

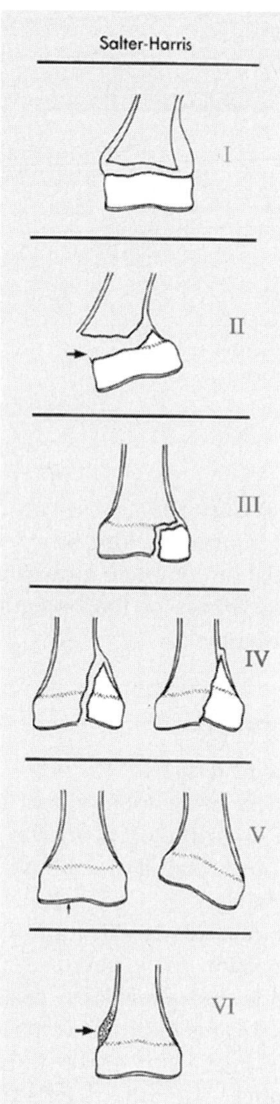

Figure 3-14 Salter-Harris classification of growth plate fractures. (From Crenshaw AH [ed]: Campbell's Operative Orthopaedics, 7th ed. St. Louis, CV Mosby, 1987, p 1057.)

Pathologic Fractures

Pathologic fractures are rare but are signs of inherent bone weakness secondary to an underlying disease process. Benign or malignant tumors and metabolic or neurologic diseases, such as OI and MM, can result in a femur fracture with minimal force.

Stress or Fatigue Fractures

Stress or fatigue fractures are a result of repetitive cyclical loading that causes microfracture without allowing enough time for healing to occur before further stress is incurred (Fig. 3-16A). These injuries often go undiagnosed and are dismissed as a muscle pull or strain. Although the proximal femur is commonly involved, diaphyseal stress injuries also occur. A high index of suspicion, prompted by a history of repetitive loading, such as running, jumping sports, or involvement in multiple sports (Box 3-4), combined with imaging studies—technetium Tc^{99m} bone scanning, radiography, MRI, or CT—can make the diagnosis (see Fig. 3-16B).

Evaluation

The evaluation begins with documentation of the history of the events leading up to the accident or injury. These details can be helpful in identifying a high-versus low-energy mechanism and may prompt the search for additional injuries. The physical examination starts with making note of the patient's general appearance followed by checking the ABCs (airway, breathing, and circulation). A complete musculoskeletal examination from head-to-toe should follow, with emphasis on the neck, spine, and pelvis, before the injured limb is examined. Once it has been established that there are no other injuries, the examiner should check for obvious deformity, swelling, tenderness, open wounds, and neurologic dysfunction. Vital sign checks and serial hematocrit evaluations should be obtained. Signs of hemodynamic instability should prompt one to look for other sources of bleeding, because it is rare for an isolated or even bilateral femur fracture to result in blood loss sufficient to cause hypotension.[14]

Management

As with any fracture, the initial management consists of splinting the limb in the field. A variety of splinting materials is commercially available; in the absence of such materials, rolled-up newspaper, cardboard, or even pieces of wood can serve as temporary support. Bandaging both lower limbs together also can be an effective temporary splint. The purposes of splinting are first to minimize pain and second to prevent potential neurovascular injury from unstable fracture ends.

Historically, definitive management of femur fractures has included a period of hospitalization for skin or skeletal traction to allow early fracture callus formation, followed by application of a spica body cast (Fig. 3-17). The cast covers the lower torso, pelvis, the entire involved leg, and the uninjured leg down to the knee. Although this treatment plan is well tolerated in the patient younger than 5 years with an isolated injury, it becomes less ideal in patients with multiple traumas involving the head, chest, and abdomen. Furthermore, spica casting is not well tolerated by older patients or for patients with preexisting bone demineralization (OI, MM, MD, CP). The treatment team for a child with multiple injuries often requires access to the chest and torso for frequent examinations, which can be limited by the cast. Moreover, subsequent radiographic studies such as CT and MRI can be suboptimal because of the inability to position the patient in a scanner. In older or larger

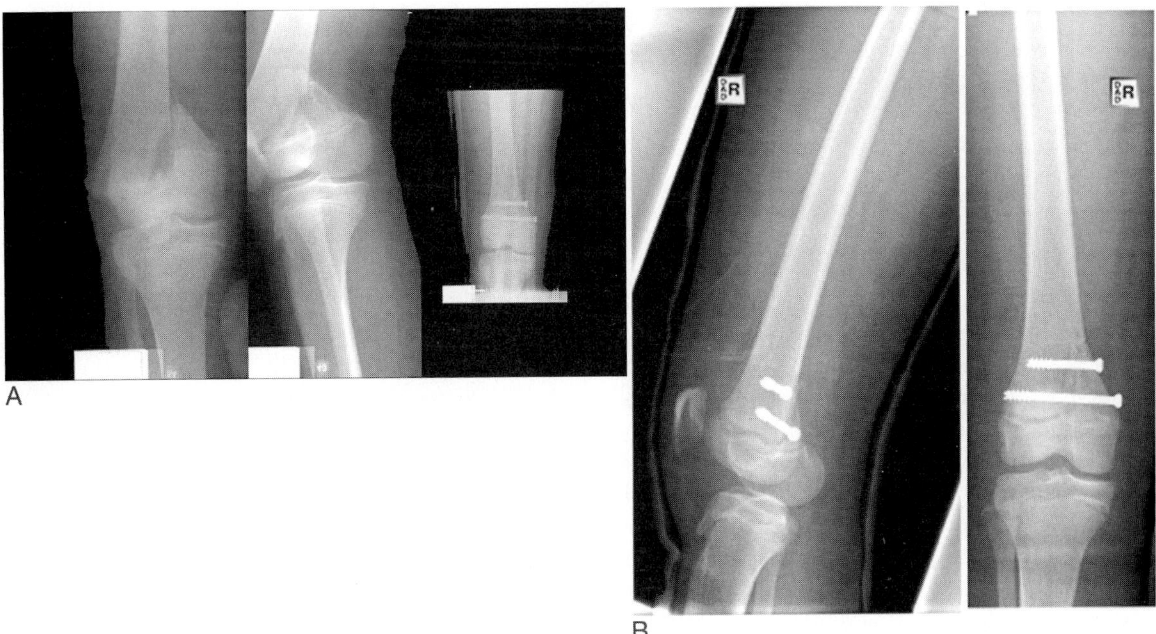

Figure 3-15 **A,** Displaced Salter-Harris type II distal femur fracture. **B,** Salter-Harris type II distal femur fracture after operative fixation.

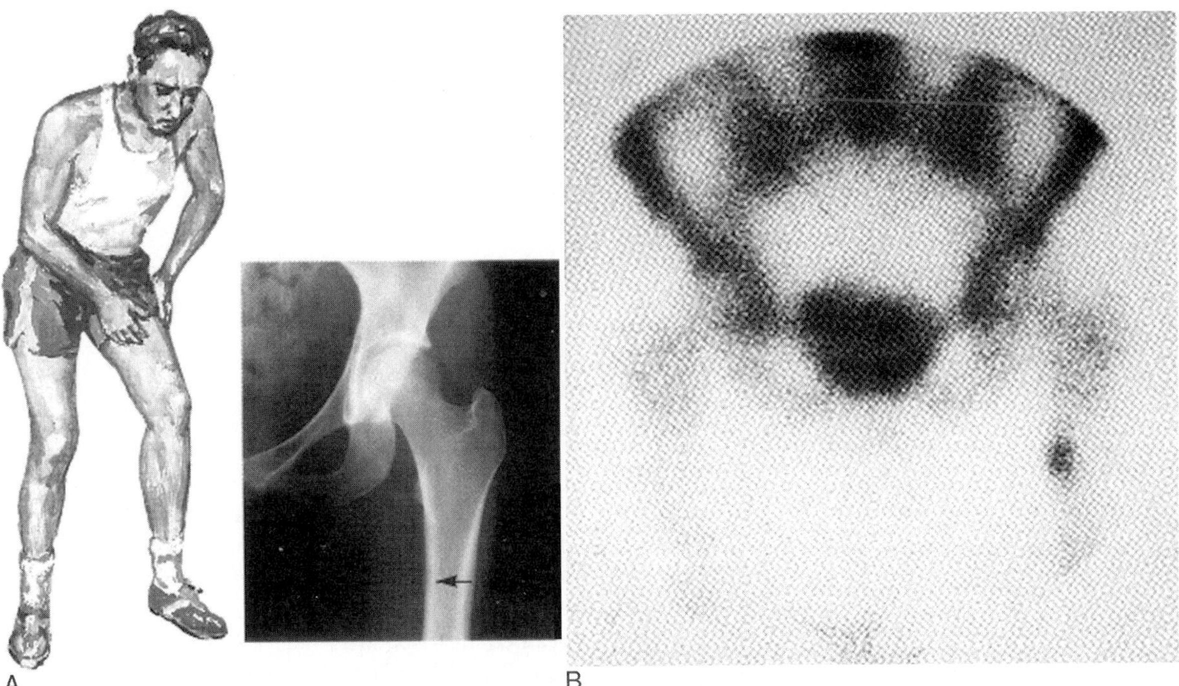

Figure 3-16 **A,** Stress fracture due to repetitive cyclical bone loading. **B,** Increased radioisotope uptake in femur consistent with stress fracture. (From Netter FH: Netter Collection of Medical Illustrations, Vol 8. Oppenheimer E (ed). ICON Learning Systems, 1997, p 139.)

Box 3-4 Historical Indicators of High Risk for Stress Fracture

- Running/jumping sports
- Participation in multiple sports year round
- Intense training after a long hiatus
- Amenorrhea in an adolescent girl
- Low-fat, high-protein diet

patients, cast immobilization presents challenges to the caretaker, such as difficulties in ambulation and transporting the child. The parent and child are typically homebound for 8 to 10 weeks (after a 2- to 3-week hospitalization, interfering with school and employment obligations. In the child with preexisting neurologic or metabolic disease, the antigravity effect of the cast contributes to further disuse osteopenia and additional weakening of the bone.

Treatment

Children Younger than 5 Years with Isolated Injury

The hospital stay for children younger than 5 years with isolated femur fractures who undergo early spica casting averages 11 days and ranges from 5 to 29 days.[15] The stay includes cast application as well as planning of home care and transportation. Most such children have uneventful healing, and the cast is removed within 6 to 8 weeks. Outcomes are excellent with low rates of leg length discrepancy and of rotatory or angular malunion.[16]

Children 5 to 10 Years Old

Treatment of femur fracture in a child 5 to 10 years old includes hospitalization with traction for 2 to 3 weeks (Fig. 3-18), followed by casting. This method poses low risk to the patient and promotes good healing potential. However there are many disadvantages to this treatment modality, not the least of which are psychosocial or body image issues related to the cast. The child will miss several weeks of school; arrangements will have to be made with the school for a home tutor, lesson plans, and so forth. Also, the child will need a caretaker in the hospital (nursing staff and parents) and at home (parents or extended family, hired help). Sometimes, a family member may have to invoke his or her rights under the federal family leave act to care for the child; the caretaker will have time off with the job preserved, but no pay. Outcomes of this treatment are good, but for some patients, healing is long and involves many psychological and social issues.

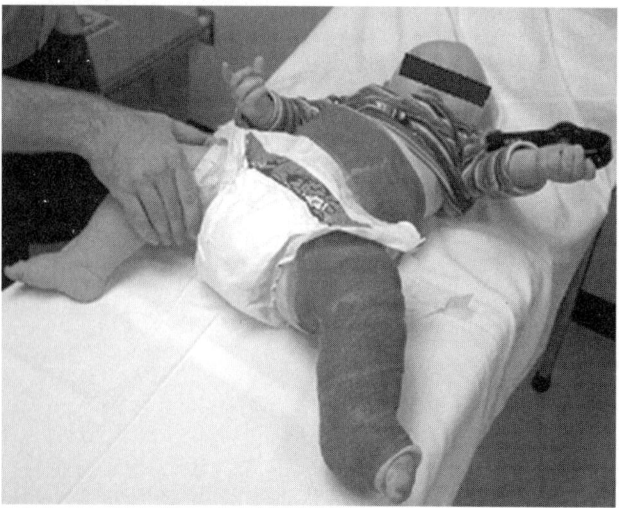

Figure 3-17 Spica cast.

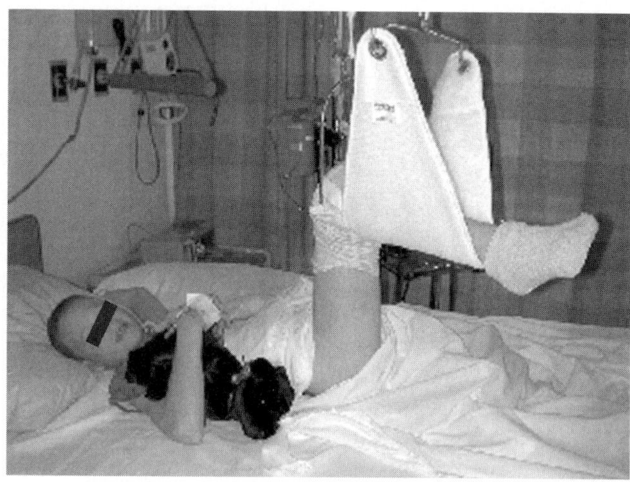

Figure 3-18 90-90 skeletal traction.

Many options exist for operative management. All facilitate earlier fracture stabilization without the need for callus formation. In the 5 to 10 year age group, treatment options include: (1) elastic intramedullary nails (Fig. 3-19A), (2) plates and screws, and (3) external fixators (see Fig. 3-19B). All of these devices facilitate early mobilization and ambulation with crutches and wheelchairs without the need for specialized vehicle transportation home and around the community. Most patients are able to return to school with limited assistance as well.

Children Older than 11 Years

Surgical options are the mainstay of treatment for femur fractures in children older than 11 years and are believed to have better long-term results than traditional traction and casting methods. In the older adolescent, traditional reamed intramedullary nails are favored for their rigid fixation. The immediate stability allows for early weight-bearing and return to function. One generally can expect fracture healing to occur within 8 to 12 weeks and the patient to return to full activity within 6 to 12 months.

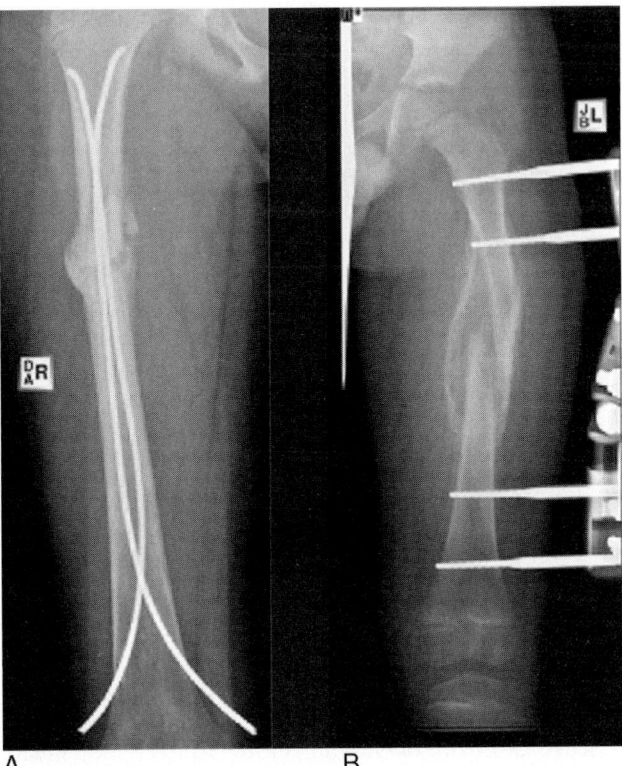

Figure 3-19 Operative management options for femur fracture in a child 5 to 10 years old include elastic intramedullary nails **(A)** and external fixators **(B).**

Special Treatment Circumstances

Child Abuse

In infants 6 months of age or younger, a Pavlik harness (Fig. 3-20) has been reported to adequately stabilize isolated femur fractures.[17] Femur fractures heal within 4 to 6 weeks and have tremendous remodeling potential. Angular deformities are better tolerated by such young patients with greater remodeling potential. In children older than 6 months, a spica cast is ideal.

Multiple Trauma

Surgical treatment of the femur fracture is favored in any child with multiple injuries. Often, uncontrolled spasms and emerging spasticity secondary to head injury in such a child worsens fracture alignment. Inadvertent manipulation of the unstable fracture causes pain, undesirably increasing intracranial pressure. The goal of operative treatment is to stabilize the fracture and counteract the deforming muscle forces. Although there are many options for treatment, such as the use of elastic intramedullary nails, percutaneous plating, and external fixation, the last is favored, for several reasons. External fixation is minimally invasive and can be quickly applied with little blood loss or operative time. Furthermore, approximately 85% of head-injured children recover functional capabilities that allow for ambulation; therefore, achieving an acceptable fracture alignment is necessary to minimize long-term functional deficit from a misaligned or foreshortened fracture.

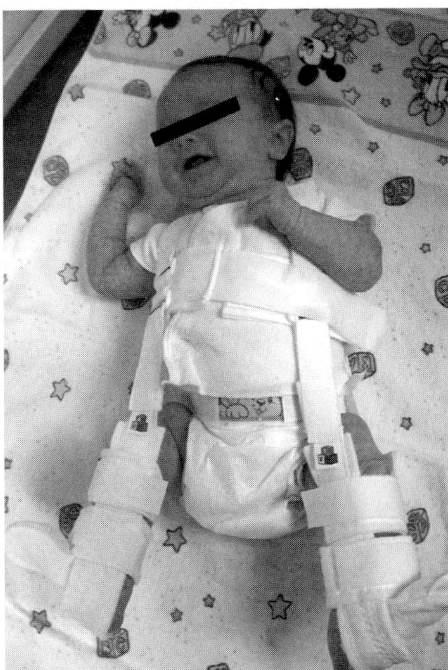

Figure 3-20 Pavlik harness.

Open Fractures

All open or compound injuries require that the bone and wound be cleansed to minimize infection and osteomyelitis. Operative stabilization is usually achieved with an external fixator that allows access to the wound for frequent examination and dressing change. Fracture stability also enhances healing of both bone and soft tissue wounds.

Floating Knee

Ipsilateral fractures of the femur and tibia are defined as a "floating knee" (Fig. 3-21). These are high-energy injuries. Operative stabilization of the femur, or often of both bones, yields the best results. Length of hospitalization, time to unsupported weight-bearing, and rates of complications (excessive limb shortening and rotatory malunion) are lower with rigid internal fixation of both bones.[18]

Complications

Leg Length Discrepancy and Angular Deformity

Limb length discrepancy is due to either overgrowth or excessive shortening of the injured leg. Two centimeters of discrepancy are well tolerated at skeletal maturity. Greater limb discrepancies can be equalized with shortening or lengthening procedures in the injured or the uninvolved limb.

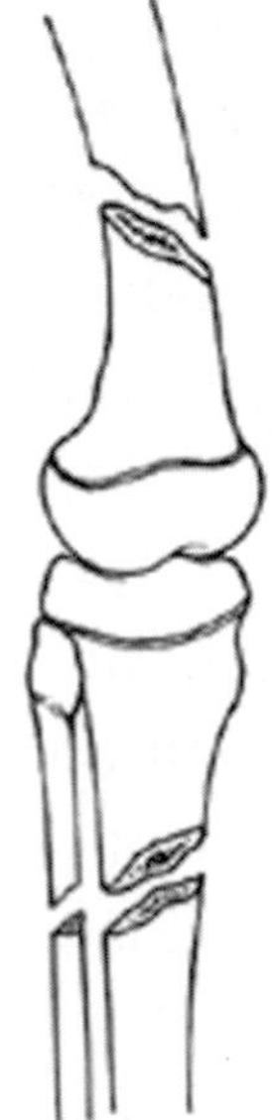

Figure 3-21 "Floating knee" fracture of the femur and ipsilateral tibia. (From Crenshaw AH [ed]: Campbell's Operative Orthopaedics, 7th ed. St. Louis, CV Mosby, 1987, p 1196.)

Avascular Necrosis

AVN of the femoral head is a serious complication resulting from damage to the blood supply of the proximal femur. It is generally an iatrogenic event secondary to antegrade insertion of intramedullary nails (Fig. 3-22) with additional injury to the peritrochanteric blood vessels in the piriform fossa. This complication can be avoided through the use of alternative techniques, such as placement of nails through the greater trochanter, retrograde nailing, plating, and external fixator application.

Growth Plate Injuries

Salter-Harris type III and type IV fractures, which are intra-articular injuries, are the most prone to growth disturbance. They require anatomic reduction and operative stabilization.[19] In addition to restoration of a congruous joint surface to minimize the development of post-traumatic arthritis, the growth plate in such fractures must be perfectly aligned to prevent future growth disturbance (Fig. 3-23). However, despite the best surgical repair effort, these injuries still can result in complete or partial growth disturbance. The amount and degree of deformity, limb shortening, or angulation can be predicted from the amount of remaining growth in the individual child. Generally, one can expect 1 cm of shortening per year of growth remaining.

Knee Stiffness

Knee stiffness occurs in about 16% of individuals with femur fractures and is especially prone to occur in patients with external fixators. The stiffness is usually transitory but may require physical therapy and may take several months to resolve after the external fixator is removed.

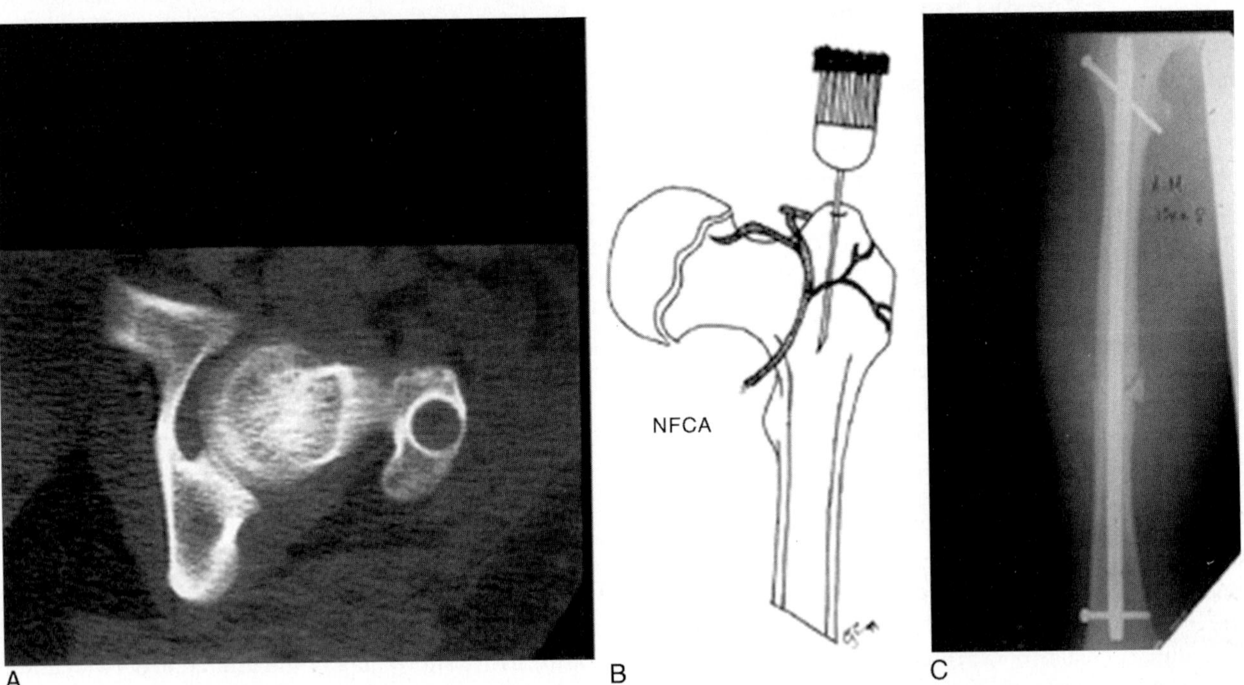

Figure 3-22 **A,** Trochanteric femoral entry point for intramedullary femoral rodding. **B,** Guidewire placement to avoid iatrogenic avascular necrosis secondary to arterial injury in femoral rodding procedures. **C,** Intramedullary rod. (**A** and **B,** From Townsend DR, Hoffinger S: Intramedullary nailing of femoral shaft fractures in children via the trochanter tip. Clin Orthop 376:113-118, 2000.)

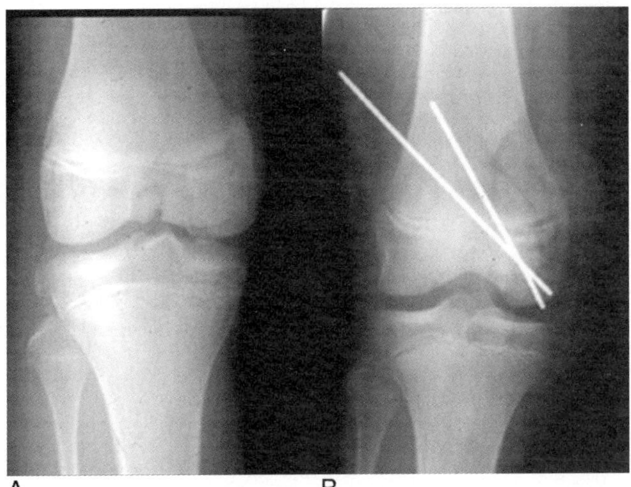

Figure 3-23 **A,** Displaced Salter-Harris type III fracture. **B,** Salter-Harris type III fracture after operative repair.

Refracture

Unfortunately, the femur can refracture after healing has occurred. With removal of load-bearing devices such as plates and external fixators, the empty screw holes can serve as stress risers (points of inherent bone weakness and stress concentration) (Fig. 3-24). It is recommended that after these devices are removed, a gradually progressive, protected weight-bearing program is implemented until the screw hole sites mature. This process generally takes another 6 to 8 weeks, during which patients are instructed to avoid vigorous high-impact sports and other activities.

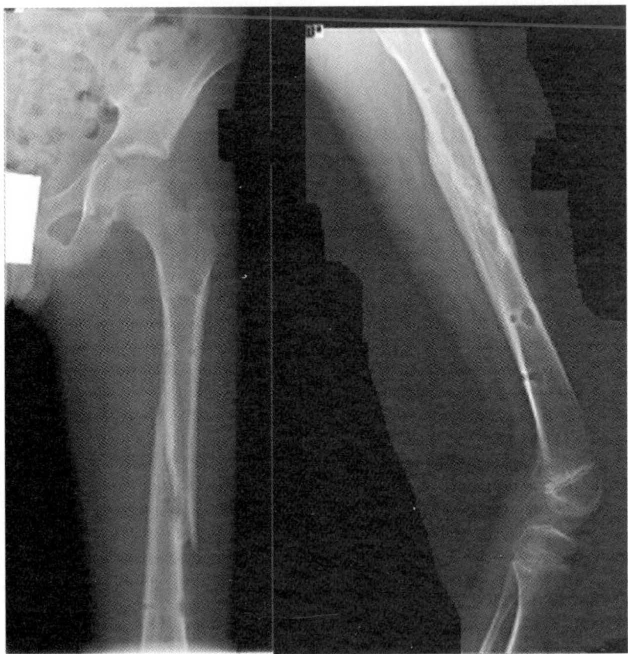

Figure 3-24 Screw-holes can act as points of stress concentration and sites of refracture.

Infection

Pin tract infections are common with external fixators. Meticulous pin site care and oral antibiotics are the treatments of choice to minimize osteomyelitis. Occasionally, pins must be removed before fracture healing to eradicate persistent pin tract infections. External fixator constructs that have multiple pin clusters allow for removal of an involved pin without compromising the fracture.

Vascular and Nerve Injuries

Vascular and nerve injuries are rare but may occur with femur fractures. The deforming forces of the gastrocnemius muscle can pull distal femur fractures into the popliteal space and injure both the common peroneal and tibial nerves as well as the popliteal artery (Fig. 3-25). When possible, femoral intramedullary rod fixation should be performed shortly after injury. A higher rate of nerve palsy has been associated with rod fixation performed 48 hours or later after injury.[20] A careful neurovascular examination detects these injuries so they can be treated.

Compartment Syndrome

Compartment syndrome can occur in conjunction with femur fractures. Tense thigh swelling and pain refractory to analgesia are early signs of compartment syndrome. With elevated compartment pressures, an urgent fasciotomy is the treatment of choice.

Summary

Femur fractures are common in children and adolescents. Fractures in younger children are typically a result of low-energy falls from playground equipment and are isolated injuries. Child abuse should be suspected in all children younger than 2 years who sustain a femur fracture. High-energy fractures are a result of motor vehicle versus pedestrian accidents or similar events and are often associated with multiple injuries. In children younger than 5 years, early spica casting is well tolerated and yields excellent results. Operative management is best for children who are older or have multiple injuries. In older children, operative treatment allows for earlier discharge from the hospital and a more rapid recovery and return to function. Improvements in the understanding and management of severe head injuries

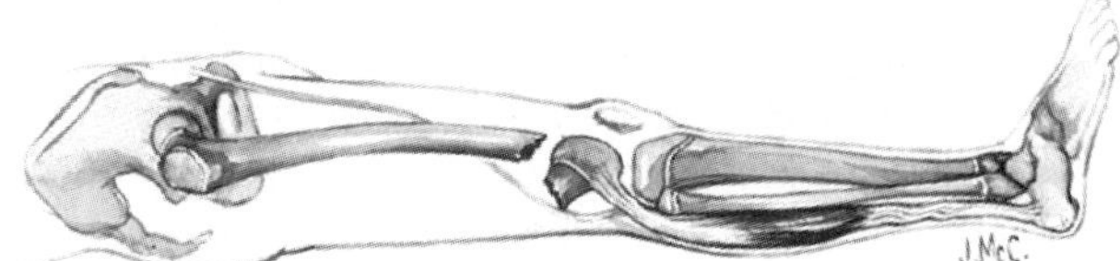

Figure 3-25 Displaced supracondylar femur fractures can cause injuries to the artery, vein, and tibial nerve in the popliteal fossa. (From Tachdjian's Pediatric Orthopaedics, vol 4, 2nd ed. Philadelphia, WB Saunders, 1990, p 3280.)

now afford many patients the chance to recover enough function to walk. It is important to align the bones of a femur fracture to allow for satisfactory union.

The overall management plan, regardless of severity of injury, should include an early assessment of family needs and resources. Identifying potential home care providers and arranging for home tutoring help ease the transition from hospital to home for a child with a femur fracture. Safety restraints and reclining wheelchairs are essential for transportation and community ambulation needs. Lastly, employing a multidisciplinary approach that involves social services, nursing, physical therapy, and the school or education system is necessary to facilitate a smooth discharge to home.

PATELLA FRACTURES

Mechanism of Injury

Patella fractures are rare, accounting for 1% of all fractures in children.[21] Most injuries are due to a direct blow to the patella that compresses it against the distal femoral condyles. These injuries occur during falls and from impact when the patella strikes the dashboard in an auto accident. Some injuries occur as a result of sudden forceful contraction of the quadriceps muscle upon a flexed knee during sporting events.

Evaluation

Patients complain of pain directly over the patella, and physical examination reveals direct point tenderness over the injured area. A palpable defect overlying the patella signifies disruption of the extensor mechanism. An inability to extend the knee against gravity (straight-leg raise) also suggests an incompetent extensor mechanism.

Fracture Pattern

The fracture pattern can range from a sleeve avulsion at either the superior or inferior pole of the patella to fracture in the midportion, either transverse or comminuted (Fig. 3-26). The patella is primarily cartilaginous in early childhood; it does not begin to ossify until a child is 6 years old. In young children, routine radiographs may not show a patella fracture because of its cartilaginous structure. Lateral radiographs are best to evaluate the patella for fracture (Fig. 3-27). Superimposition of the patella on the distal femur can often obscure fracture lines on an anteroposterior (AP) radiograph. Careful analysis should also distinguish bipartite patella from a true fracture. Bipartite patella, which is often bilateral, usually demonstrates a cleavage line in the superior lateral pole; other, less common, patterns can be present as well (Fig. 3-28). Pain with bipartite patella can indicate a fracture through its cartilaginous plate.

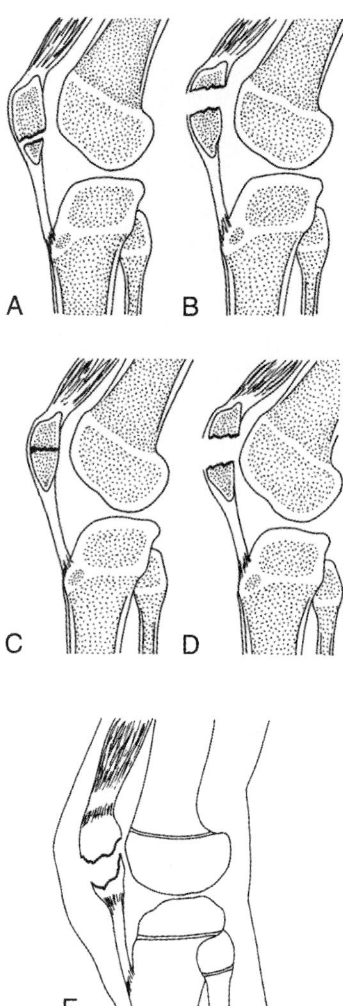

Figure 3-26 **A-D,** Types of patellar fractures: **A,** inferior pole; **B,** superior pole; **C,** transverse displaced midsubstance; **D,** transverse displaced midsubstance; **E,** substantial sleeve of avulsed cartilage when seen on radiograph appears as only a fleck of bone and looks benign. (**A** to **D,** From Ogden JA: Skeletal Injury in the Child. Philadelphia, Lea & Febiger, 1982; **E,** from Houghton GR, Ackroyd CE: Sleeve fractures of the patella in children. J Bone Joint Surg Br 61:165-168, 1979.)

Management

All displaced patella fractures associated with disruption of the extensor mechanism should be treated with operative fixation techniques similar to those used in adults (Fig. 3-29). Nondisplaced patella fractures are treated with a cylinder cast or brace (Fig. 3-30) until healing has occurred.

Summary

Patella fractures are rare in children. Most occur as a result of high-energy accidents. Careful physical examination and radiographic evaluation can identify

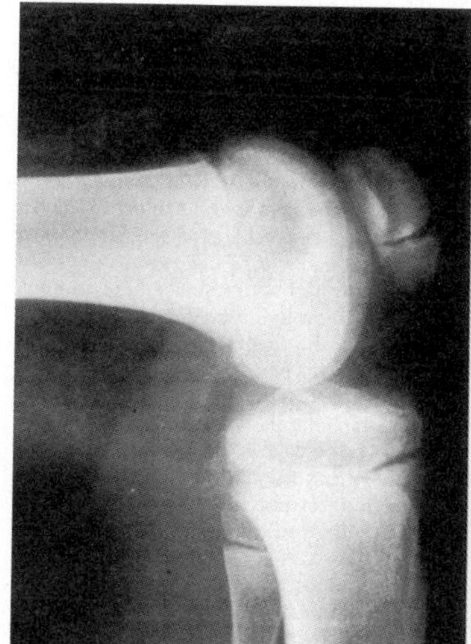
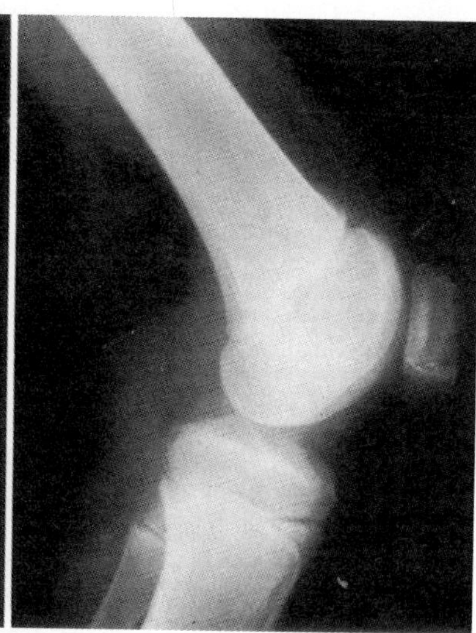

Figure 3-27 Two views of a transverse, minimally displaced patella fracture. (From Tachdjian MO: Pediatric Orthopaedics, 2nd ed. Philadelphia, WB Saunders, 1990, p 3285.)

patients with disruption of the extensor mechanism. Principles of treatment are similar to those for adult patella fractures, with emphasis on anatomic alignment of fracture ends and restoration of the extensor mechanism.

TIBIAL SPINE (INTERCONDYLAR EMINENCE) AVULSION FRACTURES

Avulsion fractures of the tibial spine are not common. They are reported most commonly in children 8 to 14 years old, and the incidence is estimated to be 3 per 100,000.[22] These injuries, pediatric equivalents of anterior cruciate ligament (ACL) injuries, are thought to occur because the incompletely ossified tibial spine of a child fails before the ACL. In addition, despite the avulsion fracture of its tibial attachment, the ACL is stressed and is often attenuated.[23] The mechanism of injury is hyperextension of the knee and occurs with sports and bicycle injuries. This injury has been associated with collateral ligament and meniscal damage.

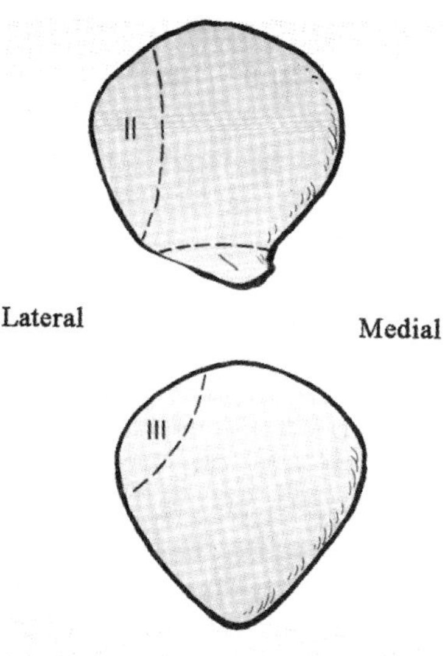

Figure 3-28 Saupe classification of bipartite patella. (From Stanitski CL, DeLee JC, Drez D Jr: Pediatric and Adolescent Sports Medicine, vol 3. Philadelphia, WB Saunders, 1994, p 312.)

Classification

Tibial spine avulsion fractures are described according to the Myers and McKeever classification system (Fig. 3-31).

The difficulty in reducing tibial spine avulsion fractures has received attention in the literature. Interposition of different soft tissues may explain the irreducibility of these fractures. The medial or lateral meniscus can be interposed between completely displaced fragments and may block reduction. The lateral meniscus is more commonly involved than the medial meniscus.[24] The transverse meniscal ligament has also been found to block reduction. Other observers discount the interposition theory and propose that the tibial spine fragment, which is attached to both the ACL and the anterior horn of the lateral meniscus, is pulled simultaneously by these ligaments in different directions and therefore cannot be reduced by manipulation.[25]

Evaluation

Physical Examination

The affected knee has a large effusion and is tender to palpation and painful with manipulation. An acutely injured knee is difficult to examine. If the patient is sufficiently relaxed, the Lachman test can be performed with the knee in about 15 degrees of flexion. Pulling

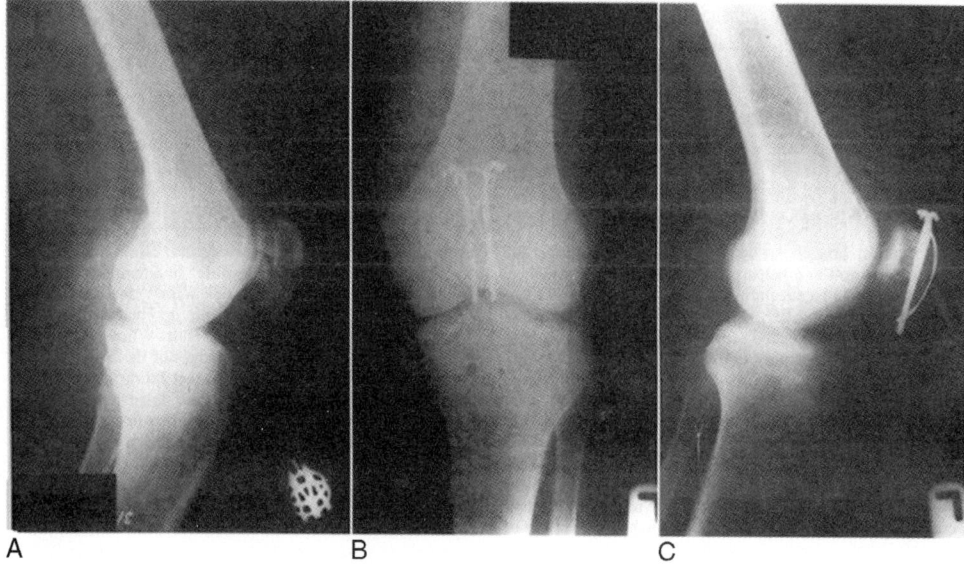

Figure 3-29 **A,** Displaced transverse fracture of the patella. **B** and **C,** Postoperative radiographs showing modified tension-band internal fixation using two anterior wire loops and two longitudinally directed Kirschner wires. (From Crenshaw AH [ed]: Campbell's Operative Orthopaedics, 7th ed. St. Louis, CV Mosby, 1987, p 1669.)

the tibia anterior to the femur in this position tests the integrity of the ACL. The uninjured knee should be compared, because there is individual variability in ligamentous laxity. More anterior displacement of the tibia in the injured than in the normal knee suggests injury to the ACL or its attachment. The examiner should rule out any other ligamentous and physeal injuries.

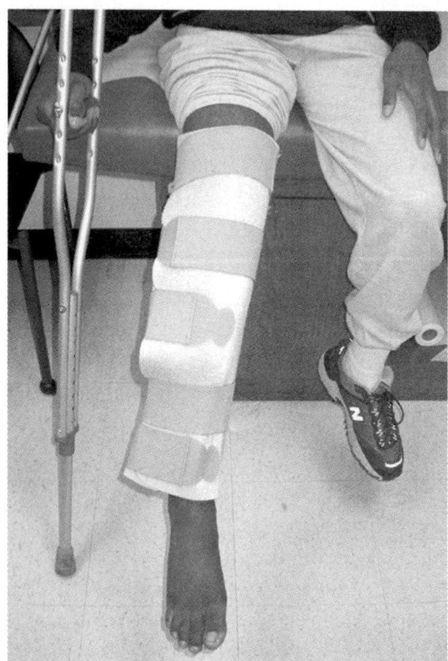

Figure 3-30 Immobilizer brace.

Imaging

AP and lateral radiographs of the knee are usually sufficient. MRI of the knee may be helpful in determining the presence of any additional intra-articular disease.

Management

Type II and type I tibial spine avulsion fractures can often be managed without an operation. Knee aspiration performed in a sterile fashion can relieve the bloody effusion. Injection of anesthetic at the same time can improve patient comfort and help the physician position the knee appropriately. Some children do not tolerate a knee aspiration without sedation.

Position of the knee for immobilization is controversial. Some believe that placing the knee in full extension or hyperextension effectively reduces the avulsion fracture by allowing the femoral condyles to push the wide base of the avulsed tibial spine down to its original position. Others contend that the knee should be immobilized in 10 to 20 degrees of flexion to put the anterior cruciate ligament in the most relaxed position, thereby allowing the fracture fragment to heal without undue traction. Regardless of position, immobilization in an above-knee cast or a cylinder cast for 3 to 4 weeks is sufficient for healing types I and II fractures (Fig. 3-32).

Type II injuries that cannot be reduced with closed manipulation can be reduced arthroscopically or with open reduction. The meniscus or a clot may be blocking the reduction.

Type III and type IV fractures require reduction of the fragment and fixation (Fig. 3-33). Both ends can usually be

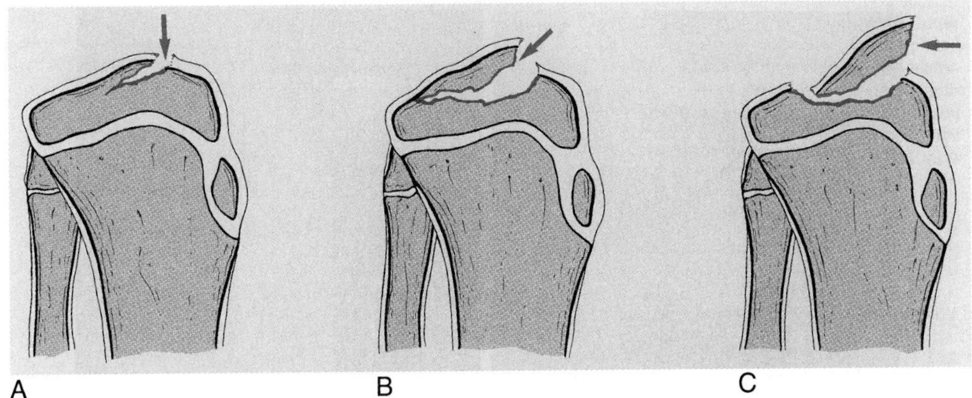

Figure 3-31 Myers and McKeever classification of tibial spine avulsion fractures. **A,** Type I—minimal or no displacement of the anterior margin of the fracture. **B,** Type II—elevation of the anterior portion of the anterior tibial spine with an intact posterior hinge. **C,** Type III—avulsed fragment is completely displaced. (From Green NE, Swiontkowski MF [eds]: Skeletal Trauma in Children, vol 3, 2nd ed. Philadelphia, WB Saunders, 1998, p 454.)

achieved with arthroscopic surgery, although an open reduction may be necessary. The meniscus may be trapped in the fracture site and thereby block reduction. The frequency of this occurrence is under debate. Fixation can be performed by a variety of methods and with a whole array of commercially available devices. Sutures can be placed through the mostly cartilaginous fragment and secured through small drill holes to the anterior tibial metaphysis. Wires may serve the same purpose. A small cannulated screw can also be placed through the tibial spine fragment and secured in the cancellous bone. Effort should be made to avoid crossing the physis if at all possible. The implants can either be bioabsorbable or metal. Proper tensioning of the ACL should be achieved by possibly even countersinking the tibial spine fragment.

Protection in a hinged knee brace allows early range-of-motion exercises. Prolonged immobilization has been associated with retropatellar chondromalacia.

In general, with appropriate treatment, results are good and non-unions rare. Mild symptomatic laxity is often present, but complaints of subjective instability are rare.[26] In fact, one study found that pathologic knee laxity was not correlated with subjectively poor knee function.[27] Anterior tibial spine injuries do not appear to be less severe in younger children and young children do not have a greater capacity for eliminating slackness of the ACL by further growth.[27]

Complications

Arthrofibrosis, an excessive scarring of the joint, is a known complication of tibial spine avulsion fracture and its treatment. Prolonged immobilization may raise the risk of this debilitating stiffness of the knee. Malunion of type III and type IV fractures can cause impingement during knee extension; this complication is treated with excision of the fragment and reattachment of the ACL.

TIBIAL TUBERCLE AVULSION FRACTURES

Avulsion fractures of the tibial tubercle are uncommon. They constitute about 1% of epiphyseal injuries. Mechanism of injury arises from athletic activities that involve jumping and landing, such as basketball and football. In addition, many patients have had Osgood-Schlatter disease. The typical clinical presentation consists of a painful "pop" in the knee upon "landing" during a basketball game. Subsequently, the patient is unable to bear weight on the leg.

A classification scheme designed by Ogden describes the fracture in terms of the distance of the fracture from the distal tip of the tibial tubercle (Fig. 3-34).

Evaluation

Physical Examination

A large swelling is noted over the anterior knee, and the tibial tubercle is exquisitely tender to palpation. The patient is unable to perform an active straight-leg raise, signifying disruption of the extensor mechanism. This mechanism comprises the entire quadriceps muscle group, the quadriceps tendon, the patella, the infrapatellar ligament, and its insertion onto the tibial tubercle. Injury to the tibial tubercle disrupts this chain at its most distal point. Furthermore, the leg may be so swollen that compartment syndrome may ensue.

Imaging

A lateral radiograph of the knee is most helpful in this situation. The Ogden classification can be used to

Text continued on page 72

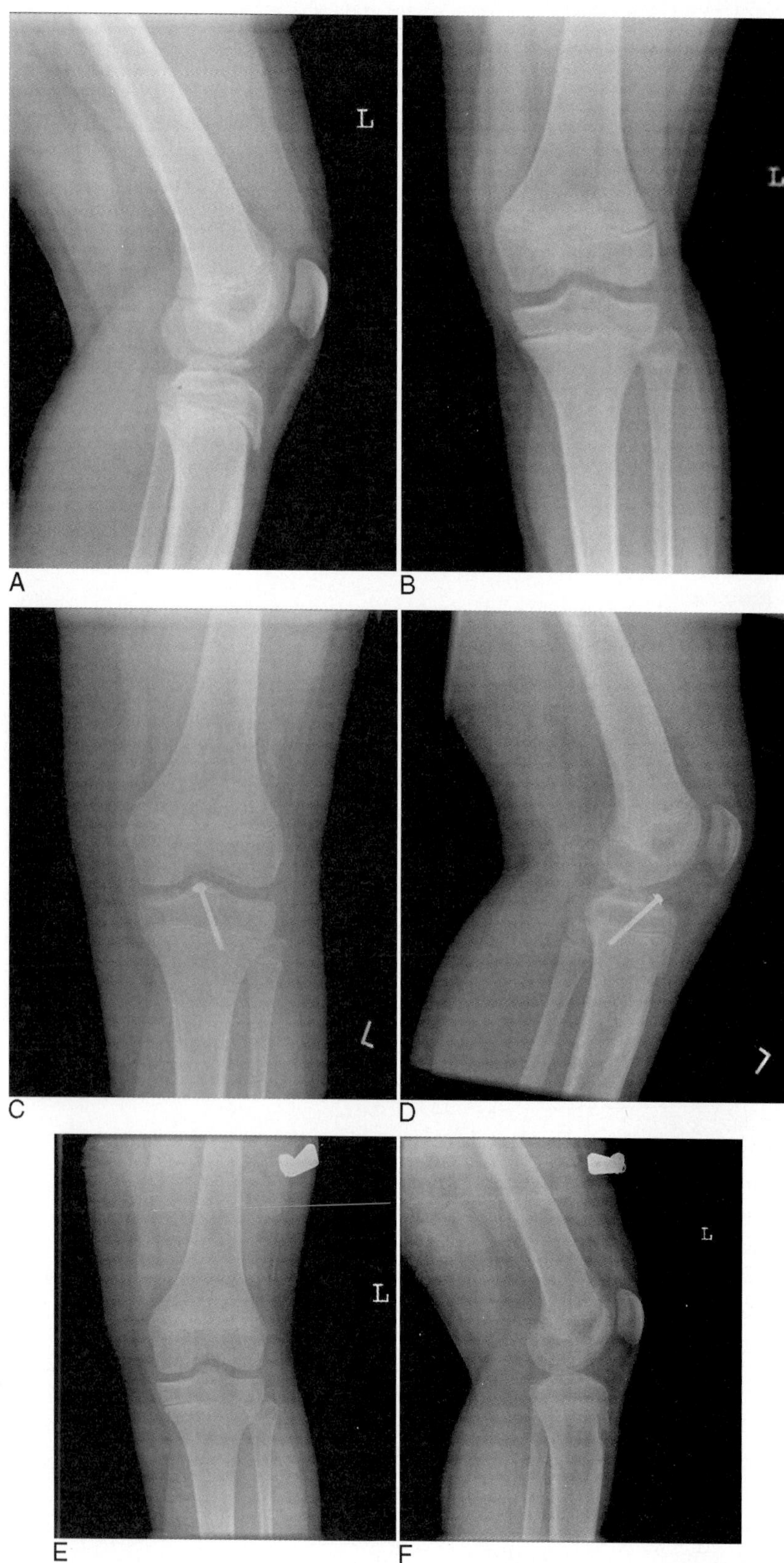

Figure 3-32 Tibial spine avulsion fracture. A and **B,** Anteroposterior and lateral radiographs of the knee of this 12-year-old boy show the displacement of the tibial spine. **C** and **D,** Arthroscopically assisted reduction with screw fixation was performed. **E** and **F,** One year later, the screw was removed. (Courtesy of Eric J. Wall, MD.)

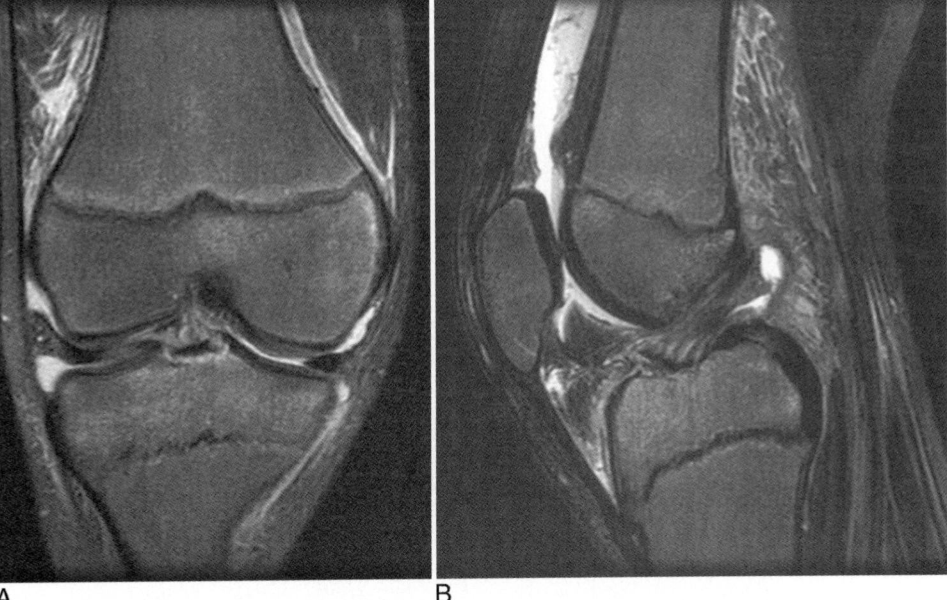

Figure 3-33 Magnetic resonance image of the knee of an 11-year-old boy shows a hinged tibial spine avulsion fracture. The injury was treated with immobilization in an above-knee cast. Lachman testing revealed asymptomatic residual laxity of the knee.

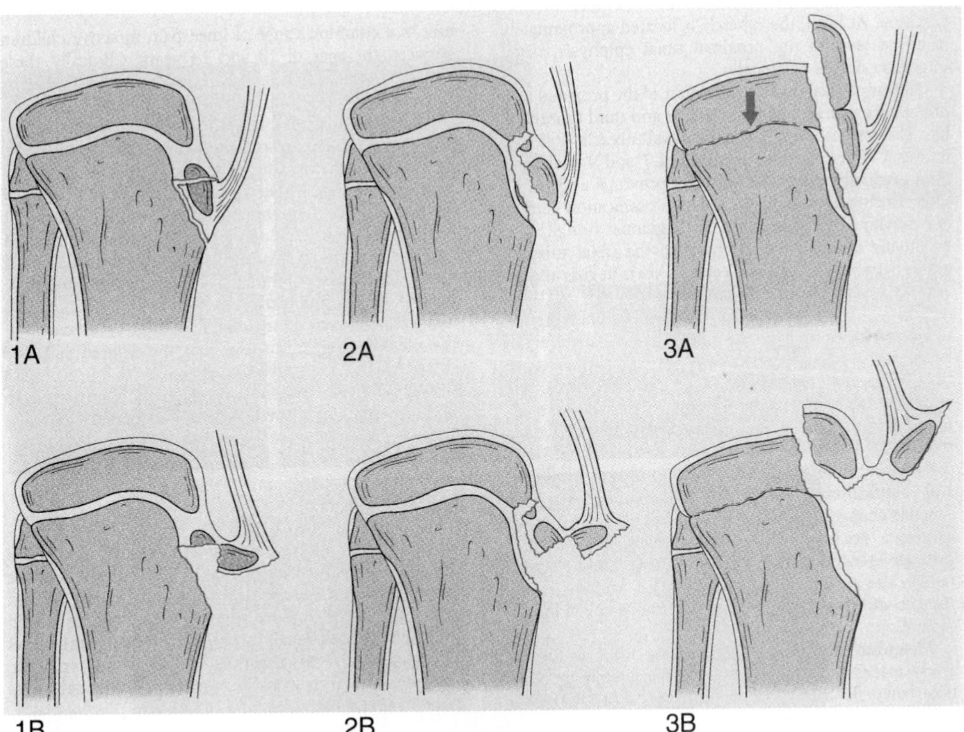

Figure 3-34 Ogden classification of tibial tubercle avulsion fractures. Type 1A: The fracture is distal to the normal junction of the ossification centers of the proximal end of the tibia and the tibial tubercle. Displacement is minimal. Type 1B: The fragment is hinged (displaced) anteriorly and proximally. Type 2: The primary fracture failure is at the junction of the ossification of the proximal end of the tibia and the tibial tubercle, essentially in line with a transverse continuation of the proximal tibial epiphysis. In Type 2B, the tubercle fragment is comminuted, and the more distal fragment may end up being more proximally displaced. Type 3: The fracture extends to the joint and is associated with displacement of the anterior fragment or fragments, leading to discontinuity of the joint surface. In Type 3A, the tubercle and the anterior aspect of the proximal tibial epiphysis are a composite unit. In Type 3B, the unit is comminuted, with the major site of fragmentation being the juncture of the ossification centers of the tubercle and proximal end of the tibia. (From Green NE, Swiontkowski MF [eds]: Skeletal Trauma in Children, vol 3, 3rd ed. Philadelphia, WB Saunders, 2003, p 458.)

determine management. CT and MRI are not necessary for diagnosis.

Management

Immobilization in an above-knee cast is appropriate for all type I and nondisplaced type II and type III fractures. Displaced type II and type III fractures require open reduction with internal fixation through a longitudinal anterior incision and placement of cannulated screws (Fig. 3-35). Periosteal sutures may also be used. Screws can be removed approximately one year later if the patient experiences subcutaneous irritation from them.

Arrest of the anterior portion of the proximal tibial physis can occur. The resulting asymmetric growth leads to a recurvatum deformity, because the posterior aspect of the proximal tibial physis outgrows the anterior portion.

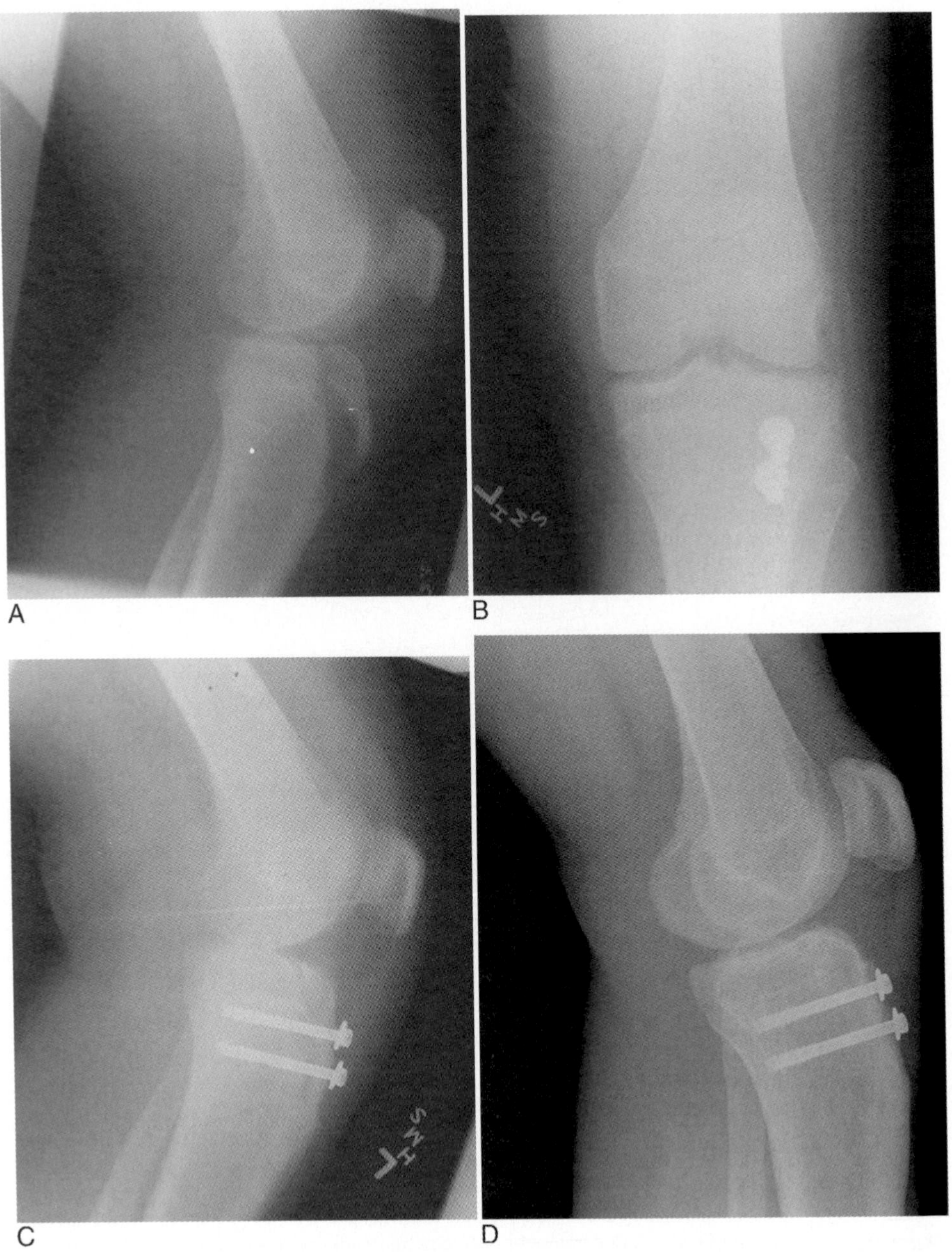

Figure 3-35 **A** and **B,** A 15-year-old boy sustained a type 3A avulsion fracture of the tibial tubercle while playing basketball. **C** and **D,** He underwent an open reduction and internal fixation. One year later, his only complaint was skin irritation from the screws, which were subsequently removed. (Courtesy of Dennis Roy, MD.)

PROXIMAL TIBIA PHYSEAL FRACTURES

Physeal fractures of the proximal tibia can result from either direct or indirect mechanisms of injury. Most of these injuries can be classified as Salter-Harris type I or type II. The most important aspect of this injury is to recognize the vascular component, as this is the pediatric equivalent of a traumatic knee dislocation (Fig. 3-36). A knee dislocation is different from a patellar dislocation and is associated with more severe ligamentous injury and disruption of surrounding soft tissues.

Evaluation

Physical Examination

The patient with proximal tibial physeal fracture is in severe pain. A thorough neurovascular examination is particularly critical in this injury. In the presence of a vascular injury, assessment of the limb for compartment syndrome is also mandatory.

Imaging

Anteroposterior and lateral radiographs of the knee are usually sufficient to diagnose this injury. A nondisplaced fracture may not be recognized without clinical suspicion of such an injury. MRI is usually not indicated.

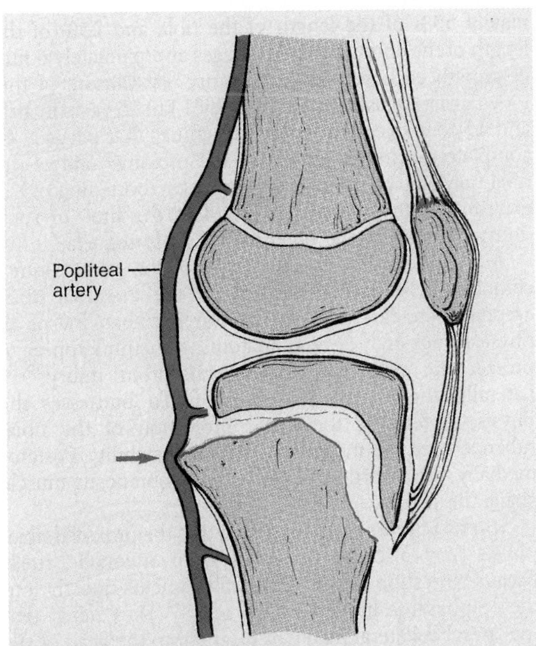

Figure 3-36 A displaced proximal tibial physeal injury can be associated with arterial injury because of the close proximity of the proximal tibial physis to the popliteal artery. (From Green NE, Swiontkowski MF [eds]: Skeletal Trauma in Children, vol 3, 3rd ed. Philadelphia, WB Saunders, 2003, p 460.)

Management

A nondisplaced proximal tibial physeal fracture should be immobilized in an above-knee cast. Displaced fractures require closed reduction with the use of general anesthesia. If the reduction seems stable under fluoroscopic evaluation, an above-knee cast will suffice. Unstable fractures may require fixation with percutaneously placed Steinmann pins and immobilization in an above-knee cast. Four weeks of immobilization without weight-bearing are followed by removal of the pins and initiation of a rehabilitation program. Close clinical follow-up is necessary to look for evidence of growth arrest or the development of angular deformity.

PROXIMAL TIBIA METAPHYSEAL FRACTURES (COZEN FRACTURES)

Definition

Fracture involving the proximal tibia metaphysis commonly occurs between the ages of 2 and 10 years.[28] This fracture is relatively uncommon but has become clinically important because of the post-traumatic development of progressive valgus deformity. This phenomenon was initially reported by Cozen in 1953; therefore, this fracture is sometimes referred to as the *Cozen fracture*, and the post-traumatic angulation as the *Cozen effect*. This deformity occurs after proximal tibial metaphyseal fractures in up to half of cases.

Etiology

The cause of the valgus deformity has been debated in the literature and is intimately tied to the treatment method (Table 3-5). It is imperative to inform the parents and caregivers of the injured child that post-traumatic

Table 3-5 Etiologies for Post-traumatic Tibia Valga

Inadequate fracture reduction	Cast immobilization without adequate correction of valgus deformity
	Soft-tissue interposition preventing reduction
Mechanical tethering	Periosteal tethering along the lateral tibial cortex
	Intact fibular tethering
Physiologic response	Preferential vascular supply to medial aspect of tibia
	Part of natural overgrowth phenomenon

valgus deformity of the tibia can occur with any form of treatment and that its development is unpredictable.

Some factors are under the control of the treating orthopaedic surgeon. They include achievement of an adequate reduction, removal of soft-tissue interposition, and close clinical follow-up with parental education.

Inadequate reduction of the fracture initially angulated by trauma has been implicated as the cause of the tibia valgus deformity. Often, the leg is placed in a bent-knee long-leg cast, which does not adequately control varus and valgus angulation (Fig. 3-37). Application of a cast with the knee fully extended allows the surgeon to better mold the cast to obtain an adequate reduction. Furthermore, anatomic reduction can be lost because of cast loosening. Therefore, the valgus angulation is not adequately corrected before fracture healing. However, this theory does not fully explain the reason for the progressive nature of the deformity, which typically occurs in the first year after fracture healing.

Another theory suggests that interposition of soft tissue in the fracture site prevents anatomic reduction. The pes anserinus (insertion of the sartorius, gracilis, and semitendinosus muscles on the medial aspect of the knee) can be torn by the trauma and flipped into the fracture site. The thick periosteum or the medial collateral ligament can get caught in the same way and prevent apposition of the fracture ends during reduction attempts. In fact, inability to obtain an adequate reduction should lead the surgeon to suspect soft tissue interposition.

Asymmetric mechanical forces across the fracture site have also been thought to contribute to the valgus deformity. Soft tissue imbalance between the medial and lateral portions of the proximal tibia is theorized to give rise to the valgus angulation. In an uninjured leg, the intact periosteum on the medial side of the proximal tibia is thought to tether the physis and thereby restrict the growth of the medial proximal tibia. Disruption of the periosteum during a fracture is then postulated to release the tether and allow less restricted growth of the medial aspect of the proximal tibia. Bony tethering of an intact fibula in the presence of a proximal tibia fracture may also explain this phenomenon. If there is no associated fibula fracture, the connections between the lateral aspect of the tibia and the fibula at the proximal tibiofibular joint near the knee and the distal tibiofibular joint at the ankle remain intact. Thus, the growth stimulation that normally occurs after children's fractures may occur preferentially on the medial side, leading to a progressive valgus angulation. However, this deformity occurs even when the fibula is fractured.[28]

Another theory suggests that unequal growth between the medial and lateral physes occurs as a result of an asymmetric vascular response.[28] This is a factor that

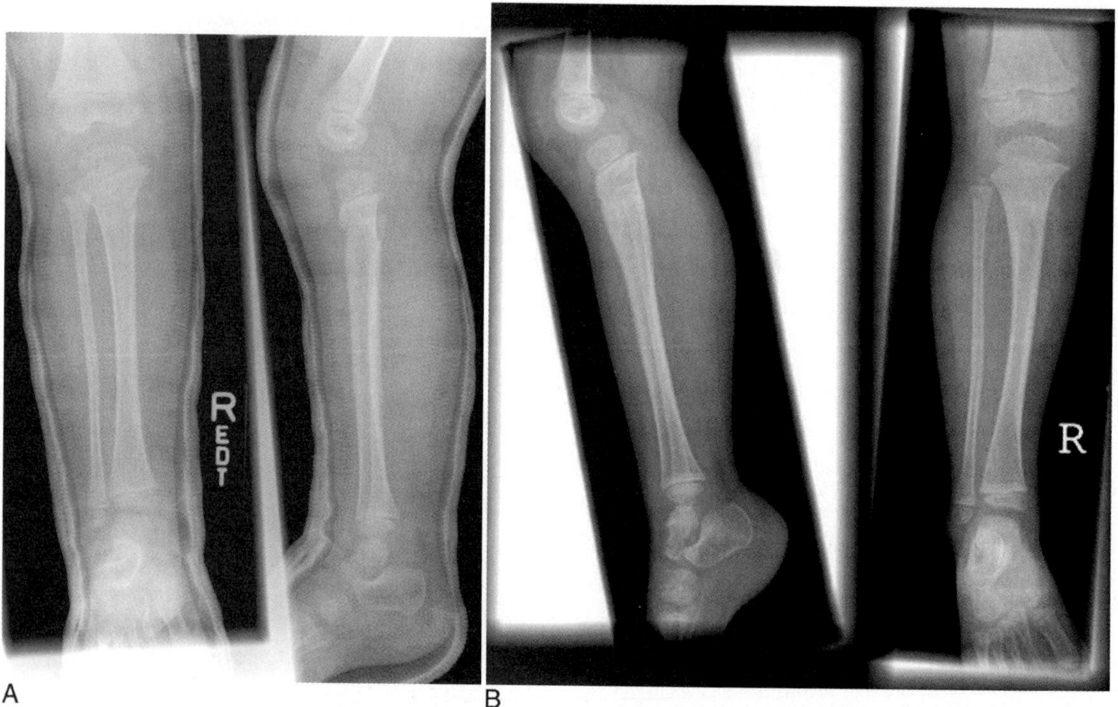

Figure 3-37 **A,** A 2½-year-old girl sustained a proximal tibial metaphyseal fracture in a sledding crash. **B,** The resulting valgus angulation was not completely corrected. The radiographs show residual valgus deformity of the proximal tibia.

cannot be controlled by the surgeon but may explain the progressive deformity phenomenon. Technetium bone scans have shown greater radioisotope uptake at the proximal tibial growth plate than in the unaffected limb, with proportionally greater uptake on the medial side. This observation suggests that the valgus deformity is due to a relative increase in vascularity and consequent overgrowth of the medial portion of the proximal tibial physis.[29]

Management

Before initiation of treatment, it is critical that the orthopaedic surgeon meet with the family to discuss the possible development of post-traumatic valgus deformity and to outline the expected course of treatment for the next few years. To minimize the development of this deformity in the child with a proximal tibia fracture, an accurate reduction must be achieved, followed by immobilization of the leg in full extension in a cast with a varus mold (Fig. 3-38). If an anatomic reduction cannot be obtained, soft tissue interposition should be suspected and addressed in the operating room. An open reduction may be necessary. A percutaneous technique can also be used to help reduce displaced and unstable fractures, followed by percutaneous pin fixation.

Once a valgus deformity develops, the treatment of choice is observation. Most of the deformity corrects spontaneously, although it may take up to 3 years to do so.[30] The valgus deformity progresses most rapidly in the first year and can continue to progress up to 20 months after injury. Reminding the parents of the nature of this condition at each office visit is helpful. Otherwise they may blame the treatment for the deformity and may pressure the surgeon to surgically correct the angulation. Results after nonoperative and operative treatment have been compared and shown to be no different; therefore, surgical correction of the valgus deformity is unwarranted in the first 2 to 3 years after a proximal tibial metaphyseal fracture.[30]

If clinically significant valgus deformity persists after 2 or 3 years, surgical options for its treatment are proximal tibial osteotomy and proximal tibial hemiepiphyseodesis. Proximal tibial osteotomy immediately corrects the valgus deformity. The proximal tibia is cut and angulated into varus, and then held together with screws or staples. This method, however, has been associated with recurrence of the valgus deformity and has not been found to change the clinical course of the condition.[30] The valgus deformity is thought to recur because the osteotomy recreates the conditions of the initial fracture. Proximal tibial hemiepiphyseodesis involves the surgical retardation or cessation of growth through the proximal tibial physis. In a young patient with many more years of growth remaining, staples placed across the medial proximal tibial physis slows growth through this area. Once adequate correction is achieved through preferential growth of the lateral portion of the physis, the staples can be removed, allowing the growth on the medial side to resume. In this way, the deformity can be corrected without permanent closure of the medial physis. In an older patient with little growth remaining, the medial physis can be surgically ablated so as to stop growth. The remaining lateral portion of the physis continues to grow, correcting the valgus deformity until closure of the physis at skeletal maturity.

TIBIAL AND FIBULAR SHAFT FRACTURES

The tibia is the most commonly fractured bone of the leg in children. Fractures involving both the tibia and fibula generally result from direct injury. The mean age of children with tibial fractures is 8 years.

Evaluation

Physical Examination

The child has pain, swelling, and deformity of the affected leg. He or she is unable to bear weight on the leg. Distal neurovascular examination must be performed.

Imaging

AP and lateral views of the tibia and fibula should include the knee and the ankle.

Management

Closed reduction and cast immobilization have been the standard method of treatment. Most fractures remodel very well, and children usually have excellent results (Fig. 3-39). Deformities that do not remodel very well include valgus angulation, apex posterior angulation (recurvatum), and rotational deformities, particularly internal rotation.[31] Casting should address all of these components so that the child's limb is in the best alignment possible. For children younger than 10 to 12 years, 15 degrees of varus angulation, 10 mm of shortening, 10 degrees of apex anterior angulation, and 15 degrees of external rotation have been well tolerated. In older children, the criteria for acceptable reduction of the tibia are more stringent. Less than 10 degrees of angulation has generally been the goal, although a long-term study of adult patients has shown that less than 5 degrees of angulation was associated with fewer degenerative changes.

Indications for internal or external fixation of tibial fractures in children are limited to open fractures, unstable closed fractures, neurovascular injuries, multiple trauma, and soft tissue abnormalities. Because open fractures must undergo several sessions of irrigation

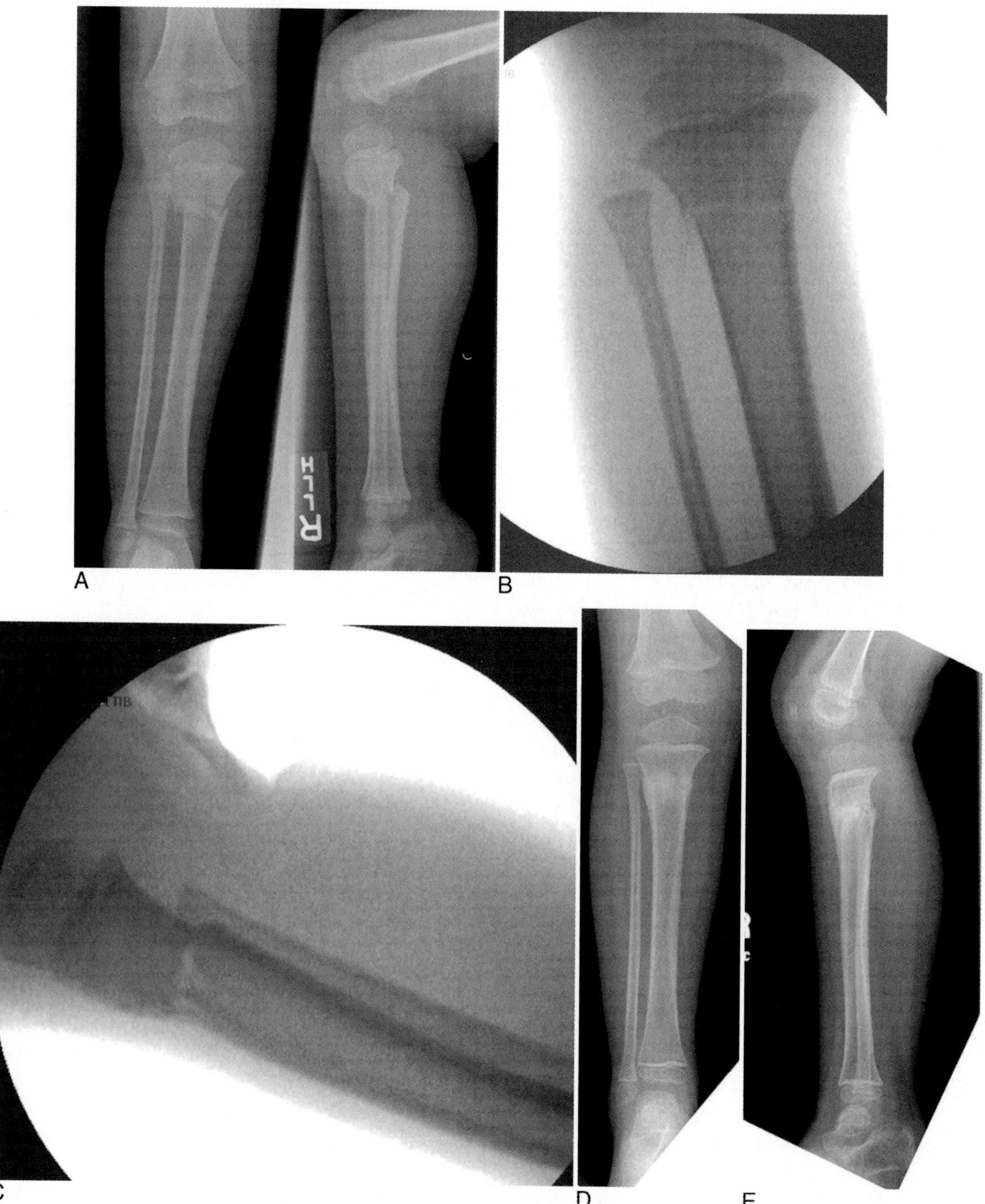

Figure 3-38 **A,** Fracture of the proximal tibial metaphysis in a 3-year-old boy. **B** and **C,** The fracture was reduced in the operating room to achieve anatomic alignment. **D** and **E,** Radiographs obtained 14 months after treatment do not show development of post-traumatic tibia valga. (Courtesy of Charles T. Mehlman, DO.)

and débridement, the wound must be easily accessible. Casting would cover the wound. Immobilization with internal fixation in an open fractures with little soft tissue injury is acceptable. In cases with more severe soft tissue injury, external fixation is more applicable. Neurovascular injuries associated with fractures require a stable bed of tissue for healing. Stable operative fixation of the bones achieves this requirement without compressing the soft tissues or preventing wound care. Patients with multiple injuries need surgical stabilization of long bone fractures to aid in mobility. Younger patients can tolerate more cast immobilization. Older patients,

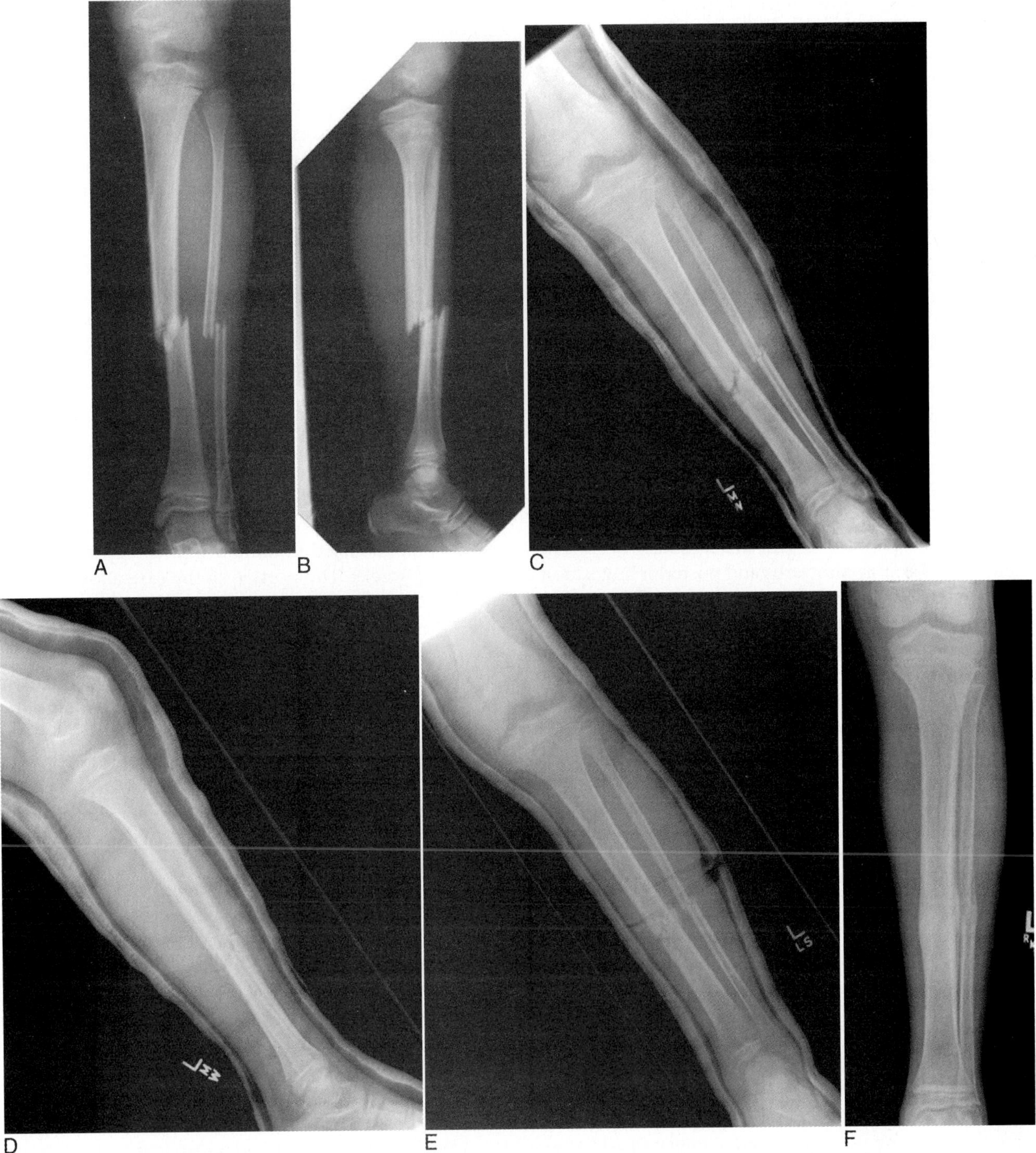

Figure 3-39 **A** and **B,** A 10-year-old boy sustained a displaced transverse fracture of the midshaft of the tibia and fibula. An above-knee cast was applied after a closed reduction. **C,** One month later, the tibia was noted to have valgus angulation. **D,** Cast wedging was performed to restore the alignment. **E** and **F,** Four months after the fracture, the tibia was healed in satisfactory alignment.

particularly adolescents, are more difficult to care for if they are immobilized with multiple casts because of their greater size and weight. In addition, prolonged cast immobilization in older patients is associated with development of joint stiffness and deep vein thrombosis.

Isolated Tibial Shaft Fractures

Isolated tibial fracture with an intact fibula is common in children. Such fractures result from an indirect rotational twisting force and do not require as much energy to produce as fractures involving both the tibia and fibula. Isolated tibia fractures often occur at the distal third of the tibial shaft. Varus angulation has been found to occur most commonly when the fracture line starts distally on the anteromedial side of the tibia and progresses in an oblique or spiral manner to the proximal posterolateral aspect of the tibia. The posterior flexor muscle groups (posterior tibialis and the toe flexors and extensors) are more concentrated medially and therefore exert a varus-producing force.

Evaluation

Physical Examination

The physical findings are similar to those in tibial and fibular shaft fractures.

Imaging

Tibia radiographs including the joints above and below the level of injury suffice.

Management

The isolated tibial fracture with an intact fibula can be difficult to reduce and maintain in the anatomic position owing to the splinting of the intact fibula. Recurrent deformities that drift into varus and posterior angulation within 3 weeks after initial injury are common (Fig. 3-40). Immobilization of the fractures is best achieved with an above-knee cast in which the knee flexed to 30 degrees and the ankle in 15 degrees of plantar flexion to minimize varus forces. Varus and posterior angulation of more than 10 degrees should be corrected, because this deformity pattern has the least capacity for remodeling.

Premature physeal closure of the ipsilateral knee, at the level of the distal femur or the proximal tibia, has been reported in adolescents after tibial diaphyseal fractures.[32]

Toddler's Fractures

Toddler's fractures occur in young ambulatory children. The age range for this fracture is typically from around 1 year to 4 years. The injury often occurs after a seemingly harmless twist or fall and is often unwitnessed. The child may not complain of pain until he or she is forced to bear weight on the affected extremity. Frequently, the child either refuses to bear weight or walks with a limp. Children in this age group are usually unable to articulate the mechanism of injury clearly or to describe the area of injury very well. Radiographs also may show no fracture, so the diagnosis is made from physical examination.

Evaluation

Physical Examination

Examining a child in this age group can be challenging. Refusal to bear weight can manifest as pulling up of the affected leg or as a florid display of protest. The most accurate way to assess the location of injury is thorough palpation of the affected lower extremity while the child is distracted.

Imaging

AP and lateral views of the tibia and fibula may show a nondisplaced spiral fracture of the distal tibial metaphysis (Fig. 3-41). An oblique view is often helpful because the fracture line may be visible in only one of three views. Fracture lines may not be visible at all, however, and the diagnosis often relies on the clinical examination. Radiographs are very helpful in excluding pathologic and metabolic conditions. A three-phase technetium bone scan can be helpful in excluding infections such as septic arthritis and osteomyelitis.

Management

Clinical suspicion of a toddler's fracture is the key to its diagnosis. A child with a history of an acute injury, inability to walk or a limp, no constitutional signs, and normal radiographic findings should be presumed to have a toddler's fracture.[33] The child with toddler's fracture is immobilized in an above knee cast for approximately 3 weeks. The portion of the case above the knee helps control rotation of the tibia and keep the cast on the leg. The child may bear weight on the leg as tolerated. Once the cast is removed, the parents and caregivers are counseled about the post-cast gait, in which a child continues to walk as if he or she were still wearing the cast. While wearing the above knee cast, the child is unable to move the knee or the ankle and therefore compensates by externally rotating the entire limb, including the foot. This adjustment allows the child to clear the ground effectively. Even after the cast is removed, this externally rotated gait persists for 1 to 2 months and becomes a major source of concern for some parents and caregivers, sometimes resulting in multiple doctor visits despite the child's painless mobility. Anticipatory counseling and reassurance are much more effective and less time-consuming than explanations offered afterwards. Toddler's fractures heal well without any adverse sequelae.

Child Abuse

Fractures are the second most common finding in child abuse after soft tissue injuries. Twenty-five percent to 50% of abused children with physical findings have fractures.

Distinguishing child abuse from accidental trauma can be challenging. A high index of suspicion is necessary to make the diagnosis. Typically, the injuries are not witnessed, and the descriptions offered by the parents and caregivers are vague. In addition, distinguishing child abuse from osteogenesis imperfecta can be difficult.

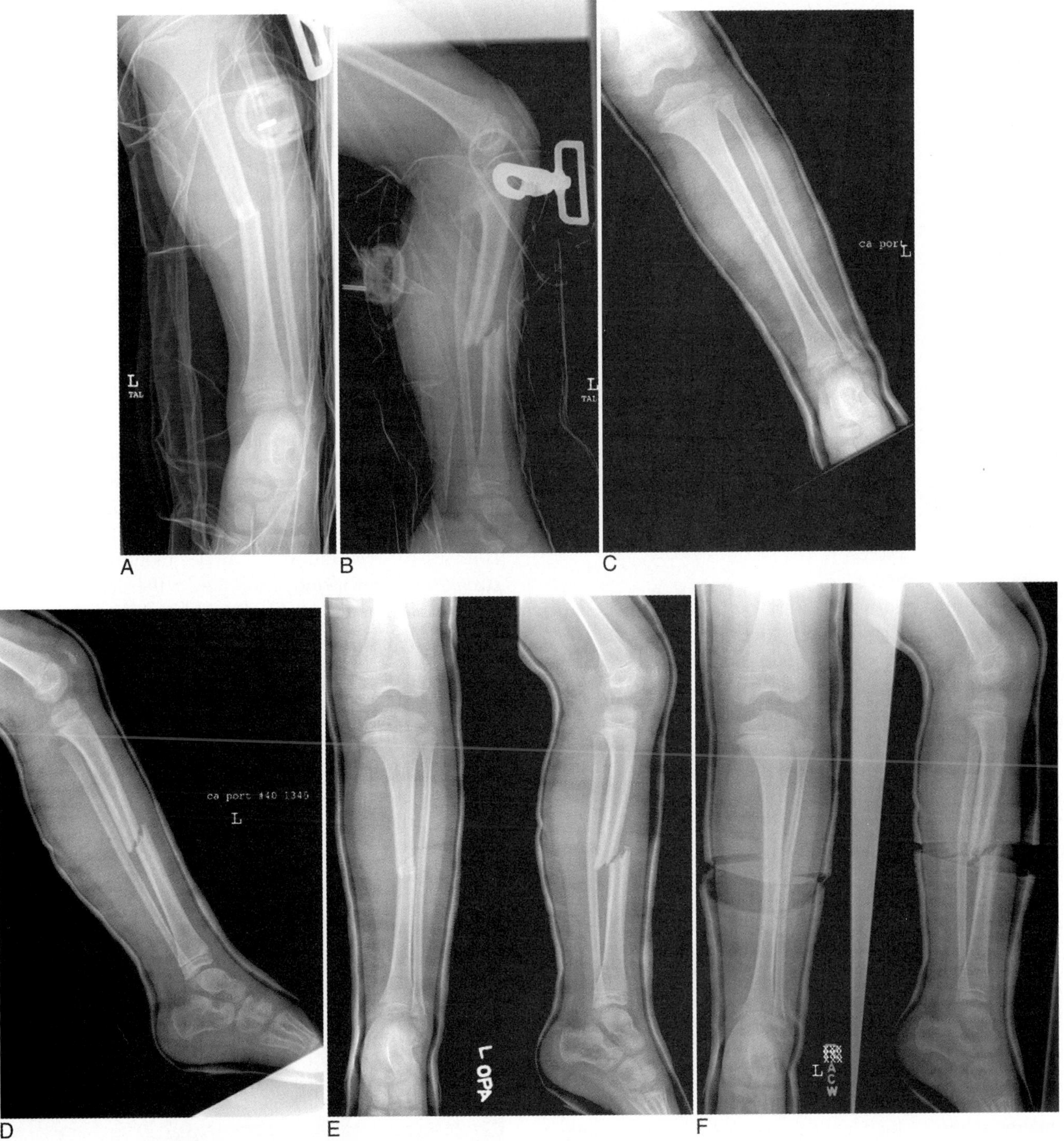

Figure 3-40 **A** and **B**, A 7-year-old boy who was hit by a car while riding a scooter sustained a displaced tibia fracture. **C** and **D**, Closed reduction performed in the operating room restored alignment with mild posterior translation. **E**, Two weeks later, the tibia had varus angulation. **F**, The cast was wedged to restore alignment.

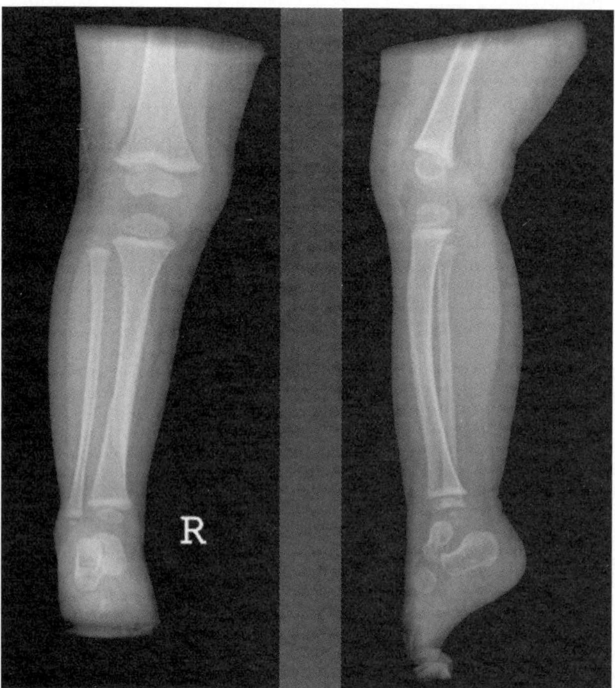

Figure 3-41 Tibia radiographs of a 2½-year-old child show the nondisplaced spiral metaphyseal fracture known as toddler's fracture.

Evaluation

Physical Examination

An abused child may have soft tissue injuries in various stages of healing, failure to thrive, and emotional problems due to deprivation and fear. Physical findings for the fracture vary with location and severity.

Imaging

Most tibia fractures in abused children are diaphyseal and transverse, not metaphyseal and spiral. A skeletal survey may be needed to assess previous healing fractures and show evidence of subperiosteal new bone formation due to blunt trauma.

Management

Closed reduction and immobilization are usually sufficient for most tibia fractures. Of paramount importance are identification of child abuse and prompt and appropriate intervention by a child abuse team.

Tibia and Fibula Stress Fractures

Stress fractures are overuse injuries associated with highly repetitive high-impact activities, such as running, basketball, volleyball, and "extreme" sports. Stress fractures often affect children unaccustomed to or not properly conditioned for these vigorous physical activities. The typical presenting complaint is diffuse aching along the proximal aspect of the tibia or the lateral aspect of the distal fibula that is worsened by increased activity. Frequently, the pain is more noticeable after the activity.

Evaluation

Physical Examination

The knees and ankles are not tender and have normal motion. Tenderness to palpation without swelling is present at either the posteromedial or posterolateral aspect of the proximal third of the tibia or the lateral aspect of the middle and distal thirds of the fibula.

Imaging

AP and lateral radiographs of the tibia and fibula may be sufficient to diagnose a stress fracture. A small lucent line may be seen across the posterior tibia or the distal third of the fibula. Sometimes, the radiographs show no obvious fracture lines but there is a sclerotic cortical thickening of the posterior tibial cortex or the fibula, suggestive of a healing stress fracture (Fig. 3-42). Bone scanning or MRI may be helpful in confirming the diagnosis.

Management

Activity modification is the key component to healing of stress fractures. Immobilization can take the form of a standard below-knee walking cast or a prefabricated removable cast boot. The patient's willingness to comply with activity modification may determine which form of immobilization would be more effective. Four to 6 weeks of immobilization are usually sufficient. Rehabilitation consists of restoration of ankle motion as well as strength and proprioception. Once the athlete has no tenderness to palpation and is able to perform exercises

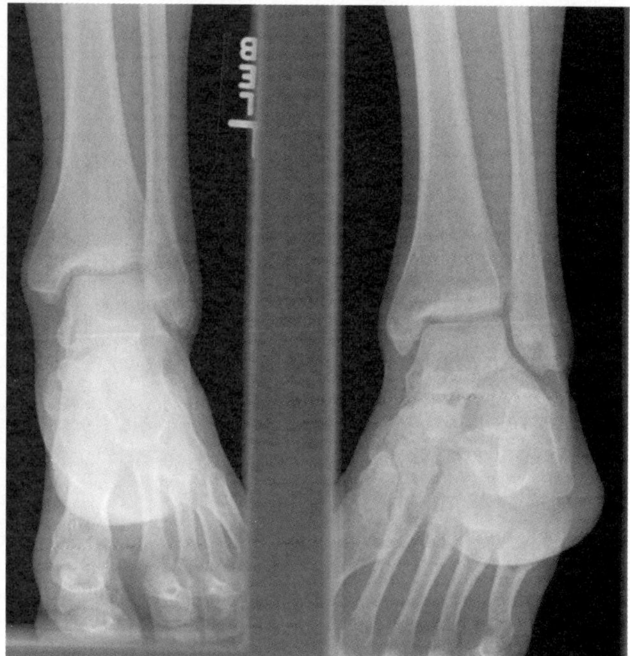

Figure 3-42 A 15-year-old girl complained of pain above her ankle that was exacerbated by soccer and running. She also had missed her menses for 3 months. Activity modification and nutritional counseling resulted in healing of a fibular stress fracture, as shown in these radiographs, and resumption of the patient's normal menstrual cycle.

without pain, he or she may resume usual activities gradually.

Special attention should be paid to adolescent female athletes. Young and adolescent girls with stress fractures may suffer from the female athlete triad, consisting of amenorrhea, anorexia, and osteoporosis (Box 3-5). Such patients usually do not volunteer information about their menstrual cycles or their eating habits; therefore, relevant questions must be asked directly and discretely. Goal-oriented, image-conscious adolescent girls may restrict food intake because they are too busy to eat or wish to lose weight. In addition, carbonated beverages, which weaken bones, tend to be particularly popular in this age group, unlike milk and soy products that contain calcium. All of these factors, coupled with intense high-impact athletic activities, create a situation in which calories and nutrients are not sufficient to keep up with the body's high energy requirements and mechanical demands. This leads to amenorrhea, osteoporosis, and stress fractures, or a combination of these conditions.

Box 3-5 Components of the Female Athlete Triad

- Amenorrhea
- Anorexia
- Osteoporosis

DISTAL TIBIA PHYSEAL FRACTURES

Ankle injuries in skeletally immature patients generally involve the growth plate. The Salter-Harris classification is used to describe fracture patterns involving the physis (Table 3-6).

Table 3-6 Salter-Harris Classification of Physeal Fractures

Type	Description
Type I	Fracture line through only the physis
Type II	Fracture involving the physis and the metaphysis
Type III	Fracture involving the physis and the epiphysis and extending to the joint surface
Type IV	Fracture extending from the joint surface through the epiphysis and physis, and exiting through the metaphysis
Type V	Crush injury to the physis
Type VI	Ablation of the perichondral ring

From Salter RB, Harris W: Injuries involving the epiphyseal plate. J Bone Joint Surg 45:537, 1963.

Evaluation

Physical Examination

The patient typically has a painful and swollen ankle that is tender to palpation over the fracture. A thorough distal neurovascular examination and soft tissue inspection should be performed. The child is usually unable to bear weight on the affected leg and needs either an assistive device or a wheelchair. Immobilizing the extremity improves comfort but may interfere with radiographic assessment.

Imaging

Ankle radiographs in AP, mortise, and lateral projections are mandatory to making an accurate diagnosis. The mortise view is obtained by internally rotating the ankle about 20 degrees so that the tibiotalar joint can be viewed directly. The ankle normally has about 20 degrees of external rotation because the fibula is slightly posterior to the tibia. An AP view of the ankle may not show the joint as well as the mortise view. CT scanning can be helpful in determining the extent of a stepoff or widening of the articular surface and for evaluating attempts at closed reduction.

Management

The goal in the treatment of distal tibia physeal injuries is restoration of articular congruity and realignment of the fractured physis. Articular stepoffs and fracture gaps have been associated with development of osteoarthritis of the ankle joint. Distortion of the growth plate can lead to growth arrest and angular deformity of the ankle.

Salter-Harris Type I Fracture

A Salter-Harris type I (SH I) fracture of the distal tibia physis is rare. This injury may be seen in neurologically impaired children and victims of child abuse.

Evaluation

Physical Examination

The patient has tenderness to palpation over the distal tibia physis with associated swelling and pain on manipulation.

Imaging

AP and lateral views of the ankle do not typically show a fracture line. Mild widening of the physis or displacement of the distal tibial epiphysis may be seen. In addition, a fibular injury may be present.

Management

Application of a below-knee walking cast for 3 to 4 weeks is sufficient immobilization. Rehabilitation to restore motion, strength, and proprioception is necessary before the child resumes regular activities. As with any fractures involving a growth plate, follow-up in 6 months to check for growth arrest is helpful.

Salter-Harris Type II Fracture

Fracture of the distal tibia physis involving the metaphysis is the most common ankle growth plate injury. The mechanism of injury involves foot supination and an external rotation force.

Evaluation

Physical Examination

The patient has a tender and swollen ankle with an obvious deformity and is unable to bear weight on it.

Imaging

AP and lateral views of the ankle show a metaphyseal spike on the distal medial or lateral aspect of the tibia. Rotational displacement may be visible only on the mortise view.

Management

Closed reduction of the fracture can usually be performed with the use of sedation (Fig. 3-43). If sufficient muscle relaxation is not achieved, the reduction may be performed in the operating room with the use of general anesthesia. An open reduction may be necessary in some cases. It is most important to correct valgus, varus, and rotational malalignments, because they do not remodel spontaneously. Repeated or delayed manipulation may increase the chance of growth plate injury and therefore should be avoided. Immobilization in an above-knee cast for 2 to 3 weeks helps control rotation of the ankle. Thereafter, a below-knee walking cast may be used. Ankle rehabilitation can begin once the below-knee cast is removed.

Salter-Harris Type III Fracture

Growth plate injury involving the articular surface often occurs in children before growth plate closure. This injury is usually the result of foot supination coupled with inversion of the ankle, which leads to fracture through the medial malleolus. Such fractures may be associated with distal fibular fractures.

Evaluation

Physical Examination

The child presents with swelling and tenderness over the medial aspect of the ankle with an isolated SH III fracture of the medial malleolus. The lateral malleolus is tender if the distal fibula is also injured.

Imaging

Multiple views of the ankle show a vertical fracture line extending from the joint surface to the distal tibial physis and exiting medially. The metaphysis is not involved.

Management

Closed reduction with the use of sedation is usually successful. However, an interfragmentary gap of more than 2 mm has been associated with growth arrest and angular deformity, making open reduction and internal fixation preferable (Fig. 3-44).[34] An anatomic reduction minimizes the development of bony bar formation across the growth plate. Care must be taken to place the screw from epiphysis to epiphysis, because a screw that crosses the physis may cause growth arrest. Immobilization in an above-knee non–weight-bearing cast for 3 to 4 weeks should follow.

Salter-Harris Type IV Fracture

The mechanism of an SH III fracture may lead to a growth plate fracture involving both the articular surface and the metaphysis; this is known as an SH IV fracture.

Evaluation

Physical Examination

The clinical presentation is the same as that of an SH III fracture.

Imaging

Radiographs show a vertical fracture line involving the metaphysis and the epiphysis. The fragment may be displaced so that the level of its physis is not congruent with the remainder of the distal tibia physis.

Management

Unlike the SH III fracture, the SH IV fracture requires open reduction to achieve an anatomic reduction. The screw or pin must be placed from metaphysis to metaphysis or from epiphysis to epiphysis (Fig. 3-45). The metaphyseal fragment may have undergone plastic deformation during the injury and therefore may have to be removed to allow the remainder of the fracture fragment to be reduced. After open reduction and internal fixation, the leg is immobilized in an above-knee, non–weight-bearing cast for 3 weeks, and then in a walking cast. Pins can be removed at the time of cast changing, and screws can be removed about a year after the operation, although screw removal is not mandatory.

Salter-Harris Type V Fracture

SH V injury to the physis is thought to result from axial compression of the growth plate. This injury is extremely rare, and its precise etiology is controversial.

Evaluation

Physical Examination

Clinical suspicion of this injury is the only way to make the diagnosis.

Imaging

Radiographs do not show any obvious injury to the epiphysis or the metaphysis. The diagnosis may be made retrospectively, when premature growth arrest is noted in follow-up films.

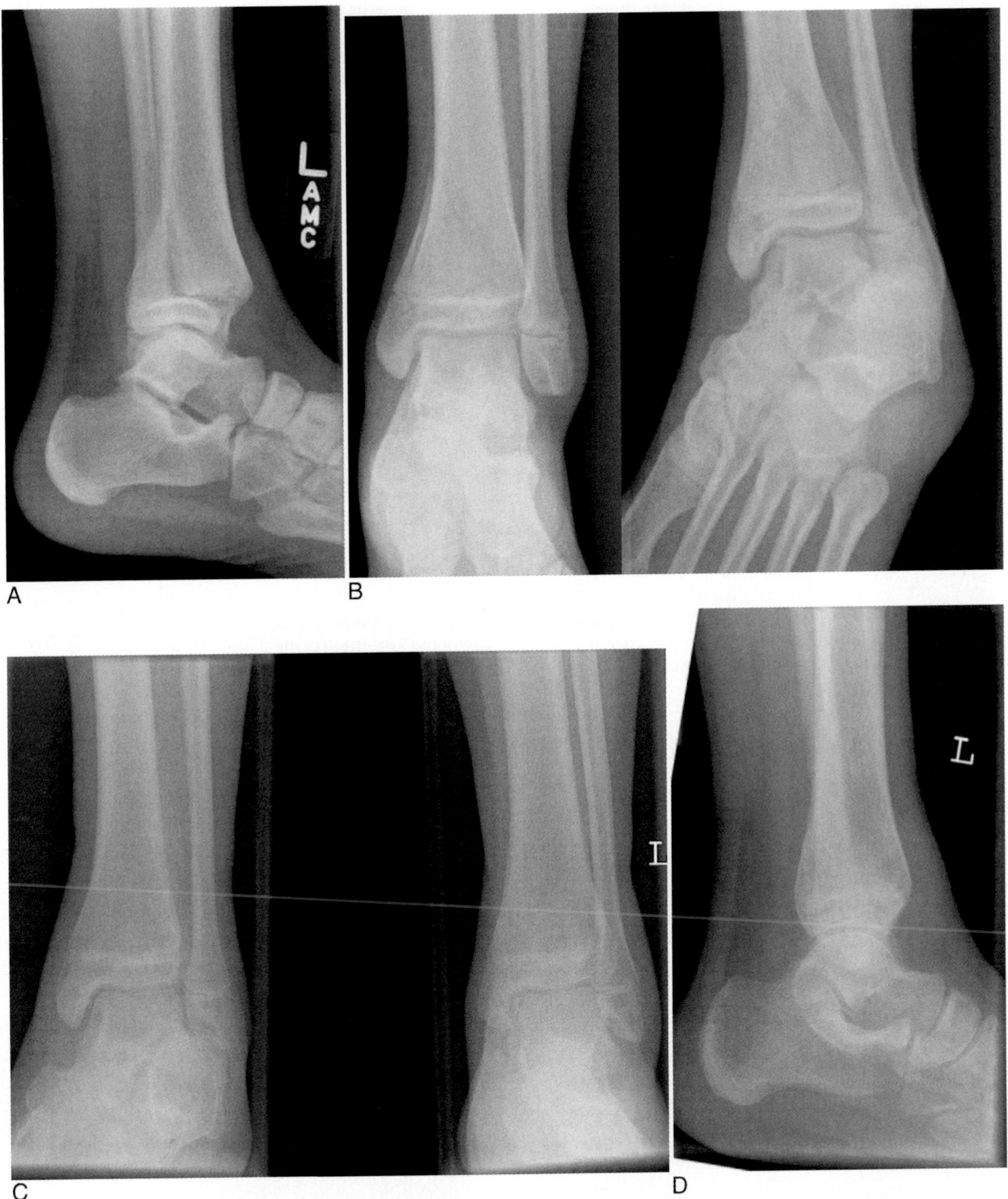

Figure 3-43 Salter-Harris type II fracture. A and **B,** Three views of the ankle of a 14-year-old boy show a displaced fracture through the distal tibial physis and the metaphysis. **C** and **D,** The patient was treated with closed reduction and application of an above-knee cast.

Management

Because the diagnosis may be retrospective, treatment involves correction of any angular deformity or leg length discrepancy. Even when this diagnosis is made early on the basis of clinical suspicion, prolonged immobilization should be avoided.

Salter-Harris Type VI Fracture and Lawnmower Injuries

Removal of the perichondral ring is classified as a Salter-Harris type VI injury. It can occur after a child's leg sustains a lawnmower injury or when the leg is dragged

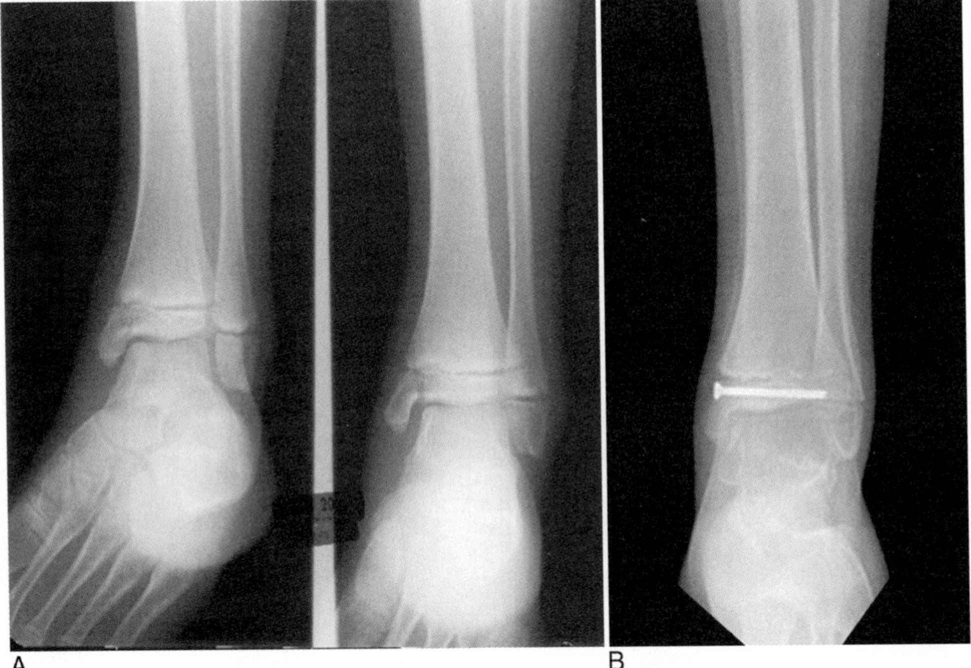

Figure 3-44 Salter-Harris type III fracture. A, Anteroposterior and mortise views in a 12-year-old boy show an intra-articular fracture involving the medial malleolus. **B,** A percutaneously placed screw was used to achieve reduction and fixation of the fracture. (Courtesy of Eric J. Wall, MD.)

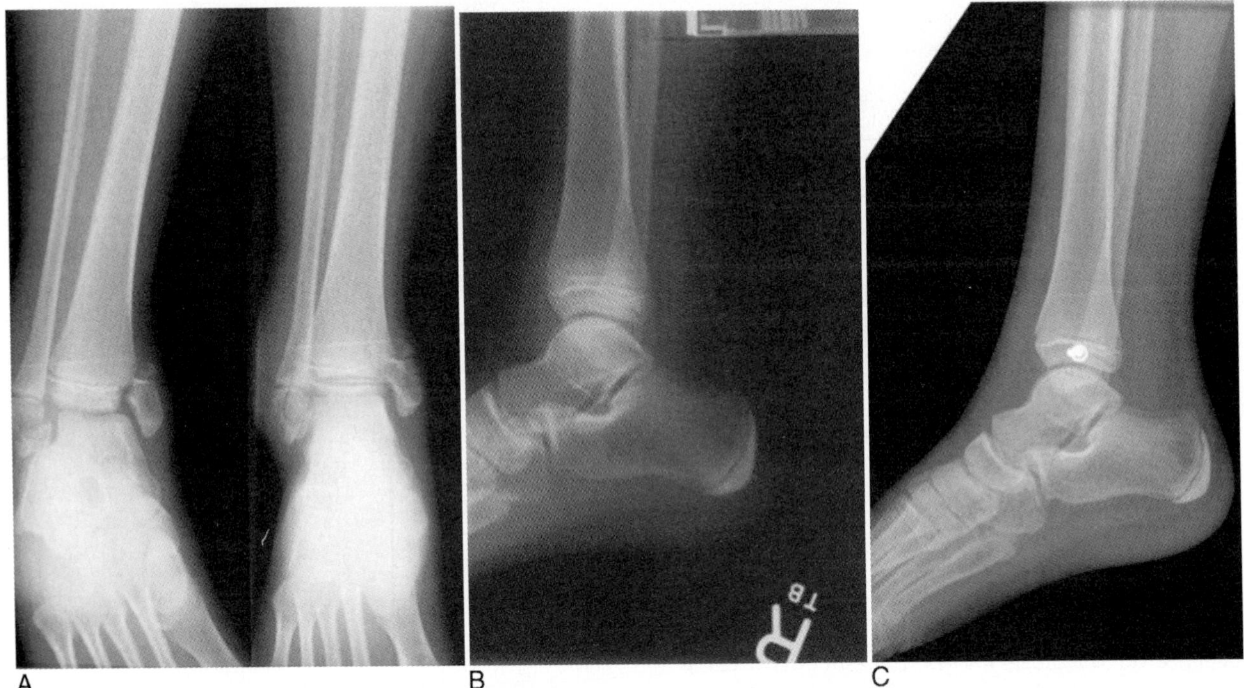

Figure 3-45 Salter-Harris type IV fracture. A, Anteroposterior and mortise views in a 10-year-old girl show a physeal fracture involving both the metaphysis and the articular surface. **B** and **C,** A screw and a washer were placed percutaneously to reduce the fracture and hold the position. (Courtesy of Charles T. Mehlman, DO.)

across concrete or pavement, resulting in a degloving injury.

Evaluation

Physical Examination

The limb's neurovascular status and the integrity of the skin must be assessed. Contamination with grass, dirt, and debris should be noted and addressed. The limb should be reexamined at regular intervals, because tissue viability and sterility may not be clear at initial presentation.

Imaging

SH VI injuries involve severe disruption of the soft-tissue envelope of the ankle. Significant portions of the ankle may be missing, and their absence may be obvious on radiographs.

Management

Wound cleansing is the primary management goal of any degloving or lawnmower injury. Multiple débridements and, often, an amputation at some level of the affected limb, are needed. The probability of subsequent growth arrests and angular deformities is high and should be clearly explained to parents and caregivers early in treatment so as to avoid later surprises.

Complications of Distal Tibia Physeal Fracture

Fractures of the distal tibia physis that occur before the beginning of physeal closure are distinct from transition fractures (Tillaux and triplane fractures) and can have bad results because of growth arrest and articular injury.

Any fracture involving the physis has the potential to cause growth arrest and to result in deformity and limb length discrepancy. Certain fracture patterns have been associated with a higher rate of growth arrest. SH II and SH IV fractures appear to have the highest rates of growth disturbance. SH IV and SH V fractures are generally the results of high-energy injuries and often result in angular and linear deformity. In one study, the patients with high-energy injuries were younger and more likely to present late. Male patients were more likely to have higher energy injuries and were also more likely to have angular and linear deformities as well as delayed treatment.[35]

Transition Fractures

Distal tibial physeal "transition" fractures occur in the adolescent with partially closed growth plates. The distal tibia physis closes over an 18-month transition period in a defined sequence: from central to medial and then lateral. The ankle is vulnerable to tibia physeal fractures during the part of the transition period when the medial physis is closed but the lateral portion is still open. The typical clinical presentation is that of a teenager who sustained an acute twisting injury after a fall from a platform (skateboard, sled, or bench) or while engaged in contact sports (sliding into base, wrestling). The main mechanism for this set of fractures is external rotation of the foot relative to the tibia. If the foot were planted on the ground, the child's leg would internally rotate relative to the foot. A loud audible "pop" and immediate pain and swelling are uniformly associated with this injury.

Tillaux and Triplane Fractures

Tillaux Fracture

A Tillaux fracture is an avulsion fracture of the unfused anterolateral epiphysis of the distal tibia by the anterior tibiofibular ligament. Forced external rotation of the foot leads to external rotation of the distal fibula (Fig. 3-46). Because the anterior inferior tibiofibular ligament is stronger than the physis at this stage in growth, the ligament pulls off a piece of the anterolateral tibial epiphysis. This is an SH III fracture because it involves the growth plate and the joint surface.

Triplane Fracture

When the fracture involves the metaphysis of the distal tibia in addition to the growth plate and joint surface (Tillaux fracture), the fracture is referred to as a triplane fracture. It can consist of two, three, or four parts. A triplane fracture, as its name implies, involves three planes:

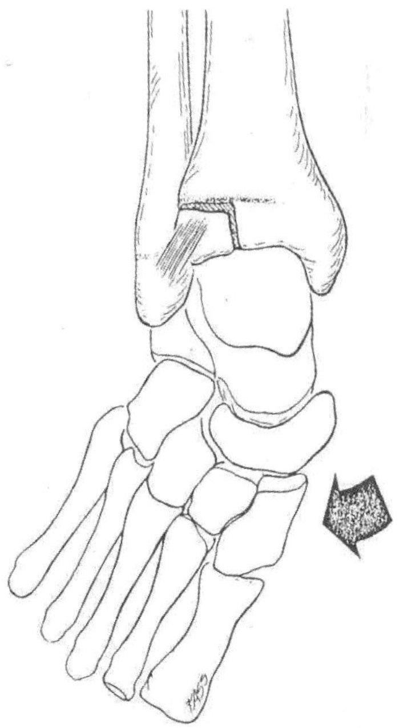

Figure 3-46 Diagram of a Tillaux fracture. Arrow demonstrates external rotation of the foot and the intact anterior tibiofibular ligament attached to the Tillaux fracture fragment. (Dias LS, Geigrich CR: Fractures of the distal tibial epiphysis in adolescence. J Bone Joint Surg Am 65:438-444, 1983.)

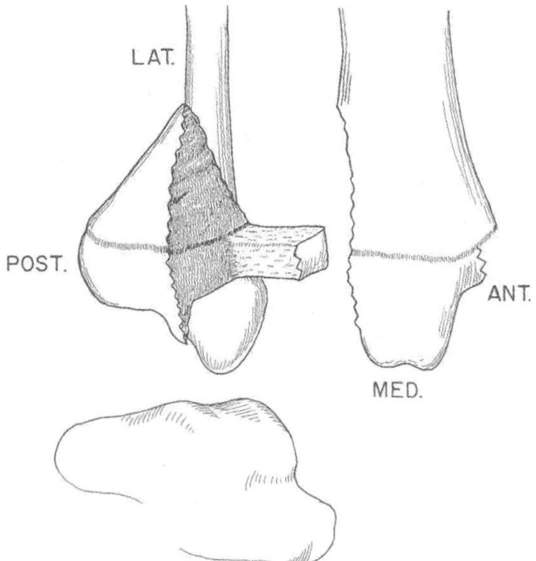

Figure 3-47 This diagram of a two-fragment triplane fracture. (From Cooperman DR, Spiegel PG, Laros GS: Tibial fractures involving the ankle in children. J Bone Joint Surg Am 60:1040-1046, 1978.)

sagittal, axial, and coronal (Fig. 3-47). The sagittal and axial components of the fracture is like those of a Tillaux fracture, in which the fracture involves the distal tibial epiphysis, extending to the articular surface, and the unfused lateral portion of the distal tibia growth plate. On AP and mortise radiographic views, a triplane fracture looks like an SH III fracture. The coronal portion involves the distal tibial metaphysis and is visible on the lateral view. Because the articular portion of the triplane fracture cannot be seen on the lateral view, the fracture pattern has the appearance of an SH II fracture on this view. The mechanism of a triplane fracture is external rotation of the foot relative to the tibia. However, the metaphyseal fracture component of a triplane fracture is usually the result of more axial energy than needed for a Tillaux fracture.

Evaluation

Physical Examination

The ankle is swollen and tender to the touch. Patients are not able to bear any weight and often are not able to ambulate at all.

Imaging

Ankle radiographs in AP, mortise, and lateral views are mandatory to make an accurate diagnosis. The mortise view is obtained by internally rotating the ankle about 20 degrees so that the tibiotalar joint can be viewed directly. The ankle normally has about 20 degrees of external rotation because the fibula is slightly posterior to the tibia. An AP view of the ankle may not show the joint as well as the mortise view. CT can be helpful in determining the extent of the stepoff and widening of the articular fractures and for evaluating attempts at closed reduction.

Tillaux fractures involve the joint and therefore are intra-articular. A small vertical fracture line on the lateral distal tibial epiphysis can be appreciated on the AP view, and anterior displacement of the anterolateral portion of the distal tibial epiphysis may be noted on the lateral view.

In the triplane fracture, the AP view shows what appears to be an SH III fracture of the distal tibial epiphysis. Lateral displacement of this piece is consistent with the three-part fracture pattern. A lateral view yields the appearance of an SH II, because it reveals the posterior metaphyseal fracture.

Management

First line of treatment for Tillaux and triplane fractures is closed manipulation to restore anatomic alignment. This procedure can be performed in the emergency department with the use of sedation or in the operating room with general anesthesia. The indication for surgery is 2 mm of displacement with articular stepoff.

The cornerstone of successful reduction of a Tillaux fracture is reversing the mechanism of injury by internally rotating the foot in relation to the ankle. Direct pressure applied to the avulsed epiphyseal fragment secures the reduction. If the closed reduction is not successful, the fracture fragments can be manipulated with a Steinmann pin introduced by a percutaneous approach (through a small incision). A lag screw can also be used to pull the fracture fragments together to reduce the articular fracture gap. An open reduction with internal fixation may even be necessary for certain Tillaux fractures (Fig. 3-48).

For triplane fractures, the foot can be internally rotated relative to the tibia, and a posteriorly directed force can be applied to the anterior tibial metaphysis. An open reduction is necessary for some triplane fractures. One or more screws are used for fracture fixation (Fig. 3-49).

Once the reduction is found to be satisfactory on radiographs or CT scans, an above-knee cast is applied, and the patient should be instructed to avoid weight-bearing for 3 to 4 weeks. Thereafter, a below-knee walking cast is applied, and the patient may bear weight on the leg as tolerated. Once the cast is removed, a comprehensive rehabilitation program focused on restoring motion, strength, and proprioception is initiated. Growth arrest is not a clinical issue in these fractures because, at the time of injury, the involved physis had already begun to close. Hence, screw violation of the growth plate has no adverse sequelae.

DISTAL FIBULA PHYSEAL FRACTURES

Distal fibula physeal fracture is one of the most common lower extremity injuries in the skeletally immature patient. In this age group, the ligaments are stronger than

Text continued on page 89

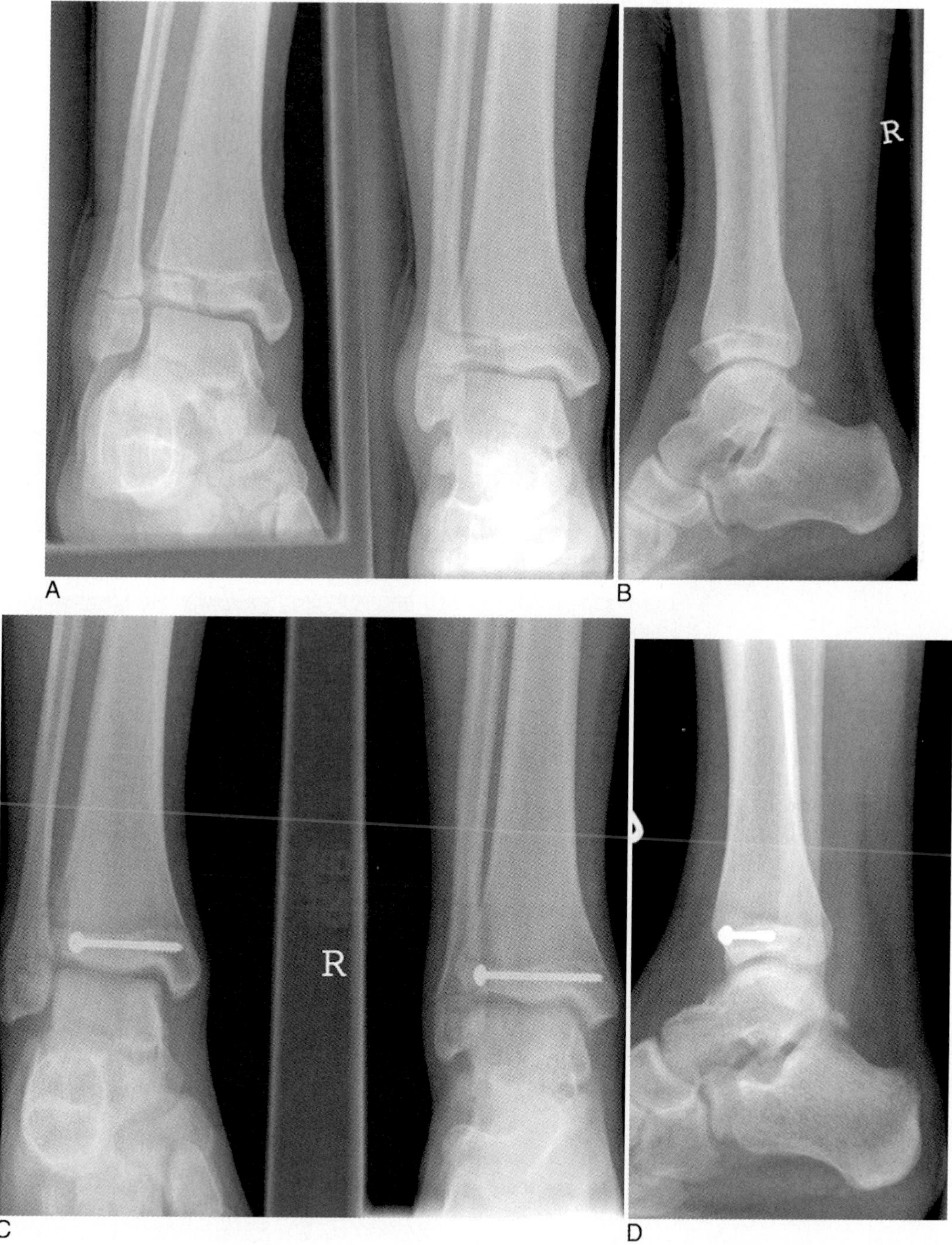

Figure 3-48 Three views of the ankle of a 14-year-old boy show an avulsion fracture of the anterolateral portion of the distal tibial epiphysis (Tillaux fracture). **A,** Mortise and anteroposterior views show the intra-articular component of the fracture. **B,** Lateral view shows the anterior displacement of the fragment. **C** and **D,** The patient underwent open reduction and internal fixation of the fracture. (Courtesy of Charles T. Mehlman, DO.)

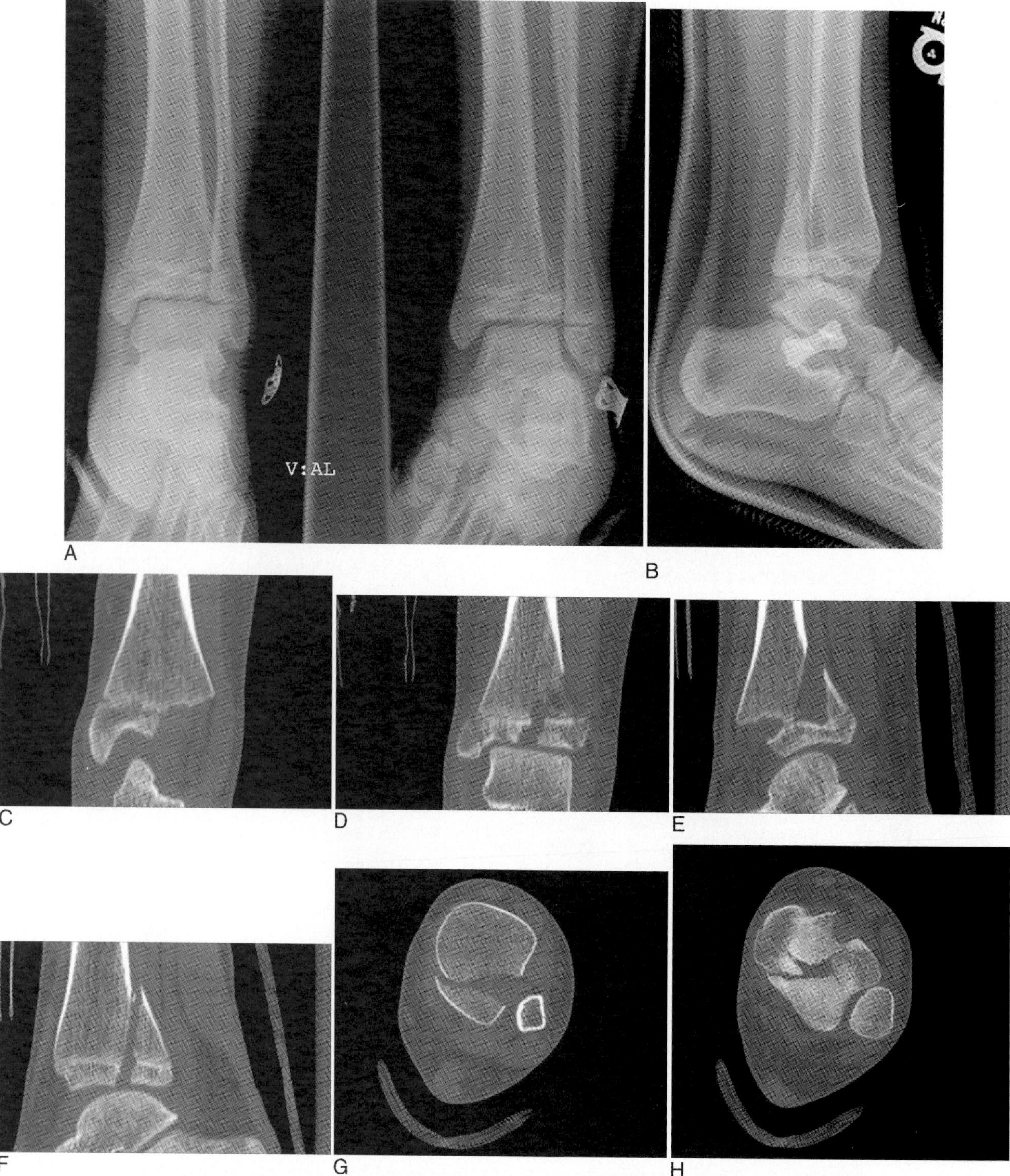

Figure 3-49 A 12-year, 11-month-old girl sustained a left ankle injury when she slid into home base during a softball game. **A,** Anteroposterior and mortise radiographs show the intra-articular triplane fracture. **B,** The lateral view shows the posterior metaphyseal fracture as well as the posterior displacement of a segment of the distal tibial epiphysis. Computed tomography scans show the fracture pattern going through three planes. **C** and **D,** Sagittal scans show the metaphyseal fracture displacement. **E** and **F,** Coronal scans show the posterior displacement of the anterolateral portion of the distal tibial epiphysis. **G** and **H,** The patient underwent a closed reduction with percutaneous screw fixation.

the physis. Therefore, instead of sustaining ankle sprains, these children have fractures at the distal fibula physis. Mechanism of injury is an ankle inversion injury associated with running on an uneven surface.

Evaluation

Physical Examination

Patients generally complain of isolated lateral ankle pain and are usually unable to fully bear weight on the leg. A large area of swelling (the size of a goose egg) overlies the distal fibula. The leg is exquisitely tender to palpation over the bony distal fibula. The anterior talofibular ligament, commonly injured during ankle sprains, is not typically tender to palpation.

Imaging

AP and lateral radiographs are routinely performed in children with complaints of ankle pain after an acute event. Most often, the radiographs do not show any displacement of the fracture, and the injury may be classified as an SH I distal fibular physis fracture. Inspection of the soft tissue outline shows a large area of swelling over the distal fibula physis (Fig. 3-50).

Management

Children generally do not abide by recommendations for activity modification. Thus, application of a below-knee walking cast (either standard or waterproof) for 3 to 4 weeks is usually necessary to allow prompt healing of the SH I distal fibula fracture. The patient may bear weight as tolerated on the leg during immobilization. Once the cast is removed, the patient is given elastic tubing and instructed in a set of exercises to regain ankle motion and restrengthen ankle stabilizers. These exercises are to be performed at least twice a day. In addition, the leg is placed in a removable ankle brace (either a stirrup or lace-up type) to protect the ankle until it regains full painless function.

Parents are instructed to allow the child to resume athletic competition only when full painless motion has been achieved. Having the patient perform a squat with both heels on the floor is one way to test for restoration of ankle motion. Hopping on one foot at a time is a reliable way to test for restoration of strength and proprioception of the injured ankle.

Long-term problems related to distal fibula physeal fractures are rare. However, premature closure of the distal fibula physis, in combination with continued growth through the distal tibia physis, can lead to asymmetric growth deformity of the ankle. This malalignment, if detected early, can be managed with surgical growth plate ablation (epiphyseodesis) of the distal tibia physis. Reinjury of the distal fibula physis is not uncommon.

FRACTURES OF THE FOOT

Most foot fractures in children can be treated nonoperatively, and they have received relatively little attention in the orthopaedic literature. There are a large number of normal variations in the appearance of a child's foot, and the clinician must be familiar with them to avoid confusing a normal variant for a traumatic injury. In addition, the child's foot remains relatively unossified for a long period, making diagnosis of fractures on plain radiographs difficult at times.

Fractures of the Talus

Fractures of the talus are rare in children. As in adults, fractures of the talus in children can result in significant complications, such as post-traumatic arthrosis and AVN, because the talus has three articular surfaces and a tenuous blood supply. Most fractures through the talus occur through the neck, and frequently they are only minimally angulated. Angulation of less than 30 degrees can generally be accepted, but patients with greater angulation should be treated with closed or open reduction as needed, followed by long-leg casting for 4 weeks. Long-term follow-up is recommended to check for AVN.

Older children and adolescents tend to have foot fracture patterns more in line with those seen in adults. Displaced talus fractures in these age groups require open reduction and internal fixation. As in younger patients, long-term follow-up is needed to carefully check for AVN subsequent to this injury.

Fractures of the lateral process of the talus may occur in conjunction with a twisting ankle injury. Lateral process fractures seem particularly prevalent in snowboarders, and these injuries frequently require CT for diagnosis.[36] Large displaced fractures should be treated by open reduction and internal fixation, and small displaced fracture fragments can be excised.[36]

AVN after talus fractures does occur in children, with a reported incidence in nondisplaced fractures as high as 29%.[37] After treatment for a talar neck fracture, radiographs should be observed for Hawkins sign, a radiolucent line beneath the dome of the talus. This sign attests to resorption of the subchondral bone beneath the talar dome, indicating an intact blood supply to the body of the talus, and carries with it a favorable prognosis regarding the development of AVN.[37] If AVN does occur, it should be treated with long-term relief of weight-bearing, typically with a patellar-tendon-bearing, molded ankle-foot orthosis with an articulating ankle.

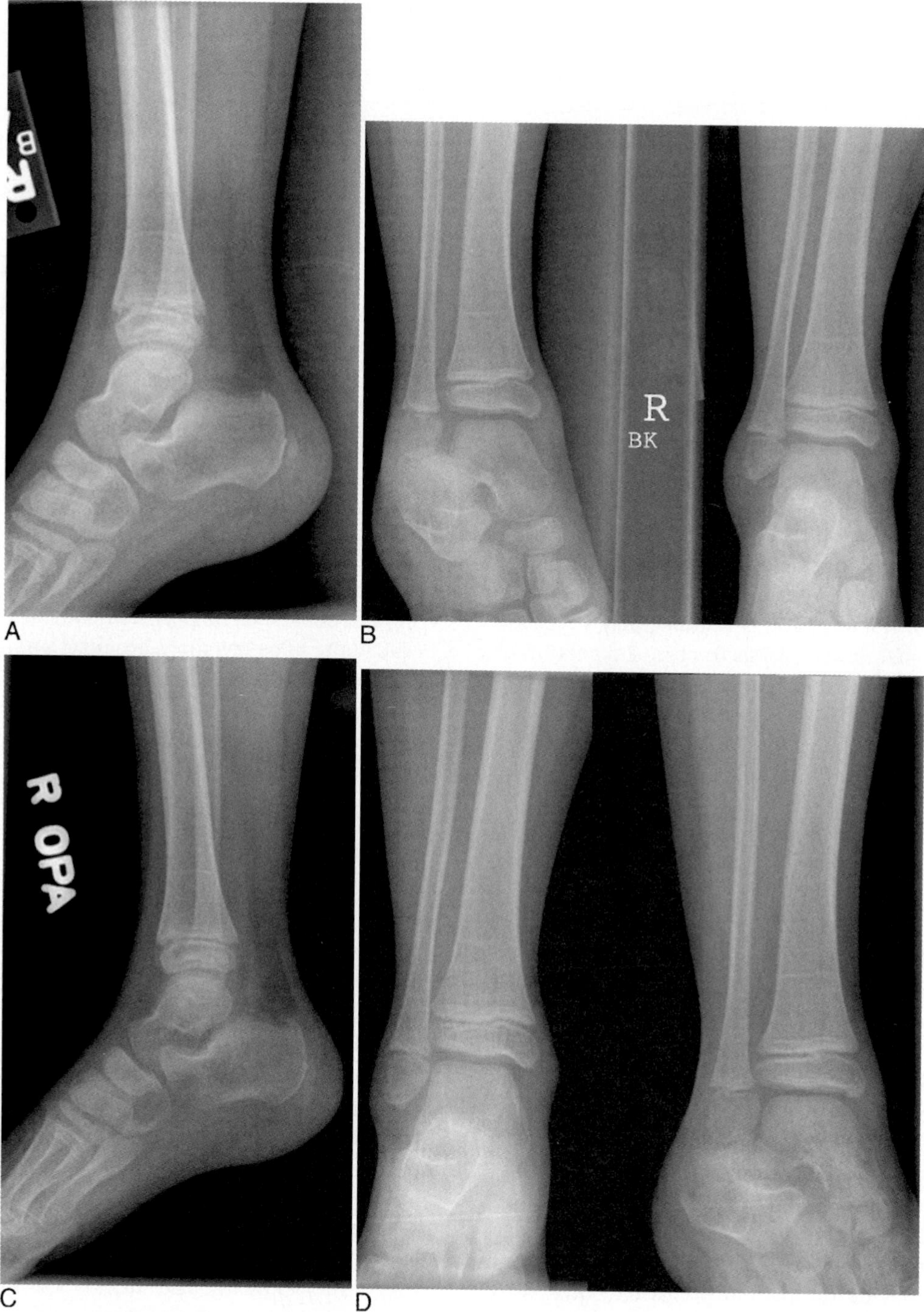

Figure 3-50 Salter-Harris type I fracture of the distal fibula physis. A 7-year-old girl sustained a twisting injury to her ankle and had swelling and tenderness over the lateral malleolus. **A** to **D,** Radiographs showed a large soft-tissue swelling over the distal fibula.

Fractures of the Calcaneus

Fractures of the calcaneus are less common in children than in adults.[38] Although most calcaneal fractures in children are isolated injuries, associated injuries, including spinal fractures, have been reported in up to a third of cases; a careful evaluation for associated injuries must be made in children with calcaneal fractures.

Treatment of calcaneal fracture varies with fracture extension and displacement. Nondisplaced or minimally displaced fractures can be treated with above-knee casts and non-weight-bearing status for 4 to 6 weeks. Displaced fractures should be treated with closed or open reduction as needed, to restore the articular surface of the subtalar joint. Displaced fractures in adolescents are best treated as in adults, with open reduction and internal fixation. Most calcaneal fractures are accompanied by extensive soft tissue swelling, which should be controlled before definitive treatment is initiated.

Midfoot Fractures

Fractures of the navicular and cuboid also occur in children. Navicular fractures commonly are avulsion fractures that represent injury to the dorsal tarsal ligament. They can be successfully treated with cast immobilization. Occult fractures of the cuboid and navicular may also occur and can be diagnosed with a technetium bone scan. CT may also be useful in evaluating these injuries, because the fracture's patterns may not be readily visible on standard radiographs. Displaced fractures may need surgical reduction and stabilization.

Tarsometatarsal fractures (Lisfranc fractures) may occur in children.[39] They are best diagnosed from a combination of AP, lateral, and oblique radiographs as well as physical evidence of swelling and tenderness over the tarsometatarsal region. MRI may aid in the diagnosis. Treatment for these injuries consists of closed reduction for displaced injuries (with percutaneous pinning if unstable) along with non-weight-bearing in a short-leg cast.

Forefoot Fractures

Metatarsal fractures account for the majority of fractures in children. They usually result from direct injury and most commonly involve the second metatarsal. Most metatarsal fractures can be treated by closed methods with below-knee casts. Displaced fractures may require closed or open reduction with internal fixation. Percutaneous smooth Kirschner wires generally provide sufficient internal fixation for these injuries.

Multiple fractures and displaced fractures at the metatarsal base may be accompanied by large amounts of swelling. Vigilance for compartment syndrome of the foot must be maintained in these situations, and compartment pressures measured if indicated. The pressures in the central and intraosseous compartments of the foot should be measured, because these compartments are the most sensitive to increased pressure in a foot compartment syndrome.[40] Treatment for compartment syndrome of the foot consists of complete release of all the compartments in the foot followed by secondary closure or skin grafting.[40]

Phalangeal fractures also commonly occur in children. They can often be managed symptomatically with buddy taping and wearing of a hard-soled shoe. Open phalangeal fractures may require irrigation and débridement. Stabilization with smooth Kirschner wires may be needed for very unstable injuries. Stubbed-toe injuries of the great toe, with bleeding from the nail margin, may indicate an occult open fracture of the physis of the distal phalanx of the great toe. This fracture may result in osteomyelitis, so prophylactic antibiotics are recommended after this injury.

MAJOR POINTS

Children may sustain unique types of fractures: birth injuries, pathologic fractures, and child abuse injuries.

Fractures suggestive of intentional injury include femur fractures in non-ambulatory children, femur fractures in children less than age 2 years, and metaphyseal corner fractures.

Hip fractures in children historically have had high complication rates, including avascular necrosis and non-union. These complications can be minimized by following principles of anatomic reduction, stable internal fixation, and spica casting.

Femur fractures in children can usually be successfully treated by a variety of different means. In children less than 5 years of age, traction and/or spica casting is frequently successful. In children older than 5, operative means may be preferred. This can include flexible intermedullary nails, rigid intermedullary nails, external fixation, and plating. Complications can be avoided by preventing excessive femoral shortening as well as avoiding antegrade, femoral intermedullary nails in children with an open proximal femoral physis.

Fractures of the proximal tibial metaphysis may overgrow into valgus. Anatomic fracture reduction and anticipatory family counseling are helpful in the management of these injuries.

Tibial shaft fractures can largely be treated non-operatively. A high index of suspicion is required to rule out compartment syndrome in these injuries.

Physeal fractures about the ankle require accurate reduction to help minimize the incidence of secondary growth disturbance.

REFERENCES

1. American Academy of Orthopaedic Surgeons Bulletin. Available online at www.aaos.org/
2. King J: Analysis of 429 fractures in 189 battered children. J Pediatr Orthop 8:585-589, 1988.
3. Watts HG: Fractures of the pelvis in children. Orthop Clin North Am 7:615-624, 1976.

4. Metzmaker JN, Pappas AM: Avulsion fractures of the pelvis. Am J Sports Med 13:349-358, 1985.

5. Torode I, Zieg D: Pelvic fractures in children. J Pediatr Orthop 5:76-84, 1985.

6. Silber JS, Flynn JM: Changing patterns of pediatric pelvic fractures with skeletal maturation: Implications for classification and management. J Pediatr Orthop 22:22-26, 2002.

7. Hamilton PR, Broughton NS: Traumatic hip dislocation in childhood. J Pediatr Orthop 18:691-694, 1998.

8. Canale ST, Bourland WL: Fracture of the neck and intertrochanteric region of the femur in children. J Bone Joint Surg Am 59:431-443, 1977.

9. Flynn JM, Wong KL, Yeh GL, et al: Displaced fractures of the hip in children: Management by early operation and immobilisation in a hip spica cast. J Bone Joint Surg Br 84:108-112, 2002.

10. Chung SM: The arterial supply of the developing proximal end of the human femur. J Bone Joint Surg Am 58:961-970, 1976.

11. Hughes LO, Beaty JH: Fractures of the head and neck of the femur in children. J Bone Joint Surg Am 76:283-292, 1994.

12. Gray D: Trauma to the hip and femur in children. In Koval KJ (ed): Orthopaedic Knowledge Update 7. Rosemont, IL, American Academy of Orthopaedic Surgeons, 2002, pp 81-91.

13. Thomas SA, Rosenfield NS, Leventhal JM, et al: Long-bone fractures in young children: Distinguishing accidental injuries from child abuse. Pediatrics 88:471-476, 1991.

14. Lynch JM, Gardner MJ, Gains B: Hemodynamic significance of pediatric femur fractures. J Pediatr Surg 31:1358-1361, 1996.

15. Wright JG: The treatment of femoral shaft fractures in children: A systematic overview and critical appraisal of the literature. Can J Surg 43:180-189, 2000.

16. Infante AF Jr, Albert MC, Jennings WB, et al: Immediate hip spica casting for femur fractures in pediatric patients: A review of 175 patients. Clin Orthop 376:106-112, 2000.

17. Stannard JP, Christensen KP, Wilkins KE: Femur fractures in infants: A new therapeutic approach. J Pediatr Orthop 15:461-466, 1995.

18. Yue JJ, Churchill RS, Cooperman DR, et al: The floating knee in the pediatric patient: Nonoperative versus operative stabilization. Clin Orthop 376:124-136, 2000.

19. Thomson JD, Stricker SJ, Williams MM: Fractures of the distal femoral epiphyseal plate. J Pediatr Orthop 15: 474-478, 1995.

20. Riew KD, Sturm PF, Rosenbaum D, et al: Neurologic complications of pediatric femoral nailing. J Pediatr Orthop 16:606-612, 1996.

21. Maguire JK, Canale ST: Fractures of the patella in children and adolescents. J Pediatr Orthop 13:567-571, 1993.

22. Skak SV, Jensen TT, Poulsen TD, et al: Epidemiology of knee injuries in children. Acta Orthop Scand 58:78-81, 1987.

23. Smith JB: Knee instability after fractures of the intercondylar eminence of the tibia. J Pediatr Orthop 4: 462-464, 1984.

24. McLennan JG: The role of arthroscopic surgery in the treatment of fractures of the intercondylar eminence of the tibia. J Bone Joint Surg Br 64:477-480, 1982.

25. Lowe J, Chaimsky G, Freedman A, et al: The anatomy of tibial eminence fractures: Arthroscopic observations following failed closed reduction. J Bone Joint Surg Am 84:1933-1938, 2002.

26. Baxter MP, Wiley JJ: Fractures of the tibial spine in children: An evaluation of knee stability. J Bone Joint Surg Br 70:228-230, 1988.

27. Janarv PM, Westblad P, Johansson C, et al: Long-term follow-up of anterior tibial spine fractures in children. J Pediatr Orthop 15:63-68, 1995.

28. Jordan SE, Alonso JE, Cook FF: The etiology of valgus angulation after metaphyseal fractures of the tibia in children. J Pediatr Orthop 7:450-457, 1987.

29. Zionts LE, Harcke HT, Brooks KM, et al: Posttraumatic tibia valga: A case demonstrating asymmetric activity at the proximal growth plate on technetium bone scan. J Pediatr Orthop 7:458-362, 1987.

30. McCarthy JJ, Kim DH, Eilert RE: Posttraumatic genu valgum: Operative versus nonoperative treatment. J Pediatr Orthop 18:518-521, 1998.

31. Shannak AO: Tibial fractures in children: Follow-up study. J Pediatr Orthop 8:306-310, 1988.

32. Navascues JA, Gonzalez-Lopez JL, Lopez-Valverde S, et al: Premature physeal closure after tibial diaphyseal fractures in adolescents. J Pediatr Orthop 20:193-1916, 2000.

33. Halsey MF, Finzel KC, Carrion WV, et al: Toddler's fracture: Presumptive diagnosis and treatment. J Pediatr Orthop 21:152-156, 2001.

34. Kling TF Jr, Bright RW, Hensinger RN: Distal tibial physeal fractures in children that may require open reduction J Bone Joint Surg Am 66:647-657, 1984.

35. Berson L, Davidson RS, Dormans JP, et al: Growth disturbances after distal tibial physeal fractures. Foot Ankle Int 21:54-58, 2000.

36. Kirkpatrick DP, Hunter RE, Janes PC, et al: The snowboarder's foot and ankle. Am J Sports Med 26:271-277, 1998.

37. Letts RM, Gibeault D: Fractures of the neck of the talus in children. Foot Ankle 1:74-77, 1980.

38. Matteri RE, Frymoyer JW: Fracture of the calcaneus in young children: Report of three cases. J Bone Joint Surg Am 55:1091-1094, 1973.

39. Wiley JJ: Tarso-metatarsal joint injuries in children. J Pediatr Orthop 1:255-260, 1981.

40. Silas SI, Herzenberg JE, Myerson MS, et al: Compartment syndrome of the foot in children. J Bone Joint Surg Am 77:356-361, 1995.

CHAPTER 4

Musculoskeletal Infection

LAWSON A. B. COPLEY
JOHN P. DORMANS

Infections of the musculoskeletal system in children comprise a broad spectrum of disorders that vary greatly in severity and complexity. At their simplest, these conditions are easily recognized and respond well to existing treatments with complete resolution. Unfortunately, circumstances commonly arise that may produce confusion in the diagnostic and treatment process, resulting in delayed treatment and adverse sequelae. Appropriate and timely evaluation may yield an accurate diagnosis and enable prompt treatment to improve outcomes, even in sequela-prone children. This chapter reviews the essential clinical, radiographic, and laboratory features of musculoskeletal infections in children and provides guidance on the fundamentals of medical and surgical management.

DEFINITIONS AND EPIDEMIOLOGY

Simply defined, *osteomyelitis* is an infection of bone, whereas *septic arthritis* is an infection of a joint. Most cases of these conditions occur from hematogenous inoculation via the metaphyseal circulation or the synovium. However, direct inoculation from penetrating trauma or surgical procedures may also initiate the process (Fig. 4-1). The vast majority of these infections are bacterial, with *Staphylococcus aureus* currently isolated as the most common causative organism in all age categories. Other organisms commonly involved in pediatric musculoskeletal infections are listed in Table 4-1.

In general, septic arthritis occurs about twice as often as osteomyelitis. A retrospective review at a large, tertiary-care medical center in Dallas found 471 cases of septic arthritis and 276 cases of osteomyelitis over a period of 26 years.[1] The evolving nature of these conditions, however, makes it difficult to establish a lasting epidemiology for geographic areas or time periods. The incidence of a specific organism as a cause of infection may be significantly altered with the advent of an immunization,

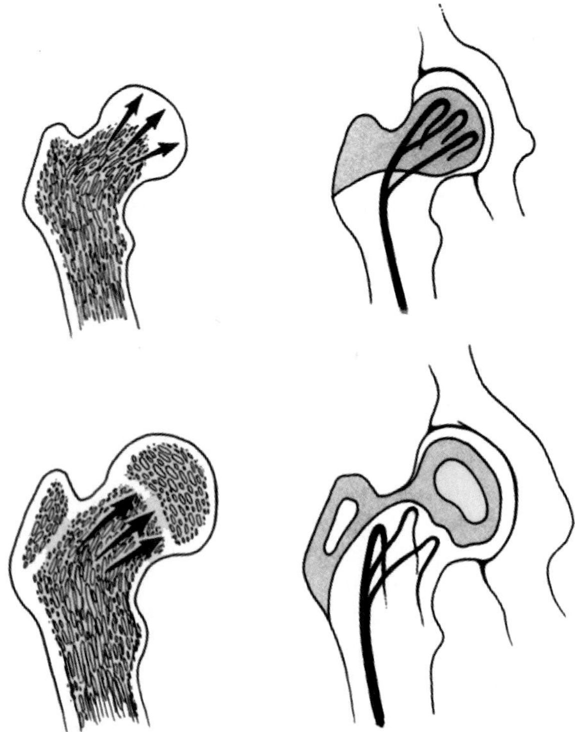

Figure 4-1 Relationship of metaphyseal and epiphyseal circulation in children younger than 18 months (*top*) versus children older than 18 months (*bottom*). (From Dormans, JP, Drummond DS: Pediatric hematogenous osteomyelitis: New trends in presentation, diagnosis, and treatment. J Am Acad Orthop Surg 2:333-341, 1994.)

as occurred with *Haemophilus influenzae*, type b, during the 1990s.[2] Other organisms might be found to have a rising incidence, as was seen with *Kingella kingae* and *Mycobacterium tuberculosis* during the late 1980s and early 1990s.[3,4]

The peak incidence of joint infections occurs during the first 5 years of life, whereas that for bone infections occurs between the ages of 5 and 10 years. The majority of cases of septic arthritis involve a single joint, most commonly the knee or hip, followed in frequency by the ankle and elbow. The metaphyses of the femur, tibia, and humerus are the most common locations of bone infection, followed by the fibula, radius, and calcaneus. However, any bone or joint may be subject to infection, which may pose a diagnostic challenge in locations like the spine and pelvis.

Occasionally there may be simultaneous infection of a bone and its adjacent joint. This situation has been thought to occur more frequently in children younger than 18 months, in whom the metaphyseal circulation is in continuity with the epiphyseal circulation (Fig. 4-2). There also appears to be a predisposition for adjacent joint infection to occur in locations in which the metaphysis of a long bone is located in an intra-articular or intracapsular location, such as the hip, ankle, and shoulder. A 2000 report identified the knee as the most common site of concurrent bone and joint involvement (31%); other principal sites are the hip (23%), ankle (18%), and shoulder (14%).[5] The reported incidence of simultaneous bone and joint infection ranges from 20% to 33% of osteoarticular infections.[5,6] Unfortunately, it is often difficult to distinguish these cases from cases of isolated septic arthritis. One study found that patients with simultaneous bone and joint infections tended to be younger, symptomatic for more than 7 days, and more likely to have received antibiotics before symptoms appeared.[6] Sequelae occurred more often in this population (62% versus 20%).[6]

EVALUATION

Clinical

The importance of obtaining a complete history and physical examination is unfortunately often overshadowed

Table 4-1 Common Causative Organisms and Empiric Antibiotic Selection for Septic Arthritis or Osteomyelitis According to Age

Age	Organism(s)	Empiric Antibiotic (Intravenous Administration)
Neonate (up to 8 weeks)	*Staphylococcus aureus, Streptococcus* sp, *Staphylococcus epidermidis, Enterococcus, Escherichia coli, Salmonella* sp, *Neisseria gonorrhoeae*	Nafcillin and gentamicin *OR* cefotaxime
Infant and Child (<3 years)	*S. aureus, Kingella kingae, Streptococcus pneumoniae,* group A streptococci	Nafcillin, oxacillin, clindamycin, or cefazolin If not immunized for *Haemophilus influenzae,* type b: cefuroxime
Children (>3 years)	*S. aureus,* group A streptococci	Nafcillin, oxacillin, clindamycin, or cefazolin
	Pseudomonas aeruginosa (foot puncture)	Ceftazidime
	Salmonella sp Sickle Cell Disease (SSD)	Cefuroxime
Adolescents	*S. aureus*	Nafcillin, oxacillin, clindamycin, or cefazolin
	N. gonorrhoeae (sexually active)	Ceftriaxone or cefotaxime

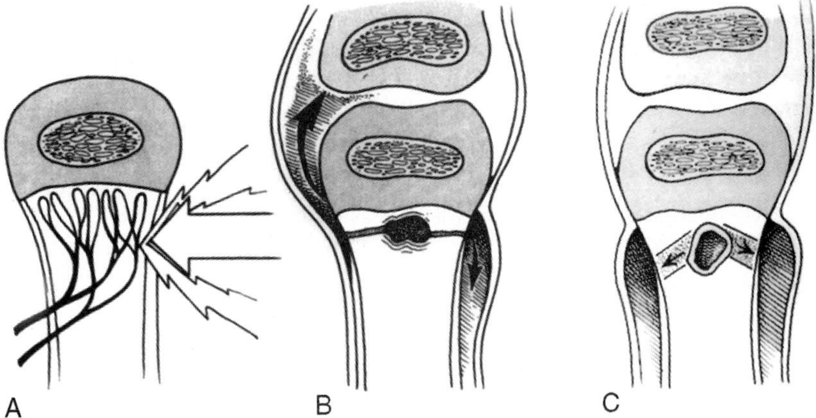

Figure 4-2 Pathophysiology of pediatric musculoskeletal infection via metaphyseal loops or direct inoculation **(A)**, contiguous spread to the adjacent joint **(B)**, and the development of subperiosteal abscess **(C)**. (From Dormans, JP, Drummond DS: Pediatric hematogenous osteomyelitis: New trends in presentation, diagnosis, and treatment. J Am Acad Orthop Surg 2:333-341, 1994.)

by the limited ability of small children to communicate and the urge to rely on laboratory or radiologic data to establish a diagnosis. However, the clinical examination and history remain paramount in the evaluation process. Frightened children can be examined on their parents' laps to reduce anxiety. The examination should be started in a location far from the suspected area of involvement, leaving the tenderest region as the last area examined. When necessary, the physician should leave the child alone with the parents after demonstrating to the parents how to elicit focal points of tenderness or limitation of joint motion. Once the child has calmed down in the absence of strangers, the parents may be better able to establish the most likely region of involvement. This knowledge is important in determining which radiologic studies will be most helpful to making the correct diagnosis.

The following aspects of the history are relevant: time of onset, nature and location of symptoms, presence of constitutional symptoms, recent infection or treatment with antibiotics, refusal to walk or bear weight, trauma, foreign travel, known recent or remote exposure to infectious disease (tuberculosis, varicella virus, Lyme disease, "strep throat"), arthralgias or myalgias, rash, subcutaneous nodules or swollen lymph nodes, and morning stiffness. Relevant physical findings that should be sought include focal tenderness, warmth, erythema, swelling, limited range of motion, pseudoparalysis, limp, synovitis, rash, and joint effusion. Even in the absence of concrete physical evidence, infection must be maintained in the differential diagnosis for children presenting with musculoskeletal pain, which may be the only symptom in subacute cases.

Laboratory

Laboratory studies are extremely useful in establishing the diagnosis of musculoskeletal infection as well as tracking the response to treatment and following the course of recovery. The studies that should be obtained initially are a complete blood count (CBC) with differential leukocyte count, measurements of erythrocyte sedimentation rate (ESR) and serum C-reactive protein (CRP) levels, and blood cultures. Other studies that may be considered when the clinical history or physical examination raises concern are listed in Table 4-2 along with the indications for ordering them.

In isolation, the white blood cell (WBC) count is a relatively poor indicator of acute hematogenous osteomyelitis (AHO), with only 25% to 35% of children showing an elevated WBC count at the time of admission.[7,8] However, the CBC with differential leukocyte count is essential during initial testing to establish a baseline as well as to look for evidence of systemic sepsis. If leukemia is considered a possible diagnosis on the basis of leukocytosis or leukopenia, anemia and thrombocytopenia, a manual inspection of the peripheral blood smear for blast cells in the circulation should be requested.

The ESR measures the rate at which erythrocytes fall through plasma. This rate principally depends on the concentration of fibrinogen but may also be increased by the presence of other acute-phase reactants found in the serum. Elevation of the ESR is a nonspecific finding in a variety of inflammatory conditions. In response to infection, however, the peak ESR has been shown to occur within 3 to 5 days of the onset with a mean peak value of 58 mm/hr.[4] This rate slowly returns to normal over approximately 3 weeks. The ESR should not be significantly elevated in response to trauma, stress reaction, or stress fracture.

Sequential determination of the serum CRP value is perhaps the most important laboratory test in the evaluation and treatment of musculoskeletal infection. C-reactive protein is an acute-phase protein synthesized by the liver in response to bacterial infection. Its serum level begins to rise within 6 hours of the triggering stimulus and increases several hundred-fold, reaching a peak within 36 to 50 hours of onset. One study showed that CRP values were elevated in 98% of children with AHO at the time

Table 4-2 Indications for Selected Additional Studies in the Evaluation for Infection

Additional Studies	Indications
Anti-streptolysin O, anti-DNAase B, or Streptozyme® test or throat swab test for group A streptococci	History of recurrent or untreated *Streptococcus* infections, migratory arthritis, arthralgias, myalgias, scarlatiniform rash
Enzyme-linked immunosorbent assay (ELISA) for Lyme antibody titer Western blot test (immunoglobulins G, M)	History of erythema chromicum migrans rash > 5 cm in diameter; tick bite; cardiac, neurologic, or orthopaedic manifestations; or travel to or residence in northeast, mid-Atlantic, and north-central United States (outdoor activity)
Antinuclear antibody (ANA) test, blood urea nitrogen (BUN) or creatine measurement, urinalysis; referral to ophthalmologist if ANA result is positive	Morning stiffness, rash, oligoarticular arthritis
HLA B-27 test	Spine stiffness and pain; sacroiliac inflammation; enthesopathy
Purified protein derivative skin test, chest radiograph	Exposure to tuberculosis or constitutional symptoms (night sweats, weight loss, fever)
Coagulation studies, liver function tests, and measurements of electrolytes, BUN/creatinine, fibrin split products, and fibrinogen	Shock, sepsis, evidence of multisystem involvement
Manual inspection of peripheral blood smear, bone marrow biopsy	Pancytopenia, leukocytosis, constitutional symptoms
Measurements of albumin, total protein, and fibrinogen, total lymphocyte count, human immunodeficiency virus test	Chronic osteomyelitis, unusual opportunistic infections, tuberculosis

of admission, with a mean value of 71 mg/L and a peak of 83 mg/L reached on day 2.[4] Because of the short half-life of CRP (47 hours), the rapid resolution to normal commonly occurs within 7 days in uncomplicated cases. One study found that serial CRP determinations combined with clinical evaluations were helpful in the detection of sequela-prone children.[8] Most of the sequelae occurred in children in whom serum CRP values remained significantly higher during the first 4 to 6 days of treatment than the mean CRP value in children without sequelae.[8]

The serum CRP level is easy to assess with a readily available laboratory nephelometer or turbidimeter and a finger-prick blood sample, and results are reported in less than an hour.[7] Consideration should therefore be given to daily or every-other-day serum CRP determinations during the early part of the illness and treatment. Serum CRP should also be monitored during the follow-up period, because a secondary rise is a warning sign of recurrent infection. Unfortunately, serum CRP may also be elevated as a result of bacterial or viral otitis media, possibly obscuring the clinical evaluation process.

Blood culture results are positive in only 30% to 50% of cases of both septic arthritis and osteomyelitis. However, the studies are indispensable because they may render the only isolate of an organism and thus serve as a guide to treatment. It is preferable that no antibiotics be administered before proper culture specimens have been obtained.

Aspiration

Aspiration has the greatest yield for diagnosis in cases of suspected septic arthritis. However, the technique is also potentially useful in cases of osteomyelitis. Joint aspiration commonly yields a volume of fluid sufficient to determine a WBC count and differential calculation of percentages of polymorphonuclear (PMN) cells. Although there are exceptions, WBC counts higher than 80,000/mL with more than 75% PMN cells suggest infection, whereas those lower than 15,000/mL with less than 25% PMN cells suggest inflammation. Counts in between these values may represent infection or an inflammatory form of arthropathy such as juvenile idiopathic arthritis (JIA). If the volume of aspirate obtained is inadequate for determination of a cell count, it should be sent only for Gram stain, culture, and sensitivity testing—the most critical studies to perform on an aspirate because they increase the likelihood of isolating an organism.

In cases of suspected osteomyelitis, bone aspiration may provide the only means of obtaining a positive culture result and therefore should be considered before initiation of antibiotic therapy. Bone aspiration or its attempt does not appear to significantly affect subsequent nuclear medicine or magnetic resonance imaging (MRI) findings.

Aspiration can be performed safely with sterile technique and intravenous sedation. The skin should be prepared carefully with povidone-iodine or alcohol. An aspiration needle of adequate size (18 gauge) should be placed on a 10- or 20-cc syringe and advanced through the skin. The plunger should then be drawn back to create a vacuum that will be released when the needle encounters a fluid collection in the deep soft tissues, subperiosteal space, or bone. The needle can then be advanced slowly first to the periosteum and then to the outer bone cortex over the metaphysis of the bone at the point of maximum tenderness. Finally, the needle may be driven into the metaphyseal region of the bone with a twisting motion. Even if only a few drops of bloody fluid are obtained, they should be sent for culture and Gram stain testing. The acquisition of a large volume of purulent material may guide the decision for surgical débridement.

IMAGING

Plain Radiography

High-quality plain radiographs are essential in all cases of suspected musculoskeletal infection. At minimum, anteroposterior and lateral projections of both the involved and uninvolved extremities should be obtained with a technique that allows for visualization of the deep soft tissues (Fig. 4-3). These films should be inspected closely for evidence of lytic or sclerotic lesions of the bone, periosteal elevation or calcification, deep soft tissue swelling, osteopenia, disk space narrowing, tumor, and fracture. Deep soft tissue swelling is the first radiographic manifestation of musculoskeletal infection. Changes in the bone secondary to osteomyelitis may not occur for 1 or 2 weeks after the onset of infection. Classic late radiographic signs include resorption of bone and periosteal new bone formation. The greatest value of the initial plain radiographs is in ruling out obvious focal disease, such as fracture or tumor that might mimic infection.

Other radiology studies may be necessary in the pursuit of a diagnosis. However, these studies should be carefully considered in light of expense, delay of definitive treatment, possible requirement for sedation, radiation exposure, and likelihood of yielding an accurate diagnosis. The decision as to which study is most appropriate to the search for a suspected condition might be better made in consultation with the radiology staff of a given facility, who will be most familiar with their capabilities. This practice also can facilitate the interpretation of the chosen study because the radiologist will be better informed about the child's clinical history.

Ultrasonography

The usefulness of ultrasonography in evaluating bone and joint infections is often overlooked in light of the availability of nuclear medicine and MRI. The advantages of ultrasonography are low cost, absence of radiation exposure, noninvasive nature without the need for sedation, ability to detect and localize joint fluid for aspiration in the hip (Fig. 4-4), and ability to detect the early changes in the deep soft tissues in osteomyelitis. Ultrasonography is also useful in identifying abscess of the psoas muscle, which may have a confusing clinical picture.

The ultrasonographic features of osteomyelitis are deep soft tissue swelling, periosteal thickening, subperiosteal fluid collection, and cortical breach or destruction.[9] These findings, in this order, correspond roughly to the duration of infection. Ultrasonography may be used to guide aspiration of a subperiosteal collection or to follow its resolution with treatment.

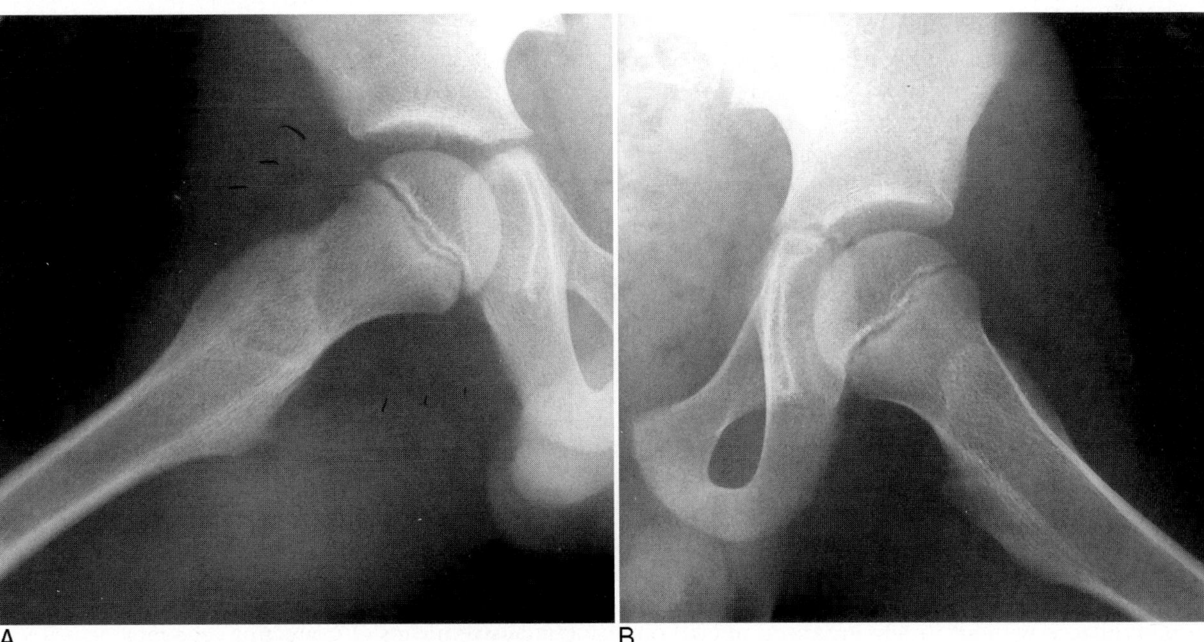

Figure 4-3 Lateral projections of the hips. A, Evidence of deep soft tissue swelling and capsular distention of the right hip. **B,** The left hip is unaffected.

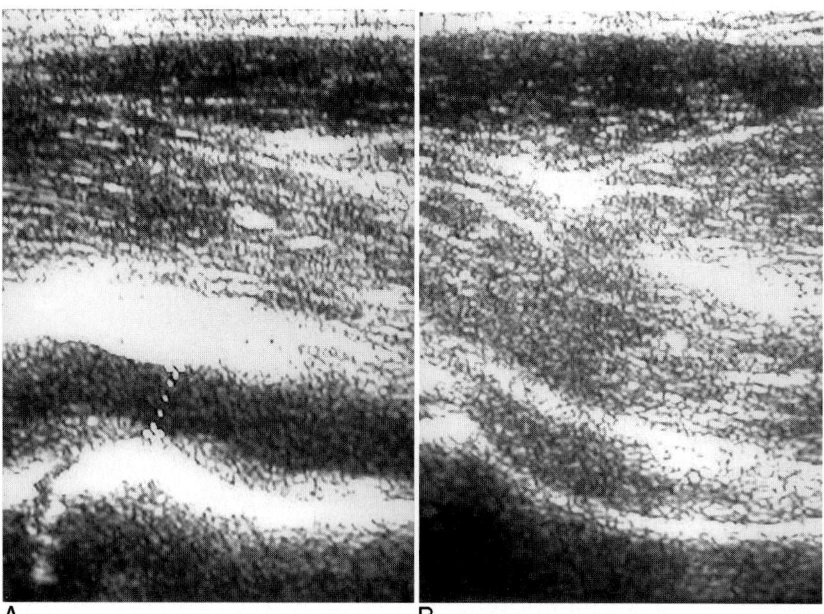

Figure 4-4 Hip ultrasonography scan in septic arthritis. Capsular thickening and joint effusion **(A)** are better appreciated when comparison is made with the unaffected hip **(B).**

Nuclear Medicine

Bone scintigraphy has several advantages over the cross-sectional imaging techniques of MRI and computed tomography (CT). It is less expensive, seldom requires sedation, and may provide evidence of multifocal osteomyelitis in neonatal infections. Technetium (^{99m}Tc) methylenediphosphonate scanning is one of the most commonly used techniques for evaluation of the skeleton for increased activity suggestive of infection. The study consists of the following three phases: (1) blood flow (essentially a radionuclide angiogram performed immediately after injection), (2) blood pool (performed after a brief period to evaluate soft tissue pooling), and (3) delayed images (performed 2 to 3 hours later to evaluate the calcium phosphate deposition in bone) (Fig. 4-5). Additional techniques are useful to differentiate the expected greater activity of the growth plate from the sometimes subtle early changes of the nearby metaphysis in cases of early osteomyelitis; they include pinhole collimation and converging collimation. Studies should be reviewed with an experienced radiologist who is familiar with the child's clinical history and skilled at the interpretation of nuclear imaging.

Generally, osteomyelitis is identified as focally increased radioactivity on all three phases of a nuclear medicine study. Cellulitis can be differentiated from osteomyelitis because cellulitis appears as diffusely increased soft tissue radioactivity on the blood flow and blood pool images without focally increased uptake on the delayed images. It may take more than 48 hours from onset for an infection to be detectable by bone scanning. A photopenic or cold bone scan (decreased uptake in bone on the delayed phase) may be obtained in approximately 8% to 20% of cases of osteomyelitis; it is thought by some physicians to be associated with a more aggressive type of infection resulting from compression of the microcirculation of the medullary canal with reduced blood flow.[10]

Properly performed with high-quality scintillation equipment, nuclear medicine studies have been reported to have a sensitivity approaching 100% for osteomyelitis,[10-12] although it may be as low as 54% to 72%.[10-12] Certain locations, such as the spine, pelvis, foot, and ankle, are more difficult to visualize with bone scans. These studies may also be difficult to interpret in neonates. The specificity of technetium bone scans for osteomyelitis is approximately 70% to 85%.[10-12] False-positive results are common because of various processes that result in greater vascularity or deposition of calcium phosphate in bone, such as tumors, stress fractures, and bone resorption due to disuse.

Septic arthritis is more difficult to diagnose with nuclear imaging. Expected findings are diffuse increased activity around a joint on the blood pool phase and either increased uptake on both sides of the joint (without focal uptake in bone) or photopenia in the epiphysis on the delayed phase. Unfortunately, the rates of false-positive results (32%) and false-negative results (30%) limit the value of this study in determining the significance of joint involvement.[12] Joint aspiration with Gram stain and culture of the fluid is a more direct and conclusive means of evaluating for septic arthritis.

Gallium (^{67}Ga) citrate scanning has been proposed as a useful adjunctive study for cases in which (1) the

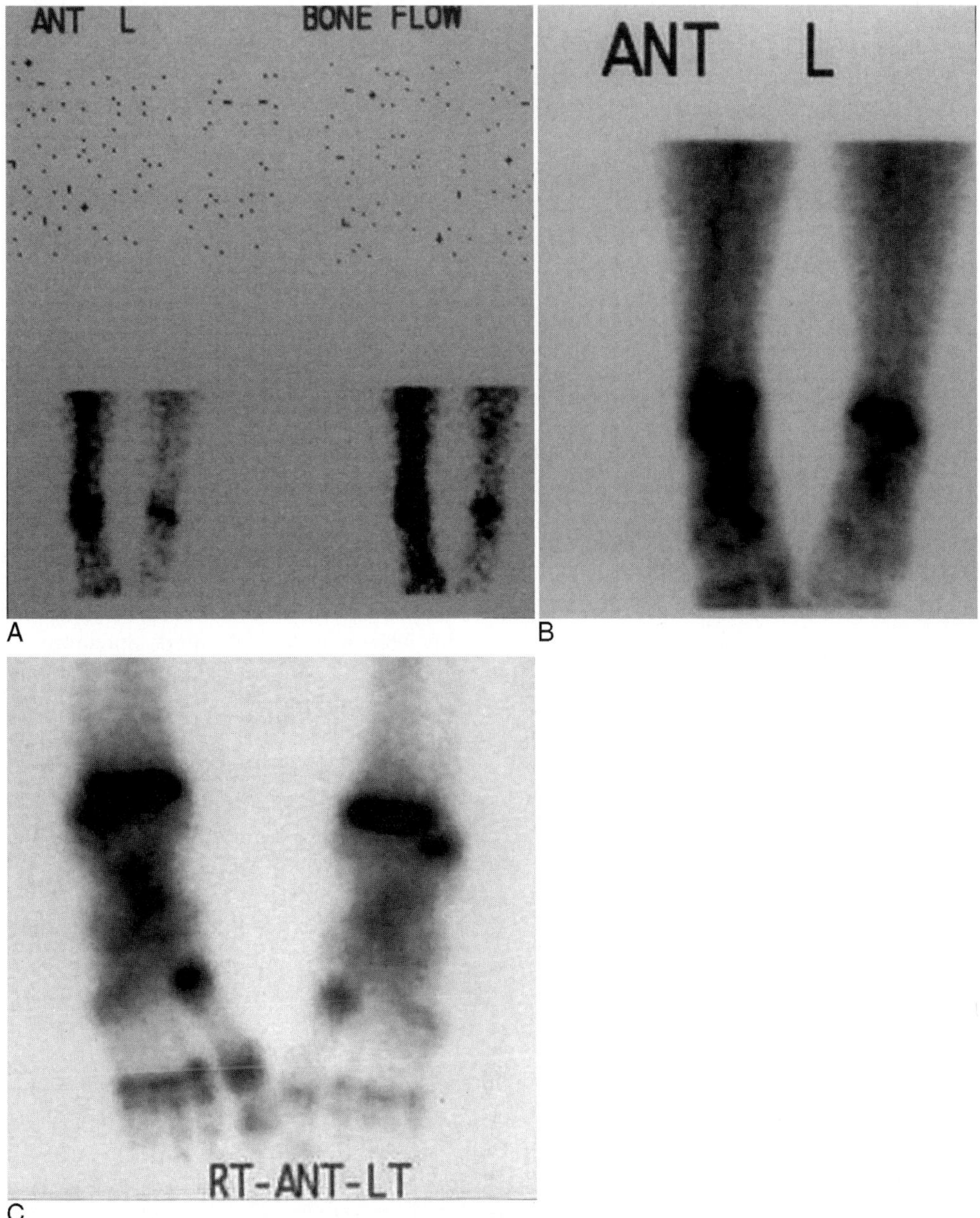

Figure 4-5 Three-phase bone scan in osteomyelitis of the fibula. Regional hyperemia on the blood flow phase **(A)** and soft tissue inflammation on the blood pool phase **(B)** are followed by focal uptake in the fibular metaphysic on the delayed images **(C)**.

technetium bone scan is normal but the clinical suspicion of osteomyelitis remains high or (2) the bone scan result is positive but an alternative cause of increased bone turnover or hyperemia exists.[11] Used in combination, technetium scanning and gallium scanning may help differentiate infarct from infection in children with sickle cell disease.[11] Because of the higher radiation dosage in gallium scanning, the technique is recommended only for cases in which the diagnosis cannot be made on the basis of clinical, laboratory, or plain radiographic criteria.

Magnetic Resonance Imaging

MRI is a powerful diagnostic tool for the evaluation of musculoskeletal infections. If not for its cost, requirement for monitored sedation in young children, and limited availability in small hospitals or rural settings, MRI would likely become the radiographic study of choice for evaluation of bone infection. In 1995, Mazur and colleagues[13] reported a sensitivity of 97% and a specificity of 92% for MRI ($1400 per study) compared with only

64% and 71%, respectively, for bone scanning ($450 per study).[13] MRI also has great utility in evaluation of the spine, shoulder girdle, or pelvis, providing high resolution and multiplane imaging in these areas, which are difficult to visualize.

Characteristics of infection seen on MRI include dark marrow on T1-weighted images and increased marrow signal intensity on T2-weighted images (Fig. 4-6). Abscess formation or subperiosteal fluid collections may also be identified as bright signals on T2-weighted images.[14] Unfortunately, a variety of field strengths and pulse sequences are frequently employed in an effort to reduce study time and cost. This practice occasionally obscures the image resolution and diminishes the specificity of the study. Another significant limitation of MRI is that up to 60% of uncomplicated septic joint effusions create abnormal marrow signal intensities that may be mistaken for adjacent osteomyelitis.[14]

OSTEOMYELITIS

Acute Hematogenous Osteomyelitis

Children with AHO, by definition, experience symptoms very quickly and are usually evaluated within the first several days of onset. The acute, focal bone pain is often, but not always, accompanied by systemic findings such as fever and malaise. The increase in awareness of this disease has resulted in earlier diagnosis of AHO, reducing the probability of sequelae when appropriate treatment is initiated. Children treated with high-dose intravenous antibiotics within 48 hours of the onset of symptoms are more likely to show a good response to nonoperative treatment than those who present more than 4 days after the onset of symptoms.

Osteomyelitis is a great imitator of other conditions leading to the acute onset of bone pain. Therefore, if a child's symptoms do not seem to respond as expected, it is especially important to consider the most relevant conditions in the differential diagnosis throughout the course of treatment. These conditions are trauma, leukemia, malignant tumors such as Ewing sarcoma and osteogenic sarcoma, and bone infarction from sickle cell crisis.

Subacute Osteomyelitis

Children with subacute osteomyelitis experience a gradual and insidious type of extremity pain without signs of systemic illness. At presentation, the pain has usually been present for at least 2 weeks and possibly for months. Laboratory test results are often unremarkable, although the ESR may be elevated. Subacute osteomyelitis is believed to result from an altered host-pathogen relationship, through either a decrease in bacterial virulence or an increase in host resistance. Alternatively, subacute osteomyelitis may be the result of partial treatment of a previously unrecognized case of AHO.

The diverse radiographic findings often present on initial studies have been used to establish methods of classification of subacute osteomyelitis. A commonly used classification, shown in Figure 4-7, divides the lesions according to location (epiphysis, metaphysis, or diaphysis)

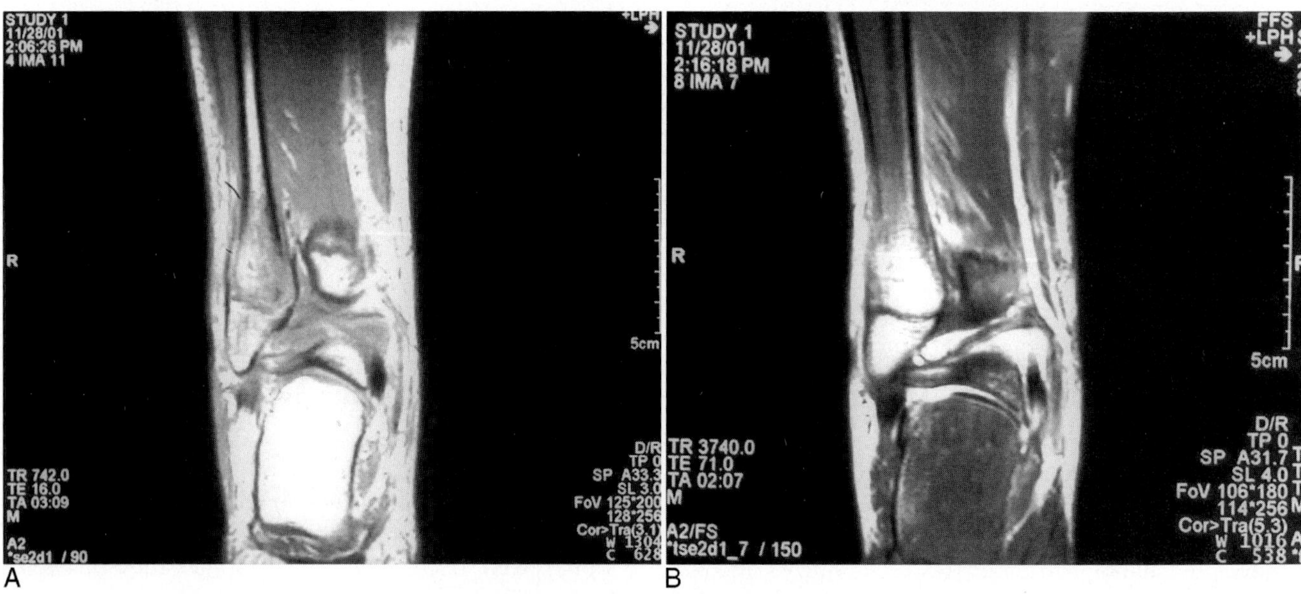

Figure 4-6 Magnetic resonance imaging findings in fibular osteomyelitis. Decreased marrow signal on T1-weighted image (**A**) with contrasting increased marrow signal on T2-weighted image (**B**).

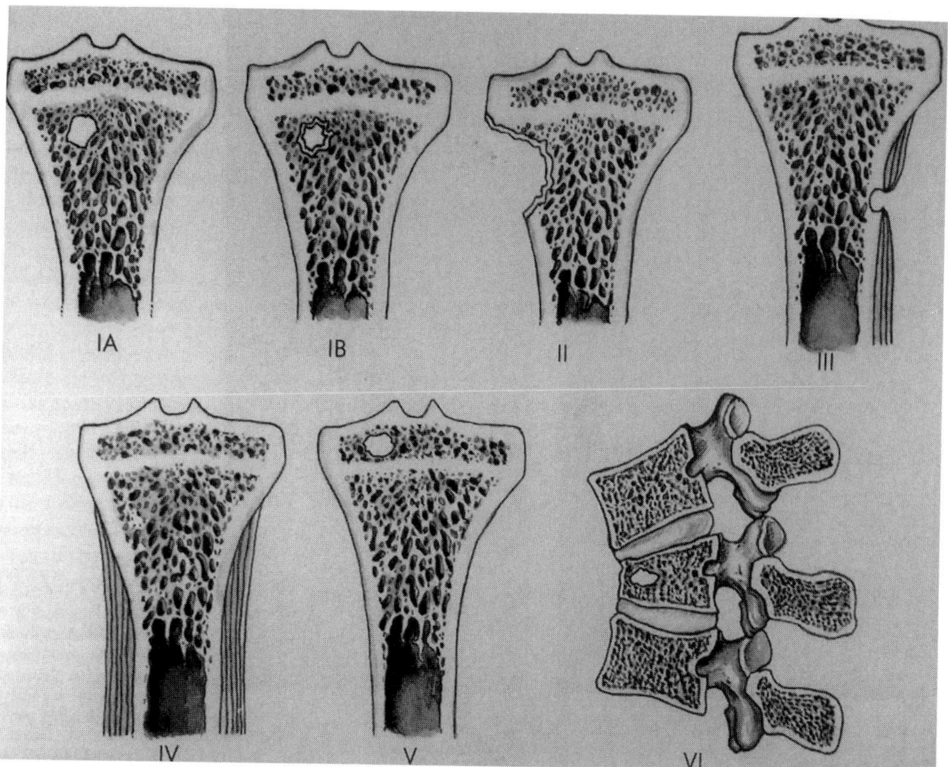

Figure 4-7 Classification of subacute osteomyelitis according to location (epiphysis, metaphysis, or diaphysis) and aggressive features (well-contained versus permeative or destructive). (From Roberts JM, Drummond DS, Breed AL, Chesney J: Subacute hematogenous osteomyelitis in children: A retrospective study. J Pediatr Orthop 2:249-254, 1982.)

and appearance (aggressive or benign).[15] The most important step in the correct treatment of this condition is to establish a differential diagnosis on the basis of clinical and radiographic features to determine the need for open biopsy. CT and MRI may help in questionable cases in which plain radiographic features suggest the malignant process of osteogenic sarcoma or Ewing sarcoma.

S. aureus is commonly cultured from the curettings from the lesions. The histologic features are often compatible with acute and chronic inflammation. Although surgical intervention has historically been preferred, Hamdy and associates[16] found that conservative management with antibiotics was successful in most cases. These investigators reserved surgery for cases either not responding to antibiotics or showing aggressive radiologic features.

Chronic Osteomyelitis

Chronic infections of the bone in children are rare in the United States because of the prompt recognition and treatment of AHO. Most often, chronic infections have been present for more than 6 weeks and have received varying degrees of treatment. The classic features of chronic osteomyelitis consist of the presence of dead bone (sequestrum) often surrounded by gross purulence and reactive new bone (involucrum). Draining sinuses may erupt as rapid expansion of infection erodes through overlying tissue planes.

The principles of treatment are surgical débridement of all necrotic tissue to leave behind viable bone and periosteum and identification of the causal organism to ensure that the most appropriate antibiotic is selected for long-term intravenous treatment. An infectious disease specialist should be consulted, and attention should be given to the nutritional status of the child to provide optimal conditions for healing and eradication of the infection. Serial surgical débridements may be necessary, and consideration may be given to temporary placement of antibiotic-impregnated cement beads to increase the antibiotic concentration in the immediate area of infection. Attempts to reconstruct bone and soft tissue deficiencies are usually made only after the infection has resolved.

Chronic Recurrent Multifocal Osteomyelitis

Chronic recurrent multifocal osteomyelitis (CRMO) is a condition of insidious onset involving multiple bone locations associated with pain and malaise. Association of CRMO with palmoplantar pustulosis has been reported. The radiographic features and histologic findings, if obtained, are suggestive of osteomyelitis. However, culture results for bone and blood are negative, and antibiotics have not been found to be necessary in treatment. Some investigators consider the condition to have an autoimmune inflammatory component and have demonstrated successful treatment with nonsteroidal anti-inflammatory medications or interferon-γ.[17] Overall, the disease is considered benign and self-limited. Proper treatment involves making the correct diagnosis without unnecessary biopsies, cultures, and surgical débridement and providing symptomatic support until the condition resolves.

SEPTIC ARTHRITIS

The major concern with septic arthritis is the potential destruction of joint cartilage from the occurrence of the exudate elicited by the presence of bacteria. A variety of proteolytic enzymes released from the WBCs and synovium begin the microscopic alteration of the joint surface in as few as 3 to 5 days. It is therefore imperative that an effort be made to reduce the joint leukocytosis as soon as possible after material has been obtained for Gram stain, culture, and sensitivity testing.

Serial aspirations of joints that are easily accessible (e.g., the knee) along with intravenous antibiotic therapy have been reported as successful and may be considered when it is not feasible to perform urgent surgery. However, most orthopaedic surgeons prefer open (or arthroscopic) joint irrigation and drainage. This procedure is a more reliable means of removing thickened or adherent exudates from the joint and allows the direct introduction of copious amounts of irrigant into the joint to quickly reduce the WBC and bacterial load. A drain may be left in place for 24 to 48 hours postoperatively to slow the reaccumulation of exudate in the joint space. Whether joint immobilization is necessary has not been clearly proven. Some children demonstrate such dramatic early restoration of joint mobility postoperatively that it is difficult to justify immobilization that may delay their recovery. Others have moderate discomfort from the surgical procedure itself and seem to benefit from a brief period of immobilization. However, it may be more difficult to evaluate clinical improvement if the joint has been immobilized.

In children in whom there is no clinical or laboratory evidence of improvement 48 hours after an initial joint irrigation and drainage procedure, a second procedure may be considered. Additionally, the possibility of adjacent osteomyelitis should be regarded as very strong. Because the duration of antibiotic treatment may be influenced by identification of a concurrent infection of bone and joint, supplemental imaging studies, such as MRI, may be indicated. Regardless, long-term radiographic and laboratory follow-up should be performed for all children with septic arthritis to ensure that sequelae are detected. Ideally, the patient should be seen weekly after discharge from the hospital, with serial serum CRP determinations to track resolution and identify recurrence. Plain radiographs and measurements of ESR and serum CRP levels should be obtained before antibiotics are discontinued at 4 weeks. This step might help identify a previously unrecognized osteomyelitis and avoid what would amount to partial treatment (sufficient for uncomplicated septic arthritis but not for osteomyelitis). It is not uncommon for the ESR to remain elevated at this time. However, it should be trending downward, and the CRP level should be normal.

TREATMENT

Delivery of the appropriate concentration of the correct antibiotic to the site of infection for long enough to completely eradicate the infection is the goal of treatment. Secondary considerations are cost, convenience to family and physician, and compliance. The protocols established to treat musculoskeletal infections has evolved rapidly in the past decade and vary significantly. Traditional use of 4 or 6 weeks of parenteral antibiotics for septic arthritis or osteomyelitis, respectively, has been commonly challenged to allow for less expensive and more convenient alternatives with equal efficacy.

Frequently, pediatric musculoskeletal infections are managed by different services within a multidisciplinary hospital, including pediatrics, infectious disease, and orthopedic surgery. Although consultation commonly includes more than one, if not all, of these groups, practice patterns and communication styles predispose to significant variability in treatment protocols within the same hospital. This fact makes it a challenge to ensure that patients with similar conditions are treated in the same manner so that outcomes can be properly assessed and treatment failures identified and understood. Under such circumstances, consideration should be given to establishing a multidisciplinary team with a unified protocol to evaluate and treat pediatric musculoskeletal infections.

Antibiotic

The importance of properly identifying the causative organism and its sensitivity to antibiotics through a diligent initial effort to obtain culture material is most evident in the selection of antibiotic. Although empiric selection can be relied on to adequately treat the most common organisms in each age category (see Table 4-1), there is obviously much greater confidence that the antibiotic selected has the appropriate spectrum of coverage if an organism is identified. The identification also reduces concerns that equivocal clinical or laboratory signs of improvement may be due to inappropriate antibiotic selection. Table 4-1 lists antibiotics commonly used for adequate empiric coverage of the expected organisms in osteomyelitis or septic arthritis according to age. An educated guess as to the causative organism, based on all of the clinical information, should be correct most of the time.

Specific antibiotic selection is determined from sensitivity data. An organism is considered susceptible to a given antibiotic if serial dilutions of the antibiotic in a ratio of 1:8 still demonstrate bactericidal properties.[18] The antibiotic with the narrowest spectrum of coverage capable of destroying the organism should be selected.

Route

Oral administration of an antibiotic is less expensive and more convenient than intravenous administration. However, although it is possible to establish adequate serum, bone, and joint bactericidal concentrations by oral means, several considerations may favor parenteral treatment. During the initial treatment period, when close monitoring of the clinical and laboratory parameters of response is necessary, intravenous delivery of antibiotics is essential. This route achieves the most immediate accumulation of antibiotics in the musculoskeletal tissues at the most critical time. Subsequently, the presence or absence of specific contraindications to oral therapy should be determined. They include, but are not limited to, uncertainty about the family's compliance with therapy, gastrointestinal disturbances that may affect absorption, and virulent or resistant organism strains that require greater degrees of confidence about treatment.

If there is any question about the efficacy of oral therapy, intravenous antibiotics should be continued. With current methods of peripheral intravenous catheter (PIC) placement, long-term antibiotic therapy at home is possible at a fraction of the cost of treatment in the hospital. A home health care team can directly monitor antibiotic therapy and the status of the intravenous site. Such a team can also periodically draw blood for laboratory studies so that results can be available at the time of follow-up appointments.

Conversion from parenteral to oral antibiotic therapy after resolution of the acute illness is safe and effective.[19] Some investigators recommend monitoring serum drug levels to maintain a peak serum bactericidal titer of at least 1:8 and a trough serum bactericidal titer of at least 1:2, to ensure adequate treatment during oral therapy.[18] Others have found this step to be unnecessary with appropriate use of high-dose oral antistaphylococcal agents in cases of culture-negative AHO.

Duration

Variation also exists as to the appropriate duration of treatment. Generally, joint infections require shorter treatment than bone infections. The possibility of a chronic bone infection necessitates a longer period to ensure eradication of disease. Generally, the duration of antibiotic therapy for uncomplicated osteomyelitis is approximately 6 weeks, and that for uncomplicated septic arthritis approximately 4 weeks.[1,19] Close monitoring of clinical signs and laboratory parameters during the treatment course, but especially near the end of treatment, is helpful in identifying patients who may benefit from longer treatment or a change in the regimen.

SURGERY

Surgery often plays a key role in the early treatment of septic arthritis. However, the role of surgery in osteomyelitis is less clear. Most cases in children respond well to medical treatment alone. One ultrasonography study found that subperiosteal elevations as great as 3 mm resolved completely with antibiotic treatment alone, a finding that questions the absolute necessity of surgical drainage when such a process is identified.[9] Most physicians would agree that in children with radiographically demonstrable deep soft tissue or intraosseous abscess formation, surgical decompression is necessary to allow for clinical and laboratory improvement and eventual resolution of the infection. Some would suggest that if significant improvement has not resulted within 48 hours, regardless of radiographic evidence of abscess, surgical exploration and decompression should be considered. Clearly, these decisions must be made on an individual basis, with all clinical, laboratory, and radiologic information for the patient taken into account. In borderline or complex cases, close communication should be established among the physician primarily responsible for the patient, the orthopaedic surgeon, the infectious disease specialist, and the radiologist, to enable objective and informed decisions to be made.

Generally, children older than 1 year who present within 48 hours of the onset of illness do well with antibiotic treatment alone. Infections in children older than 1 year who present 5 or more days after the onset of illness as well as in children younger than 1 year are more likely to need surgical drainage for resolution.[7,8]

SPECIAL CONSIDERATIONS

Neonatal and Infantile Infections

Although the neonatal period is defined as the first 4 weeks of life, the pathogenesis of neonatal infections extends over the first 8 weeks. The immaturity of the immune system during that period predisposes the neonate to infection by a wide range of organisms that are less virulent in other circumstances. Neonatal infection can be regarded as taking two distinct forms. The first occurs in premature infants, who spend substantial time in the intensive care unit in the presence of nosocomial pathogens while undergoing frequent invasive procedures (including umbilical vessel catheterization) for intravenous access, monitoring, and hyperalimentation. Almost half of infants demonstrating sepsis under these circumstances have multiple sites of infection. Therefore, a high index of suspicion should be maintained when there is any evidence of sepsis in the premature infant. Consideration should be given to evaluation of each hip, and any other suspicious joint, with ultrasonography or aspiration, because of the severe consequences of a missed infection and the lack of clear clinical, laboratory, and radiographic signs to indicate the foci of infection. Likely causative organisms are *S. aureus* and gram-negative bacteria. *Candida albicans* may also be involved in neonates undergoing prolonged broad-spectrum antibiotic treatment for sepsis.

The second form of neonatal infection occurs in term infants who have been routinely discharged from the hospital after delivery. Manifestation of their musculoskeletal infection usually occurs between 2 and 4 weeks of life but can occur up to 8 weeks after delivery. These infections are most commonly monoarticular and caused by group B *Streptococcus*.

Because of the immaturity of the immune system in neonates, signs and symptoms of infection are largely absent. Swelling, pseudoparalysis, and tenderness may be subtle. Radiographic and laboratory studies may offer little guidance because of the lack of inflammatory response to infection in such patients. Bone scans have been reported to yield positive findings in as few as 32% of cases of neonatal osteomyelitis.[11]

Selection of antibiotic should be carefully considered through close communication with an infectious disease specialist and a neonatal intensivist, especially for hospital-acquired sepsis. Blood culture results are positive in 50% of neonates with proven infection and may be the only indication of a specific organism. Empiric antibiotic selection should cover penicillin-resistant forms of *S. aureus*, group B *Streptococcus*, and gram-negative enteric organisms. Hepatic and renal function as well as body weight are important considerations in choosing the correct antibiotic and dose.

Sickle Cell Disease

Despite great concerns about the possibility of infection in children with sickle cell disease, the actual incidence of musculoskeletal involvement is quite low (0.2% to 5%).[20] The difficulty in differentiating the extremely common crises from infection on the basis of clinical, laboratory, and radiographic data has led to the frequent attention this issue has received in the literature. In one review of 2000 children with sickle cell disease, only 14 musculoskeletal infections (10 osteomyelitis, 4 septic arthritis) were identified over a 22-year period.[20] The majority of infections occurs in children who are homozygous for the hemoglobin S gene. Although *Streptococcus pneumoniae* is a common pathogen in children with sickle cell disease because of impaired splenic function, it is uncommon in bone and joint infections. The most common causative organisms are *Salmonella* species and *S. aureus*. Empiric antibiotic selection should cover both organisms until specific guidance from culture results is available. Cefotaxime or ceftriaxone is considered appropriate for this purpose.

The initial management of musculoskeletal pain in children with sickle cell disease should include oxygen, hydration, and analgesics. Failure to show improvement within 2 to 4 days, along with fever and the appearance of systemic illness, should elevate the possibility of infection as the underlying cause. Blood cultures and aspiration or open biopsy of the area of involvement are the next steps in the evaluation process, because these procedures have the highest diagnostic yields. One report found that 75% of tissue biopsy specimens and 70% of aspirates had positive results, compared with 58% of blood culture findings.[20] Antibiotics should be withheld until after all culture specimens have been obtained.

The expense, radiation exposure, and lack of proven efficacy of radionuclide scans should limit their use to those cases in which the diagnosis is still uncertain after these initial efforts of evaluation and treatment. In such cases, consideration should be given to combined technetium scanning and gallium scanning.[11] The expected finding in osteomyelitis is (1) decreased or normal uptake on technetium scan along with increased uptake on gallium scan in the same spatial distribution or (2) increased uptake on both scans in an incongruent spatial distribution.

SIGNIFICANT ORGANISMS

Group A Streptococci

Group A streptococci is responsible for several types of musculoskeletal infection in children. The most serious is a toxic shock–like syndrome characterized by severe local tissue destruction and life-threatening systemic manifestations. Musculoskeletal complaints have been noted in up to 87% of cases.[21] Affected children typically have a febrile and toxic presentation with evidence of multisystem disease (cardiac, hepatic, renal, central nervous system, hematologic, and musculoskeletal).[21] Aggressive resuscitation is necessary along with timely surgical decompression of foci of infection in the musculoskeletal system after a vigilant search for such sites. *Streptococcus pyogenes* may also cause osteomyelitis or septic arthritis via hematogenous inoculation in the absence of systemic shock.

Group A streptococcal pharyngitis may be followed by acute rheumatic fever (ARF) or, less commonly, by a post-streptococcal reactive arthritis (PSRA).[22] Although these forms of arthritis are not likely to be confused with bacterial infection of a joint, they should be included in the differential diagnosis of a warm, erythematous joint in children older than 4 years. Salicylates and antibiotic treatment and prophylaxis appear to have significant roles in the management and prevention of long-term sequelae in both ARF and PSRA.

The orthopedic manifestations of rheumatic fever classically include a migratory polyarthritis that usually affects the lower extremities first. The modified Jones criteria are useful in establishing a diagnosis. At least two major criteria (carditis, polyarthritis, subcutaneous nodules, erythema marginatum, and chorea) or one major and two minor criteria (fever, arthralgia, increased ESR or serum CRP levels, and prolonged PR interval on electrocardiogram) along with evidence of preceding streptococcal infection are necessary. Post-streptococcal reactive arthritis is believed to be a variant of ARF in which the Jones criteria are not otherwise satisfied. A 10-day course of an antistreptococcal antibiotic along with salicylate therapy until the arthralgias resolve serves as initial therapy.[22] Long-term prophylaxis is helpful in preventing recurrent streptococcal infections and reducing the likelihood of sequelae.

Kingella kingae

Within the past three decades, reports have surfaced of osteomyelitis and septic arthritis caused by *Kingella kingae*, a fastidious gram-negative diplococcus. In 1998, Lundy and Kehl[3] reported that 17% of the musculoskeletal infections in children younger than 3 years involved *K. kingae*, which replaced *H. influenzae* as the most common gram-negative organism in this age group. The natural habitat of *K. kingae* is the upper respiratory tract mucous membranes, and the suspected pathogenesis is hematologic dissemination. Growing awareness of the potential role of *K. kingae* in musculoskeletal infections in children younger than 3 years as well as recognition of the need for specific specimen acquisition methods and culture conditions may lead to better identification of this pathogen in osteomyelitis or septic arthritis.

Neisseria meningitidis

Although *Neisseria meningitidis* is not known for direct infection of the musculoskeletal system, it is significant as a causal organism in purpura fulminans, which has devastating musculoskeletal consequences. This disorder is characterized by the acute onset of progressive dermal vascular thrombosis, disseminated intravascular coagulation, and shock. The pathogenesis is described as a Shwartzman-like reaction provoked by the endotoxin from gram-negative bacteria. The peripheral cutaneous lesions are initially sterile, but they may become superinfected and gangrenous. The affected areas gradually heal with demarcation of the necrotic tissues followed by scarring and autoamputation.

Principles of treatment for purpura fulminans involve initial resuscitation efforts with appropriate antibiotics effective against the causal organism, which is *N. meningitidis* in the majority of cases. A third-generation cephalosporin, such as ceftriaxone, is usually effective. Aggressive fluid management, which is given in either an intensive care unit or burn center, may require pulmonary artery catheterization to monitor the delicate balance of the child's volume status. Fresh frozen plasma and vitamin K are used initially to correct possible deficiencies of coagulation factors, antithrombin III, protein C, and protein S. Early use of cardiac inotropic agents along with normalization of circulating protein C levels through the use of purified protein C concentrates have also been shown to improve outcomes.[23] Successful surgical reconstruction, which is often delayed until a clear demarcation between viable and nonviable tissues is apparent, requires a multidisciplinary team approach involving plastic and orthopaedic surgeons.

Streptococcus pneumoniae

Although more commonly associated with pneumonia or meningitis, *S. pneumoniae* has been reported in osteomyelitis and septic arthritis in children between the ages of 3 and 24 months. In one institution during a 15-year period, 23 of 184 children (13%) had musculoskeletal infections due to *S. pneumoniae*.[24] This group represented approximately 5% of those children hospitalized with a systemic pneumococcal infection during the same period. It was previously thought that these infections were indistinguishable from those caused by *H. influenzae*.[24] However, this situation has changed with the significant decrease in *H. influenzae* infections in the United States after the introduction of a conjugated vaccine in the 1990s.[2]

Pneumococcal infection has been identified as another cause of purpura fulminans in children.[25] Although *S. pneumoniae* is not an endotoxin-producing organism, the pneumococcal autolysin is thought to play this role.[25]

Neisseria gonorrhoeae

Pediatric patients are affected by gonococcal arthritis in the following three situations: (1) in a neonate passing through the birth canal of an infected mother, (2) through sexual abuse of a child or adolescent, and (3) in an adolescent who is sexually active. The onset of disseminated disease may occur anywhere from days to months after the initial infection. Commonly, dissemination is identified as polyarthritis involving the knee, ankle, or wrist. Associated findings are fever, chills, rash, and tenosynovitis of the dorsum of the hand.

When gonococcal infection is suspected, culture specimens should be obtained from the joint fluid, cervix of postpubertal girls, urethral or prostatic discharge of males, and also from the vagina, pharynx, and rectum in a child suspected to be a victim of sexual abuse. Because *Neisseria gonorrhoeae* is difficult to culture, special specimen handling instructions must be given to the laboratory to increase the potential of positively identifying the organism. Specific culture tubes for transport should be requested from the laboratory. Sterile culture specimens are plated on chocolate blood agar, and nonsterile culture specimens on Thayer-Martin medium, which contains antibiotics to inhibit growth of oropharyngeal and anorectal flora. Cultures of *N. gonorrhoeae* require a 5% to 10% carbon dioxide atmosphere. Gram staining may demonstrate intracellular gram-negative diplococci.

Treatment of gonococcal arthritis involves local aspiration and irrigation of the joint and intravenous administration of a third-generation cephalosporin (because of the prevalence of penicillin-resistant strains). The decision for surgical arthrotomy and drainage of a joint should be made for each patient. For infection of a hip joint or joints with large amounts of purulent material, open treatment may be required to facilitate rapid resolution.

Mycobacterium tuberculosis

Tuberculosis infections have been rising in incidence in the United States since 1985.[26] Extrapulmonary tuberculosis is more common in children younger than 5 years, occurring in approximately 5% to 10% of children with the disorder.[26] Osteomyelitis, dactylitis, or septic arthritis may take 1 to 3 years to manifest after the initial infection. More than half of all cases of tubercular osteomyelitis involve the spine, followed in incidence by infections around the hip and knee.

Spinal involvement usually occurs in the anterior third of the vertebral body. The lower thoracic and upper lumbar regions are commonly affected. The bone lesions are destructive, creating collapse and kyphosis when they progress. Paravertebral abscess and calcification are almost pathognomonic of spinal tuberculosis. Skeletal tuberculosis is associated with characteristic round cystic lesions in the epiphysis or metaphysis with centrifugal, ill-defined margins. The lack of sclerotic margins or periosteal response is a typical finding. The growth plate does not offer significant resistance to the spread of infection.

Diagnosis of *M. tuberculosis* infection of a joint or digit requires a high index of suspicion, with skin testing for tuberculosis using purified protein derivative and identification of the organism in culture material. Positive culture results can be obtained in approximately 80% of children with extrapulmonary disease.[26] The WBC count is frequently normal, but the ESR is often elevated.

Current recommendations for the treatment of skeletal tuberculosis call for four-drug therapy with isoniazid, rifampin, pyrazinamide, and streptomycin for 2 months followed by isoniazid and rifampin for 10 months. Surgical decompression of foci of infection is rarely necessary. Indications for spinal surgery include neurologic involvement, spinal instability, and failure of medical treatment. Surgical treatment for kyphotic deformity should be performed on a case-by-case basis. Some investigators have shown that surgical débridement combined with anterior strut grafting and posterior instrumentation leads to a higher union rate and less residual spinal deformity. The rising incidence of resistant strains due, in part, to inadequate treatment of the initial infection may serve to increase the need for surgical débridement in the future.

Borrelia burgdorferi (Lyme Disease)

Lyme disease, caused by the spirochete *Borrelia burgdorferi*, was named after the Connecticut town in which it was first identified. Most commonly it occurs in children in the northeast, mid-Atlantic, and north-central regions of the United States. The common vector is the deer tick. After inoculation, by means of a tick bite that may go unnoticed, the period before the appearance of systemic manifestations ranges from 2 to 30 days. The multisystem infection may be mistaken for juvenile arthritis or septic arthritis. However, the U. S. Centers for Disease Control and Prevention (CDC) have established diagnostic criteria helpful in making the correct diagnosis. They are the presence of a characteristic erythema migrans rash with a diameter of at least 5 cm and one cardiac, neurologic, or musculoskeletal manifestation of the disease. Laboratory testing utilizes the immunoglobulin (Ig) M enzyme-linked immunosorbent assay (ELISA), but the result may not be positive for the first 3 to 6 weeks of infection. All positive or equivocal results must be confirmed with a Western blot test. During the first 4 weeks of suspected infection, both the IgM and IgG Western blot procedures should be used.

The treatment of Lyme disease initially consists of 10 to 30 days of oral antibiotics (amoxicillin or doxycycline). In patients with severe neurologic or cardiac manifestations or recurrence after oral therapy, 14 to 28 days of intravenous ceftriaxone may be necessary.

A post–Lyme disease syndrome, consisting of recurrent arthralgias, myalgias, headache, neck pain, and fatigue, has been described. Treatment with antibiotics is controversial, and spontaneous resolution within 6 months is common. Overdiagnosis of Lyme disease, due to the inordinate attention that this condition has received in the media, is a significant problem. Therefore, a careful evaluation should proceed according to CDC recommendations.

CHALLENGING LOCATIONS

Spine

With the use of modern imaging techniques, particularly MRI, the continuity of discitis and vertebral osteomyelitis is more clearly understood. Although this condition is classically described as a refusal to walk associated with back pain, the presentation is found in fewer than 50% of children and adolescents.[27] An insidious onset is typical, with minimal signs or symptoms of infection. Older adolescents may even present with abdominal pain or poor appetite. Results of laboratory and plain radiographic studies may be equivocal, with the exception of elevations of ESR and serum CRP. As a result, delay in diagnosis is not uncommon.[27]

Supplemental studies that may help locate the specific site of disease and differentiate infection from tumor or fracture are single-photon emission computed tomography (SPECT), CT, and MRI. Resolution of SPECT is superior to that of technetium scanning in the spine. MRI offers the greatest amount of information to aid in this process.[13] Destruction of bone or marrow edema located in adjacent vertebrae with involvement of one or two disk spaces suggests infection. A larger amount of destruction of adjacent vertebrae, which would likely be visible on plain radiographs, is suggestive of tuberculosis.[26] The differential diagnosis of vertebral collapse includes eosinophilic granuloma, Ewing sarcoma, osteogenic sarcoma, and leukemia. In these conditions, the disk spaces remain unaffected, a feature that differentiates these disorders from infection.

Because of the morbidity risk of open spine biopsy to obtain culture specimens, the procedure is rarely considered necessary. Blood cultures should be performed, but have less yield than those obtained to evaluate infection in the extremities. Because *S. aureus* is the most likely causative organism, empiric therapy consists of a semisynthetic penicillin or first-generation cephalosporin for 4 weeks. Initial parenteral therapy may be switched to the oral route after adequate clinical and laboratory evidence of improvement (usually 4 to 7 days). Bracing is usually unnecessary. Destructive lesions, which are nevertheless rare, may require structural support to prevent kyphosis from vertebral collapse until some reconstitution of vertebral height occurs. Studies have now suggested that the long-term effect of infection and its sequela on the disk space is that of persistent narrowing or fusion rather than restitution. Children with persistent radiographic changes have been more prone to backache. It is relevant to inform the child's family of this possibility at the initiation of treatment.

Pelvis

Another common site of diagnostic dilemmas and delay is the pelvis, which may be involved in approximately 6% of pediatric musculoskeletal infections.[28] The wide variety of symptoms, equivocal nature of physical findings, and negative findings of routine radiographs often lead to uncertainty of diagnosis. Laboratory indices of infection may be only mildly elevated. The most important step in the evaluation process is to maintain an open mind and include pelvic osteomyelitis and sacroiliac septic arthritis in the differential diagnosis for children or adolescents who present with hip, lumbosacral, buttock, or abdominal pain. A thorough examination involves palpation of the pelvic crests, spines, tuberosities, and rami; range-of-motion testing of both hips consisting of flexion, abduction, and external rotation (FABER); and inspection of gait. A rectal examination may be necessary to test for tenderness along the inner margins of the pelvis or sacrum. CT or MRI is useful to evaluate these areas with greater resolution than that of plain radiographs.[13] As in the spine, when nuclear imaging is considered, SPECT is the procedure of choice.

Most cases respond to antibiotic treatment alone. Although surgery was considered necessary in 24% of patients in one series involving 82 pelvic infections,[28] later experience suggests that nonsurgical management is effective in the majority of cases. The fact that *S. aureus* is the most common organism should guide empiric treatment if blood culture results are negative (50%). *Salmonella* is not uncommon and may be cultured from the stool, if it is regarded as a possible pathogen.[28] Initial parenteral antibiotic treatment may be switched to oral therapy when the serum CRP begins to fall and the clinical findings improve (usually 4 to 7 days). The duration of treatment is 6 weeks.

Abscess of the psoas muscle is another condition engendering diagnostic uncertainty, because it may mimic a variety of conditions—septic arthritis of the hip, pelvic infection, appendicitis, and spinal infection. Although rare, psoas abscess should be included in the differential diagnosis for children and adolescents with vague abdominal, genitourinary, spinal, or hip complaints accompanied by laboratory evidence of infection. Although there are no consistently unique features of psoas abscess allowing for diagnosis, femoral nerve dysfunction and elevation of serum creatinine kinase levels may guide the diagnostic process to performance of ultrasonography or CT of the region (Fig. 4-8).[29]

Once psoas abscess has been identified, the treatment involves open débridement or ultrasound-guided needle aspiration and placement of a drain (see Fig. 4-8). Antibiotics can be selected on the basis of culture result. However, empiric therapy should be effective against *S. aureus* because it is the most common causative organism.

Foot

The two types of foot infections that are clinically important are puncture wounds of the foot and hematogenous calcaneal osteomyelitis. Although puncture wounds are extremely common in children, development of osteomyelitis or septic arthritis as a result of such wounds is extremely rare (<1%). The majority of children with early evidence of a soft tissue infection (cellulitis) experience prompt resolution with soaks, rest, elevation, and oral antistaphylococcal antibiotics. The rare child in whom osteomyelitis or septic arthritis ultimately develops most likely has sustained a deep penetration of the bone or joint. When such an infection does occur, *Pseudomonas aeruginosa* is the most likely cultured organism.

A reasonable protocol for management of nail puncture wounds consists of initial superficial cleansing, tetanus prophylaxis, radiographs to ensure the absence of retained foreign body, and recommendation for rest and elevation with close outpatient follow-up after counseling about the signs and symptoms of infection. With established infection, an attempt at antistaphylococcal antibiotic treatment under close observation is reasonable as long as there is no clinical or radiographic evidence of a deep infection of the bone or joint. Children with a deep infection that does not respond to an intravenous antipseudomonal antibiotic should undergo surgical exploration for irrigation and débridement. Change of therapy to an oral fluoroquinolone antibiotic, such as ciprofloxacin, may be considered after clinical and laboratory signs of improvement. Studies have now suggested that, when necessary, ciprofloxacin may be safely used in the pediatric population without the concern about cartilage toxicity previously observed experimentally in animals.[30]

Hematogenous calcaneal osteomyelitis is responsible for up to 8% of bone infections in children.[31] The significance of this condition is found in the diagnostic challenge it poses. A variety of other common childhood conditions may mimic calcaneal infection, such as stress fracture, contusion, apophysitis, and enthesopathy. The clinical and laboratory findings can be less dramatic than those seen in long bone infections, leading to delay of treatment and adverse sequelae. The universal site of involvement is the metaphyseal-equivalent portion of the posterior tuberosity (Fig. 4-9).[31] The alteration of the apophyseal plate in this region may result in growth arrest with secondary deformity and loss of calcaneal length.[31]

A high index of suspicion should be maintained about focal heel pain in a child with elevation of ESR or serum CRP. MRI may be useful as the diagnostic study of choice to identify an infection as well as evaluate for

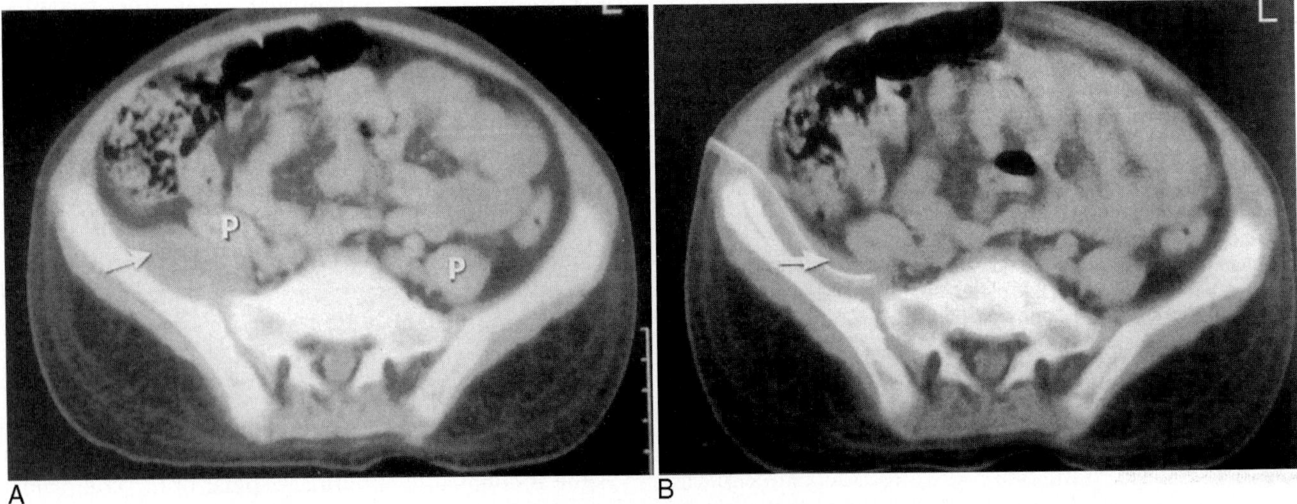

Figure 4-8 Psoas abscess **(A)** and result of percutaneous drainage guided by computed tomography **(B).** (From Herring JA [ed]: Tachdjian's Pediatric Orthopaedics, vol 3, 3rd ed. Philadelphia, WB Saunders, 2002, pp 1841-1877.)

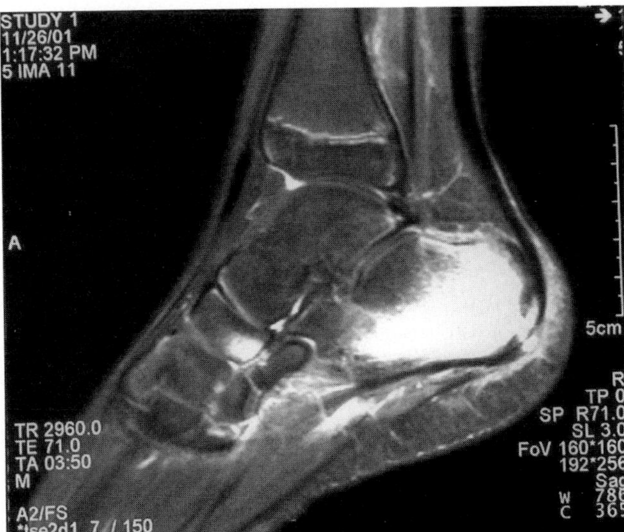

Figure 4-9 Typical appearance of hematogenous calcaneal osteomyelitis in the metaphyseal region of the posterior tuberosity.

intraosseous abscess formation that may require surgical decompression (see Fig. 4-7).[13,31] *S. aureus* is the most common organism, and empiric antibiotic therapy should be chosen accordingly. Most children seen within 48 hours of the onset of symptoms have good response to medical treatment alone. Sixty percent to 75% of those who present more than 5 days after onset of symptoms require surgical decompression.[31] Aspiration should be performed in cases that do not respond to antibiotics after 24 to 48 hours. The duration of antibiotic treatment is 6 weeks, with a change from intravenous to oral therapy considered after clinical and laboratory evidence of improvement has been obtained.

SUMMARY

Pediatric musculoskeletal infections are associated with a diverse presentation ranging in spectrum from obvious and acute to insidious and chronic. Thorough history and physical examination, supplemented by appropriately selected radiographic and laboratory studies, should result in a timely and correct diagnosis in most cases. Every effort should be made to properly identify the causative organism by obtaining blood cultures and aspirating the involved bone and joint. A high index of suspicion for musculoskeletal infection must be maintained in the neonate as well as in the child who has vague complaints associated with the spine, pelvis, or foot. Vigilant evaluation in these circumstances likely reduces diagnostic delay and avoids adverse sequelae.

MAJOR POINTS

Staphylococcus aureus remains the most common causative organism in musculoskeletal infection for all age categories.

The incidence of simultaneous osteomyelitis and septic arthritis is 20% to 33% of osteoarticular infections.

The white blood cell (WBC) count may be elevated in only 25% to 35% of children with osteomyelitis.

The peak erythrocyte sedimentation rate (ESR) occurs within 3 to 5 days of the onset of infection and slowly returns to normal over approximately 3 weeks.

The serum C-reactive protein (CRP) level begins to rise within 6 hours of the onset of infection, peaking at 36 to 50 hours and resolving within 7 days.

Blood cultures should be obtained whenever infection is suspected.

Antibiotics should not be administered until after proper culture specimens have been obtained.

A joint aspirate with a WBC count greater than 80,000/mL and more than 75% polymorphonuclear (PMN) leukocytes suggests infection.

Deep soft tissue swelling is the first radiographic manifestation of musculoskeletal infection.

Magnetic resonance imaging (MRI) has great utility in evaluation of areas that often obscure the diagnosis of infection, such as the spine, pelvis, and shoulder girdle.

Children with acute hematogenous osteomyelitis (AHO) who are treated within 48 hours of symptom onset respond better to nonoperative treatment than those who present longer than 4 days after the onset of symptoms.

Every reasonable effort should be made to identify a causative organism, and antibiotic selection should be directed to an agent with the narrowest spectrum of coverage and bactericidal properties against the specific organism.

The pathogenesis of neonatal infections extends over the first 8 weeks of life.

Bone scans yield positive results in as few as 32% of cases of neonatal osteomyelitis.

Group A streptococci may cause a life-threatening systemic illness, with musculoskeletal involvement in up to 87% of cases.

Although puncture wounds of the foot are extremely common in children, osteomyelitis and septic arthritis rarely occur (<1%).

REFERENCES

1. Jackson MA, Nelson JD: Etiology and medical management of acute suppurative bone and joint infections in pediatric patients. J Pediatr Orthop 2:313-323, 1982.

2. Bowerman SG, Green NE, Mencio GA: Decline of bone and joint infections attributable to *Haemophilus influenzae* type b. Clin Orthop 341:128-133, 1997.
3. Lundy DW, Kehl DK: Increasing prevalence of *Kingella kingae* in osteoarticular infections in young children. J Pediatr Orthop 18:262-267, 1998.
4. Unkila-Kallio L, Kallio MJT, Eskola J, Peltola H: Serum C-reactive protein, erythrocyte sedimentation rate, and white blood cell count in acute hematogenous osteomyelitis of children. Pediatrics 93:59-62, 1994.
5. Perlman MH, Patzakis MJ, Kumar PJ, Holtom P: The incidence of joint involvement with adjacent osteomyelitis in pediatric patients. J Pediatr Orthop 20:40-43, 2000.
6. Jackson MA, Burry VF, Olson LC: Pyogenic arthritis associated with adjacent osteomyelitis: Identification of the sequela-prone child. Pediatr Infect Dis J 11:9-13, 1992.
7. Roine I, Arguedas A, Faingezicht I, Rodriguez F: Early detection of sequela-prone osteomyelitis in children with use of simple clinical and laboratory criteria. Clin Infect Dis 24:849-853, 1997.
8. Unkila-Kallio L, Kallio MJT, Peltola H: The usefulness of C-reactive protein levels in the identification of concurrent septic arthritis in children who have acute hematogenous osteomyelitis. J Bone Joint Surg 76A:848-853, 1994.
9. Mah ET, LeQuesne GW, Gent RJ, Paterson DC: Ultrasonic features of acute osteomyelitis in children. J Bone Joint Surg 76B:969-974, 1994.
10. Pennington WT, Mott MP, Thometz JG, et al: Photopenic bone scan osteomyelitis: A clinical perspective. J Pediatr Orthop 19:695-698, 1999.
11. Lewin JS, Rosenfield NS, Hoffer PB, Downing D: Acute osteomyelitis in children: Combined Tc-99m and Ga-67 imaging. Pediatr Radiol 158:795-804, 1986.
12. Sundberg SB, Savage JP, Foster BK: Technetium phosphate bone scan in the diagnosis of septic arthritis in childhood. J Pediatr Orthop 9:579-585, 1989.
13. Mazur JM, Ross G, Cummings RJ, et al: Usefulness of magnetic resonance imaging for the diagnosis of acute musculoskeletal infections in children. J Pediatr Orthop 15:144-147, 1995.
14. Erdman WA, Tamburro F, Jayson HT, et al: Osteomyelitis: Characteristics and pitfalls of diagnosis with MR imaging. Radiology 180:533-539, 1991.
15. Roberts JM, Drummond DS, Breed AL, Chesney J: Subacute hematogenous osteomyelitis in children: A retrospective study. J Pediatr Orthop 2:249-254, 1982.
16. Hamdy RC, Lawton L, Carey T, et al: Subacute hematogenous osteomyelitis: Are biopsy and surgery always indicated? J Pediatr Orthop 16:220-223, 1996.
17. Gallagher KT, Roberts RL, MacFarlane JA, Stiehm ER: Treatment of chronic recurrent multifocal osteomyelitis with interferon gamma. J Pediatr 131:470-472, 1997.
18. Marshall GS, Mudido P, Rabalais GP, Adams G: Organism isolation and serum bactericidal titers in oral antibiotic therapy for pediatric osteomyelitis. South Med J 89:68-70, 1996.
19. Kim HKW, Alman B, Cole WG: A shortened course of parenteral antibiotic therapy in the management of acute septic arthritis of the hip. J Pediatr Orthop 20:44-47, 2000.
20. Chambers JB, Forsythe DA, Bertrand SL, et al: Retrospective review of osteoarticular infections in a pediatric sickle cell age group. J Pediatr Orthop 20:682-685, 2000.
21. Jackson MA, Burry VF, Olson LC: Multisystem group A β-hemolytic streptococcal disease in children. Rev Infect Dis 13:783-788, 1991.
22. Moon RY, Greene MG, Rehe GT, Katona IM: Poststreptococcal reactive arthritis in children: A potential predecessor of rheumatic heart disease. J Rheumatol 22:529-532, 1995.
23. White B, Livingstone W, Murphy C, et al: An open-label study of the role of adjuvant hemostatic support with protein C replacement therapy in purpura fulminans-associated meningococcemia. Blood 96:3719-3723, 2000.
24. Jacobs NM: Pneumococcal osteomyelitis and arthritis in children. Am J Dis Child 145:70-74, 1991.
25. Cnota JF, Barton LL, Rhee KH: Purpura fulminans associated with *Streptococcus pneumoniae* infection in a child. Pediatr Emerg Care 15:187-188, 1999.
26. Vohra R, Kang H, Dogra S, et al: Tuberculous osteomyelitis. J Bone Joint Surg 79B:562-566, 1997.
27. Song KS, Ogden JA, Ganey T, Guidera KJ: Contiguous discitis and osteomyelitis in children. J Pediatr Orthop 17:470-477, 1997.
28. Mustafa MM, Saez-Llorens X, McCracken GH, Nelson JD: Acute hematogenous pelvic osteomyelitis in infants and children. Pediatr Infect Dis J 9:416-421, 1990.
29. Song J, Letts M, Monson R: Differentiation of psoas muscle abscess from septic arthritis of the hip in children. Clin Orthop 391:258-265, 2001.
30. Redmond AO: Risk-benefit experience of ciprofloxacin use in pediatric patients in the United Kingdom. Pediatr Infect Dis J 16:147, 1997.
31. Jaakkola J, Kehl D: Hematogenous calcaneal osteomyelitis in children. J Pediatr Orthop 19:699-704, 1999.

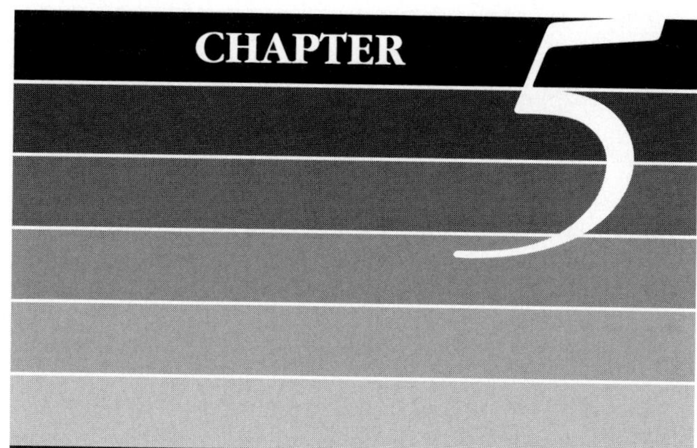

Skeletal Dysplasias and Metabolic Disorders of Bone

BULENT EROL
JOHN P. DORMANS
LISA STATES
FREDERICK S. KAPLAN

SKELETAL DYSPLASIAS

The *skeletal dysplasias*, also known as *osteochondrodysplasias*, are a group of genetic disorders characterized by generalized disorders of growth and development of bone and cartilage. About 200 conditions are recognized to date. The skeletal dysplasias are rare; for both lethal and nonlethal forms, the incidence is about five affected fetuses in 10,000 pregnancies. Generalized disturbances in the development of the skeleton affect the skull, spine, and extremities to varying extents. There are often abnormalities in the facial structures. The resulting alterations in the size and shape of the limbs and trunk are frequently associated with disproportionate short stature (*dwarfism*). Disproportionate short stature is characteristic of the skeletal dysplasias, a feature differentiating these conditions from endocrine (e.g., absence of growth hormone) and metabolic (e.g., rickets) disorders that cause proportionate short stature.

Dwarfing conditions are frequently referred to as *short-limb* or *short-trunk dysplasias*, according to whether trunk or limbs are more extensively involved (Box 5-1). In short-limb dysplasias, the extremities are disproportionately short compared with the trunk. In contrast, short-trunk dysplasias produce greater shortening of the spine relative to the limbs. Disproportionate involvement of the trunk is known as *microcormia*. Disproportionate involvement of the limbs is known as *micromelia*. Micromelia divides into the following subtypes according to the segment of the limb with the greatest involvement: rhizomelic (proximal), mesomelic (middle), and acromelic (distal); these terms refer to the arm, forearm, and hand or to the thigh, leg, and foot, respectively.

Box 5-1 Dwarfing (Disproportionate Short Stature) Conditions in Skeletal Dysplasias

- Short-limb dwarfism—micromelia
  - Rhizomelia; proximal segment (arm, thigh)
  - Mesomelia; middle segment (forearm, leg)
  - Acromelia; distal segment (hand, foot)
- Short-trunk dwarfism—microcormia

The diversity of the skeletal dysplasias and the heterogeneity that may exist within a specific disorder have made classification difficult. These disorders have been classified according to the pattern of bone involvement, as in the International Classification of Osteochondrodysplasias (Box 5-2).[1] The newer trend, however, is to group them according to the specific causative protein, enzyme, or gene defect, if known (Box 5-3). Management of the skeletal dysplasias involves accurate genetic counseling as well as the recognition and treatment of musculoskeletal abnormalities and associated intrinsic medical problems.

Achondroplasia

Achondroplasia is the most common form of short-limb dwarfism, with an estimated prevalence of approximately 1 in 30,000 to 1 in 50,000.[2] It is characterized by disproportionate short-limb rhizomelic dysplasia. Achondroplasia is an autosomal dominant condition, although two thirds of cases arise from spontaneous new mutations. The mutation of achondroplasia, an activating missense mutation in the gene encoding fibroblast growth factor receptor 3 (FGFR3), is the most common single-point mutation in the human genome.[3] The mutation has been mapped to chromosome 4. Normally, the FGFR3 gene is expressed in articular chondrocytes, and the gene product functions to restrain cell division in the proliferative cells of the growth plate. The activating mutations in the FGFR3 gene lead to further retardation of cell division in the proliferative zone of the growth plates, resulting in phenotypic features of achondroplasia. The primary defect is abnormal endochondral bone

Box 5-2 International Classification of Skeletal Dysplasias, 1992 (A Partial List)

A. Defects of the tubular bones and flat bones and axial skeleton
  - Achondroplasia group
    - Achondroplasia
    - Hypochondroplasia
    - Thanatrophic dysplasia
  - Metatropic dysplasia group
  - Atelosteogenesis/diastrophic dysplasia group
  - Osteogenesis imperfecta
  - Kniest-Stickler dysplasia group
  - Spondyloepiphyseal dysplasia congenita group
  - Other spondyloepi-(meta)-physeal dysplasias group
    - X-linked spondyloepiphyseal dysplasia tarda
    - Pseudoachondroplasia
  - Dysostosis multiplex group
    - Mucopolysaccharidoses
    - Mucolipidoses
  - Epiphyseal dysplasias
    - Multiple epiphyseal dysplasia
  - Chondrodysplasia punctata
  - Metaphyseal dysplasias
  - Mesomelic dysplasias
    - Dyschondrosteosis
  - Dysplasias with significant (but not exclusive) membranous bone involvement
    - Cleidocranial dysplasia
  - Multiple dislocations with dysplasias
    - Larsen syndrome
  - Dysplasias with decreased bone density
    - Osteogenesis imperfecta (several types)
    - Idiopathic juvenile osteoporosis
  - Dysplasias with defective mineralization
    - Hypophosphatasia
    - Hypophosphatemic rickets
  - Dysplasias with increased bone density

B. Disorganized development of cartilaginous and fibrous components of the skeleton
  - Dysplasia epiphysealis hemimelica
  - Hereditary multiple exostoses
  - Enchondromatosis
  - Fibrous dysplasia

C. Idiopathic osteolyses

Box 5-3 Classification of Skeletal Dysplasias Based on Etiology

- Fibroblast growth factor receptor-3 (FGFR3) group (local regulator of cartilage growth)
  - Achondroplasia
  - Hypochondroplasia
  - Thanatophoric dysplasia
- Sulfate transporter protein group (sulfate transportation)
  - Diastrophic dysplasia
- COL2A1 group (type II collagen, structural cartilage protein)
  - Kniest syndrome
  - Spondyloepiphyseal dysplasia congenita
- Collagen oligomeric matrix protein (COMP) group (structural cartilage protein)
  - Pseudoachondroplasia
  - Multiple epiphyseal dysplasia
- Storage disorders
  - Mucopolysaccharidoses
  - Mucolipidoses
- COL1A1 group (type I collagen, structural osseous protein)
  - Osteogenesis imperfecta

formation. Periosteal and intramembranous ossification processes are normal. The risk of having a child with achondroplasia rises with paternal age.

Clinical Findings

Achondroplasia is recognizable at birth as a disproportionate short-limbed rhizomelic dysplasia. The trunk length is normal, but the limbs are short (Fig. 5-1). Developmental motor milestones are frequently delayed, although normal motor coordination is achieved in later childhood, with independent ambulation typically occurring at 18 to 24 months.[4]

Frontal bossing, flattening of the nasal bridge, and midface hypoplasia are typical facial features of children with achondroplasia (see Fig. 5-1).[5] The digits of the hand have extra space between the third and fourth rays, so the digits are separated into three groups—the "trident hand." Elbow flexion contracture or radial head dislocation may occur. Kyphosis at the thoracolumbar junction may be seen in infancy. This kyphosis improves spontaneously with independent ambulation. Ligamentous laxity is present in achondroplastic patients, leading to external rotation of the lower limbs and genu recurvatum in infancy. Genu varum occurs in some patients after they begin walking.

Radiographic Features

Foramen magnum stenosis, common because of disproportionate growth of the chondrocranium and neurocranium, is measured most accurately on computed tomography (CT) or magnetic resonance imaging (MRI) (Fig. 5-2). There is distinct narrowing of the interpedicular

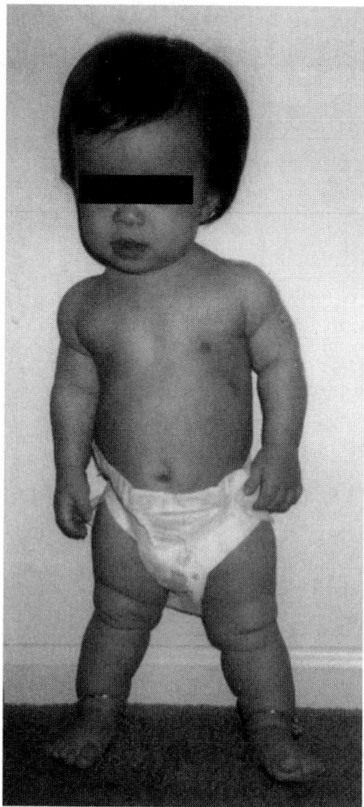

Figure 5-1 An 18-month-old girl with achondroplasia. The trunk length is normal, but the proximal segments of the limbs are short (rhizomelic pattern). The elbows have a mild flexion contracture. Note the typical facial features: frontal bossing, flattening of the nasal bridge, and midface hypoplasia.

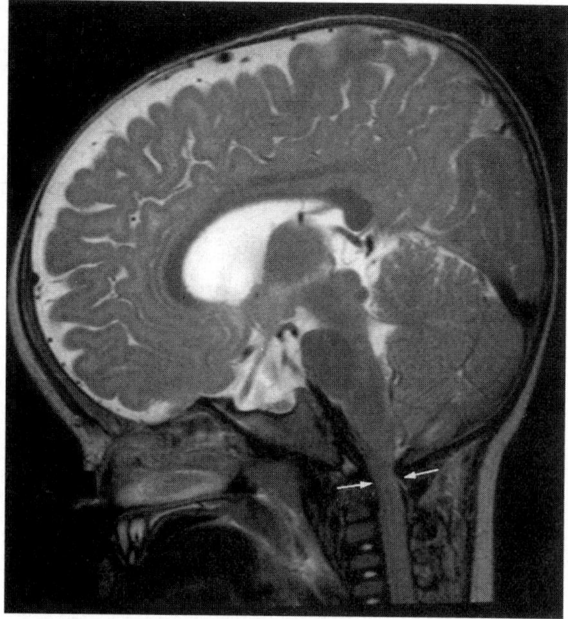

Figure 5-2 Magnetic resonance image of a 6-month-old child with achondroplasia shows the characteristic narrow foramen magnum *(arrows)*.

distances from upper to lower lumbar spine. Before walking age, a kyphosis at the thoracolumbar junction may be seen (Table 5-1). The pelvis is typically broad and short, and the ilium has a square appearance. The acetabular roof is horizontal, and the femoral heads are well covered. The long bones are short and thick with metaphyseal flaring. Angulations at both the distal femoral and proximal tibial metaphyses contribute to varus alignment of the knee (Fig. 5-3).

Medical Problems

Obesity typically begins in early childhood and is a lifelong problem for people who have achondroplasia.[4] Frequent ear infections occur secondary to underdevelopment of the midfacial skeleton. These recurrent infections may lead to hearing loss. The chest wall diameter is narrowed in achondroplasia, so pulmonary function, particularly vital capacity, is reduced. Narrowing of the foramen magnum is a typical problem in the first several

Table 5-1 Spinal Abnormalities Seen in Various Skeletal Dysplasias

Dysplasia	Cervical Spine	Thoracolumbar Spine
Achondroplasia	Foramen magnum stenosis	Stenosis; kyphosis at the thoracolumbar junction
Metatropic dysplasia	Atlantoaxial instability	Kyphosis; scoliosis
Diastrophic dysplasia	Cervical kyphosis	Kyphosis; scoliosis
Kniest syndrome	Atlantoaxial instability	Kyphosis; scoliosis
Spondyloepiphyseal dysplasia (congenita tarda)	Atlantoaxial instability	Kyphosis; scoliosis
Pseudoachondroplasia	Atlantoaxial instability	
Mucopolysaccharidoses	Cervical instability	Kyphosis; scoliosis
Chondrodysplasia punctata	Atlantoaxial instability	Kyphosis; scoliosis
Metaphyseal chondrodysplasia (McKusick type)	Atlantoaxial instability	
Cleidocranial dysplasia		Scoliosis (with syringomyelia in some)
Larsen syndrome	Cervical kyphosis; midcervical instability	Scoliosis

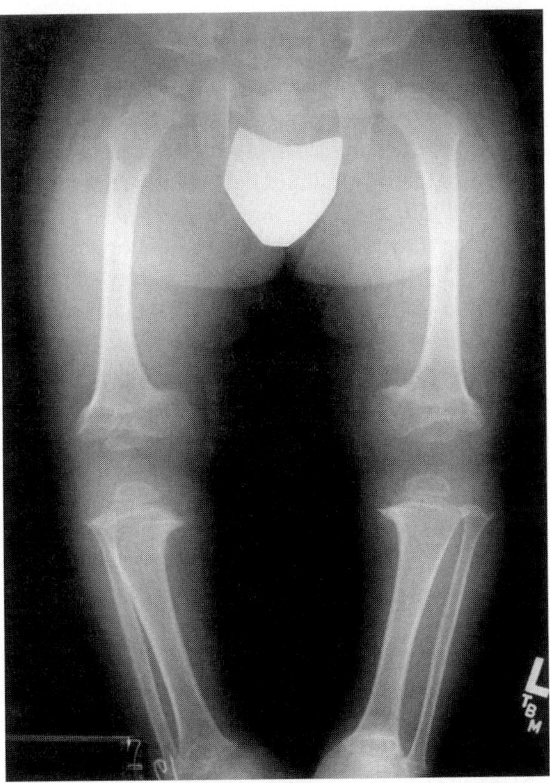

Figure 5-3 The lower extremities in a young walking child with achondroplasia show abnormal metaphyseal flaring and broadening throughout all the long bones. Medial tibial spurs are related to mild genu varum. Also note the deep acetabula.

years of life and may result in a variety of neurologic signs, including developmental delay, hypotonia, sleep apnea, and feeding difficulties. Decompression of the brainstem often leads to improvement of neurologic symptoms. Enlargement of head circumference (*megacephaly*) is common but does not necessarily indicate hydrocephalus that requires shunting. Although patients with achondroplasia are among the most stable and healthy of patients with skeletal dysplasias, mortality rates are nevertheless high in all age groups. The most common causes are sudden death in young infants, central nervous system events or respiratory problems in older children and young adults, and cardiovascular problems in older adults.

Orthopaedic Implications

Thoracolumbar spinal stenosis is the most common and disabling problem in the adult with achondroplasia (see Table 5-1). Onset of symptoms in the third decade of life is typical, but earlier presentation may be seen and symptoms usually occur in the lumbar spine. The presenting symptoms are low back pain, leg pain, paresthesia, paraparesis, incontinence, and neurogenic claudication. Diagnosis is best made on MRI. Spinal decompression by multiple-level laminectomies is indicated.

Thoracolumbar kyphosis is extremely common in the first years of life, although most patients experience improvement in kyphosis without treatment when they begin independent ambulation. Kyphosis does not improve in 10% to 15% of patients, however (Fig. 5-4). Bracing and avoidance of unsupported sitting have been recommended for these patients. For children in whom bracing fails, posterior spinal fusion without instrumentation (fusion in situ) is performed. A halo body cast is applied after fusion in situ.

Genu varum affects at least 50% of people who have achondroplasia. It is usually progressive and requires treatment. There is no evidence that use of bracing in children with achondroplasia is effective. The treatment of genu varum usually involves surgical correction by proximal tibiofibular realignment osteotomy.

Limb lengthening of the arms and legs may be considered in patients with achondroplasia. Gradual distraction of the bone with special external fixators has resulted in substantial elongation of up to 30 cm in overall height between femur and tibia. The use of human growth hormone for short stature in achondroplasia has no scientific basis, although it continues to undergo clinical trials.

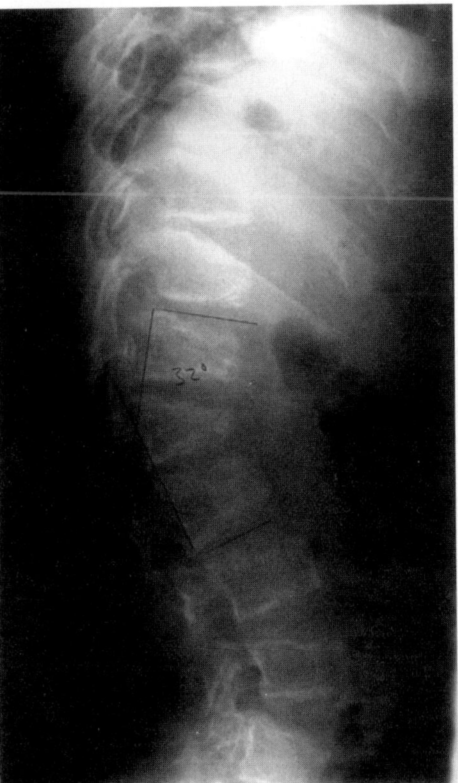

Figure 5-4 **A 4-year-old boy with achondroplasia.** This lateral radiograph of the spine shows a kyphosis with a sharp apex centered at a wedge-shaped first lumbar vertebra. Diffuse irregularity of the vertebral body end plates and rib ends is shown. The spinal deformity in this patient required bracing.

Hypochondroplasia

Hypochondroplasia is similar to achondroplasia phenotypically and genotypically, but the two disorders are nevertheless distinct. Hypochondroplasia is characterized by mild short-limb dwarfism. It is an autosomal dominant allelic variant of achondroplasia. The mutation occurs in the tyrosine kinase domain of the gene in hypochondroplasia, but in the transmembrane domain in achondroplasia.[3] There does not appear to be a relationship between hypochondroplasia and later paternal age.

Clinical Findings

Hypochondroplasia is one of the most subtle of the skeletal dysplasias. Generally, the diagnosis is not made before the child is 2 years old. The trunk height is almost normal, and the shortening of the upper and lower limbs is symmetrical in a mesomelic pattern. Except for mild frontal bossing, the facial appearance is normal. Spinal deformities are rarely seen in patients with hypochondroplasia, although mild ligamentous laxity persists. Varus angulation of the knees is mild and may resolve with growth. Significant genu varum occurs in less than 10% of patients.

Radiographic Features

Radiographic findings are usually mild in hypochondroplasia. Primary and secondary criteria have been proposed. The primary criteria are narrowing of the lumbar interpedicular distances; short, square iliac crests; short, broad femoral necks; mild metaphyseal flaring; and shortening of the long tubular bones (Fig. 5-5). Secondary criteria are shortening of the lumbar pedicles, concavity of the posterior vertebral bodies, elongation of the distal fibula, and shortening of the distal ulna.[6]

Differential Diagnosis

Hypochondroplasia has more phenotypic variation in severity than achondroplasia. In the severe form, hypochondroplasia may resemble achondroplasia. Conversely, the mild form may be mistaken for constitutionally short stature. In its classic presentation with mild short stature and mild genu varum deformity, hypochondroplasia may resemble Schmid metaphyseal dysplasia.

Orthopaedic Implications

The skeletal abnormalities seen in hypochondroplasia are usually mild and rarely require surgical intervention. Spinal stenosis may be seen in about one third of patients, but it is usually mild and does not require sur-

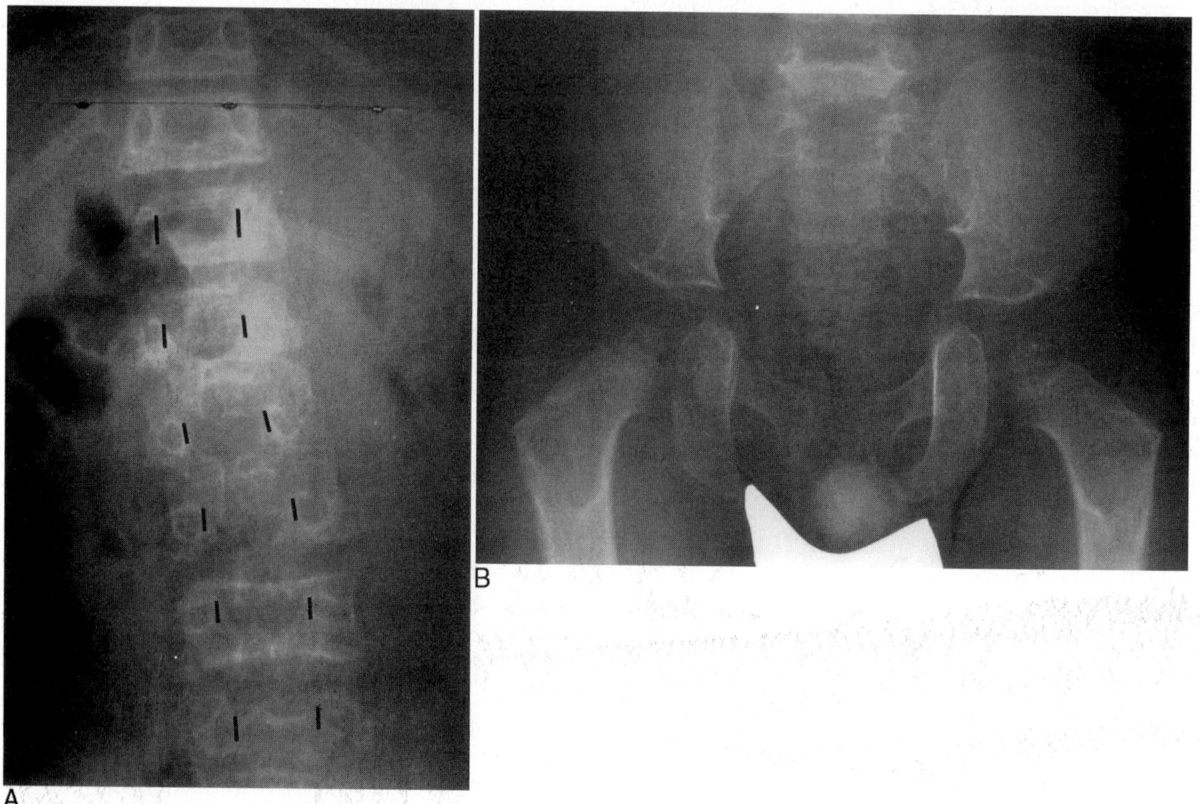

Figure 5-5 A 7-year-old boy with hypochondroplasia. A, A primary criterion for hypochondroplasia is a decrease in the interpedicular distance in the lower lumbar spine. **B,** The pelvis in this patient shows square iliac wings; short, broad femoral necks; and deep acetabula.

gical treatment. If there is significant genu varum, realignment osteotomy may be indicated.

Metatropic Dysplasia

Metatropic dysplasia is a rare skeletal dysplasia characterized by a change in body proportions with growth. It is transmitted in an autosomal dominant or recessive manner. The cause of metatropic dysplasia has not been elucidated, but it is thought to result from a defect in endochondral ossification. Some histologic abnormalities of the growth plate, causing developmental arrest, have been studied and appear to be characteristic. In a study by Boden and colleagues,[7] the major histologic findings were (1) the absence of formation of normal primary spongiosa in the metaphysis, (2) the presence of a thin seal of bone at the chondro-osseous junction, with abnormal metaphyseal vascular invasion and arrest of endochondral growth, and (3) normal-appearing perichondral ring structures with persistence of circumferential growth. These findings suggested an uncoupling of endochondral and perichondral types of growth, offering an explanation for the dumbbell-shaped morphologic structure of the osseous metaphysis seen in patients with metatropic dysplasia.

Clinical Findings

During infancy, short limbs and a relatively long trunk are characteristic of metatropic dysplasia. With growth, a severe kyphoscoliosis typically develops, resulting in apparent shortening of the trunk as well as an apparent reversal in body proportions.[4] Many patients with metatropic dysplasia have a small tail-like appendage overlying the lower sacrum. It is usually a few centimeters long and arises from the gluteal fold. The facial appearance is usually normal. The limbs are significantly short, with bulbous enlargement of the metaphyses of the long bones and severe joint contractures (e.g., flexion contractures up to 30 or 40 degrees).

Radiographic Features

Odontoid hypoplasia with upper cervical spine instability (atlantoaxial instability) commonly occurs in patients with metatropic dysplasia (see Table 5-1). Spinal involvement is characterized by severe *platyspondyly* (flatness of the vertebral bodies) and anterior wedging of the vertebral bodies. Kyphosis and scoliosis are typically present early in life and are usually progressive (Fig. 5-6A). Flaring of the metaphyseal regions of the long bones gives them a dumbbell shape (Fig. 5-6B). Joint incongruity may be seen as a result of delayed epiphyseal

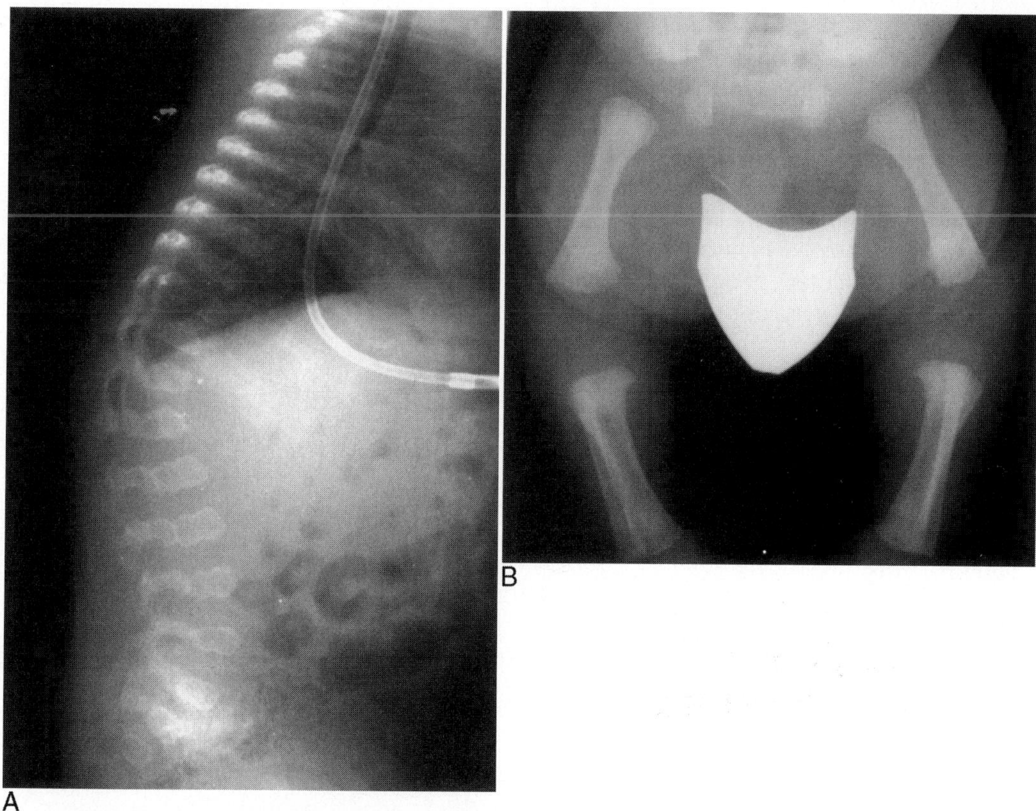

Figure 5-6 A 5-month-old patient with metatropic dysplasia. A, A thoracolumbar kyphosis is centered at a hypoplastic first lumbar vertebra. The lower thoracic vertebrae and lumbar vertebrae are abnormally shaped as well. **B,** All the long bones are short and broad with flaring of the metaphyses, creating the characteristic dumbbell shape in this patient. Note the deep acetabula.

ossification, and premature osteoarthritis of major weight-bearing joints is a common sequela.

Medical Problems

Patients with metatropic dysplasia commonly have severe restrictive pulmonary disease that is life threatening. Such children have a small stiff thorax that may be further compromised by the development of spinal deformities. Death can occur in infancy from pulmonary insufficiency. A high incidence of upper cervical spine (C1-C2) abnormalities occurs in metatropic dysplasia, which may lead to myelopathic changes. Ventriculomegaly or hydrocephalus has been reported in up to 25% of patients.

Orthopaedic Implications

Stability of the upper cervical spine should be evaluated periodically (at 1-year intervals in a growing child) with lateral flexion-extension radiographs. An atlantodens interval (ADI) larger than 5 mm indicates instability, although many patients with such an interval are asymptomatic. For asymptomatic patients with radiographic evidence of instability, flexion-extension MRI should be performed to evaluate cord compression. ADI larger than 5 mm may require posterior spinal fusion (occipitocervical fusion) with or without decompression, if there are neurologic signs and symptoms or MRI evidence of cord compression.[4] Prophylactic cervical fusion is also recommended for the asymptomatic patients with instability of 8 mm or more. Halo vest immobilization is used for 8 to 12 weeks postoperatively.

Kyphoscoliosis may progress rapidly during the first few years of life. For curves smaller than 45 degrees, bracing should be instituted. Spinal fusion is advisable for more severe, progressive curves. Anterior as well as posterior spinal fusion is recommended, because of the high rate of pseudoarthrosis in this condition. Spinal stenosis makes instrumentation difficult, so fusion in situ usually is preferred. A halo body cast is applied after spinal fusion.

The hip and knee flexion contractures in metatropic dysplasia commonly need surgical intervention, including soft tissue releases and, rarely, osteotomies. Premature osteoarthritis of the hips and knees is a common problem. Total joint arthroplasty is successful for severely symptomatic adult patients.

Chondroectodermal Dysplasia

Chondroectodermal dysplasia, also known as *Ellis-van Creveld syndrome*, is characterized by short-limb disproportionate dwarfism, polydactyly, hypoplasia of the nails, dental deficiencies, and congenital heart disease. It is transmitted in an autosomal recessive manner and is more common in inbred populations, most notably in the Pennsylvania Amish community. A novel gene located on the short arm of chromosome 4, Ellis-van Creveld syndrome gene (EVC), has been identified in individuals with chondroectodermal dysplasia.[3] Investigators detected low levels of EVC expression in developing bone, heart, kidney, and lung. In bone, EVC was expressed in the developing vertebral bodies, ribs, and both upper and lower limbs. The EVC gene encodes a 992-amino acid protein that has no homology to known proteins other than in a short region that may be a leucine zipper.

Clinical Findings

Chondroectodermal dysplasia is recognizable at birth. The patients have shortening of the limbs in an acromelic pattern. Postaxial (small finger-sided) polydactyly of the hands is typical, occasionally involving the feet as well. Syndactyly (webbed digits) and dysplastic nails of the fingers and toes may also occur. Spinal deformities have been reported rarely in patients with chondroectodermal dysplasia. The valgus alignment of the knees is usually progressive, producing a significant deformity with patellar dislocation.

Radiographic Features

Patients with chondroectodermal dysplasia have a narrow chest with short ribs. The bones of the forearm are disproportionately short, with hypoplasia of the proximal radius and distal ulna. Fusions between carpal bones of the hand are common. The pelvis has small iliac crests and sciatic notches. The hip joints are congruous, but the femoral necks are generally in valgus position (Fig. 5-7). Bilateral valgus deformity of the knees usually is relatively symmetric.

Medical Problems

One third of infants with chondroectodermal dysplasia are stillborn or die of cardiorespiratory complications in

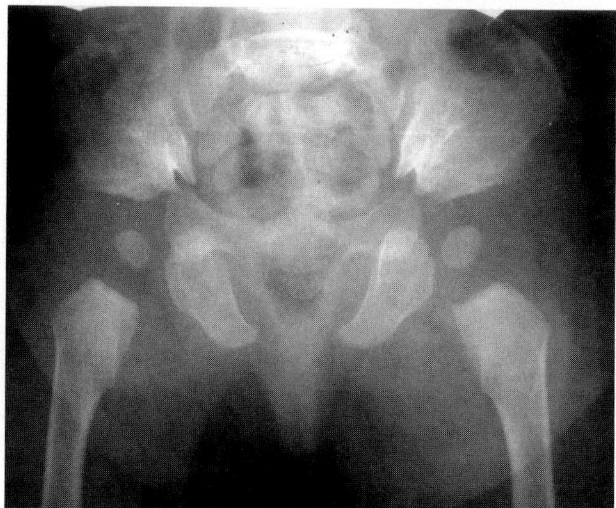

Figure 5-7 The pelvis of a 9-month-old patient with chondroectodermal dysplasia has small iliac bones and narrow sciatic notches. This child also has bilateral coxa valga (increased femoral neck angle).

the first 2 weeks of life. Congenital cardiac defects, the most common a defect of primary atrial septation producing a common atrium, occur in 60% of affected individuals. The teeth are conical with wide spaces and are lost early. Genitourinary system abnormalities, such as hypospadias, epispadias, and undescended testes, may occur.

Orthopaedic Implications

The cardiac status of the patient with chondroectodermal dysplasia should be evaluated carefully before any surgical intervention is undertaken. Excision of the postaxial digits and release of syndactylies are the only treatments needed for the arms in most patients. Progressive genu valgum usually requires surgical intervention; realignment osteotomy is indicated for valgus deformity of more than 20 degrees. The deformity may recur after osteotomy because of the continued growth disturbance of the lateral proximal tibial epiphysis, so continued follow-up until skeletal maturity is required.

Diastrophic Dysplasia

Diastrophic dysplasia is a rare, autosomal recessive, skeletal dysplasia characterized by severe short-limb dwarfism with extensive spinal deformities and specific hand, foot, and ear abnormalities. The disease occurs in most populations but it is particularly prevalent in Finland owing to an apparent founder effect. The responsible gene, located on the long arm of chromosome 5, encodes a sulfate transporter protein ("diastrophic dysplasia sulfate transporter").[3] Impaired function of this protein is thought to lead to undersulfation of proteoglycan in the cartilage matrix, thus affecting hydration of growth plate cartilage, articular cartilage, nasal and auricular cartilage, and intervertebral disks. Histopathologic analysis shows that chondrocytes appear to degenerate prematurely and that collagen is present in excess.

Clinical Findings

Diastrophic dysplasia is recognizable at birth, being characterized by extreme short stature with micromelia. The head is normocephalic, and the facial appearance is characteristic, with a narrow nasal bridge, broadened midnose, and flared nostrils. Cleft palate and cauliflower ear deformities are common. Specific hand and foot malformations are universal in patients with diastrophic dysplasia.[5] Symphalangism (stiffness of the interphalangeal joints) of the fingers, the "hitchhiker thumb," and rigid bilateral equinovarus deformities of the feet are characteristic. Flexion contractures of the elbow, hip, and knee joints are common and further compromise the functional length of the limbs. These joints also have marked limitation of motion. Lumbar lordosis may develop secondary to hip flexion contractures. Severe cervical kyphosis or thoracic kyphoscoliosis with a progressive pattern is also common.[5]

Radiographic Features

The metacarpophalangeal joint of the thumb is typically subluxated or dislocated, giving rise to a widely abducted thumb, also called "hitchhiker thumb." The vertebral bodies may show some irregularities or wedging. Cervical kyphosis is a common finding in patients with diastrophic dysplasia. Kyphosis or scoliosis of the thoracolumbar spine occurs in more than 80% of patients and commonly develops into a severe, progressive structural curve (see Table 5-1). Exaggerated lumbar lordosis may also be detected (Fig. 5-8). Long bones are usually short and broad with metaphyseal flaring. Appearance of the epiphyseal centers of ossification is delayed for all major joints. Severe coxa vara and incongruity of the hip joints may cause secondary hip dislocation and osteoarthritis. The feet usually have a severe equinovarus deformity.

Medical Problems

Early comprehensive medical attention is required for respiratory difficulties due to diastrophic dysplasia. Some patients die in infancy of respiratory failure, but most have a normal life span unless there are cardiopulmonary sequelae from severe scoliosis or quadriplegia secondary to cervical kyphosis. Cleft palate may contribute to respiratory difficulties, because of aspiration

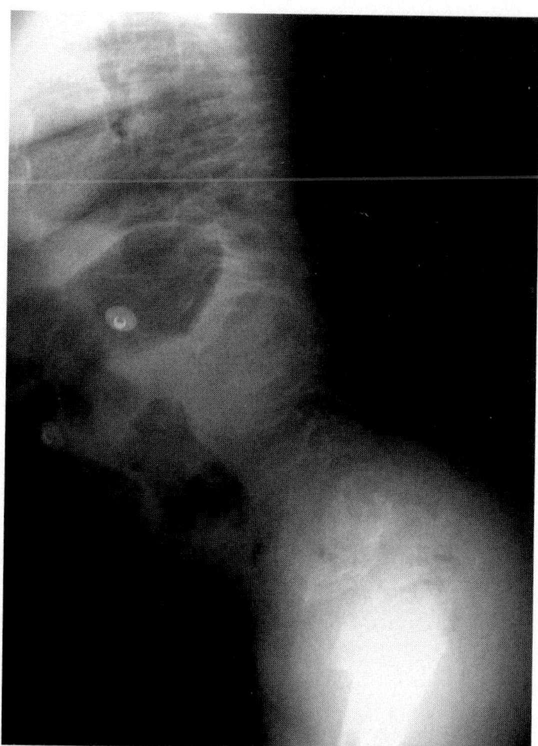

Figure 5-8 A thoracolumbar kyphosis with an exaggerated lumbar lordosis is seen in this young child with diastrophic dysplasia. There is generalized platyspondyly with anterior beaking of the lumbar vertebrae. A hypoplastic first lumbar vertebra is seen at the apex of the kyphosis. Note the flared ribs with irregular rib ends.

during feeding. Surgical repair is required in most patients. Hearing impairment may develop secondary to stenosis of the external auditory canal.

Orthopaedic Implications

Cervical kyphosis develops during the first 2 years of life in about 30% of patients with diastrophic dysplasia. Lateral flexion-extension radiographs and, sometimes, flexion-extension MRI of the cervical spine should be obtained. If the cervical kyphosis is not progressive and there is no instability or neurologic signs, the kyphosis can be observed, and it may improve spontaneously. Progressive deformities with instability should be treated surgically by posterior cervical fusion and halo vest immobilization. If neurologic involvement is present, anterior decompression and fusion should be considered along with posterior fusion.

Scoliosis affects about half of patients with diastrophic dysplasia and often begins early in childhood. For the curves smaller than 45 degrees, bracing is recommended. Large curves often continue to progress in adulthood. Surgical intervention is required to prevent progression for curves larger than 45 degrees. Posterior spinal fusion is the mainstay of the treatment. In the presence of associated kyphosis exceeding 50 degrees, anterior spinal fusion may be performed as well.

Hip and knee flexion contractures should be assessed together. Physical therapy and splinting should be instituted early for the management of these joint contractures. Realignment osteotomies are performed for residual contractures, improving function. Osteoarthritis of the hip joint reduces walking ability in patients with diastrophic dysplasia. Total joint arthroplasty is successful for the severely symptomatic adult.

In diastrophic dysplasia, equinovarus foot deformity is common. The feet are rigid and resistant to conservative treatment by serial casting. Surgical treatment is required in most patients to achieve a plantigrade foot.

Kniest Dysplasia

Kniest dysplasia is a severe skeletal dysplasia characterized by disproportionate short-trunk dwarfism, kyphoscoliosis, flat facies, large stiff joints with contractures, and hearing and visual impairments.[5] This disorder resembles classic metatropic dwarfism in many respects but is transmitted in an autosomal dominant manner. Mutations in the gene that encodes type II collagen (COL2A1), the predominant protein of cartilage, have been identified in a number of individuals with Kniest dysplasia.[3] Most mutations are between exons 12 and 24 of the COL2A1 gene.

Histopathologic findings include a disorganized physeal growth plate, soft crumbly cartilage with a "Swiss cheese" appearance, and diastase-resistant intracytoplasmic inclusions in the resting chondrocytes. Scanning electron microscopy demonstrates striking fragmentation and disintegration of collagen fibrils, resulting in large open cystlike spaces, and deficiency and disorganization of the collagen fibrils.[8]

Clinical Findings

Kniest dysplasia can be recognized at birth in most patients, but in patients with mild involvement, its recognition may be delayed. By the time an affected patient is 1 year old, contractures of the elbows, hips, and knees are evident. Limited motion at the joints, particularly at the hips and fingers, is common. Contractures and joint stiffness cause delayed motor development. In a 3-year-old patient, all of the usual manifestations of Kniest dysplasia are evident. The face is flat with widely spaced, prominent eyes, and flat nasal bridge. Significant disproportionate short-trunk dwarfism and rhizomelic involvement of the limbs are present. The trunk is short and broad. Kyphoscoliosis and marked lumbar lordosis with hip flexion contractures further contribute to the short stature. The elbows, wrists, knees, and ankles are enlarged and prominent.

Radiographic Features

Osteoporosis of the spine and limbs is evident from birth in patients with Kniest dysplasia. Hand involvement is significant, with generalized osteoporosis as well as narrowing of the intercarpal and interphalangeal joints of the fingers and thumbs. Abnormalities of the odontoid with atlantoaxial instability and hypoplasia of the cervical vertebrae may be seen (see Table 5-1). Generalized platyspondyly, vertical clefting in the vertebral bodies, and kyphoscoliosis are common in the thoracic and lumbar spine (Fig. 5-9A). The pelvic appearance is characteristic, consisting of short, broad iliac crests and small, insufficient acetabula. The dumbbell-shaped long bones have very short, broad metaphyses, giving the appearance of joint enlargement (see Fig. 5-9B).

Medical Problems

Severe respiratory distress and recurrent pulmonary infections, requiring appropriate treatment, may occur frequently during infancy in a child with Kniest dysplasia. Cleft palate is found in at least 50% of patients and usually requires surgical treatment. Hearing losses are common and appear to be related to chronic otitis media. Frequency of severe myopia and retinal detachment makes ophthalmologic examination essential.

Orthopaedic Implications

Evaluation of upper cervical spine instability is essential. It can be accomplished through examination of lateral flexion-extension radiographs and, if required, flexion-extension MRI. In a patient with significant instability or neurologic signs, posterior cervical fusion should be performed. Thoracic kyphoscoliosis is usually not severe, and

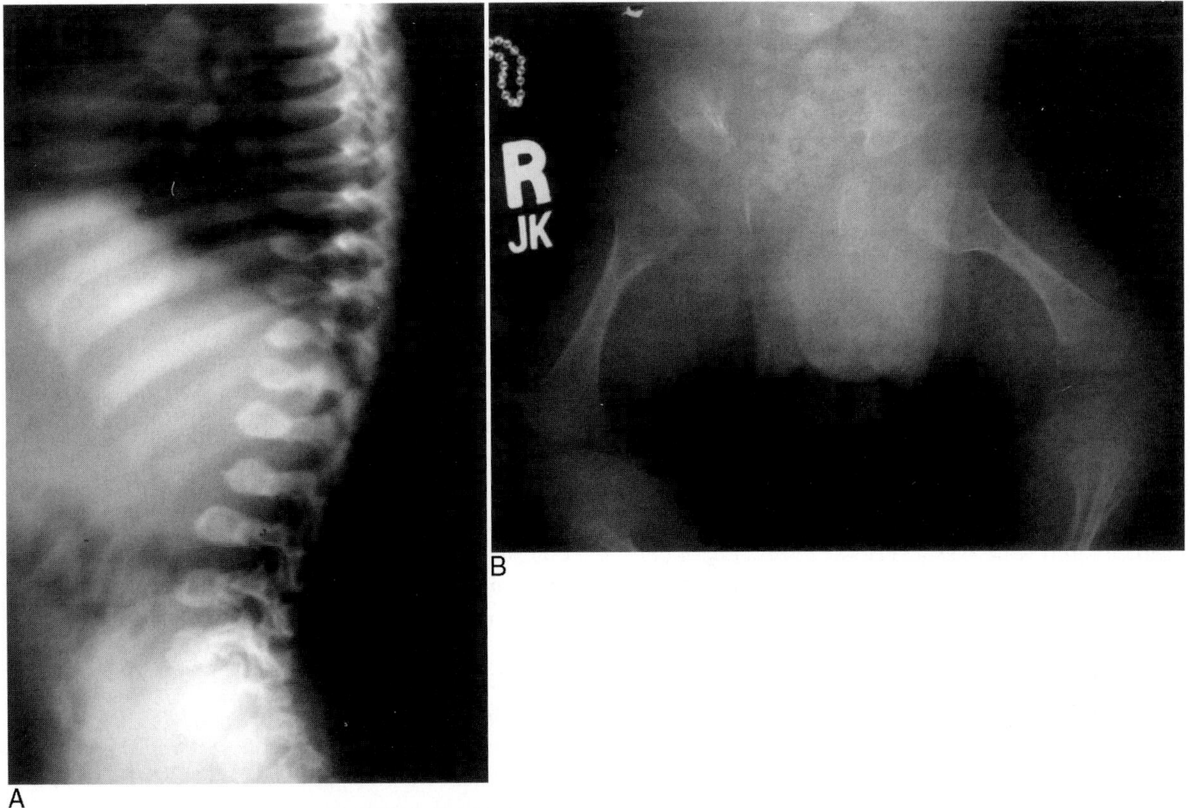

Figure 5-9 A 3-month-old patient with Kniest dysplasia. A, A lateral view of the spine shows anterior beaking of the vertebrae throughout the spine. **B,** The pelvis is characteristic, with short and broad iliac crests and small, insufficient acetabula. The long bones are dumbbell-shaped, with short diaphyses and broad, flared metaphyses.

surgical treatment is not required. Early physical and occupational therapy is needed for joint stiffness and contractures to enable the patient to gain and maintain motion, especially in the small joints of the hands, hips, knees, and ankles. Osteoarthritis of the hip is common in the second or third decade of life, and total hip arthroplasty is the only reasonable alternative for symptomatic hips.

Spondyloepiphyseal Dysplasia Congenita

Spondyloepiphyseal dysplasia is a descriptive term for a group of rare disorders characterized by disproportionate short-trunk dwarfism with primary involvement of the vertebrae and epiphyseal centers. Spondyloepiphyseal dysplasia congenita (SEDC) is the most common type, with an estimated prevalence of about 3 to 4 per million. It is transmitted in an autosomal dominant manner, but most patients acquire the disease through a new mutation. The gene defect has been linked to a deletion at the type II collagen gene locus, COL2A1, on chromosome 12.[3] Type II collagen is the predominant protein of cartilage, and mutations have been observed in the alpha-1 chain, resulting in alteration in length. Electron microscopy has demonstrated intracellular inclusions, which are probably due to intracellular retention of procollagen.

Clinical Findings

SEDC can be diagnosed in infancy. Findings are disproportionate short-trunk dwarfism and rhizomelic involvement of the limbs (Fig. 5-10A and B). Head circumference is normal with flattened facies and wide-set eyes. The neck is short, and the chest is barrel-shaped in combination with pectus carinatum deformity (Fig. 5-11A).[5] Thoracic scoliosis and kyphosis may be evident in adolescence. The patient usually has increased lumbar lordosis, either primary or secondary to hip flexion contractures. Genu valgum and equinovarus deformities are common lower limb problems seen in patients with SEDC.

Radiographic Features

The development of ossification centers is delayed in patients with SEDC. The extent of platyspondyly varies. The vertebral bodies are initially biconvex but become progressively flattened with age, and the end plates become irregular. The odontoid may be hypoplastic or absent, leading to atlantoaxial instability that may cause neurologic compromise, even in early childhood (see Fig. 5-11B and C and Table 5-1). Progressive kyphoscoliosis may develop in late childhood (see Fig. 5-10C and D). Iliac crests are short and small with horizontal acetabular roofs. Ossification of the capital femoral epiphysis is usually delayed, and coxa vara of varying severity is seen (see Fig. 5-10E).[9] The ossification centers of the distal femur and proximal tibia are also delayed, with flattening and irregularity of the articular surfaces (see Fig. 5-10F). Genu valgum is commonly seen.

Medical Problems

Patients with SEDC may experience restrictive lung disease in infancy because of their small thorax, but most such children survive. Retinal detachment or severe myopia is common in patients with SEDC, so ophthalmologic surveillance is indicated. Cleft palate may occur and usually requires surgical treatment.

Orthopaedic Implications

Upper cervical spine instability or spinal stenosis may be associated with cord compression and myelopathic changes in children with SEDC. Periodic evaluation of cervical instability with lateral flexion-extension radiographs and flexion-extension MRI is essential. MRI is also very helpful for evaluation of spinal stenosis. Posterior cervical fusion should be performed in any patient with instability or cord compression (see Fig. 5-11D). Decompression may be considered if there is significant stenosis.

The initial treatment should include bracing for kyphoscoliotic curves smaller than 45 degrees. Progressive curves that are larger than 45 degrees commonly require posterior spinal fusion and instrumentation, with the addition of anterior fusion for large or rigid curves. The canal size is typically adequate for instrumentation, but preoperative MRI should be performed for assessment.

Coxa vara is usually associated with hip flexion contracture and lumbar lordosis. The procedure of choice is the proximal femoral valgus-extension osteotomy. Severe angular deformities around the knee are treated with realignment osteotomies. Total joint replacement may be considered for selected adult patients with symptomatic osteoarthritis of the hips and knees. Equinovarus deformity is usually resistant to conservative treatment, so surgical correction with soft tissue releases is required in most patients.

Spondyloepiphyseal Dysplasia Tarda

Spondyloepiphyseal dysplasia tarda (SEDT) is a disorder of endochondral bone formation characterized by disproportionate short stature with short neck and trunk. It occurs in approximately two of every 1 million people. It is distinguished from SEDC because of later age at diagnosis and milder involvement. Several genetic patterns of transmission have been reported. The most common is X-linked, in which boys and men are more commonly and more severely affected. Generally, obligate female carriers are clinically and radiographically indistinguishable from the general population, although some have phenotypic changes consistent with expression of the gene defect. A recessive form has also been reported. X-linked SEDT can be caused by mutations in the sedlin (SEDL) gene, which is localized to the X chromosome.[3] SEDL is widely expressed in tissues, including fibroblasts, lymphoblasts, and fetal cartilage, and encodes a protein (sedlin) with a putative role in endoplasmic reticulum-to-Golgi vesicular transport.

Clinical Findings

Patients with SEDT are usually diagnosed at about 4 years of age. Stature is mildly shortened. SEDT primarily affects the spine and the large joints, in which the changes become evident when patients are between 10 and 14 years old. Thoracic kyphoscoliosis associated with back pain may be seen. Patients usually have hip pain, and they initially may be diagnosed as having bilateral Perthes disease. Progressive osteoarthritis of the hips and knees may be seen by early adolescence. Angular deformities of the lower extremities are rare.

Radiographic Features

Symmetrical involvement of the shoulders, hips, and knees is seen in patients with SEDT. Radiographic changes in the hip are very typical, including abnormal femoral heads (with coxa magna, flattening, and subluxation), acetabular insufficiency, and premature osteoarthritis (Fig. 5-12A). These features may mimic those of bilateral Perthes disease. Mild genu varum or genu valgum may be seen, with flattening of the femoral condyles and deformation of the tibial articular surfaces (see Fig. 5-12B). Spinal involvement, including platyspondyly and anterior wedging of the vertebral bodies, usually affects the thoracic spine and may lead to kyphoscoliosis (see Fig. 5-12C). Odontoid hypoplasia may cause atlantoaxial instability (see Fig. 5-12D and Table 5-1).

Orthopaedic Implications

All patients with SEDT should be evaluated for atlantoaxial instability, and cervical fusion should be considered if significant instability is detected. Scoliotic curves are usually mild to moderate and are managed with observation or bracing. Hip problems commonly require surgical intervention, such as proximal femoral osteotomy to provide joint congruity or total joint arthroplasty (in adults) to achieve symptomatic relief. Angular deformities of the knees usually do not require treatment.

Pseudoachondroplasia

Pseudoachondroplasia is one of the most common skeletal dyplasias with a prevalence of four per 1 million. Although first described as a form of spondyloepiphyseal dysplasia, pseudoachondroplasia is a distinct dwarfing condition readily differentiated from that disorder.

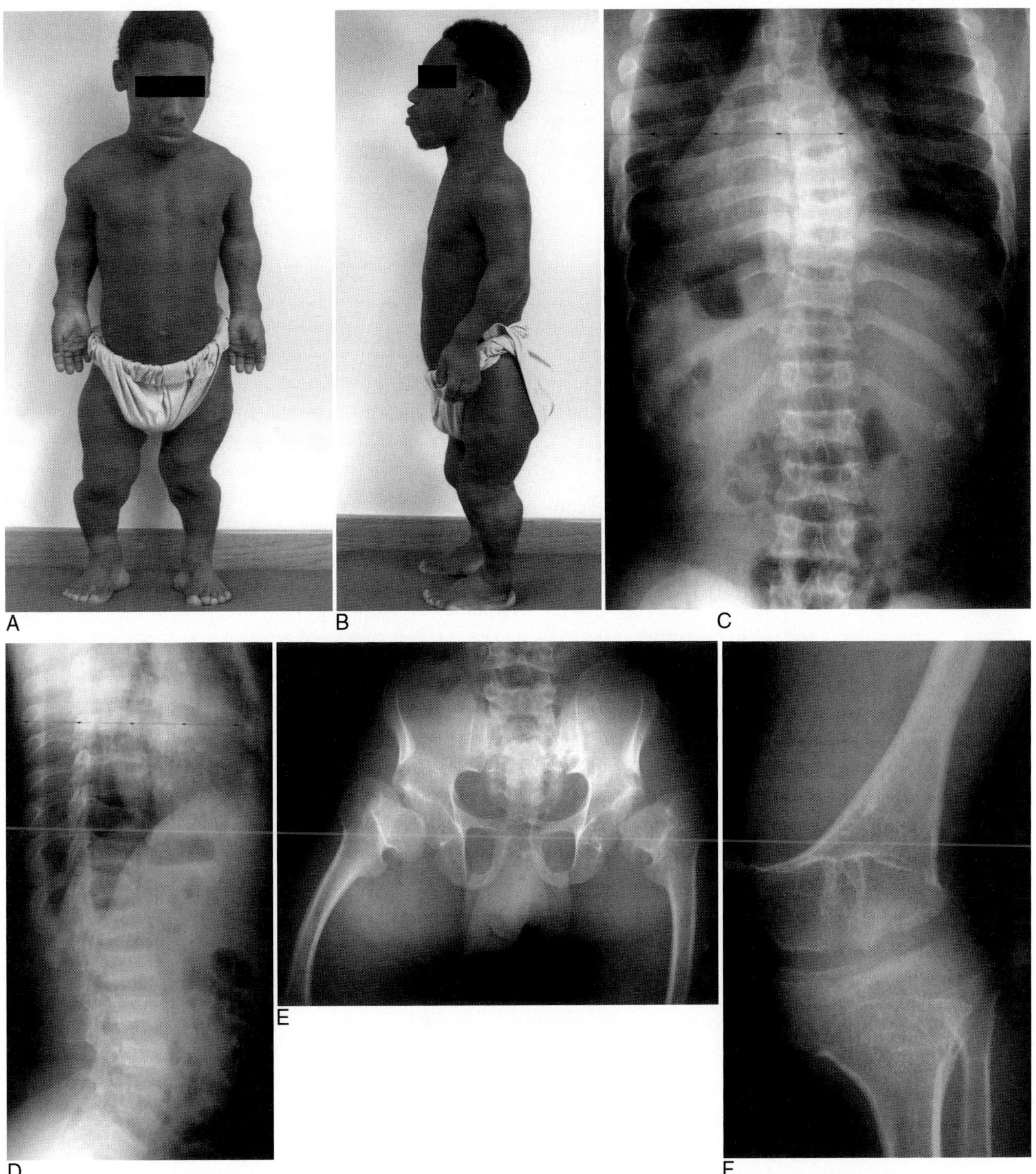

Figure 5-10 A 19-year-old patient with spondyloepiphyseal dysplasia congenita. **A** and **B,** Note the markedly short stature with short trunk and rhizomelic involvement of the limbs. There are angular deformities of the lower limbs, including bilateral genu valgum and bowing of the femur and tibia. The elbows have a flexion contracture. **C,** On a posteroanterior (PA) radiograph of the spine, a thoracic scoliosis is seen. The ribs are broad and short, resulting in a small thorax. **D,** A lateral radiograph of the spine shows diffuse platyspondyly and mild kyphosis centered at a hypoplastic T11. **E,** This patient has marked coxa vara associated with hip flexion contractures. As shown on the anteroposterior radiograph, the femoral necks are short, the heads are broad, and there is overgrowth of the greater trochanters. These abnormalities lead to the shallow, dysplastic acetabula seen here. Note the small, vertical iliac wings. **F,** At the knee, a valgus deformity results from a hypoplastic lateral femoral condyle. Both femoral and tibial epiphyses are abnormally flattened and broad.

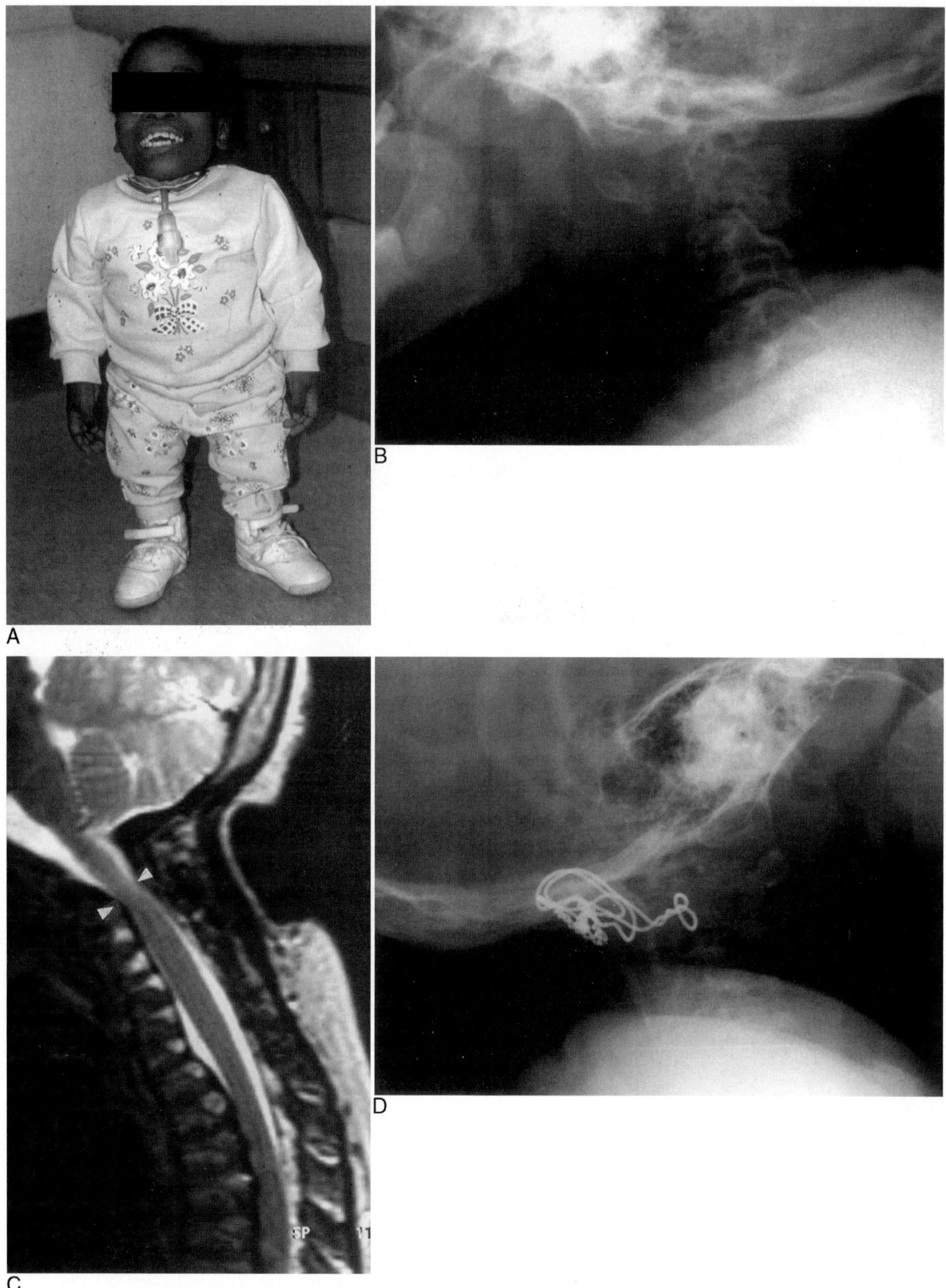

Figure 5-11 A 10-year-old girl with spondyloepiphyseal dysplasia congenita. A, Note the markedly short stature and short neck. **B,** A lateral cervical spine radiograph depicts a hypoplastic, barely visible odontoid and a significantly widened atlantodens interval (ADI), characteristic of cervical instability. **C,** Magnetic resonance image of the cervical spine shows narrowing of the spinal canal at the level of the atlas (C1) *(arrows)*. The spinal cord appears thinned at and just above this level. **D,** This patient underwent posterior cervical fusion (occiput to the first, second, and third cervical vertebrae) and decompression. Wires and a bone graft can be seen on this lateral radiograph.

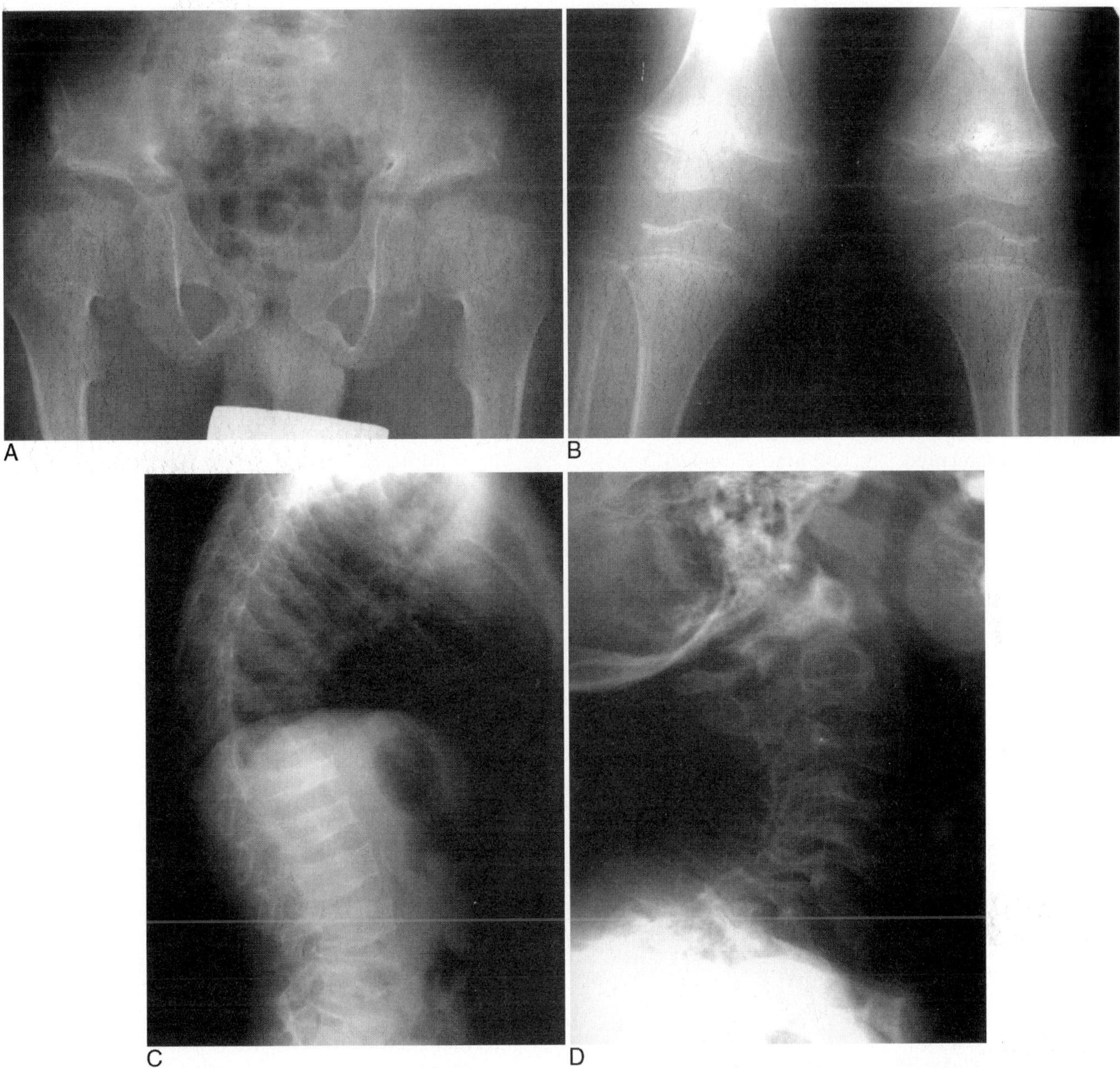

Figure 5-12 An 8-year-old patient with spondyloepiphyseal dysplasia tarda. **A,** Radiographic findings in the proximal femurs include small femoral head with delayed ossification and enlargement of the metaphyses (coxa magna). Note the deep acetabula with horizontal acetabular roof. **B,** At the knees, the long bones have irregular, flattened epiphyses and enlarged metaphyses. Mild genu valgum is present. **C,** The thoracolumbar spine has significantly flattened and elongated vertebrae throughout, characteristic of diffuse platyspondyly. A moderate thoracolumbar kyphosis is also present. **D,** A lateral view of the cervical spine shows a hypoplastic odontoid and platyspondyly.

Pseudoachondroplasia is characterized by rhizomelic short-limb dwarfism usually associated with epiphyseal and metaphyseal changes and mild spinal involvement. It is transmitted as an autosomal dominant condition. A gene for this disorder has been localized to chromosome 19 and appears to encode the cartilage oligomeric matrix protein (COMP), a glycoprotein that is found in matrix surrounding chondrocytes.[3] Accumulation of an abnormal form of COMP in the rough endoplasmic reticulum of chondrocytes, rather than absence of COMP, causes pseudoachondroplasia. COMP is also expressed in tendons and ligaments, and the presence of abnormal COMP in these tissues is plausibly responsible for the loose joints that are a consistent feature of this disorder. Pseudoachondroplasia resembles achondroplasia because of its rhizomelic pattern but otherwise has little in common with it.

Clinical Findings

Patients with pseudoachondroplasia appear normal at birth, and growth retardation is seldom recognized until the second year of life or later, at which time body proportions resemble those of persons with achondroplasia.[4] Unlike in achondroplasia, however, the head and face are normal. The trunk is normal, except for mild scoliosis and exaggerated lumbar lordosis in some patients. Varus, valgus, and recurvatum deformities of the knees are common and result from osseous changes and marked ligamentous laxity.

Radiographic Features

Odontoid hypoplasia and atlantoaxial instability may be observed in patients with pseudoachondroplasia (see Table 5-1). The radiographs of the spine usually show a mild platyspondyly with oval vertebral bodies and, rarely, a mild scoliosis. The long bone involvement is characterized by metaphyseal flaring and epiphyseal irregularity (Fig. 5-13). Ossification of the epiphyses is delayed and fragmented. The epiphyseal irregularity may lead to degenerative joint disease.

Orthopaedic Implications

Periodic evaluation of upper cervical spine instability is essential for patients with pseudoachondroplasia. Lateral flexion-extension radiographs and, when required, flexion-extension MRI should be obtained, and cervical fusion should be considered if significant instability is detected. Scoliotic curves are usually mild (smaller than 25 degrees), and are monitored periodically without treatment. Occasionally, a patient may have a larger curve (between 25 and 45 degrees) that requires bracing. Angular deformities of the knee do not usually respond to conservative treatment modalities, and surgical correction with multiple level osteotomies is performed. Recurrence of angular deformities is common, and further surgery may be needed. Total joint arthroplasty is the treatment of choice for premature osteoarthritis of the knee and hip joints.

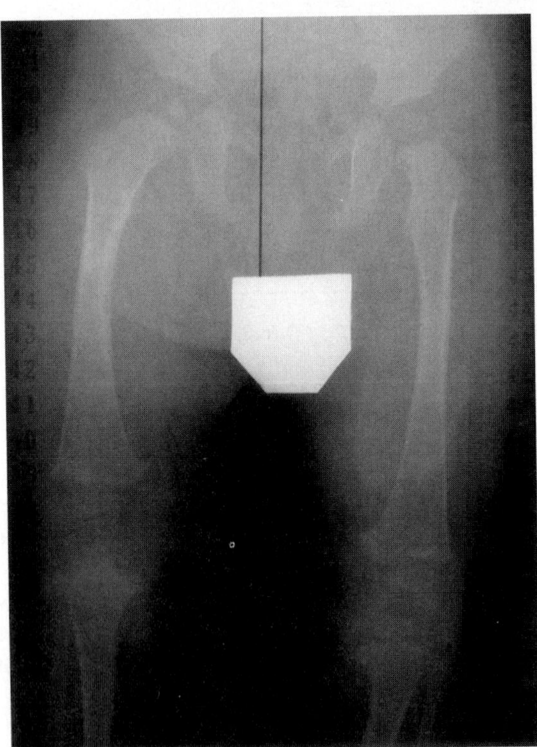

Figure 5-13 A young child with pseudoachondroplasia has asymmetric widening of the metaphyses, greater on the right than the left, and shortening of the right femur.

Mucopolysaccharidoses

The mucopolysaccharidoses (MPSs) are a group of inherited metabolic disorders caused by deficiencies of specific lysosomal enzymes that result in intracellular accumulation of partially degraded glycosaminoglycans. Several different disorders are described on the basis of the clinical, radiographic, and biochemical defects (Table 5-2). Although there is phenotypic variability, these disorders have some common clinical features, such as facial dysmorphism, short stature, organomegaly, cardiac problems, and joint contractures.[5] Mental retardation may be associated with some types. Most of the MPSs show similar changes in the cartilage; resting cartilage consists of uniformly stained matrix, with chondrocytes that are larger than normal and stain positively for glycosaminoglycans.[3]

Although the MPSs can be diagnosed biochemically after birth, clinical diagnosis usually is made in patients between 6 months and 6 to 10 years old, depending on the type. A flat nasal bridge, hypertelorism, and corneal clouding are typical facial features seen in children with MPS (Fig. 5-14). Short stature, short neck, and joint contractures occur almost in all types (Fig. 5-15). Cervical instability, thoracolumbar kyphoscoliosis, dysplasia of the pelvis, and broadening and shortening of the long bones may be seen. The patients with MPS I (Hurler syndrome) and MPS IV (Morquio syndrome) are usually more severely affected than those with other types of MPS.

Genetic counseling is essential for all children diagnosed with MPS. Medical problems require appropriate treatment. Orthopaedic treatment usually consists of symptomatic corrective measures, such as fusion of cervical spine instability and conservative or surgical treatment of spinal curvatures and joint contractures.

Multiple Epiphyseal Dysplasia

Multiple epiphyseal dysplasia (MED), one of the most common skeletal dysplasias, is characterized by delayed epiphyseal ossification and limb deformities. It is broadly categorized into more severe Fairbank and milder Ribbing types. MED is transmitted as an autosomal dominant condition, and mutations have been found in the gene for COMP on chromosome 19, as in pseudoachondroplasia.[3] In other cases of MED, however, abnormali-

Table 5-2 Mucopolysaccharidoses and Specific Enzyme Deficiencies

Mucopolysaccharidoses (MPSs)	Enzyme Deficiency	Gene Locus
MPS I (Hurler syndrome)	Alpha-L-iduronidase	Chromosome 4
MPS II (Hunter disease)	Iduronate-2-sulfatase	X chromosome
MPS III (Sanfilippo syndrome)		
Type A	Heparan sulfate sulfatase	
Type B	Alpha-*N*-acetylglucosaminidase	
Type C	Acetyl CoA: alpha-glucosaminide-*N*-acetyltransferase	
Type D	*N*-acetyl-glucosaminide-6-sulfatase	Chromosome 12
MPS IV (Morquio syndrome)		
Type A	Galactosamine-6-sulfate sulfatase	
Type B	β-galactosidase	
MPS VI (polydystrophic dysplasia)	Arylsulfatase B	Chromosome 5

ties have been found in the alpha-2 fibers of type IX collagen (COL9A2).[3] Type IX collagen is a cartilage-specific fibril-associated collagen located on the fibril surfaces. It may form a macromolecular bridge between type II collagen fibrils and other matrix components—and thus may be important for the adhesive properties of cartilage.

Clinical Findings

The stature of the patient with MED is often within normal limits. The head and face are normal. The spine is minimally involved and usually asymptomatic. Children with MED are usually referred to orthopaedic surgeons, later in childhood, for joint pain in the lower limbs, decreased range of motion of the hips and knees, or gait disturbance. Angular deformities of the lower limbs, including coxa vara, genu varum, and genu valgum, are common. There may be flexion contractures of the knees and elbows. Shortening of the digits of the hands and feet is the only clinical feature typical of patients with MED.

Radiographic Features

Delayed epiphyseal ossification with subsequent irregular ossification and joint surface deformation is typical in MED. Upper extremity involvement is mild; there may be irregularities in the proximal and distal humerus and radius (Fig. 5-16). The tubular bones of the hands are often shortened, with maximal involvement of the

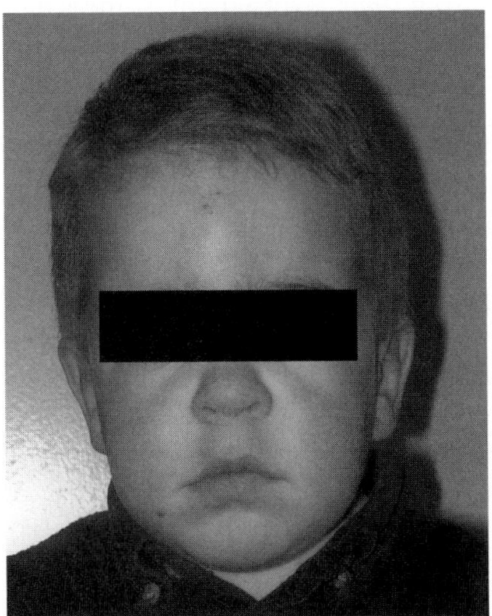

Figure 5-14 A 2-year-old boy with mucopolysaccharidosis type II (Hunter disease). Note the typical facial features, including a flat nasal bridge and hypertelorism.

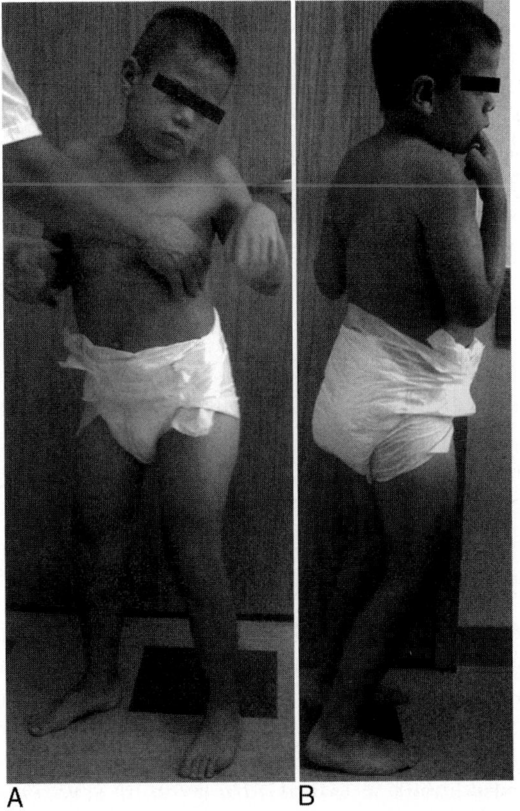

Figure 5-15 A 6-year-old boy with mucopolysaccharidoses type III (Sanfilippo syndrome). **A** and **B,** Note the short stature, short neck, and joint contractures (knees and elbows).

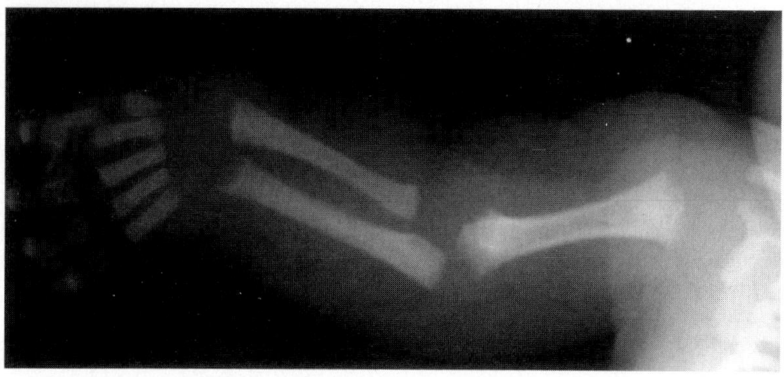

Figure 5-16 Ossification centers are delayed in this 6-month-old patient with multiple epiphyseal dysplasia. The long bones are broad and have flared ends, especially the humerus and ulna. Both ends of the bones are abnormal.

middle and distal phalanges. Angular deformities of the lower limbs may occur as a result of asymmetrical physeal growth. Severe, symmetric involvement of the hips is common, with deformed femoral heads, poor acetabular coverage, and avascular necrosis. Premature osteoarthritis of the hips is commonly seen.[4] Radiographs of the knees show angular deformities with flattened femoral condyles. The ankles in the patient with MED are usually in valgus alignment; changes occur more in the talus than in the distal tibia.

Orthopaedic Implications

Patients with MED are often referred to orthopaedic surgeons for suspicion of bilateral Perthes disease. Several radiographic clues may be helpful. In MED, abnormalities in the acetabulum are primary and are more pronounced. The radiographic changes are symmetric and fairly synchronous. It is also helpful to obtain radiographs of the knees, ankles, shoulders, and wrists. If motion of the hips is in satisfactory range and there are no significant degenerative changes, realignment osteotomies may be considered. For patients whose MED was diagnosed late and who have premature osteoarthritis, total joint arthroplasty may be the only reasonable treatment option.

Valgus alignment of the knees and ankles usually requires surgical correction by realignment osteotomies. These deformities may recur after surgical correction because of asymmetric physeal and epiphyseal growth. Therefore, realignment osteotomies are usually performed closer to skeletal maturity.

Chondrodysplasia Punctata

Chondrodysplasia punctata is a rare skeletal dysplasia characterized by short-limb dwarfism and multiple punctate epiphyseal calcifications that are present at birth and resolve over the first year of life. It has been subclassified into three groups: the most common X-linked dominant type, also known as *Conradi-Hünermann syndrome,* an autosomal recessive rhizomelic type, and rare X-linked recessive type.[3] Four additional subtypes have been described that are even more rare.

The cause of Conradi-Hünermann syndrome was unknown until identification of mutations in the gene encoding emopamil-binding protein (EBP), which catalyzes an intermediate step in cholesterol biosynthesis. EBP mutations that produce truncated proteins result in typical Conradi-Hünermann syndrome, whereas phenotypes resulting from missense mutations are not always typical for this disorder.[3] Rhizomelic chondrodysplasia punctata type 1 is caused by mutations in the peroxin 7 gene (PEX7), which encodes receptors required for the importation of matrix proteins into peroxisomes. Rhizomelic chondrodysplasia punctata type 2 shows deficiency of the enzyme acyl–coenzyme A:dihydroxyacetonephosphate acyltransferase; the disorder is often (but not always) fatal in the first year of life. Finally, X-linked recessive chondrodysplasia punctata (CDPX) is caused by mutations in the arylsulfatase E (ARSE) gene, resulting in a sulfatase deficiency. The nature of the CDPX phenotype suggests that ARSE may be essential for the correct composition of cartilage and bone matrix during bone development. The importance of several lysosomal sulfatases in cartilage and bone development is evident from their involvement in the catabolic pathway of sulfated glycosaminoglycans, which are essential components of the extracellular matrix of cartilage.

Clinical Findings

Conradi-Hünermann syndrome is characterized by typical facial features consisting of a depressed nasal bridge, a bifid nasal tip, and alopecia. Common findings in the rhizomelic form are microcephaly, growth retardation, psychomotor retardation, feeding difficulties, and spasticity. Patients with chondrodysplasia punctata have symmetrical shortening of the arms and thighs. Limb-length inequality, coxa vara, and multiple joint contractures are common.[4,5] Spinal findings include atlantoaxial instability, congenital scoliosis, and kyphosis. Equinovarus and other foot deformities may be seen.

Radiographic Features

The characteristic punctate calcifications are observed radiographically at birth and usually disappear by the

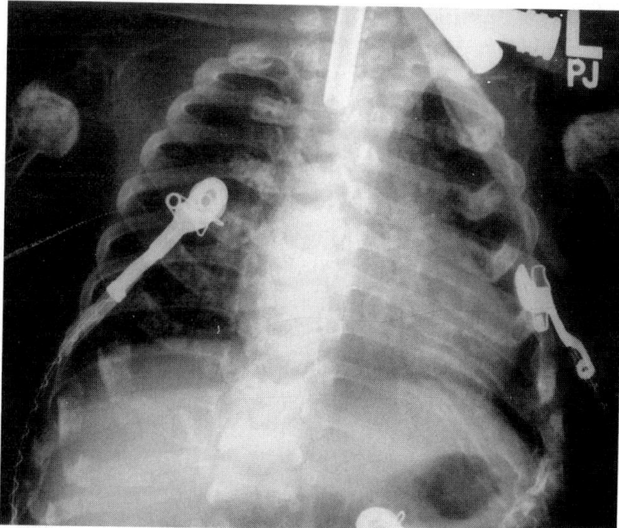

Figure 5-17 A 3-month-old patient with chondrodysplasia punctata has dense, punctate calcifications in the humeral heads and anterior rib ends, characteristic of this disorder. A small thorax has resulted in restrictive lung disease.

time a patient is 1 year old (Fig. 5-17). Unilateral or bilateral coxa vara deformity is frequently associated with asymmetric shortening of the femur (Fig. 5-18). Congenital vertebral anomalies (i.e., hemivertebra, unilateral unsegmented bar, block vertebra) that cause congenital spinal deformities are common (see Table 5-1).

Medical Problems

Patients with the rhizomelic type of chondrodysplasia punctata usually die of respiratory complications or seizure-related disorders during the first year of life. Frequency of bilateral congenital cataract and optic atrophy makes ophthalmologic consultation essential for patients with chondrodysplasia punctata. The possibilities of renal abnormalities and congenital heart disease require careful evaluation.

Orthopaedic Implications

Spinal problems with this disorder commonly require surgical intervention. Atlantoaxial instability must be assessed by means of lateral flexion-extension radiographs and, if required, flexion-extension MRI. If significant instability is present, posterior cervical fusion should be performed. In most patients, congenital scoliosis and kyphosis can progress rapidly during the first 1 or 2 years of life, and the best results are obtained by early spinal fusion.

Limb-length inequalities of more than 3 to 4 cm may occur, and limb lengthening may be considered in some patients. Discrepancies are not treated by epiphyseodesis, because the heights of patients with chondrodysplasia punctata are already below the third percentile. Most flexion contractures are not severe enough to require surgical intervention and are well treated by physical therapy. If coxa vara is significant, proximal femoral realignment osteotomy is considered.

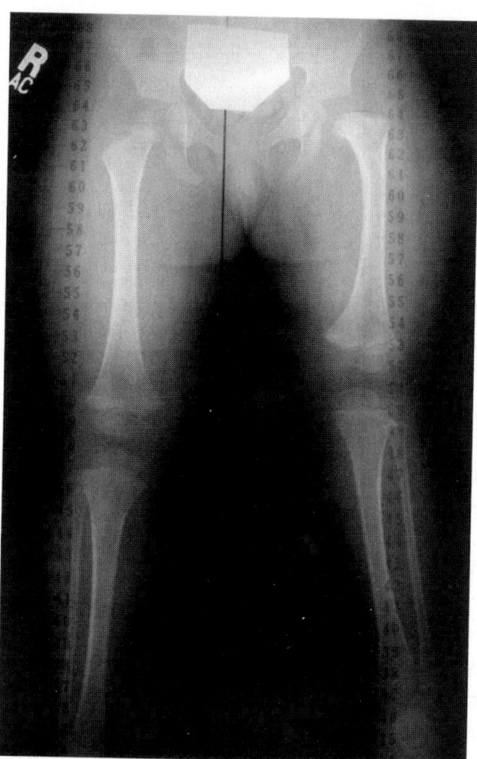

Figure 5-18 During development, the epiphyses take on a more normal appearance, as seen in this 18-month-old patient with chondrodysplasia punctata. The long bones are broad. A delay in ossification of the left femoral head and significant shortening of the left femur have resulted in a limb-length inequality, a common finding in children with this disorder. Coxa vara, seen in the left proximal femur, may develop from flexion contractures.

Metaphyseal Chondrodysplasia

The metaphyseal chondrodysplasias are a group of disorders characterized by metaphyseal deformity and irregularity adjacent to the physes, with little or no epiphyseal involvement. The real defect is in the growth plate itself; the metaphyseal changes are the end results. Schmid metaphyseal chondrodysplasia and McKusick metaphyseal chondrodysplasia are the most common types. Schmid metaphyseal chondrodysplasia is an autosomal dominant disorder with a mutation in the gene for the alpha-1 chain of type X collagen (COL10A1).[3] Type X collagen is synthesized specifically and transiently by hypertrophic chondrocytes at sites of endochondral ossification, such as growth plates. However, the precise function of type X collagen is unknown. McKusick metaphyseal chondrodysplasia, also known as *cartilage-hair hypoplasia*, is common in the Amish community of Lancaster County, Pennsylvania, as well as in Finland. It is an autosomal recessive disorder, and the gene defect is located on chromosome 9. Mutations in the RMRP gene, which encodes the RNA component of mitochondrial RNA-processing endoribonuclease (RNase MRP), have been shown to be responsible for this disorder.[3] The RNase MRP consists of an RNA molecule bound to several proteins. It has at least two functions—cleavage of RNA in mitochondrial DNA synthesis and nucleolar cleaving of pre-ribosomal RNA. The mutations in the RMRP gene cause McKusick metaphyseal chondrodysplasia by disrupting a function of this enzyme that affects multiple organ systems.

Schmid Metaphyseal Chondrodysplasia

Clinical Findings

Patients with Schmid metaphyseal chondrodysplasia are normal at birth and are diagnosed when 2 to 3 years of age. They have rather minimal clinical abnormalities, and the adult height is minimally shortened. The head and face are not affected, and the upper extremity involvement is mild. The thorax and the spine have a normal appearance, except for increased lumbar lordosis in some patients. The patients usually present to the orthopaedic surgeon with leg pain, a waddling gait, varus angulation of the knee, or short stature.

Radiographic Features

Spinal changes occur infrequently in patients with Schmid metaphysial chondrodysplasia. Radiographic changes characteristically occur at the metaphyseal regions of the long bones; the metaphyses are widened and scalloped and may have cysts. Some widening of the physis occurs, but not to the extent observed in rickets. Shortening and bowing of the long bones and genu varum may be seen.

McKusick Metaphyseal Chondrodysplasia

Clinical Findings

McKusick metaphyseal chondrodysplasia is diagnosed when affected children are 2 to 3 years of age. Patients with the disorder have light-colored, sparse hair. Microscopic examination shows the hair to be smaller in diameter than normal hair and, often, to lack pigmentation. Progressive dwarfing results in markedly short adult stature. Patients have generalized ligamentous laxity, but the elbows actually have flexion contractures. Pectus excavatum or carinatum may be observed. Mild genu varum is common.

Radiographic Features

Atlantoaxial instability and some minimal changes in the thoracolumbar spine that are not of much clinical importance may be seen in McKusick metaphyseal chondrodysplasia (see Table 5-1). The metaphyseal involvement is more evenly distributed, and there is more shortening and less varus angulation of the long bones than seen in the Schmid type. Radiographic changes in the thorax, including changes at the costochondral junctions and Harrison grooves as well as a prominent sternum, occur in two thirds of patients.

Medical Problems

Immunologic abnormalities are found in more than half of patients with McKusick metaphyseal chondrodysplasia.[4] An alteration in T-cell immunity makes patients susceptible to viral infections in childhood, with a predisposition to severe varicella zoster infections. Continued antibiotic prophylaxis in the first 6 months of life is recommended. Patients with this disorder have a greater tendency for hematologic problems, including lymphopenia, neutropenia, and anemia. There is an increased risk of malignancy, such as lymphoma, sarcoma, and skin cancer. Hirschsprung disease, intestinal malabsorption, and megacolon may also develop.

Differential Diagnosis

Metaphyseal chondrodysplasia must be differentiated from vitamin D metabolism disorders. The radiographic changes in the metaphyseal regions of the long bones and angular deformities of the lower limbs may resemble those seen in various types of rickets. However, unlike in rickets, epiphyseal and physeal involvement is not severe in metaphyseal chondrodysplasia. Also, biochemical abnormalities are not found in metaphyseal chondrodysplasia.

Orthopaedic Implications

Patients with McKusick metaphyseal chondrodysplasia should be evaluated for atlantoaxial instability, and if significant instability is found, posterior cervical fusion should be performed. Genu varum usually improves with growth during the first decade. Rarely, it does not improve, instead progresses to a severe deformity that requires surgical correction consisting of proximal tibiofibular osteotomy.

Jansen Metaphyseal Chondrodysplasia

Jansen metaphyseal chondrodysplasia is a rare autosomal dominant disorder characterized by abnormal growth plate maturation and laboratory findings that are indistinguishable from those in hyperparathyroidism. This disorder is caused by activating mutations in the receptor for parathyroid hormone (PTH) and parathyroid hormone-related peptide (PTHrP).[3] Through somatic cell hybrid analysis, the mutations in the PTHR gene have been mapped to chromosome 3 in humans.

Severe shortening of the limbs, frontal bossing, and micrognathia are the characteristic clinical findings at birth. Bowing of the long bones occurs with growth as a result of the elongation of the abnormal metaphyses. Flexion contractures may develop in the major joints. The abnormal laboratory findings typical in this disorder include hypercalcemia, hypophosphatemia, and increased renal excretion of phosphate, cyclic adenosine monophosphate (cAMP), and hydroxyproline, despite normal or undetectable levels of PTH and PTHrP.

Dyschondrosteosis (Leri-Weill Syndrome)

Dyschondrosteosis is an autosomal dominant skeletal dysplasia characterized by disproportionate short stature with predominantly mesomelic limb shortening. Expression is variable and consistently more severe in females, who commonly display the Madelung deformity of the forearm (shortening and bowing of the radius with dorsal subluxation of the distal ulna). The disorder is caused by a mutation in the short stature homeobox-containing gene (SHOX) or the SHOX, Y-linked, gene (SHOXY) located on the X and Y chromosomes.[3] SHOX gene has previously been described as the short stature gene implicated in Turner syndrome. It functions as a repressor for growth plate fusion and skeletal maturation in the distal limbs and, thus, counteracts the skeletal maturing effects of estrogens.

Clinical Findings

The diagnosis of dyschondrosteosis is usually made in late childhood or adolescence on the basis of either short stature or wrist pain and deformity. The growth disturbance of the middle segments of the extremities is most notable in the distal radius, causing a Madelung deformity. Patients have bowed forearms with wrist pain and limited wrist, elbow, and forearm motion. Lower limb changes are usually less severe, consisting of only a mild genu varum or ankle valgus.

Radiographic Features

Radiographic changes are found in the ulna, radius, tibia, and fibula in patients with dyschondrosteosis. In the presence of Madelung deformity, there is shortening, bowing, and broadening of the radius (Fig. 5-19A). The ulna is also shortened, but not as much as the radius. The dorsal subluxation of the distal ulna is also detected (see Fig. 5-19B). The tibia and fibula are short, with the fibula longer than tibia in most patients. Mild genu varum or valgus angulation of the ankle may be seen.

Differential Diagnosis

The differential diagnosis of dyschondrosteosis includes other disorders associated with bilateral Madelung deformity, such as Turner syndrome, hereditary multiple exostoses, and Ollier disease. Trauma (e.g., epiphyseal fractures) may cause premature closure of the ulnar-volar portion of the distal radial epiphysis, producing a similar deformity, although most cases are unilateral.

Orthopaedic Implications

Patients concerned about short stature may be referred to an endocrinologist for discussion of human growth hormone treatment. Patients with wrist pain may be treated initially with a wrist splint and nonsteroidal anti-inflammatory agents. If the pain persists, surgical treatment may be considered. Surgical treatment of the Madelung deformity consists of realignment osteotomy of the distal radius in combination with shortening of the distal ulna. Genu varum and ankle valgus usually do not require surgical correction.

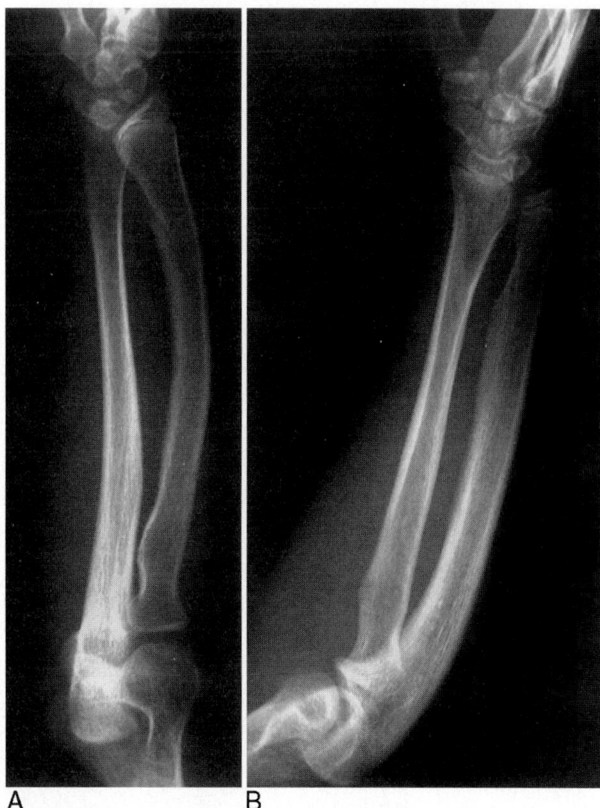

Figure 5-19 Madelung deformity in the forearm of a patient with dyschondrosteosis. A, The radius is shortened, bowed, and broadened. **B,** The ulna is also shortened. Note the dorsal subluxation of the distal ulna.

Cleidocranial Dysplasia

Cleidocranial dysplasia is an autosomal dominant skeletal dysplasia characterized by abnormal clavicles, patent sutures and fontanelles, supernumerary teeth, short stature, and a variety of other skeletal changes. The prevalence is estimated at 1 in 200,000. The disease gene has been mapped to chromosome 6 within a region containing core-binding factor alpha subunit 1 (CBFA1), a member of the runt family of transcription factors.[3] CBFA1 controls differentiation of precursor cells into osteoblasts and is thus essential for intramembranous as well as endochondral bone formation.

Clinical Findings

Cleidocranial dysplasia is recognized at birth. Affected patients have mildly to moderately diminished stature, with heights in most female and some male patients below the fifth percentile for age. Large, broad and short cranium, frontal bossing, hypertelorism, depressed nasal bridge, and midface hypoplasia are typical facial findings. Fontanelles and open sutures persist for years or for life. Dental abnormalities are common. The upper thorax is narrow, with absence of or poorly defined superior and inferior clavicular depressions. Palpable defects of the clavicles are present. Hypermobility of the shoulders is very typical; many patients are able to completely appose the shoulders anteriorly (Fig. 5-20A).[4,5] Hand abnormalities include short, tapered fingers and thumb. Kyphoscoliosis, which occurs in a minority of patients, has been reported in association with syringomyelia in several cases (see Fig. 5-20B). Developmental coxa vara is a common problem for patients with cleidocranial dysplasia.

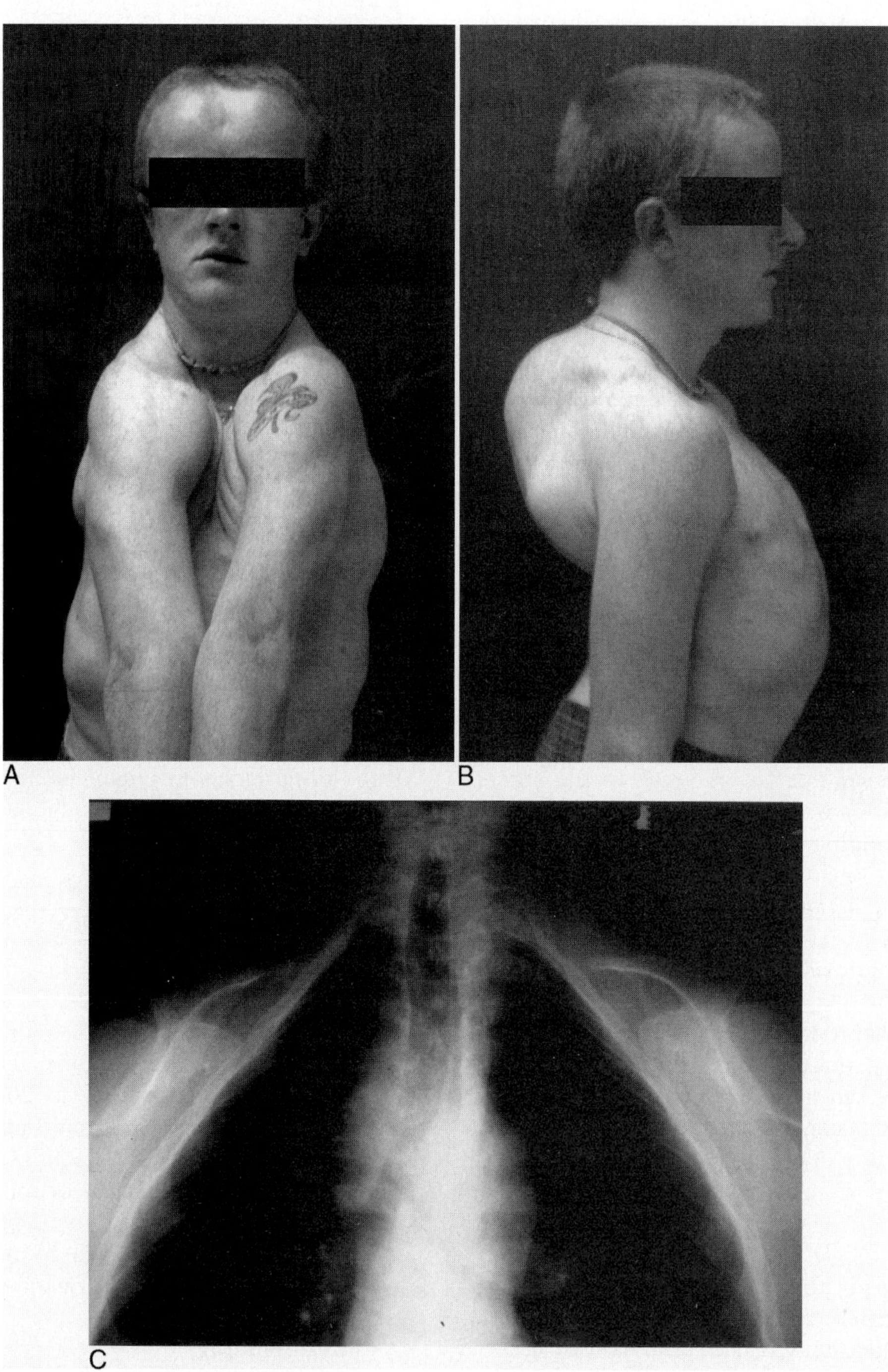

Figure 5-20 **A,** A 20-year-old patient with cleidocranial dysplasia has excessive shoulder mobility. **B,** The patient has thoracal kyphoscoliosis and increased lumbar lordosis. **C,** Complete absence of both clavicles contributes to the abnormal appearance of the bell-shaped thorax.

Radiographic Features

Abnormalities of the clavicle consist of complete absence, hypoplasia, and, most commonly, absence of the central portion with rudimentary medial and lateral portions (see Fig. 5-20C). Spinal deformities, including scoliosis, may occur as a result of abnormal development of ossification centers (see Table 5-1). Involvement of the pelvis is typical, with delayed ossification of the pubic symphysis. Hip abnormalities, such as unilateral or bilateral coxa vara and shortening and broadening of the femoral head and neck, are commonly detected. The distal phalanges of fingers may be underdeveloped.

Orthopaedic Implications

Clavicular defects found in patients with cleidocranial dysplasia do not require surgical intervention. These defects are asymptomatic, and attempts to reconstruct the clavicles are not recommended. Coxa vara is usually progressive, surgical correction with proximal femoral valgus osteotomy must be performed.

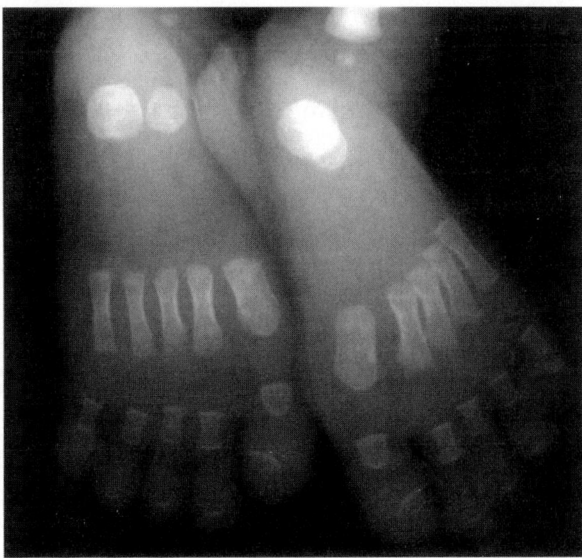

Figure 5-21 Both feet in this infant with Larsen syndrome have short terminal phalanges. The middle phalanges are not ossified. Equinovarus is seen on the right foot, and equinovalgus on the left foot.

Larsen Syndrome

Larsen syndrome is characterized by multiple congenital joint dislocations, facial dysmorphism, and ligamentous laxity. Autosomal dominant as well as recessive forms have been described. Through linkage analysis, the gene for autosomal dominant Larsen syndrome (LAR1) has been mapped to chromosome 3, but the biochemical defect is unknown.[3]

Clinical Findings

Larsen syndrome is recognizable at birth. A broad face with hypertelorism, depressed nasal bridge, and prominent forehead is typical. Congenital spinal deformities are frequently seen in patients with Larsen syndrome.[10] The cervical spine is most commonly and most severely affected; severe cervical kyphosis or instability may be associated with significant neurologic alterations. Scoliosis may affect the thoracic and lumbar spine. Ligamentous laxity and congenital joint dislocations, especially of the hips, knees, and elbows, are very common. Cubitus varus and limited extension of the elbows may be seen. The thumb has a wide distal phalanx, and the fingers are cylindrical with broad ends and short nails. Characteristic foot deformities include equinovarus and equinovalgus.

Radiographic Features

Congenital defects of the cervical, thoracic, and lumbar spine occur frequently in patients with Larsen syndrome (see Table 5-1). Cervical spinal defects, including vertebral body hypoplasia, posterior element dysraphism, and segmentation abnormalities, may result in severe cervical kyphosis or midcervical instability. Thoracolumbar scoliosis secondary to congenital vertebral anomalies may be seen. Congenital dislocations of the hips, knees, and elbows are frequently detected. Accessory carpal bones and short terminal phalanges are characteristic radiographic findings in Larsen syndrome (Fig. 5-21).

Orthopaedic Implications

Cervical spine problems should be evaluated carefully in patients with Larsen syndrome. Surgical stabilization is indicated for patients with severe cervical kyphosis or instability. It is usually achieved by posterior cervical fusion, but in some patients with severe cervical kyphosis, anterior and posterior fusion may be required. Congenital scoliosis and kyphosis are commonly progressive, and early spinal fusion should be considered to obtain the best results.

Hip, knee, and foot problems in patients with Larsen syndrome usually resist conservative treatment. Reduction of the knee dislocations should be completed before treatment of the hips, because at least 45 degrees of knee flexion is desirable to relax the hamstrings and maintain the reduction of the hip. Open reduction associated with some soft tissue procedures, including lengthening or release of capsular, ligamentous, or muscular structures around the knee, are usually required. After reduction of the knee is accomplished and motion is regained, reduction of the hip dislocation should be considered; in general, this reduction must also be open.

Hereditary Multiple Exostoses

Hereditary multiple exostoses is one of the most common skeletal dysplasias seen by orthopaedic surgeons, with an estimated prevalence of approximately 1 in 18,000. It is characterized by cartilage-capped prominences that develop from the epiphyses of the long bones. A genetically heterogeneous autosomal dominant disorder, hereditary multiple exostoses has been associated with mutations in at least three different genes, termed *exostosin* (EXT) genes. The three described EXT loci have been mapped—EXT1 to chromosome 8, EXT2 to chromosome 11, and EXT3 to chromosome 19.[3,11] According to linkage analysis, the EXT1 and EXT2 loci appear to be altered in the majority of families, whereas EXT3, which has not been fully isolated and characterized, is probably less commonly affected. EXT1 and EXT2 function as tumor-suppressor genes and encode two homologous glycoproteins that are expressed throughout the musculoskeletal system. Both glycoproteins are glycosyltransferases located in the membrane of the endoplasmic reticulum and have roles in modifying and enhancing the synthesis and expression of heparan sulfate. Heparan sulfate is a complex polysaccharide that has been implicated in a variety of cellular processes, including cell adhesion, growth factor signaling, and cell proliferation.

Clinical Findings

The exostoses usually appear after age 3 or 4 years. Statures of affected patients are at the low end of normal for age. Problems caused by this condition may be divided into the following four categories: (1) local prominence and impingement by the exostoses; (2) asymmetric growth of two-bone segments, such as the forearm and the leg; (3) limb-length inequality; and (4) late degeneration into chondrosarcoma. Local prominence may cause pressure on muscles, tendons, or nerves, resulting in pain, limited motion (e.g., forearm motion), or nerve palsy (e.g., peroneal palsy from a proximal fibular lesion). Asymmetric growth often leads to angular deformities of the upper and lower limbs (Fig. 5-22). Limb-length inequality, due to more involvement of one limb than of the other, is common. Malignant transformation in children and adolescents with hereditary multiple exostoses is very rare and difficult to monitor. The most practical way is to educate patients and their parents about signs of malignant transformation, such as increased growth of an exostosis and pain over an exostosis.

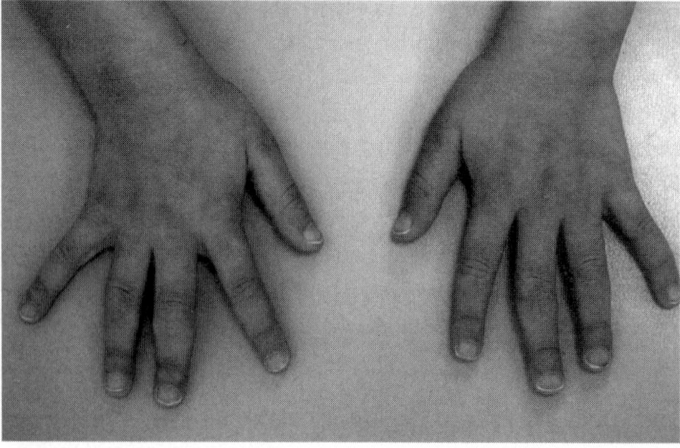

Figure 5-22 A 7-year-old boy with hereditary multiple exostoses. Note the angular deformities of the fingers.

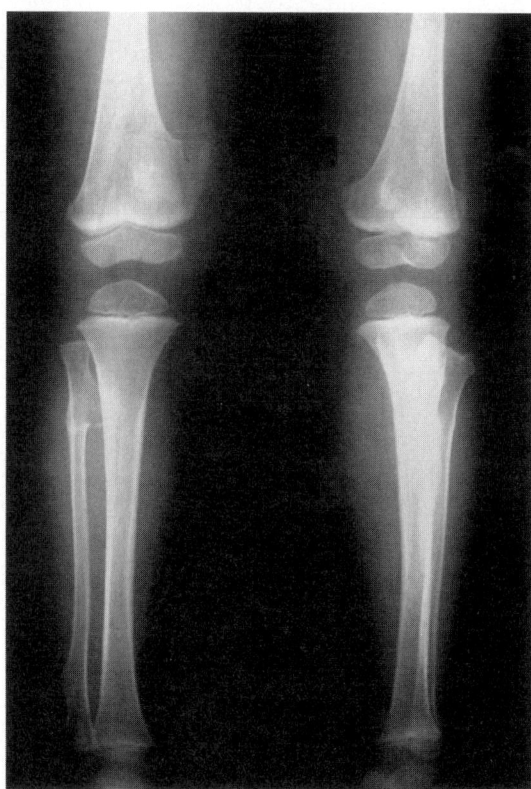

Figure 5-23 Wide-based, bony protuberances are seen in both distal femurs and proximal fibulae. The cortex is continuous with the bone. A normal trabecular pattern is seen.

Radiographic Features

The exostoses may grow perpendicular to the bone in a sessile or pedunculated fashion (Fig. 5-23). The cortex of the exostosis is contiguous with that of the bone itself. The femoral necks are usually wide and in valgus angulation (Fig. 5-24). Genu valgum, ankle valgus, and radial head subluxation with ulnar shortening are frequently seen.

Orthopaedic Implications

Because the lesions are numerous and multiple bones are affected, a careful evaluation of the upper and lower limbs, including range of motion of the joints, neurologic examination, and measurement of the angular deformities, should be performed. Any exostoses causing significant symptoms should be excised. Angular deformities of the knee, ankle, and wrist are treated with hemiepiphyseodesis in young patients and corrective osteotomy

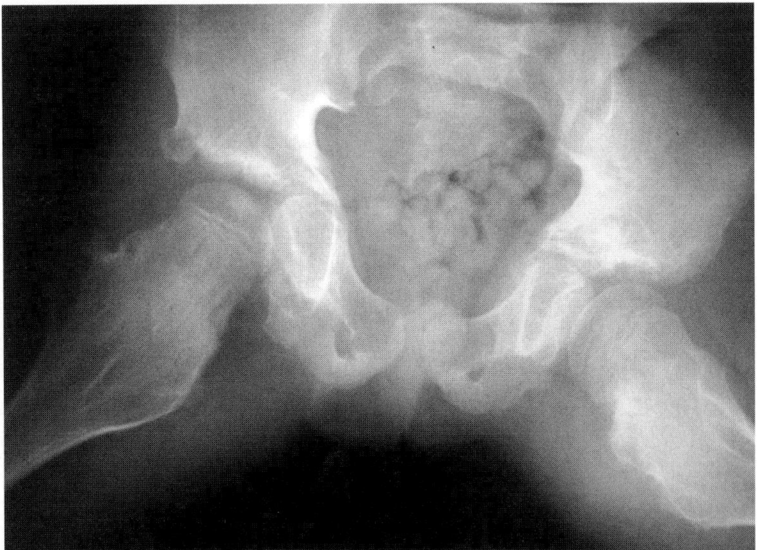

Figure 5-24 In both proximal femora, multiple exostoses cause widening of the femoral necks. Bilateral coxa valga is seen. Irregularities of the bones of the pelvis are due to small exostoses.

in older patients. Epiphyseodesis is the most appropriate treatment for significant limb-length inequality. Painful radial head dislocation may be treated with excision of the radial head at skeletal maturity.

METABOLIC DISORDERS OF BONE

Metabolic bone disease can be defined as impairment of the shape, strength, and composition of bone due to alteration of bone mineral homeostasis. The major factors affecting this homeostasis are the ions, hormones, and signal transduction pathways. Intracellular and extracellular levels of three ions—calcium, phosphorus, and magnesium—which are regulated by three hormones—parathyroid hormone, calcitonin, and 1,25-dihydroxyvitamin D—act upon three tissues—bone, intestine, and kidney—to provide this homeostasis. Other minerals, hormones, and target tissues are involved as well, making these diseases a complex interaction of many exogenous and endogenous factors. Common clinical features are electrolyte disturbances, fractures, bone deformities, abnormal gait, and short stature. The most common forms of metabolic bone disease in children are the various types of rickets and renal osteodystrophy.

Mineral Metabolism

Calcium and Phosphorus Homeostasis

Three principles govern calcium and phosphate shifts in the body.[12] First, if the concentrations of Ca^{++} and HPO_4^- exceed the critical solubility product, ectopic calcification will occur. The solubility of the $CaHPO_4$ salt is increased (and, consequently, the tendency for ectopic calcification is decreased) by mild to moderate acidosis. Second, the irritability and conductivity of nervous tissue and muscle tissue (smooth and skeletal muscle) are inversely proportional, and the irritability and conductivity of cardiac muscle directly proportional, to the concentrations of Ca^{++}. The margin of safety is small. Hypocalcemia leads to hypertonia, hyperreflexia, convulsions, and death in diastole. Hypercalcemia leads hypotonicity, hyperreflexia, obtundation, and death in systole. Third, calcium can not cross cell membranes without a transport system. The cell barrier-transport system for calcium consists of 1,25-dihydroxyvitamin D (activated vitamin D), cytosolic phosphate, and, to a lesser extent, PTH. 1,25-dihydroxyvitamin D increases the synthesis of calcium-binding proteins, such as calbindin or cholecalcin, whereas cytosolic phosphate acts at the membrane transport level; PTH acts via adenyl cyclase-cyclic adenosine monophosphate to increase calcium entry to the intracellular space and to activate the release of calcium from the mitochondria. The major controller is 1,25-dihydroxyvitamin D; phosphate acts only by turning off the entry of calcium at a critical level (and therefore is protective against ectopic calcification). The role of PTH is primarily to balance the action of vitamin D, through its differential effects on calcium and phosphorus metabolism.

Biology of Vitamin D

The provitamins D consist of ergosterol, ingested in the form of animal fats, and 7-dehydrocholesterol, synthesized in the liver. Both of these metabolically inactive sterols are stored in the skin and, in the presence of ultraviolet light, are converted to ergocalciferol (vitamin D_2) and cholecalciferol (vitamin D_3). After transportation to the liver, they are converted to 25-hydroxyvitamin D. The final and most critical conversion

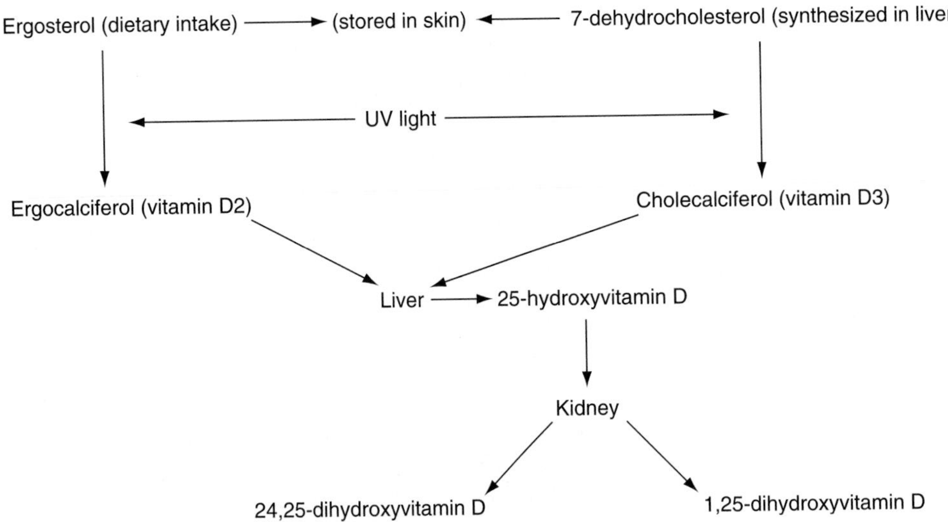

Figure 5-25 Biology of vitamin D. The provitamins D (ergosterol and 7-dehydrocholesterol) are stored in the skin and, in the presence of ultraviolet (UV) light, are converted to ergocalciferol (vitamin D_2) and cholecalciferol (vitamin D_3). In the liver, vitamin D_2 and vitamin D_3 are converted to 25-hydroxyvitamin D. The final step occurs in the kidney, where 25-hydroxyvitamin D is converted to less active 24,25-dihydroxyvitamin D or highly active 1,25-dihydroxyvitamin D.

occurs in the kidney, where 25-hydroxyvitamin D is converted to either the less active 24,25-dihydroxyvitamin D or the highly active 1,25-dihydroxy form (Fig. 5-25). A low serum calcium level, a low serum phosphate level, and a high PTH level favor conversion to the 1,25 analogue. On the other hand, a high serum calcium level, a high serum phosphate level, and a low PTH level favor formation of the less potent 24,25-dihydroxyvitamin D.

1,25-dihydroxyvitamin D controls calcium metabolism in the gut, proximal tubule, and bone. The major function is to increase the efficiency of the small intestine to absorb dietary calcium and transfer it into the circulation. It also increases calcium absorption from the proximal tubules. In bone, vitamin D enhances the mobilization of calcium stores when dietary calcium is inadequate to maintain serum blood calcium levels within the normal range.

Biology of Parathyroid Hormone

PTH is synthesized in the parathyroid glands from a biosynthetic precursor, pro-PTH. Serum calcium levels carefully regulate release of the hormone: The lower the serum calcium level, the more PTH is synthesized and elaborated. Maintenance of extracellular calcium homeostasis is the primary role of PTH. Its actions are synergistic with those of 1,25-dihydroxyvitamin D, which are to increase calcium transport from the gut and renal tubules and to promote calcium release from the bone (lysis of hydroxyapatite crystals). PTH acts independently of vitamin D to activate the osteoclast population to resorb bone. Another action of PTH (also independent of vitamin D) is to diminish the tubular reabsorption of phosphate.

Maintenance of Serum Calcium

Multicellular organisms require a highly regulated concentration of calcium in the extracellular fluid. The absorption of calcium from the gastrointestinal tract, reabsorption of calcium from the renal tubule, and bone-blood exchange are the three major components of the calcium control system. All are under the control of the 1,25-dihydroxyvitamin D and PTH synergistic transport system. The lowered serum calcium level stimulates the production and release of PTH, which activates the synthesis of 1,25-dihydroxyvitamin D. Together, the two agents act to increase calcium absorption from the gut, tubular reabsorption of filtered calcium in the kidney, and resorption of bone (Fig. 5-26). Bone resorption occurs by lysis of the crystalline apatite through osteoclastic resorption. Any excess phosphate that appears as a result of the breakdown of bone, under the influence of PTH, is rapidly excreted by the kidney by means of a marked decrease in the tubular reabsorption of phosphate. In this manner, short-term calcium deficits, even if profound, may be rapidly corrected by a highly effective balance system.[13]

Rickets

Rickets is a syndrome rather than a specific disease entity. Despite the numerous etiologic pathways, the main cause of the disorder is the lack of available extracellular calcium, phosphorus, or both, which interferes with physeal growth and mineralization of the skeleton, resulting in clinical deformities in the growing child. This lack of calcium and phosphorus may be due to inadequate intake of calcium and vitamin D, impaired

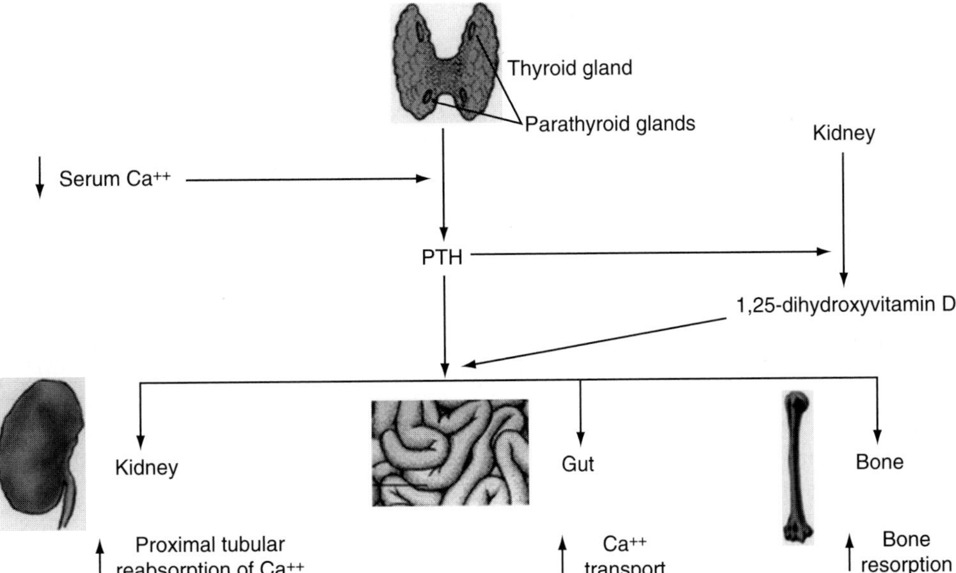

Figure 5-26 Maintenance of serum calcium (Ca^{++}). The lowered serum calcium level stimulates the production and release of parathyroid hormone (PTH) from parathyroid glands. PTH activates the synthesis of 1,25-dihydroxyvitamin D in the kidney. These agents act together to increase tubular reabsorption of filtered calcium in the kidney, calcium transport in the gut, and resorption of bone. UV, ultraviolet.

absorption of phosphorus or vitamin D, decreased conversion of vitamin D to its active form, end-organ insensitivity to vitamin D, impaired release of calcium from bone, and phosphate wasting (Box 5-4). The clinical presentation, histologic abnormalities, and radiographic changes are similar for many of the different causes of rickets, with the exception of renal osteodystrophy (see later discussion). Evaluation of patients with rickets consists of a careful history including family history, physical examination, radiographic evaluation, and laboratory tests.

Vitamin D–resistant rickets is commonly seen by pediatric orthopaedic surgeons. Hypophosphatemic rickets, also known as *phosphate diabetes*, is the common form of vitamin D–resistant rickets and is characterized by a renal tubular defect in phosphate transport. It is commonly transmitted as an X-linked dominant disorder. The gene responsible for this disorder was identified through positional cloning and designated PHEX (formerly PEX), to indicate a phosphate-regulating gene with homology to endopeptidases on the X chromosome. This enzyme appears to play an important role in cleaving endogenous fibroblast growth factor-23 (FGF23), a potent phosphaturic hormone.[3] X-linked dominant hypophosphatemic rickets is fully expressed in hemizygous males. Isolated hypophosphatemia may signify the presence of the trait in heterozygous females. With full expression, the condition consists of hypophosphatemia, lower limb deformities, and stunted growth.

Box 5-4 Causes of Rickets

- Deficiency diseases
  - Vitamin D–deficient rickets (inadequate intake of vitamin D ± no sunlight)
  - Chelators in the diet (i.e., phytates, oxylates)
  - Phosphorus deficiency
- Gastrointestinal disorders
  - Gastric rickets
  - Hepatobiliary rickets (free fatty acids in gut bind calcium)
  - Enteric rickets (i.e., inflammatory bowel disease)
- Vitamin D–resistant rickets
  - Hypophosphatemic rickets (decreased tubular reabsorption of phosphate)
  - Decrease in 1,25-dihydroxyvitamin D production
  - End-organ insensitivity to autogenous 1,25-dihydroxyvitamin D
  - Renal tubular acidosis
- Unusual forms of rickets
  - Rickets in association with soft tissue and bone tumors
  - Rickets in association with fibrous dysplasia
  - Rickets in association with neurofibromatosis
  - Rickets in association with anticonvulsant medications
- Renal osteodystrophy

Clinical Findings

Children with rickets usually have short stature, often less than the third percentile. Muscle weakness of the abdomen and extremities may be seen. Frontal bossing and enlargement of the suture lines (e.g., caput quadratum) are common. Delayed dentition, enamel defects, and extensive caries are common dental anomalies. Examination of the chest is likely to show enlargement of the costal cartilages (rachitic rosary), indentation of the lower ribs where the diaphragm inserts (Harrison groove), and, occasionally, pectus carinatum. The spine is commonly affected, most characteristically with a long thoracic kyphosis.

Ligamentous laxity is a common finding in children with rickets. The long bones are deformed and shortened, usually with bowing in the lower limbs. A general guideline is that if the disease manifests during the stage of physiologic bowing (age 1 to 2 years), the result will be varus deformity, and that active disease during the stage of physiologic genu valgum (age 2 to 4 years) produces valgus deformity.[13] Upper limbs usually do not have significant deformities. Apparent enlargement of the elbows, wrists, knees, and ankles may be detected by physical examination and is due to metaphyseal enlargement.

Radiographic Features

Plain radiographs are most useful for evaluation of rickets. In milder forms of the syndrome, radiographic findings may be subtle. General radiographic findings are osteopenia, thin cortices, and small trabeculae with an overall decrease in bone mass. The osteopenia is more marked in the metaphyses, giving a "washed-out" appearance. The cortices, vertebral end plates, and trabeculae often appear fuzzy and indistinct. The appearance of the growth plates, including irregular widening or cupping, is the most classic finding (Fig. 5-27). Looser lines, ribbon-like linear radiolucencies extending transversely from one cortex across the medullary canal, represent areas of weakening or incomplete fractures. They may become complete transverse fractures, sometimes with only minor trauma. Bowing of the femur and tibia and angular deformities of the lower extremities, including coxa vara, genu varum, and genu valgum, are common radiographic findings (Fig. 5-28).

Laboratory Tests

The main diagnostic laboratory tests are measurements of serum calcium, phosphate, and alkaline phosphatase levels. Also helpful are determinations of serum 25-hydroxyvitamin D, 1,25-dihydroxyvitamin D, and PTH levels and of urine calcium and phosphate levels. Abnormal laboratory values may be the only findings in an infant with rickets. Children with classic or vitamin D–deficient rickets usually have low to low-normal levels of serum calcium, low levels of serum phosphorus, elevated levels of serum alkaline phosphatase and PTH, low concentrations

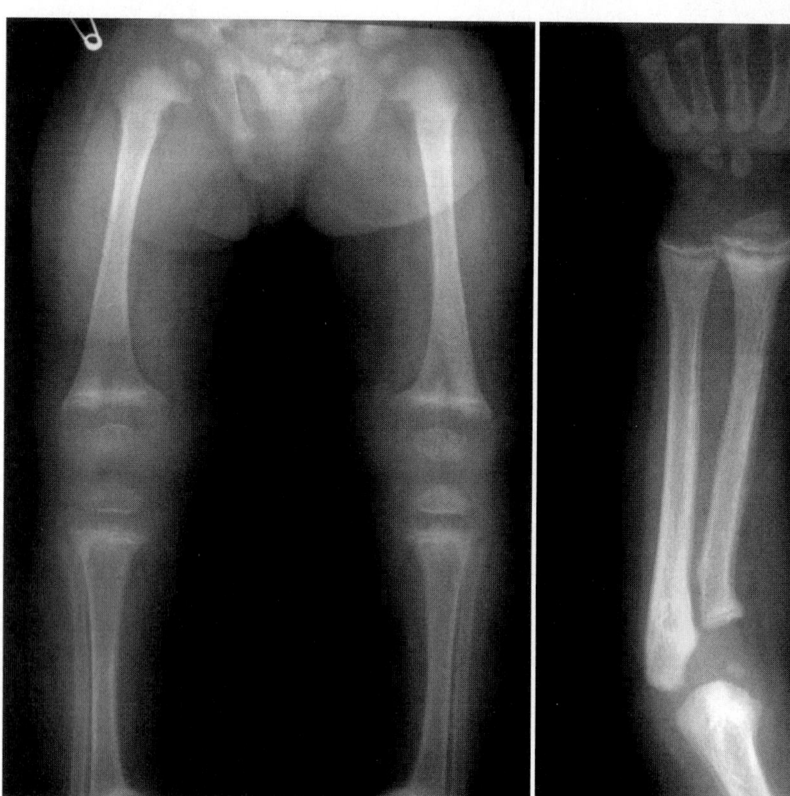

Figure 5-27 The radiographic findings in rickets are most easily seen at the sites of most active growth, the knees and wrists. A, In a 3-year-old boy with active rickets, all the long bones at the knees have widened growth plates with washed-out, irregular metaphyses. Some of the metaphyses have a feathery, "paintbrush" appearance. Note the characteristic cupping of the metaphyses and generalized osteopenia. **B,** The forearm and wrist of a different child have dense metaphyseal bands, indicating a period of healing. Subcortical tunneling can be seen along the radius, ulna, and metacarpals. Generalized osteopenia is present.

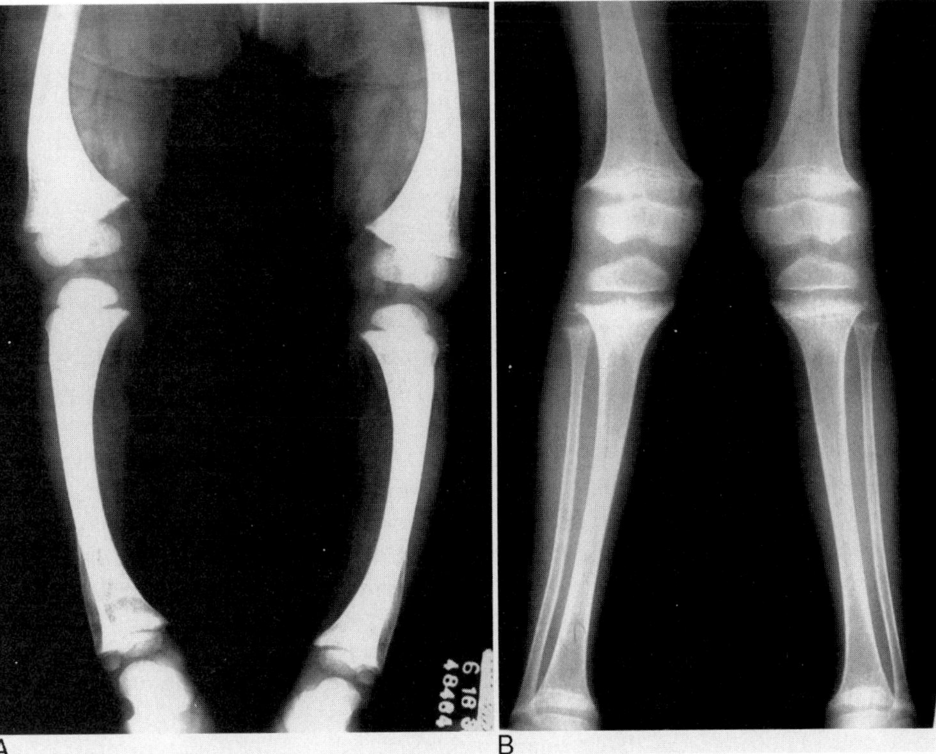

Figure 5-28 **A,** Genu varum in a 2-year-old patient with rickets. Both femora, tibiae, and fibulae are bowed. **B,** Genu valgum in a 4-year-old patient with active rickets. The physes are widened, and the metaphyses are cupped and irregular.

of 25-hydroxyvitamin D and 1,25-dihydroxyvitamin D, diminished levels of urinary calcium, and markedly diminished tubular reabsorption of phosphate.

Differential Diagnosis

Osteomalacia, the adult counterpart of rickets, is also characterized by the presence of excessive amounts of unmineralized osteoid, resulting in skeletal deformity. However, it occurs only after the physes have closed and lacks the growth disturbances seen in patients with rickets. Physiologic genu varum or valgum, Blount disease, and some skeletal dysplasias with angular deformities of the knee should be considered in the differential diagnosis of rickets. The child with physiologic genu varum or valgum and Blount disease has no other findings, and the stature and development are within normal ranges. Metaphyseal, epiphyseal, or other skeletal dysplasias, such as achondroplasia and hypochondroplasia, may be associated with short stature and multiple skeletal abnormalities, including angular deformities of the knee.

Renal Osteodystrophy

Renal osteodystrophy includes bone diseases that occur as a result of renal failure. Improved management of renal bone disease has lowered the incidence of renal osteodystrophy.[12,13] In renal osteodystrophy, glomerular damage leads to phosphate retention, and tubular injury causes decreased production of 1,25-dihydroxyvitamin D, the active form of vitamin D. These two factors severely inhibit the gut's ability to absorb calcium. The resultant hypocalcemia triggers severe secondary hyperparathyroidism, which remains ineffective in increasing intestinal absorption of calcium. Therefore, the body's only means of raising serum calcium levels is through bone resorption.

Patients with chronic renal disease are hyperphosphatemic, and even when pH is reduced, shifting the solubility product, they depend on a decreased serum calcium level to avoid precipitation of the relatively insoluble $CaHPO_4$. If for any reason (e.g., dietary indiscretion, spontaneous improvement, or dialysis) calcium increases to near-normal levels, calcium salts may be precipitated at a variety of ectopic sites.[13]

Clinical Findings

Patients with renal osteodystrophy may have all the features of rickets. The bones are fragile, and fractures occur frequently with minor trauma. The presence of calcification in the conjunctivae and skin can produce significant irritation and itching. The periarticular calcification and ossification can cause severe limitation and pain in one or more joints. Ligamentous laxity and muscle weakness may be seen. Slipped epiphyses, especially in the proximal femur, are common.

Radiographic Features

Radiographic changes seen in renal osteodystrophy are unique, consisting of "salt-and-pepper" skull, absence of the cortical outline of the outer centimeter of the clavicles, and subperiosteal resorption of the ulnas, terminal tufts of the distal phalanges, and medial proximal tibias. Slipped epiphyses are also frequently seen in patients with renal osteodystrophy.

Brown tumors, which appear as expanded destructive bone lesions, are usually round or ovoid with indistinct margins. They are due to secondary hyperparathyroidism and are most common in cases of severe and long-standing renal osteodystrophy. Brown tumors may be present in the long bones or pelvis and, when associated with thinning of the cortex, may be the sites of pathologic fractures.

Management

The role of the orthopaedic surgeon in the treatment of rickets and renal osteodystrophy has shifted considerably with the understanding of the basic science of the disorders associated with both entities. Medical treatment of the underlying metabolic disturbance, coordinated by a pediatrician or a pediatric endocrinologist, is the necessary first step in management, because (1) it alone may be curative, (2) the general health of the individual depends on it, and (3) orthopaedic intervention without it will prove disappointing. Medical treatment aims to correct the alteration in physiology with the use of agents such as vitamin D, 1,25-dihydroxyvitamin D, calcium infusions, neutral phosphate solutions, and other dietary and pharmacologic interventions. The extent of remodeling that is likely to occur depends on the growth remaining after correction of the physiologic abnormality. It is usually possible to achieve a cure in many patients with rickets, with expectations of normal growth and lifestyle.

In the presence of fracture or when deformity exceeds the physiologic range and predisposes the individual to progressive deformity or altered mechanical alignment, orthopaedic treatment is indicated. Fractures require appropriate treatment by closed methods (i.e., casting) or surgical intervention. Lower limb deformities can be managed with bracing or surgery. Progressive deformities of more than 15 to 20 degrees and failure of brace treatment are the indications for surgical intervention. Realignment of lower limb deformities is the goal of surgical treatment. Multiple-level osteotomies are usually required and are fixed with intramedullary rods; the deformed segment of the bone is divided into multiple straight, smaller segments, which are realigned over the rod. Healing time can be quite prolonged. Recurrence risk is about 20% to 25%.

Hypophosphatasia

In most classification systems, hypophosphatasia is included as a cause of rickets because of its similar clinical and radiographic features. However, it has a different pathophysiology and should be differentiated from rickets.[13] The three different types of hypophosphatasia are adult, infantile, and childhood. Severe infantile and childhood types are transmitted in an autosomal recessive manner, whereas the mild adult type may be transmitted as a dominant or recessive trait. Hypophosphatasia results from a genetic error, which has been mapped to chromosome 1, in the synthesis of alkaline phosphatase in liver, bone, or kidney.[3] This enzyme is necessary for the maturation of the primary spongiosa in the physes, and its deficiency leads to normal production of bone (osteoid) but inadequate mineralization, with resultant skeletal deformities that mimic those in rickets.

Clinical Findings

Patients with hypophosphatasia usually show the characteristic changes early in life. Absence of calcification of the calvaria (craniotabes), late closure of the fontanelles and sutures, and craniosynostosis are common findings. Dentition may be markedly delayed. Bowing of the long bones and knock-knee deformities are common. Fractures after minor trauma may occur.

Radiographic Features

Radiographic changes in hypophosphatasia are similar to those in rickets. Generalized osteopenia, most marked

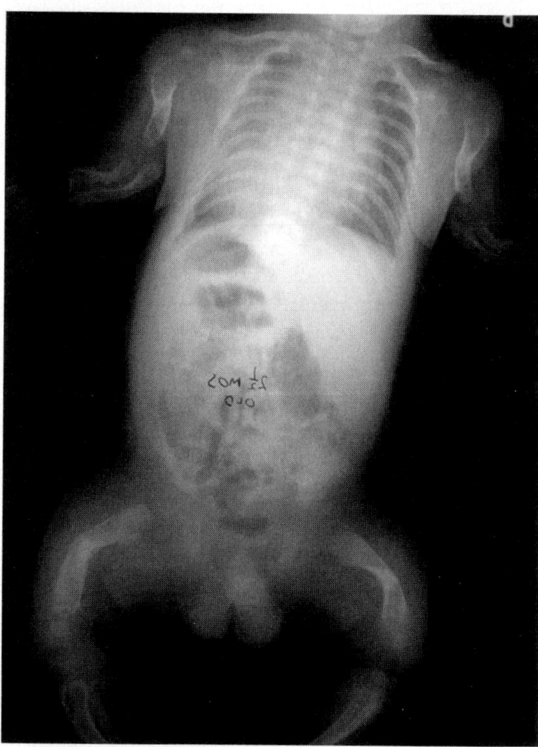

Figure 5-29 A 3-month-old patient with hypophosphatasia has bowing of the long bones. Focal round or wedge-shaped lucencies, representing islands of cartilage, are seen in the metaphyses, a finding unique to hypophosphatasia. In addition, the ribs are short, and the thorax is small.

in the calvarium and the metaphyseal regions of the long bones, is seen. Broad metaphyses and central cup- or wedge-shaped ossification defects of the central physes are typical (Fig. 5-29). Bowing of the long bones and angular deformities of the lower extremities may be seen.

Management

There is no definitive therapy for hypophosphatasia. Pathologic fractures may be a difficult problem because of the poor quality of the bone. Closed treatment methods are usually employed. If closed treatment fails, surgical intervention is required. Bowing of the long bones and angular deformities of the lower extremities may require treatment if they are progressive and exceed the physiologic range. They are managed with bracing or, if indicated, surgical treatment.

Osteogenesis Imperfecta

Osteogenesis imperfecta (OI) is a genetically transmitted disease resulting in fragility of the entire skeleton. It is seen with varying levels of severity, from multiple fractures in an infant to only a few fractures before maturity in a child. The clinical variation is due to differences in the causative mutation. OI is due to a defect in type I collagen. Type I collagen is present in bone, skin, tendon, ligament, cornea, sclera, and dentin. It is a triple helix, composed of two alpha-I chains and one alpha-II chain. The mutations in OI involve one of the two genes that encode the chains of type I collagen. The COL1A1 gene on chromosome 17 encodes the alpha-1 chain, and COL1A2 gene on chromosome 7 encodes the alpha-2 chain.[3] Mild forms of OI often result from reduced amounts of type I collagen of normal composition, and severe forms from structural abnormalities in type I collagen.

Numerous classifications have been proposed for OI. The Sillence classification system is most commonly used (Table 5-3).[14] It divides OI into 4 types: types 1 and 4 are transmitted in an autosomal dominant manner, and types 2 and 3 are transmitted in an autosomal recessive manner. Dental findings are used to further subtype OI, into A without and B with dentinogenesis imperfecta. Although the Sillence classification remains the most helpful system for the geneticist in ordering the many features of this entity, it may be less helpful for the pediatric orthopaedic surgeon consulted in the perinatal period to estimate the musculoskeletal prognosis for an affected child. To address this issue, Shapiro advanced a congenita-tarda classification (Box 5-5).[15]

Table 5-3 Sillence Classification of Osteogenesis Imperfecta

Type 1A–B	Most common, mild type Mild to moderate bone fragility, little or no deformity
Type 2	Perinatal, lethal type; patients rarely survive infancy Extremely fragile bones, severe deformity
Type 3	Severe, progressively deforming type Moderate to severe deformity at birth with progressive, neonatal fractures
Type 4A–B	Moderately severe type Mild to moderate bone fragility and long bone/spine deformity

Clinical Findings

Patients with OI characteristically have fragile bones and short stature. Many patients have small, triangular faces. The sclera may be blue in many but not all cases. The defective dentinogenesis of deciduous or permanent teeth or both may be seen. Hearing may be impaired owing to defects in the bones of the middle ear. The laxity of the ligaments results in hypermobile joints and a higher incidence of joint dislocation. Spinal deformities such as scoliosis may be seen in some patients. Deformities of the long bones due to fractures or microfractures usually develop (Fig. 5-30A).

Radiographic Features

Some degree of generalized osteopenia is detected in almost all patients with OI. It is evident from visual inspection in most patients, but in even the mildest cases, bone densitometry shows at least a 25% decrease in mineralization. The osteopenic vertebrae may fracture easily, resulting in a flattened or biconcave shape. Thoracic or thoracolumbar scoliosis is commonly detected. The pelvis may show acetabular protrusion. The long bones may be thin and bowed with thin cortices and a poorly developed trabecular pattern (see Fig. 5-30B). Deformities may result from multiple fractures (Fig. 5-31).

Differential Diagnosis

The differential diagnosis of OI includes child abuse, idiopathic juvenile osteoporosis, and fibrous dysplasia (rare). History is extremely helpful in differentiating OI

Box 5-5 Shapiro Classification of Osteogenesis Imperfecta

Congenita; implies that fractures occurred in utero or at birth, diagnosed at birth
- A. Crumpled femurs or ribs
- B. Normal bone contours but with fractures

Tarda; diagnosed later
- A. Fractures before walking
- B. Fractures after walking

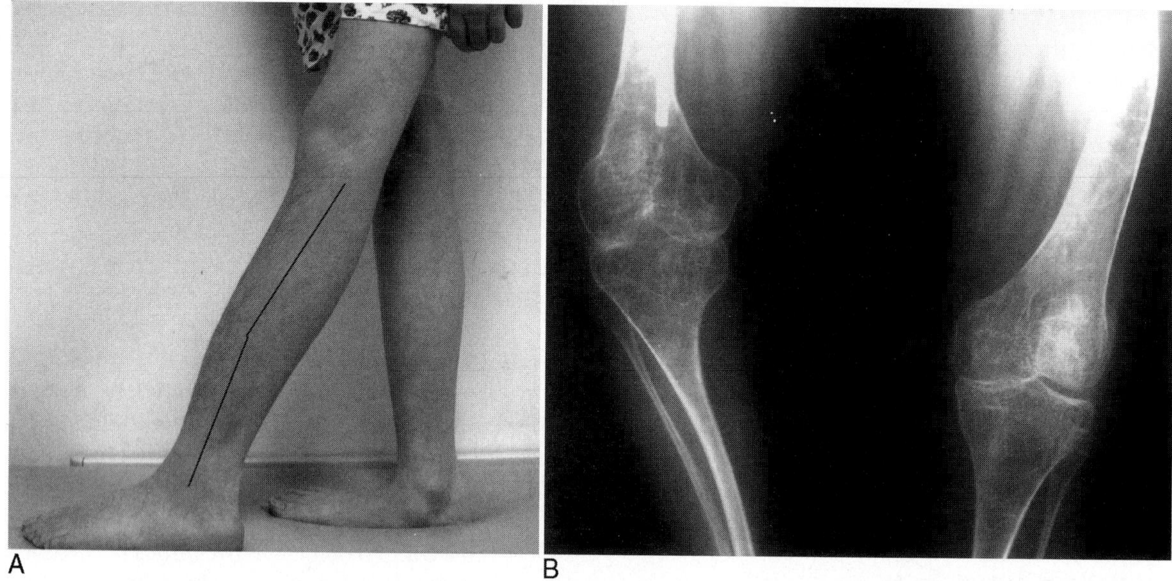

Figure 5-30 A 14-year-old boy with osteogenesis imperfecta. A, Note the angular deformity (apex anterior angulation) of the left leg secondary to recurrent fractures of the tibia. **B,** The radiograph of the lower extremities shows severe demineralization and bowing of the long bones. Note the thin cortices and poorly developed trabecular pattern.

from child abuse. Fractures occurring with relatively mild injury, a positive family history, the presence of abnormalities of the teeth, sclera, or hearing, and a systemic osteopenia revealed by radiography may all suggest OI. Idiopathic juvenile osteoporosis may manifest as spontaneous or pathologic fractures, but is usually a transient, self-limited disorder. Fibrous dysplasia causes bone deformities and fractures, but the bones are not as tapered and thin as in OI, and many of the bones in a patient with fibrous dysplasia are totally free of disease.

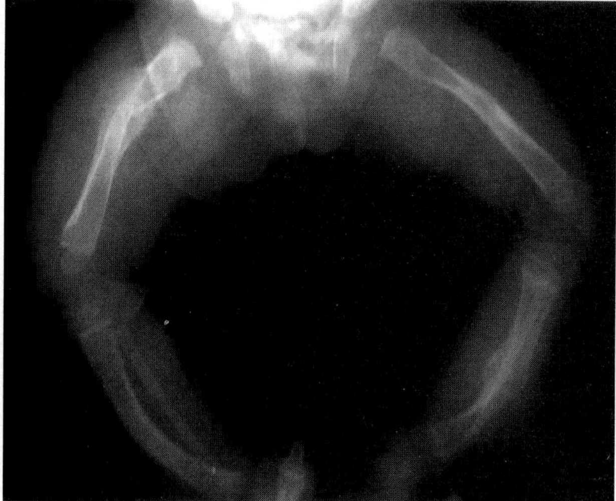

Figure 5-31 A 10-month-old patient with osteogenesis imperfecta has characteristic findings: diffusely decreased mineralization, bowing of the long bones, and multiple healing fractures.

Management

Many systemic treatment modalities have been attempted for OI, but none is widely accepted. Investigators have used calcium, vitamin C, vitamin D, fluoride, calcitonin, and magnesium without benefit. Biphosphonates, potent inhibitors of bone resorption, have been suggested in clinical trials to have a protective effect, but research is still ongoing.[16] Allogeneic bone marrow transplantation is being tried for the most severe cases in young infants.[17]

Orthoses for the lower extremities may help young patients stand. Lightweight hip-knee-ankle-foot orthoses (HKAFOs) or pneumatic trousers, although seldom used, may prevent fractures in patients who are at risk but who have not undergone rod stabilization. Treatment of fractures is a major problem in patients with OI (Fig. 5-32). Callus formed in response to the fracture is identical in

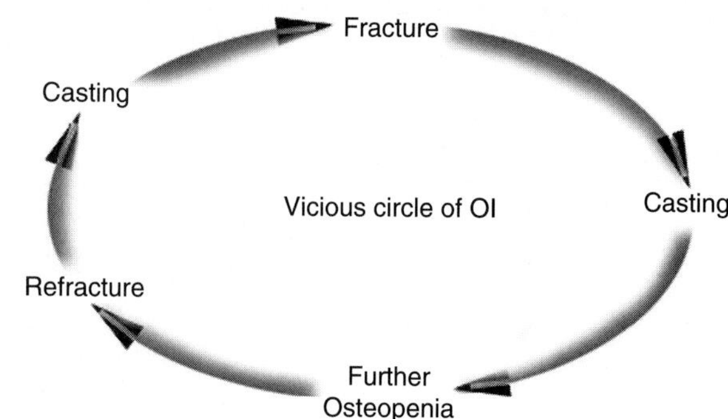

Figure 5-32 The "vicious circle" of osteogenesis imperfecta (OI).

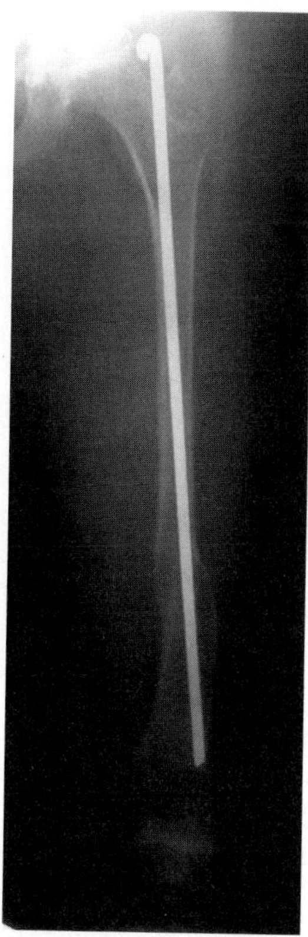

Figure 5-33 An intramedullary rod transfixes a healing fracture in a child with osteogenesis imperfecta.

structure with the rest of the skeleton; it is plastic and easily deformed by mechanical forces. Closed treatment methods are usually employed. If management by closed means proves difficult, treatment with internal fixation may be considered (Fig. 5-33). Intramedullary rods (load-sharing devices) are preferable to plates and screws, which tend to become dislodged from the weakened bone.[18]

Deformities of the long bones may require surgical treatment. The indications are severe diaphyseal bowing (usually, anterolateral bowing of the femur, and anterior bowing of the tibia) that prevents standing, recurrent fractures in a given region, and, occasionally, cosmesis. Realignment of the deformed bone is achieved with multiple osteotomies and intramedullary fixation with expansile rods. Pseudoarthrosis develops in up to 20% of patients postoperatively.

Scoliosis is a difficult problem to treat in OI as in other disorders involving osteopenia. The curves tend to progress relentlessly, and bracing is ineffective in controlling progression of the deformity. Segmental instrumentation is performed because of the poor quality of bone. Spinal curves may be fused early (at 40 degrees) to halt the relentless progression.

Basilar invagination is evident radiographically in up to one quarter of patients with OI. The deformable bones are unable to withstand the increasing weight of the head. Symptoms include cranial nerve palsies, headaches, respiratory depression, spasticity, nystagmus, and weakness, and may lead to early death. There is no completely satisfactory treatment for this complication. Conservative treatment with full-time use of a brace may provide partial symptomatic relief. Surgical therapy also is an option.

Idiopathic Juvenile Osteoporosis

Idiopathic juvenile osteoporosis is a rare, self-limited disorder of unknown cause that affects previously healthy children. The age of onset is usually between 8 and 14 years, and resolution usually occurs spontaneously within 2 to 4 years after onset or after puberty. It must be differentiated from other osteopenic conditions affecting children.

Clinical Findings and Radiographic Features

Idiopathic juvenile osteoporosis is characterized initially by bone and joint pain due to spontaneous fractures in previously healthy children. Back pain may also be present. Generalized osteopenia of varying levels is seen; osteopenia is more marked at the metaphyseal regions of the long bones (Fig. 5-34). Collapse of the vertebral bodies and spinal deformities, especially kyphosis, occur frequently.

Differential Diagnosis

Idiopathic juvenile osteoporosis must be differentiated from other conditions resulting in osteopenia and bone fragility during childhood, such as OI, hematologic malignancies, thyroid disorders, Cushing disease, steroid-induced osteopenia, and disuse osteopenia. The diagnosis is usually made through demonstration of the features of this disease and ruling out of other conditions with similar manifestations. Rapid progression after many years of normality differentiates idiopathic juvenile osteoporosis from osteogenesis imperfecta.

Management

Idiopathic juvenile osteoporosis is a self-limited disorder that tends to resolve spontaneously.[13] It has been difficult to demonstrate the efficacy of any treatment regimen in altering the natural history of the disease. For kyphosis, antikyphotic bracing has been recommended. Surgical intervention is rarely required. Metaphyseal fractures should receive appropriate orthopaedic management. Prolonged disuse or immobilization can worsen the osteoporosis and clinical symptoms.

Osteopetrosis

Osteopetrosis is a rare metabolic bone disease characterized by a diffuse increase in skeletal density and obliteration of marrow spaces. Histologic analysis shows the skeleton to contain cores of calcified cartilage

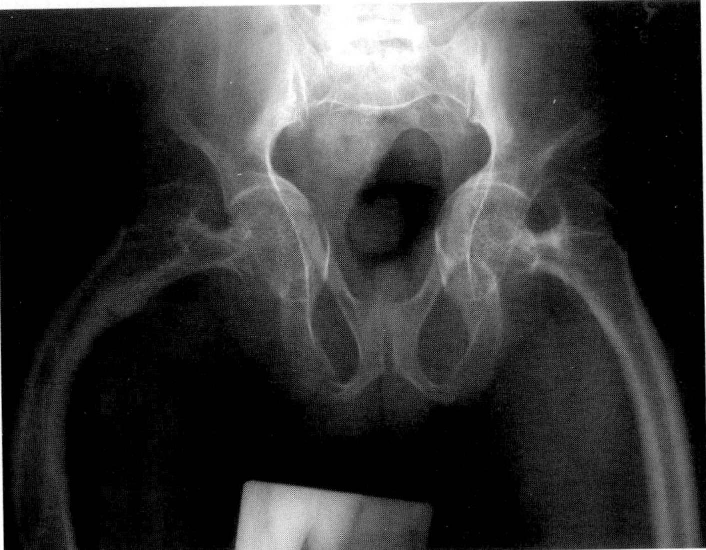

Figure 5-34 A teenager with idiopathic juvenile osteoporosis has diffuse osteopenia and resultant deformities of the pelvis and femurs. Protrusio acetabuli is severe.

surrounded by areas of new bone; this new bone formation is normal but there is a deficiency of bone and cartilage resorption, resulting in exceedingly dense bones. The osteoclasts are abnormal and lack a functional ruffled border.

The three different forms of osteopetrosis are an autosomal recessive infantile malignant form, an autosomal recessive intermediate form, and an autosomal dominant adult (tarda) form.[19] The infantile form is characterized by severe anemia, thrombocytopenia, hepatosplenomegaly, cranial and optic nerve palsies, multiple fractures, and a compromise of the immune system. Death may occur at a young age from anemia or sepsis. The intermediate form is usually diagnosed in later childhood, after a fracture. It may have some features of the infantile form, but presentation is milder. Although the general health and life span of patients with the adult form of osteopetrosis are usually unaffected, a lifelong history of fractures and osteomyelitis usually characterizes the clinical picture. Generalized increased density of the bones is the main radiographic feature in osteopetrosis (Fig. 5-35). Deformities secondary to fractures may be seen.

Treatment for infantile osteopetrosis is bone marrow transplantation at a young age with marrow from an appropriately HLA-matched donor.[13] A successful transplant may resolve the hematologic abnormalities and can result in gradual restoration of patent marrow cavities. High-dose 1,25-dihydroxyvitamin D therapy with a low-calcium diet has been employed because of its ability to stimulate osteoclasts and bone resorption.

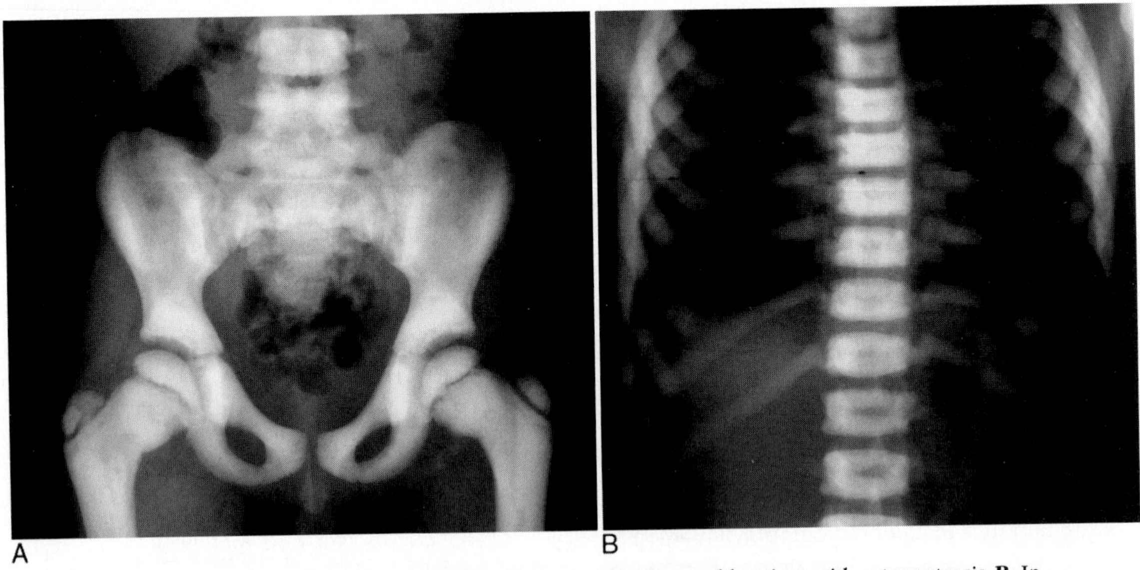

Figure 5-35 **A,** The bones are diffusely dense in this 10-year-old patient with osteopetrosis. **B,** In the spine, the centers of the vertebral bodies are relatively lucent, giving a "rugger jersey" (horizontally striped shirt) appearance on radiography.

Fractures in the intermediate and adult forms of osteopetrosis are common and require appropriate treatment. Healing does occur but may be delayed. Deformities due to fractures may need corrective osteotomies. Intramedullary fixation is desirable but may be difficult to apply because of the abnormal structure of the bone. Osteomyelitis is common as a result of the diminished vascularity and defective immune response in patients with this disease.

Fibrodysplasia Ossificans Progressiva

Fibrodysplasia ossificans progressiva (FOP) is a rare autosomal dominant disorder characterized by congenital malformations of the great toes and progressive heterotopic ossification of soft tissues. The causative genetic defect remains unknown. Lymphoblastoid cell lines derived from patients with FOP overexpress bone morphogenetic protein-4 (BMP4) and underexpress potent BMP antagonists in response to a BMP stimulus. BMP4 attracts mononuclear cells, induces angiogenesis, stimulates fibroproliferation (from putative mesenchymal stem cells) and apoptosis, and provokes endochondral bone induction, leading to the formation of mature ossicles of heterotopic bone that replace skeletal muscle and other connective tissues.[20]

Biopsy specimens of developing FOP lesions are exceedingly rare, because surgical trauma often leads to exacerbation of ossification. Histologic examination of *early* FOP lesions reveals an intense perivascular B-cell lymphocytic infiltration and also a mixed B- and T-cell infiltrate (the cells weakly coexpress BMP4) within muscle. Whether the early lymphocytic infiltrate is a causative event is uncertain. The *intermediate-stage* lesions are histologically indistinguishable from those in aggressive fibromatosis. Tissue from FOP lesions at a *late stage* shows endochondral ossification and formation of marrow elements.

Heterotopic ossification usually appears within the first decade of life after spontaneous or trauma-induced flare-ups. Progressive episodes of heterotopic ossification lead to ankylosis of all major joints of the axial and appendicular skeleton, rendering movement impossible. Most patients are confined to a wheelchair by their early 20s and require lifelong assistance in performing activities of daily living. Severe restrictive disease of the chest wall puts patients at an increased risk of associated cardiopulmonary problems.

There is no established medical treatment for FOP; medical intervention is currently supportive. Physical therapy to maintain joint mobility may be harmful if pursued aggressively and may provoke or exacerbate lesions. Surgical release of joint contractures is generally unsuccessful and risks new, trauma-induced heterotopic ossification. Creative use of BMP technology will probably have important applications in the inhibition of heterotopic ossification in diseases such as FOP.

SUMMARY

Skeletal dysplasias are disorders of the growth and remodeling of bone and its cartilaginous precursor. Although they are rarely seen, it is important to review them, because (1) they require effective treatment once diagnosed and (2) improving our understanding of each provides additional insight into skeletal development. The pathogenesis of many of these conditions is slowly being worked out, teaching us little by little about the growth of the skeleton. Future advances in molecular biology may also yield more effective treatment options for metabolic bone disorders, which are currently managed principally with symptomatic treatment.

MAJOR POINTS

Disproportionate short stature (dwarfism) is characteristic of the skeletal dysplasias, a feature differentiating these conditions from endocrine and metabolic disorders that cause proportionate short stature.

Generalized disturbances in the development of the skeleton affect the skull, spine, and extremities to varying extents.

Management of the skeletal dysplasias consists of accurate genetic counseling and the recognition and treatment of musculoskeletal abnormalities and associated intrinsic medical problems.

Achondroplasia, the most common form of short-limb dwarfism, is recognizable at birth as a disproportionate short-limbed rhizomelic dysplasia.

Thoracolumbar kyphosis is extremely common in patients with achondroplasia in the first years of life, most of whom show improvement without treatment once they start walking independently.

Cervical spine instability is a common feature of most skeletal dysplasias. Stability of the upper cervical spine should be evaluated with lateral flexion-extension radiographs and, if needed, flexion-extension magnetic resonance imaging.

Specific hand and foot malformations, including symphalangism of the fingers, the "hitchhiker thumb," and rigid bilateral equinovarus deformities, are universal in patients with diastrophic dysplasia.

Patients with spondyloepiphyseal dysplasia tarda or multiple epiphyseal dysplasia frequently experience hip pain, and radiographic findings in their hip joints are abnormal. These patients are often referred to orthopaedic surgeons with a diagnosis of bilateral Perthes disease.

(Continued)

MAJOR POINTS—cont'd

Mucopolysaccharidoses have some common clinical features, including facial dysmorphism, short stature, organomegaly, cardiac problems, and joint contractures.

The patients with chondrodysplasia punctata have multiple epiphyseal calcifications that are present at birth and resolve over the first year of life.

Patients with dyschondrosteosis (Leri-Weill syndrome) often have Madelung deformity in late childhood or adolescence.

Hypermobility of the shoulders due to abnormal clavicles is very typical in patients with cleidocranial dysplasia.

Congenital dislocations of the hips, knees, and elbows are frequently detected in patients with Larsen syndrome.

Plain radiographs are very helpful in the diagnosis of rickets. The classic radiographic findings are generalized osteopenia, thin cortices, and irregular widening or cupping of the growth plates.

Osteomalacia, physiologic genu varum or valgum, Blount disease, and some skeletal dysplasias with angular deformities of the knee should be considered in the differential diagnosis of rickets.

Medical treatment of the underlying metabolic disturbance, coordinated by a pediatrician or a pediatric endocrinologist, is the necessary first step in the management of both rickets and renal osteodystrophy.

Osteogenesis imperfecta should be differentiated from child abuse. A positive family history, fractures occurring with relatively mild injury, the presence of abnormalities of the teeth, sclera, or hearing, and systemic osteopenia may suggest osteogenesis imperfecta.

Idiopathic juvenile osteoporosis is a self-limited disorder that tends to resolve spontaneously.

REFERENCES

1. Beighton P, Geidon A, Garlin R, et al: International classification of osteochondrodysplasias. Am J Med Genet 44:223, 1992.
2. Dietz FR, Matthews KD: Current concepts review: Update on the genetic bases of disorders with orthopaedic manifestations. J Bone Joint Surg 78A:1583, 1996.
3. Online Mendelian Inheritance In Man, OMIM. McKusick-Nathans Institute for Genetic Medicine, John Hopkins University (Baltimore, MD) and National Center for Biotechnology Information, National Library of Medicine (Bethesda, MD), 2000. Available online at: http://www.ncbi.nlm.nih.gov/omim/
4. Sponseller PD: The skeletal dysplasias. In Morrisy RT, Weinstein SL (eds): Lovell and Winter's Pediatric Orthopaedics, 5th ed. Philadelphia, Lippincott Williams & Wilkins, 2001.
5. Jones KL: Smith's Recognizable Patterns of Human Malformations, 5th ed. Philadelphia, WB Saunders, 1997.
6. Fasanelli S: Hypochondroplasia: Radiological diagnosis and differential diagnosis. In Nicoletti B (ed): Achondroplasia: Human Achondroplasia: A Multidisciplinary Approach. New York, Plenum, 1999.
7. Boden SD, Kaplan FS, Fallon MD, et al: Metatropic dwarfism: Uncoupling of endochondral and perichondral growth. J Bone Joint Surg 69A:174, 1987.
8. Gilbert-Barnes E, Langer LO: Kniest dysplasia: Radiologic, histopathologic, and scanning EM findings. Am J Med Genet 63:34, 1996.
9. Wynne-Davies R, Hall C: Two clinical variants of spondyloepiphyseal dysplasia congenita. J Bone Joint Surg 64B:435, 1982.
10. Laville JM, Lakermore P, Limouzy F: Larsen's syndrome: Review of the literature and analysis of thirty-eight cases. J Pediatr Orthop 14:63, 1994.
11. Stieber JR, Pierz KA, Dormans JP: Hereditary multiple exostoses: A current understanding of clinical and genetic advances. The University of Pennsylvania Orthopaedic Journal 14: 39, 2001.
12. Mankin HJ: Review article: Rickets, osteomalacia and renal osteodystrophy: An update. Orthop Clin North Am 21:81, 1990.
13. Zaleske DJ: Metabolic and endocrine abnormalities. In Morrisy RT, Weinstein SL (eds): Lovell and Winter's Pediatric Orthopaedics, 5th ed. Philadelphia, Lippincott Williams & Wilkins, 2001.
14. Sillence DO: Osteogenesis imperfecta: An expanding panorama of variance. Clin Orthop 159:11, 1981.
15. Shapiro F: Consequences of an osteogenesis imperfecta diagnosis for survival and ambulation. J Pediatr Orthop 5:456, 1985.
16. Glorieux FH, Bishop NJ, Plotkin H, et al: Cyclic administration of pamidronate in children with severe osteogenesis imperfecta. N Engl J Med 339:947, 1998.
17. Marini JC: Osteogenesis imperfecta: Managing brittle bones [editorial]. N Engl J Med 339:947, 1998.
18. Dormans JP, Flynn JM: Pathologic fractures associated with tumors and unique conditions of the musculoskeletal system. In Beaty JH, Kasser JR (eds): Rockwood and Wilkins' Fractures in Children, 5th ed. Philadelphia, Lippincott Williams & Wilkins, 2001.
19. Shapiro F: Osteopetrosis: Current clinical considerations. Clin Orthop 294:34, 1993.
20. Kaplan FS, Delatycki M, Gannon FH, et al: Fibrodysplasia ossificans progressiva. In Emery AEH (ed): Neuromuscular Disorders: Clinical and Molecular Genetics. Chichester, UK, John Wiley & Sons, 1998.

CHAPTER 6

Spinal Disorders

KRISTAN A. PIERZ
JOHN P. DORMANS

Pediatric spinal disorders may be associated with pain, deformity, neurologic changes, or a combination of these factors. By identifying such signs and symptoms, one can initiate or facilitate the appropriate evaluation and treatment of a variety of conditions of the spine. Some disorders of the pediatric spine may be detected as early as in utero or during infancy, and others may not be apparent until later childhood or adolescence. This chapter highlights the key features of the pediatric back evaluation and then provides an overview of frequently encountered conditions of the spine and offers information useful for their diagnosis and treatment.

The following terms used throughout the chapter are defined here for reference:

- *Scoliosis*: lateral curvature of the spine; includes coronal plane deviation and rotation
- *Kyphosis*: posterior curvature of the spine in the sagittal plane; usually seen in the thoracic spine
- *Lordosis:* anterior curvature of the spine in the sagittal plane; usually seen in the cervical or lumbar spine
- *Structural curve*: spinal segment with a fixed lateral curvature that fails to correct with bending or traction

HISTORY

As with any medical condition, a complete history should be obtained for any patient with a potential spinal disorder. It consists of a history of the present illness, past medical and surgical experiences, and a family history. Such information is essential to developing a differential diagnosis, determining which tests to order, and instituting an appropriate treatment plan.

During history taking, certain information should be obtained. For example, does the patient experience pain, and is it localized or diffuse, is it related to activity, or does it occur at night? Idiopathic scoliosis is rarely associated with pain. However, in conditions such as tumors, infections, and spondylolysis pain may be the primary complaint. Is there an associated deformity? If so, is it progressive? When was it first noticed? How was it detected (during school screening; as a limb length inequality, gait abnormality, pain)? Has the patient experienced a recent injury or repetitive microtrauma? Spondylolysis, for example, may occur in athletes, such as gymnasts and football linemen, who frequently place excessive hyperextension forces on the lumbar spine. Are there associated symptoms? Fevers and weight loss may be associated with infectious or malignant conditions, whereas weakness, bowel or bladder changes, and sensory deficits may suggest an underlying neurologic problem. Poor pulmonary function may signify a neuromuscular disease or a severe thoracic deformity.

The perinatal history and previous medical history are also important. The majority of organ systems are formed simultaneously in the embryonic period, between the third and eighth weeks of pregnancy. Therefore, malformations in one organ system should engender suspicion about malformations in other systems, including the musculoskeletal system. Delays in achieving developmental milestones may suggest conditions potentially associated with spinal deformities, such as cerebral palsy. Knowing whether a girl has started her menses or a boy has begun shaving allows one to assess a patient's maturity level and predict whether sufficient growth remains to affect a spinal deformity. Previous surgery, such as a laminectomy, may result in progressive kyphosis. It is also helpful to obtain old medical records and prior radiographs.

The family history can also provide useful information. Conditions such as Duchenne muscular dystrophy, which is transmitted in a sex-linked recessive manner, or spinal muscular atrophy, transmitted as an autosomal recessive trait, often have known inheritance patterns. This information is useful to making the diagnosis as well as in counseling the family. Many patients with idiopathic scoliosis have a positive family history; however, this inheritance has variable expressivity.

PHYSICAL EXAMINATION

The physical examination of the spine involves much more than simply looking at the back. If there is spinal deformity, the severity of such deformity and how it affects the rest of the body must be assessed. Additionally, one must examine the entire patient, looking for clues to a possible underlying disease process. The examination should be carried out in a private, well-lit room. A hospital gown (open at the back) worn over underpants or shorts is recommended. Although the examiner must be sensitive to the patient's modesty, one cannot adequately assess a patient through layers of clothing. A general overview of the physical examination follows; the remainder of the chapter focuses on specific conditions of the spine and highlights features unique to them.

General Examination

The examination begins with observations about the patient's overall condition. Is the child mature enough to participate in his or her own care and comprehend the goals of treatment? Is the child well nourished and well developed? Can the child walk independently? Is there a limp or gait abnormality, which may suggest a limb length inequality or a weakness due to a neurologic condition?

The general body habitus should also be noted. Height and weight should be measured and plotted on standardized graphs. Poor posture may account for mild spinal deformities, and obesity may hide even rather large curves. Very tall, thin individuals with large arm spans may have Marfan syndrome, a condition that can be associated with scoliosis or spondylolisthesis as well as cardiovascular abnormalities and ocular findings. At the other extreme, dwarfism encompasses a wide variety of bone dysplasias, many of which can be associated with scoliosis, kyphosis, or cervical instability. Global ligamentous laxity, as demonstrated by knee or elbow hyperextension or the ability to touch the thumb to the volar forearm (Fig. 6-1), may indicate a connective tissue disorder such as Ehlers-Danlos syndrome.

Assessment of breast and pubic hair development is useful in determining a patient's physical maturity and may be graded according to the Tanner staging system.[1] Development of a child who has not yet experienced pubertal changes is Tanner stage 1, whereas that of an adult is Tanner stage 5. A patient with Tanner grade 2 or 3 development is usually in the adolescent growth spurt. This fact is critical, because a mild curve may progress quickly during the growth spurt.

The skin examination can also offer diagnostic information. Hyperelasticity is associated with connective tissue disorders. Café au lait spots, often considered by patients to be simple birthmarks, may be seen with neurofibromatosis (Fig. 6-2). Such a diagnosis should be considered if the marks are large, more than five in number, or located in the axilla. *Spina bifida*, a term used to describe a wide range of spinal cord defects, may

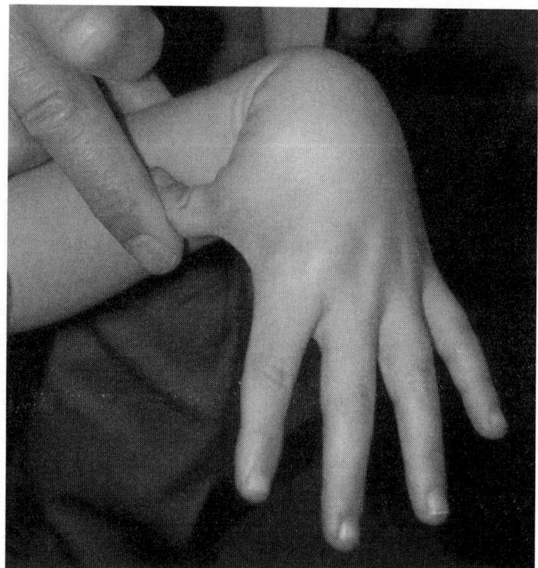

Figure 6-1 Clinical example of ligamentous laxity, demonstrated by the ability to touch the thumb to the volar forearm.

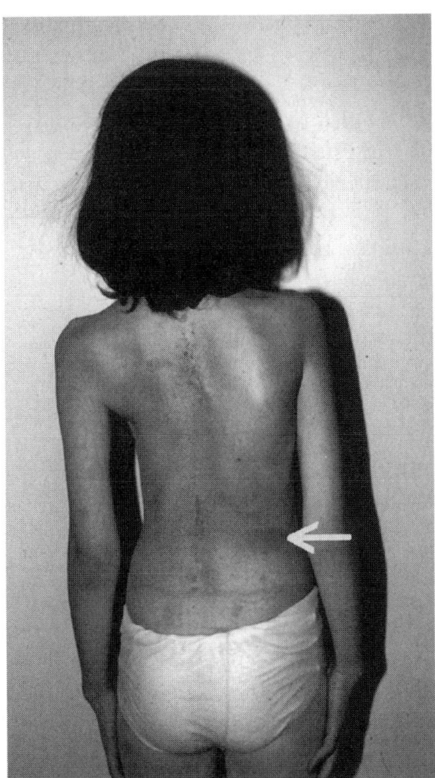

Figure 6-2 Clinical photograph of a patient with neurofibromatosis. Note the multiple café au lait spots (*arrow*) and healed incisional scar from previous spine surgery.

manifest as a very obvious herniation of the meninges and neural contents protruding from the back of a newborn. Alternatively, the appearance may be much more subtle, with the only external evidence as a hairy patch, a subcutaneous lipoma, or a dermal sinus located on the back.

Evaluation of the Spine

Examination of the back should proceed in an organized manner. If there is a history of pain, the patient should be asked to point to the area of concern. Initial inspection of the standing patient, from behind, may reveal a deformity such as scoliosis or abnormal kyphosis or lordosis. Long hair should be lifted to allow clear visualization of the neck and upper back. A low hairline or webbed neck may suggest Klippel-Feil syndrome, a condition consisting of multiple abnormal cervical segments and possible associated renal or cardiac abnormalities. One should document the direction and location of the deformity (e.g., left thoracic, right thoracolumbar). Is there an associated shoulder or pelvic asymmetry? If the iliac crests are not level, placing a block under the foot of the lower side may correct a scoliosis due to a limb length discrepancy. Additionally, a scoliosis due to a limb length discrepancy should be corrected if the spine is examined with the patient seated.

Scoliosis may or may not produce decompensation. With a compensated spine, the head is centered over the middle of the pelvis; a decompensated spine may result in a lateral lean of the torso. This can be documented by dropping a plumb line from over the seventh cervical vertebra (Fig. 6-3). Normally, this line passes through the gluteal cleft. Deviation of the line to the left or right, as measured in centimeters, quantifies the decompensation.

The Adams forward bend test allows one to assess spinal asymmetries.[2] With the feet together and the legs straight, the patient is instructed to bend forward from the waist. The arms are allowed to hang freely with the palms opposed (Figs. 6-4 and 6-5A to D). The patient should be viewed from the front, from behind, and from the side. A rib prominence suggests a rotational abnormality. The height of this prominence can be measured in centimeters, or a scoliometer can be used to quantify the extent of rotation (see Fig. 6-4).[3] When this test is used as a school-screening tool, identifying seven degrees of trunk rotation as possible scoliosis results in few false-positives and a referral rate of 3%.[4]

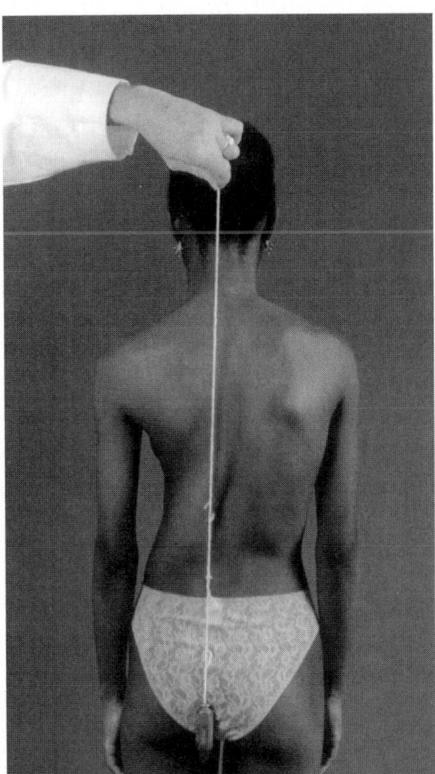

Figure 6-3 Clinical photograph of a patient with scoliosis. A plumb line hung from the base of the neck passes to the left of the gluteal cleft, demonstrating mild decompensation. Note also the shoulder asymmetry and right scapular prominence.

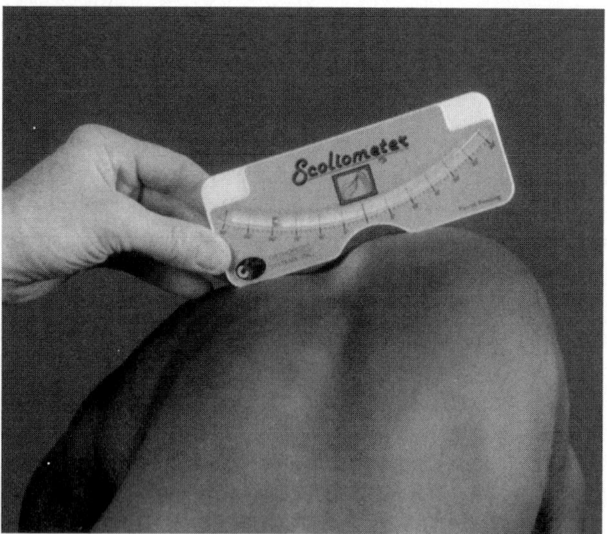

Figure 6-4 Clinical photograph of the same patient viewed in Figure 6-3, now performing an Adams forward bend test and demonstrating 20 degrees of trunk rotation as measured with a scoliometer.

Neurologic Examination

A neurologic examination is essential to evaluation of the spine. One can quickly assess lower extremity weakness by having the patient ambulate on the heels, on the toes, and in a squatting position. Difficulty getting up from the seated position (abnormal Gower test result) may be due to proximal muscle weakness, as seen in conditions such as Duchenne muscular dystrophy. Balance and gait can also be assessed to rule out ataxic conditions.

The upper and lower extremity reflexes, including the Babinski reflex, should be examined. Additionally, the umbilical reflex can be elicited through stroking of the abdomen toward the umbilicus in all four quadrants. A normal response is symmetrical deviation of the umbilicus toward the stimulus. Abnormal umbilical reflexes may be the first sign of intraspinal disease such as a syrinx or spinal cord tumor. The patient should also be told to perform straight-leg raises to rule out nerve root tension.

Abnormal findings on the examination of the extremities may also indicate intraspinal anomalies. For example, a cavus foot, clubfoot, or vertical talus may suggest spinal dysraphism. Clawing of the digits suggests muscular imbalance. Calf or thigh circumferences can be determined with a tape measure to check for muscular atrophy.

IMAGING

Radiography

When a curvature of the spine is initially suspected, 36-inch extended-length radiographs, showing the spine from the shoulders to the pelvis, should be obtained. Standing radiographs (or sitting films for those unable to stand) of the spine in the coronal and sagittal planes are recommended (see Fig. 6-5E and F). The tube-to-film distance is kept constant at 72 inches to allow for uniform comparison between serial films. Posteroanterior (PA) views expose the breasts and thyroid to less radiation than anteroposterior (AP) views. Lateral views are indicated if there is a history of pain or sagittal deformity.

To keep the radiation exposure low, the number of films obtained should be limited. Initial films should be obtained without breast and gonadal shields, which would obscure associated anomalies. Subsequent films, however, may be taken with breast or gonadal shields if they would not obscure the area of interest. The flexibility of a spinal deformity can be evaluated by obtaining a supine film with the patient bending against the deformity or with the addition of traction (Fig. 6-6). Such information is useful if surgery is being considered; however, these films are not necessary for monitoring of small curves. Fast films, filters, and beam collimation are modern techniques that help limit radiation scatter.

By convention, the radiograph is viewed as if the patient is being viewed from behind, with the heart and stomach bubble on the left. Curves are described by location (cervical, thoracic, thoracolumbar, or lumbar), direction (left or right convexity), and size. Curves are routinely measured with the Cobb technique (see Fig. 6-6A and Fig. 6-7). On either the PA or lateral radiograph, the end vertebrae are identified as those most tilted from the horizontal. A line is then drawn along the upper end plate of the most cranial end vertebra, and a perpendicular line is extended down from this line. Next, a line is drawn along the lower end plate of the most caudal end vertebra, and a perpendicular line is extended proximally from this third line. The intersection of the two perpendicular lines forms the Cobb angle, which describes the severity of scoliosis or kyphosis. In a patient with more than one curve, the lowest end vertebra of the upper curve serves as the upper end vertebra of the lower curve and is referred to as the *transitional vertebra*.

On a PA radiograph of a normal spine, the vertebral bodies form a column centered over the sacrum. Imaginary perpendicular lines extending up from the lumbosacral facets form an area referred to as the *stable zone of Harrington* (see Fig. 6-7).[5] As curves bend away from the vertical axis (also known as the "center sacral vertical line"), the apical vertebrae tend to deviate out of this zone. In the normal spine, a line extending up from the center sacral vertical line bisects the pedicles. In scoliotic curves, however, lateral translation is associated with rotation as the vertebral bodies deviate away from the midline. As a curve returns to the midline, the vertebra that is most closely bisected by the center sacral

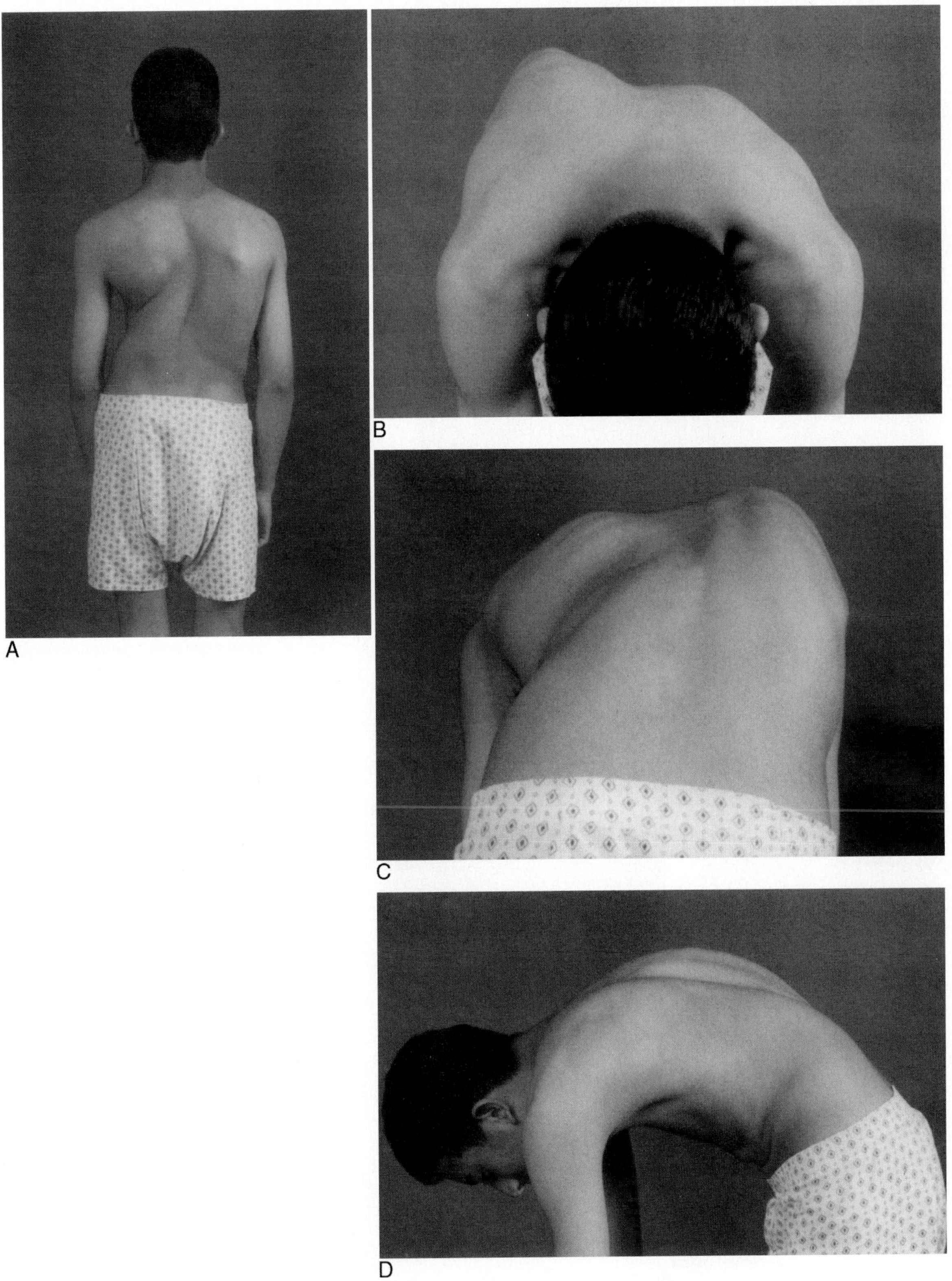

Figure 6-5 **A,** Clinical photograph of a patient with scoliosis. The same patient performing an Adams forward bend test and viewed from the front **(B)** from the back **(C),** and from the side **(D).** Note the large right rib prominence.

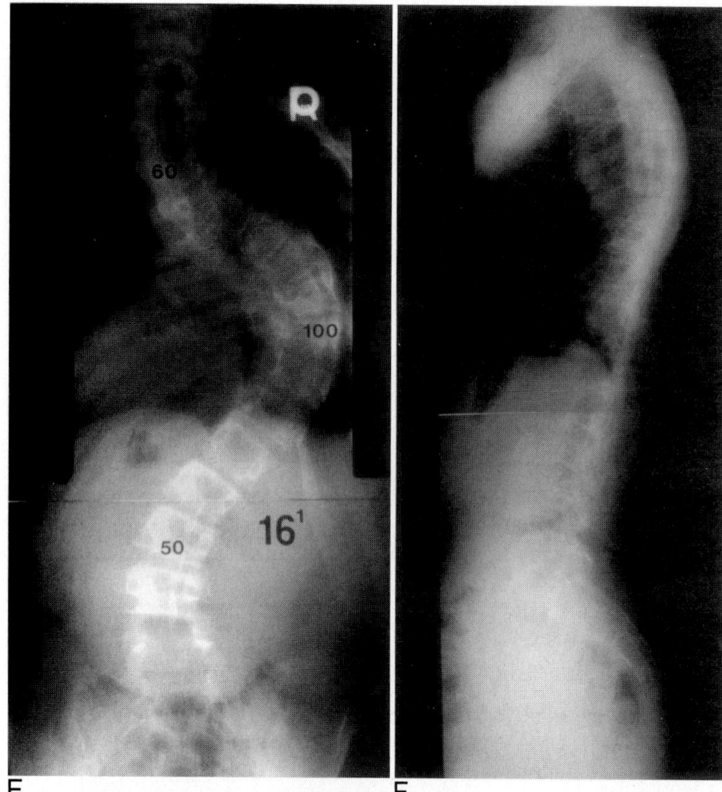

Figure 6-5 (Cont'd) **E,** Posterolateral radiograph of the same patient with the Cobb angle measurements of each curve written on the apical vertebrae. **F,** Lateral radiograph of the same patient. Note the apparent flattening of the spine with loss of thoracic kyphosis.

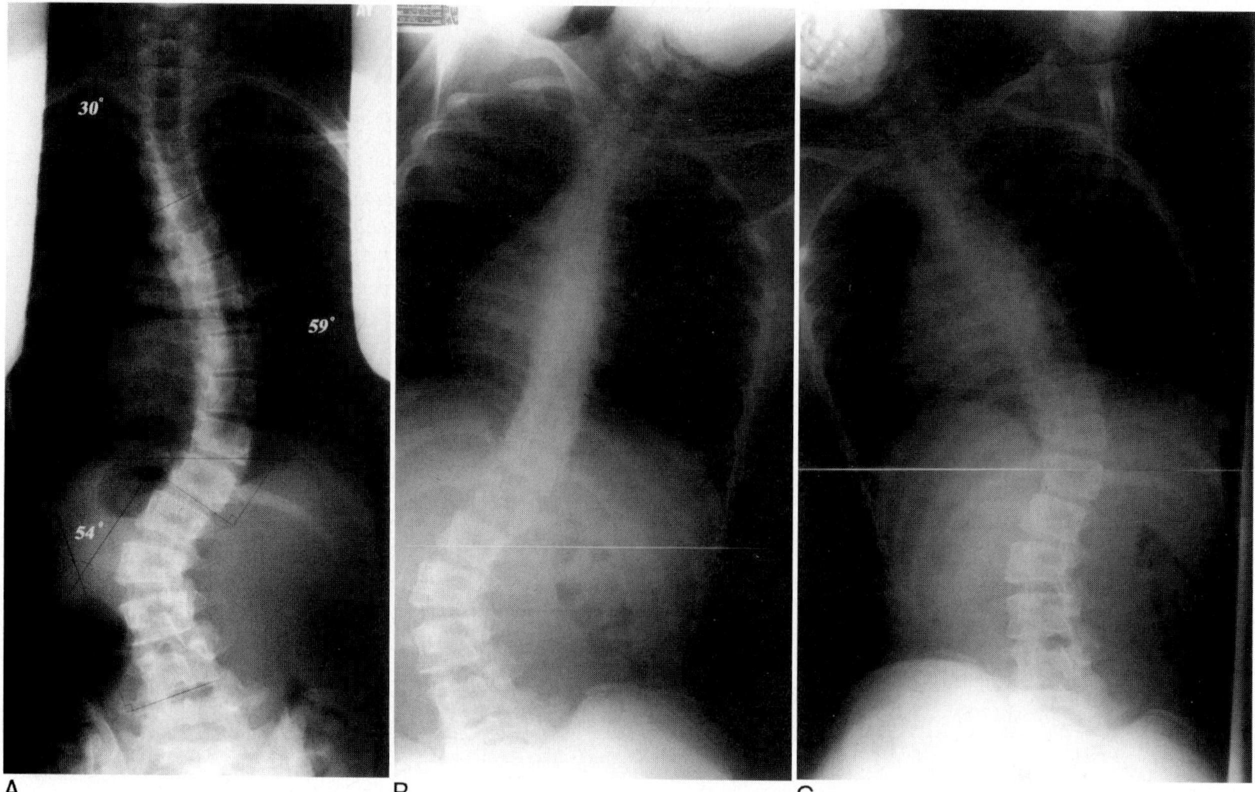

Figure 6-6 **A,** Posteroanterior radiograph of a patient with adolescent idiopathic scoliosis. Lines have been drawn to demonstrate calculation of the Cobb angle. The Cobb angle values have been written alongside each curve. Bending to the right **(B)** and left **(C)** demonstrates the flexibility of the curves. On the basis of the iliac apophyses, ossification in this patient is Risser stage 4.

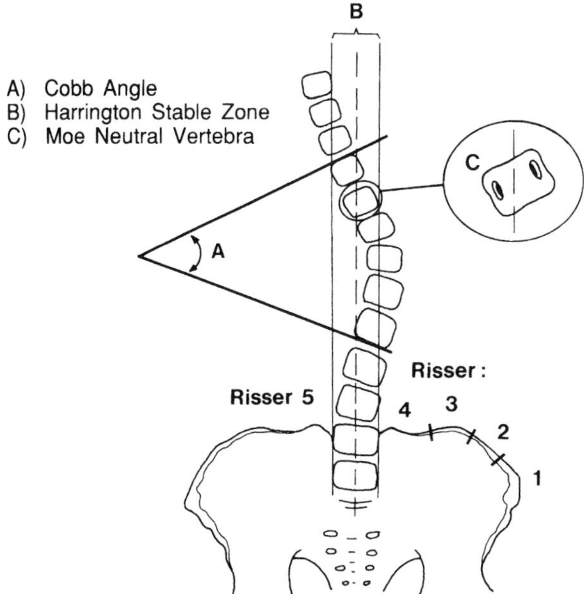

Figure 6-7 Cartoon illustrating the radiographic tools used to describe spinal irregularities: Cobb angle, Harrington stable zone, Moe neutral vertebra, and Risser stages, all of which are described in the text. (From Stefko RM, Erickson MA: Pediatric orthopaedics. In Miller MD [ed]: Review of Orthopaedics, 3rd ed. Philadelphia, WB Saunders, 2000, p 165.)

vertical line is referred to as the *stable vertebra* (see Fig. 6-7).[5] The stable zone of Harrington and the stable vertebra define the portion of the spine that is well-compensated and are useful for determining how far to extend a fusion when spinal surgery is indicated.

Radiographs that include the iliac crests are useful for assessment of skeletal maturity (see Fig. 6-6B and C). Ossification of the crests begins anteriorly and progresses posteriorly (see Fig. 6-7). When seen on the PA radiograph, the apophysis appears to proceed from lateral to medial. The Risser stage is determined by dividing the crest into quarters and identifying which portions of the apophysis have ossified.[6] In Risser stage 0, there is no ossification; Risser stages 1 to 4 correspond to the successive ossification of each quarter; in Risser stage 5, the apophysis has fully ossified and fused with the ilium. The most rapid skeletal growth spurt occurs during Risser stage 1, whereas most growth has ceased by Risser stage 4. Cessation of vertebral body growth is also heralded by the fusion of the vertebral ring apophyses with the vertebral end plates. Skeletal maturity can also be assessed by comparing a radiograph of the left hand and wrist with the standards in Greulich and Pyle's *Radiographic Atlas of Skeletal Development of the Hand and Wrist*.[7]

Magnetic Resonance Imaging

Magnetic resonance imaging (MRI) can be very useful in identifying spinal cord disease and should be obtained whenever neurologic changes are found by physical examination. Conditions that may not be apparent on plain radiographs, such as syringomyelia, tumors, Arnold-Chiari malformations, and tethered spinal cord, are easily visualized by MRI (Fig. 6-8). Additionally, patients with atypical curve patterns (such as a left thoracic curve), rapidly progressing curves, or infantile or juvenile idiopathic scoliosis should be evaluated with MRI.

Computed Tomography

Computed tomography (CT) scans are useful when fine bony detail is necessary. Acute fractures, spondylolysis, and bone tumors, such as an aneurysmal bone cyst, osteoid osteoma, and osteoblastoma, are better characterized by CT than by standard radiography (Fig. 6-9). Three-dimensional reconstructions can be created to help visualize complex deformities (Fig. 6-10).

Myelography

In myelography, injection of contrast material into the subarachnoid space is followed by imaging with CT scanning or radiography. This method helps localize spinal cord tumors, spinal dysraphism, and spinal cord impingement due to deformity. MRI, which is less

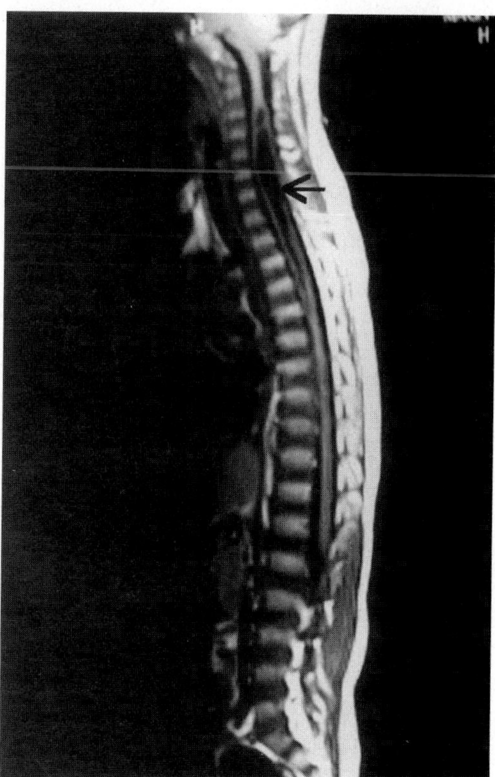

Figure 6-8 Magnetic resonance image showing syringomyelia. The *arrow* highlights the syrinx, a cyst within the spinal cord.

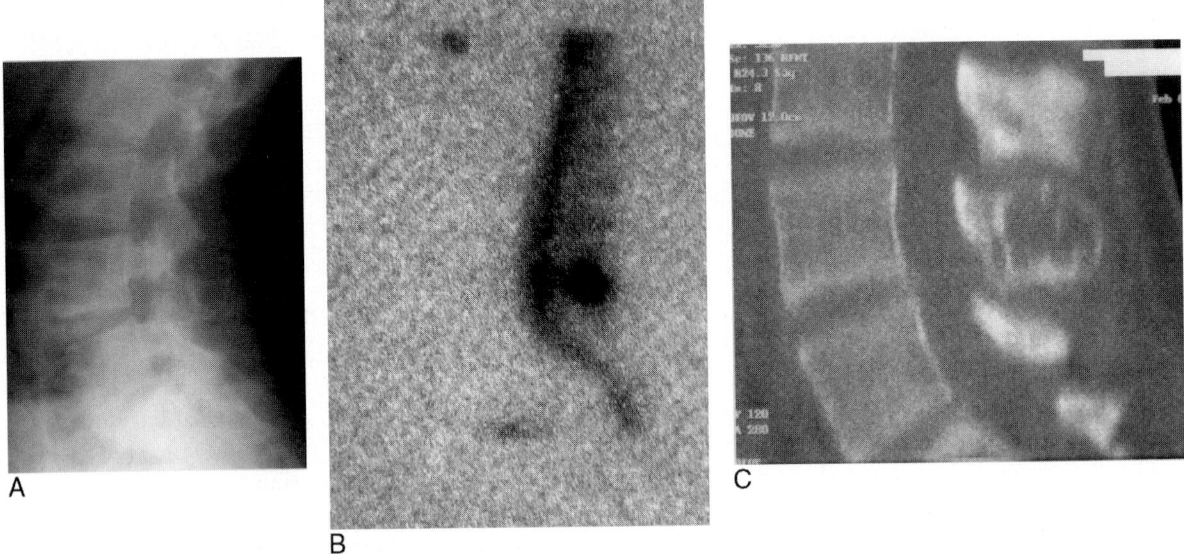

Figure 6-9 **A,** Lateral radiograph of an aneurysmal bone cyst of the posterior elements of the lumbar spine. A bone scan **(B)** highlights the area of interest, but a computed tomography scan **(C)** shows more detail.

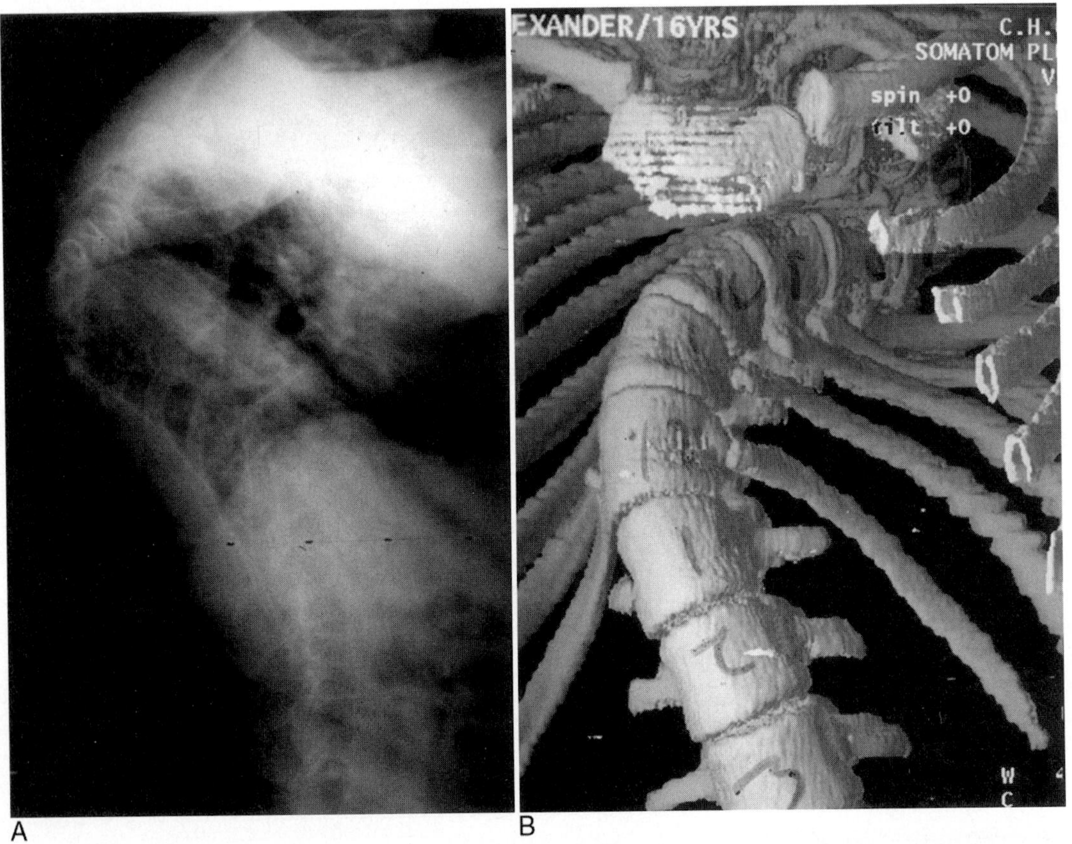

Figure 6-10 **A,** Radiograph of a severe spinal deformity. The vertebral rotation and overlapping of the ribs make it difficult to visualize the anatomic detail. **B,** A three-dimensional reconstruction created from computed tomography scanning allows a better understanding of the spinal anatomy.

invasive, has replaced myelography for most problems, but myelograms are still used occasionally to elucidate complex deformities.

Bone Scanning

Scintigraphy, or bone scanning, involves intravenous injection of a radionuclide, usually technetium (^{99m}Tc) methylenediphosphonate. Gallium (^{67}Ga) citrate or indium In111-labeled white blood cells may also be used to detect infection. Scans are then performed to identify areas of increased uptake (see Fig. 6-9B). Single-photon emission computed tomography (SPECT) has better spatial resolution than planar imaging and has gained acceptance for imaging of low back pain. Radionuclide bone imaging, although sensitive for identifying and localizing areas of increased bone activity, can be nonspecific, and follow-up imaging may be needed to truly characterize the area of interest.

LABORATORY STUDIES

Laboratory studies are not required for all patients with spinal disorders, but they can be useful in certain situations. A complete blood count (CBC) with differential leukocyte count and an erythrocyte sedimentation rate (ESR) determination are useful screening tests for patients who complain of night pain or have constitutional symptoms suggesting an infectious or neoplastic condition. A serum C-reactive protein (CRP) quantification can also be added if infection is suspected. If a rheumatologic source is likely, testing for rheumatoid factor (RF), antinuclear antibody (ANA), and HLA B27 may be helpful. In areas endemic for Lyme disease, a Lyme titer determination should also be considered.

BACK PAIN

Back pain is less common in childhood and adolescence than in adulthood but is more likely to have an identifiable cause.[8] A list of common potential causes of back pain in children is given in Box 6-1. The lifetime prevalence of back pain appears to increase with advancing age, reported as 12% at 11 years and as high as 50% at 15 years.[9]

In the evaluation of a child with back pain, the patient's history is extremely important. Overuse injuries, although less common than in adults, can cause backaches in children. Activity-related pain usually resolves after a few days of rest. Certainly, the patient who has experienced acute trauma should be immobilized until appropriate imaging studies can be obtained. Children and adolescents can sustain fractures, disk herniations, and ligamentous injuries to their spinal columns. The pediatric spine, however, has greater elasticity than the mature spine. Because the bones and ligaments of the pediatric spine can tolerate more stretch than the spinal cord, children are at risk of having neurologic injuries even if radiographic findings are normal; this pattern of injury is referred to as spinal cord injury without radiographic abnormality (SCIWORA).

Infections should be suspected in patients who present with back pain or refuse to walk. Erythrocyte sedimentation rate and C-reactive protein values are usually

Box 6-1 Differential Diagnoses of Back Pain in Childhood and Adolescence

- Mechanical/traumatic
  - Muscle strain/overuse injuries
  - Fracture
  - Spondylolysis/spondylolisthesis
  - Herniated disk
  - Slipped vertebral apophysis
- Developmental
  - Spondylolysis/spondylolisthesis
  - Scheuermann kyphosis
  - Painful scoliosis
- Inflammatory
  - Diskitis/vertebral osteomyelitis
  - Tuberculous spondylitis
  - Disk space calcification
  - Ankylosing spondylitis
  - Juvenile rheumatoid arthritis
  - Other rheumatologic conditions
- Neoplastic
  - Benign
    - Anterior
      - Langerhans cell histiocytosis/eosinophilic granuloma
      - Giant cell
    - Posterior
      - Aneurysmal bone cyst
    - Osteoid osteoma/osteoblastoma
  - Malignant
    - Leukemia/lymphoma
    - Ewing sarcoma
    - Metastatic (neuroblastoma, Wilms tumor, etc.)
    - Spinal cord/meningeal/epidural tumors
    - Rhabdomyosarcoma
- Visceral
  - Appendicitis
  - Pyelonephritis
  - Retroperitoneal abscess
- Psychological
  - Rare—consider this diagnosis only after complete evaluation for other sources

elevated in infections, but the white blood cell (WBC) count and culture results are of variable reliability. Infections of the pediatric spine may involve the disk space (*diskitis*) or the vertebral body (*osteomyelitis*). Frequently, however, it is difficult to determine where the initial bacterial seeding began, and an entire vertebra-disk-vertebra unit becomes involved (*spondylitis*). Spondylosis is best seen on MRI. The most common pathogen is *Staphylococcus aureus*, and treatment usually involves antibiotics. Rarely is surgery necessary.

Tumors also may manifest as back pain, which often occurs at night.[10] The most common tumors are listed in Box 6-1. If the patient also has constitutional symptoms, such as fever and malaise, malignancy must be considered. If laboratory test results are normal and pain is the only symptom, a benign bone lesion is the more likely diagnosis. Imaging studies help with the diagnosis, but a biopsy is often necessary for confirmation. Aneurysmal bone cysts, although histologically benign, can be locally aggressive and cause painful expansion of the posterior bony elements, requiring surgical excision for relief of symptoms (Fig. 6-11). Another benign bone tumor, the osteoid osteoma, tends to arise in the posterior spine. Classically, the pain associated with osteoid osteomas increases at night and may be relieved with aspirin or nonsteroidal anti-inflammatory agents. Complete relief, however, may be achieved only by surgical excision of the lesion.

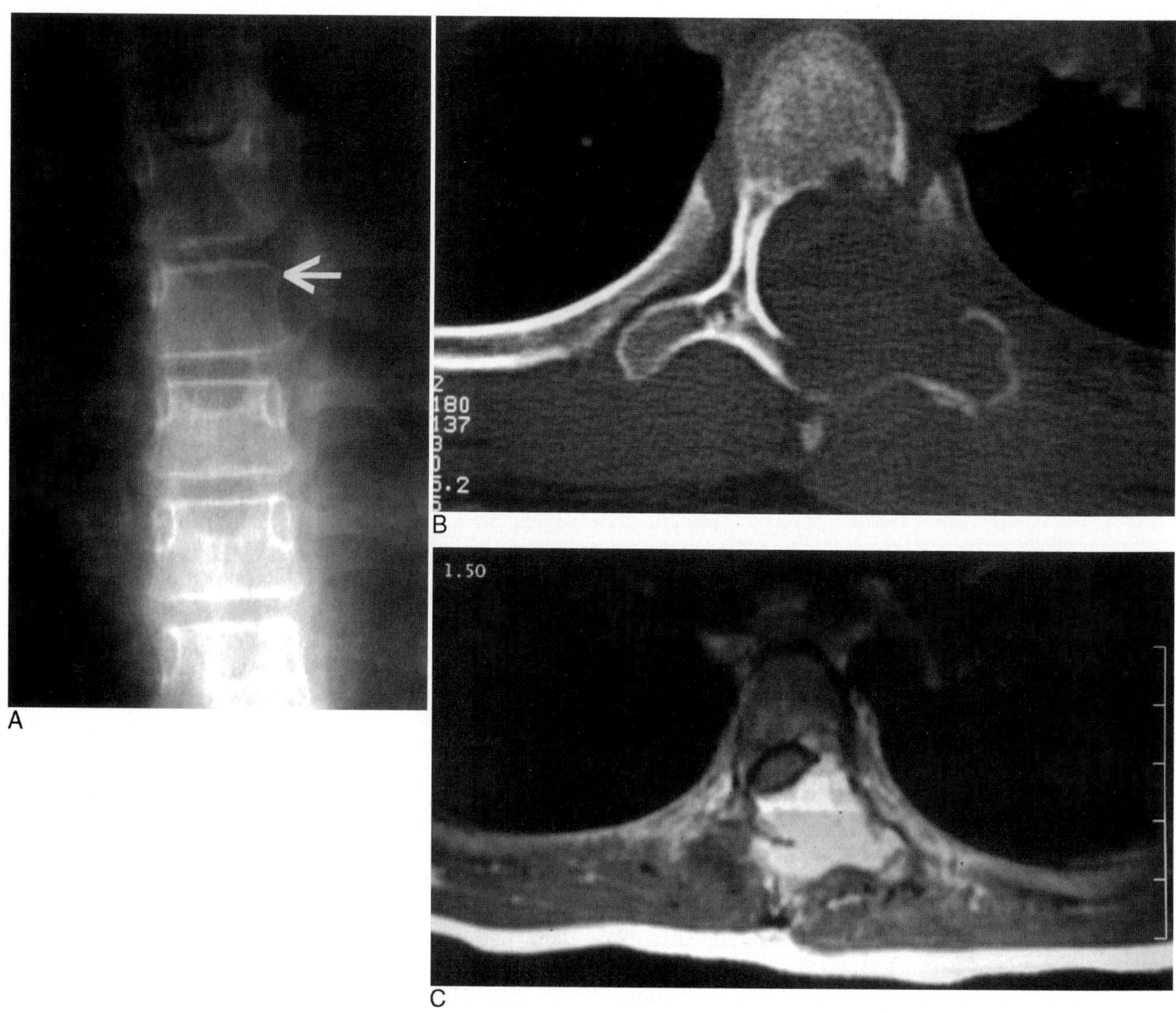

Figure 6-11 **A,** Anteroposterior radiograph of a patientwith an aneurysmal bone cyst. Note the apparent absence of the pedicle (*arrow*). The axial computed tomography scan **(B)** and the axial **(C)**

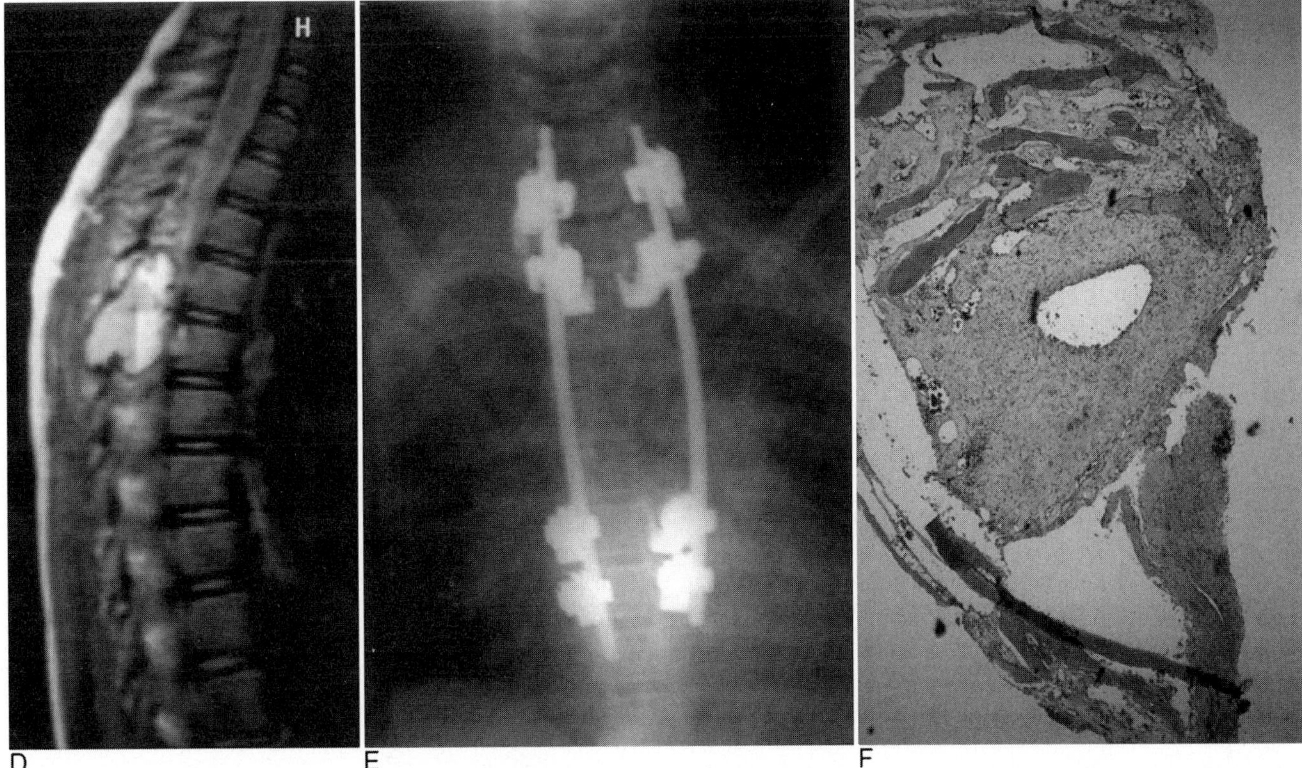

Figure 6-11 (Cont'd) and sagittal **(D)** magnetic resonance images provide greater detail. **E,** Treatment consisted of surgical excision with posterior instrumentation for stabilization. **F,** Histologic analysis confirmed the diagnosis of an aneurysmal bone cyst.

Deformity associated with back pain may be due to true structural changes in the bony architecture or may be caused by a muscular spasm in response to the pain. Deformity may exist, however, in the absence of pain. This situation is common in idiopathic scoliosis and in neuromuscular diseases.

IDIOPATHIC SCOLIOSIS

Idiopathic scoliosis is defined as scoliosis not associated with any other condition. On a standing radiograph, the lateral curvature of the spine should measure at least 10 degrees using the Cobb technique before being labeled true scoliosis. Long, gentle, flexible curves that disappear with forward bending and are not associated with a rib hump or rotational changes may be due to postural changes rather than true scoliosis. A curve should be classified as idiopathic only after other causes have been excluded. Curves associated with neurologic symptoms, excessive pain, or atypical patterns should raise suspicion of an underlying cause.

Idiopathic scoliosis can be classified according to the age of onset. The subtypes are infantile (onset between birth and 3 years), juvenile (onset between 3 and 10 years), and adolescent (onset after age 10, or postpubescent onset). In addition to differing with age of onset, these subtypes vary in risk factors, rate of progression, and treatment options.[11,12]

Before addressing the differences among the subtypes of idiopathic scoliosis, we offer a brief overview of the natural history of scoliosis. Such information is necessary to understanding why some curves can be observed, whereas others require intervention. In one natural history study, Weinstein and Ponseti[13] noted that progression of curves after skeletal maturity was greatest for curves larger than 50 degrees, especially in the thoracic spine. Conversely, curves smaller than 30 degrees tended to be stable. Large curves have been implicated in pulmonary dysfunction, decreased self-image, and a higher incidence of back pain in adulthood.[14]

In a long-term follow-up study in Sweden, Pehrsson and colleagues[12] found that although the mortality rate for patients with adolescent idiopathic scoliosis was the same as that for the general population, the rate for patients with infantile or juvenile idiopathic scoliosis was higher. Branthwaite[15] showed that cardiopulmonary compromise was possible if the age of onset of scoliosis was less than 5 years. This relationship can most likely be explained by the fact that the number of alveoli is incomplete at birth and continues to increase until about 8 years of age. The age of onset of deformity, therefore, may be more critical than its actual severity in predicting mortality risks.

Infantile Idiopathic Scoliosis

Infantile idiopathic scoliosis manifests in children 3 years or younger. This condition is rarely seen in the United States and is more common in Europe. It has been postulated that supine or semisupine infant positioning may contribute to the deformity. Boys are affected more frequently than girls, and plagiocephaly is frequently noted. Left thoracic curves are most common, followed by thoracolumbar curves. Mehta[16] has studied this condition and identified the rib-vertebral angle difference (RVAD) as a predictor of curve progression (Fig. 6-12). To calculate RVAD, the angle between a rib on the convex side of the curve and a line perpendicular to the vertebral end plate is subtracted from the same angle measured on the concave side of the curve. Curves with RVADs greater than 20 degrees are likely to progress and have a worse prognosis. Mehta[16] also subdivided progressive curves into benign and malignant forms, with the malignant form undergoing more severe progression during the first 5 years of life.

Infantile idiopathic curves that are nonprogressive rarely need treatment and tend to resolve spontaneously. However, progressive curves do require treatment. Koop[10] reviewed the literature and summarized treatment based on the RVAD value (Fig. 6-13). Active treatment usually begins with early casting followed by bracing. For relentlessly progressing curves, surgery may be indicated. The *crankshaft phenomenon* has been described in patients who underwent early posterior spinal fusions and experienced subsequent rotational deformity because of continued anterior vertebral growth.[17] Crankshaft phenomenon can be prevented (1) through delay of surgery until the child is older than 10 years, (2) with the addition of an anterior fusion, or (3) with special instrumentation that allows subsequent expansion.

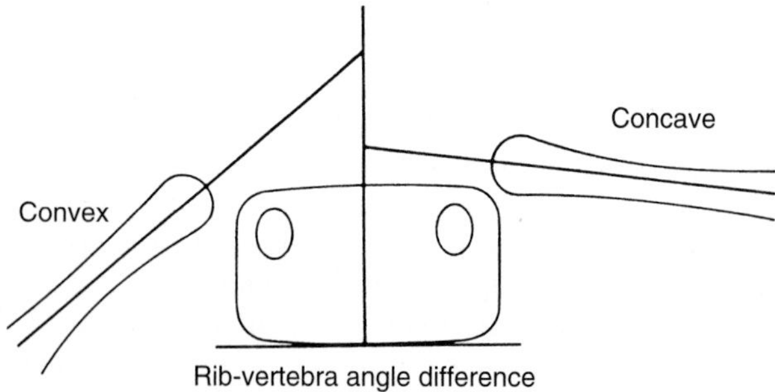

Figure 6-12 Example of how to construct the rib-vertebra angle difference (RVAD) as defined by Mehta. (From Koop SE: Infantile and juvenile idiopathic scoliosis. Orthop Clin North Am 19:332, 1988.)

Juvenile Idiopathic Scoliosis

Juvenile idiopathic scoliosis, which manifests in children between 3 and 10 years of age, accounts for between 12% and 21% of all cases of idiopathic scoliosis.[11] The proportion of girls to boys increases with age, and right thoracic curves predominate. Some cases of infantile scoliosis are not detected until children are older than 3 years, being classified as the juvenile subtype. For this reason, initial treatment is similar to that for infantile idiopathic scoliosis, especially for left thoracic curves.

With increasing age, however, curve behavior tends to become more like that seen in adolescent idiopathic scoliosis. Highly flexible curves larger than 25 degrees may be treated with Milwaukee bracing, and less flexible curves should be corrected with casting before bracing. Curves smaller than 25 degrees may be merely observed unless they progress. Surgery may be needed for curves that do not stabilize. As with infantile cases, instrumentation without fusion may be performed in an attempt to delay definitive fusion until the spine has grown adequately.

Adolescent Idiopathic Scoliosis

Adolescent idiopathic scoliosis has a prevalence of approximately 25 per 1000; however, this prevalence decreases with increasing curve magnitude (Table 6-1). The female-to-male ratio increases from about 1.4:1 for curves less than 20 degrees to about 10:1 for curves more than 40 degrees.[14] Although no single gene or mode of inheritance has been identified, hereditary patterns are thought to exist, with autosomal dominance or multifactorial inheritance being the most likely. Family history is positive for approximately 30% of patients with adolescent idiopathic scoliosis. The family history, however, is not usually helpful in predicting magnitude of curves or rate of progression. Growth hormone, calmodulin, vestibular-ocular-proprioceptive functions, and alterations in connective tissues have all been investigated for their contributions to the etiology and progression of idiopathic scoliosis. To date, no single theory has gained full acceptance.

School screening has been advocated for the diagnosis of scoliosis and has been endorsed by the American Academy of Orthopaedic Surgeons and the Scoliosis Research Society. Such screening is recommended for girls at ages 11 and 13 years and for boys at age 13 or 14 years. Currently, an Adams forward bend test, with or without the use of the scoliometer, is used by most screening programs (see Figs. 6-4 and 6-5). The prevalence of scoliosis has been reported to be approximately

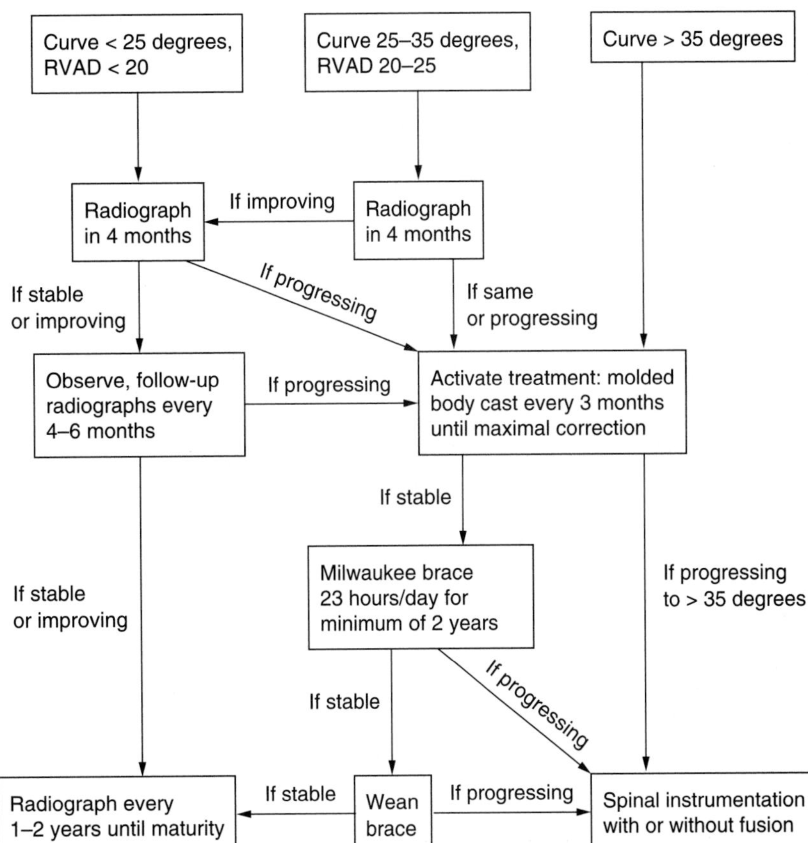

Figure 6-13 Algorithm for the treatment of infantile idiopathic scoliosis. (Based on Koop SE: Infantile and juvenile idiopathic scoliosis. Orthop Clin North Am 19:331-337, 1988.)

2% to 3%; however, the prevalence of curves larger than 30 degrees is only about 0.3%. The goals of screening should be to identify a treatable condition in a cost-effective way and to alter the natural history of the condition. Bunnell[3] found that referral based on 5 degrees of trunk inclination resulted in a 12% referral rate with many false-positive results, whereas use of a 7-degree inclination decreased the referral rate to 3% and improved the positive predictive value. In 1993, the U.S. Preventive Services Task Force summarized existing literature on school screening for scoliosis and found the evidence not sufficiently conclusive for formal recommendations to be made.[18]

Curve patterns in adolescent idiopathic scoliosis may be thoracic, lumbar, thoracolumbar, or double major curves. The King-Moe classification system, described in 1983, has gained acceptance as a descriptive tool as well as a basis for surgical correction (Fig. 6-14).[5] Lenke and associates[19] offered a new classification system that uses lumbar spine and thoracic sagittal spine modifiers (Fig. 6-15). The surgical implications of these classification systems are beyond the scope of this chapter; the figures illustrating them are presented here to provide a reference for the terms frequently used to characterize curve patterns.

The goals of treatment for adolescent idiopathic scoliosis are to halt the progression of curves and to prevent a patient from entering adulthood with a large deformity. Characteristics such as maturity and curve size at the time of presentation have been associated with curve progression (Tables 6-2 and 6-3). After reviewing the literature, Weinstein[14] identified the following curve patterns and growth factors as indicators of higher risks for curve progression: double curve patterns, larger curve magnitude at presentation, younger age at presentation, presentation of curve before menarche, lower Risser

Table 6-1 Prevalence of Adolescent Idiopathic Scoliosis

Cobb Angle (degrees)	Female-to-Male Ratio	Prevalence
>10	1.4-2:1	2-3
>20	5.4:1	0.3-0.5
>30	10:1	0.1-0.3
>40		<0.1

(From Weinstein SL: Adolescent idiopathic scoliosis: natural history. In Weinstein SL [ed]: The Pediatric Spine: Principles and Practice, 2nd ed. Philadelphia, Lippincott Williams & Wilkins, 2001, p 356.)

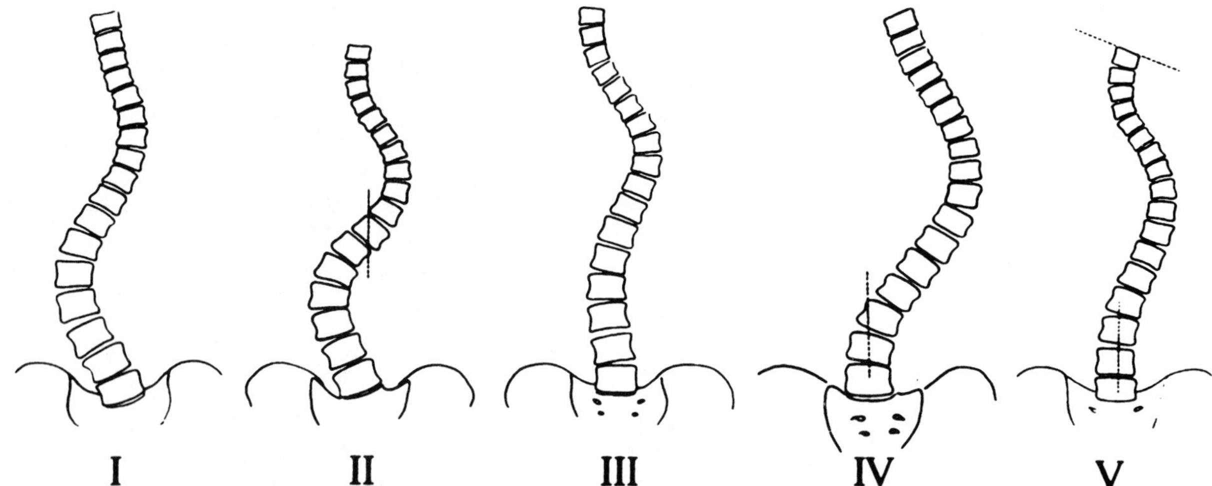

Figure 6-14 Illustration of the five King-Moe deformity patterns of adolescent idiopathic scoliosis. In type I, the S-shaped thoracolumbar curve crosses the midline, and the lumbar curve is larger or less flexible than the thoracic. In type II, the S-shaped thoracolumbar curve crosses the midline, and the thoracic curve is larger or less flexible than the lumbar. In type III, the thoracic curve predominates, and any lumbar curve is highly flexible and does not cross the midline. In type IV, a long sweeping thoracic curve extends well into the lumbar region, with L4 tilted into the curve. In type V, there is a double thoracic curve. These curve patterns have implications for the choice of levels to fuse when surgery is indicated. (Adapted from King HA, Moe JH, Bradford DS, et al.: The selection of fusion levels in thoracic idiopathic scoliosis. J Bone Joint Surg Am 65:1302-1313, 1983.)

stage at time of curve detection, and female gender when (compared with boys with comparable curves). Recommended treatment options are based on an understanding of the natural history of idiopathic scoliosis and an identification of curves that are at risk of progressing.

Physical therapy, electrical stimulation, bracing, and surgery have all been proposed as potential treatment options, yet only bracing and surgery are believed to affect the natural history of scoliosis. Although physical activity is encouraged for all patients, physical therapy by itself has not been shown to affect curve progression. In a prospective multicenter study, Nachemson and Peterson[20] found that bracing does have a significant effect on curve progression but that electrical stimulation does not. The current treatment recommendations are summarized in Table 6-4.

Immature patients with curves between 25 degrees and 40 degrees are commonly treated with bracing (Fig. 6-16). The goal of bracing is to prevent curve progression during the adolescent growth spurt. Bracing initially began in the 1940s as a way of providing postoperative immobilization. In the 1950s and 1960s, orthopaedists began to use the Milwaukee brace, a cervical-thoracic-lumbar-sacral orthosis (CTLSO), as a nonoperative treatment for adolescent idiopathic scoliosis. The Milwaukee brace consists of a molded pelvic portion with metallic upright supports, a throat mold, and an occipital upper portion. Pressure pads are attached to exert counter-pressure on the thoracic curve apices. Because of the poor compliance associated with the Milwaukee brace's clearly visible cervical extension, the Boston brace system was designed in the 1970s; it is probably still the most commonly used brace. This thoracic-lumbar-sacral orthosis (TLSO) is created from prefabricated pelvic and thoracolumbar modules, and it controls curves via pressure from lateral pads and by decreasing lumbar lordosis. Other TLSOs are the Wilmington brace, the Miami brace, and the Charleston bending brace. The Charleston bending brace is unique in that it is molded with pressure at the curve apex but provides a bending force against the curve. It is designed for nighttime use only because it holds the body in an awkward position.

Once brace treatment has been selected, a protocol must be followed, and the patient's course must be documented with serial office visits and radiographs, usually at 4- to 6-month intervals, until maturity. Full-time brace wear is defined as at least 22 hours per day, with 1 or 2 brace-free hours allowed for bathing or athletic activities. In an effort to improve patient compliance and decrease the psychosocial effects of bracing, some orthopaedists advocate part-time use of bracing. In 1997, Rowe and colleagues[21] published a meta-analysis of the efficacy of nonoperative treatment on idiopathic scoliosis. They found 23-hour daily bracing regimens to be the most successful at controlling curves and the Milwaukee brace to be slightly more effective than TLSOs.

Curve Type

Type	Proximal Thoracic	Main Thoracic	Thoracolumbar / Lumbar	Curve Type
1	Non-Structural	Structural (Major*)	Non-Structural	Main Thoracic (MT)
2	Structural	Structural (Major*)	Non-Structural	Double Thoracic (DT)
3	Non-Structural	Structural (Major*)	Structural	Double Major (DM)
4	Structural	Structural (Major*)	Structural	Triple Major (TM)
5	Non-Structural	Non-Structural	Structural (Major*)	Thoracolumbar / Lumbar (TL/L)
6	Non-Structural	Structural	Structural (Major*)	Thoracolumbar / Lumbar - Main Thoracic (TL/L - MT)

*Major = Largest Cobb Measurement, always structural
Minor = all other curves with structural criteria applied

STRUCTURAL CRITERIA
(Minor Curves)

Proximal Thoracic: - Side Bending Cobb ≥ 25°
- T2 - T5 Kyphosis ≥ +20°

Main Thoracic: - Side Bending Cobb ≥ 25°
- T10 - L2 Kyphosis ≥ +20°

Thoracolumbar / Lumbar: - Side Bending Cobb ≥ 25°
- T10 - L2 Kyphosis ≥ +20°

LOCATION OF APEX
(SRS definition)

CURVE	APEX
THORACIC	T2 - T11-12 DISC
THORACOLUMBAR	T12 - L1
LUMBAR	L1-2 DISC - L4

Modifiers

Lumbar Spine Modifier	CSVL to Lumbar Apex
A	CSVL Between Pedicles
B	CSVL Touches Apical Body(ies)
C	CSVL Completely Medial

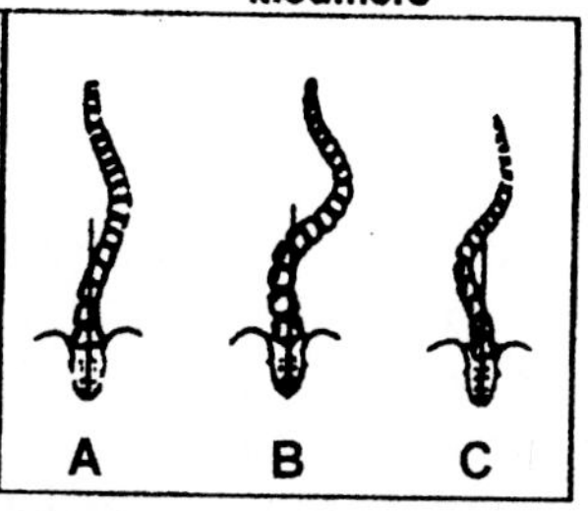

A B C

Thoracic Sagittal Profile T5 - T12	
– (Hypo)	< 10°
N (Normal)	10°- 40°
+ (Hyper)	> 40°

Curve Type (1-6) + Lumbar Spine Modifier (A, B, or C) + Thoracic Sagittal Modifier (–, *N*, *or* +)
Classification (e.g. 1B+):__________

Figure 6-15 Summary of the Lenke classification system for spinal deformity. As with the King-Moe system, the main curve types (1 through 6) are based on the location and flexibility of the curves. Location is defined by the location of the apex of the curve, as described by the Scoliosis Research Society (SRS). The lumbar modifier (A through C) defines where the center sacral vertical line (CSVL) falls with respect to the lumbar vertebrae. The thoracic modifier (+, N, –) refers to the amount of sagittal kyphosis. (From Lenke LG, Betz RR, Harms J, et al: Adolescent idiopathic scoliosis: A new classification to determine extent of spinal arthrodesis. J Bone Joint Surg Am 83:1172, 2001.)

Table 6-2 Incidence of Progression as Related to Risser Stage and Curve Magnitude at Detection

	Percentage of Curves that Progressed	
Risser Stage	5- to 19-Degree Curves	20- to 29-Degree Curves
0 or 1	22	68
2 through 4	1.6	23

(Adapted from Lonstein JE, Carlson JM: The prediction of curve progression in untreated idiopathic scoliosis during growth. J Bone Joint Surg Am 66:1061, 1984.)

Table 6-3 Incidence of Progression as Related to Patient Age at Presentation and Curve Magnitude

	Percentage of Curves that Progressed	
Age When First Seen (Years)	5- to 19-Degree Curves	20- to 29-Degree Curves
≤ 10	45	100
11-12	23	61
13-14	8	37
≥ 15	4	16

(With permission from Lonstein JE, Carlson JM: The prediction of curve progression in untreated idiopathic scoliosis during growth. J Bone Joint Surg Am 66:1061, 1984.)

Table 6-4 Treatment Algorithm for Adolescent Idiopathic Scoliosis

Curve Magnitude (Degrees)	Maturity (Risser Stage*)	Treatment
0–25	Immature	Observation
25–30	Immature	Bracing†
30–40	Immature	Bracing
>40	Immature	Surgery
>50	Mature	Surgery

*Risser stages 0–2 indicate immaturity, and stages 2–5, maturity. If patient is 1 year past menarche, treat as mature.
†If curve has demonstrated ≥ 5 degrees of progression; otherwise observation.

Clearly, many variables are involved in determining the success of brace treatment. The choice of brace type, the length of time in the brace (full-time versus part-time use), compliance of the patient, and the curve pattern being treated are only some to consider. An analysis of all treatment options is beyond the scope of this chapter; but certain generalizations can be made. For example, bracing can be used to control many curves between 20 and 40 degrees in the skeletally immature child. Once started, successful bracing should be continued until the patient has reached at least Risser ossification grade 4 or is 1.5 to 2 years beyond menarche. Full-time bracing may be more successful than part-time bracing. Bracing may be less successful if a curve demonstrates hypokyphosis. Also, a curve with an apex above T7 may not be controllable without a superstructure like that seen in the Milwaukee brace. The initial correction achieved with bracing may be lost over time. Finally, for patients whose curves cannot be controlled by nonoperative means, there are surgical options that vary according to curve pattern, curve flexibility, and surgeon preference.

CONGENITAL SPINAL DEFORMITIES

Congenital scoliosis refers to a lateral curvature of the spine that is due to vertebral anomalies that develop in the embryonic period. Sagittal plane deformities, such as congenital kyphosis and lordosis, may also occur. Although by definition a congenital anomaly is present at birth, the actual clinical deformity may not be detected until later in life. Anomalies that do not produce significant deformity may escape detection altogether, leaving the true incidence of congenital scoliosis unknown.

The classification system for congenital scoliosis is based on the embryologic development of the spine. Normally, during the fourth week, the mesenchymal column of embryonic tissue is arranged into sclerotomic segments. With further development, the formed segments proliferate and condense, with the caudal half of one sclerotome merging with the cranial half of the adjacent sclerotome to form a new segment, the precartilaginous vertebral body. Congenital anomalies are classified into two groups, those caused by failures of formation and those caused by failures of segmentation (Fig. 6-17).[22]

A failure of formation results in incomplete formation of a vertebra. Depending on how much of the vertebra is lacking, various degrees of deformity may occur. For example, if only a partial failure of formation occurs on one side of the vertebra, both pedicles may exist and only a mild wedging may be present (i.e., wedge vertebra). If, however, there is a complete absence of half of a vertebra's structure, a hemivertebra is formed (Fig. 6-18). The level of segmentation around the hemivertebra determines its potential for growth and subsequent deformity. A fully segmented hemivertebra has growth potential on both ends, whereas a semisegmented or nonsegmented hemivertebra is synostosed to one or both of its adjacent vertebrae, thus limiting its potential for growth and deformity. An incarcerated hemivertebra is smaller than a fully segmented hemivertebra and is tucked into a niche between adjacent vertebrae, thus causing less ultimate deformity.

A failure of segmentation may be unilateral or bilateral and may involve two or more vertebrae. If only one side is affected, a unilateral unsegmented bar arises that forms a bony bridge, and the other side may continue to grow and create a convexity. If, however, both sides fail to segment, a block vertebra forms, resulting in a shortened segment; this process occurs in Klippel-Feil syndrome. Unless there is asymmetry in the growth arrest, block vertebrae rarely produce angular deformity.

Through studying the natural history of congenital scoliosis, McMaster[23] determined which patterns are at the greatest risk of progression and helped develop treatment recommendations. The unilateral unsegmented bar with a contralateral, fully segmented hemivertebra has the worst prognosis and should be treated surgically once recognized. Unilateral unsegmented bars also progress rapidly and should be treated operatively. Posterior fusion in situ is usually recommended. For unilateral unsegmented bars in a girl younger than 10 years or a boy younger than 13 years, an anterior fusion may be added to prevent the crankshaft phenomenon. A fully segmented hemivertebra has growth potential on each surface; therefore, resulting curves tend to progress in a steady fashion and frequently require surgery. Curves due to partially segmented hemivertebra tend to progress less rapidly. Curves due to nonsegmented hemivertebrae, incarcerated hemivertebrae, and block vertebrae may progress

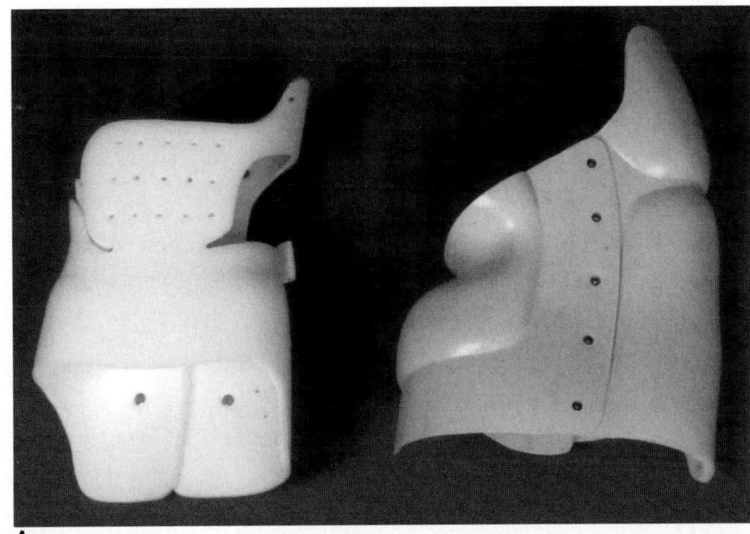

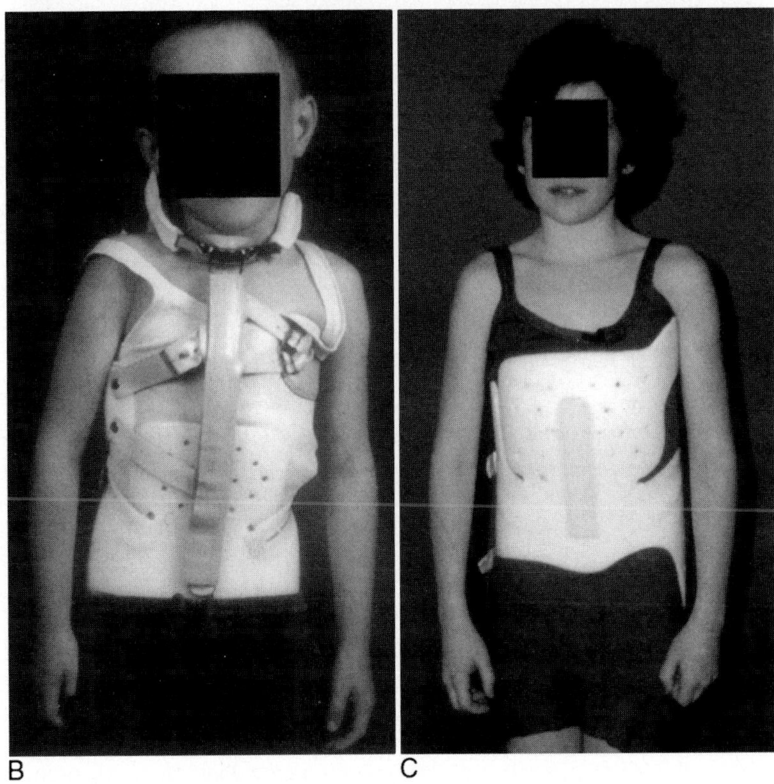

Figure 6-16 **A,** Two thoracic-lumbar-sacral orthoses (TLSOs) available for treating adolescent idiopathic scoliosis. The Boston brace *(left)* can be worn full-time. The Charleston bending brace *(right)*, which holds the body in an overcorrected position, is reserved for nighttime use. **B,** The Milwaukee brace is still used today to gain control of upper thoracic curves, but its cervical extension makes it less appealing than the TLSOs. **C,** The lower profile of the Boston brace is more cosmetically appealing and is acceptable for curves with apices below T7.

slowly or not at all and can usually be observed. Kyphosis due to failure of formation of anterior structures tends to progress and is associated with a high risk of neurologic involvement. Bracing is ineffective for controlling congenital curves.

The embryonic period consists of weeks 3 through 8 of fetal development, and weeks 4 through 6 are the most critical for spinal formation. At this time, the three germ layers are giving rise to specific tissues and organs. Because development of the spinal cord also occurs and is closely associated with the development of the vertebral column, it is not surprising that intraspinal anomalies may coexist with congenital deformities. Such deformities are most commonly associated with the unilateral unsegmented bar with contralateral hemivertebra. Bradford and coworkers[24] found that 38% of patients with congenital spinal deformities had an associated intraspinal defect, such as tethered cord, diastematomyelia, diplomyelia, low-lying conus, teratoma, or syringomyelia. A *diastematomyelia* is a localized split in

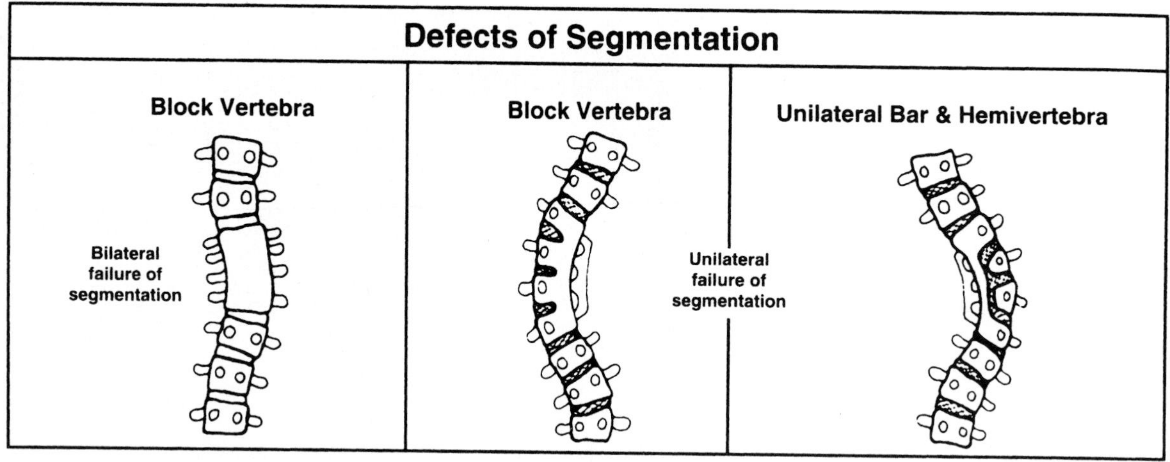

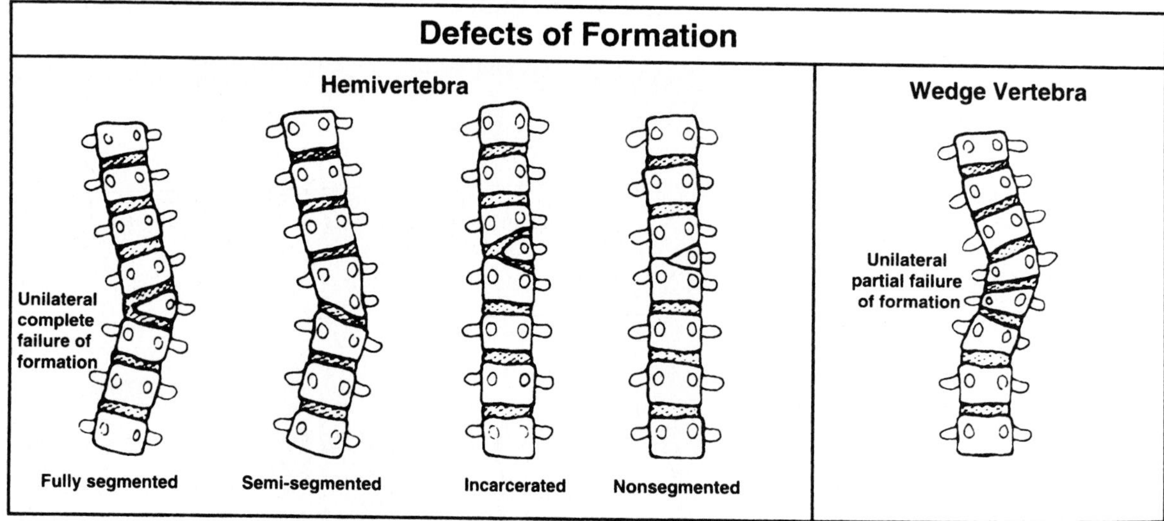

Figure 6-17 The defects of segmentation and formation that can occur during spinal development. (See text for description.) (From McMaster MJ: Congenital scoliosis. In Weinstein SL [ed]: The Pediatric Spine: Principles and Practice, 2nd ed. Philadelphia, Lippincott Williams & Wilkins, 2001, p 163.)

the spinal cord or cauda equina caused by a posteriorly projecting osseous or fibrocartilaginous spur from a vertebral body (Fig. 6-19), a *diplomyelia* is a true division or duplication of the cord, and a *syringomyelia* is a cyst within the cord. Congenital cervical vertebral anomalies can also be present, often referred to as Klippel-Feil syndrome, and may cause dangerous instability.

MRI may not be necessary for every patient with congenital scoliosis; however, the modality may be performed for any suspicious clinical or radiologic findings or in a patient about to undergo surgery to correct the deformity. With respect to other organs, Beals and associates[25] found that 61% of patients with vertebral malformations had anomalies affecting seven other systems. The genitourinary system is involved in approximately 25% of patients, and congenital heart disease may affect approximately 10%. Renal ultrasonography or intravenous pyelography as well as cardiac evaluation may be necessary to identify potentially life-threatening problems.

SPONDYLOLYSIS AND SPONDYLOLISTHESIS

The terms spondylolysis and spondylolisthesis stem from Greek words; *spondylos* means vertebra, *lysis* means break or defect, and *olisthesis* means movement or slipping. *Spondylolysis* refers to a defect in the pars interarticularis that may be unilateral or bilateral. *Spondylolisthesis* refers to the forward slippage of one vertebra on another. These conditions can occur at any age and are not specific to the pediatric population.

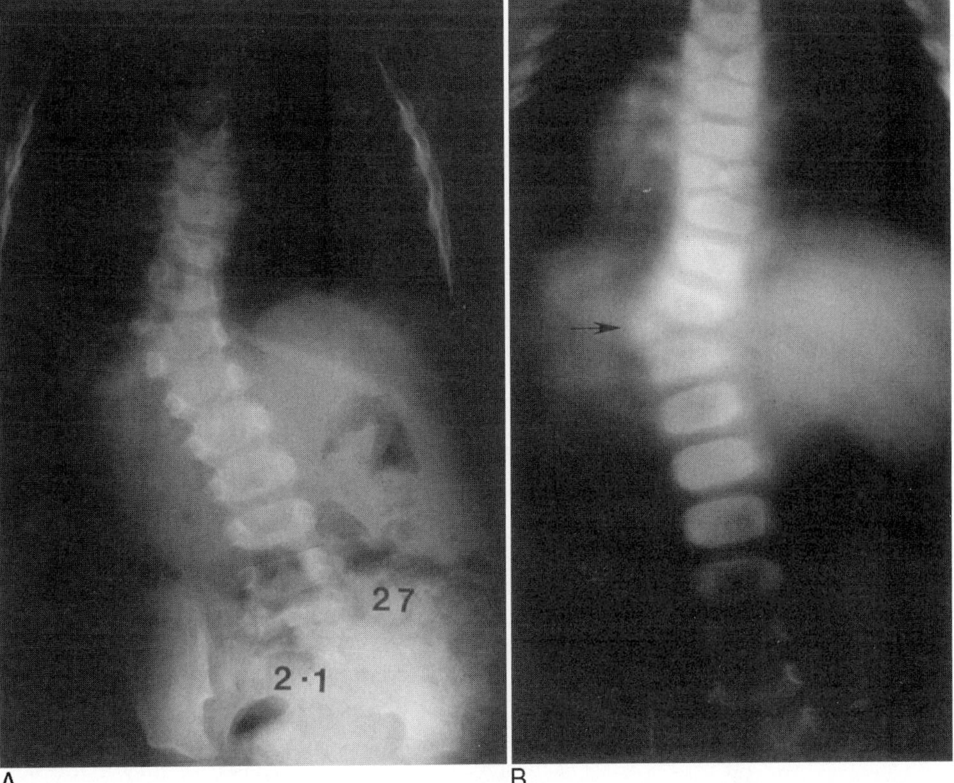

Figure 6-18 Standard radiograph **(A)** and tomogram **(B)** of a hemivertebra resulting in a congenital scoliosis. Note the more proximal incompletely formed vertebrae.

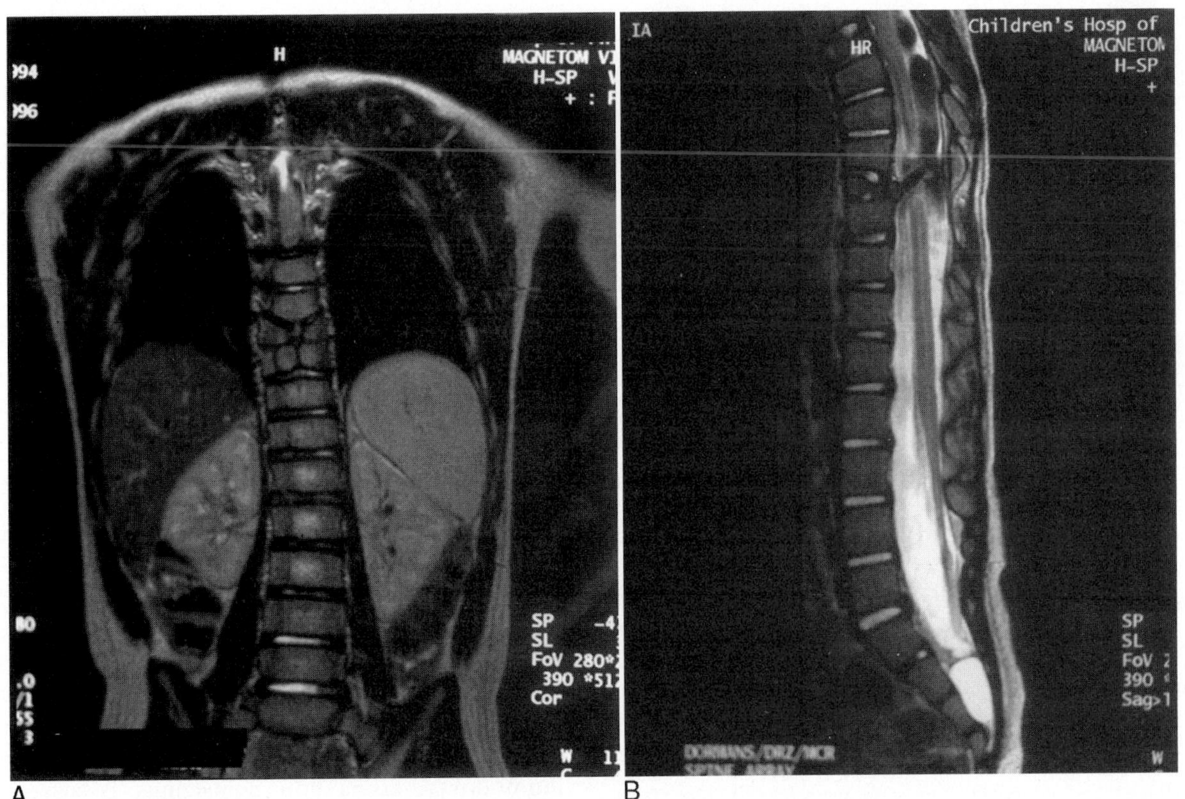

Figure 6-19 Coronal **(A)** and sagittal **(B)** magnetic resonance images depicting a diastematomyelia. Note the osseous projection extending from the vertebral body into the spinal cord.

The Wiltse classification, commonly used to describe spondylolysis and spondylolisthesis (Fig. 6-20),[26] can be briefly summarized as follows:

- Type 1: congenital or dysplastic—dysplastic posterior elements result in deficient articular processes of the facet joints, usually at L5-S1, allowing L5 to slip on S1. This type may be associated with spina bifida.
- Type 2: isthmic—lesion exists in the pars interarticularis, and the facets remain normal. The pars defect may be (A) a lytic stress fracture, (B) an elongated pars (which may represent a healed fracture), or (C) an acute pars fracture.
- Type 3: degenerative—degenerative arthritis affecting the facet joints.

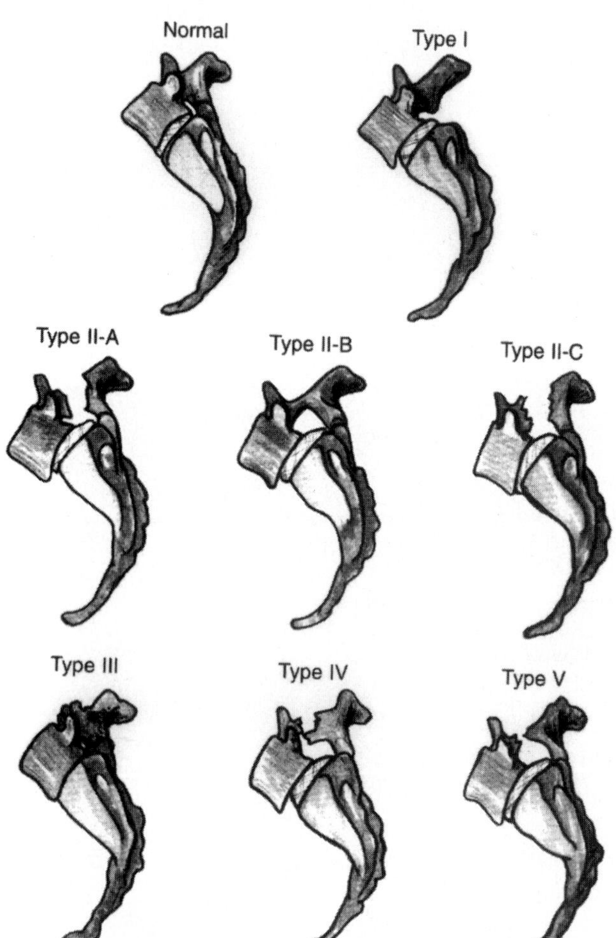

Figure 6-20 The types of defects that can occur in the pars interarticularis as described by Wiltse. Type I is dysplastic and has a congenitally deficient facet joint. Type II is isthmic and involves a lesion within the pars. Type III results from a degenerative process. Type IV results from acute trauma to an area other than the pars. Type V occurs after generalized or local bone disease, such as osteoporosis or tumor. (From Hu SS, Bradford DS: Spondylolysis and spondylolisthesis. In Weinstein SL [ed]: The Pediatric Spine: Principles and Practice, 2nd ed. Philadelphia, Lippincott Williams & Wilkins, 2001, p 434.)

- Type 4: post-traumatic—acute fracture and/or ligamentous injury in an area other than the pars interarticularis, resulting in slippage of one vertebra on another.
- Type 5: pathologic—generalized or local bone disease resulting in destruction of posterior elements and allowing forward slippage.
- Type 6: postoperative—sometimes included to account for the loss of posterior elements secondary to surgery.

Types 1 and 2 are most commonly seen in children and adolescents. Isthmic spondylolisthesis is not seen at birth; however, the incidence increases to 5% in children 6 years old. The incidence is much higher in certain populations, such as the Alaskan Eskimos.

The suggested causes of spondylolysis and spondylolisthesis have included repetitive microtrauma, upright posture, and increased lordosis. Sports such as gymnastics, football (especially in line positions), wrestling, and ice hockey may put athletes at higher risks for hyperlordotic positions and, therefore, increase their risk for pars defects. Although boys are more frequently affected, the rate of progression is higher in girls.

Spondylolysis and spondylolisthesis may be asymptomatic or may manifest as pain. Patients frequently have tight hamstrings and walk with a bent-knee, flexed-hip gait. Nerve root impingement, usually of the L5 root, can occur. Radiographically, spondylolysis may be seen as a pars defect on lateral or oblique views of the lumbar spine. Those defects not seen on a plain radiograph may be detected with bone scanning, single photon emission computed tomography, or CT (Fig. 6-21A).

The amount of spondylolisthesis can be expressed as a percentage, according to the Meyerding classification, through measurement of the amount of anterior slippage, in millimeters, of the superior vertebra on the inferior vertebra and division of this number by the anteroposterior width of the inferior vertebra (Fig. 6-22).[27] Multiplying the resulting value by 100 yields a percentage. Grade 1 spondylolisthesis is defined as 0 to 25% slippage, grade 2 as 26% to 50%, grade 3 as 51% to 75%, and grade 4 as 76% to 100%. A slippage of more than 100% is either grade 5 spondylolisthesis, or spondyloptosis.

Treatment of spondylolysis without slippage is based on symptoms. For asymptomatic patients, no treatment is necessary. If the patient experiences pain that is aggravated by a specific activity, avoidance of that activity is recommended until symptoms cease. For patients experiencing pain, full-time wearing of a brace for 3 to 6 months, followed by gradual weaning, may relieve symptoms. Physical therapy that emphasizes abdominal strengthening and stretching of the lumbodorsal fascia and hamstrings is also recommended. Refractory pain can be treated with in situ posterior spinal fusion. If the pars defect is at L4 or

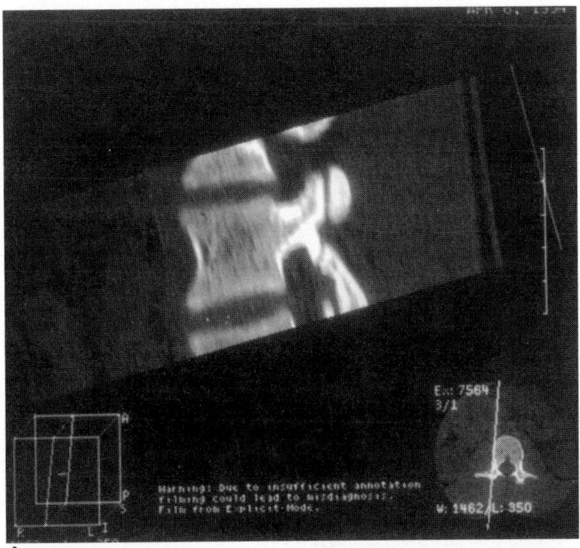

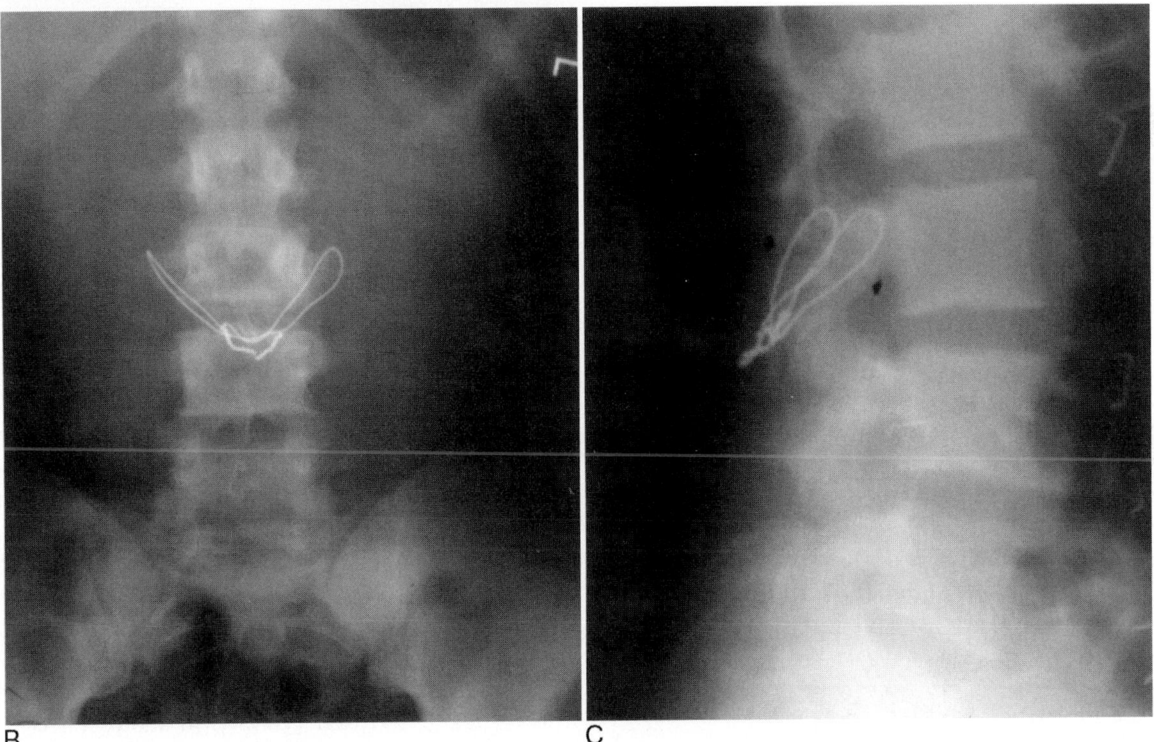

Figure 6-21 **A,** Computed tomography scan of an isthmic spondylolysis. Because of persistent pain, this lesion was treated with in situ wiring. Anteroposterior **(B)** and lateral **(C)** radiographs show the postoperative repair. The *arrows* highlight the lucency on the lateral image that represents the pars defect.

higher, one can consider direct repair techniques using screws or wires (see Fig. 6-21).

Treatment of spondylolisthesis is based on symptoms and extent of slippage. Surgery should be considered for patients with refractory pain, slip progression, more than 50% slippage, or neurologic changes (Fig. 6-23). Nerve root irritation may resolve after stabilization of a spondylolisthesis with an in situ fusion, obviating formal decompression. If a laminectomy is performed, a fusion should be added to avoid destabilization of the spine. Although most low-grade slips can be stabilized with a single-level fusion, higher-grade slips may require multiple-level fusions (e.g., L4 to the sacrum) to overcome the tension placed on the fusion mass. Reducing a high-grade

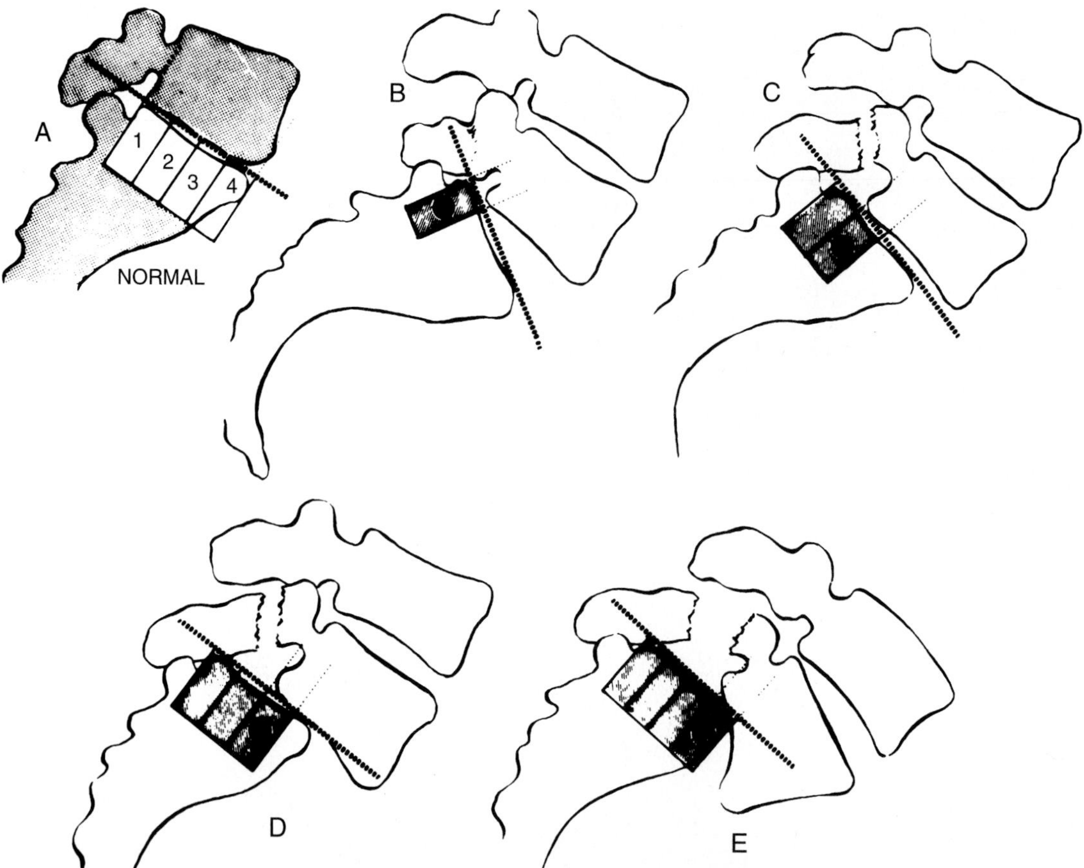

Figure 6-22 Meyerding classification of spondylolisthesis. **A,** Normal. **B,** Type I spondylolisthesis, or 0 to 25% slippage. **C,** Type II spondylolisthesis, or 26% to 50% slippage. **D,** Type III spondylolisthesis, or 51% to 75% slippage. **E,** Type IV spondylolisthesis, or 76% to 100% slippage. (From Hu SS, Bradford DS: Spondylolysis and spondylolisthesis. In Weinstein SL [ed]: The Pediatric Spine: Principles and Practice, 2nd ed. Philadelphia, Lippincott Williams & Wilkins, 2001, p 436.)

slip before fusion remains controversial because of the potential risk of neurologic injury. Table 6-5 summarizes the treatment of spondylolisthesis.

SCHEUERMANN KYPHOSIS

Unlike the coronal plane, in which the normal spine is straight, the spine demonstrates both thoracic kyphosis and lumbar lordosis in the sagittal plane. The extent of normal kyphosis, as viewed on a lateral radiograph, varies by individual, but ranges between 20 and 45 degrees. Excessive rounding of the back can be caused by postural changes or structural abnormalities. Patients, and frequently parents, may find the cosmetic aspects of kyphosis disturbing. One can distinguish postural round back from true Scheuermann kyphosis by assessing the flexibility of the curve and looking for vertebral changes. Postural round back is corrected with hyperextension, demonstrates no structural changes in the vertebral bodies or intervertebral disks, and tends to improve with hyperextension exercise programs. Scheuermann kyphosis, however, is a more rigid condition.

In 1920, Holger Scheuermann[28] described the radiographic characteristics of the condition that now bears his name—increased kyphosis in adolescence, wedging of vertebral bodies, and irregularities of vertebral end plates (Fig. 6-24). In 1964, Sorensen[29] added the criterion vertebral wedging of 5 degrees or more at three or more adjacent levels. Protrusion or herniation of disk material into the vertebral body, called Schmorl nodes when visualized on radiographs, can be seen in the kyphotic areas as well as in unaffected areas. Scheuermann[28] believed that the condition was due to aseptic necrosis of the ring apophyses. Other theories as to the causes of Scheuermann kyphosis are mechanical weakening of the cartilaginous vertebral end plates, familial predisposition, elevated growth hormone levels, collagen defects, juvenile osteoporosis, and even vitamin deficiencies. To date, the true etiology remains unclear.

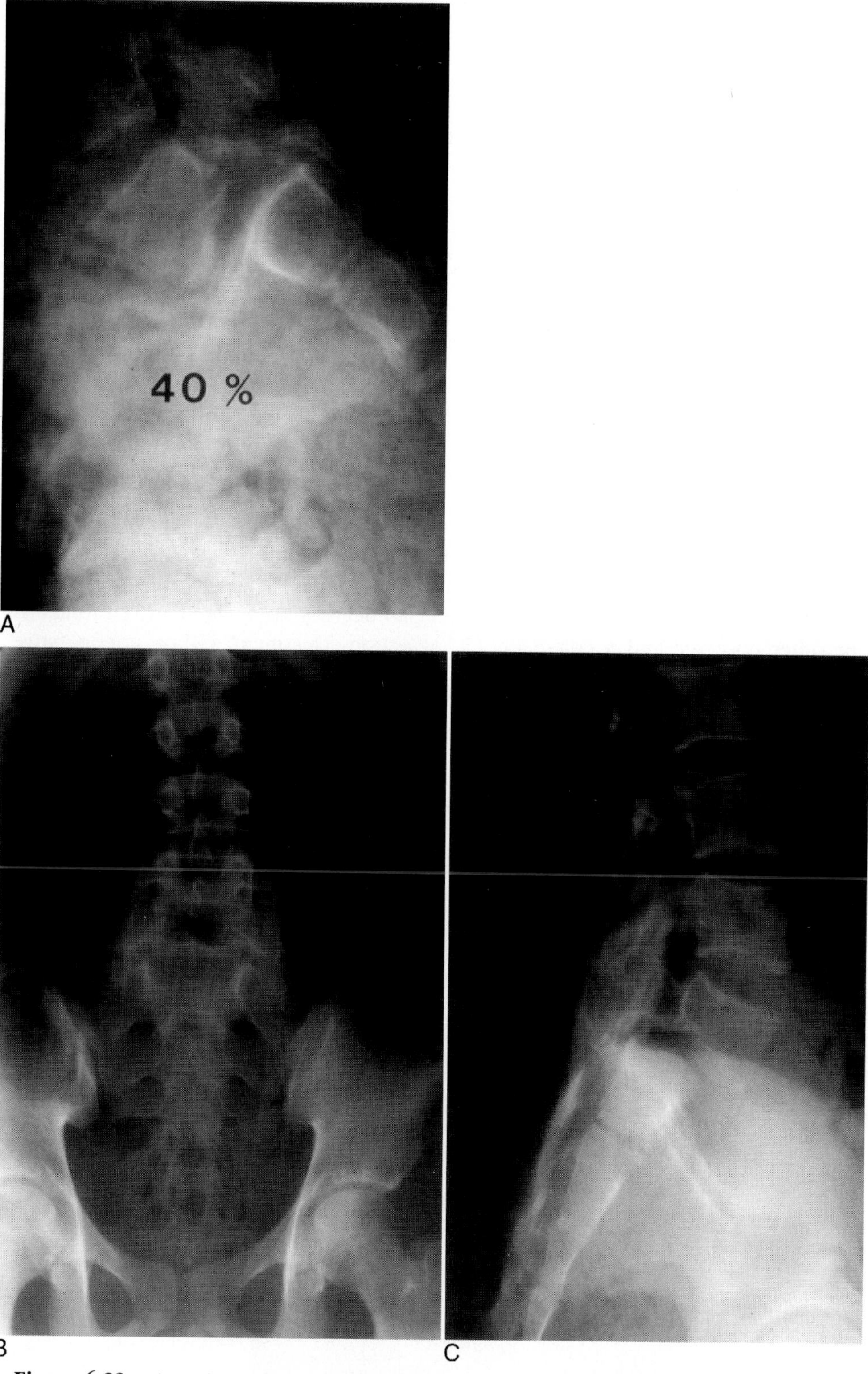

Figure 6-23 **A,** Radiograph showing type II, 40% spondylolisthesis that was not responsive to conservative treatment. Because of persistent pain, a posterior spinal fusion in situ was performed to stabilize the slip. Note the consolidation of the bone graft mass extending between L4 and the sacrum on the anteroposterior **(B)** and lateral **(C)** postoperative views.

Table 6-5 Treatment of Spondylolisthesis

Grade (% of Slippage)	Symptoms	Treatment
1 (0–25)	No pain	Observation
	Pain	Bracing
	Refractory pain	In situ fusion
2 (25–50)	No pain	Observation (fusion if symptoms progress)
	Pain	Fusion of L5-S1
3 (51–75)		Fusion of L4-S1
4 (76–100)		Fusion of L4-S1

Scheuermann kyphosis has an incidence of 0.4% to 8%[29] and appears to have a male preponderance. Although Scheuermann[28] reported a male-to-female ratio of 7.3:1, the ratio is more likely closer to 2:1. Patients tend to present during adolescence, and radiographic changes consistent with Scheuermann kyphosis have not been seen in patients younger than 10 years. Clinical findings consist of observation of a cosmetic deformity by the patient or other observer, and a complaint of back pain, especially toward the end of the adolescent growth spurt. Ascani and colleagues[30] have noted that, in younger patients, pain frequently localizes to the periapical region with paravertebral radiation. As patients become older, the pain tends to manifest as a low backache. Even in patients presenting without subjective complaints of pain, direct palpation of the skin overlying the paravertebral muscles may elicit tenderness.

Scheuermann kyphosis usually occurs in the thoracic region, with an apex localized to between T7 and T9. Mild scoliosis may be associated with the deformity. A thoracolumbar form, with an apex between T10 and T12, also occurs. The radiologic evaluation should include a standing left lateral projection of the entire spine, a standing PA view, and a passive hyperextension test, in which the radiograph is obtained with the patient lying supine on a wedge placed just below the apex of the deformity. CT and MRI can also be used if greater detail is required or in a patient with neurologic symptoms.

Scheuermann kyphosis may progress during the adolescent growth spurt as well as later in life. The amount of progression varies, however, and a patient's subjective pain may not correlate with the magnitude of the curve. For patients with stable curves smaller than 60 degrees, the natural history of Scheuermann kyphosis tends to be rather benign. Adolescents with curves smaller than 50 degrees rarely need any treatment other than observation. Treatment, either nonoperative or surgical, is reserved for patients with rapidly progressing kyphosis or vertebral wedging, unrelenting pain, and respiratory dysfunction due to deformity.

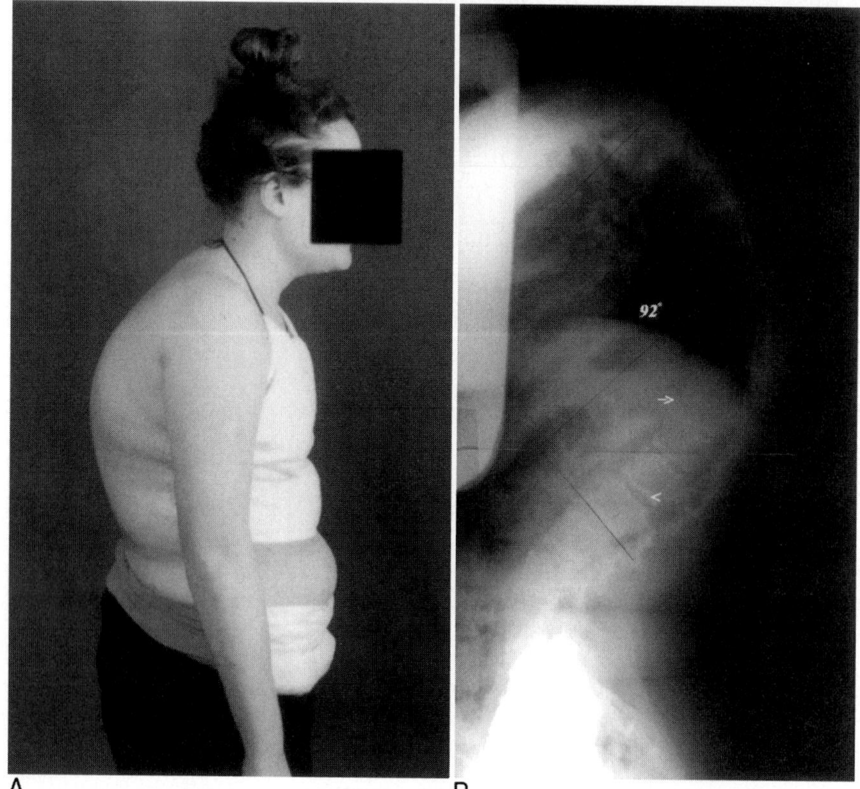

Figure 6-24 **A,** Clinical photograph of a 14-year-old girl with Scheuermann kyphosis. **B,** Lateral radiograph of the same patient. Note the wedging of the vertebrae (*arrow*) and the Schmorl node (*arrowhead*) associated with irregularities in the end plates.

Physical therapy alone cannot correct structural changes; however, it is a useful adjunct to other treatments. Through better muscle tone and flexibility, posture can be improved and pain can be reduced in some patients. Physical therapy is commonly recommended for patients with postural round backs, but its role in treating Scheuermann kyphosis is limited.

Bracing is the most common treatment for Scheuermann kyphosis. It can be effective in skeletally immature patients with curves between 50 degrees and 75 degrees that demonstrate at least 40% passive correctability. If curves are very rigid, a series of corrective casts may be tried before bracing. Once a patient approaches skeletal maturity, not enough growth time is left for reconstitution of the vertebral end plates. The Milwaukee brace is the most widely used brace for curves with apices between T6 and T9 (Fig. 6-25). Unfortunately, the occipital chin ring is highly visible and makes compliance an issue. Only curves with more caudal apices are amenable to the lower-profile TLSOs. The brace is usually worn full-time for 12 to 18 months, followed by weaning to a part-time wear if no curve progression is noted. Bracing may be continued until the patient reaches skeletal maturity. Surgery may be indicated for a curve that is larger than 75 degrees or that rapidly progresses despite bracing.

NEUROMUSCULAR DISEASES

Spinal deformities are commonly associated with neuromuscular disorders. Cerebral palsy and myelodysplasia are the most common, but conditions such as muscular dystrophies, spinal muscular atrophy, Friedreich ataxia, and neurofibromatosis also occur and cause spinal changes. Any condition that interrupts or interferes with control of distal motor units by the central nervous system can affect neuromuscular balance, thus causing weakness, contractures, or deformity. Table 6-6 lists the average percentages of patients with various neurovascular disorders who also have spinal deformities.

Cerebral palsy is a generic term that refers to the brain's abnormal control of motor function. Intelligence may or may not be affected. Insult to the immature brain, before the age of 2 years, can result in a permanent brain lesion that leads to an upper motor neuron syndrome causing spasticity. The extent of involvement varies and, when described anatomically, can manifest as quadriplegia (affecting all four extremities), diplegia (affecting the lower extremities more than the upper), or hemiplegia (affecting one side of the body). Spinal deformities, especially scoliosis, are more common in patients with cerebral palsy than in the general population, and the

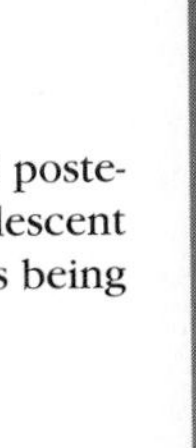

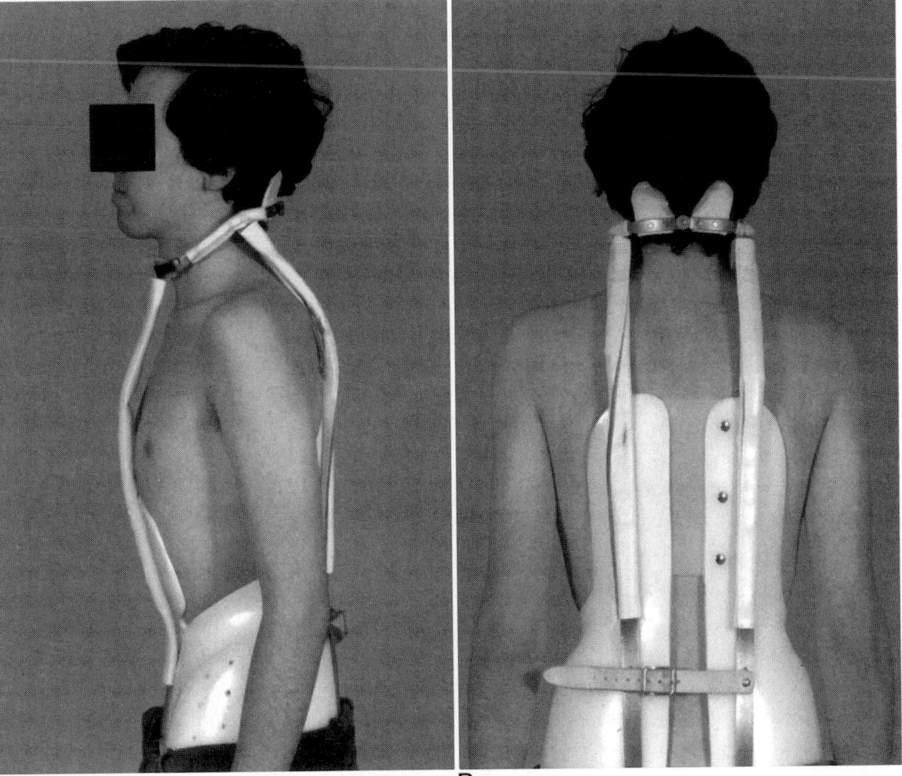

Figure 6-25 Lateral **(A)** and posterior **(B)** radiographs of an adolescent boy with Scheuermann kyphosis being treated in a Milwaukee brace.

Table 6-6 Spinal Deformities in Neuromuscular Disorders

Neuromuscular Disorder	Percentage of Patients with Spinal Deformity*
Cerebral palsy	25
Myelodysplasia	60
Spinal muscular atrophy	65
Friedreich ataxia	80
Duchenne muscular dystrophy	90
Neurofibromatosis	25
Traumatic paralysis	Approaches 100 for high level of injury

*Note: These are averages. The percentage of patients with spinal deformities varies according to the severity of disease involvement or the level of the spinal cord affected.

incidence rises with severity of involvement. The treatment of scoliosis depends on the magnitude of the curve. Small curves may be observed, but curves larger than 45 degrees commonly require surgical stabilization. Bracing is usually unsuccessful.

Myelodysplasia, also known as spina bifida and spinal dysraphism, refers to defects that occur during formation of the neural tube. In its simplest form, spina bifida occulta, incomplete closure of the vertebral elements results in a minimal bony gap in the posterior vertebral arch. This condition may be completely asymptomatic with no clinical findings, or there may be a small tuft of hair or skin dimpling over the level of the lesion. In more severe cases, failure of closure of the neural tube can result in herniation of the spinal cord and meninges (myelomeningocele) or the meninges alone (meningocele) through the posterior spine, manifesting as a sac of neural contents protruding from the patient's back. Neurologic function below the level of the lesion is compromised, and the risk of spinal deformity is greater with more proximal lesions. Patients with thoracic level lesions almost always experience scoliosis; whereas those with sacral level lesions may have no spinal deformity.

Duchenne muscular dystrophy, a sex-linked recessive abnormality associated with the absence of dystrophin protein, results in progressive weakness as muscle is gradually replaced with connective tissue. Without the support of truncal musculature, scoliosis progresses rapidly in early adolescence. Affected patients commonly die of cardiopulmonary complications by their early twenties. Surgical spinal fusion with instrumentation is recommended for curves between 25 degrees and 30 degrees before pulmonary function fails, to enable patients to maintain the ability to sit.

Friedreich ataxia, or spinocerebellar degenerative disease, involves motor and sensory defects; whereas spinal muscular atrophy, due to the loss of anterior horn cells from the spinal cord, produces progressive motor loss. These as well as other myopathies and neuropathies can result in truncal weakness and spinal deformities. As with other neuromuscular disorders, bracing does not usually control progression.

Neurofibromatosis is an autosomal dominant disorder of neural crest origin in which neural crest cells migrate to the skin, brain, spinal cord, peripheral nerves, and adrenal glands. Cutaneous lesions (café au lait spots; see Fig. 6-2), plexiform or cutaneous neurofibromas (Fig. 6-26), axillary or inguinal freckling, optic gliomas, Lisch nodules (hamartomas of the iris), and osseous lesions may be present in patients with neurofibromatosis. Scoliosis is common in these patients, and the curves can be classified as either idiopathic-like or dystrophic. The idiopathic-like curves can be managed like those in adolescent idiopathic scoliosis. The dystrophic curves, however, are short, sharply angulated, and relentlessly progressive; they need prompt surgical stabilization.

There are also a variety of conditions affecting the components of specific body tissues that may result in spinal deformity. For example, bone dysplasias, such as achondroplastic dwarfism and spondyloepiphyseal dysplasia, result from abnormal bone development and can affect the spine. Collagen abnormalities, such as those associated with osteogenesis imperfecta or Marfan syndrome, can cause spinal deformities in 20% to 80% of affected patients. Clearly, it is beyond the scope of this discussion to examine all of the possible developmental conditions that can affect the spine. Human development is extremely complex, and the spine can be

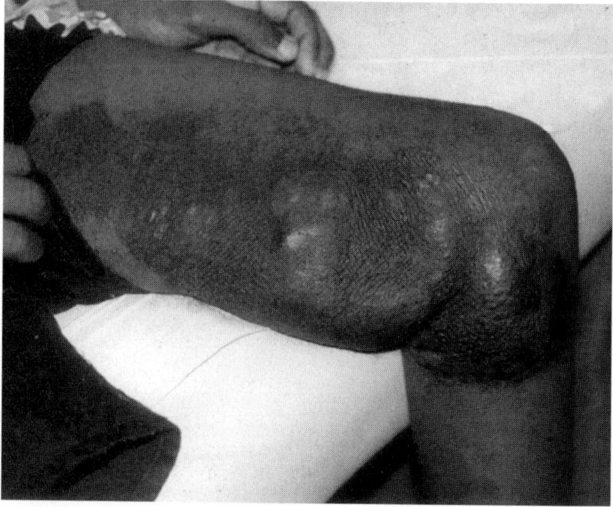

Figure 6-26 Plexiform neurofibroma in a patient with neurofibromatosis.

affected at any stage. From embryologic beginnings to the rapid growth phase of adolescence, the spine continues to grow and to respond to internal and external stimuli.

MAJOR POINTS

Evaluation of spinal disorders requires a careful history, physical examination, radiographic evaluation, and laboratory studies. Back pain in pediatric patients usually has an identifiable source.

Treatment for adolescent idiopathic scoliosis is based on the severity of curvature and the patient's skeletal maturity. For patients in whom 2 or more years of growth remain and the curve is between 25 and 40 degrees, bracing is the recommended treatment.

Congenital spinal deformities may be due to failures of formation or segmentation.

Spondylolysis refers to a defect in the pars interarticularis, and *spondylolisthesis* is the slippage of one vertebra on another.

Scheuermann kyphosis is a structural deformity that may manifest as back pain during adolescence. Unlike postural round back, this disorder is unlikely to improve with physical therapy.

Many neuromuscular disorders are commonly associated with spinal deformity. Surgery is usually required to stabilize progressive curves in patients with such disorders.

REFERENCES

1. Tanner J: Growth and endocrinology of the adolescent. In Gardener L (ed): Endocrine and Genetic Diseases of Childhood. Philadelphia, WB Saunders, 1975.
2. Adams W: Lectures on Pathology and Treatment of Lateral and Other Forms of Curvature of the Spine. London, Churchill Livingstone, 1865.
3. Bunnell W: An objective criterion for scoliosis screening. J Bone Joint Surg Am 66:1381-1387, 1984.
4. Bunnell W: Outcome of spinal screening. Spine 18: 1572-1580, 1993.
5. King HA, Moe JH, Bradford DS, et al: The selection of fusion levels in thoracic idiopathic scoliosis. J Bone Joint Surg Am 65:1302-1313, 1983.
6. Risser J: The iliac apophysis: An invaluable sign in the management of scoliosis. Clin Orthop 11:111-119, 1958.
7. Greulich W, Pyle S: Radiographic atlas of skeletal development of the hand and wrist, 2nd ed. Stanford, Stanford University Press, 1959.
8. Turner P, Green J, Galasko C: Back pain in childhood. Spine 14:812-814, 1989.
9. Burton AK, Clarke RD, McClune TD, et al: The natural history of low back pain in adolescents. Spine 21: 2323-2328, 1996.
10. Dormans JP, Pill SG: Benign and malignant tumors of the spine in children. In Spine: State of the Art Reviews 14:263-280, 2000.
11. Koop SE: Infantile and juvenile idiopathic scoliosis. Orthop Clin North Am 19:331-337, 1988.
12. Pehrsson K, Larsson S, Oden A, et al: Long term follow-up of patients with untreated scoliosis: A study of mortality, causes of death, and symptoms. Spine 17:1091-1096, 1992.
13. Weinstein SL, Ponseti IV: Curve progression in idiopathic scoliosis. J Bone Joint Surg Am 65:447-455, 1983.
14. Weinstein SL: Adolescent idiopathic scoliosis: natural history. In Weinstein SL (ed): The Pediatric Spine: Principles and Practice, 2nd ed. Philadelphia, Lippincott Williams & Wilkins, 2001.
15. Branthwaite MA: Cardiorespiratory consequences of unfused idiopathic scoliosis. Br J Dis Chest 80:360-369, 1986.
16. Mehta M: The rib-vertebral angle in the early diagnosis between resolving and progressive infantile scoliosis. J Bone Joint Surg Br 54:230-243, 1972.
17. Dubousset J, Herring JA, Shufflebarger H: The crankshaft phenomenon. J Pediatr Orthop 9:541-550, 1989.
18. US Preventive Services Task Force: Screening for adolescent idiopathic scoliosis. JAMA 269:2667-2672, 1993.
19. Lenke LG, Betz RR, Harms J, et al: Adolescent idiopathic scoliosis: A new classification to determine extent of spinal arthrodesis. J Bone Joint Surg Am 83:1169-1181, 2001.
20. Nachemson AL, Peterson LE: Effectiveness of treatment with a brace in girls who have adolescent idiopathic scoliosis: A prospective, controlled study based on data from the Brace Study of the Scoliosis Research Society. J Bone Joint Surg Am 77:77:815-822, 1995.
21. Rowe DE, Bernstein SM, Riddick MF, et al: A meta-analysis of the efficacy of non-operative treatments for idiopathic scoliosis. J Bone Joint Surg Am 79:664-674, 1997.
22. McMaster MJ: Congenital scoliosis. In Weinstein SL (ed): The Pediatric Spine: Principles and Practice, 2nd ed. Philadelphia, Lippincott Williams & Wilkins, 2001.
23. McMaster MJ, Ohtsuka K: The natural history of congenital scoliosis: A study of 251 patients. J Bone Joint Surg Am 64:1128-1147, 1982.
24. Bradford DS, Heithoff KB, Cohen M: Intraspinal abnormalities and congenital spine deformities: A radiographic and MRI study. J Pediatr Orthop 11:36-41, 1991.
25. Beals RK, Robbins JR, Rolfe B: Anomalies associated with vertebral malformations. Spine 18:1329-1332, 1993.
26. Wiltse LL, Newman PH, MacNab I: Classification of spondylolysis and spondylolisthesis. Clin Orthop 117:23-29, 1976.
27. Hu SS, Bradford DS: Spondylolysis and spondylolisthesis. In Weinstein SL (ed): The Pediatric Spine: Principles and Practice, 2nd ed. Philadelphia, Lippincott Williams & Wilkins, 2001.

28. Scheuermann HW: Kyphosis dorsalis juvenilis. Ugeskr Laeger 82:385-393, 1920.
29. Sorensen KH: Scheuermann's Juvenile Kyphosis: Clinical Appearances, Radiography, Aetiology and Prognosis. Copenhagen, Munksgaard, 1964.
30. Ascani E, La Rosa G, Ascani C: Scheuermann kyphosis. In Weinstein SL (ed): The Pediatric Spine: Principles and Practice, 2nd ed. Philadelphia, Lippincott Williams & Wilkins, 2001.

CHAPTER 7

Hip Disorders

JUNICHI TAMAI
BULENT EROL
JOHN P. DORMANS

Although hip disorders are common in children and adolescents, the clinical presentation of a child with a hip disorder may not be straightforward. The child or caregiver may report complaints of pain, a limp or an abnormal gait. Alternatively, the child may complain of knee rather than hip pain. This chapter provides an overview of the history-taking and physical examination for the pediatric hip followed by a detailed description of the principal orthopaedic hip disorders of childhood (Box 7-1).

Box 7-1 Hip Disorders in Children

Developmental dysplasia of the hip (DDH)
Legg-Calvé-Perthes disease (LCP)
Slipped capital femoral epiphysis (SCFE)
Idiopathic chondrolysis of the hip
Coxa vara
Femoral anteversion

HISTORY

Careful attention should be paid to any reported changes in gait. The caregiver can often describe a limp accurately. Having the caregiver mimic the gait may be helpful if the child is currently unable to walk. A description of the severity and time course for the gait change, as well as activities that worsen it, are also essential. Pain is the most common presenting complaint in older children with a hip disorder. The clinician should ask the patient to describe the quality, location, severity, time course, and frequency of the pain. Exacerbating and mitigating factors should also be elucidated. The clinician must also inquire about previous episodes of pain, the presence of a similar condition on the other side (including both knee and hip), previous associated injuries, operations, hospitalizations, and musculoskeletal conditions.

PHYSICAL EXAMINATION

Observation and Inspection

A careful observation of the patient's posture can detect hyperlordosis of the spine, which may accompany bilateral hip dislocations (Fig. 7-1). Having the patient stand on one foot forces the hip abductors to work to keep the pelvis level. A patient with a hip disorder may exhibit a positive *Trendelenburg sign*, in which the abductors of the affected hip fail to keep the pelvis level, so the contralateral hip is lower than the affected hip (Fig. 7-2).

To assess gait, the clinician should have the patient walk in the examination room or the hallway. A patient with a unilateral hip disorder may have *Trendelenburg gait,* in which the child leans over the affected hip with each step to compensate for weak hip abductors. A patient with pain in one hip or lower limb may exhibit *antalgic gait*, in which the stance phase is shorter for the affected limb in order to unload that side more quickly, so the unaffected limb appears to be taking quicker steps. Other tests to evaluate the overall function of the lower extremities involve asking patients to walk on the toes and then the heels. Toe walking tests the strength of the calf muscles, and heel walking tests the anterior tibialis muscles and the peroneal nerves that innervate them. Both heel walking and toe walking assess balance, coordination, and range of motion. Having the patient rise from a squatting position (deep-knee bend) tests buttock and thigh muscle strength and screens for limitations in ranges of motion for the hips, knees, and ankles. A more difficult task for some children is hopping on one foot at a time, which requires high levels of balance and strength.

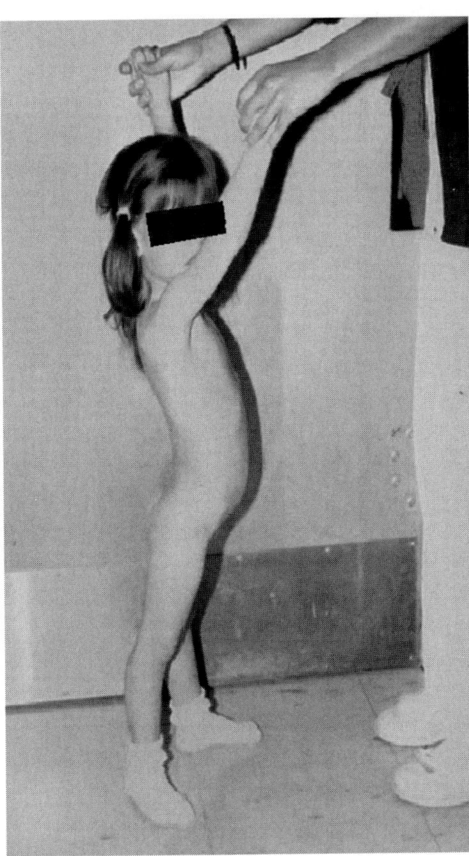

Figure 7-1 A patient with bilateral dislocated hips typically has a swayback appearance characterized by hyperlordosis of the lumbar spine. (Photograph courtesy of Dennis Roy, MD.)

All children should be screened for deformities. Deformities may be due to a genetic syndrome that manifests as characteristic features of the face, skin, trunk, or extremities. Any asymmetry of the face, the shoulders, or extremities, particularly leg length discrepancy, should be noted and evaluated further. Hemihypertrophy may suggest the presence of a genetic or neurologic disorder and should be distinguished from swelling, which may be associated with an injury, infection, or a tumor.

Palpation and Manipulation

During the examination, the clinician should ensure that the patient is in the most comfortable position possible. The caregiver of a young or apprehensive child can assist in the examination by holding the child in his or her lap.

The patient or caregiver should be asked to help localize the area of pain or discomfort by pointing to it with one finger. The clinician should first examine areas that do not hurt to rule out any other disease. Gentle palpation should be used to search for effusion, spinal disease, or masses of the extremity and trunk. The clinician must also be careful to isolate each joint during range-of-motion manipulation. For example, the knee can be isolated from the hip by holding the thigh securely and allowing the leg to hang over the edge of the examination table. Moving the knee in this position prevents inadvertent movement of the hip, thereby helping to distinguish between knee pain due to a knee problem and referred pain caused by a hip disorder. Hip pain can be elicited by the log-roll test, in which the examiner gently rolls the supine patient's entire lower limb (internal and external hip rotation) by holding the thigh. The log-roll test effectively isolates the hip by preventing irritation of the knee and back during the movement.

Clinical Pearl

Knee pain may be due to referred pain to the knee from underlying hip disease, including osteoarthritis, osteonecrosis, Legg-Calvé-Perthes disease, and slipped capital femoral epiphysis (SCFE). Hip pain may be due to spine disease, such as a herniated intervertebral disk or diskitis. The spine, hips, and lower extremities should always be examined in the patient with a limp.

DEVELOPMENTAL DYSPLASIA AND HIP DISLOCATION

Historical Background

Until recently, dislocation of the hip seen in newborns was referred to as "congenital dislocation of the hip" (CDH). The term *developmental dysplasia of the hip* (DDH) has replaced the former name to reflect the evolutionary nature of hip problems in the first few months of life.[1] About 2.5 to 6.5 cases per 1000 live births develop hip dysplasia, and a significant percentage of these cases are not evident on neonatal screening examinations.[2] Because the pathologic processes leading to hip dysplasia may not be present or identifiable at birth, periodic examination of every infant's hip is essential at each routine well-baby examination until the child is 1 year old.[1,3]

Definition

DDH encompasses the entire spectrum of abnormalities involving the growing hip, ranging from simple dysplasia to dysplasia plus subluxation or dislocation of the hip joint. *Dysplasia* refers to the abnormal development of tissues, organs, or cells. Therefore, developmental dysplasia of the hip is a progressive condition in which the hip structures do not develop adequately. The condition has the following three characteristic components: (1) varying levels of abnormality in the slope of the acetabulum, (2) excessive laxity of the hip joint that

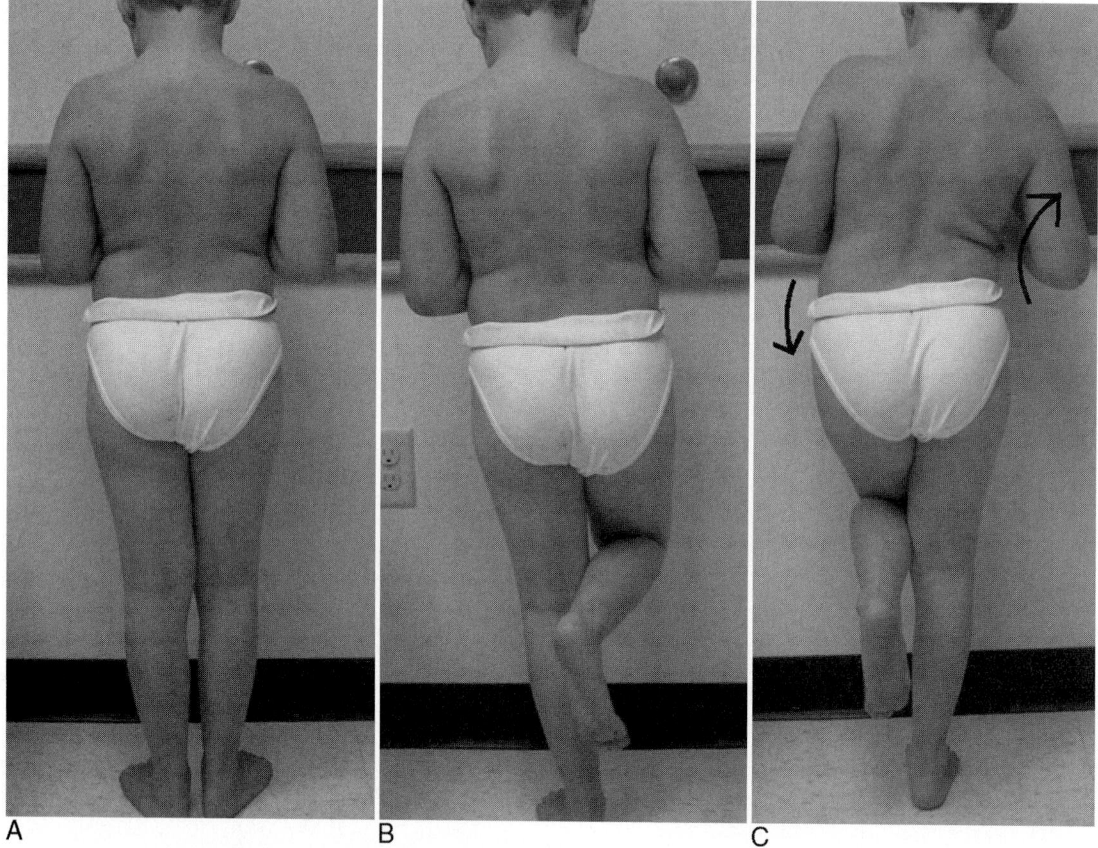

Figure 7-2 Trendelenburg sign: In a patient with a hip disorder, the abductor muscle mechanism of the affected hip is not able to keep the pelvis stable when the patient stands only on the affected limb. A, When the patients stands on both feet, the shoulders and pelvis are level. **B,** When the patients stands on the unaffected left limb, the level positions of the shoulders and pelvis are maintained. **C,** However, when the patient stands on the affected right limb, the pelvis tilts down to the left (*arrow*) and there is compensatory leaning (to the right) of the trunk (*arrow*) over the affected hip to maintain balance.

allows the femoral head to slide upward and laterally out of its normal relationship with the acetabulum, and (3) abnormal rotation of the upper end of the femoral shaft, leading to a malalignment of the femoral head and the acetabulum.

When *dislocation*—displacement of adjoining parts from their usual relationship—occurs in the hip, the head of the femur has completely lost contact with the articular surface of the acetabulum. The dislocated femur is most commonly displaced from the acetabulum in the posterior and superior direction. Three stages of DDH can be identified, as follows: (1) the femoral head may be retained within an inadequate acetabulum (dysplasia only), (2) the femoral head may move slightly away from the acetabular medial wall (dysplasia with subluxation), and (3) the femoral head may slip out of the acetabulum, resulting in a complete loss of contact between the femoral head and acetabulum (dysplasia with dislocation). When *subluxation*—incomplete dislocation of a bone in a joint—occurs in the hip, the head of the femur has not completely lost contact with the articular surface of the acetabulum. Physical findings for a subluxated hip may be normal, or the *Barlow test* (the examiner attempts to passively dislocate the flexed hip by holding the thigh and gently pushing the femoral head out of the acetabulum) may reveal some laxity.

Teratologic hip dislocations have identifiable causes and occur before birth (Box 7-2). Conditions associated with teratologic dislocations may be neurologic disorders (e.g., myelomeningocele), connective tissue disorders (Ehlers-Danlos syndrome), myopathic disorders (e.g., arthrogryposis multiplex congenita), or syndromic conditions (e.g., Larsen syndrome). Most dislocations that are irreducible at birth have defined causes and are therefore considered teratologic.[4]

Natural History

Although some studies suggest that a high percentage of newborns with DDH may spontaneously improve

Box 7-2 Conditions Associated with Teratologic Dislocations of the Hip

Neurologic disorders
- Myelomeningocele (spina bifida)

Connective tissue disorders
- Ehlers-Danlos syndrome
- Puerto Rican syndrome
- Other connective tissue disorders

Myopathic disorders
- Arthrogryposis multiplex congenita
- Others

Syndromic conditions
- Larsen syndrome
- Eagle-Barrett syndrome (prune-belly syndrome)

without treatment,[3] many untreated cases of unilateral DDH progress, with development of a leg length discrepancy and a painless Trendelenburg gait (limp) in childhood or young adulthood. Osteoarthritis may occur in later life (fourth to sixth decade). In fact, up to 20% of cases of adult hip osteoarthritis may be due to DDH. Hip fusion and total hip replacement may be considered for the treatment of the symptomatic hip in young adults with unilateral DDH. A hip that has been fused is immobile but pain free. A total hip replacement can provide a mobile, pain-free hip; however, this procedure is associated with risk of infection as well as loosening and degradation of the artificial joint.

Older children with bilateral DDH often have no leg length discrepancy and no appreciable limp but may exhibit a waddling gait. Children with bilateral DDH tend to walk with hyperextension of the lumbar spine (hyperlordosis) and often have a swayback appearance when viewed from the side (see Fig. 7-1). Like patients with unilateral DDH, these patients often experience early osteoarthritis. Total hip arthroplasty is the treatment of choice for adults with symptomatic bilateral DDH. Bilateral hip fusion is not an acceptable treatment option in the ambulating patient who would be unable to walk after the procedure.

Risk Factors and Incidence

About 1% of infants have dislocated, dislocatable, or subluxatable hips. Risk factors for DDH are well documented; they include female gender, breech presentation, positive family history, and reduced space in utero. Seventy percent of hip dislocations occur in girls. This gender preponderance is thought to be due to the greater susceptibility of girls to maternal relaxin hormone which increases ligamentous laxity.

Although only 2% to 3% of all babies are born in breech presentation, the rate is 16% to 25% for patients with DDH (Fig. 7-3). This fact is probably related to the strong hamstring forces on the hip that result from the knee extension that occurs during breech birth. The greater tension on the hamstrings pushes the femoral head out of the acetabulum, resulting in hip instability.[5]

A family history of DDH is also a strong risk factor. The risk to subsequent children is 6% in a family with one affected child, 12% with one affected parent, and 36% with one affected child and one affected parent. Twin concordance was documented in monozygotic twins as 43%, and in dizygotic twins as 3%.[6]

Any condition that leads to a tighter uterine space and, consequently, less room for normal fetal motion, may

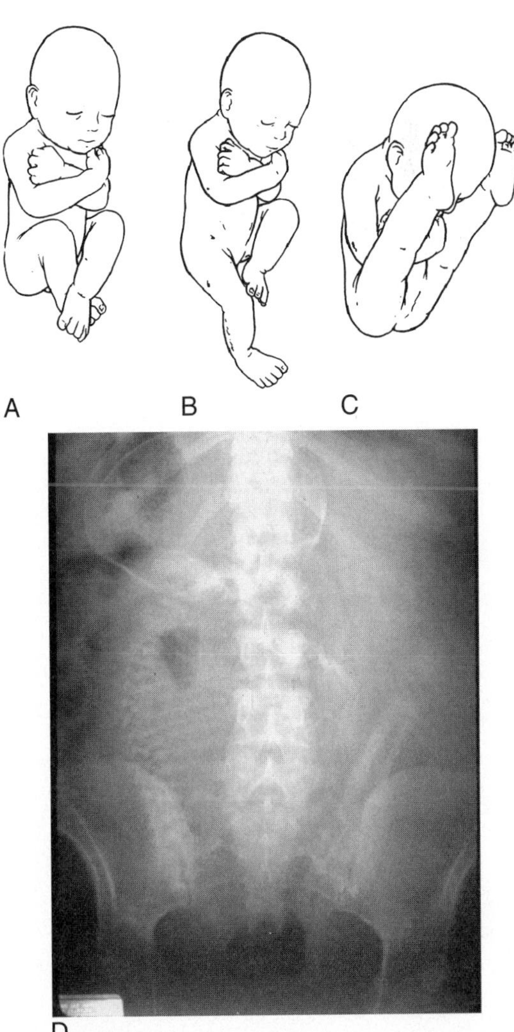

Figure 7-3 **A** to **C**, Breech birth position raises the risk of developmental dysplasia of the hip, particularly the frank breech position **(C)**. **D**, Plain radiograph of a pregnant mother with an infant in breech position. (**A** to **C** from Herring JA: Developmental dysplasia of the hip. In Herring JA [ed]: Tachdjian's Pediatric Orthopaedics. Philadelphia, WB Saunders, 2002, pp 513-654.)

be associated with DDH. These conditions include oligohydramnios, large birth weight, first pregnancy, and premature rupture of membranes. Other children with a higher incidence of DDH are infants delivered by cesarean section and those cared for in special care units after birth.

A child with DDH should be examined for other "molding" or "packing" deformities, such as congenital muscular torticollis (head tilt) (Fig. 7-4), plagiocephaly (flat portion of head), metatarsus adductus (Fig. 7-5), and congenital hyperextension of the knee.[5] Conversely, a child with any of the previously mentioned deformities should be examined for DDH.[7]

The incidence of DDH varies among different ethnic groups. The incidence per 1000 in one study was noted to be 188 in indigenous Canadian Indians, 75 in Yugoslavians, 20 in American Navajo Indians, 0 in Chinese, and 0 in Africans. In contrast, the incidence in white newborns is 1.0% for hip dysplasia and 0.1% for hip dislocation.[4] These differences may be due to environmental factors, such as child-rearing practices, rather than to genetic predisposition. African and Asian caregivers have traditionally carried babies against their bodies in a shawl so that a child's hips are flexed, abducted, and free to move.[8] This keeps the hips in the optimum position for stability and for dynamic molding of the developing acetabulum by the cartilaginous femoral head. On the other hand, children in Native American and Eastern European cultures, which have a relatively high incidence of DDH, have historically been swaddled in confining clothes that bring their hips into adduction and extension positions.[8] This position increases the tension of the psoas muscle-tendon unit and may predispose the hips to displace, and eventually dislocate, laterally and superiorly.

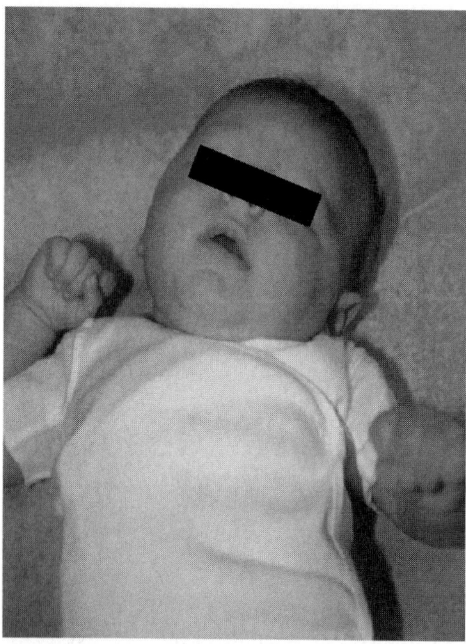

Figure 7-4 Congenital torticollis is associated with facial asymmetry and unilateral shortening of the sternocleidomastoid (SCM) muscles. This child's left SCM muscle is shortened, causing the left ear to tilt to the left shoulder and the chin to point toward the right side. (Photograph courtesy of Dennis Roy, MD.)

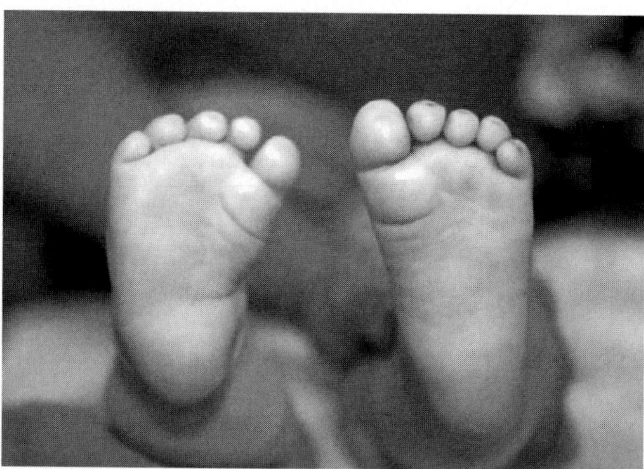

Figure 7-5 Metatarsus adductus varus can be associated with developmental dysplasia of the hip. Note the varus deformity of the child's right foot. (Photograph courtesy of Dennis Roy, MD.)

Sixty percent of cases of DDH involve only the left hip. The right hip is affected unilaterally in only 20% of cases, and DDH is bilateral in 20%. This propensity to affect the left side can best be explained by the fact that the fetus's left hip is commonly adducted against the mother's lumbosacral spine in the left occiput anterior (LOA) intrauterine position.[1]

Physical Findings

The most reliable clinical methods of DDH detection in the newborn are the Ortolani and Barlow (provocative) maneuvers (Figs. 7-6 and 7-7). The examination must be carried out with the infant unclothed and placed supine on a flat examination table in a warm, comfortable setting.

Both the Ortolani and Barlow maneuvers begin with the hips and knees flexed to 90 degrees. For the *Ortolani maneuver*, reduction and dislocation occur in sequence (i.e., ball moving over ridge in and out of acetabulum). The hip is gently abducted, and the greater trochanter is gently elevated. This movement allows a dislocated femoral head to glide back into the acetabulum. A palpable "clunk" (rather than an audible one) corresponds to reduction of the femoral head and was described by Ortolani as the *segno della scata*, or "sign of the ridge." A reducible hip, therefore, is deemed "Ortolani positive." The result of the Ortolani maneuver may be negative with a completely dislocated, irreducible hip; a

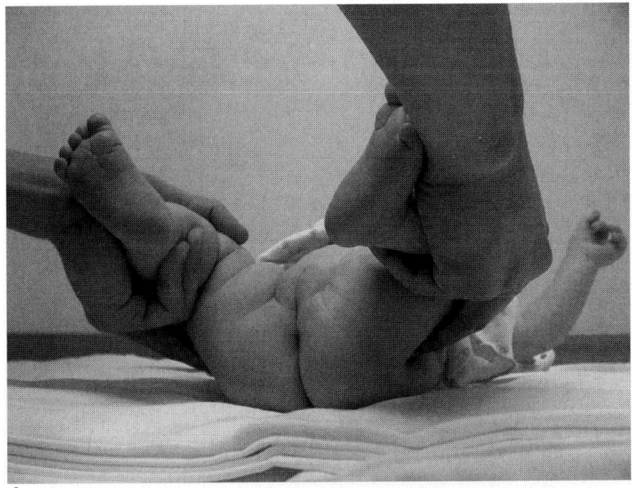

A

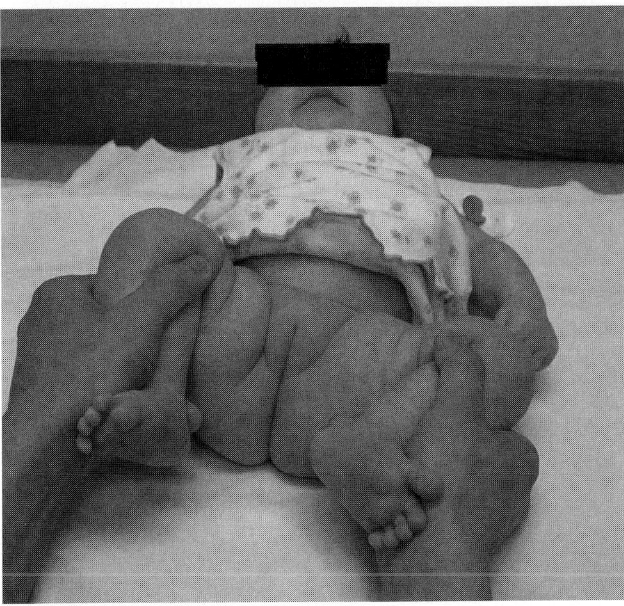

B

Figure 7-6 **A** and **B,** In the Ortolani maneuver (sign of the ridge—ball of femoral head moving in and out of the acetabulum), the examiner holds the patients thighs in abduction and, with the fingertips, applies an anteriorly directed force to the greater trochanter. If a dislocated hip is dislocating and reducible, the result is positive. If the hip is dislocated but irreducible, the result is negative. Note the asymmetric abduction in this child. The right hip is dislocated and therefore does not allow full hip abduction.

negative result in this case is simply a sign that the hip is firmly dislocated and cannot be reduced with manipulation in the nonanesthetized child. The Barlow or provocative maneuver assesses the potential for dislocation of a nondisplaced hip. The examiner adducts the flexed hip and gently pushes the thigh posteriorly in an effort to dislocate the femoral head. This motion may or may not be accompanied by a palpable clunk or jerking sensation as the femoral head slides out of the acetabulum. Therefore, a positive Barlow test result signifies a dislocatable hip; if the femoral head is already dislocated, the result is negative.[9,10]

A *hip click* is the high-pitched sensation felt at the very end of abduction during testing for DDH with Barlow and Ortolani maneuvers. It occurs in up to 10% of newborns. Classically, a hip click is differentiated from a hip "clunk," which is heard and felt as the hip goes in and out of joint. Most experts consider hip clicks benign, although the origin is unclear. Possible origins of hip clicks are movement of either the ligamentum teres or the synovium between the femoral head and acetabulum (hip capsule), sliding of the iliopsoas tendon over the crest of the ilium, and movement of the iliotibial band over the cartilaginous greater trochanter. Worrisome features that may warrant further evaluation (e.g., hip ultrasonography, hip radiograph) are late-onset click, associated orthopaedic abnormalities, and other clinical features suggestive of developmental dysplasia (e.g., asymmetric skin folds or creases, leg length discrepancy).

The *Galeazzi test* is an evaluation of apparent thigh length (Fig. 7-8). With the patient supine and the hips and knees flexed at 90 degrees, the levels of the knees are inspected. The Galeazzi sign is present if the level of the knees is uneven and is cause for concern. This apparent shortening of one femur may be due to unilateral hip dislocation, to proximal femoral focal deficiency (PFFD), a disorder in which the proximal femur does not develop normally, or to a mild leg length discrepancy. The Galeazzi sign is absent, however, if the child's condition is bilateral (i.e., bilateral hip dislocations).

Asymmetry of thigh and gluteal skin folds may be present in 10% of normal infants but is suggestive of DDH. A short thigh with multiple skin folds on the medial thigh is consistent with proximal migration of the skeletal structures in a patient with a unilateral hip dislocation (Fig. 7-9). The perineum on the side of the dislocation may be broadened because of the lateral displacement of the femoral head.

In addition, hip abduction may be limited (Fig. 7-10). In a dislocated hip, the high-riding femoral head shortens the distance between the hip adductor muscles and their insertions on the medial aspect of the femur. The shorter distance leads to tightening of the hip adductor muscles and contributes to the limitation in hip abduction. Another helpful test is the *Klisic test*, in which the examiner places a long finger over the greater trochanter and the index finger of the same hand on the anterior superior iliac spine (Fig. 7-11). In a normal hip, an imaginary line drawn between the two fingers points to the umbilicus. In the dislocated hip, the trochanter is elevated, and the line projects halfway between the umbilicus and the pubis.[5]

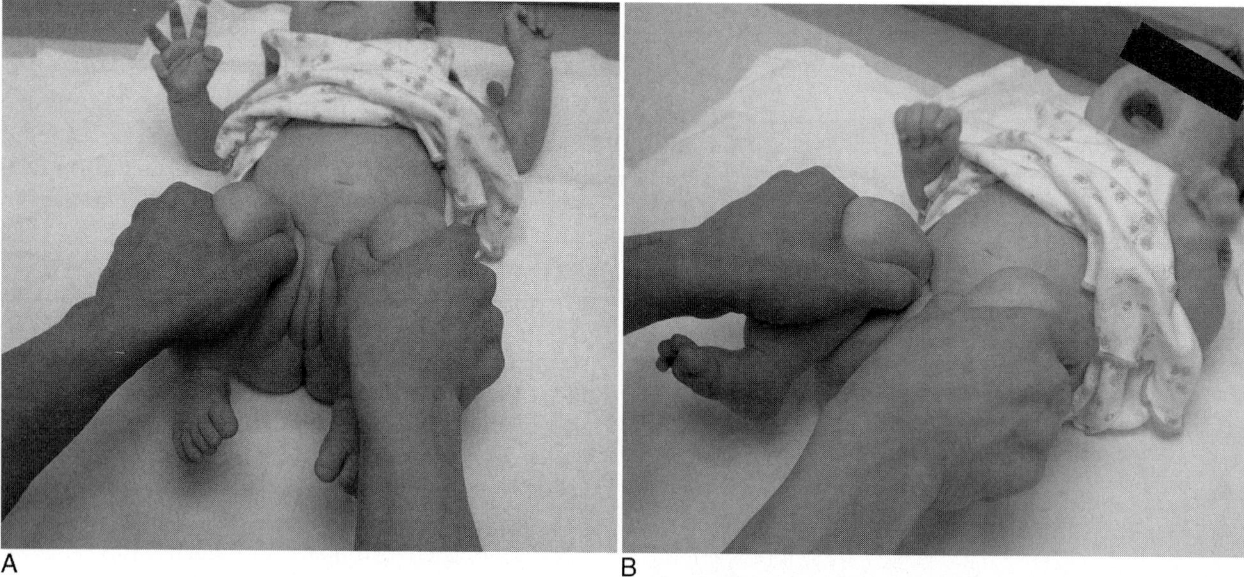

Figure 7-7 **A** and **B,** The Barlow test (provocative maneuver demonstrating dislocation of hip) is performed with the patient's hips and knees flexed. Holding the patient's limbs gently, with the thigh in adduction, the examiner applies a posteriorly directed force. This result is positive in a dislocatable hip.

Recommendations

All infants should undergo a clinical examination by a physician or physician equivalent on at least two occasions in the first 3 months of life. Barlow, Ortolani, and Galeazzi tests, as well as assessment of hip abduction, should be performed during the newborn period.

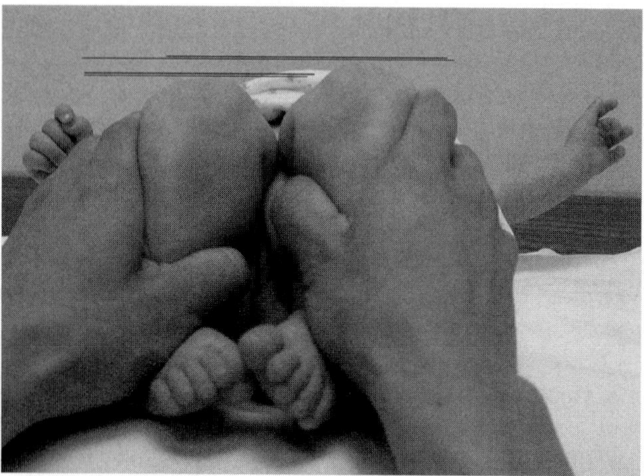

Figure 7-8 **The Galeazzi test is performed with the patient's hips and knees flexed at right angles.** The patient must be placed supine on a flat firm surface. An asymmetry in the apparent knee height indicates a difference in the length of the femur or a dislocation of one of the hips. The result would be negative for a patient with bilateral dislocation of the hips. A Galeazzi test performed on this patient shows that the right knee is lower than the left. Which hip is more likely dislocated?

Limitation of abduction becomes the most important sign of DDH in infants 8 to 12 weeks of age, because results of the Barlow and Ortolani tests may be negative in older infants with DDH. The Galeazzi test and evaluation for limb length discrepancy continue to be useful in children older than 12 weeks.

Imaging Studies

In infants younger than 6 months, the acetabulum and proximal femur are predominantly cartilaginous and thus not visible on plain radiographs. In this age group, these structures are best visualized with ultrasound.[11,12] In addition to morphologic information, ultrasound provides dynamic information about the stability of the hip joint.[13]

Real-time Ultrasound Examination

The advantages of real-time ultrasound examination (Fig. 7-12) are (1) lack of irradiation, (2) noninvasiveness, (3) ability to directly visualize the cartilaginous femoral head, and (4) ability to provide information on hip position, stability, and morphology during a dynamic examination. The ultrasound examination can be used to monitor acetabular development, particularly of infants undergoing Pavlik harness treatment; this modality can minimize the number of radiographs taken and may allow the clinician to detect failure of treatment earlier.

The disadvantages of using ultrasonography are high cost, limited availability, and a paucity of expert ultrasonographers and qualified test interpreters. Moreover, the test may be limited by inadequate specificity and

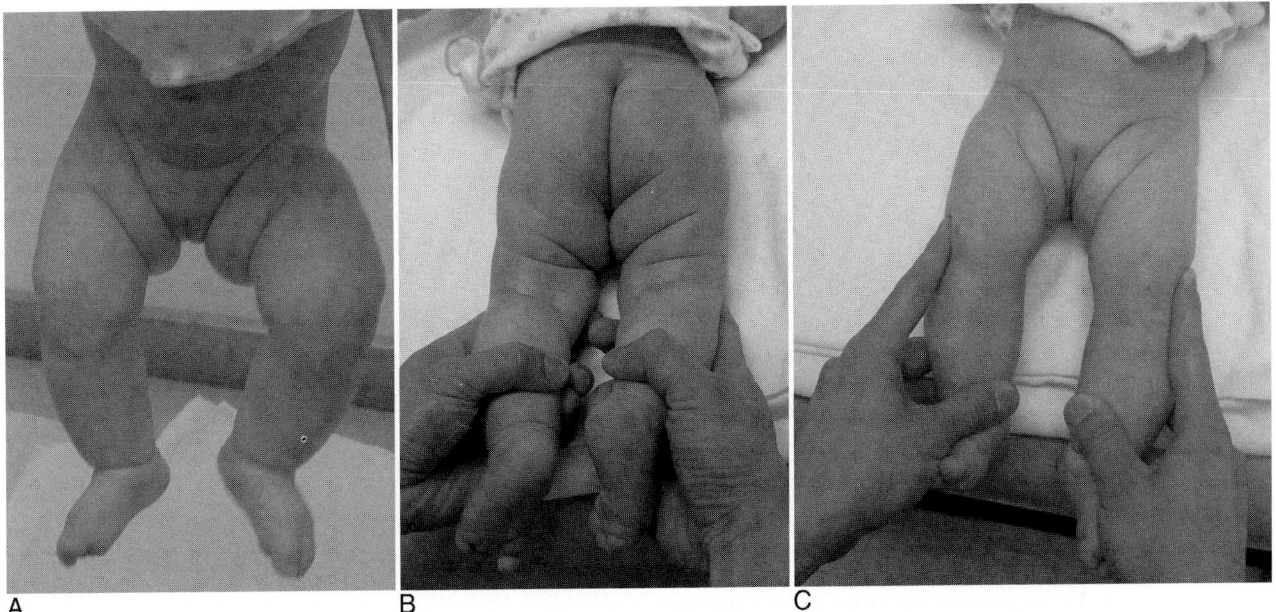

Figure 7-9 Asymmetric skin folds suggest proximal migration of the underlying skeletal structures. A and **B,** Note the differences in the proximal thigh folds both anteriorly and posteriorly. **C,** In addition, the left leg appears longer than the right. These findings are suggestive of a right hip dislocation.

sensitivity, resulting in both overtreatment of benign conditions and failure to lower the incidence of late diagnosis.

Indications

Because physical examination is not completely reliable and late diagnosis of DDH still occurs, some investigators have recommended routine ultrasonographic screening.[14] Others argue, however, that universal ultrasonographic screening can lead to overdiagnosis and overtreatment. At present, the issue remains controversial. Universal screening is more commonly conducted in Europe; in the United States, the decision to

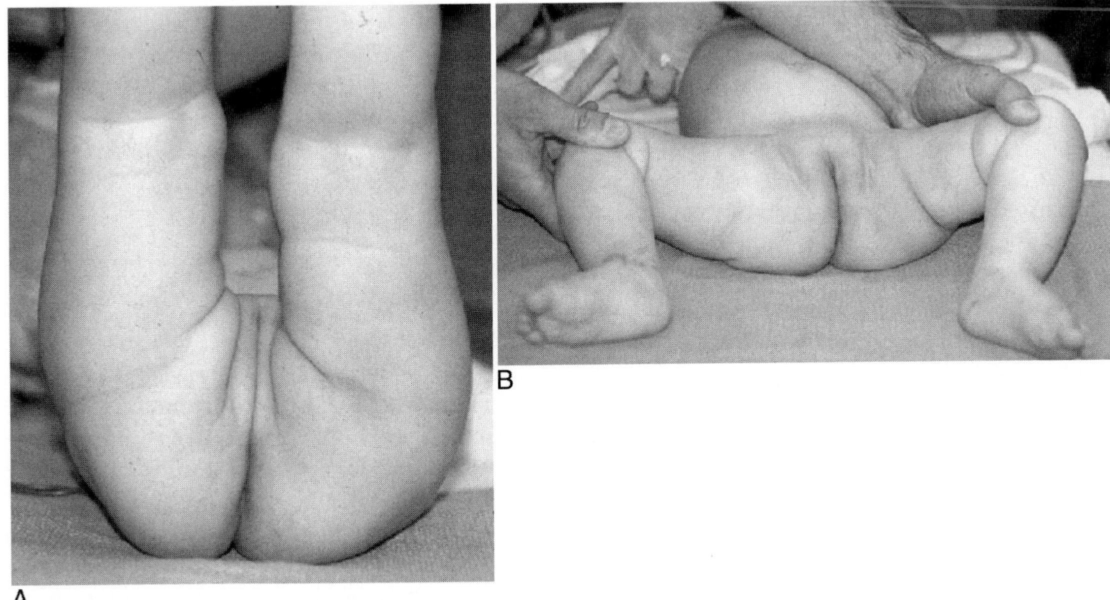

Figure 7-10 **A** and **B,** Decreased abduction of the left hip in an older child is indicative of left hip dislocation.

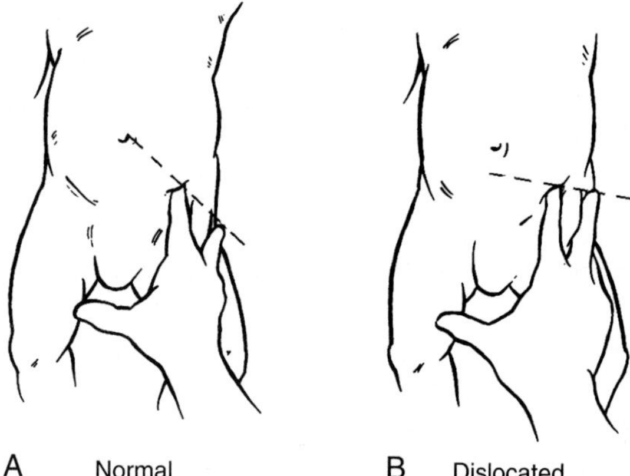

Figure 7-11 Klisic test. A, In a normal hip, an imaginary line drawn through the tip of an index finger placed on the patient's iliac crest and the tip of the long finger placed on the patient's greater trochanter should point to the umbilicus. **B,** In a dislocated hip, the imaginary line drawn through the two fingertips runs below the umbilicus because the greater trochanter is abnormally high. (From Herring JA: Developmental dysplasia of the hip. In Herring JA [ed]: Tachdjian's Pediatric Orthopaedics. Philadelphia, WB Saunders, 2002, pp 513-654.)

screen a child for DDH is based on risk factors and physical findings.[2,15]

Interpretation of Ultrasound Study

To more easily understand the ultrasound study of the newborn, it is helpful to first evaluate it in the same way as one would a hip radiograph of a newborn. The anteroposterior (AP) view of the hip is similar to the coronal ultrasonograph (Fig. 7-13). The ilium seen on the radiograph is similar to the lateral part of the ilium seen on the ultrasonograph. The shallow acetabular socket can be seen with both modalities. The femoral head, which cannot be seen on a radiograph, can be identified on an ultrasonograph. An ultrasound study of a normal hip shows the femoral head seated in the acetabulum with about half of the head covered by the acetabular roof (like a ball of ice cream in an ice cream scoop). In a dynamic ultrasound study of an unstable hip, the operator performs the Barlow maneuver during the study, and the femoral head can be seen as it is pushed out of the acetabulum (like a ball of ice cream falling off the ice cream scoop). As with all imaging tests, a pediatric radiologist should be consulted for the definitive interpretation of the ultrasound study.

Radiographs

Radiographs are recommended for an infant once the proximal femoral epiphysis ossifies, usually by 4 to 6 months. In infants this age, the radiographic examination has proved to be more effective, less costly, and less operator-dependent than ultrasound examination. An AP view of the pelvis can be interpreted through the use of several lines drawn on it.

The *Hilgenreiner line* is a horizontal line drawn through the top of the triradiate cartilage (the clear area in the depth of the acetabulum) (Fig. 7-14). The *Perkins line*, a vertical line through the most lateral ossified margin of the roof of the acetabulum, is perpendicular to the Hilgenreiner line (see Fig. 7-14). The ossific nucleus of the femoral head should be located in the medial lower quadrant of the intersection of the two lines.[16] The *Shenton line* (Fig. 7-15) is a curved line drawn from the medial aspect of the femoral neck to the lower border of the superior pubic ramus. In a child with normal hips, this line is a continuous contour. In a child with DDH, this line consists of two separate arcs and therefore is described as "broken." The *acetabular index* is the angle formed between the Hilgenreiner line and a line drawn from the depth of the acetabular socket to the most lateral ossified margin of the roof of the acetabulum. This angle measures the development of the osseous roof of the acetabulum. In the newborn, this index can be up to 40 degrees; by 4 months in the normal infant, it should be no more than 25 degrees.

Radiographs of the hip in abduction and internal rotation should also be obtained, as these views show whether the hip dislocation is reducible.

Screening

Clinical screening for DDH in the newborn nursery still does not detect some cases. Garvey and associates[17] have shown that in at-risk children with normal hip findings, hip radiographs taken at 4 months were often abnormal. Of 375 children with abnormal radiographs at 4 months in their study, radiographs at 15 months were abnormal in 46. However, no child with normal radiographs at 4 months had abnormal radiographs at 15 months. Therefore, there is no evidence that a child with normal hip radiographs at 4 months will experience hip dysplasia by 15 months. For this reason, all patients screened for DDH as newborns should undergo subsequent examination at 4 to 6 months to verify that radiographic findings are normal.[4,17]

Management

Nonoperative Management

The goal in management of DDH is to achieve and maintain a concentric reduction of the femoral head within the acetabulum in order to provide the optimal environment for normal development of both the femoral head and acetabulum. The reduction is maintained by keeping the hips flexed and abducted and the knees flexed. Wide abduction of the hips can cause osteonecrosis of the femoral epiphysis by stretching the vessels to the femoral head. Therefore, positioning the hip in the "safe position"—between full abduction

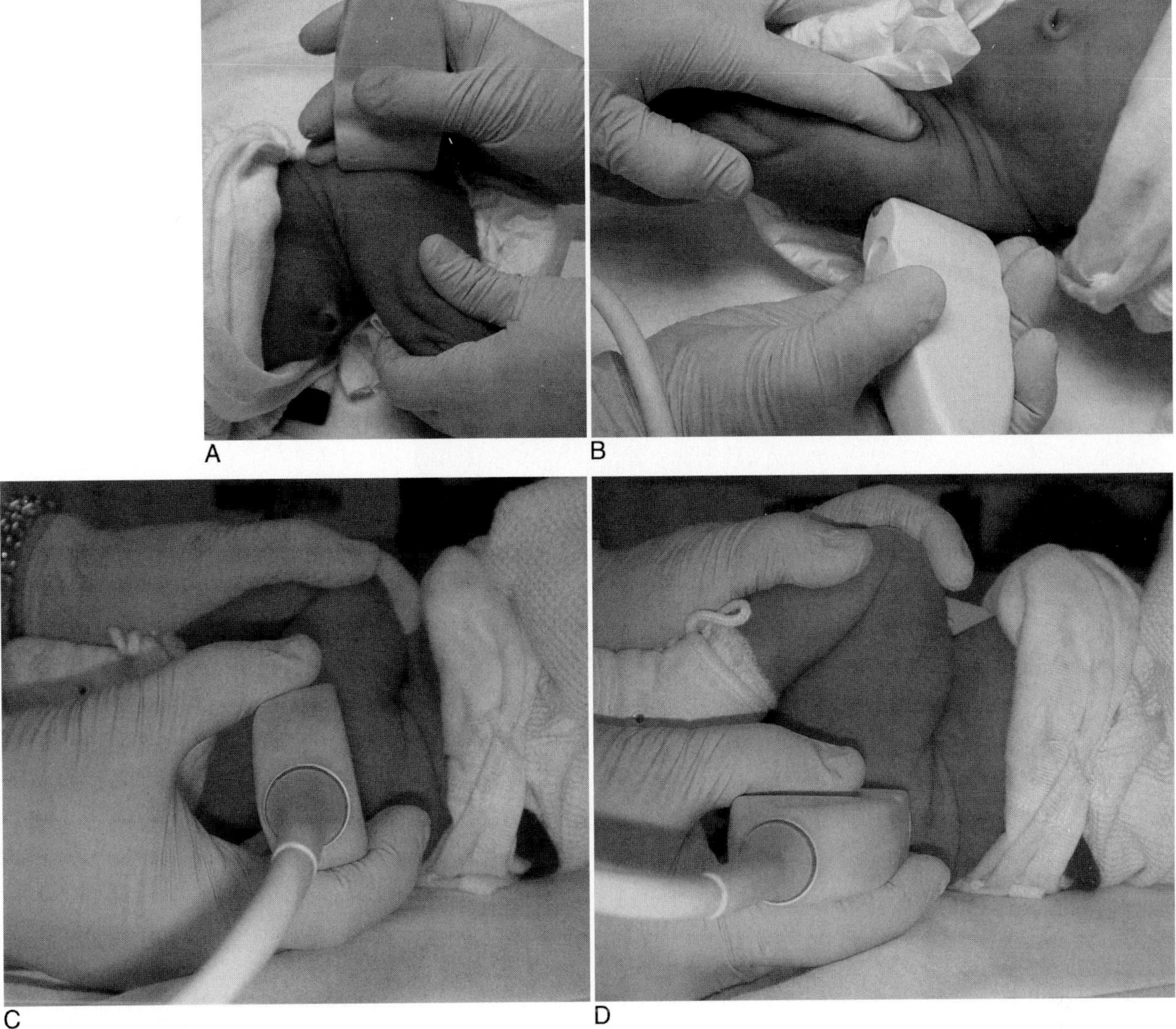

Figure 7-12 **A** to **D,** In the newborn child, an ultrasound examination by an experienced ultrasonographer is the most accurate method of detecting hip dysplasia. Ultrasound images can provide dynamic information when the ultrasonographer performs a Barlow test. The femoral head can be visualized sliding in and out of the acetabulum.

and the position in which the femoral head dislocates in extreme adduction—is imperative.

The Pavlik harness is the most commonly used device for the treatment of DDH (Fig. 7-16). Triple diapers have no role in the treatment of DDH, as they give the parents a false sense of security and do not provide reliable stabilization or positioning.[10]

Pavlik Harness

Infants up to 6 months old with "unstable" and reducible ("Ortolani-positive") hips must be treated to ensure proper hip development. Pavlik harness treatment does not rigidly immobilize the hips and therefore allows dynamic molding of the acetabulum by the cartilaginous femoral head. Frequent examinations and readjustments are necessary to ensure that the harness is applied correctly. A 6-week course of treatment is begun after an ultrasound examination confirms reduction of the hips. Success of Pavlik harness treatment is likely if the patient is otherwise normal and the caregivers are both well-educated about DDH and compliant with use of the harness.

Use of the Pavlik harness should be discontinued if no reduction of the hip can be documented after 3 to 4 weeks of use. A teratologic cause for hip dislocation must be considered at this time. Furthermore, use of the Pavlik harness is contraindicated in any hip condition

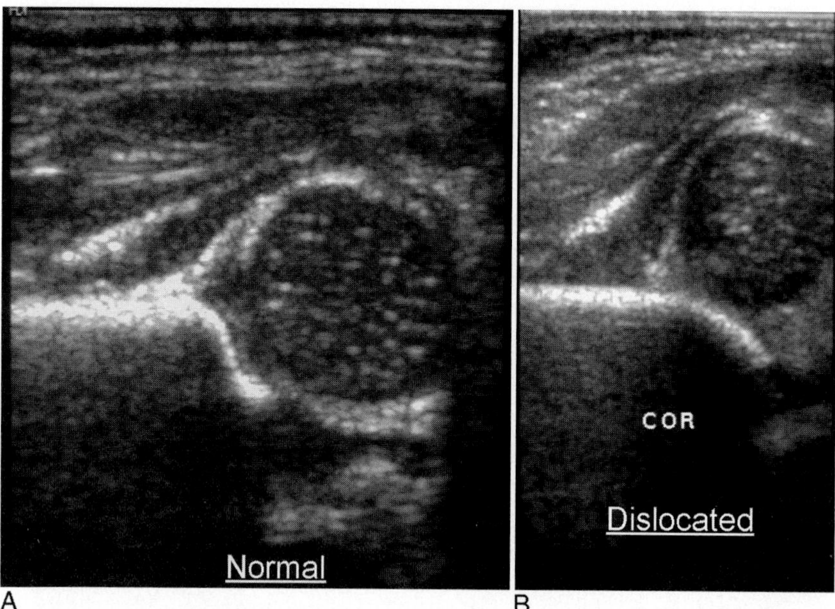

Figure 7-13 **A,** An ultrasound image in the coronal plane of a normal hip shows a femoral head well reduced in the acetabulum. **B,** A similar image from another patient shows the femoral head displaced proximally out of a shallow acetabulum. (Images courtesy of Richard Bella, MD.)

associated with myelomeningocele, arthrogryposis, or marked ligamentous laxity.

Problems associated with the Pavlik harness include avascular necrosis (AVN) (due to excessive hip flexion and abduction) and failure of hip reduction. In addition, worsening of acetabular dysplasia can occur if the unreduced femoral head is held against the posterior wall of the developing acetabulum. An inferior dislocation of hip may be due to overzealous tightening of the Pavlik harness with excessive hip flexion. Femoral nerve palsy from compression of the nerve may result. Brachial plexus palsy can also occur when the harness is applied improperly. Skin maceration may also result when any immobilization device is not kept clean and dry at all times.

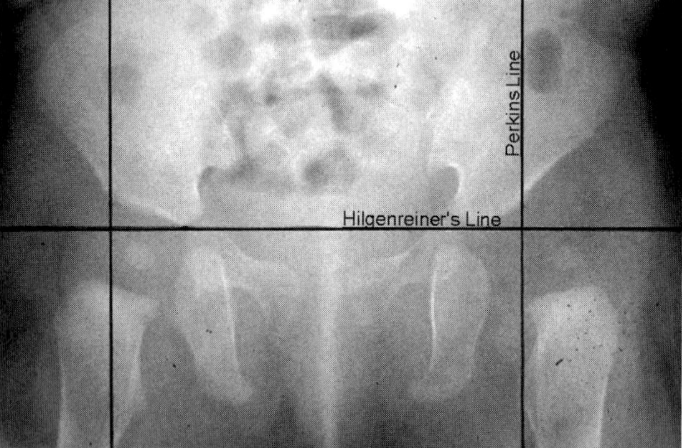

Figure 7-14 On an anteroposterior radiograph of the hips, a Hilgenreiner line is drawn horizontally through the triradiate cartilage of the acetabulum. A Perkins line is perpendicular to this, crossing the lateral edge of the acetabulum. In this 6-month-old child, the ossific nucleus of the left hip is not in the proper lower medial quadrant but, instead, in the lower lateral quadrant.

Success rates for treatment with a Pavlik harness are approximately 98% for children with hip dysplasia or subluxation and approximately 85% for children with complete hip dislocation.

Closed Reduction and Spica Casting

If Pavlik harness treatment fails, the child can be taken to the operating room for an examination under anesthesia (EUA), an attempt at closed reduction, and an arthrogram. An arthrogram of the affected hip is used for visual confirmation of hip reduction (Fig. 7-17A and B). The patient is positioned under a fluoroscopic machine, and a radiopaque dye is injected into the hip joint. The dye helps outline the cartilaginous (and therefore radiolucent) femoral head as well as the cartilaginous border of the developing acetabulum. An adductor tenotomy may be needed to allow adequate hip abduction to reduce the femoral head.

Once the femoral head is reduced, the patient is immobilized in a spica cast (Fig. 7-18A and B) in the "safe position" (between full abduction and the position at which the head dislocates in adduction) (Fig. 7-19). A postreduction radiograph and computed tomography (CT) scan are used to assess the adequacy of the reduction. The spica cast treatment is continued for up to 6 months. Because the child will grow substantially during this period, cast changes are usually made every 6 weeks. Each cast change is performed with the patient under general anesthesia and in the operating room, where the reduction of the hip can be monitored each time with an arthrogram.

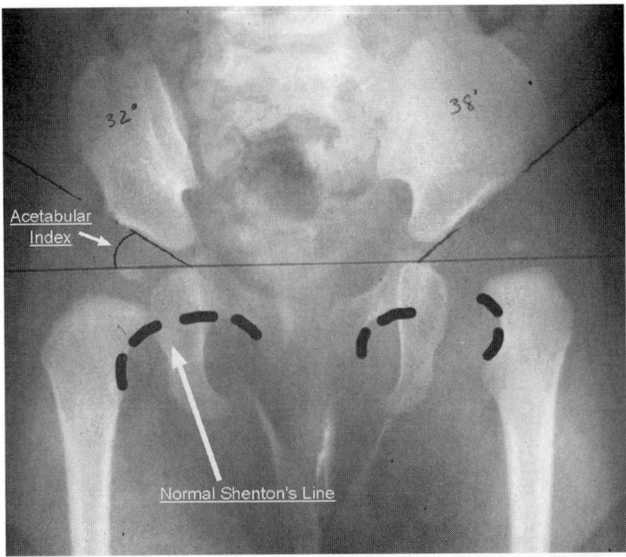

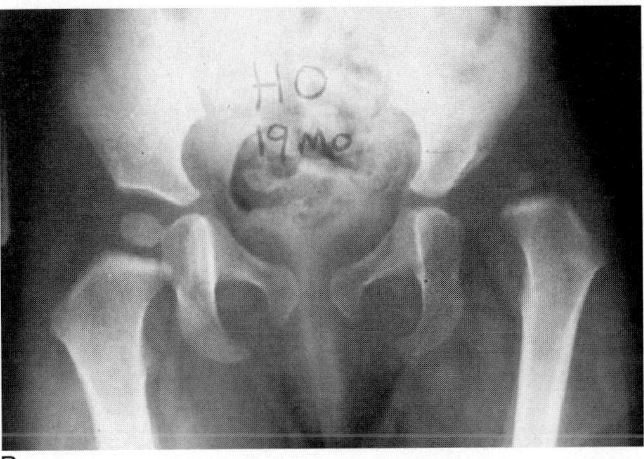

Figure 7-15 A Shenton line is a curved line drawn along the inferior border of the superior pubic ramus to the medial border of the femoral neck on an anteroposterior radiograph. A, Note the smooth continuous contour on the normal right hip. The Shenton line on the dysplastic left hip is described as "broken." The acetabular index measures the slope of the ossified acetabular roof. The acetabular index on the normal right hip is 32 degrees. The dysplastic left hip has a larger index. **B,** In an older patient, the diagnosis of a left hip dislocation can be made more easily.

Abduction Bracing

Once the patient is found to have a stable, well-reduced hip, the spica cast treatment is discontinued. An abduction brace can be applied to help keep the hip in a stable position (Fig. 7-20).

Operative Management

Failure of closed reduction and immobilization necessitates an open reduction with postreduction spica cast immobilization. An important step of the operation is removal of the ligamentum teres and the fibrofatty pulvinar, with division of the transverse acetabular ligament and the iliopsoas tendon to allow the femoral head to seat deeply into the dysplastic shallow acetabulum. The surgeon may need to perform a shortening varus femoral osteotomy to facilitate reduction of the femoral head into the acetabulum. If the acetabular coverage is inadequate, a pelvic realignment procedure may be needed to help keep the femoral head reduced. A postreduction radiograph and CT scan are performed to confirm the reduction of the femoral head. The spica cast treatment is subsequently continued for several months.

Indications for Referral to the Orthopaedic Surgeon

An infant in whom physical findings are suspicious for DDH and imaging findings are consistent with hip dysplasia should be referred to an orthopaedic surgeon. The patient should be evaluated with an ultrasound if younger than 4 to 6 months, and with radiography if older than 4 to 6 months.

Developmental Dysplasia of the Hip after Walking Age

Clinical Presentation

The ambulatory child with a previously undetected dysplastic or dislocated hip often presents to the physician after the family has noticed a limp, a waddling gait, or a leg length discrepancy.

Physical Findings

The most reliable physical finding for DDH in the walking child is limited hip abduction. Subluxation or dislocation of the hip leads to a high-riding femoral head with respect to the acetabulum. This causes shortening of the adductor muscles, which in turn limits abduction. The Ortolani and Barlow tests are usually not helpful in a child of walking age. A patient with a unilateral dislocation demonstrates the Galeazzi sign and telescoping of the affected extremity. Asymmetric skin folds may be present for the same reason.

The patient is likely to have a painless Trendelenburg sign and a Trendelenburg gait. A Trendelenburg sign results from functionally weakened hip abductor muscles; it is commonly seen in the child with a dislocated hip. With a dislocated hip, the abductor muscles are at a mechanical disadvantage and are effectively weakened because the proximal femoral insertions of the abductor muscles are relatively close to the muscles' origins on the ilium. The muscles, therefore, do not have adequate tension to exert maximum force. These muscles are unable to properly support the child's body weight when the contralateral foot is off the floor. As a result, the pelvis tilts away from the affected hip. Thus, when a child with

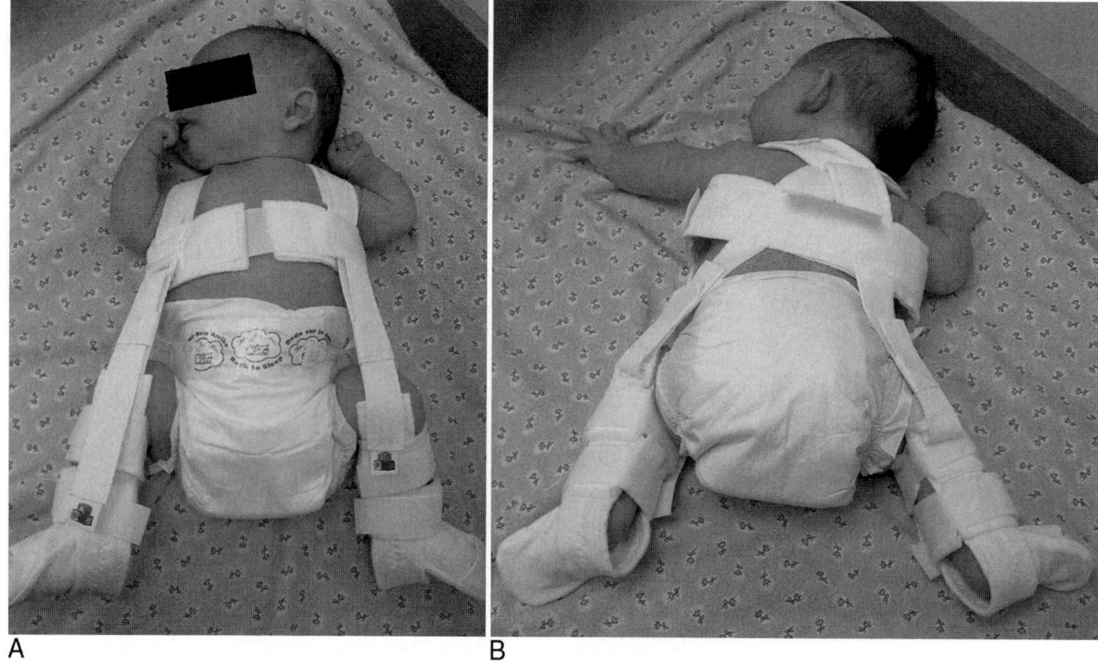

Figure 7-16 **A** and **B**, The Pavlik harness is applied to keep the hips flexed and abducted. Diaper changes can be performed without the removal of the device. Care must be taken to set the lengths of the straps properly and to check them regularly. Note that the child is free to move the hips and knees within the harness.

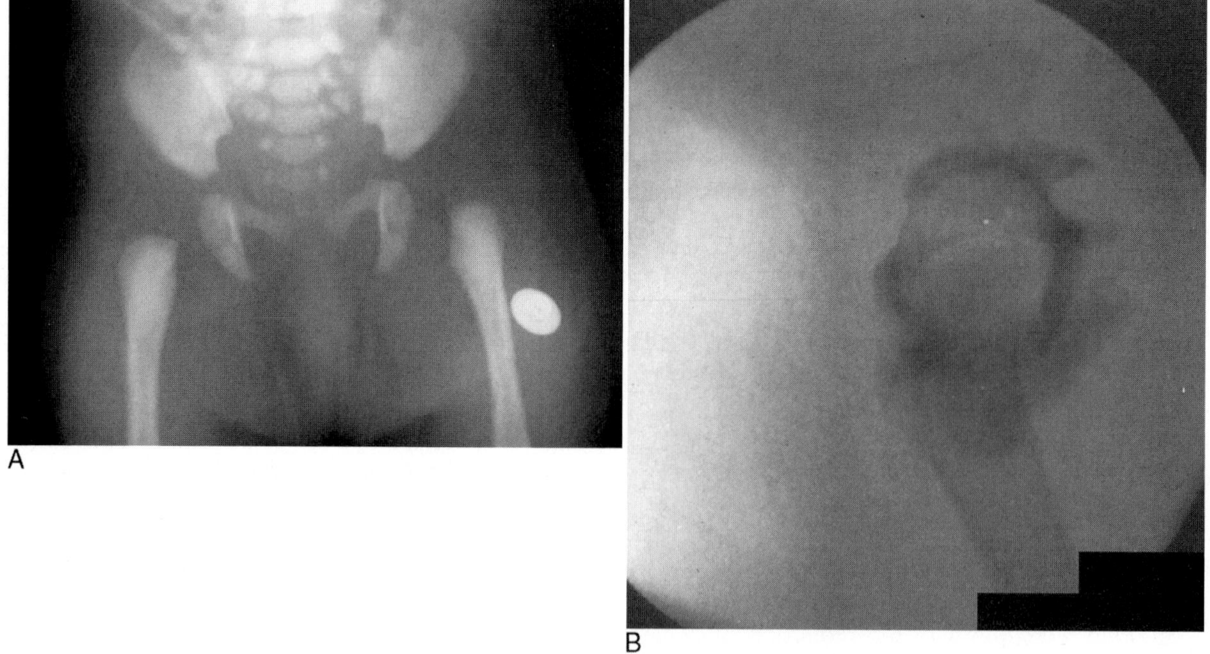

Figure 7-17 **A**, When the femoral heads have not yet ossified, they are not visible on plain radiographs. (Photograph courtesy of Dennis Roy, MD.) **B**, Injecting radiopaque dye into the hip joint (arthrogram) allows the cartilaginous head to be well visualized.

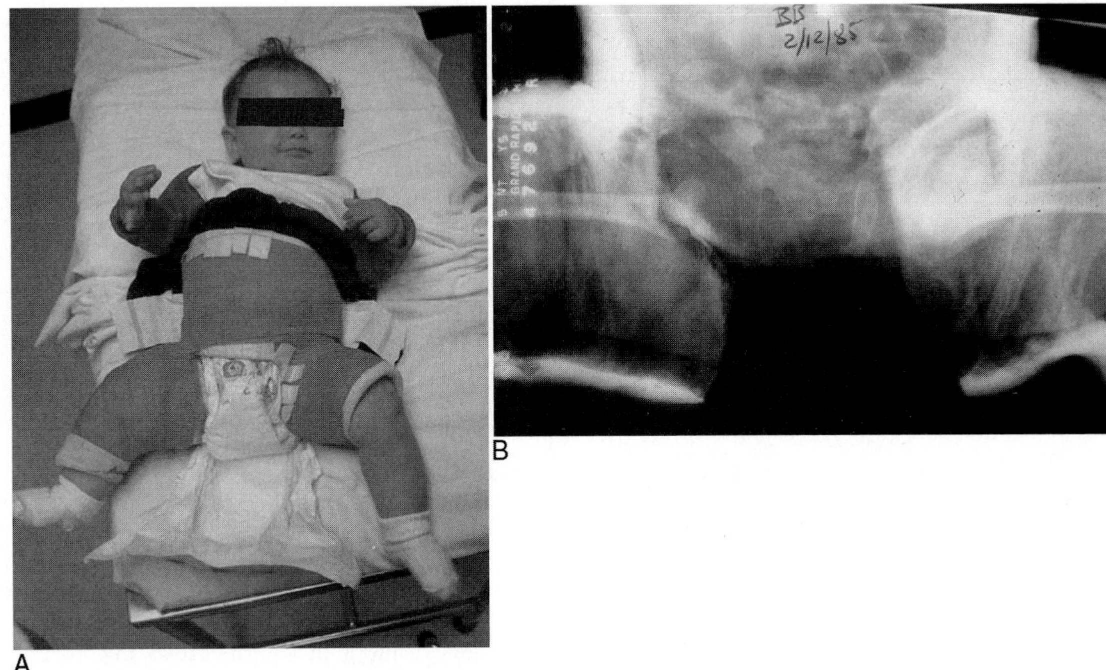

Figure 7-18 **A,** A spica cast is applied in the operating room after an examination under anesthesia, an arthrogram, an adductor longus tenotomy, and a closed reduction. **B,** After closed reduction and application of the cast, a postreduction radiograph is taken.

a right hip dislocation stands on the right foot, the left hip drops to a lower level.

The gait cycle consists of the stance phase and the swing phase. A child with a dislocated hip walks with a Trendelenburg gait because the hip abductors are unable to keep the pelvis level when the affected limb is in the stance phase of the gait cycle and the contralateral limb is in the swing phase. To avoid falling in the direction of the contralateral limb, the child compensates by leaning over the affected hip (the "abductor lurch"). For example, a child with a right hip dislocation will tilt his or her torso over the right hip when the left foot leaves the ground, leading to the characteristic "abductor lurch" of the Trendelenburg gait.

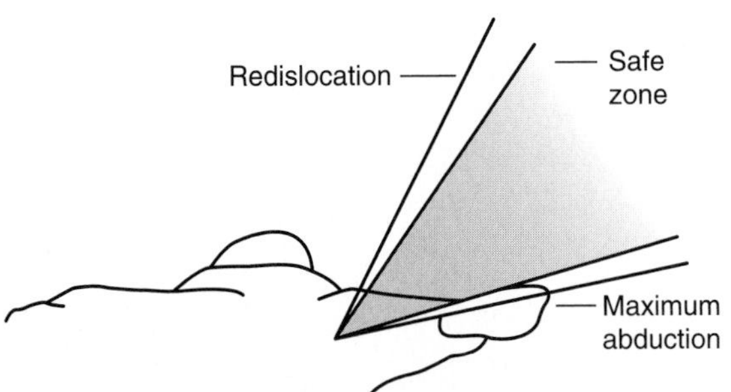

Figure 7-19 **The safe zone of Ramsey.** (From Ramsey PL, Lasser S, MacEwen GD: Congenital dislocation of the hip: Use of the Pavlik harness in the child during the first six months of life. J Bone Joint Surg Am 58:1000-1004, 1976).

The walking child with bilateral dislocations may be more difficult to recognize (Fig. 7-21). Such a child has a wide perineum and a waddling gait, lurching in both directions. Flexion contracture of the hips leads to a characteristic swayback (hyperlordosis of the lumbar spine) deformity.

Imaging Studies

Radiographs

AP and frog-leg lateral views of both hips are required. The lines used for the evaluation of infants are applicable

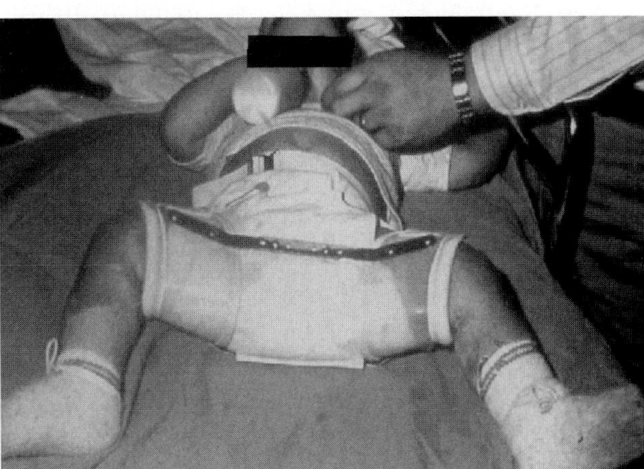

Figure 7-20 **Abduction bracing.** Once the spica cast is removed, the patient can be placed in an abduction brace to keep the hip in a stable position. (Photograph courtesy of Dennis Roy, MD.)

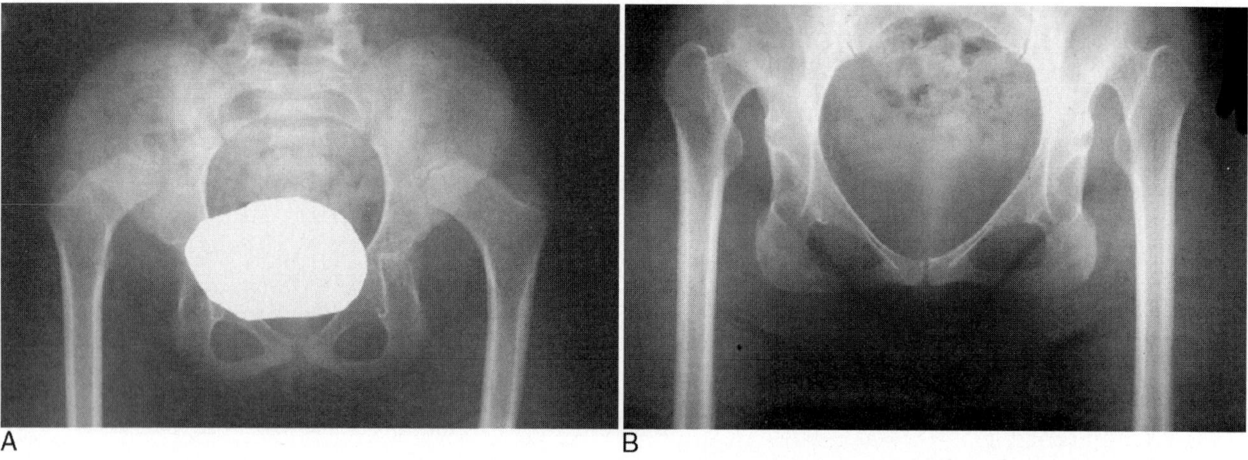

Figure 7-21 Plain radiographs of a young child **(A)** and an older child **(B)** with complete bilateral hip dislocations.

for use on an AP view in a walking child. A false profile view can show the amount of anterior coverage of the femoral head.

Computed Tomography

CT scans are not typically used in the diagnosis of hip dysplasia. However, axial CT scans are useful in confirming the concentric reduction of a hip after a closed or open reduction. A CT scan is routinely ordered for a child who has undergone an open reduction of a dislocated hip and application of a spica cast. A CT scan also may be helpful for planning reconstructive pelvic osteotomies (Fig. 7-22).

Magnetic Resonance Imaging

Magnetic resonance imaging (MRI) can also be used to confirm the concentric reduction of a hip after a closed or open reduction.

Management

The goals of management are (1) to obtain an atraumatic concentric reduction of the femoral head, (2) to maintain the reduction, providing an optimum environment for femoral and acetabular development, and (3) to avoid AVN. In addition, care must be taken to avoid the development of osteonecrosis due to extreme hip abduction.

Delay in diagnosis makes achieving these treatment goals more difficult, because an older child has less potential for acetabular and femoral remodeling (Fig. 7-23). The older the child is at the time of diagnosis, the more complex treatment becomes. The management of older children with DDH is more likely to be complicated by osteonecrosis of the femoral head.

Closed Reduction

In patients 6 to 12 months old, a 2- to 3-week course of traction may help bring the dislocated femoral head closer to the acetabulum. Although the efficacy of traction is debatable, it continues to be used in many centers.

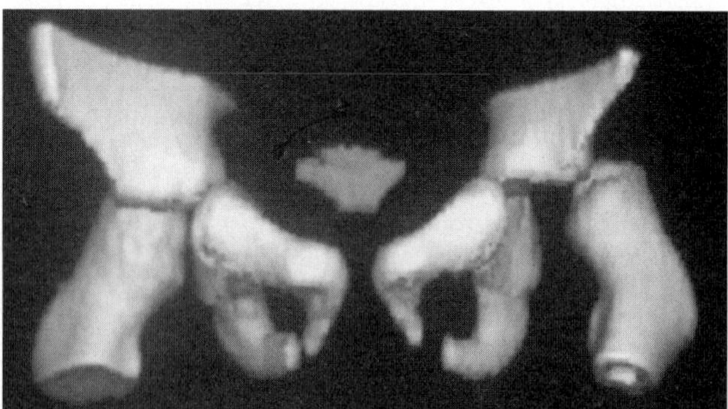

Figure 7-22 A three-dimensional computed tomography scan can be helpful for planning pelvic reconstruction or for confirming reduction of a dislocated hip after surgery or closed reduction.

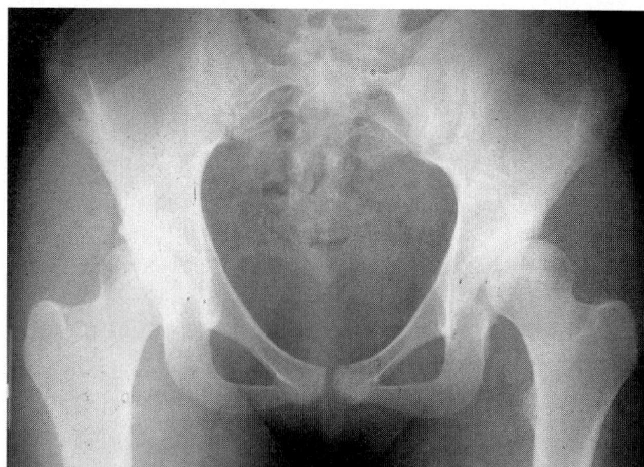

Figure 7-23 Anteroposterior (AP) plain radiograph of an older child showing subluxation and dysplasia of the left hip and mild dysplasia of the right hip.

A closed reduction can be performed under general anesthesia in the operating room with the aid of fluoroscopy. An arthrogram can help determine the reducibility of the hip by outlining the contours of the developing acetabulum and the femoral head. An adductor tenotomy—which involves releasing the tendons of the abnormally tight adductor muscles—can improve the success rate of closed reduction by allowing for greater hip abduction. Once a satisfactory reduction is achieved, the patient is immobilized in a spica cast.[18]

Open Reduction

Once the child is older than 12 months, the success rate for closed reduction of a dislocated hip begins to decline. Children older than 2 years almost always require surgical reduction because, by this age, the tightened hip capsule and the shortened hip musculature prevent a closed reduction.

Open reduction of the hip involves removing any structures blocking a concentric reduction of the femoral head into the dysplastic acetabulum. The "loose" redundant hip capsule can also be "tightened" to help secure a reduction (i.e., capsulorrhaphy). Femoral or pelvic osteotomies may be necessary to effectively realign the previously dislocated or dysplastic hip. Reduction can be confirmed using an arthrogram, and the patient should be immobilized in a spica cast. The duration of immobilization varies according to the underlying disease, age of the patient, and type of operation.[5]

Indications for Referral to the Orthopaedic Surgeon

An ambulatory child with a painless limp and a leg length discrepancy is likely to have undetected DDH and should be referred for further orthopaedic evaluation after radiographs have been obtained.

LEGG-CALVÉ-PERTHES DISEASE

Definition

Legg-Calvé-Perthes Disease (LCPD) is a disorder of the femoral head of unclear etiology. It involves temporary interruption of the blood supply to the bony nucleus of the proximal femoral epiphysis that leads to impairment of epiphyseal growth and an increase in bone density. The dense bone is subsequently replaced by new bone, resulting in a flattened and enlarged femoral head. Once new bone is in place, the femoral head slowly remodels until skeletal maturity.[19,20]

Epidemiology

LCPD generally affects children 4 to 12 years old. Boys are more commonly affected than girls by a ratio of 4 or 5 to 1. The incidence of bilaterality is 10% to 12%. There is no clear evidence that LCPD is an inherited disorder.

Etiology

The etiology of LCPD is not completely understood. LCPD may be an avascular phenomenon of the femoral head, although it is different from the osteonecrosis of the femoral head that develops after a femoral neck fracture or the systemic administration of corticosteroids. Another proposed etiology is an endocrine-related[21] or trauma-induced loss of interosseous or extraosseous blood supply. It has also been suggested that LCPD may be a local manifestation of a systemic epiphyseal disease.

Factors related to the development of LCPD are (1) coagulation abnormalities involving proteins C and S,[22,23] (2) arterial compromise of the femoral head, (3) abnormal venous drainage of the femoral head and neck,[24] (4) abnormal growth and development, and (5) trauma, particularly in the predisposed child. Other associated factors are hyperactivity or attention deficit disorder,[25] hereditary influences,[26] and environmental influences (including nutrition). One "unifying" hypothesis for the etiology of LCPD suggests that lack of thrombolysis in the venous drainage of the femoral neck increases pressure in the femoral head circulation, resulting in osteonecrosis. Antecedent trauma might precipitate this event in the highly active predisposed child.[19]

Natural History

The course of LCPD varies considerably from patient to patient. The age of the child at the onset of disease is the most important factor affecting its course. The younger child has a milder course and a better outcome. In addition, a child with a shorter course of disease has a more favorable outcome.

The clinical course of LCPD can be broken down into four pathologic phases: (1) the incipient, or synovitis, phase, (2) the osteonecrosis phase, (3) the fragmentation phase, and (4) regeneration and revascularization (healing) phase.

The incipient, or synovitis, phase of LCPD lasts 1 to 3 weeks. It is characterized by reduced movement due to increased hip joint fluid and a swollen synovium. The hip radiographs are typically normal.

During the osteonecrosis phase of LCPD, which lasts 6 months to 1 year, the blood supply is interrupted to part or all of the femoral head. The ischemic portion of the bone dies, but the contour of the femoral head remains unchanged.

The fragmentation phase typically lasts less than 1 year but can last up to 3 years. During this period, limping and pain are more pronounced, and a greater degree of motion is lost.

The regeneration and revascularization phase is the last and longest pathologic phase of LCPD, lasting 1 to 3 years. The blood supply returns, causing both resorption of necrotic bone and laying down of new immature bone. Permanent hip deformity can occur in this phase.[10,19]

Prognosis

The main favorable prognostic factors for LCPD are young age of the child (<6 years), less than 50% epiphyseal involvement,[27] and short duration of disease.

Children who experience signs and symptoms of LCPD before they are 5 years old tend to recover without residual problems. Patients older than 9 years at presentation usually have a poor prognosis. The reason for this difference is not clear. Because the femoral head in a younger child is mostly cartilage, ischemic destruction and subsequent collapse of the bony portion of the femoral head probably do not destroy the entire structure. The femoral head of an older child, however, would have a more global collapse because it is mostly bone. The collapsed femoral head of the older child is less likely to be reconstituted to its original shape.

Additional factors associated with poor prognosis are greater epiphyseal involvement, persistent loss of range of motion, premature physeal closure, lateral subluxation or extrusion of the femoral head, and longer duration of disease.

Clinical Presentation

Children with LCPD usually present with a limp accompanied by hip pain or pain referred to the thigh or knee. The limp and the pain are reported to be exacerbated by strenuous activities and are worse at the end of the day. The child may occasionally have night pain. The time course for the pain is characterized by periods of exacerbation and alleviation. The patient or caregiver may also recall a traumatic event preceding the limp or hip pain.

The classic portrait of a child with LCPD is that of a small, thin, extremely active child who is always running and jumping. The typical patient with LCPD also limps after strenuous physical activities.[19]

Physical Findings

The child with LCPD who presents with knee pain experiences exacerbation of pain on isolated range-of-motion assessment of the ipsilateral hip. Isolated palpation and manipulation of the knee usually do not cause discomfort.

In the early phase of LCPD, muscle spasm may be the cause of restriction in motion. Gentle examination may elicit greater range of motion. As the disease progresses, the range of motion of the affected hip becomes progressively limited, particularly in abduction and medial rotation. Hip adduction or flexion contractures may even develop.

The LCPD limp is a combination of the antalgic gait, the Trendelenburg gait, and the Trendelenburg sign. In an attempt to decrease the pressure within the hip joint, the child leans over the affected hip, thereby decreasing the force of the abductor muscles. An antalgic gait may be particularly prominent after strenuous activity at the end of the day.

Shortening of the affected extremity can occur in LCPD if the patient has a significant femoral head deformity.

Imaging Studies

AP and frog-leg lateral views of both hips are necessary for the evaluation of suspected LCPD. LCPD has been divided into the following radiographic stages: (1) initial (osteonecrosis), (2) fragmentation, (3) reossification, and (4) residual (Table 7-1).[19]

Table 7-1 Radiographic Stages of Legg-Calvé-Perthes Disease

Stage	Findings
Initial (osteonecrosis)	Early signs: lateralization of the femoral head and smaller ossific nucleus Later signs: subchondral fracture, increased density of the femoral head, and metaphyseal lucencies
Fragmentation	Lucent areas appear in the femoral head Segments of femoral head are demarcated Increased density resolves Acetabular contour is more irregular
Reossification (healing)	New bone formation occurs in the femoral head Lucencies are replaced by new (woven) bone
Residual	Femoral head is fully reossified; gradual remodeling of head shape occurs until skeletal maturity; the acetabulum also remodels.

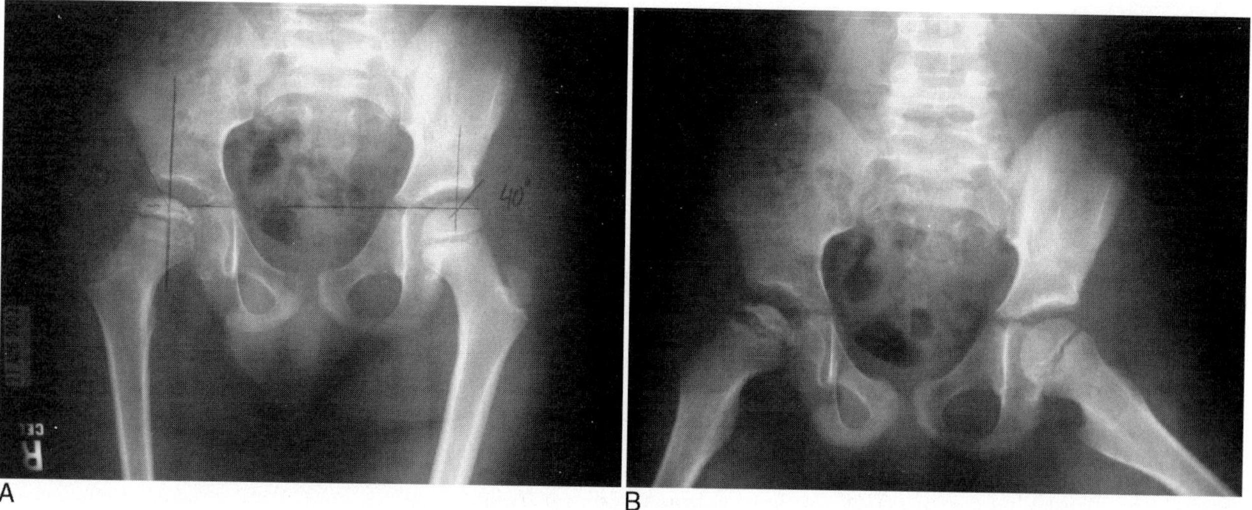

Figure 7-24 Anteroposterior **(A)** and frog-leg **(B)** radiographs of a child with Legg-Calvé-Perthes disease of the right hip in the osteonecrosis phase.

Early signs of the initial stage are lateralization of the femoral head and smaller ossific nucleus. Later findings include subchondral fracture, increased density of the femoral head, and metaphyseal lucencies (Fig. 7-24).[28]

In the fragmentation stage (Fig. 7-25), lucent areas appear in the femoral head, segments of the femoral head demarcate, increased density resolves, and the acetabular contour becomes more irregular.

During the reossification (healing) stage, new bone formation occurs in the femoral head and lucencies are replaced by new (woven) bone.

The residual stage is marked by the reossification of the femoral head, gradual remodeling of head shape until skeletal maturity, and remodeling of the acetabulum (Fig. 7-26).

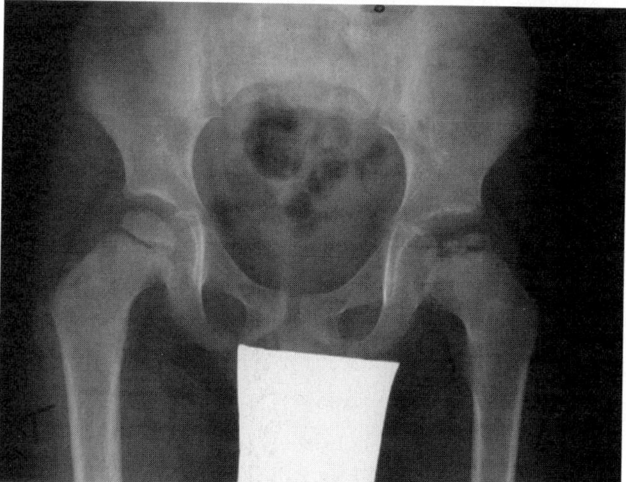

Figure 7-25 Radiograph shows the epiphyseal fragmentation characteristic of Legg-Calvé-Perthes disease in the left hip.

It is important to note that radiographic findings in LCPD may lag behind the progression of the disorder by as much as 3 to 6 months. Radionucleotide bone scans may be better for following the course of LCPD. Early ischemia and AVN are visualized as decreased localizations of isotope on bone scans.

The lateral pillar classification system for Legg-Calvé-Perthes disease evaluates the shape of the femoral head epiphysis on the AP radiograph (Fig. 7-27). The head is divided into three sections, or pillars. The lateral pillar occupies the lateral 15% to 30% of the head width, the central pillar about 50% of the head width, and the medial pillar 20% to 35% of the head width. The extent of involvement of the lateral pillar can be subdivided into three groups. In group A, the lateral pillar is radiographically normal. In group B, the lateral pillar has some lucency but more than 50% of the lateral pillar height is maintained. In group C, the lateral pillar is more lucent than in group B, and less than 50% of the pillar height remains. This classification has been found to be easy to apply during the active stage of the disease and can predict the amount of flattening of the femoral head at skeletal maturity. When combined with age of onset, it can be used to predict the natural history of the disease. In one study employing this system, children whose hips classified as group A all had spherical femoral heads at skeletal maturity. Outcomes for children with group B hips were better for those younger than 9 years at the onset of disease. In group C, the majority of femoral heads became aspherical at skeletal maturity.[29]

Management

The goal of treatment of LCPD is to promote a spherical, well-covered femoral head with hip range of motion

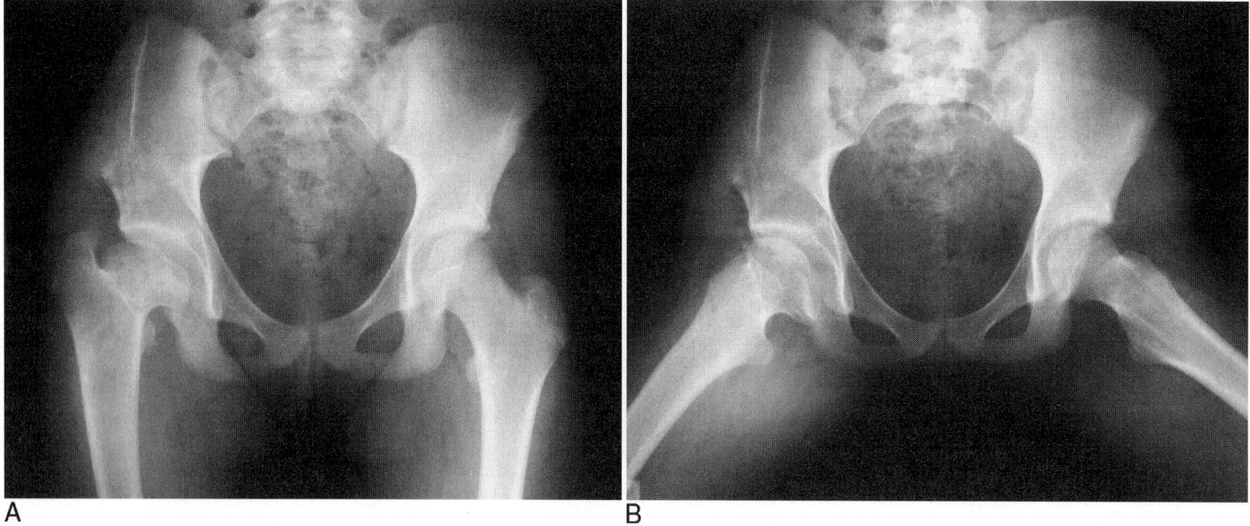

Figure 7-26 Anteroposterior **(A)** and frog-leg **(B)** radiographs showing long-term follow-up of a 12-year-old girl with Legg-Calvé-Perthes disease of the right hip, 5 years after an acetabular realignment operation. Though the right hip is deformed, the patient is active and asymptomatic.

that is normal or close to normal. The two main principles of LCPD treatment are (1) maintenance of range of motion and (2) acetabular containment of the femoral head during the active period of the process.

Nonoperative Management

The two primary means of treating pain related to LCPD are bed rest and traction. A traction apparatus can be set up in the home. Nonsteroidal anti-inflammatory drugs (NSAIDs) and crutches (to reduce weight-bearing) may also be helpful in minimizing pain. Once the patient is comfortable, physical therapy, with an emphasis on maintaining range of motion, is a crucial element of LCPD management.

Abduction devices, such as the Petrie cast (Fig. 7-28) and hip abduction orthoses, have been used to keep the femoral epiphysis contained in the acetabulum. These devices may be used while the patient is either bearing weight on the affected limb or restricted from weight-bearing. It should be noted, however, that weight-bearing abduction orthoses are not effective in changing the natural history of severely involved hips.[30,31]

An alternative nonoperative treatment option reserved for milder cases is restriction of activity without the use of braces or casts. The clinician monitors the patient regularly and watches for signs of contracture or subluxation.

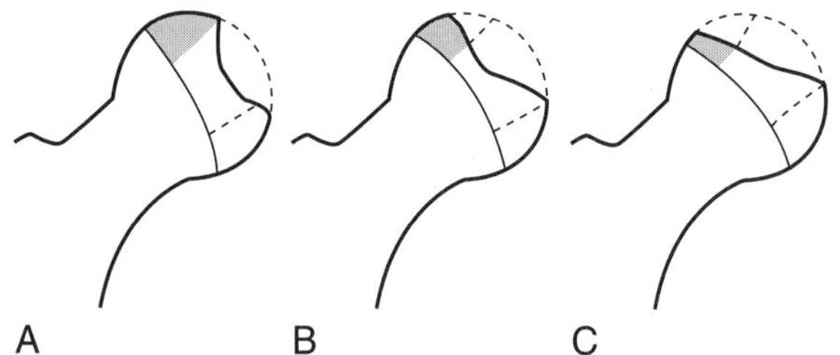

Figure 7-27 Lateral pillar classification for Legg-Calvé-Perthes disease. A, In group A, there is no involvement of the lateral pillar. **B,** In group B, more than 50% of the lateral pillar height is maintained. **C,** In group C, less than 50% of the lateral pillar height is maintained. (From Herring JA, Neustadt JB, Williams JJ, et al: The lateral pillar classification of Legg-Calvé-Perthes disease. J Pediatr Orthop 12:143-150, 1992.)

Operative Management

The goals of surgical treatment are no different from those of conservative management (i.e., maintaining range of motion and achieving containment of the femoral head). An adductor tenotomy, sometimes supplemented by a medial capsular release, allows the hip to be sufficiently abducted and the femoral head to be reduced into the acetabulum. In addition, an osteotomy of the proximal femur can be performed to position the femoral head deeper into the acetabulum while maintaining the limb in a weight-bearing position. Another alternative is a pelvic osteotomy to rotate the acetabulum into a better position to contain the femoral head.[32-34]

Differential Diagnosis

The differential diagnosis of LCPD includes conditions that can produce osteonecrosis, such as hemoglobinopathies, leukemia, lymphoma, idiopathic thrombocytopenic purpura, and hemophilia. Radiographic

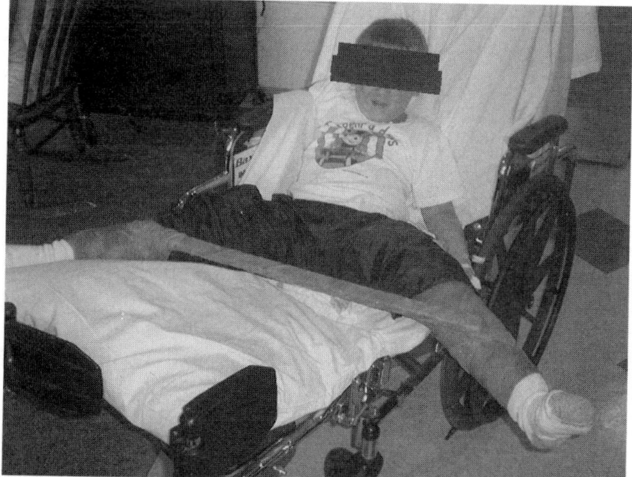
A

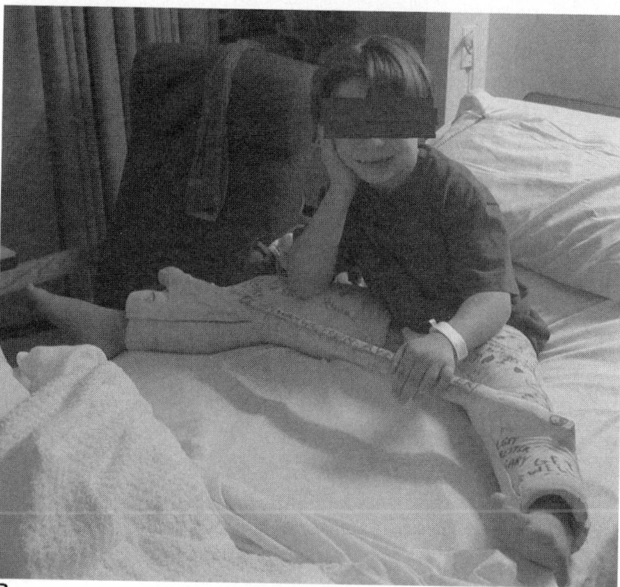
B

Figure 7-28 **A** and **B,** A Petrie cast consists of two cylinder casts connected by an abduction bar to maintain hip abduction. After the initial phase of treatment, the cylinder casts can be bivalved (split longitudinally) to serve as removable braces that the patient wears only while in bed.

findings in the hips in hypothyroidism are similar to those in LCPD, but patients with hypothyroidism have bilateral hip involvement. A strong family history of hip abnormalities suggests the presence of an epiphyseal dysplastic condition.

Indications for Referral to the Orthopaedic Surgeon

After other conditions that mimic LCPD are ruled out, any child with suspected Legg-Calvé-Perthes disease should be referred to an orthopaedic surgeon.

SLIPPED CAPITAL FEMORAL EPIPHYSIS

Definition

Slipped capital femoral epiphysis is a well-known hip disorder that affects adolescents, most often between ages 12 and 15. It involves displacement of the capital femoral epiphysis from the metaphysis through the zone of the hypertrophy layer of the physeal plate. The term *slipped capital femoral epiphysis* is actually a misnomer, because the femoral head is held in the acetabulum by the ligamentum teres; thus, it is actually the femoral neck that comes upward and outward while the head remains in the acetabulum.

Classification

The clinical classification for SCFE depends on the patient's ability to walk. SCFE is considered "stable" if the child is able to walk with or without crutches. A child with "unstable" SCFE is unable to walk, with or without crutches. This classification is helpful in predicting prognosis. Patients with unstable SCFE have a much higher prevalence of osteonecrosis (up to 50%) than those with stable SCFEs (nearly 0%).[58] This difference is most likely due to the vascular injury caused at the time of initial displacement. A "cold" bone scan (demonstrating an absence of vascularity) is seen only in unstable cases; in such cases, the risk of subsequent development of osteonecrosis is 80% to 100%.[35]

The imaging classification depends on the presence or absence of a hip effusion on ultrasonograph. An ultrasound study demonstrating the absence of metaphyseal remodeling and the presence of an effusion is consistent with an acute event, the inability to walk, and an unstable SCFE. Metaphyseal remodeling and the absence of an effusion are ultrasonographic findings consistent with the ability to walk and therefore with stable SCFE.

Epidemiology

The annual incidence of SCFE has been reported to average 2 per 100,000 in the general population. Globally, incidence has ranged from 0.2 per 100,000 in eastern Japan to 10.08 per 100,000 in the northeastern United States.[41] African-American and Polynesian populations have been reported to have higher incidences of SCFE.

Obesity is the most closely associated factor in the development of SCFE. In close to two thirds of the patients, the body weight is above the 90th percentile in weight-for-age profiles. Furthermore, obese children tend to present with this condition at an earlier age. Obesity, rather than race or geography, may be the underlying factor predisposing certain populations to the development of SCFE.[42]

SCFE is related to puberty; close to 80% of cases of SCFE occur during the adolescent growth spurt. Age at presentation is generally between 10 and 16 years for boys, and between 9 and 15 years for girls. SCFE has a male predilection at a rate of 1.43:1. The left hip is more often affected in unilateral cases.[42]

Etiology

Although certain endocrinologic disorders have been linked to SCFE, the etiology is unknown in the vast majority of cases. For idiopathic SCFE, a combination of factors, both biomechanical and biochemical, result in a weakened physis that subsequently fails.

Children with SCFE are anatomically predisposed to failure of the growth plates at the proximal femur. Obese children often have retroverted femoral necks that are directed more posteriorly than those of other children.[36] The proximal femoral physis is also more vertical in heavy children. Furthermore, the acetabula of obese children are deeper and have a more secure relationship with the capital femoral epiphyses. These anatomic features of the proximal femur and acetabulum, coupled with the excessive weight of these children, result in greater sheer stresses across this growth plate, culminating in "slipped" femoral epiphysis.[37]

SCFE is a disease of puberty and, thus, hormonal and endocrinologic changes. During puberty, growth hormone increases the physiologic activity of the physis, leading to rapid longitudinal growth of the physis and a widened and weakened proximal femoral growth plate. The higher prevalence of SCFE in children who are receiving growth hormone supplementation and who have hypothyroidism,[38-40] hyperthyroidism, hypogonadism, hypopituitarism, or renal osteodystrophy also suggests an association between this disorder and an endocrine derangement. Although most children with SCFE do not have a demonstrable endocrine disorder, some experts theorize that a subtle endocrinopathy may be present.[41]

The effect of gonadotropins may explain the male preponderance of SCFE. Estrogen reduces physeal width and increases physeal strength, whereas testosterone reduces physeal strength.

Natural History

The natural history of SCFE without treatment is difficult to ascertain. The two main concerns are (1) progression of the slip and (2) the development of degenerative joint disease. One Swedish study reported that few untreated patients with SCFE experienced restrictions in work capacity or social life as a result of the disease after 20 to 60 years of follow-up.[43] In contrast, an American study found that close to one third of patients required surgery after sustaining an acute episode superimposed on a chronic SCFE.[44] Overall, some mild cases of SCFE stabilize on their own. However most patients with SCFE, especially those with unstable conditions, experience progression.

The risk of osteoarthritis in patients with untreated SCFE depends on the severity of the displacement.[45] Patients with greater displacement have a higher likelihood of osteoarthritis. Those with mild or moderate slips have positive clinical outcomes because the congruity of the femoral head with the acetabulum is maintained. Patients with an untreated, unstable SCFE may experience limitations in hip range of motion due to residual deformity of the proximal femur. Whether subclinical forms of SCFE lead to early osteoarthritis is debatable.[43]

Long-term studies of the available treatment options have shown that patients with SCFE who underwent in situ screw fixation had the best results, regardless of the severity of the slip. In situ screw fixation is associated with the best long-term function, the lowest risk of complications, and the most effective delay of degenerative arthritis.[46]

Clinical Presentation

A high level of clinical suspicion for SCFE is warranted; prompt treatment makes a significant difference in the child's prognosis.

The child with SCFE often complains of knee or distal thigh pain. Because hip pain may be referred to the knee via the obturator and femoral nerves, distinguishing true knee pain from referred pain is critical in identifying a patient with SCFE. The clinician who performs an isolated examination of the knee can miss the diagnosis of SCFE.

Eliciting information about timing of the appearance of a limp and the onset of hip, thigh, or knee pain can often be challenging. In SCFE, pain may be acute or chronic. One child may be able to state the exact moment the pain began, but another may present with intermittent or constant, hip, thigh, or knee pain that has lasted weeks to months.

Although traumatic injuries can be associated with SCFE, the vast majority of patients with the disease have a long-standing problem with no acute change in the level of pain or the quality of the limp. In about 10% of cases, an acute slip occurs during a seemingly harmless activity. An acute exacerbation of chronic SCFE can also occur.

Assessing whether the child with SCFE can walk is crucial to understanding the prognosis. A child who is unable to walk has an unstable SCFE and a greater risk of osteonecrosis. The child who is able to walk has a stable SCFE and a more favorable prognosis.

The physician must look for problems with both hips, because 25% of patients with SCFE have bilateral involvement. Half of those with bilateral SCFE (one eighth of all patients with SCFE) present with symptoms on both sides; and a substantial number of the remaining patients have symptoms within 18 months. Younger patients are particularly at risk for development of a slip on the contralateral hip because more time will elapse before closure of their proximal femoral physes.[47,48]

A careful physical examination and review of systems are necessary to identify any concomitant endocrine abnormalities (Table 7-2). Systemic conditions associated with SCFE include hypothyroidism, panhypopituitarism, hypogonadism, rickets, and exposure to radiation.[49]

Physical Findings

The classic patient with SCFE is an obese African-American boy with delayed skeletal and sexual maturity who walks with a waddling gait and a laterally rotated leg (Fig. 7-29). Patients with unstable SCFE are unable to walk.

In the patient with SCFE, hip flexion often causes obligatory lateral rotation of the thigh with associated pain (Fig. 7-30). Isolated motion of the knee should not cause discomfort in SCFE. Medial rotation of the affected thigh is limited or absent. A hip flexion contracture may be present.

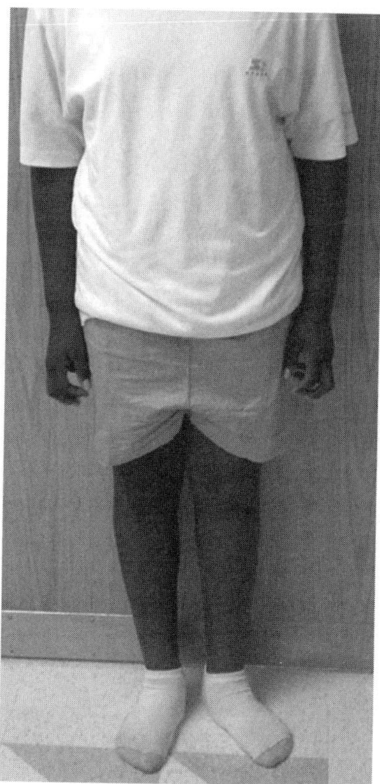

Figure 7-29 This 13-year-old boy with slipped capital femoral epiphysis has the typical body habitus. Note the lateral rotation of the affected left lower extremity.

Imaging Studies

AP and frog-leg lateral radiographs of both hips are the imaging studies most commonly ordered for patients in whom SCFE is suspected. The AP view usually demonstrates widening and irregularity of the physis. A crescent-shaped area of increased density can frequently be identified in the proximal portion of the femoral neck. This "metaphyseal blanch sign" corresponds to the double density created from the anteriorly displaced femoral neck overlying the femoral head.[50] In an unaffected patient, the *Klein line*—drawn through the superior cortex of the femoral neck—intersects the epiphysis.[42] In a patient with SCFE, the Klein line no longer intersects the epiphysis because the femoral neck has moved proximally and anteriorly relative to the epiphysis (Fig. 7-31A).

The frog-leg lateral view usually demonstrates the posterior displacement and stepoff of the epiphysis on the femoral neck (see Fig. 7-31B). The analogy of an ice cream scoop falling off the cone is often used to describe this disorder to patients and their caregivers.

Table 7-2 Systemic Abnormalities Associated with Slipped Capital Femoral Epiphysis

Hypothyroidism	Panhypopituitarism
Hyperthyroidism	Rickets/renal osteodystrophy
Hypogonadism	Radiation exposure

Data from Loder RT, Hensinger RN, Alburger PD, et al: Slipped capital femoral epiphysis associated with radiation therapy. J Pediatr Orthop 18:630-636, 1998.

Management

Nonoperative Management

Nonoperative treatment is not a successful definitive management option for patients with SCFE. A patient diagnosed with SCFE should be restricted from bearing weight on the affected limb (through use of a wheelchair or bed rest) and should be hospitalized promptly in preparation for surgery. Ideally, he or she should be started on bed rest to minimize the risk of further progression of the slip.

Operative Management

In situ screw fixation with one screw is the treatment of choice for SCFE.[44,51,52] As the term *in situ* implies, no effort is made to reduce the displacement between the epiphysis and femoral neck. Screw fixation is performed to prevent any further displacement by hastening the closure of the physis (Fig. 7-32).[53]

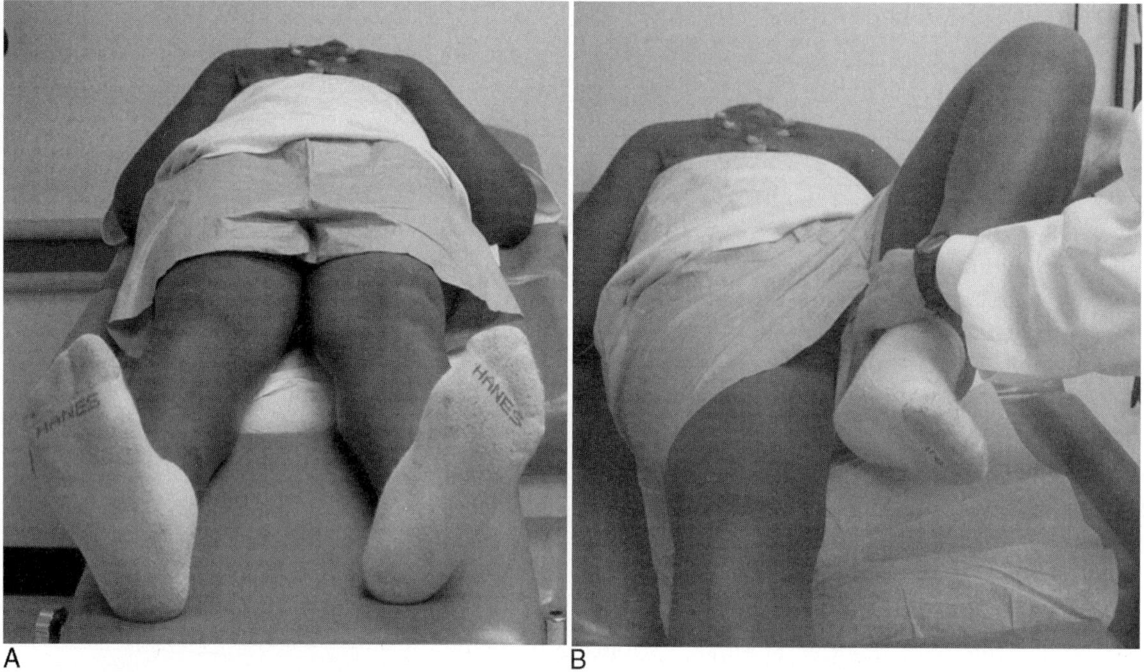

Figure 7-30 Physical examination of a patient with slipped capital femoral epiphysis. A, Note the lateral rotation of the affected limb when the patient is lying supine. **B,** Passive hip flexion results in obligatory lateral rotation of the hip due to the distorted morphology of the proximal femur in this disorder.

Although spontaneous reduction of the slip may occur, intentional reduction is not recommended. Attempts at forceful reduction of a SCFE have been associated with the development of osteonecrosis. However, for patients with severe slips and associated limitations in motion or persistent pain, a realignment osteotomy of the proximal femur can be performed once the physis is closed.[54]

After in situ fixation of the hip, patients are generally instructed to use crutches and begin toe-touch

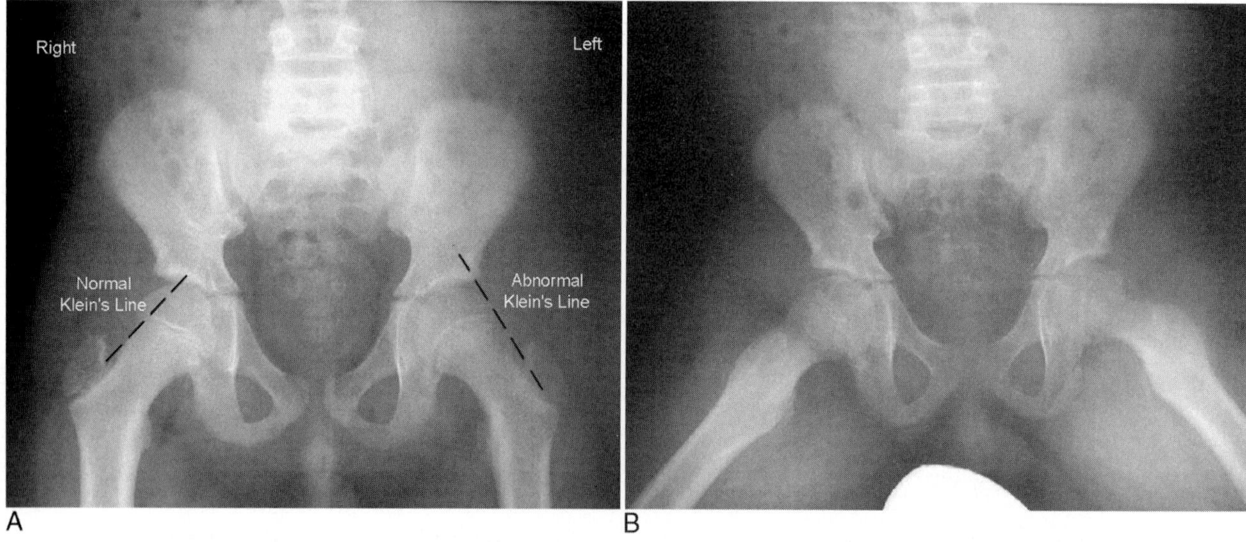

Figure 7-31 A, Klein line, drawn along the superior cortex of the femoral neck on the anteroposterior view of the pelvis, normally intersects the epiphysis. The right hip in this patient is normal. The left hip has slipped capital femoral epiphysis. The femoral neck has moved proximally and anteriorly relative to the epiphysis, so the Klein line no longer intersects the epiphysis. **B,** The "slip" is more easily noted on the frog-leg view.

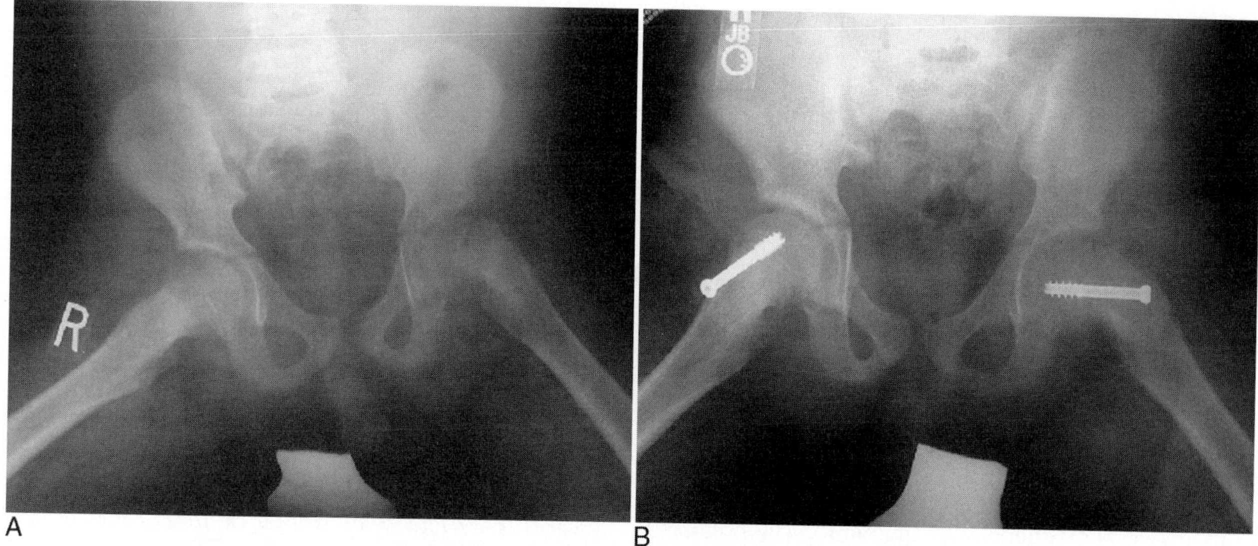

Figure 7-32 This patient underwent an in situ screw fixation of the left hip for treatment of slipped capital femoral epiphysis. A, Note that the displacement of the epiphysis was not reduced before placement of the screw. **B,** The right hip underwent screw fixation prophylactically. The goal of screw fixation is to prevent slip progression and to promote closure of the physis.

weight-bearing only on the affected extremity. A spica cast may be necessary for immobilization in selected children who are unable to comply with activity restrictions. Range of motion of the operated hip improves over time.[55]

The two major adverse outcomes associated with SCFE are osteonecrosis and chondrolysis.[56] Severe slips, which may involve greater insults to the femoral head vascular supply at the time of physeal displacement, are associated with a higher rate of osteonecrosis.[57] As noted previously, patients who are unable to walk, and therefore have unstable SCFE, have a much higher rate of osteonecrosis (47% vs. 0%) than ambulatory patients with stable hips.[58] Iatrogenic injury to the lateral epiphyseal vessels can also occur with placement of the screw in the lateral aspect of the femoral head. However, rates of osteonecrosis (AVN) have diminished significantly because of improvements in slip stabilization techniques.

Chondrolysis—the acute dissolution of articular cartilage in the hip—is associated with hip stiffness and pain. The etiology of this condition is unknown, but proposed causes include immunologic or autoimmune disorders within the hip joint. Although chondrolysis can occur in the untreated hip with SCFE, the vast majority of cases have been reported to follow surgical treatment. Improper placement of the screw that goes unrecognized can result in violation of the joint surface by the screw tip, ultimately leading to articular damage. An alternative operative technique involving the insertion of bone graft across the growth plate had been proposed to promote early fusion and to avoid screw penetration problems.[59] Improvement in screw placement technique has led to a decline in the rate of chondrolysis.[60]

Indications for Referral to the Orthopaedic Surgeon

An adolescent with a presentation suspicious for SCFE should either be instructed to use crutches or placed in a wheelchair, then sent immediately to the pediatric orthopaedic surgeon or the emergency department.

IDIOPATHIC CHONDROLYSIS OF THE HIP

Definition

Chondrolysis of the hip is characterized by progressive destruction of the articular cartilage of both femoral and acetabular surfaces, resulting in joint space narrowing and stiffness. Known causes of chondrolysis of the hip include infection, trauma, prolonged immobilization,[61,62] and treatment of SCFE[63] complicated by unrecognized placement of the screw in the hip joint.[64,65] Idiopathic chondrolysis of the hip (ICH) is an acute and rapidly progressive chondrolysis seen most commonly in adolescents, with isolated involvement of the hip joint and no demonstrable cause.[66-69]

Differential Diagnosis

The differential diagnosis for ICH includes pyogenic arthritis, tuberculous arthritis, juvenile rheumatoid arthritis (JRA), seronegative spondyloarthropathy, and pigmented villonodular synovitis (PVNS). A patient with a septic hip is usually febrile and systemically ill. The hip pain is acute and is associated with intense guarding against passive movement of the hip. Laboratory values such as white blood cell (WBC) count, erythrocyte sedimentation rate (ESR), and serum C-reactive protein (CRP) levels are generally elevated in cases of infection. Purified protein derivative (PPD) test results are positive in immunocompetent patients with tuberculous arthritis. Patients with seronegative spondyloarthropathy generally test positive for the HLA-B27 marker. Chondrolysis associated with tuberculous arthritis and JRA occur only after a prolonged period of symptoms. Furthermore, monoarticular JRA rarely involves the hip; when it does, disease does not progress to destruction of the joint and fibrous ankylosis.[68] Patients with pigmented villonodular synovitis often have a more chronic clinical course, with radiographs demonstrating more cystic erosions in the subchondral bone on both sides of the joint.[60]

Epidemiology

ICH is rare, and its true incidence is unclear. The disorder generally affects girls more frequently than boys, but the ratio varies from study to study. The reported age at the onset of symptoms averages 12.5 years for girls and 14.5 years for boys. ICH appears to affect either hip at equal rates. Bilateral involvement has been reported. Approximately half of patients with ICH are of African descent,[66] and this group has been found to have the worst outcomes.[68]

Etiology

Chondrolysis is thought by many to be autoimmune in origin. Synovial tissue from involved hip joints has routinely demonstrated a higher content of chronic inflammatory cells, including lymphocytes, plasma cells, and monocytes concentrated in a perivascular pattern. In addition, immunocomplex deposition of immunoglobulin (Ig) M and the C3 component of complement in the synovium of involved joints have been demonstrated in patients with chondrolysis associated with SCFE.[70] Other causal explanations for ICH are nutritional abnormalities, mechanical injury, ischemia, abnormal capsular pressure, and an inherently abnormal chondrocyte metabolism within the articular cartilage.[60]

Natural History

The prognosis of ICH is highly variable and unpredictable. The course of this condition appears to have two stages, acute and chronic. The acute stage, lasting 6 to 16 months, begins with the onset of symptoms. An inflammatory state leads to a painful hip with a reduced range of motion and concentric loss of articular cartilage. Histologic studies have shown articular fibrillation with loss of the superficial layer of the articular cartilage with areas of chondrocyte degeneration.[66] Over time, the synovium shows a decrease in inflammation and an increase in fibrous tissue deposition. The chronic stage, which may last 3 to 5 years, is characterized by one of three possible outcomes. Some hips continue to deteriorate and ultimately become fused and painful. Other hips may become painlessly ankylosed in a position that causes some limitation of hip function. In the third group, the involved hip may have resolution of pain, with a partial or complete return of motion and improved joint space width on plain radiographs. The extent of joint space restoration, however, does not necessarily correlate with return of function.[66] It is still unclear which patient characteristics are associated with more favorable outcomes.[60]

Clinical Presentation

The typical presentation in ICH is that of an afebrile African-American premenarchal adolescent girl with insidious onset of pain in the anterior aspect of the affected hip. The hip joint has become progressively stiff and she has a limp. Development of hip contractures in flexion and abduction or adduction may cause pelvic obliquity and an apparent limb length discrepancy.

Physical Findings

Examination of the chondrolytic hip demonstrates significant restriction of motion in all planes associated with muscle spasm. In the most common pattern of contracture, the hip is fixed in flexion, abduction, and lateral (external) rotation.[60]

Laboratory Studies

In ICH, values reported for complete blood count (CBC), urinalysis, rheumatoid factor, antinuclear antibody, and HLA-B27 marker measurements are usually within normal limits. Results of blood culture and tuberculin skin testing are negative. The erythrocyte sedimentation rate may be slightly elevated but rarely exceeds 30 mm/hr.[60,66]

Imaging Studies

The radiographic hallmark of ICH is narrowing of the involved hip joint space from its normal 4 to 5 mm[71] to a value less than 3 mm (Fig. 7-33). Complete obliteration of the joint space rarely occurs. Osteopenia of the surrounding bones and changes in sizes of the femoral head

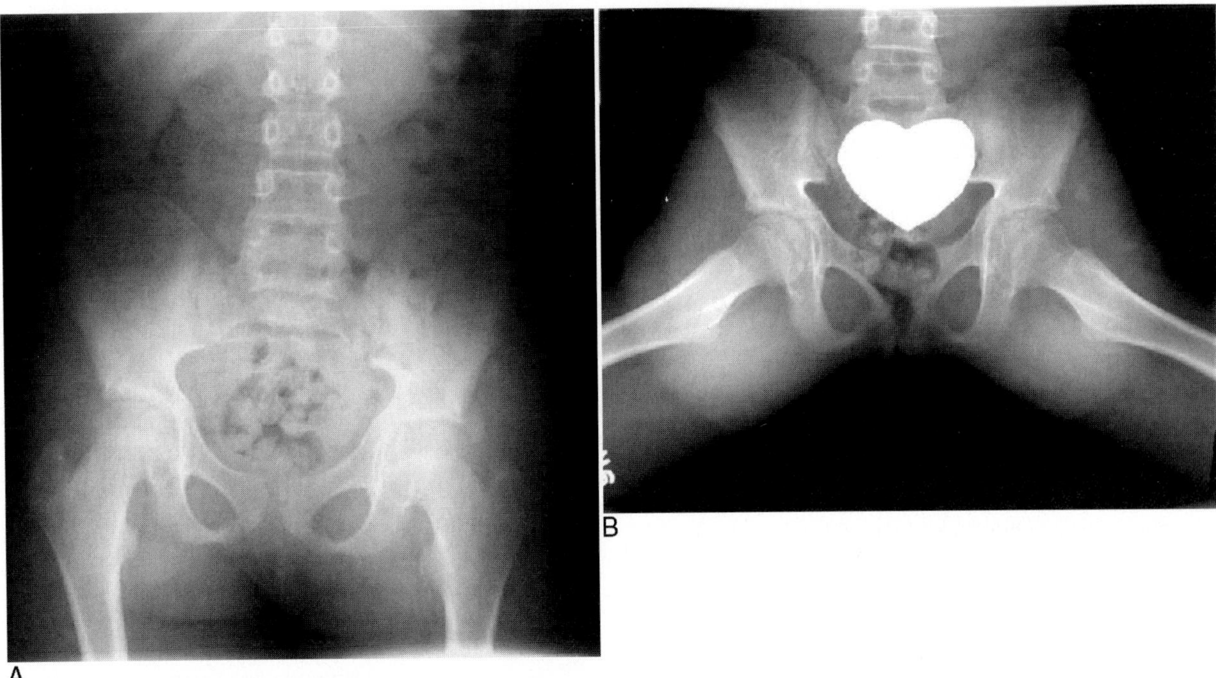

Figure 7-33 Anteroposterior **(A)** and frog-leg **(B)** radiographs showing idiopathic chondrolysis of bilateral hips. Note the narrow articular space between the femoral head and the acetabulum. The prognosis for this condition is poor. (Images courtesy of Charles T. Mehlman, DO.)

and neck are common early findings. In addition, half of patients with ICH demonstrate a mild protrusio acetabuli—a medial bulging of the acetabulum—associated with osteophyte formation on the lateral margin of the acetabulum. Later radiographic findings are partial joint space restoration, lateral femoral head overgrowth, and premature physeal closure.[66,72]

The diagnosis of ICH need not be one of exclusion. In the majority of cases, the diagnosis can be made from the patient's characteristic clinical presentation and plain radiographs. The routine use of arthrography, scintigraphy, CT scanning, and magnetic resonance imaging in this condition is not recommended. However, these modalities may be helpful in making the correct diagnosis when ICH is clinically suspected but cannot be confirmed from plain radiographs.

Management

Current recommendations for the management of ICH focus on control of synovial inflammation, maintenance of hip motion, and prolonged relief from weightbearing on the involved joint. Nonsteroidal anti-inflammatory drugs can help limit the inflammation. Periodic use of skin traction and bed rest can also provide relief during acute exacerbation of joint pain and motion loss. The use of crutches to allow the patient to bear partial or no weight on the affected hip is also an essential part of the management plan. Cases recalcitrant to nonoperative management may require hip fusion. Surgical release of persistent contractures and an aggressive physical therapy program may help restore motion to the affected hip.[73]

COXA VARA

Classification

Coxa vara is a varus deformity of the proximal femur. The neck-shaft angle, drawn between the line of the femoral neck and the line of the femoral shaft viewed on an AP radiograph, measures between 130 and 145 degrees in normal children. In coxa vara, the angle is decreased, typically less than 110 degrees. The classification of coxa vara varies among investigators.[60,74,75] In the classification scheme proposed by Beals,[74] varus deformity of the hip can be roughly classified as developmental, congenital, dysplastic, or traumatic (Box 7-3).

Developmental Coxa Vara

Definition

Developmental coxa vara, also called infantile or cervical coxa vara, involves the proximal femoral physis. This deformity is not present at birth. It develops in early childhood and is typically associated with mild limb shortening and characteristic radiographic features. The varus deformity, indicated by the femoral neck-shaft

Box 7-3 Classification of Coxa Vara

DEVELOPMENTAL COXA VARA

Physeal involvement
Postnatal onset
Unilateral or bilateral
Often progressive
Does not remodel

CONGENITAL COXA VARA (CONGENITAL FEMORAL DEFICIENCY WITH COXA VARA)

Subtrochanteric area
Present at birth
Unilateral
Not progressive
Does not remodel
May be associated with proximal femoral focal deficiency, congenital short femur, or congenital bowed femur

DYSPLASTIC COXA VARA

Metaphyseal or subtrochanteric regions
Bilateral
Often progressive
Does not remodel
Associated with generalized dysplasia and diseases
Metaphyseal region: spondylometaphyseal dysplasia, spondyloepiphyseal dysplasia, sponastrime dysplasia, and cleidocranial dysplasia
Subtrochanteric region: vitamin D-resistant rickets, fibrous dysplasia, Paget disease, osteogenesis imperfecta, and osteopetrosis

TRAUMATIC COXA VARA

Physeal involvement
Not associated with generalized dysplasia
Progressive deformity (no spontaneous remodeling)
Physeal insufficiency and trochanteric overgrowth
Septic hip (destruction of the femoral head)
Vascular injuries to the physis and epiphysis
Legg-Calvé-Perthes disease
Osteonecrosis (femoral neck fracture, traumatic hip dislocation, and complication after reduction of developmental dysplasia of the hip)
Spontaneous remodeling (with non-progressive deformity)
Perinatal epiphyseal separation (associated with difficult breech delivery)
Fracture or osteotomy of the proximal femur

angle, worsens over time. Developmental coxa vara is different from dysplastic coxa vara, which may be associated with skeletal dysplasias and diseases.

Differential Diagnosis

The differential diagnosis of developmental coxa vara includes the other forms of coxa vara—congenital, dysplastic, and traumatic.

Epidemiology

Developmental coxa vara is a rare entity, with a reported incidence of 1 in 25,000 live births worldwide. Involvement is bilateral in one third to one half of patients. There is no predilection for one hip over the other. Rates in the two sexes are equal. A familial pattern has been suggested but not proven.[60,74]

Etiology

The cause of developmental coxa vara remains unclear. The most widely accepted hypothesis postulates a primary ossification defect in the femoral neck. This ossification defect predisposes the local dystrophic bone to fatigue in response to weight-bearing shearing stresses, leading to a progressive varus deformity. Histologic studies have shown that abnormal chondrocyte development in the growth plate cartilage prevents the formation of a solid connection between the physis and the adjacent metaphyseal bone, leading to progressive varus deformity of the femoral neck. Unlike in SCFE, however, there is no slippage between the epiphysis and the metaphysis.[76]

Natural History

Patients with developmental coxa vara are at risk for stress fracture-related non-union of the femoral neck and premature osteoarthritis of the hip. Studies have shown that patients with a relatively vertically oriented physis (more than 45 degrees from the horizontal plane) have a poor prognosis. Patients with a more horizontally oriented physis experience spontaneous healing of the femoral neck defect and associated arrest progression of the deformity.[60]

Clinical Presentation

Most patients with developmental coxa vara present sometime between the initiation of ambulation and 6 years. The most common complaint is a progressive gait abnormality. Pain is rarely reported.

Physical Findings

In developmental coxa vara, the greater trochanter is noted to be somewhat prominent and elevated. The patient with unilateral involvement exhibits a Trendelenburg sign because of weak abductor muscles (Fig. 7-34). In bilateral involvement, the patient walks with a waddling gait and has increased lumbar lordosis,

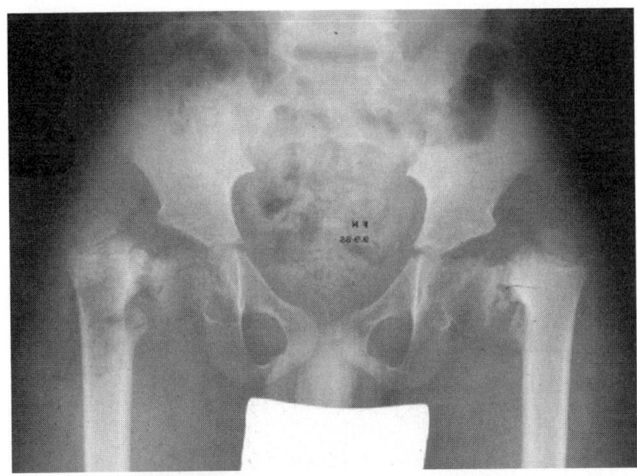

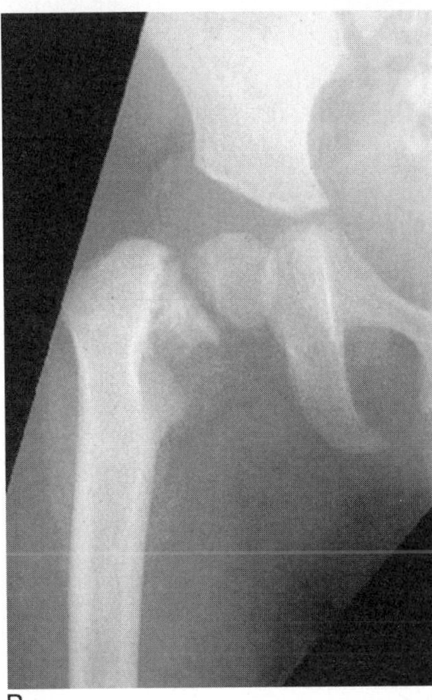

Figure 7-34 Plain radiographs showing two typical cases of coxa vara, one bilateral **(A)** and the other of only the right hip **(B)**.

similar to that seen in bilateral developmental hip dislocations (see Fig. 7-34).

There may be a mild leg length discrepancy in developmental coxa vara. Range of motion is limited, particularly in hip abduction and medial rotation, because of the altered anatomy of the hip.

Imaging Studies

AP and frog-leg lateral views of both hips are required to evaluate cases of suspected coxa vara. The femoral neck-shaft angle (the angle formed between the line of the femoral neck and the femoral shaft on the AP view) of the hip is 130 to 145 degrees in normal children. This angle is decreased to less than 110 degrees, and typically found to be about 90 degrees, in a child with coxa vara. The *Hilgenreiner-epiphyseal* (H-E) *angle*—the angle formed between the Hilgenreiner line (see Fig. 7-14) and a line drawn parallel to the epiphysis—is normally less than 25 degrees. In coxa vara, the H-E angle is greater than 25 degrees, typically progressing to between 45 and 60 degrees.[77] The AP view demonstrates vertical position of the physis (Fig. 7-35A). An inverted Y pattern in the inferior femoral neck is the hallmark of this condition. The lucencies are in the shape of the letter Y and represent the widened physes. The interposed triangular segment is an area of dystrophic bone.

Management

Nonoperative management has not resulted in satisfactory outcomes for developmental coxa vara. Indications for surgery are an abnormal gait associated with a Hilgenreiner-epiphyseal angle greater than 45 degrees[77,78] or a femoral neck-shaft angle of less than 90 to 100 degrees. Operative management involves realignment with a proximal femoral osteotomy (see Fig. 7-35B).[77,79] The goal of the operation is to overcorrect the deformity so that the physis is nearly horizontal.[74] Overcorrection consists of decreasing the Hilgenreiner-epiphyseal angle to less than 30 to 40 degrees or increasing the neck-shaft angle to more than 160 degrees. This orientation reduces the shearing forces across the physis and helps prevent recurrence of the deformity.[78,80] Patients who undergo operations during early childhood have the best outcomes.[81] Proper treatment of developmental coxa vara can result in a painless and functional hip without Trendelenburg gait. A mild, clinically insignificant limb length discrepancy may result from surgery.

Congenital Coxa Vara (Congenital Femoral Deficiency with Coxa Vara)

Definition

Congenital coxa vara is more accurately described as "congenital femoral deficiency with coxa vara." The condition is present at birth and is thought to be caused by an embryonic limb-bud abnormality. It is nearly always unilateral. The deformity involves the subtrochanteric region of the femur and generally does not progressively worsen or spontaneously improve. Congenital musculoskeletal abnormalities associated with congenital coxa vara include proximal femoral focal deficiency (PFFD), congenital short femur, and congenital bowed femur. Proximal femoral focal deficiency, the primary cause of congenital coxa vara, is the focus of this section.

PFFD has been classified in many ways. The Aitken classification has gained the widest acceptance. It describes PFFD from the least severe form (class A), in which the femoral head and acetabulum are both present and adequate, to the most severe form (class D), in which the femoral head and acetabulum are both

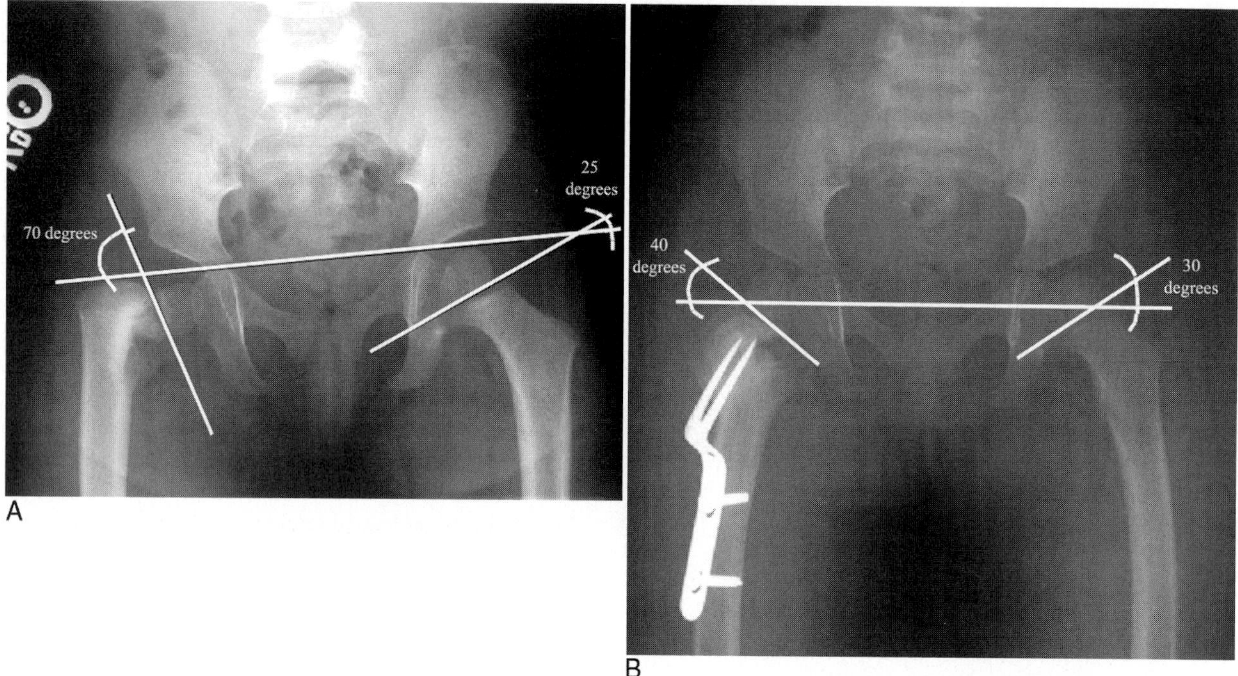

Figure 7-35 A 5-year-old boy with leg length discrepancy was noted to have right hip coxa vara. A, Measurement of the Hilgenreiner-epiphyseal (H-E) angle is close to 90 degrees. **B,** The H-E angle has been corrected by surgery.

absent. The classification proposed by Gillespie complements this scheme by setting guidelines for surgical management. Of note, the clinician caring for a child with PFFD must understand that multiple psychosocial issues related to the disorder must be addressed in a careful and compassionate manner.

Classification of Proximal Femoral Focal Deficiency

Aitken Classification

The Aitken classification is the most widely used system for classifying femoral deficiencies.[82] PFFDs are categorized as class A, B, C, or D (Fig. 7-36 and Table 7-3).

In Class A, the femoral shaft is short but present. The femoral head is also present, and the acetabulum is normal. A bony connection exists between all components of the femur. A varus deformity of the subtrochanteric region of the femur (coxa vara), often due to a pseudoarthrosis, is characteristic of this condition. The femoral shaft may be positioned proximal to the femoral head.

Class B PFFD is characterized by a shorter femoral shaft with a bony tuft at the proximal end of the femur. The femoral head is present but cannot be visualized until the head ossifies. The acetabulum is dysplastic. The proximal end of the femoral shaft is proximal to the acetabulum. Even at maturity, there is no bony continuity between the femoral head and the shaft.

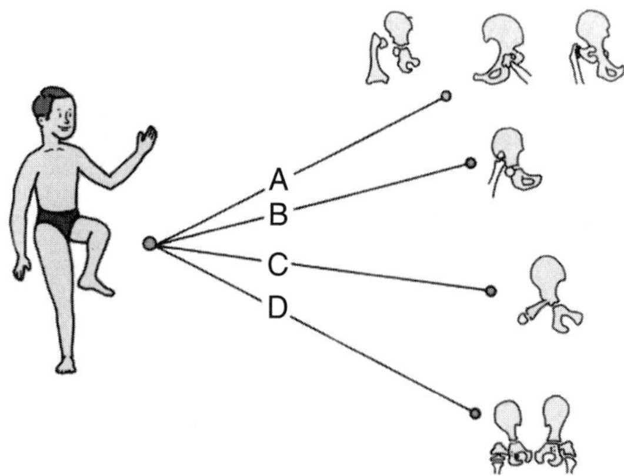

Figure 7-36 Aitken classification for proximal femoral focal deficiency (PFFD). In class **A,** all proximal femoral components eventually ossify with severe subtrochanteric varus, often with pseudoarthrosis. In class **B,** the head of the femur is in a competent acetabulum, but there is never bony or cartilaginous continuity between the shaft and head. Class **C** disease consists of complete absence of the head, acetabulum, and apophysis at the proximal end of the femur. In class **D,** in addition to absence of the acetabulum and femoral head, the femoral segment is abnormally short and severely flexed with no proximal femoral apophysis. The majority of bilateral cases of PFFD are class D. (From Aitken GT: The child amputee: An overview. Orthop Clin North Am 3:447-472, 1972.)

Table 7-3 Aitken Classification of Proximal Focal Femoral Deficiency

Class	Femoral Head	Acetabulum	Femoral Segment	Relationship Between Femur and Acetabulum
A	Present	Normal	Short	Bony connection between components Femoral head in acetabulum Subtrochanteric varus angulation
B	Present	Moderately dysplastic	Short Proximal bony tuft	No bony connection between head and shaft Femoral head in acetabulum
C	Absent or represented by ossicle	Severely dysplastic	Short Proximal tapering	May be bony connection between shaft and proximal ossicle No articular relationship between femur and acetabulum
D	Absent	Absent	Short Deformed	None

In class C, there is a short femoral segment with proximal tapering. The femoral head is either absent or represented by an ossicle. The acetabulum is severely dysplastic.

In class D, the shaft of the femur is extremely short or absent, there is no femoral head, and the acetabulum is either poorly developed or absent as well.

Gillespie Classification

The Gillespie classification, which divides femoral deficiencies into three groups, is useful for planning surgical treatment (Fig. 7-37).[83]

The patient with group A PFFD is considered a candidate for limb lengthening because the length of the affected femur is at least 60% that of the normal femur. The foot of the affected limb is at mid-tibia level or below compared with the unaffected limb, even with the presence of a flexion contracture in the shorter limb. Knee function may be either good or bad.

In group B disease, the length of the affected femur is less than 50% of that of the normal side. The foot of the affected limb is at the level between the knee and mid-tibia of the unaffected limb. A surgical conversion, such as a knee fusion or a van Nes rotation, followed by prosthetic fitting would be most suitable in children with group B PFFD.

Group C PFFD is characterized by virtual absence of the femur with the affected foot positioned at the level of the unaffected knee or above. Patients with this deformity should be managed with prostheses. Retaining the foot within the socket of the prosthesis may improve suspension and control.

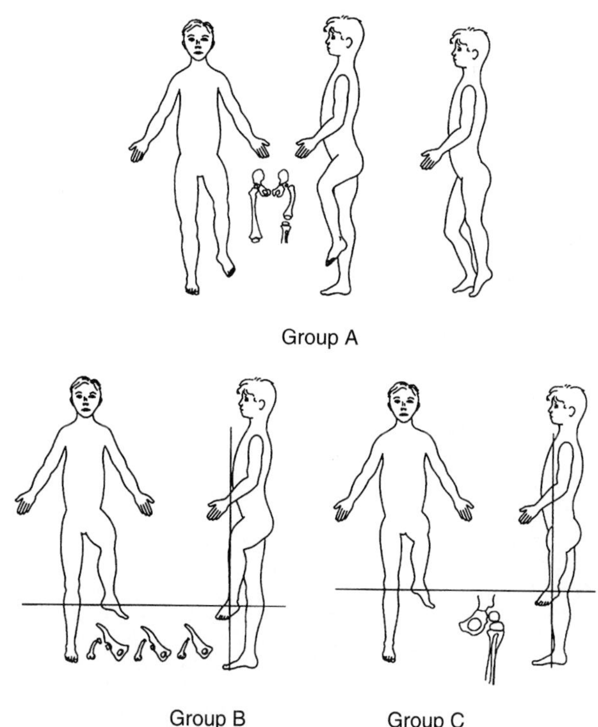

Figure 7-37 Gillespie classification for proximal femoral focal deficiency (PFFD). The vertical line in each view indicates anterior displacement of weight-bearing axis of tibia, and the horizontal line indicates length relationship to the other leg. **A,** In a congenitally short femur (group A) the child can bear weight on the leg by extending the hip and knee; the child does have a sense of proximal stability, and leg-length discrepancy is around 20%. **B,** In group B PFFD (Aitken classes A, B, and C), the leg-length discrepancy is around 40%, with characteristic anterior projection of the thigh and flexed knee. In group **C** (Aitken class D), the thigh is short and bulbous, and the leg is externally rotated with the foot at or proximal to the level of the other knee. (From Gillespie R: Classification of congenital abnormalities of the femur. In Herring JA, Birch JG: The Child with a Limb Deficiency. Rosemont IL, American Academy of Orthopaedic Surgeons. 1998, p 63.)

Differential Diagnosis

The differential diagnosis for congenital coxa vara includes other types of coxa vara—developmental, dysplastic, and post-traumatic coxa vara. Marked limb length discrepancy may help identify PFFD and congenital short femur.

Etiology

The specific causes of congenital limb deficiencies are unknown in most cases and may be multifactorial. Lower limb embryogenesis begins between the fourth and sixth weeks of gestation. Femoral defects probably occur from developmental disturbances during this time of limb bud growth and differentiation.[84] Altered proliferation and maturation of chondrocytes may play roles in disturbing normal mineralization, vascular flow, and endochondral growth of the proximal femur.[85] Environmental and genetic factors may play roles in the development of some limb deficiencies. Thalidomide is one teratogenic drug associated with a large number of limb abnormalities.[86]

Clinical Presentation and Physical Findings

Congenital coxa vara is associated with PFFD and congenital shortening of the femur, but the hip deformity is generally not the presenting complaint.

Patients with PFFD typically present with an extremely short and bulky thigh, a flexed and abducted hip, and a laterally rotated limb. The affected foot is usually at the level of the unaffected knee. Because of hip and knee flexion contractures, the limb often appears shorter than it actually is anatomically. An ipsilateral fibular hemimelia—failure of proper formation of the fibula—may be present in a large proportion of patients with PFFD. A good clue is the absence of the lateral malleolus, detected by palpation of the lateral aspect of the ankle.

Patients with *congenital shortening of the femur*, a disorder related to PFFD, have a more subtle clinical presentation. The affected thigh is shorter than the contralateral thigh and the leg (tibia/fibula) may also be shorter. The femur may have an anterolateral bow, and the overlying skin may be dimpled. Other features are femoral retroversion (lateral rotation of the femur), valgus deformity of the knee, and ipsilateral fibular hemimelia.

The deformity in congenital coxa vara does not resolve spontaneously. The percentage of shortening of the femur compared with the unaffected side is constant.[74] For example, if the femur is 20% shorter than the unaffected side during early childhood, it will continue to be 20% shorter than the normal side in adulthood.

Imaging Studies

The diagnosis of congenital coxa vara can usually be made from plain radiographs (Fig. 7-38). Attention to the acetabulum, the femoral head, and the femoral shaft can help classify the limb deficiency. Scanograms or orthoroentgenograms, radiographs taken with a ruler, can determine the overall limb length discrepancy. The clinician should be aware that hip or knee flexion contractures may influence the measurement of limb lengths.

Management

Many treatment options are available for patients with PFFD.[74,84,86-88] Each patient must be evaluated carefully to enable development of an appropriate management plan.

The "abductor lurch" (Trendelenburg gait) associated with congenital coxa vara and PFFD can be

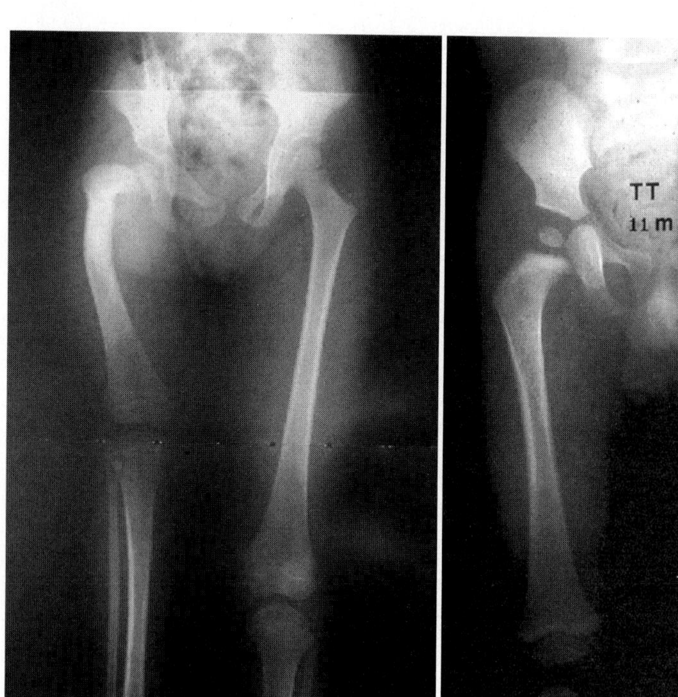

Figure 7-38 Plain radiographs showing two patients with proximal femoral focal deficiency. **A,** Note the shortening of the right femur with associated coxa vara of the right hip. **B,** This patient has more severe involvement with near-complete absence of the left femur.

addressed with fusion of the femur to the ilium. This procedure can stabilize the hip and prevent trunk swaying. A valgus-producing proximal femoral osteotomy may also help improve hip mechanics.

Limb length discrepancy in PFFD can be treated either with or without an operation. Many patients, particularly those with Gillespie group 3 deficiencies, are candidates for prosthetic fitting. Indications for limb lengthening include prediction of the affected femur length to be at least half the length of the normal femur at maturity, with a predicted limb length discrepancy of 17 to 20 cm. Correction should be achieved with no more than three separate procedures. Hip abnormalities, such as coxa vara and hip retroversion, should be corrected prior to lengthening to avoid iatrogenic hip dislocations. In addition to hip stability, knee stability is important. Crossing the knee joint with the external fixator frame (such as the Ilizarov frame) and performing soft tissue lengthening may prevent knee joint subluxation.

A Syme amputation (amputation at the ankle joint) with a knee arthrodesis can be performed at the same time to create a long bone consisting of a short femur fused to a tibia. This has the advantage of providing an effectively longer femur with an end-bearing limb suitable for prosthetic fitting after a single operation. The drawbacks, however, are that the limb is often too long and that it lacks knee motion and control.

The van Nes rotationplasty creates a knee joint by attaching the ankle backwards to the distal femur, thus creating a knee joint with a backwards ankle joint (the heel is pointing forward). Motor control and sensory feedback are excellent after this technically challenging procedure. Prosthesis fitting and training allow the patient to walk without significant gait disturbances or excessive energy expenditure.[87] The disadvantage of this option is poor cosmesis and derotation (loss of rotated position) over time. Contraindications for this operation include severe foot and ankle deformities and bilateral femoral deficiency.

Dysplastic Coxa Vara

Definition

Many generalized skeletal dysplasias and diseases are associated with coxa vara. The deformity in these conditions is generally progressive and does not spontaneously resolve. This form of coxa vara can involve the metaphyseal or the subtrochanteric regions of the femur.

Metaphyseal deformities have been associated with spondylometaphyseal dysplasia, spondyloepiphyseal dysplasia, sponastrime dysplasia, cleidocranial dysplasia, metaphyseal dysostosis, chondrodysplasia punctata, and multiple epiphyseal dysplasia.[74,75]

Subtrochanteric varus deformity with generalized bowing of the femur have been associated with skeletal diseases, such as vitamin D–resistant rickets, fibrous dysplasia, Paget disease, osteogenesis imperfecta, and osteopetrosis.

Differential Diagnosis

The differential diagnosis of dysplastic coxa vara is similar to that of other forms of coxa vara. The most important distinction in this type of hip deformity is to identify and correct the underlying disease.

Epidemiology

The generalized skeletal dysplasias and diseases already mentioned are associated with coxa vara. The precise rate of varus hip deformity in each condition is not clear.

Etiology

The etiology of the varus femoral deformity lies in the overall malformation of skeletal structures in these generalized skeletal dysplasias and diseases.

Natural History

Deformity in these conditions is progressive and does not resolve spontaneously.

Clinical Presentation and Physical Findings

Patients present with generalized deformity or disease, not specifically a hip problem. Bilateral involvement of the hips is common. Physical findings such as short stature, other deformities, dysmorphisms, other skeletal abnormalities, and bilateral involvement suggest the presence of a generalized skeletal dysplasia.

Imaging Studies

The varus hip deformity is seen on plain radiographs of the pelvis. A skeletal survey may help determine the type of skeletal dysplasia or disease.

Management

The selection of treatment options for dysplastic coxa vara can be complicated by the nature of the underlying condition. Appropriate therapy can be initiated once the femoral head ossifies and the rate and magnitude of progression of varus deformity are determined. Prognosis varies from condition to condition. A subtrochanteric valgus osteotomy of the femur can be helpful in preventing the progression of deformity.

Traumatic Coxa Vara

Definition

Traumatic coxa vara involves the physis and is not associated with any generalized skeletal dysplasias. Coxa vara can result from direct injury to the proximal femoral physis and the proximal femur from infections, vascular injuries, and fractures.[74]

Differential Diagnosis

The differential diagnosis for traumatic coxa vara includes developmental and congenital coxa vara.

Epidemiology

The incidence of traumatic coxa depends on the rate of complications associated with conditions such as septic hip, osteonecrosis of the femoral head, Legg-Calvé-Perthes disease, perinatal epiphyseal separation, proximal femoral fractures, and varus-producing proximal femoral osteotomies.

Etiology

Conditions leading to progressive varus hip deformity include hip infection, Legg-Calvé-Perthes disease, and osteonecrosis. A septic hip, if not treated promptly, can lead to septic necrosis of the hip and complete destruction of the femoral head. Femoral neck fractures and traumatic hip dislocations can cause osteonecrosis of the femoral head by disrupting its vascular supply. In a child with DDH, reduction of a dislocated hip and application of a spica cast in excessive abduction can also lead to acquired coxa vara by compromising blood flow to the femoral head. When the normal growth through the proximal femoral physis is compromised, varus deformity develops because of the continued disproportionate growth of the greater trochanter.

Coxa vara can also occur after a perinatal epiphyseal separation associated with a difficult breech delivery. The deformity associated with this event has been found to remodel spontaneously. A varus hip position can result from malunion of a femoral neck or intertrochanteric fracture or from a varus-producing femoral osteotomy. These injuries heal well, and the proximal femur undergoes spontaneous correction.

Natural History

The natural course of acquired traumatic coxa vara depends on the natural history of the underlying conditions. In general, osteonecrosis of the femoral head has a poor prognosis.

Clinical Presentation and Physical Findings

Patients with traumatic coxa vara are generally older than those with developmental or congenital coxa vara. They are usually ambulatory and are noted to have limps and associated limb length discrepancies, both of which may be more severe if the initial insult occurred earlier in life. A Trendelenburg sign or gait may be present because of altered hip abductor mechanics. Limb length discrepancy may be present as a result of altered growth through the proximal femoral physis.

Imaging Studies

Plain radiographs usually yield sufficient evidence from which to make the diagnosis of coxa vara. Vascular injury to the proximal femoral epiphysis and the physis are suggested by failure of growth of the ossific nucleus, fragmentation and deformity of the femoral head, and failure of growth of the femoral neck. Relative overgrowth of the greater trochanter may be noted. Comparison with the unaffected hip may be helpful.

Management

Alteration of hip mechanics because of trochanteric overgrowth can be corrected with epiphysiodesis of the greater trochanter physis once the apophysis becomes visible at age 5. In children older than 9 years, the greater trochanter can be transferred distally to increase the length of the hip abductors, improving their mechanics to allow them to keep the pelvis level throughout the gait cycle.[74] Osteonecrosis of the hip typically leads to a painful, arthritic hip joint and may require surgery. However, management decisions should be made on an individual basis. Even with marked deformity and advanced degenerative changes, a patient's function may be adequate to forestall an operation. A total hip replacement can provide a pain-free mobile joint. However, in a young person, such a procedure may have to be revised multiple times during a lifetime, because the prosthesis can wear out in active people. In a patient with a history of septic necrosis of the hip, the risk of prosthesis infection may make total hip replacement a less attractive treatment strategy.

Indications for Referral to the Orthopaedic Surgeon

Any child with a limb length discrepancy and an abnormal gait should be evaluated for a hip disorder or a limb deficiency by an orthopaedic surgeon. Pelvic radiographs and a scanogram or orthoroentgenogram should be obtained if coxa vara is suspected.

FEMORAL ANTEVERSION

Definition

Femoral anteversion, or medial femoral torsion, is a common cause of in-toeing in younger children. The deformity is not in the tibia or the foot but rather in the proximal femur. In the normal child, the femoral head is directed approximately 15 degrees anterior to the shaft of the femur, and therefore has 15 degrees of femoral anteversion. A larger femoral anteversion forces the entire limb to be medially rotated to maintain the normal relationship between the acetabulum and the femoral head. This leads to in-toeing.

Clinical Presentation

The child is typically brought in by the caregiver with the chief complaint of in-toeing or clumsiness. Although these children tend to fall quite often, they are usually good sprinters.

Physical Examination

With the child lying prone and knees flexed at 90 degrees, the examiner rotates the thigh medially (i.e., feet pushed outwards) and laterally (i.e., feet pushed inwards) to assess range of motion of the hip. Medial rotation of more than 60 degrees and limited lateral rotation of the thigh to less than 20 degrees are highly suggestive of femoral anteversion. Femoral anteversion may be confused with internal tibial torsion. Observation of the orientation of the patella helps distinguish these two conditions. In internal tibial torsion, the patellae are in typical anatomic alignment, but in femoral anteversion, they are medially rotated. Alignment of the patellae with the second metatarsals rules out internal tibial torsion.

A child with femoral anteversion is often observed sitting in the reverse tailor position (i.e., the W position) (Fig. 7-39).

Management

The patient and the caregiver should be encouraged to adopt a different sitting style, such as the "Indian-style" position. The natural course of femoral anteversion is improvement over time. Also, as the child's pelvis grows in width, the medially rotated feet will not collide as much during ambulation.

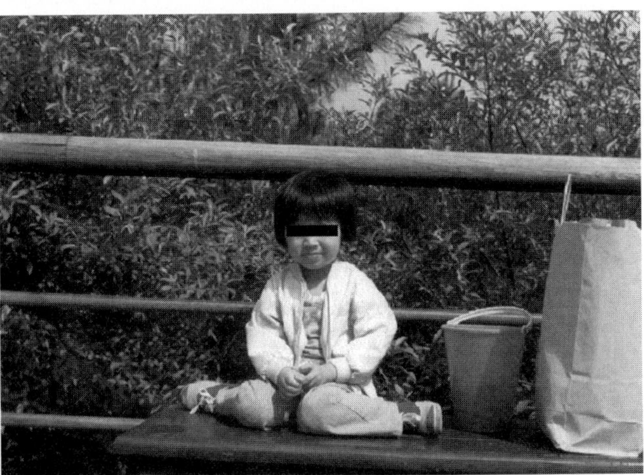

Figure 7-39 The typical W sitting position of a boy with femoral anteversion.

Indications for Referral to the Orthopaedic Surgeon

A patient with a persistent problem of "clumsiness" should undergo a neurologic as well as an orthopaedic evaluation (as described previously) by the primary care provider. If neurologic disease has been ruled out and the physical findings are consistent with femoral anteversion, a referral to an orthopaedic surgeon is not necessary, because the natural course of this condition is improvement over time. However, cases of extreme and persistent rotational deformities of the extremities may benefit from corrective surgery.

MAJOR POINTS

A child with a gait abnormality should undergo a thorough hip evaluation.

Knee pain in a child may be due to hip disease.

Certain hip disorders are common in each age group.

Risk factors for developmental dysplasia of the hip are female gender, breech position, positive family history, and reduced intrauterine space.

Developmental dysplasia of the hip may not be present at birth, so children at risk for the disorder must be monitored closely.

Teratologic hip dislocations have identifiable causes and often are irreducible at birth.

Children with Legg-Calvé-Perthes disease typically present with knee pain and a limp.

The goal in the treatment of Legg-Calvé-Perthes disease is containment of the femoral head and maintenance of hip range of motion.

A patient with slipped capital femoral epiphysis needs prompt surgical attention.

Unstable slipped capital femoral epiphysis is associated with a high risk for development of osteonecrosis of the hip.

Slipped capital femoral epiphysis can affect both hips.

Idiopathic chondrolysis of the hip is a rare disorder that may manifest as pelvic obliquity and apparent leg length discrepancy.

Coxa vara and proximal femoral focal deficiency should be included in the differential diagnosis for gait abnormality and limb length discrepancy.

Bilateral femoral anteversion is a benign condition.

REFERENCES

1. Aronsson DD, Goldberg MJ, Kling TF Jr, et al: Developmental dysplasia of the hip. Pediatrics 94:201-8, 1994.

2. Lehmann HP, Hinton R, Morello P, et al: Developmental dysplasia of the hip practice guideline: Technical report. Committee on Quality Improvement, and Subcommittee on Developmental Dysplasia of the Hip. Pediatrics 105:E57, 2000.

3. Bialik V, Bialik GM, Blazer S, et al: Developmental dysplasia of the hip: A new approach to incidence. Pediatrics 103:93-99, 1999.

4. Haynes RJ: Developmental dysplasia of the hip: Etiology, pathogenesis, and examination and physical findings in the newborn. Instr Course Lect 50:535-540, 2001.

5. Herring JA: Developmental dysplasia of the hip. In Herring JA (ed): Tachdjian's Pediatric Orthopaedics. Philadelphia, WB Saunders, 2002, pp 513-654.

6. Wynne-Davies R: Acetabular dysplasia and familial joint laxity: Two etiological factors in congenital dislocation of the hip: A review of 589 patients and their families. J Bone Joint Surg Br 52:704-716, 1970.

7. MacEwen GD, Millet C: Congenital dislocation of the hip. Pediatr Rev 11:249-252, 1990.

8. Wenger DR: Developmental dysplasia of the hip. In Wenger DR, Rang M (eds): The Art and Practice of Children's Orthopaedics. New York, Raven Press, 1993, pp 256-296.

9. Huurman WW: Pediatric hip disease. In Brown DE, Neumann, RD (eds): Orthopedic Secrets. Philadelphia, Hanley & Belfus, 1999, pp 214-220.

10. Hyman JE, Lee FY, Dormans JP, et al: Orthopedics. In Polin RA, Ditmar MF (eds): Pediatric Secrets, Philadelphia, Hanley & Belfus, 2001, pp 613-640.

11. Bellah R: Ultrasound in pediatric musculoskeletal disease: Techniques and applications. Radiol Clin North Am 39:597-618, 2001.

12. Harcke HT, Kumar SJ: The role of ultrasound in the diagnosis and management of congenital dislocation and dysplasia of the hip. J Bone Joint Surg Am 73:622-628, 1991.

13. Weintroub S, Grill F: Ultrasonography in developmental dysplasia of the hip. J Bone Joint Surg Am 82:1004-1018, 2000.

14. Godward S, Dezateux C: Surgery for congenital dislocation of the hip in the UK as a measure of outcome of screening. MRC Working Party on Congenital Dislocation of the Hip, Medical Research Council. Lancet 351(9110):1149-1152, 1998.

15. Patel H: Preventive health care, 2001 update: Screening and management of developmental dysplasia of the hip in newborns. CMAJ 164:1669-1677, 2001.

16. Guille JT, Pizzutillo PD, MacEwen GD: Development dysplasia of the hip from birth to six months. J Am Acad Orthop Surg 8:232-242, 2000.

17. Garvey M, Donoghue VB, Gorman WA, et al: Radiographic screening at four months of infants at risk for congenital hip dislocation. J Bone Joint Surg Br 74:704-707, 1992.

18. Vitale MG, Skaggs DL: Developmental dysplasia of the hip from six months to four years of age. J Am Acad Orthop Surg 9:401-411, 2001.

19. Herring JA: Legg-Calvé-Perthes disease. In Herring, JA (ed): Tachdjian's Pediatric Orthopaedics. Philadelphia, WB Saunders, 2002, pp 655-709.

20. Weinstein SL: Legg-Calvé-Perthes syndrome. In Morrissey RT, Weinstein SL (eds): Lovell and Winter's Pediatric Orthopaedics. Philadelphia, Lippincott Williams & Wilkins, 2000, pp 957-998.

21. Neidel J, Boddenberg B, Zander D, et al: Thyroid function in Legg-Calvé-Perthes disease: Cross-sectional and longitudinal study. J Pediatr Orthop 13:592-597, 1993.

22. Glueck CJ, Crawford A, Roy D, et al: Association of antithrombotic factor deficiencies and hypofibrinolysis with Legg-Perthes disease. J Bone Joint Surg Am 78:3-13, 1996.

23. Kealey WD, Mayne EE, McDonald W, et al: The role of coagulation abnormalities in the development of Perthes' disease. J Bone Joint Surg Br 82:744-746, 2000.

24. Glueck CJ, Freiberg RA, Crawford A, et al: Secondhand smoke, hypofibrinolysis, and Legg-Perthes disease. Clin Orthop 352:159-167, 1998.

25. Loder RT, Schwartz EM, Hensinger RN: Behavioral characteristics of children with Legg-Calvé-Perthes disease. J Pediatr Orthop 13:598-601, 1993.

26. Gallistl S, Reitinger T, Linhart W, et al: The role of inherited thrombotic disorders in the etiology of Legg-Calvé-Perthes disease. J Pediatr Orthop 19:82-83, 1999.

27. Catterall A: The natural history of Perthes' disease. J Bone Joint Surg Br 53:37-53, 1971.

28. Hoffinger SA, Henderson RC, Renner JB, et al: Magnetic resonance evaluation of "metaphyseal" changes in Legg-Calvé-Perthes disease. J Pediatr Orthop 13:602-606, 1993.

29. Herring JA, Neustadt JB, Williams JJ, et al: The lateral pillar classification of Legg-Calvé-Perthes disease, J Pediatr Orthop 12:143-150, 1992.

30. Martinez AG, Weinstein SL, Dietz FR: The weight-bearing abduction brace for the treatment of Legg-Perthes disease. J Bone Joint Surg Am 74:12-21, 1992.

31. Meehan PL, Angel D, Nelson JM: The Scottish Rite abduction orthosis for the treatment of Legg-Perthes disease: A radiographic analysis. J Bone Joint Surg Am 74:2-12, 1992.

32. Crawford AH, Bowen JR, Green NE, et al: Symposium: Legg-Calvé-Perthes disease. Contemp Orthop 11:65-108, 1985.

33. Herring JA: The treatment of Legg-Calvé-Perthes disease: A critical review of the literature. J Bone Joint Surg Am 76:448-458, 1994.

34. Thompson GH, Price CT, Roy D, et al: Legg-Calvé-Perthes disease: Current concepts. Instr Course Lect 51:367-384, 2002.

35. Rhoad RC, Davidson RS, Heyman S, et al: Pretreatment bone scan in SCFE: A predictor of ischemia and avascular necrosis. J Pediatr Orthop 19:164-168, 1999.

36. Gelberman RH, Cohen MS, Shaw BA, et al: The association of femoral retroversion with slipped capital femoral epiphysis. J Bone Joint Surg Am 68:1000-1007, 1986.

37. Pritchett JW, Perdue KD: Mechanical factors in slipped capital femoral epiphysis. J Pediatr Orthop 8:385-388, 1988.

38. Crawford AH, MacEwen GD, Fonte D: Slipped capital femoral epiphysis co-existent with hypothyroidism. Clin Orthop 122:135-140, 1977.

39. Wells D, King JD, Roe TF, et al: Review of slipped capital femoral epiphysis associated with endocrine disease. J Pediatr Orthop 13:610-614, 1993.

40. Zubrow AB, Lane JM, Parks JS: Slipped capital femoral epiphysis occurring during treatment for hypothyroidism. J Bone Joint Surg Am 60:256-258, 1978.

41. Loder RT, Aronsson DD, Dobbs MB, et al: Slipped capital femoral epiphysis. Instr Course Lect 50:555-570, 2001.

42. Kehl DK: Slipped capital femoral epiphysis. In Morrissey RT, Weinstein SL (eds): Lovell and Winter's Pediatric Orthopaedics. Philadelphia, Lippincott Williams & Wilkins, 2000, pp 999-1033.

43. Ordeberg G, Hansson LI, Sandstrom S: Slipped capital femoral epiphysis in southern Sweden: Long-term result with no treatment or symptomatic primary treatment. Clin Orthop 191:95-104, 1984.

44. Carney BT, Weinstein SL, Noble J: Long-term follow-up of slipped capital femoral epiphysis. J Bone Joint Surg Am 73:667-674, 1991.

45. Carney BT, Weinstein SL: Natural history of untreated chronic slipped capital femoral epiphysis. Clin Orthop 322:43-47, 1996.

46. Dobbs MB, Weinstein SL: Natural history and long-term outcomes of slipped capital femoral epiphysis. Instr Course Lect 50:571-575, 2001.

47. Hurley JM, Betz RR, Loder RT, et al: Slipped capital femoral epiphysis: The prevalence of late contralateral slip. J Bone Joint Surg Am 78:226-230, 1996.

48. Loder RT, Aronson DD, Greenfield ML: The epidemiology of bilateral slipped capital femoral epiphysis: A study of children in Michigan. J Bone Joint Surg Am 75:1141-1147, 1993.

49. Loder RT, Hensinger RN, Alburger PD, et al: Slipped capital femoral epiphysis associated with radiation therapy. J Pediatr Orthop 18:630-636, 1998.

50. Steel HH: The metaphyseal blanch sign of slipped capital femoral epiphysis. J Bone Joint Surg Am 68:920-922, 1986.

51. Aronson DD, Loder RT: Slipped capital femoral epiphysis in black children. J Pediatr Orthop 12:74-79, 1992.

52. Dormans JP, Crawford AH, Loder RT, et al: Symposium: Slipped capital femoral epiphysis. Contemp Orthop 31:369-380, 1995.

53. Dormans JP: A simple model for illustrating screw fixation of high-grade slipped capital femoral epiphysis. J Orthop Techniques 3:47-54, 1995.

54. Crawford AH: The role of osteotomy in the treatment of slipped capital femoral epiphysis. Instr Course Lect 38:273-279, 1989.

55. Siegel DB, Kasser JR, Sponseller P, et al: Slipped capital femoral epiphysis: A quantitative analysis of motion, gait, and femoral remodeling after in situ fixation. J Bone Joint Surg Am 73:659-666, 1991.

56. Crawford AH: Slipped capital femoral epiphysis. J Bone Joint Surg Am 70:1422-1427, 1988.

57. Herman MJ, Dormans JP, Davidson RS, et al: Screw fixation of Grade III slipped capital femoral epiphysis. Clin Orthop 322:77-85, 1996.

58. Loder RT, Richards BS, Shapiro PS, et al: Acute slipped capital femoral epiphysis: The importance of physeal stability. J Bone Joint Surg Am 75:1134-1140, 1993.

59. Bloom ML, Crawford AH: Slipped capital femoral epiphysis: An assessment of treatment modalities. Orthopedics 8:36-40, 1985.

60. Kehl DK: Developmental coxa vara, transient synovitis, and idiopathic chondrolysis of the hip. In Morrissey RT, Weinstein SL (eds): Lovell and Winter's Pediatric Orthopaedics. Philadelphia, Lippincott Williams & Wilkins, 2000, pp 1035-1057.

61. Frymoyer JW: Chondrolysis of the hip following Southwick osteotomy for severe slipped capital femoral epiphysis. Clin Orthop 99:120-124, 1974.

62. Pellicci PM, Wilson PD Jr: Chondrolysis of the hips associated with severe burns: A case report. J Bone Joint Surg Am 61:592-596, 1979.

63. Heppenstall RB, Marvel JP Jr, Chung SM, et al: Chondrolysis of the hip. Clin Orthop 0(103):136-142, 1974.

64. Stambough JL, Davidson RS, Ellis RD, et al: Slipped capital femoral epiphysis: An analysis of 80 patients as to pin placement and number. J Pediatr Orthop 6:265-273, 1986.

65. Walters R, Simon S: Joint destruction: A sequel of unrecognized pin penetration in patients with slipped capital femoral epiphysis. In Riley LH Jr (ed): The Hip: Proceedings of the Eighth Open Scientific Meeting of the Hip Society. St. Louis, CV Mosby, 1980, p 145.

66. Daluga DJ, Millar EA: Idiopathic chondrolysis of the hip. J Pediatr Orthop 9:405-411, 1989.

67. del Couz Garcia A, Fernandez PL, Gonzalez MP, et al: Idiopathic chondrolysis of the hip: Long-term evolution. J Pediatr Orthop 19:449-454, 1999.

68. Duncan JW, Nasca R, Schrantz J: Idiopathic chondrolysis of the hip. J Bone Joint Surg Am 61:1024-1028, 1979.

69. Wenger DR, Mickelson MR, Ponseti IV: Idiopathic chondrolysis of the hip: Report of two cases. J Bone Joint Surg Am 57:268-271, 1975.

70. Eisenstein A, Rothschild S: Biochemical abnormalities in patients with slipped capital femoral epiphysis and chondrolysis. J Bone Joint Surg Am 58:459-467, 1976.

71. Hughes LO, Aronson J, Smith HS: Normal radiographic values for cartilage thickness and physeal angle in the pediatric hip. J Pediatr Orthop 19:443-448, 1999.

72. Bleck EE: Idiopathic chondrolysis of the hip. J Bone Joint Surg Am 65:1266-1275, 1983.

73. Roy DR, Crawford AH: Idiopathic chondrolysis of the hip: Management by subtotal capsulectomy and aggressive rehabilitation. J Pediatr Orthop 8:203-207, 1988.

74. Beals RK: Coxa vara in childhood: Evaluation and management. J Am Acad Orthop Surg 6:93-99, 1998.

75. Herring JA: Congenital coxa vara. In Herring, JA (ed): Tachdjian's Pediatric Orthopaedics. Philadelphia, WB Saunders, 2002, pp 765-781.

76. Bos CF, Sakkers RJ, Bloem JL, et al: Histological, biochemical, and MRI studies of the growth plate in congenital coxa vara. J Pediatr Orthop 9:660-605, 1989.

77. Weinstein JN, Kuo KN, Millar EA: Congenital coxa vara: A retrospective review. J Pediatr Orthop 4:70-77, 1984.

78. Desai SS, Johnson LO: Long-term results of valgus osteotomy for congenital coxa vara. Clin Orthop 294:204-210, 1993.

79. Cordes S, Dickens DR, Cole WG: Correction of coxa vara in childhood: The use of Pauwels' Y-shaped osteotomy. J Bone Joint Surg Br 73:3-6, 1991.

80. Carroll K, Coleman S, Stevens PM: Coxa vara: Surgical outcomes of valgus osteotomies. J Pediatr Orthop 17:220-224, 1997.

81. Serafin J, Szulc W: Coxa vara infantum, hip growth disturbances, etiopathogenesis, and long-term results of treatment. Clin Orthop 272:103-113, 1991.

82. Aitken GT: The child amputee: An overview. Orthop Clin North Am 3:447-472, 1972.

83. Gillespie R: Classification of congenital abnormalities of the femur. In Herring JA, Birch JG (eds): The Child with a Limb Deficiency. Rosemont IL, American Academy of Orthopaedic Surgeons, 1998, p 63.

84. Bryant DD 3rd, Epps CH Jr: Proximal femoral focal deficiency: Evaluation and management. Orthopedics 14:775-784, 1991.

85. Boden SD, Fallon MD, Davidson R, et al: Proximal femoral focal deficiency: Evidence for a defect in proliferation and maturation of chondrocytes. J Bone Joint Surg Am 71:1119-1129, 1989.

86. Epps CH Jr: Proximal femoral focal deficiency. J Bone Joint Surg Am 65:867-870, 1983.

87. Alman BA, Krajbich JI, Hubbard S: Proximal femoral focal deficiency: Results of rotationplasty and Syme amputation. J Bone Joint Surg Am 77:1876-1882, 1995.

88. Herring JA: Limb deficiencies. In Herring JA (ed): Tachdjian's Pediatric Orthopaedics. Philadelphia, WB Saunders, 2002, pp 1745-1810.

CHAPTER 8

Upper Extremity Disorders

BENJAMIN CHANG
BONG. S. LEE

INJURY

Initial assessment of the injured upper extremity in a child, as in an adult, begins with obtaining a history and proceeds to the physical examination and special studies as necessary. However, one must give special consideration to the child's age and maturity in order to obtain the requisite information without unduly alarming the patient. The goal of the initial assessment is to determine what structures have been injured so that one can initiate appropriate and timely treatment.

History

The history of the injury can provide important clues as to what has been injured. In addition to questioning the child, one should interview the parents and other adult witnesses to the injury. Essential elements of the history are listed in Box 8-1.

Physical Examination

The purpose of the physical examination is to determine which structures have been injured. One must test all structures within the zone of injury systematically to avoid missing an injury. The examination is begun distally

Box 8-1 Essential Elements of History in Hand Injuries

GENERAL HISTORY

- Age
- Sex
- Hand dominance
- Significant medical history
- Past surgical history
- Medications
- Allergies

HISTORY OF INJURY

- Mechanism
- Time
- Symptoms
- Functional deficits
- Previous injuries
- Prior treatment
- Associated injuries

and proceeds proximally; functional deficits distal to the zone of injury point to injured proximal structures. To obtain useful information, one must minimize the discomfort to the patient during the examination. One way to allay the patient's fears is to demonstrate the examination on the uninjured side first. This also allows one to compare the injured with the uninjured side. One gains the patient's trust by starting with observation and then proceeding to manipulation *in the following order:* gentle palpation, tests of active motion, and exploration. Open wounds should be explored only after establishment of adequate anesthesia. One can often gain all the necessary information by testing the parts of the extremity distal to the level of injury, without ever probing the wound.

The upper extremity examination should proceed in the following order: circulation, sensibility, soft tissues, skeleton, and motor function. Circulation is first because it is the most critical component and can be checked with minimal discomfort to the patient. Motor function is tested last because it requires the patient's cooperation and depends on intact musculotendinous units, stable bones, and mobile joints. All symptomatic areas and at least one joint proximal and distal to the level of injury should be examined. Table 8-1 summarizes the elements of the upper extremity examination.

Circulation

In a well-perfused hand, the fingertips and nail beds are pink, the hand is warm, and capillary refill time is 2 seconds or less. One can usually palpate the radial and ulnar pulses easily at the wrist unless there is proximal occlusion or vasoconstriction (e.g., from hypothermia). Doppler ultrasonography and pulse oximetry can be helpful adjuncts to physical examination in equivocal cases.

Sensibility

In older children, one can test sensibility with light touch ("look away and tell me which finger I am touching") or two-point discrimination. Normal static two-point discrimination is 5 mm or less in the fingertips. There are three autonomous sensory zones in the hand (Fig. 8-1) corresponding to the three major sensory nerves: index fingertip (median), small fingertip (ulnar), and dorsum of the thumb–index finger web space (radial).

Sensibility can be hard to assess in a young child with these standard tests because they require the patient's understanding and cooperation. Two signs of sensory denervation that do not rely on the patient's accurate response are (1) anhidrosis of the skin and (2) lack of skin wrinkling with immersion in water.[1] Compare these signs with those in the uninjured hand.

Table 8-1 Upper Extremity Examination

Physical Examination	Observation	Manipulation	Special Tests
Circulation	Color	Temperature Capillary refill Pulse	Doppler ultrasonography Pulse oximetry
Sensibility	Anhidrosis	Immersion test Light touch Two-point discrimination	Nerve conduction
Soft tissues	Open wounds	Exploration	
Skeleton	Deformity	Palpation Range of motion	Radiography
Motor function	Spontaneous motion	Tenodesis effect Squeeze test Range of motion Strength	Nerve conduction Electromyography

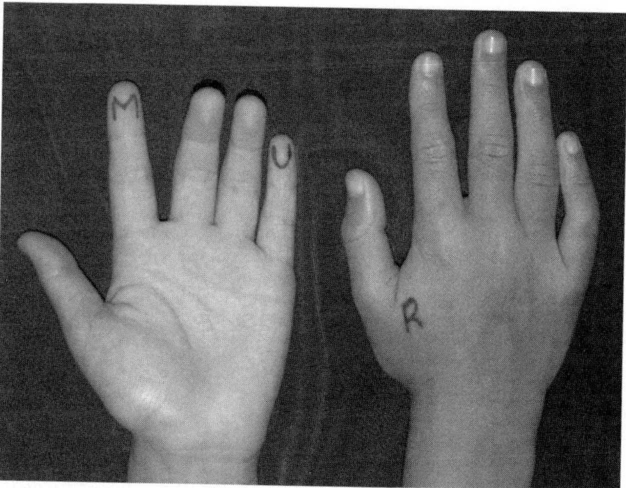

Figure 8-1 Autonomous sensory zones of the hand: median (M), ulnar (U), and radial (R).

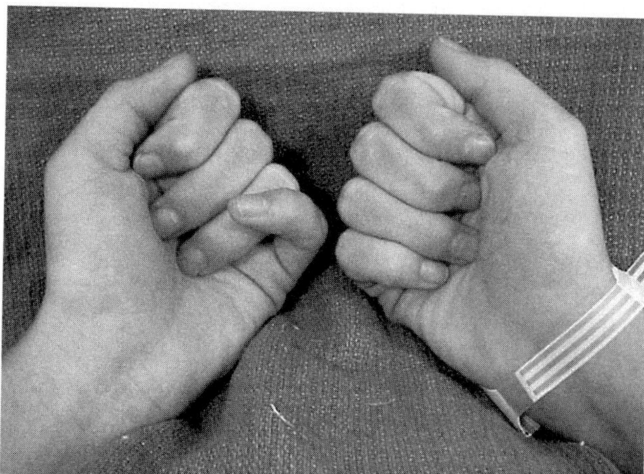

Figure 8-2 Rotational deformity of small finger after proximal phalanx fracture.

Soft Tissues

If there is an open wound, one should look for exposed bone, joint, or tendon. If any of these structures is exposed, there is more urgency in closing the wound. Irrigate, débride, and close the wound in the emergency room if definitive repair of underlying injuries will not occur for more than 8 hours. Simple closure is not appropriate, however, if a skin deficit, devitalized area, or contamination is present. For repair of these more complex wounds, the patient should be taken to the operating room as soon as can be arranged. A simple sketch of the original wound, including old scars, is an important part of the medical record. One should note any swelling, erythema, or other signs of infection. The muscles should be palpated to make sure that a compartment syndrome is not overlooked. Last, the wound should not be probed or explored without anesthesia, and local anesthetic should not be infiltrated into the wound until one has completed the sensory examination.

Skeleton

Obvious angular or rotational deformities indicate a dislocated joint or a displaced fracture (Fig. 8-2). Although skeletal injuries can cause loss of motion, the "rule" that if a patient can move a bone, it is not broken is utterly unreliable. In fact, fractures and dislocations can allow *abnormal* mobility. Point tenderness is a much more accurate sign of skeletal injury, especially when accompanied by swelling and bruising, and should trigger appropriate radiographic examination. One should request posteroanterior (PA), true lateral, and oblique radiographs of all injured hands. The part that is to be examined should be specified on the order for radiographs: If the long finger is injured, requesting a radiograph of the hand invariably produces a lateral projection with overlapped fingers, thus obscuring the injured finger. All three views are necessary because a fracture may be visible in only one view. (Treatment of specific upper extremity fractures is covered in Chapter 2.)

Motor Function

Evaluation of motor function should begin with observation of the child's resting posture and spontaneous movements. Normally, the fingers are held in slight flexion at rest because of the resting tone of the flexor muscles, which are stronger than the extensors. A complete flexor tendon laceration disrupts the normal cascade, with the injured digit being more extended than the uninjured ones (Fig. 8-3). Lack of spontaneous movement can be an indication of nerve, muscle, or tendon injury but can also be a response to pain. Painful skeletal

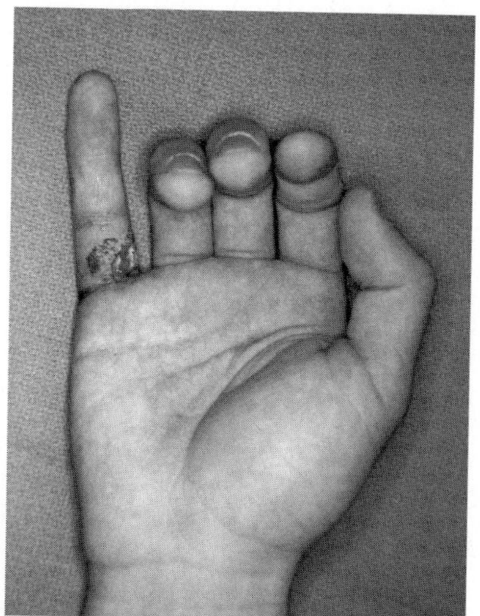

Figure 8-3 Complete flexor tendon laceration.

injuries, such as fractures, dislocations, and sprains, and soft tissue injuries, such as lacerations and even contusions, can all cause guarding.

One can gain additional information about motor function by performing tests that require some manipulation. In older cooperative patients, standard motor testing is performed. Table 8-2 lists the motor function and innervation of upper extremity muscles. Each muscle group on the uninjured side should be tested first to make sure that the patient understands what to do and to allow one to compare the strength of the injured and normal sides. In addition, any deficits in active or passive range of motion are noted. In younger or uncooperative patients, the tenodesis effect and the squeeze test can be used to test the digital flexor and extensor tendons. Resting muscle tone causes the fingers to flex as the wrist is extended and extend as the wrist is flexed (tenodesis effect; Fig. 8-4); because they also cross the wrist joint, wrist extension tightens the digital flexors, and wrist flexion extends the distal flexors. Direct compression of the finger and thumb flexors in the distal forearm tightens those tendons and will cause the digits to flex (squeeze test).[2] These last two tests also work when general anesthesia has been established. Nerve conduction studies and electromyography (EMG) can provide objective information about the level, severity, and chronicity of nerve injury.

Soft Tissue Injury

Skin

Skin on children is very elastic, and simple lacerations without tissue loss may look like large, open wounds. If irregularities along the two sides of the wound margin

Table 8-2 Upper Extremity Motor Function

Action	Muscles (Primary)	Chapter Figure No.	Nerves	Roots
Elbow				
Flexion	Biceps brachii, brachialis		Musculocutaneous	C5-C6
	Brachioradialis		Radial	C6-C7
Extension	Triceps brachii		Radial	C6-C7
Wrist				
Flexion	Flexor carpi radialis		Median	C6-C7
	Flexor carpi ulnaris		Ulnar	C8-T1
Extension	Extensor carpi radialis longus	8-10	Radial	C6-C7
	Extensor carpi radialis brevis	8-10	PIN	C6-C7
	Extensor carpi ulnaris	8-13	PIN	C6-C7
Forearm				
Pronation	Pronator teres		Median	C6-C7
	Pronator quadratus		AIN	C8-T1
Supination	Biceps brachii		Musculocutaneous	C5-C6
	Supinator		PIN	C6-C7
Thumb				
Flexion	Flexor pollicis longus	8-5	AIN	C8-T1
Extension	Extensor pollicis longus	8-11	PIN	C6-C7
Abduction	Abductor pollicis longus	8-9	PIN	C6-C7
Adduction	Adductor pollicis		Ulnar	C8-T1
Palmar abduction	Abductor pollicis brevis	8-14	Median	C8-T1
	Opponens pollicis			
Finger				
PIP flexion	Flexor digitorum superficialis	8-7	Median	C7-C8
DIP flexion	Flexor digitorum profundus	8-6	AIN (index, long)	C7-C8
			Ulnar (ring, small)	C7-C8
MP extension	Extensor digitorum communis	8-12	PIN	C6-C7
	Extensor indicis proprius	8-12	PIN	C6-C7
	Extensor digiti minimi	8-12	PIN	C7-C8
MP flexion, IP extension	Interossei, lumbricals		Ulnar	C8-T1
	Lumbricals		Median	C8-T1
Abduction	Dorsal interossei	8-16	Ulnar	C8-T1
	Abductor digiti minimi	8-17	(Small)	
Adduction	Volar interossei		Ulnar	C8-T1

AIN, anterior interosseous nerve, branch of median nerve; DIP, distal interphalangeal joint; MP, metacarpophalangeal joint; PIN, posterior interosseous nerve, branch of radial nerve; PIP, proximal interphalangeal joint.

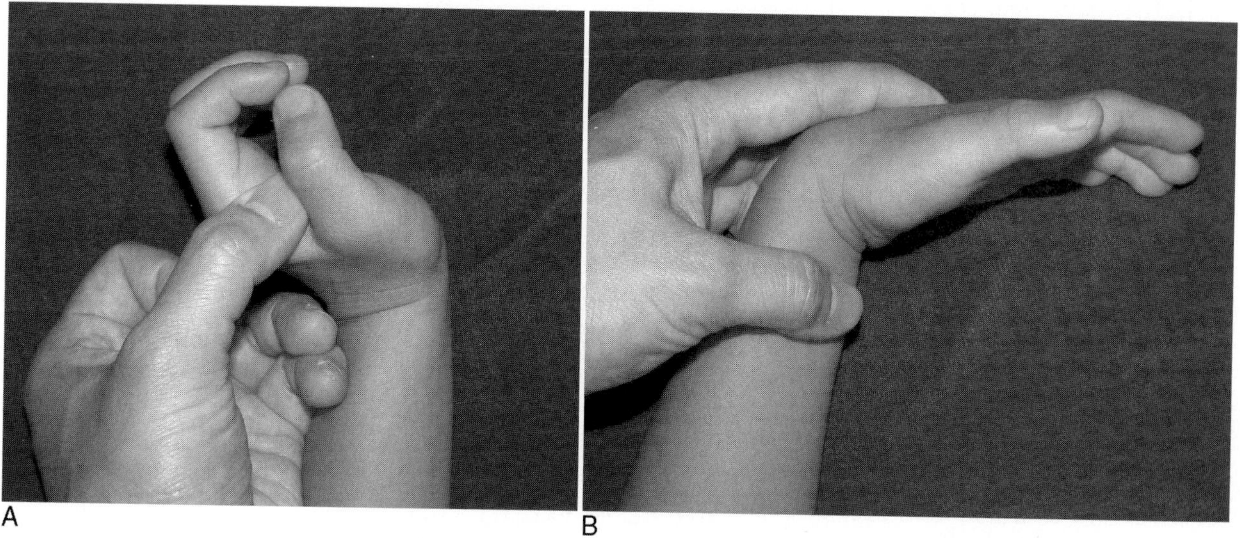

Figure 8-4 Tenodesis effect. A, Fingers passively flex with extension of the wrist. **B,** Fingers passively extend with flexion of the wrist.

match up, it is likely that no skin has been lost. Lacerations without skin loss can be irrigated, débrided, and closed primarily if there are no injuries to underlying structures. Before closure, the wound is explored to ensure that all structures within the zone of injury are indeed intact and that there are no foreign bodies in the wound. Radiographs can be helpful in identifying radiopaque foreign bodies and fractures. Lacerations that cross the digital flexion creases should be closed with a Z-plasty to avoid a flexion contracture after healing. Contaminated wounds can be débrided and treated with moist saline dressings, which are applied for 48 hours and changed twice daily, then closed if there are no signs of infection. Delayed primary closure is also useful for cases in which edema precludes primary closure without tension.

A single-layer closure with absorbable suture such as 5-0 plain gut is preferable in the fingers and palm, because (1) these areas usually heal with minimal visible scarring, even with absorbable suture, and (2) removal of nonabsorbable sutures can be as traumatic to the patient (and physician) as their insertion! On the dorsum of the hand and proximal to the wrist, scarring is more prominent; therefore, one should consider a subcuticular closure with an absorbable monofilament suture such as Monocryl®. This is a two-layer closure, consisting of buried interrupted sutures in the deep dermis to bring the wound edges together and a superficial running subcuticular suture to accurately align the skin edges.

Lacerations that create skin flaps can also be closed primarily. There is a risk of ischemia and necrosis of the flap, however, particularly if it is long and has a narrow base. If the flap is narrow, it should be excised and the wound closed primarily. To reduce tension on a larger flap, the wound is partially closed at the end near the tip of the flap before the flap is sutured back in place. Tension on a skin flap can reduce its viability. For degloving injuries, obviously nonviable skin is débrided, and the remaining skin is sutured down to the underlying tissues *under no tension*. This procedure maximizes the chance for survival of the degloved skin. The patient should returned to the operating room the next day for a "second look," excision of additional nonviable skin, and coverage of all open areas with skin graft. In major degloving injuries, the skin graft is harvested from the degloved skin with a dermatome and used for immediate coverage of the open wound at the initial operation.

Skin avulsion injuries create a true deficit in soft tissue coverage. The size of the defect and the nature of the wound bed determine the most appropriate method for coverage. Elevating and rearranging skin immediately adjacent to the wound can close smaller wounds. These *local flaps* can be advanced, transposed or rotated into the wound. The V-Y advancement flap is an example of a local flap that is particularly useful for closing fingertip defects (Fig. 8-5). A V-shaped incision is made in the skin adjacent to the open wound with the wound at the top of the V. The skin in the V is left attached to the subcutaneous tissues, from which it derives its blood supply. Advancing the skin flap into the open wound closes the primary defect, and suturing the skin together at the apex of the V to form a Y-shaped closure closes the resulting donor defect. By distributing the tension from closing a defect over a larger area, use of local flaps enables closure of defects that are too large for primary closure. Nevertheless, the flaps depend on the elasticity of skin adjacent to the defect, making them insufficient for large wounds.

Skin grafts can close large wounds that have a well-vascularized bed and no exposed bone, tendon, or joint. Full-thickness skin grafts provide better skin coverage

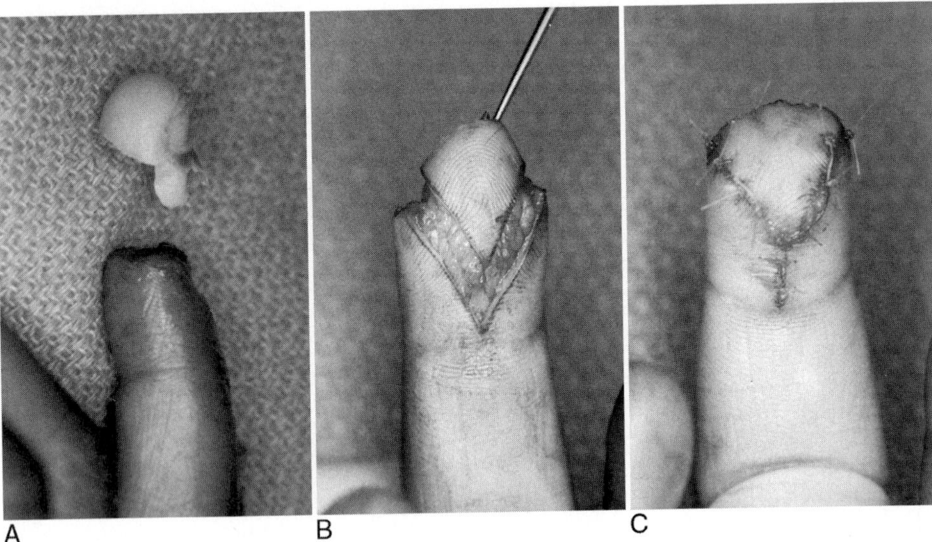

Figure 8-5 V-Y flap closure of fingertip amputation. A, Fingertip amputation. **B,** V-shaped advancement flap. **C,** Y-shaped closure.

because they contain the full thickness of the epidermis and dermis. The full-thickness skin graft contracts less during healing and is more durable and supple after it has healed than the split-thickness skin graft. For these reasons, full-thickness skin grafts are preferred over split-thickness grafts in the hand, where contraction of the graft would limit motion. However, because of the thickness of the graft, the nutrients from the wound bed have a longer distance to diffuse during the first few days after grafting, before capillary ingrowth occurs. Full-thickness skin grafts thus have a lower rate of survival ("take"). Potential donor sites for full-thickness skin grafts, in decreasing order of size, are the lower abdomen, groin, elbow flexion crease, and wrist flexion crease.

Split-thickness skin grafts contain the epidermis and a partial thickness of the dermis (Fig. 8-6). The thickness can be adjusted fairly accurately with modern dermatomes. Because some dermis is left behind at the donor site, the site will eventually reepithelialize just like a second-degree burn, leaving a scar. This feature allows one to harvest split-thickness grafts of much larger size than is possible with full-thickness skin grafts, which are limited by the need to close the donor site.

If a wound is too large for closure with local flaps and the bed is not suitable for skin grafting, one can chose a regional, distant, or free skin flap to close the wound. Such flaps can contain skin but also subcutaneous tissue, muscle, bone, nerve, and even tendon. They provide soft tissue coverage and restore function as well.

Regional flaps utilize tissue that is not immediately adjacent to the wound but can be transferred over to cover the wound while remaining attached to its blood supply. The radial forearm flap is an example of a regional flap that can be used to cover defects from the metacarpophalangeal joints to the elbow; it is based on its vascular pedicle, consisting of the radial artery and veins (Fig. 8-7).

A *distant flap* brings tissue from distant parts of the body to the hand but is left attached to the donor site for approximately 2 weeks to allow for ingrowth of blood supply to the flap from the hand. The flap is then divided from the distant donor site and survives on its new blood supply entering the flap around the periphery from the native hand skin. Unlike the skin graft, which derives its blood supply from the wound bed under the graft, a distant flap can be used to cover tissue not suitable for skin grafting (e.g., tendon) as long as the skin around the wound is well vascularized. The groin flap can supply a fairly large area of skin and subcutaneous tissue and still allow for primary closure of the donor site. It is very useful for coverage of soft tissue defects in the hand and wrist (Fig. 8-8).

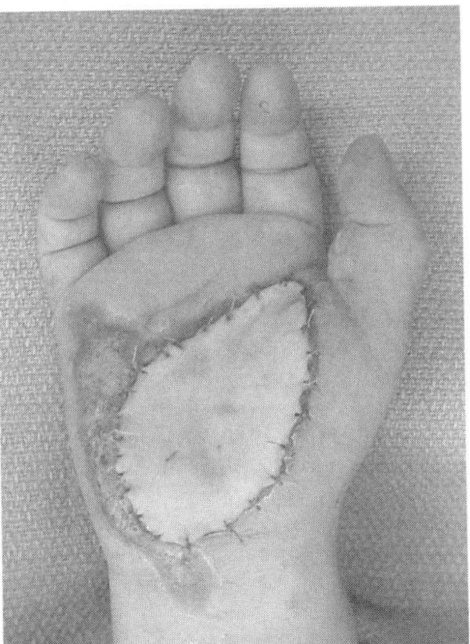

Figure 8-6 Split-thickness skin graft covering a palm abrasion wound.

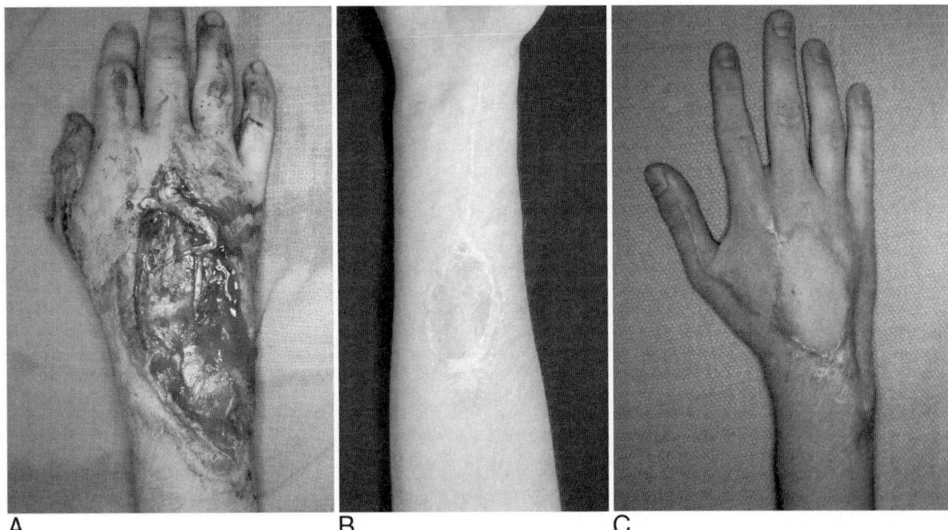

Figure 8-7 Radial forearm flap. A, Dorsal hand avulsion wound. **B,** Flap donor site covered with skin graft. **C,** Healed flap.

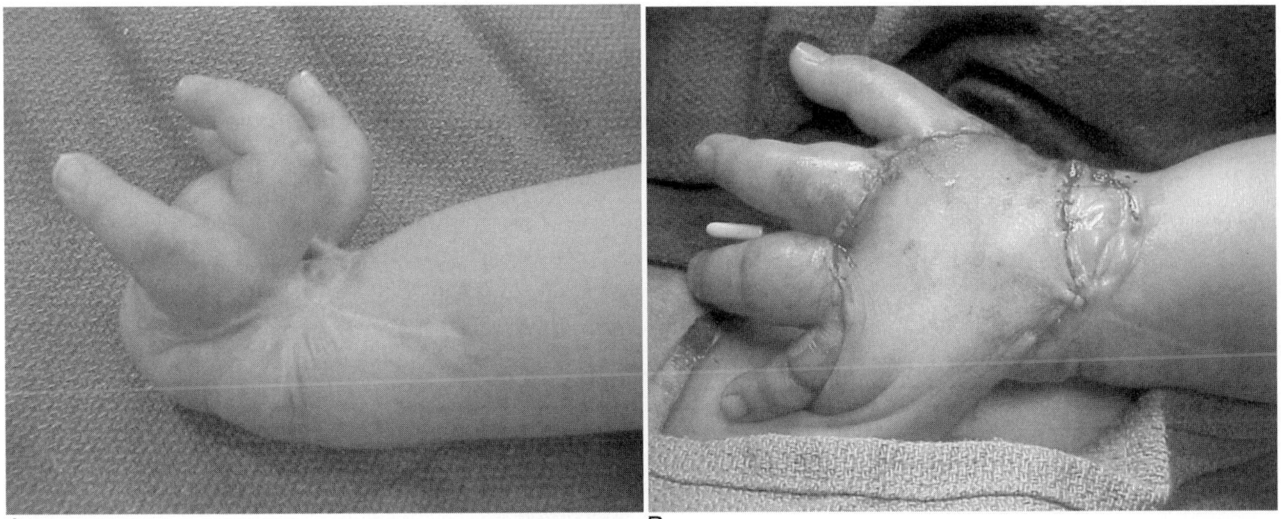

A

B

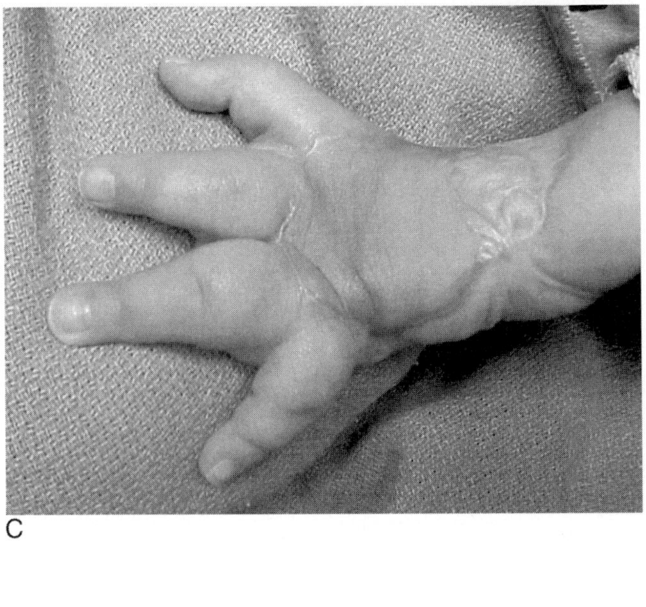

C

Figure 8-8 Groin flap. A, Wrist contracture from severe intravenous infiltration. **B,** First stage of groin flap. **C,** Healed flap.

Free flaps are the most versatile flaps for soft tissue coverage of the hand. Any area of tissue with a single dominant artery and vein can be transferred as a free flap to cover a soft tissue defect, as long as a suitable recipient artery and vein can be found near the defect to anastomose with the flap's vessels. Unlike regional flaps, free flaps are not tethered to a limited "arc of rotation." Unlike distant flaps, free flaps do not force the hand to be tied to another part of the body for 2 weeks. Use of a free flap is technically more demanding, however, especially in very young children, because of the need to perform microvascular anastomoses. Nevertheless, only a free flap can cover some extensive soft tissue defects. Figure 8-9 shows the arm of a 4 year-old patient who was dragged by a car and suffered deep abrasion injuries exposing the elbow joint. A scapular free flap was transferred from the patient's back to cover the joint, and skin grafts were harvested to cover the exposed muscle.

Vascular

Exsanguinating hemorrhage, although rare, is one of only two hand emergencies that can be truly life threatening (the other being necrotizing infection). Partial laceration of a major artery is almost always the source, because a completely transected vessel usually undergoes retraction and thrombosis. To control bleeding, one elevates the extremity and applies direct pressure to the bleeding vessel with a gloved finger. Because of collateral circulation, both ends of the lacerated vessel must be compressed. In most cases, bleeding stops after 10 minutes of *constant* pressure. Applying pressure with a large wad of gauze diffuses the pressure and is less effective. Wrapping an elastic bandage over a large wad of gauze to create a pressure dressing should also be avoided because the bandage becomes a tourniquet, causing venous engorgement and distal ischemia. If bleeding cannot be controlled by direct pressure alone, one can apply pressure to the brachial artery proximal to the injury to diminish the arterial inflow while continuing to apply direct pressure to the bleeding vessel.

As a last resort, a pneumatic tourniquet can be applied proximal to the bleeding vessel, and the patient rapidly transported to the operating room for surgical control of the bleeding. Without anesthesia, most patients have unbearable ischemic pain after a tourniquet has been inflated for 15 to 20 minutes, and the tourniquet will have to be released for at least 5 minutes before re-inflation. The arm can be exsanguinated by elevation before inflation of the tourniquet to 100 mm Hg above systolic pressure. A blood pressure cuff wrapped with tape can substitute for a pneumatic tourniquet, but the tubes on the cuff must be clamped to maintain pressure. A belt or

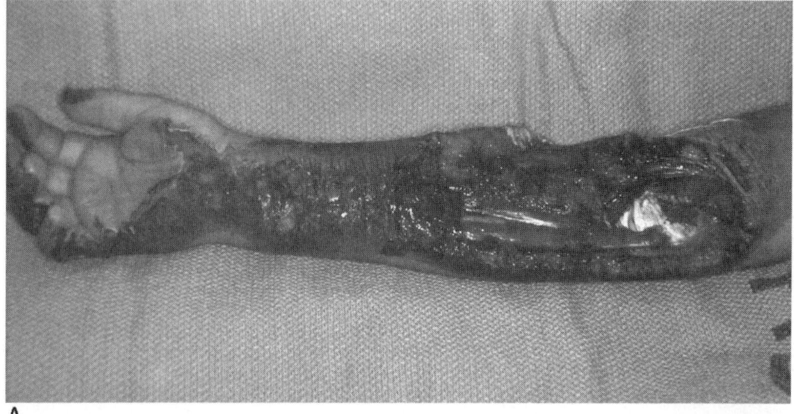
A

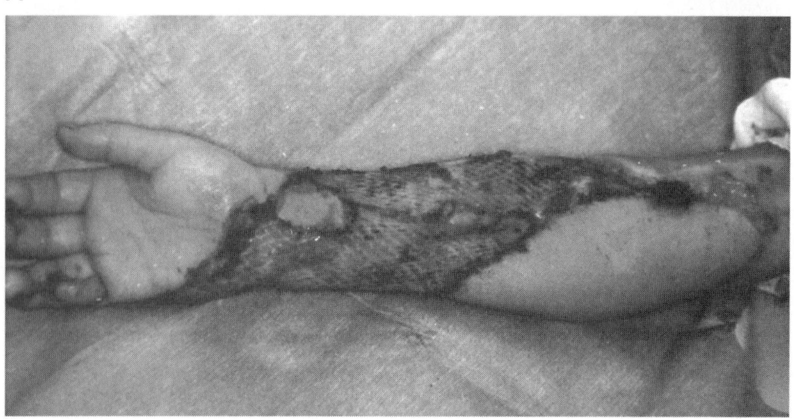
B

Figure 8-9 Scapular free flap. A, Deep abrasion injury with exposed elbow joint. **B,** Joint covered with a scapular flap.

Box 8-2 Ways to Stop Bleeding

Direct pressure
Elevation
Pneumatic tourniquet
Not clamping

other narrow band should not be used as a tourniquet because it applies pressure over a very small area and can cause permanent injury to underlying nerves. Bleeding vessels should never be blindly clamped, because nerves accompany most major blood vessels. Box 8-2 summarizes ways to stop bleeding.

In addition to bleeding, vascular injuries can also cause ischemia of the hand or arm. Collateral circulation is usually excellent in children, but occlusion of both digital arteries to a digit or both the radial and ulnar arteries in the forearm can produce ischemia. If the palmar arch is incomplete, occluding either the radial or ulnar artery can cause part of the hand to become ischemic. Because of collateral circulation, occluding the brachial artery may or may not cause ischemia, depending on the length and location of the occluded segment. Once a lacerated artery has been identified and occluded, one can assess the distal perfusion and decide whether to repair or ligate the vessel.

If distal perfusion is adequate, both the proximal and distal cut ends of the artery should be ligated. Sometimes, the patient is no longer bleeding when examined but has a history of pulsatile bleeding immediately after injury. In this instance, one must still identify and ligate the injured artery to prevent delayed hemorrhage, arteriovenous fistulas, and pseudoaneurysm formation.

If distal perfusion is inadequate, prompt restoration of perfusion is essential. Muscle suffers permanent damage after 6 hours of warm ischemia. In most cases of penetrating trauma, the patient should be taken directly to the operating room for exploration and repair of the injured vessel. A fractured limb with ischemia should be reduced and splinted to see whether perfusion improves with better alignment. If the ischemia persists, the patient should undergo emergency angiography followed by operative repair. Usually one finds that the vessel is trapped in the fracture site or that the vessel has a segmental thrombosis from intimal damage. In the upper extremity, vascular injury is most common after a supracondylar humeral fracture, which can damage the brachial artery (Fig. 8-10). The damaged segment of artery should be resected and replaced with an interposition vein graft. Prophylactic fasciotomy should be performed if ischemia time exceeds 4 to 6 hours.

Radial artery cannulation for hemodynamic monitoring, especially if the patient is hypotensive or receiving vasopressors, can also cause hand ischemia (Fig. 8-11). The initial treatment is to remove the cannula and improve cardiac output. Anticoagulation or thrombolytic therapy may be helpful if ischemia persists and threatens tissue loss. Surgical revascularization is another option, but many patients who need radial arterial lines for monitoring are not stable enough for a long microsurgical procedure. An Allen test (Box 8-3) should be performed before a radial artery cannula is placed, to ensure that the hand will be adequately perfused by the ulnar artery. If all of the digits do not promptly reperfuse with only the ulnar artery open, the palmar arterial arch is incomplete, and the thumb may become ischemic if a radial arterial line is inserted.

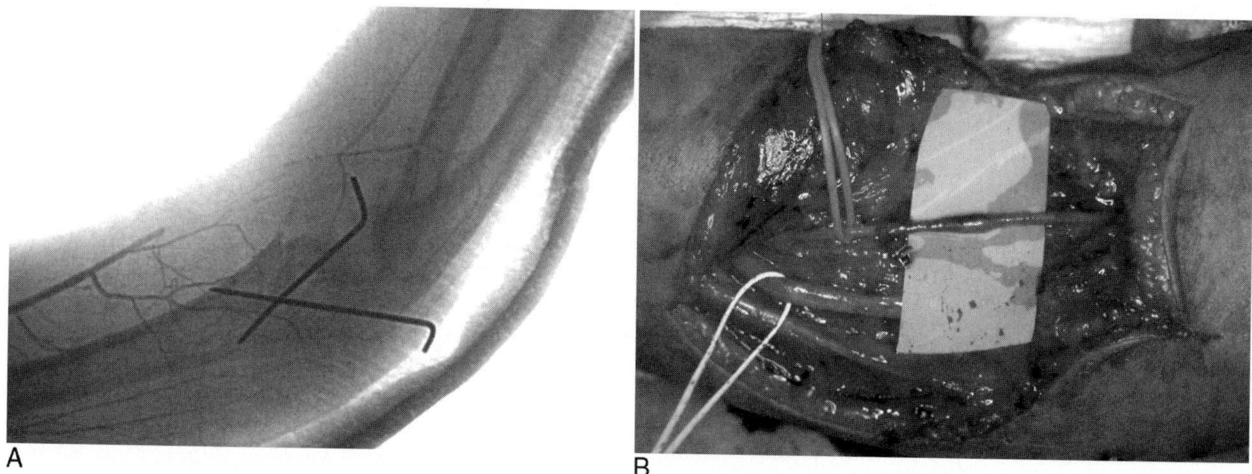

Figure 8-10 Brachial artery occlusion after supracondylar humeral fracture. **A,** Angiogram. **B,** Thrombosed segment.

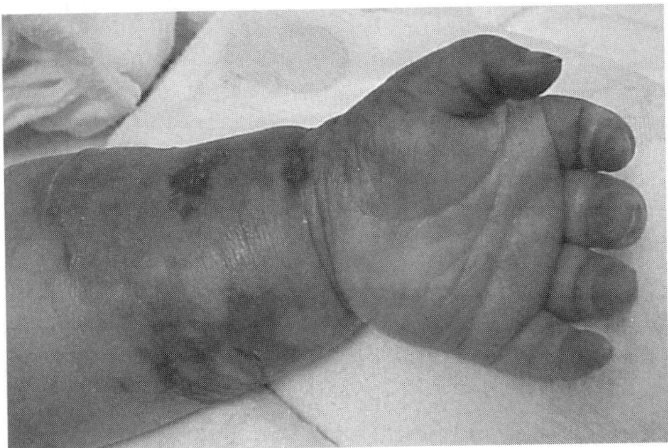

Figure 8-11 Hand ischemia after radial artery cannulation.

Nerve

Nerve injuries in children occur usually after penetrating trauma. Lacerations with broken glass seem especially prone to involve deep neurovascular and tendinous structures, even when the skin laceration appears small and innocuous. One should suspect a nerve laceration if there are motor or sensory deficits distal to the level of injury or if there is an arterial injury, because many nerves travel with arteries in the upper extremity (Table 8-3). Nerve injuries from sharp penetrating trauma should be treated with exploration and repair. If there are other associated injuries that require immediate exploration (e.g., vascular), nerve repair can be performed at the same time. Otherwise, the wound can be irrigated and closed, and a delayed primary nerve repair can be performed within a week. Repair of lacerations to small, purely sensory nerves (e.g., digital nerves) can be delayed for up to 3 weeks without compromise of the final outcome. Nerve deficits after gunshot wounds are best observed for 3 weeks to see whether there is any spontaneous recovery of nerve function, which can occur if the nerve has not been directly transected by the bullet. If the nerve has been transected, the delay allows for clear demarcation of the zone of injury by fibrosis, so that this segment of the nerve can be débrided before nerve repair (which usually requires nerve graft).

Box 8-3 Allen's Test

1. Elevate and squeeze the hand to exsanguinate.
2. Compress radial and ulnar arteries at the wrist.
3. Release the radial artery with the hand open, and check for capillary refill.
4. Repeat steps 1 and 2, then release the ulnar artery and check capillary refill.

Table 8-3 Nerves in Close Proximity to Arteries

Artery	Adjacent Nerve(s)
Axillary	Brachial plexus
Brachial	Median and ulnar
Ulnar	Ulnar
Digital	Digital

Blunt trauma can cause nerve injury by direct crush, compartment syndrome, or traction. The extent of injury determines the potential for recovery. *Neurapraxia* produces a localized conduction block with no Tinel sign (tingling with percussion over a nerve) at the site of injury. Recovery should begin by 3 weeks and be complete by 3 months.[3] *Axonotmesis* produces axonal damage with loss of the axoplasm and myelin distal to the injury (Wallerian degeneration). The nerve regenerates at a rate of 1 mm/day through axonal sprouting into the empty Schwann cell tubes. Tinel sign is present at the site of injury and advances with the regenerating nerve. The time to recovery is determined by the distance between the site of injury and the end organ. *Neurotmesis* is complete transection of the nerve. A neuroma forms at the end of the transected nerve and may cause dysesthesia. Because nerve function does not recover without surgery, repair of the transected nerve is the best way to avoid neuroma symptoms. These specific levels of nerve injury are discrete points along a continuum. In many nerve injuries, the extent of injury is different in different parts of the same nerve.

Electrodiagnostic testing can be a useful adjunct to clinical tests in determining the severity of injury and following the progress of recovery. The presence of denervation changes on electromyography, such as fibrillations or positive sharp waves, signifies a level of injury higher than neurapraxia. Nerve conduction studies can help to determine the severity and location of injury but may not identify partial nerve injuries.

Good prognosis for recovery after nerve repair is associated with nerves with pure motor or sensory function, patient age less than 10 years, sharp mechanism of injury, more distal location of injury, and delay of repair less than 6 months. With prolonged delay in nerve repair, recovery of motor and sensory function is limited by degeneration of the end organs. After denervation, muscle becomes atrophied by 2 months, fibrotic by 1 year, and fragmented by 3 years. The motor end plates are gone after 2 years; therefore, recovery of motor function is not expected after 2 years of denervation. With sensory function, there is no clear correlation between timing of repair and prognosis for recovery, except that after

1 year, one can expect recovery of only protective sensibility. The total delay in reinnervation is the sum of the delay in repair plus the time needed for the nerve to regrow from the point of injury to the end organ (roughly 1 month for each inch).

Tendon

Tendon injuries are primarily caused by penetrating trauma, and the diagnosis is usually clear from the history and physical findings. A common mechanism of tendon injury in children is laceration from broken glass or a knife. One must assume that any tendon deep to a skin laceration may have been injured, and every tendon in the zone of injury should be tested. A tendon injury should be suspected if there is evidence of nerve or arterial injury in the hand, because nerves, arteries, and tendons lie in close proximity. The level of the tendon injury may be different from the level of the skin laceration, depending on the position of the hand during injury. For example, if a flexor tendon laceration occurs with the fingers in a fully flexed position, the tendon laceration retracts distal to the skin laceration when the hand is examined in an open position.

The hand is first observed in the resting posture: All of the fingers should be in a gently flexed posture with the small finger most flexed and the index finger least flexed. A *complete* tendon laceration causes the affected finger to fall outside this normal cascade (see Fig. 8-3). Each tendon should then be tested by active motion both without and with resistance (Fig. 8-12). In a finger with a partial tendon laceration, resting posture and active motion are normal, but resisted motion produces pain. Young children may not cooperate with active motor testing because of anxiety, pain, or inability to understand the directions. Magnetic resonance imaging (MRI) and high-resolution ultrasonography can demonstrate tendon lacerations but are currently not reliable in partial tendon lacerations. Surgical exploration may be the only way to determine whether a tendon or nerve has been injured. Exploration in the emergency room should be discouraged, because visualization is usually inadequate because of poor lighting as well as lack of proper instruments, anesthesia, and exposure.

Flexor tendon injuries are divided in to five zones (Fig. 8-13). The level of the tendon injury with the finger extended, not the level of the skin laceration, determines the zone of injury. Zone 2, extending from the distal palmar flexion crease to the middle of the middle phalanx, is often referred to as "no man's land" because results of repair are poorest in this area. The flexor digitorum superficialis (FDS) and profundus (FDP) tendons are enclosed in a tight flexor tendon sheath in zone 2, and they tend to adhere to each other and to the surrounding sheath after repair. Flexor tendon injuries are best explored and repaired within 1 week, before the proximal end of the tendon retracts and the tendon sheath fills with scar tissue. If treatment is delayed, a primary repair may not be possible, necessitating a two-stage repair with tendon grafting, which carries a much worse prognosis.

In addition to partial lacerations, flexor tendon injuries are most often missed in the palm (zone 3) and wrist (zone 5). The FDS lies superficial to the FDP in the palm and can be completely transected, leaving the FDP intact. The finger will still flex at all three joints but flexion of the proximal interphalangeal joint will be weak and cause pain. The wrist flexors, flexor carpi ulnaris (FCU) and flexor carpi radialis (FCR), are superficial and may be

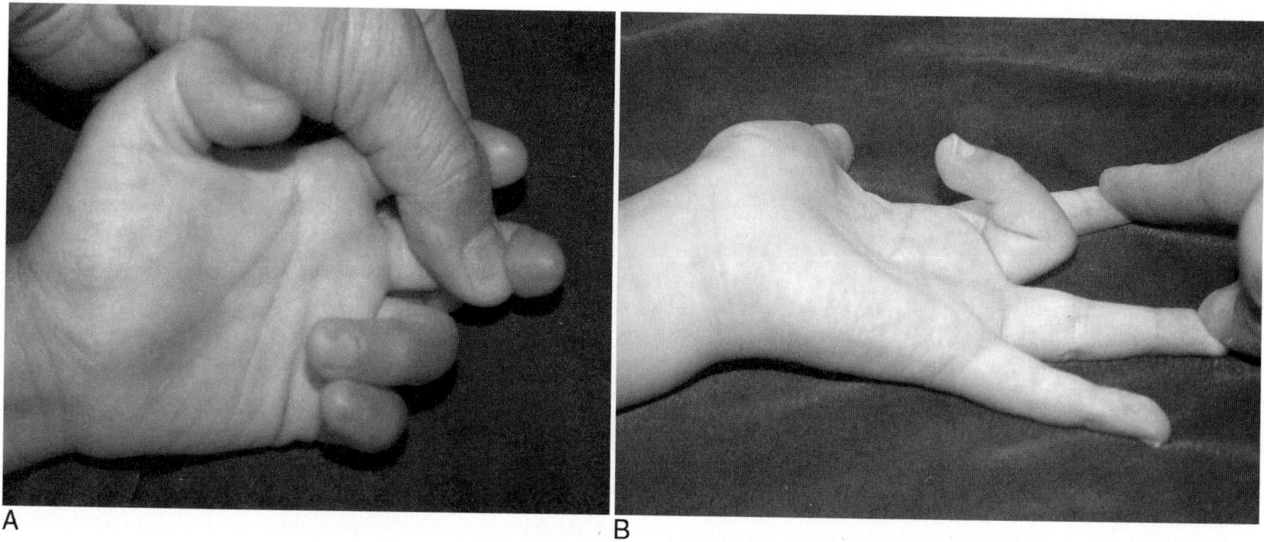

Figure 8-12 **A,** Flexor digitorum profundus. **B,** Flexor digitorum superficialis.

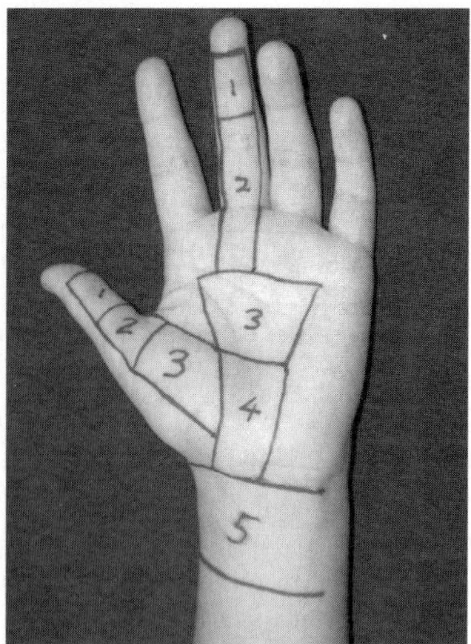

Figure 8-13 Zones of flexor tendon injury.

lacerated without injury to the deeper digital flexors. The wrist still flexes actively with just the digital flexors intact, but flexion against resistance causes pain.

A flexor tendon injury can occur without laceration of the skin. The patient usually gives a history of grabbing an opponent's jersey while playing ball, and feeling a sharp pain or snapping sensation in the long finger. Afterwards, the patient is unable to actively flex the distal interphalangeal (DIP) joint (Fig. 8-14) and may attribute the injury to a sprain or dislocation. However, the injury is actually an avulsion of the FDP from its insertion on the distal phalanx (jersey finger), caused by forced flexion against resistance. The avulsed tendon may retract proximally into the palm and should be repaired within a week to prevent excessive shortening of the tendon-muscle unit and scarring of the tendon sheath.

Extensor tendon injuries, if not recognized and repaired, can cause flexion deformities of underlying joints. The deformity may not be immediately apparent but instead may develop over time and may involve adjacent joints as the finely balanced extensor mechanism is thrown out of balance. As with flexor tendon injuries, diagnosis is usually apparent on physical examination. Resisted extension is weak compared with the uninjured side and produces pain. Extensor tendons usually do not retract as much as flexor tendons, and the cut ends may be clearly visible in the wound. If both ends are visible, the tendon is repaired in the emergency room. Otherwise, the wound should be irrigated and closed, and the patient referred to a hand surgeon for tendon repair within 3 weeks. Independent extensor tendons, such as the thumb extensors, extensor indicis proprius (index finger), and extensor digiti minimi (small finger), should be repaired within 1 to 2 weeks because they are not tethered to adjacent tendons via juncturae tendinum and tend to retract when lacerated. Lacerations to dorsal radial and ulnar sensory nerves are common and should be repaired at the time of tendon repair.

A *mallet finger* deformity (inability to extend the DIP joint) develops after injury to the terminal portion of the digital extensor tendon (Fig. 8-15). The mechanism of injury can be a laceration of the tendon over the DIP joint or, more commonly, a blunt axial load injury to the end of the finger, which causes avulsion of the tendon from its insertion at the base of the distal phalanx. The closed injury can cause avulsion of a fragment of bone from the distal phalanx articular surface; therefore, radiographs are essential. In the child, the fracture may involve the growth plate. Most closed mallet injuries, even with fracture, are best treated with 6 weeks of constant (24 hours/day) splinting in extension. One can use a straight dorsal padded aluminum splint secured by

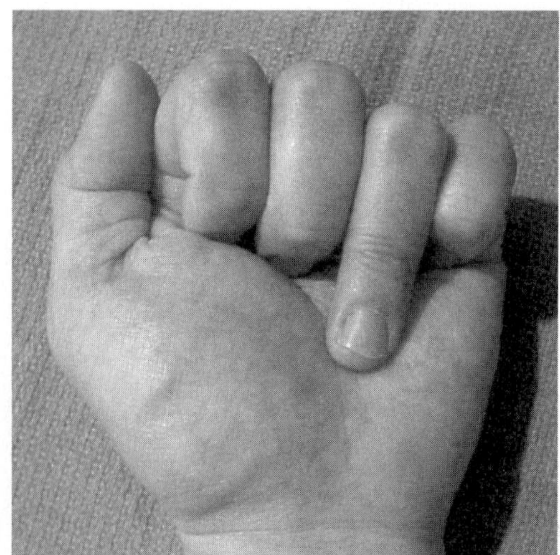

Figure 8-14 Jersey finger (flexor digitorum profundus avulsion).

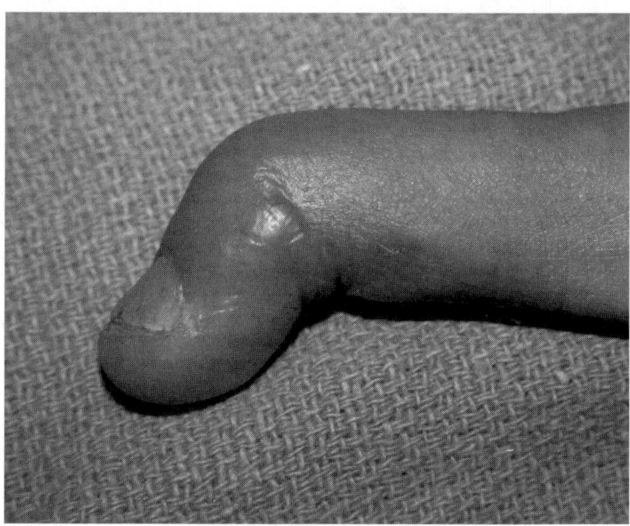

Figure 8-15 Mallet finger.

tape or a specially designed splint like the Stack splint. The DIP joint should be kept in extension without hyperextension to avoid ulceration of the skin on the dorsum of the digit. Splinting can be used successfully to treat a mallet injury even if the patient presents as late as 6 months after injury.[4] The proximal interphalangeal (PIP) joint is left free; active motion is encouraged at the PIP and metacarpophalangeal (MP) joints to avoid stiffness. Displaced mallet fractures that are associated with subluxation of the DIP joint or that are seen on the lateral radiograph to involve more than one third of the articular surface should be treated with anatomic reduction and internal fixation. Lacerations to the terminal extensor tendon should be repaired with suture and immobilized in extension for 4 weeks. Untreated terminal extensor injuries can lead to a fixed flexion deformity of the DIP joint and hyperextension at the PIP joint, the *swan neck deformity* (Fig. 8-16).

Injury to the extensor tendon over the PIP joint allows unopposed flexion at the joint by the FDS tendon and over time can lead to the *boutonnière deformity* (Fig. 8-17), which consists of hyperextension of the DIP joint, fixed flexion of the PIP joint, and hyperextension of the MP joint. The portion of the extensor tendon over the PIP joint, the central slip, inserts dorsally at the base of the middle phalanx and can be injured by laceration or by dislocation of the PIP joint. Central slip injury is often missed and should be suspected if the patient has pain and weakness on resisted extension of the PIP joint, even if he or she can actively extend the joint immediately after injury. The boutonnière deformity may not develop for several weeks after injury, until the lateral bands on either side of the central slip subluxate palmar to the axis of the PIP joint and become flexors of the joint rather than extensors. This deformity is treated with splinting the finger in extension at the PIP joint for a minimum of 4 weeks, leaving the MP and DIP joints free. Open central slip injuries should be sutured and then splinted.

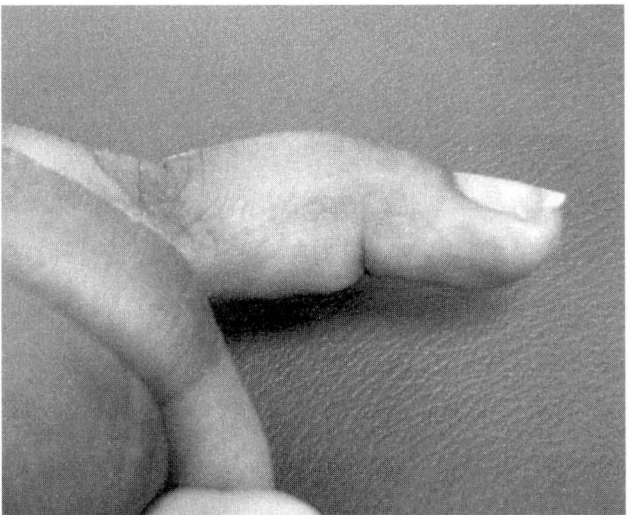

Figure 8-16 Swan neck deformity.

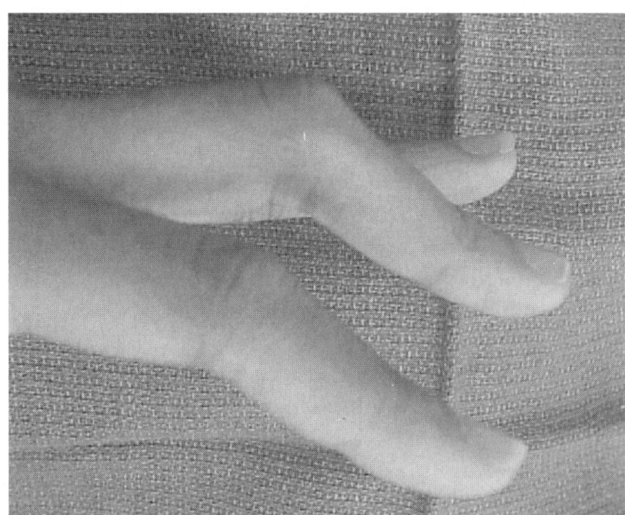

Figure 8-17 Boutonnière deformity.

The extensor mechanism over the MP joint is made up of a thick central portion and a thin extensor hood that encircles the dorsum of the proximal phalanx. Lacerations are typically partial but should be repaired by direct suture within 3 weeks. (The skin should be closed in the emergency room, and the hand placed in a volar splint.) Laceration of the central extensor tendon causes pain on resisted extension and an extensor lag at the MP joint. Lacerations over the MP joint are often "fight bites," caused by a striking of clenched fist on an opponent's tooth, and are at high risk for septic arthritis (discussed later). Laceration of the extensor hood may lead to subluxation of the central extensor tendon to either the radial or ulnar side of the joint, making it difficult for the patient to initiate extension of the MP joint from a flexed position.

Overall, extensor tendon injuries have a better prognosis than flexor tendon injuries. It is imperative that flexor tendon injuries be recognized and repaired promptly, because primary repair carries a much better prognosis. Prognosis is worse in tendon injuries associated with extensive soft tissue trauma, fracture, and neurovascular injury. In these combined injuries, the priority for repair is revascularization, skeletal stabilization, and then soft tissue coverage.

Compartment Syndrome

One of the true emergencies in hand surgery, *compartment syndrome*, is excessive pressure in the subfascial muscle compartments that results in irreversible loss of muscle and nerve function if left untreated. Causes include severe crush injuries, bleeding after arterial puncture, fractures, burns, muscle ischemia, and excessively tight casts. Any mechanism that causes swelling of the muscle raises compartment pressure and reduces venous outflow, so can initiate a positive-feedback loop whereby increased pressure decreases venous outflow, thus further increasing pressure within the tight fascial compartment, ultimately causing ischemic necrosis of the muscles and nerves within the compartment. Compartment syndrome may affect the volar or dorsal compartments of the forearm and the intrinsic muscle compartments of the hand (Fig. 8-18). The hand and forearm compartments are listed in Table 8-4.

Pain in the involved muscle compartment out of proportion to injury is usually the first symptom. Pain on passive stretch of those muscles is pathognomonic. The compartment becomes tense and painful to palpation. Compression of the nerves in the compartment causes paresthesias and later leads to paralysis. Pallor and loss of distal pulses are late findings that may not be present in all cases of compartment syndrome. Symptoms of compartment syndrome are listed in Table 8-5. If this disorder is left untreated, the muscles and nerves in the compartment undergo ischemic necrosis, leaving the extremity paralyzed, contracted, and insensate (*Volkmann's contracture*).

If the diagnosis of compartment syndrome remains equivocal after physical examination, the compartment pressure can be measured with an arterial line setup and an 18-gauge needle or a commercially available device specifically made for measuring compartment pressure. A pressure higher than 30 mm Hg, or within 30 mm Hg of the mean arterial pressure in a hypotensive patient, warrants fasciotomy.[5] Serial measurements of compartment pressure may be useful in obtunded patients. Compartment pressure measurement is contraindicated in patients who have coagulopathies and in patients with clear signs and symptoms of compartment syndrome.

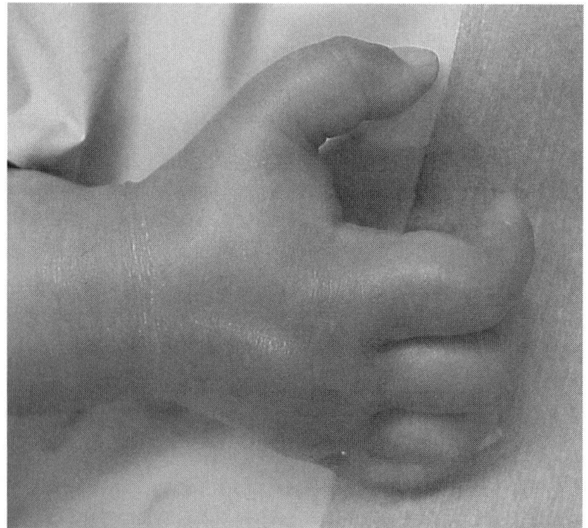

Figure 8-18 Compartment syndrome of the hand after crush injury.

Table 8-4 Forearm and Hand Compartments

Forearm	Hand
Volar	Thenar
Dorsal	Hypothenar
Radial (mobile wad)	Interosseous

Treatment of compartment syndrome consists of urgent fasciotomy of all affected compartments with débridement of devitalized tissues. In severe cases, the wound may be left packed open until the swelling subsides, and then closed with skin grafting. The carpal tunnel should also be decompressed, but the skin can be closed to protect the median nerve and flexor tendons. Prophylactic fasciotomy should be considered for obtunded patients with a mechanism of injury appropriate to compartment syndrome or with injuries that have caused a period of ischemia to the limb. Early hand rehabilitation is essential to restore maximal range of motion.

Compartment syndrome is a problem that responds readily to early treatment and is irreversible when found late. The presence of compartment syndrome should be actively sought in every patient with a high-energy injury to the limb. If signs and symptoms are not present at the initial examination, they can appear later, when swelling increases as a response to injury. Serial examinations are warranted until the swelling subsides. Complaints of growing pain after application of a dressing or cast should prompt removal of the entire dressing or cast and examination for compartment syndrome. Missed diagnosis and late diagnosis are the main pitfalls associated with compartment syndrome.

Fingertip and Nail Bed Injuries

Fingertip injuries are very common in children, most often occurring from crushing of the finger in a door. Initial examination should note the level of injury, presence of nail bed injury, and whether there is exposed

Table 8-5 Symptoms of Compartment Syndrome

Timing	Symptom
Early	Pain
	Paresthesias
Late	Paralysis
	Pallor
	Pulselessness

bone. If the fingertip is still attached, the distal tip color, capillary refill, and sensibility should be checked. Radiographs are essential.

The level of injury determines the choice of treatment for complete amputations. Amputation distal to the bone heals well with daily dressing changes. The parents must be reassured that fingertip amputation wounds less than 1 cm in diameter, with no exposed bone, heal better by secondary intention than surgical closure. Amputations through the distal phalanx require closure with a local fingertip flap or a thenar flap to cover the bone and maintain length (Fig. 8-19). Amputations proximal to the nail fold but distal to the DIP joint are best treated with shortening and primary closure. In children younger than 2 years, the fingertips are so small that amputated fingertips can survive as composite grafts if they are sutured back on with a few absorbable sutures to approximate the skin. Amputations proximal to the DIP joint should be considered for replantation, which is discussed in the following section.

Incomplete amputations are often associated with nail bed lacerations and distal phalanx fractures (Fig. 8-20). These injuries can usually be treated in the emergency room with use of sedation and digital nerve block. A Penrose drain is used as a digital tourniquet to achieve a bloodless field. The nail plate should be dissected free of the nail bed with a fine hemostat or smooth periosteal elevator to fully expose the laceration. The nail bed is then repaired with 6-0 or 7-0 absorbable sutures, and the nail plate is replaced to protect the repair. Realignment and repair of the nail bed laceration is usually sufficient treatment for the underlying fracture as well. Lacerations of the adjacent skin can be repaired with 6-0 absorbable sutures.

A laceration through the most proximal portion of the nail bed can be associated with an open Salter-Harris type 1 fracture of the distal phalanx growth plate (Seymour fracture). Such a fracture should be treated in the operating room with irrigation, reduction, and percutaneous pinning (Fig. 8-21), which bring the nail bed laceration together without the need for suturing.

Isolated subungual hematomas from a crush injury to the fingertip can be very painful and can be drained by trephination of the nail plate with an ophthalmic cautery or heated paper clip. The nail plate should be removed and nail bed explored if there is a displaced fracture of the distal phalanx, laceration of the skin adjacent to the nail, or displacement of the proximal portion of the nail plate from the nail fold. These three findings are more accurate predictors of nail bed laceration than the size of the hematoma.

Amputations

Amputations in children are most often caused by a crush or avulsion mechanism such as from a bicycle chain or spoke. Replantation of the amputated part is the ideal reconstruction, because it restores both form and function without any donor site morbidity and maintains growth potential. By definition *replantation* is reattachment of a completely amputated part, whereas *revascularization* is reattachment of an incompletely amputated part requiring vascular reconstruction (Fig. 8-22). If there are no life-threatening injuries and replantation is technically feasible, all amputated parts should be replanted in children.

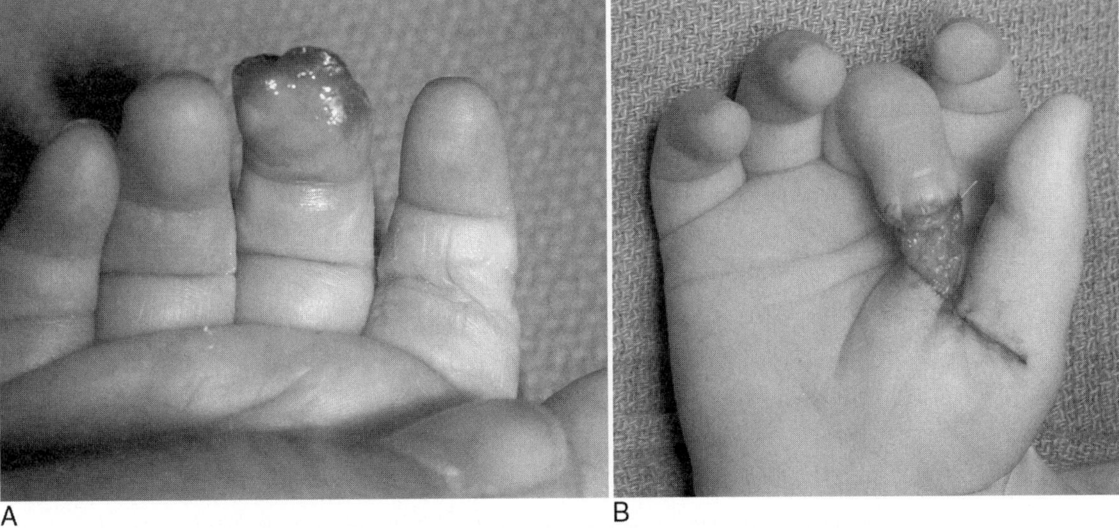

Figure 8-19 **A,** Fingertip amputation with exposed bone. **B,** Thenar flap attached.

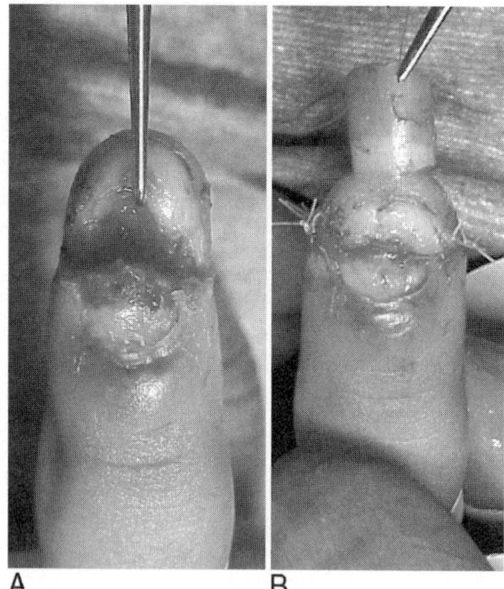

Figure 8-20 **A,** Nail bed laceration. **B,** Nail bed after repair.

Initial treatment for a child with an amputation begins with a complete trauma survey to identify other, potentially life-threatening injuries. An intravenous line is established, cephalothin is administered, and tetanus prophylaxis is given. The amputation stump is irrigated, bleeding is stopped, and a sterile dressing is applied. Radiographs of the stump and the amputated part are obtained. The part is then irrigated, wrapped in moist saline gauze, and placed in a sterile watertight container. The container is placed in mixture of ice and water to cool the part, thus delaying the onset of ischemic necrosis. Partially amputated parts should be immobilized with a splint and cooled with an ice pack over the dressing. *The amputation should NOT be completed.* If the patient is stable, prompt transfer should be arranged to a replantation center. One should avoid the temptation to reassure the patient or family that the part can be replanted. Only the surgeon, after exploration in the operating room, can determine whether a part can be replanted. Contraindications to replantation include multilevel injury (Fig. 8-23), prolonged ischemia time, and severe crush or avulsion.

Replantation entails 4 to 8 hours of surgery for a single digit. The replanted part is monitored by continuous pulse oximetry and hourly checks of color and capillary refill for the first 48 to 72 hours after surgery. Any sign of decreased perfusion or venous insufficiency should prompt a return to the operating room for reexploration. The patient remains hospitalized for approximately 1 week after replantation. The hemoglobin level should be monitored; children require transfusion after replantation more commonly than adults.

Approximately 70% to 85% of upper extremity replantations in children survive, a lower percentage than that for adults. However, children achieve better function if the part survives, because of superior nerve regeneration, bone healing, and joint mobility. Functional outcome after replantation is poorest for crush and avulsion injuries and best for partial amputations. The functional outcome also depends on the level of the amputation: Replantation at the upper arm or proximal forearm carries the worst prognosis, whereas replantation at the wrist, the palm, or the finger distal to the insertion of the FDS carries the best prognosis.

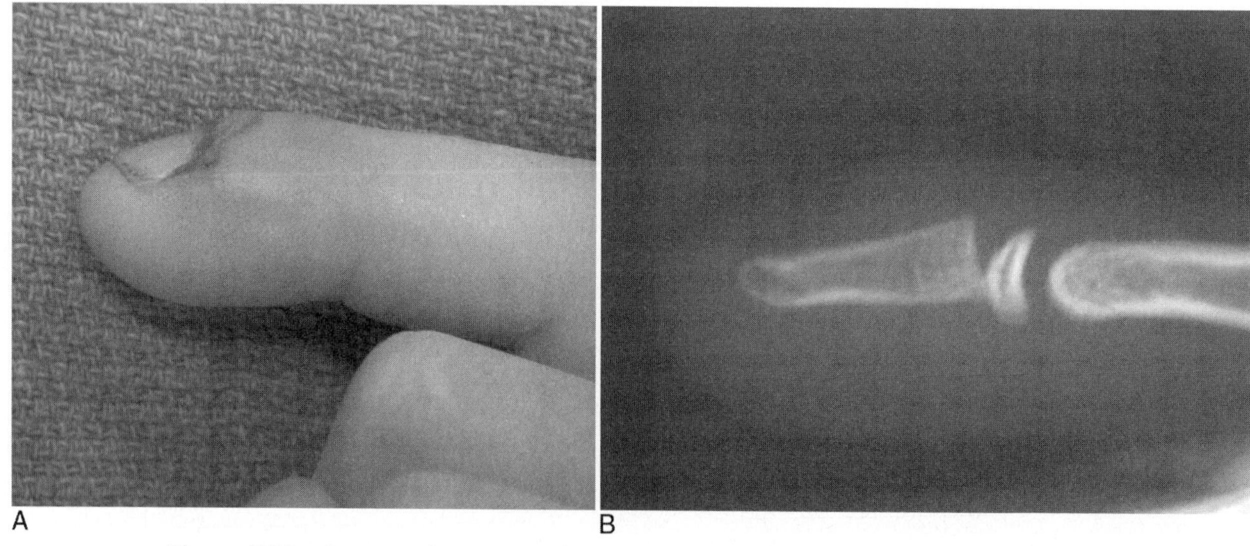

Figure 8-21 **Seymour fracture. A,** Gross appearance. **B,** Radiograph demonstrating growth plate fracture of distal phalanx.

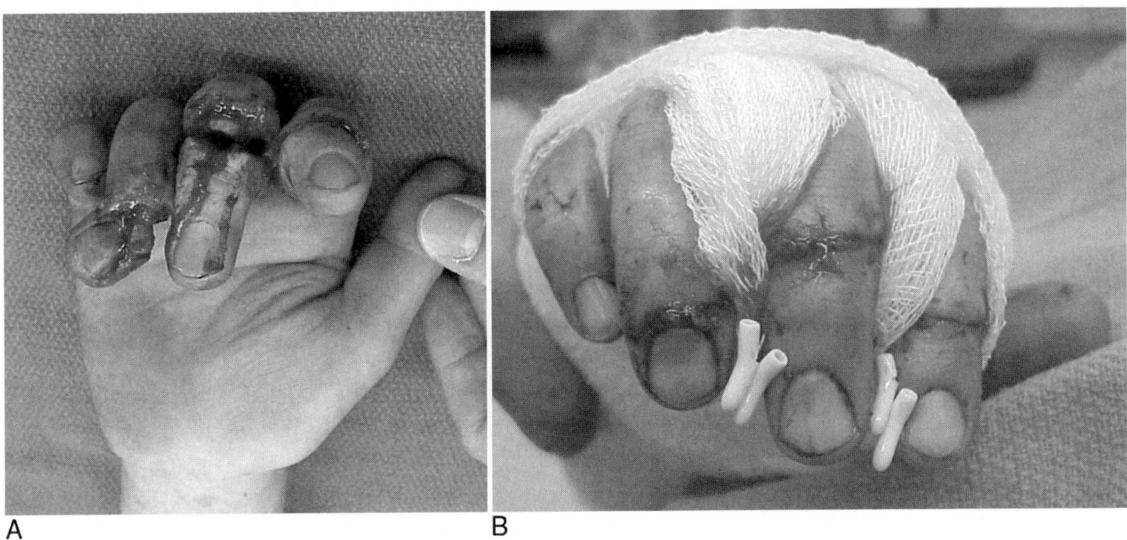

Figure 8-22 **A,** Partial amputation of digit from crush injury. **B,** Digits after revascularization.

Burns

Burns can be caused by thermal, mechanical, chemical, or electrical injury. In children, thermal injury is most common because most chemical and electrical burns are occupational. Direct contact with a hot surface, scalding, and an open flame can cause thermal burns. Typical examples are touching a fireplace glass enclosure, scalding from pulling down a hot pot of water, and burning by clothing in a house fire. Scalding and contact burns in infants who are still unable to walk should raise the suspicion of child abuse.

Thermal burns are classified according to depth of injury. First-degree burns produce erythema but no skin necrosis. Second-degree burns exhibit painful blistering with loss of the epidermis and part of the dermis. Third-degree burns involve the full thickness of the skin, leaving the skin dry, pale, and insensate. First- and second-degree burns heal by reepithelialization from the skin appendages, as long as infection and desiccation are avoided. Third-degree burns heal by scarring and contraction, which can restrict motion in the hand. A joint contracture develops if a third-degree burn crosses a flexion crease and is allowed to heal by scar contraction.

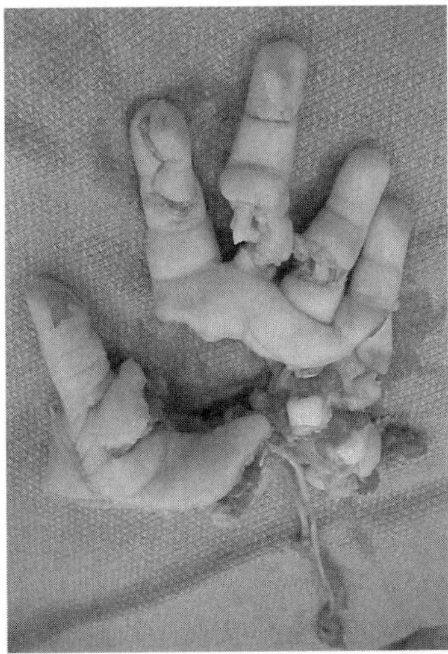

Figure 8-23 Multilevel injury by a meat grinder in a 4 year old.

First- and second-degree burns are treated with a topical antimicrobial ointment, usually silver sulfadiazine, which is soothing, minimizes the chance of infection, and keeps the wound moist. These more superficial burns typically reepithelialize in 1 week. If the burn crosses a joint flexion crease, the hand should be splinted with the involved joints in extension. Third-degree burns are best treated with early tangential excision and full-thickness skin graft to prevent joint contracture. The hand is then splinted in the "safe" position (MP joints flexed, PIP and DIP joints extended). Range-of-motion exercises begin as soon as the grafts are adherent. Once the grafts are healed, custom compression gloves are fitted to reduce edema and the formation of hypertrophic scars. It may be difficult to differentiate a deep second-degree burn from a third-degree burn, but any hand burn that has not healed by 2 weeks is probably best treated with excision and skin graft. Exposed tendon or bone requires pedicled or free flaps for coverage.

Mechanical abrasions from contact with a rough surface can occur from child versus motor vehicle collisions and from exercise treadmills (Fig. 8-24). Many of these injuries are equivalent to deep second-degree or third-degree thermal burns. Treatment is identical to that for thermal burns, except that more extensive cleansing and débridement are usually needed.

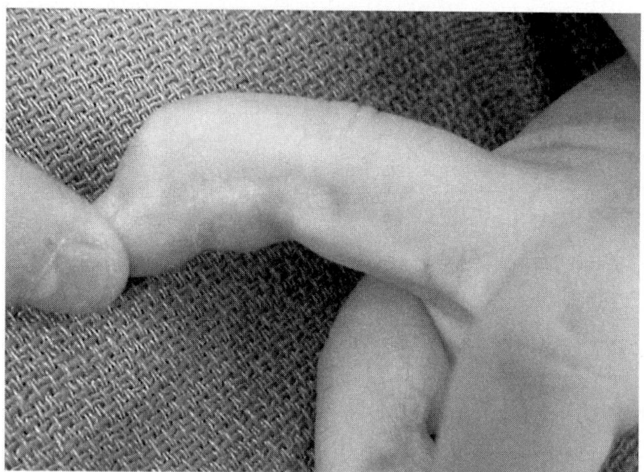

Figure 8-24 Treadmill abrasion injury healed with contracture.

Children can suffer *chemical burns* by coming in contact with household products containing strong acids (e.g., toilet cleaners) and alkalis (e.g., bleach). Initial treatment consists of removal of all clothing contaminated by the chemical and copious irrigation of the affected skin with tap water for at least 20 minutes. Specific neutralizing agents may be indicated (e.g., calcium gluconate for hydrofluoric acid burns).

Electrical burns in children are most often from 110-volt household current, which rarely causes the problems associated with high-voltage (>1000-volt) injuries, such as cardiac arrhythmias, renal failure, seizures, and compartment syndrome. Most burns occur when the child sticks a conductive object into an electric socket and suffers a flame burn to the hand from the electric arc. Such injuries usually heal with topical silver sulfadiazine dressings.

CONGENITAL HAND DIFFERENCES

Congenital hand differences are present in about 1 of 626 newborns, of which 10% have significant functional or cosmetic deformities.[6] The etiology of congenital anomalies is not known in about 50% of cases, but some of them are genetic, caused by chromosome abnormalities and teratogenic changes in the first 6 to 7 weeks of gestation. Because the etiology of hand anomalies is not known in so many cases, the most commonly used classification system is based primarily on morphology (Table 8-6); it was devised by the International Federation of Societies for Surgery of the Hand (IFSSH).[7]

Table 8-6 Classification of Congenital Hand Differences

Group	Description	Examples
1	Failure of formation	Radial clubhand, cleft hand
2	Failure of differentiation	Syndactyly, trigger finger
3	Duplication	Polydactyly
4	Overgrowth	Macrodactyly
5	Undergrowth	Hypoplastic thumb
6	Congenital constriction band syndrome	Amniotic band syndrome
7	Generalized skeletal abnormalities	Arthrogryposis

Group 1—Failure of Formation

After congenital amputation at different levels, the *radial clubhand* is the most common complex deformity in this group (Fig. 8-25). The radial clubhand deformity manifests as radial deviation of the hand due to partial or complete absence of the radius in the forearm and is often associated with absence of the thumb, limited motion of the elbow joint, and a short, bowed ulna. Fifty percent of cases are bilateral. The etiology is unknown, but radial clubhand is not hereditary. This disorder is frequently associated with other malformations and syndromes, including VATER (vertical defects, imperforate anus, tracheoesophageal fistula, and radial and renal dysplasia) syndrome, Holt-Oram syndrome (associated cardiac defects), and Fanconi anemia (progressive pancytopenia).[2]

Early intervention for treatment is important to avoid any fixed joint contracture, which is much more difficult to correct later in life. The newborn's arm should be immobilized with serial casting followed by splinting to passively correct the radial deviation of the wrist. Surgical intervention with centralization of the hand to

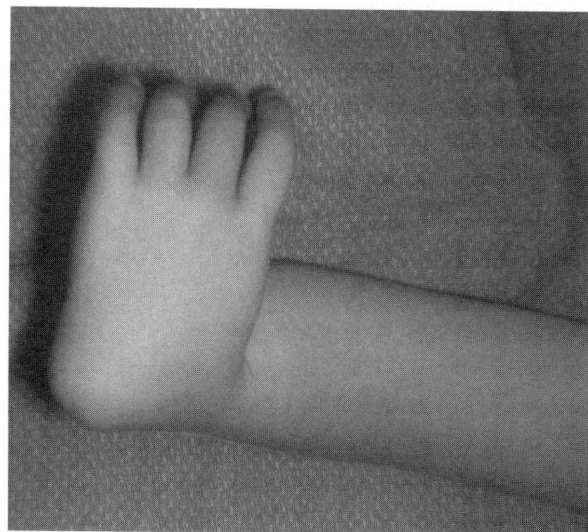

Figure 8-25 Untreated 1-year-old child with radial clubhand.

the distal ulna is performed at the age of 6 to 12 months, followed by pollicization of the index finger 6 months later if the thumb is absent. Long-term follow-up is essential because of the very frequent recurrence of flexion deformity and radial deviation of the wrist.

Most children with unilateral radial clubhand become functionally independent, but in those with bilateral deformity, significant functional impairment often remains even after surgery. Most of the functional difficulties in bilateral cases are with washing, dressing, and feeding.

Ulnar clubhand, much less common than radial clubhand, is usually associated with absence of the ulnar ray digits and syndactyly of the radial digits (Fig. 8-26).[8] The problem joint is the elbow rather than the wrist. Surgery involves separation of the syndactyly at 6 to 12 months and fusion of the proximal ulna to the distal radius to make a one-bone forearm at when the child is 5 years or older.

Cleft hand deformity is a rare anomaly (Fig. 8-27). The cleft hand is a functional triumph and a social disaster. Patients with such hands can perform almost any function that they wish, but more often than not they hide their hands because of the grotesque appearance. There are two types, typical and atypical. Typical cleft hand has a V-shaped defect in which the entire long finger ray is missing. This type is usually bilateral, is strongly familial, and is usually inherited as an autosomal dominant trait. The feet are often also involved. The atypical type of cleft hand is unilateral and nongenetic, without associated involvement of the feet. The cleft is U-shaped with several rays absent, but the metacarpals are usually present. Most patients with cleft hands require multiple reconstructive operations, including cleft closure, first web space widening, and rotational osteotomy.

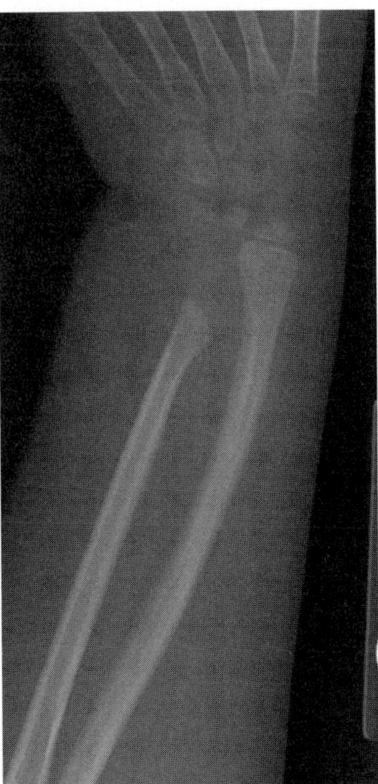

Figure 8-26 Ulnar clubhand.

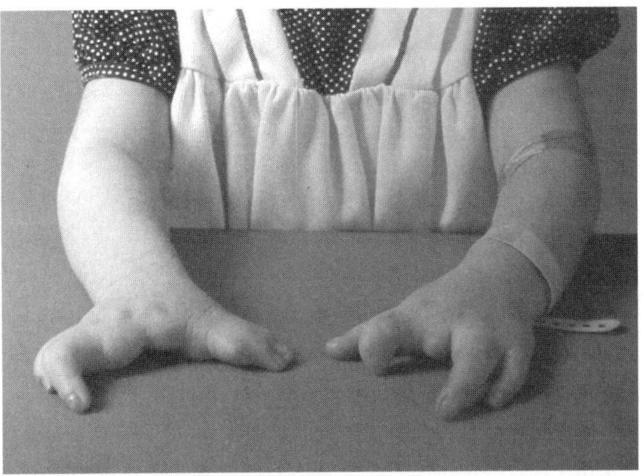

Figure 8-27 Bilateral cleft hands.

Group 2—Failure of Differentiation (Separation of Parts)

Syndactyly is the most common hand congenital deformity after polydactyly (Fig. 8-28). A family history is presented in 10% to 40% of patients, depending on the reporting series. Half of cases are bilaterally symmetrical. The rays most commonly involved are the middle and ring fingers (third web space). Simple syndactyly involves only soft tissues and *complex syndactyly* involves the bones as well (Fig. 8-29). Syndactyly is a commonly associated anomaly in Poland, Chotzen, and Down syndromes. The timing of syndactyly correction depends on the type. For simple and incomplete syndactyly, the best surgical result can be achieved when the child is older, but usually before school starts. However, early separation during the first year of age is indicated in cases of complex syndactyly associated with Apert syndrome or syndactyly between rays of unequal lengths (e.g., thumb and index finger) to avoid secondary angular deformity. Most cases require full-thickness skin grafts in addition to local flaps. Adjacent syndactylies should be repaired in stages to avoid devascularization of the intervening digit. The most common complication is partial recurrence of the syndactyly, so-called web creep.

Radioulnar synostosis is a condition that occurs at the proximal forearm in the large majority and is bilateral in 60% of cases (Fig. 8-30). Because of this severe pronation deformity of the forearms, daily living activities, such as catching a ball, are difficult. Parents do not usually recognize this deformity until the child becomes active. The only treatment option is supination derotational

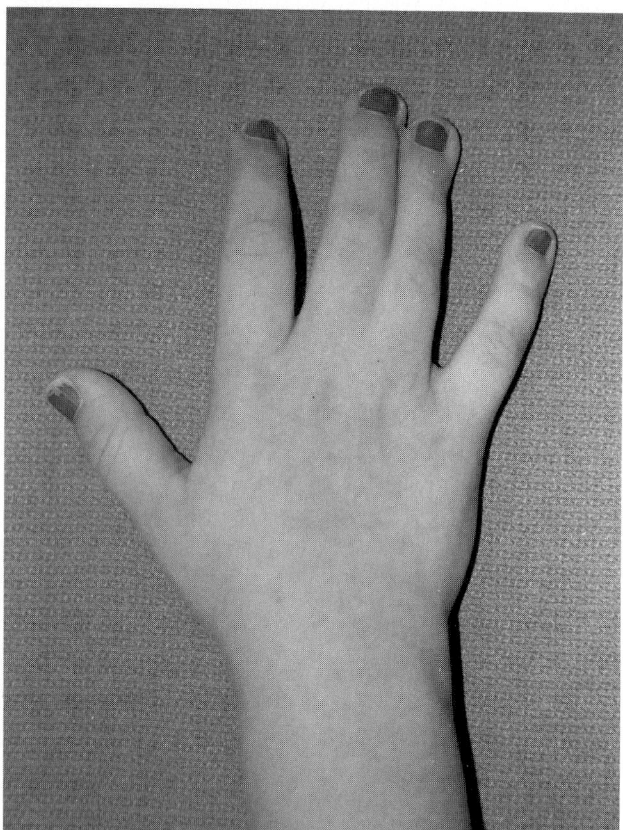

Figure 8-28 Simple, incomplete syndactyly.

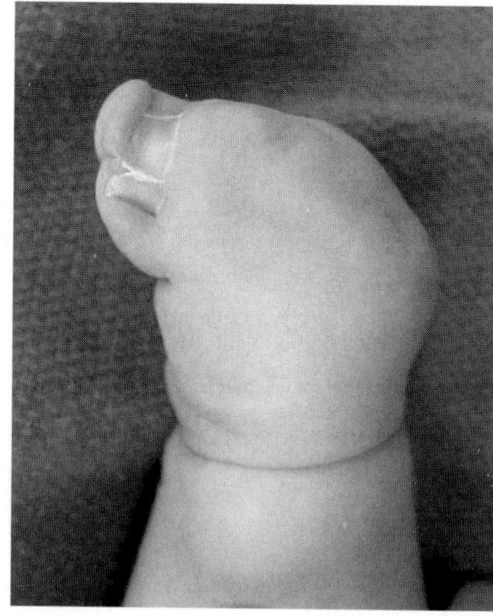

Figure 8-29 Complex syndactyly with Apert syndrome.

osteotomy of the nondominant side, because all attempts to restore active rotation by a variety of methods have proved unsuccessful.

Camptodactyly is a congenital flexion deformity of the digit, usually at the proximal interphalangeal joint of the small finger (Fig. 8-31). It is commonly bilateral and either is transmitted by autosomal dominant trait or occurs sporadically. *Adolescent camptodactyly* first manifests in early adolescence and is more common in girls. Both types of camptodactyly may become much more marked during the adolescent growth spurt. Most cases of camptodactyly can be treated conservatively, with stretching and splinting, but if the deformity progresses to an angle of more than 60 degrees, surgery is recommended. Severe cases are best treated with dorsal angular osteotomy of the neck of the proximal phalanx to decrease the flexion deformity; however, the PIP joint loses some range of motion in flexion with this procedure.

Clinodactyly (Fig. 8-32) is a curvature of the digit in the radial-ulnar plane, most commonly seen in the small finger and less commonly in the triphalangeal or delta phalangeal thumb. A wedge osteotomy, the treatment of choice for functionally significant angulation (greater than 30 degrees), is usually performed around the age of 4 years, before the child starts school.

Congenital trigger thumb (Fig. 8-33) is a flexion deformity of the interphalangeal joint caused by an idiopathic swelling in the flexor tendon at the level of the metacarpophalangeal (MCP) joint. This nodule prevents free excursion of the flexor tendon into and out of the tendon sheath, causing the thumb to “pop” or trigger when brought from a fully flexed to a fully extended

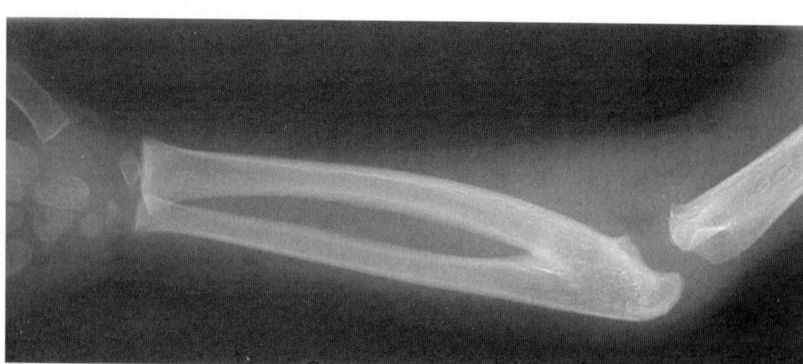

Figure 8-30 Radioulnar synostosis.

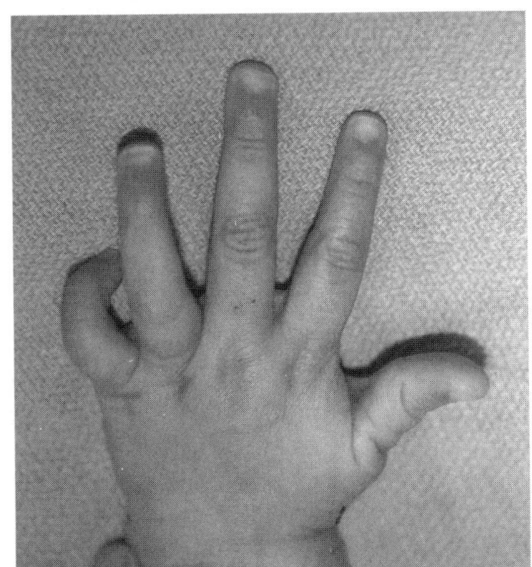

Figure 8-31 Camptodactyly involving the little finger.

position. Although this triggering may be painful, the nodule is usually not tender to palpation. Some children keep the thumb in extension to avoid the pain of triggering. Most commonly, however, the patient presents with a fixed flexion deformity at the thumb interphalangeal joint that cannot be corrected passively. Trigger thumb can be differentiated from congenital clasped thumb, which involves a flexion deformity at the MCP joint. Trigger thumb can be present at birth but often is not noticed or does not develop until later in infancy. Trigger thumb can resolve spontaneously in about 30% of cases manifesting at birth.[9] Those that are initially diagnosed in children between 6 and 30 months old have only a 12% chance of spontaneous resolution within 6 months. If the trigger thumb does not resolve by itself, surgical release of the tendon sheath effectively restores normal range of motion unless repair is delayed beyond the age of 3 or 4 years. Triggering of digits other than the thumb can occur in children but is much less common.

Group 3—Duplication

Polydactyly is the most common congenital hand deformity, accounting for 14.6% of the total in a series at Iowa University Hand Center.[6] Polydactyly most commonly affects the border digits and is extremely rare in the central digits. *Thumb (radial) polydactyly* can occur in isolation or as part of a syndrome (Fig. 8-34). Isolated thumb polydactyly is unilateral and sporadic. Thumb polydactyly, when part of a syndrome (e.g., Noack, Carpenter, Holt-Oram, Down, VATER), is usually transmitted as an autosomal dominant trait. Its' presence should signal the need for a thorough physical evaluation, because it may indicate concealed malformations or a possibility of abnormalities arising later in life (Fanconi anemia). Wassel[10] classified thumb polydactyly into seven different types according to the level of duplication. The most common form of duplicate thumb is complete duplication of the proximal and distal phalanges, Wassel type IV. Surgical correction, which can be carried out when the child is between 1 and 3 years old, usually involves deletion of the smaller thumb. Earlier surgery can damage the epiphysis of the remaining normal parts, resulting in premature epiphysial closure and a shortened digit. Long-term follow-up is also essential because there is a tendency for development of deviation deformities, especially during the adolescent growth spurt.

Ulnar polydactyly (Fig. 8-35) usually occurs in isolation and is ten times more prevalent than thumb polydactyly in African Americans. It can be inherited as a

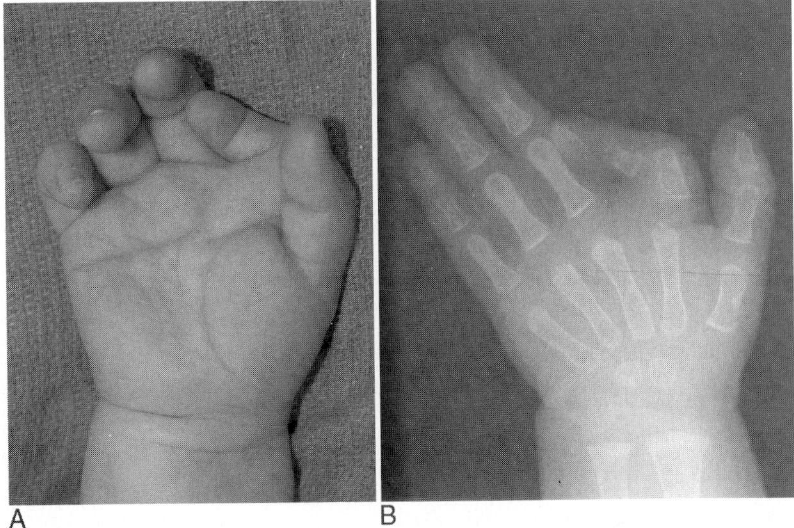

Figure 8-32 **A,** Clinodactyly of index finger, **B,** Radiograph of clinodactyly.

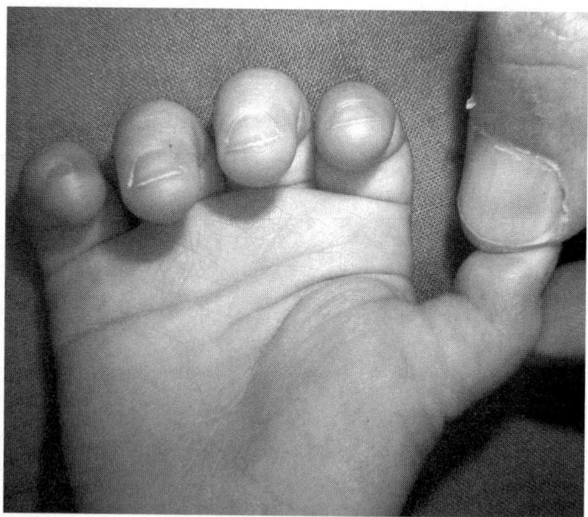

Figure 8-33 Congenital trigger thumb with interphalangeal flexion deformity.

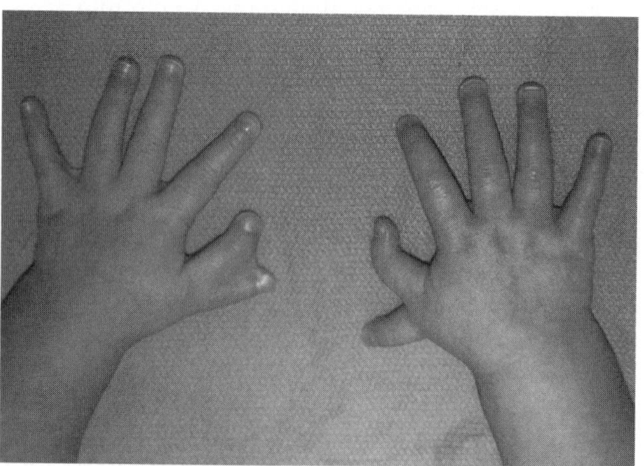

Figure 8-34 Thumb polydactyly.

dominant trait with variable penetrance but usually occurs sporadically. Ulnar polydactyly can be associated with a variety of other anomalies and (mostly recessive) syndromes. Although many extra digits are "tied off" in the nursery, excision of the ulnar duplicate is preferred to avoid leaving a soft tissue remnant that can be a source of irritation later in life. Extra digits attached only by a narrow soft tissue bridge can be excised in the nursery with the use of local anesthesia and closed with one or two absorbable sutures. Those attached by a wider base or by bone should be excised in the operating room after the patient's first birthday, when general anesthesia is safer.

Group 4—Overgrowth

Macrodactyly is a nonhereditary congenital enlargement of the digit (Fig. 8-36). It is unilateral in 90% of cases. Seventy percent of cases of unilateral macrodactyly affect more than one digit, usually those on the radial side of the hand. Most involve the phalanges rather than the metacarpals. The most common type of macrodactyly is a lipofibromatosis involving digits in the median nerve distribution and demonstrating two patterns of growth. Static macrodactyly is presented at birth, and enlargement keeps pace with growth of the normal digits. Progressive macrodactyly is sometimes not apparent until as late as 2 years of age; it is a more aggressive form in which the enlargement progresses more quickly than the adjacent digits, and it involves the adjacent palm. Treatment is very difficult (epiphysiodesis, debulking of the soft tissues, or both) and very often ends in amputation. Macrodactyly can also be associated with neurofibromatosis and vascular conditions.

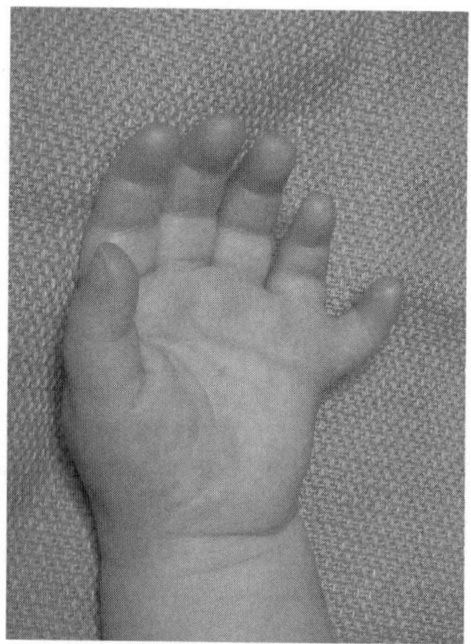

Figure 8-35 Ulnar polydactyly.

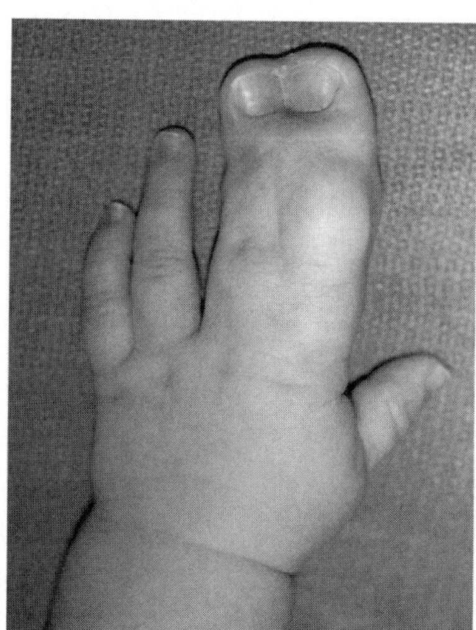

Figure 8-36 Macrodactyly involving long and index fingers with syndactyly.

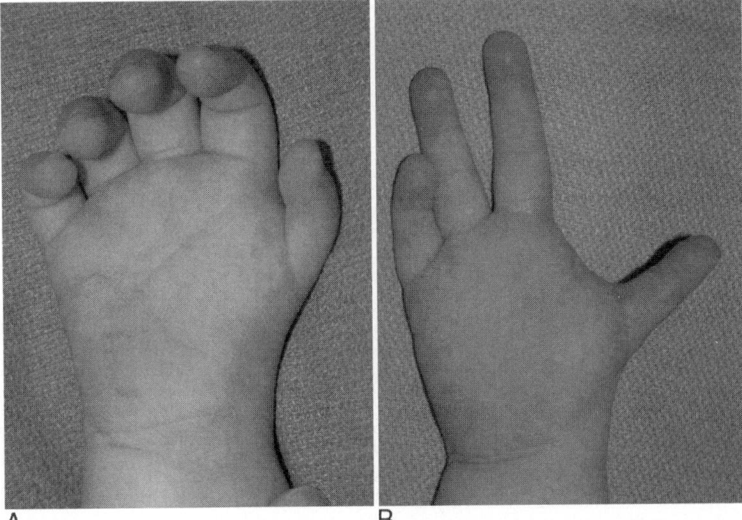

Figure 8-37 **A,** Hypoplastic thumb with unstable carpometacarpal joint. **B,** After pollicization.

Group 5—Undergrowth

The most common (and difficult) type of undergrowth is *thumb hypoplasia*. The extent of undergrowth is variable, from complete absence (aplasia) to very minor hypoplasia. Treatment depends on the severity of hypoplasia of the thumb. If the patient has a stable thumb carpometacarpal (CMC) joint, the thumb can be preserved, but multiple stages of reconstruction, including skin rearrangement, tendon transfer, MCP joint stabilization, and bone lengthening, are required. If the CMC joint of the thumb is unstable, the preferred treatment is deletion of the hypoplastic thumb and pollicization of the index finger to create a new thumb (Fig. 8-37). Pollicization is best performed early in childhood, at 6 month to 3 years, to take advantage of the young child's ability to learn the new pattern of prehension.

The *clasped thumb* is a hypoplastic thumb with underdevelopment of the extensor tendon and thenar muscles with a resulting flexion deformity is at the MCP joint (Fig. 8-38), rather than the interphalangeal joint (as seen in trigger thumb). The clasped thumb is usually treated first with splinting of the thumb in extension at the MCP joint. If the patient does not have sufficient active extension of the MCP joint when 3 years old, tendon transfer of the extensor indicis proprius to the thumb extensor is indicated.

Brachydactyly, or short fingers, is the delight of geneticists and the despair of the surgeon (Fig. 8-39). Most cases of brachydactyly are associated with other malformation syndromes, such as Poland, Holt-Oram, Silver, and Apert. Most of the short fingers also have stiff interphalangeal joints; therefore, not many of them benefit from lengthening, despite entreaties from parents of affected children.

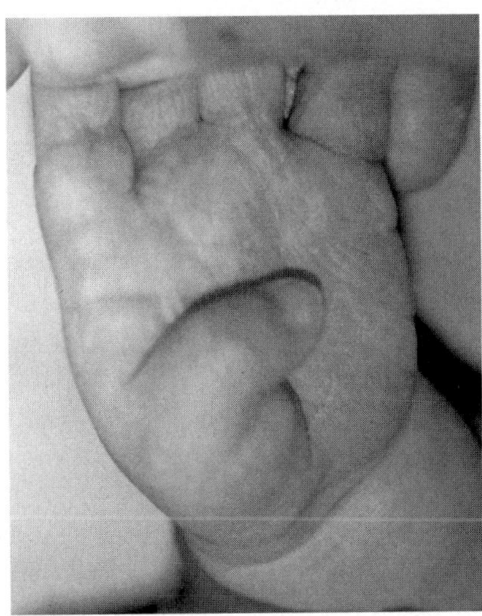

Figure 8-38 Clasped thumb deformity with metacarpal joint flexion and hypoplastic thumb.

Group 6—Congenital Constriction Band Syndrome

Congenital constriction band syndrome occurs sporadically and is thought to occur from external constriction of the limb by an amniotic band that can produce varying degrees of constriction deformity or even intrauterine amputation (Fig. 8-40). Constriction bands can be found in association with club foot, craniofacial clefts, visceral omphaloceles, and a variety of genitourinary anomalies. Release of the constriction ring is required immediately after birth if there is marked edema distal to the constriction ring, a sign of vascular compromise to the veins and lymphatic vessels. Most constriction bands are not a threat to circulation and,

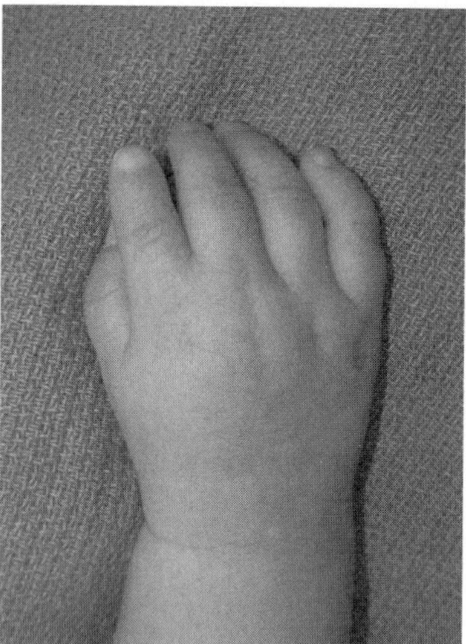

Figure 8-39 Brachydactyly associated with Poland syndrome.

therefore, can be treated electively after the patient's first birthday. Surgical treatment consists of excision of the tight constriction ring and rearrangement of the skin and subcutaneous tissues by multiple Z-plasty incisions. Hands with severe constriction bands that have caused fusion of the distal ends of the fingers (acrosyndactyly) should undergo early release of the syndactyly, within the first 6 months of life, to prevent progressive angulation deformity of the fingers with growth.

Group 7—Generalized Skeletal Abnormalities

Arthrogryposis is a congenital neuromuscular disorder involving both upper and lower extremities. It is characterized by multiple joint contractures and decreases in muscle bulk and number. Arthrogryposis is a sporadically occurring condition with systemic nonprogressive contracture and weakness of the limbs. The upper extremities in arthrogryposis have fixed joint contractures with internal rotation of the shoulder, extension of the elbow, flexion and ulnar deviation of the wrist, flexed digits, and thumb-in-palm deformity (Fig. 8-41). Milder cases can involve just the hand and wrist with extension contracture of varying severity at the elbow. Most children with arthrogryposis are of above-average intelligence. There are no associated visceral abnormalities, and life expectancy is normal. The consistent goal of any treatment should be to enhance the quality of life and facilitate functional independence. Treatment usually starts with splinting and occupational therapy. When the child is 3 to 6 months old, the wrist and elbow contractures are released and tendon transfers are performed in the left upper extremity, followed 3 months later by a similar procedure on the right side. The goal of the surgery is to allow for full flexion at the elbow and 40 degrees of extension at the wrist. Although this is not a progressive disease, the joint contracture commonly recurs after surgery without long-term splinting and therapy.

TUMOR

Hand tumors in children are rare, and the majority of tumors are benign. The relative frequency of surgically excised pediatric hand tumors in Colon and Upton's[11] series of 349 cases are listed in Table 8-7. For any child with a hand tumor, a careful history and physical examination can suggest a likely diagnosis. Imaging studies can be helpful with the diagnosis of bony tumors. Ultrasonography can differentiate cystic from solid tumors. However, pathologic examination of the speci-

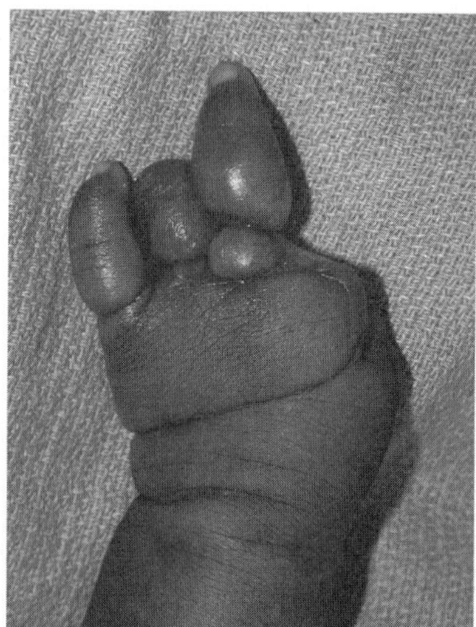

Figure 8-40 Constriction band syndrome in a newborn infant.

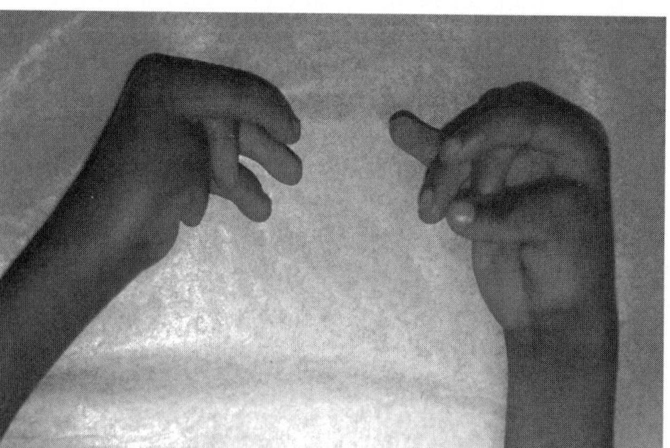

Figure 8-41 Arthrogryposis. Ulnar drifting and flexion contracture of the digits.

Table 8-7 Pediatric Hand Tumors

Tumor	Frequency (%)
Cysts	27
Foreign body	21
Vascular malformations	14
Enchondroma	9
Epidermal inclusion cysts	7
Fibrous tumors	6
Nodular tenosynovitis	3
Exostoses	3
Pseudoaneurysm	3
Glomus tumor	2
Lipoma	2
Malignant tumors	2

Adapted from Colon F, Upton J: Pediatric hand tumors: A review of 349 cases. Hand Clin 11:224, 1995.

men is the only way to definitively exclude malignancy. Exclusion of malignancy is probably the most common indication for surgery.

The history should include the following details about the tumor: duration, changes in size, changes in pigmentation for cutaneous lesions, antecedent trauma, pain, and functional problems. A long duration of existence with no growth favors a benign lesion but is insufficient to exclude malignancy. Changes in pigmentation or contour can signify malignant change in cutaneous nevi. A history of penetrating trauma before onset of a tumor suggests foreign body, pseudoaneurysm, or epidermal inclusion cyst as the likely diagnosis. Pain and functional impairment may be indications for excision. A family history should also be obtained because some conditions are inherited, such as multiple hereditary exostoses.

Physical examination should note the size, location, presence of tenderness, texture, firmness, and fixation to surrounding tissues. A complete neuromuscular and vascular examination of the extremity should be performed. Functional impairments should be measured and recorded.

Plain radiographs should be obtained for all bony tumors. If there are any unusual radiographic or clinical features, additional imaging with MRI or computed tomography (CT) can help with diagnosis and staging of the lesion. Soft tissue tumors that are not obviously ganglion cysts or vascular malformations should undergo MRI before excision unless they are small, superficial, and easily excised for diagnosis. Magnetic resonance angiography (MRA) and MRI can identify the extent and flow characteristics of vascular tumors, such as malformations and pseudoaneurysm.

If the diagnosis is still not certain from the history, physical findings, and imaging features, the mass should be excised for pathologic examination. If the mass is large, an incisional biopsy may be performed first, and definitive excision deferred until the pathologic diagnosis is available.

Benign Soft Tissue Tumors

Cysts

Fluid-filled cysts are the most common soft tissue hand tumors in children, as in adults. The most common location is the wrist (ganglion cysts; Fig. 8-42), followed by the flexor tendon sheath (retinacular cysts). Both types are firm and rubbery in consistency, fixed to the underlying joint or tendon sheath, and covered by normal, mobile skin. Tenderness may or may not be present; most cysts are asymptomatic. If the appearance or location is atypical, ultrasonography can confirm the diagnosis. Wrist ganglion cysts arise from the joint, and retinacular cysts from the tendon sheath. Synovial cysts, the least common, arise from the extensor tendons on the metacarpal portion of the hand. Cysts may fluctuate in size, and some may spontaneously regress. Cysts may appear at any age from infancy to adolescence. Mucous cyst of the DIP joint is not found in children because it is caused by osteoarthritis.

Immobilization, traumatic rupture, and aspiration are not recommended. Aspiration was effective in only 20% of Colon and Upton's[11] cases. Observation is the preferred treatment unless the cyst causes pain or functional impairment. Surgical excision involves removal of the entire cyst wall along with a small portion of the wrist capsule or tendon sheath to prevent recurrence.

Foreign Body

Foreign bodies are most often found in the palmar surface of the hand and should be suspected when there is a history of a puncture wound or the patient presents

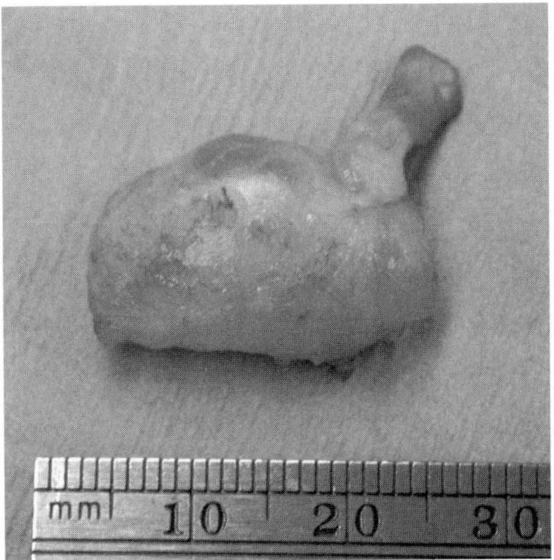

Figure 8-42 Ganglion cyst with stalk.

with a mass and infection unresponsive to antibiotics. Many younger children do not give a history of antecedent trauma. Imaging with plain radiographs can demonstrate metal, stone, and some glass foreign bodies. Radiolucent foreign bodies, such as wood splinters and pencil lead, can be detected on ultrasonography, but such an evaluation is not mandatory. Treatment is by removal of the foreign body and curettage of the cavity. The incision should be left open if there is any evidence of infection.

Vascular Tumors

Vascular tumors represent nearly 20% of tumors in the upper extremity. Hemangiomas and vascular malformations are the most common pediatric vascular tumors and occur with equal frequency in the upper extremity. Other vascular tumors, in descending order of frequency, are pyogenic granuloma, pseudoaneurysm, and glomus tumor.

Hemangiomas can arise anywhere on the hand and are the most common vascular tumor in children (Fig. 8-43). They rapidly proliferate during the first 2 years of life and spontaneously involute by 5 to 7 years. Therefore, surgery is rarely necessary.

Vascular malformations are usually present at birth, grow proportionately with the patient, and do not involute.[12] Prognosis is strongly determined by whether the malformation is a slow-flow or fast-flow type. Slow-flow malformations have a good prognosis and are further categorized as capillary, venous, or lymphatic (Fig. 8-44). Fast-flow malformations have a palpable pulsation or thrill (Fig. 8-45). They contain arteriovenous fistulae, which progressively enlarge and can produce a distal vascular steal. Initial treatment in all malformations involves the use of compression garments, although these are not well tolerated by many patients. Surgical indications include pain, excessive bulk, functional impairment, bleeding, and vascular steal. MRI and MRA should be obtained before surgery to define the extent and flow characteristics of the malformation. Low-flow malformations and some high-flow malformations can be debulked in stages. High-flow malformations that exhibit vascular steal are the most difficult to treat and eventually must undergo amputation in 90% of cases.[13] Selective embolization has been used instead of surgery or before surgery in the high-flow type. Surgery is reserved for the specific indications already listed and should not be performed prophylactically.

Pyogenic granulomas are rapidly growing polypoid tumors composed of highly vascular granulation tissue that bleeds easily (Fig. 8-46). They arise from small wounds that fail to heal. In the hand, they are most often found on the palm and palmar side of the digits. Small pyogenic granulomas may resolve with silver nitrate cautery. Larger granulomas should be excised, and the defects closed. Curettage or shave excision commonly results in recurrence.

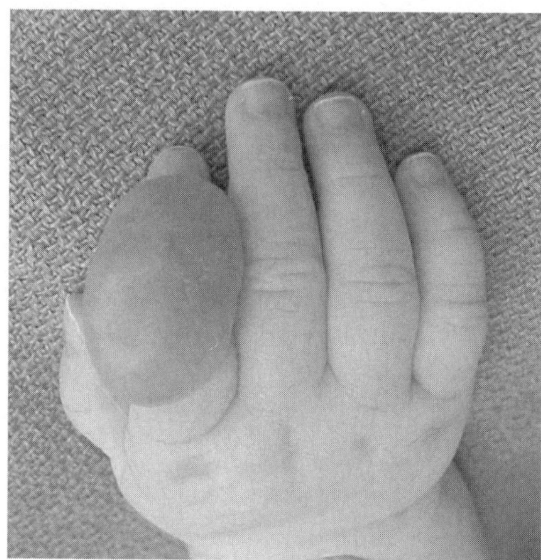

Figure 8-44 Low-flow lymphatic-venous vascular malformation.

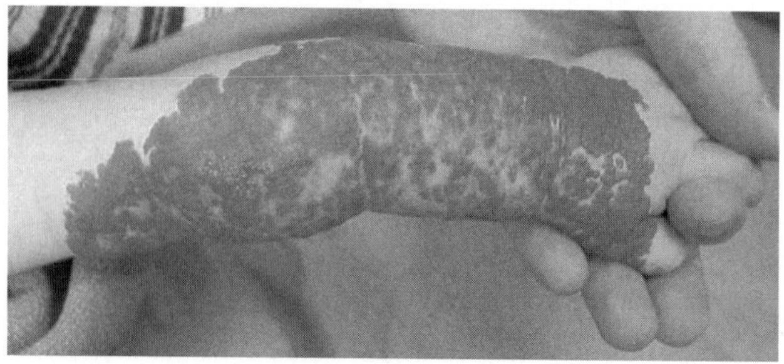

Figure 8-43 Hemangioma with areas of regression.

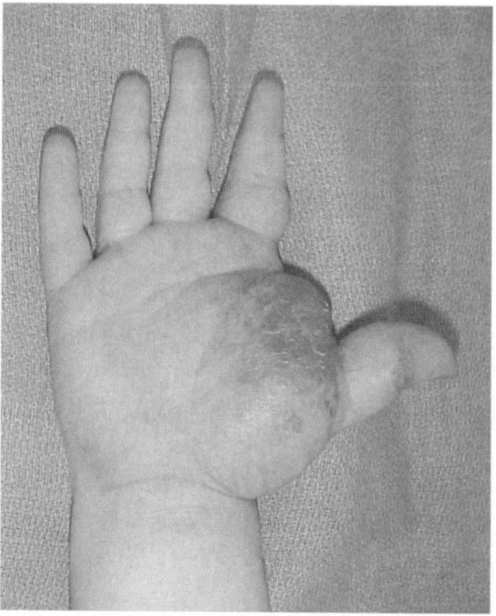

Figure 8-45 High-flow arteriovenous malformation.

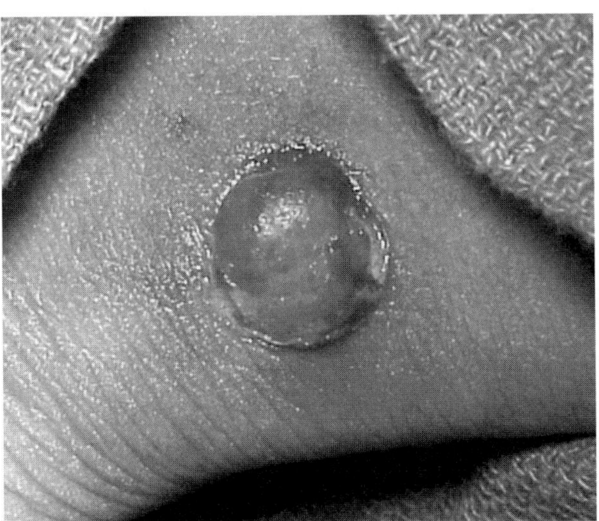

Figure 8-46 Pyogenic granuloma.

Pseudoaneurysms (Fig. 8-47) of the upper extremity manifest as slowly enlarging pulsatile masses weeks to months after a puncture wound. Typically, pulsatile bleeding was noted at the time of injury and stopped with direct pressure. MRA or Doppler ultrasonography confirms the diagnosis. If distal perfusion is adequate, the pseudoaneurysm can simply be excised, and the artery ligated. Revascularization with a vein graft is necessary if there are any signs of ischemia after excision of the pseudoaneurysm.

Glomus tumors are very rare but can be the source of unexplained pain in the hand. In a child with pain that is worse with exposure to cold or with pressure, one should suspect a glomus tumor. Visible as small bluish tumors, these lesions are most often found on the glabrous surface of the hand or in a subungual location. A glomus tumor may be hard to palpate because of its smallness. MRI can aid in diagnosis but is usually not necessary. Treatment is complete excision.

Epidermal Inclusion Cyst

A firm, fixed, nontender mass, epidermal inclusion cyst is most commonly found in the palm and the volar pads of the fingers. The cyst usually follows an episode of penetrating trauma by months to years, but the history of trauma may not be elicited in every case. Fragments of epithelium or germinal matrix are left in the subcutaneous tissue after the penetrating trauma and continue to produce keratin, forming a cystic collection. The cyst grows very slowly and can erode the underlying distal phalanx; thus, radiographs may aid in diagnosis. Complete excision is curative. Epidermal inclusion cyst can recur if part of the cyst wall is left behind.

Fibrous Tumors

Fibrous tumors are rare but create anxiety in parents of affected children because the lesions are hard and immobile and they grow. *Infantile digital fibroma* is found on the sides or dorsal surfaces of the ulnar three digits in young children. It grows rapidly and can infiltrate the skin. *Juvenile aponeurotic fibroma* is usually found in the palm. Stippled calcifications are apparent on radiographs. Fibromas can be found in other locations, such as between the extensor tendon and the proximal phalanx. Treatment for all fibromas is complete excision. Recurrence rates are high because complete excision is often impossible.

Nodular Tenosynovitis

Like fibroma, nodular tenosynovitis is also hard, immobile, and expansile, but it is also multilobulated (Fig. 8-48). Other names for nodular tenosynovitis are giant cell tumor and xanthoma. These lesions are yellowish brown

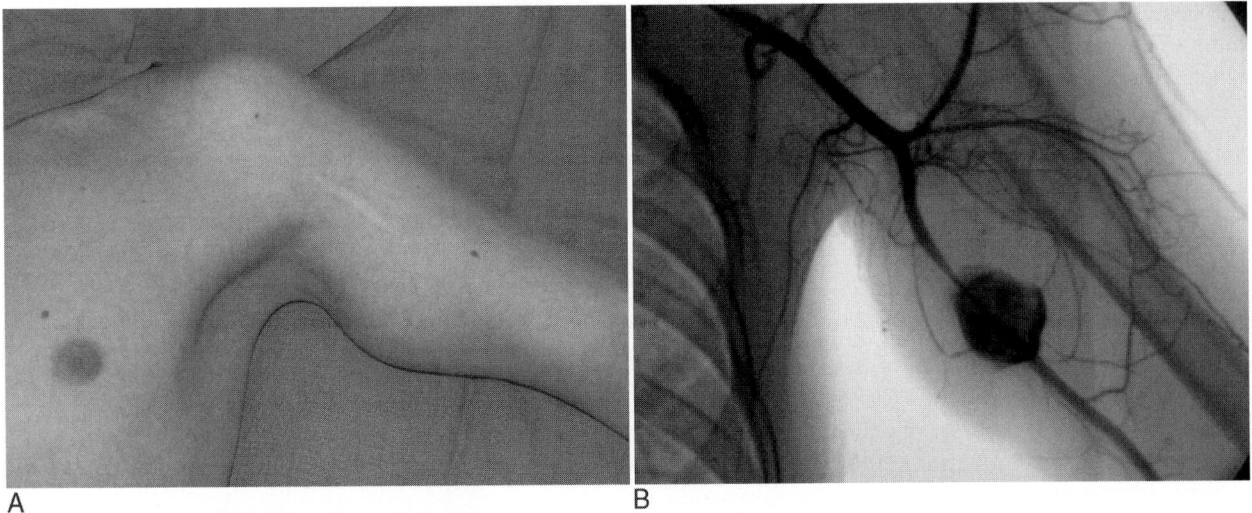

Figure 8-47 **A,** Pseudoaneurysm of brachial artery 13 years after excision of an osteochondroma. **B,** Angiogram of pseudoaneurysm.

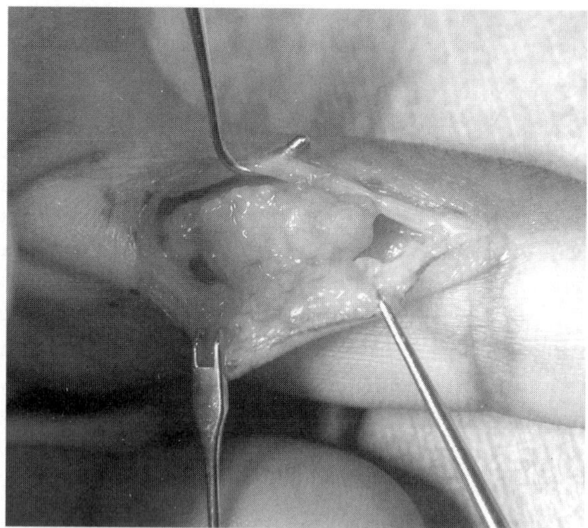

Figure 8-48 Nodular tenosynovitis of the digit with single hook retracting the digital nerve.

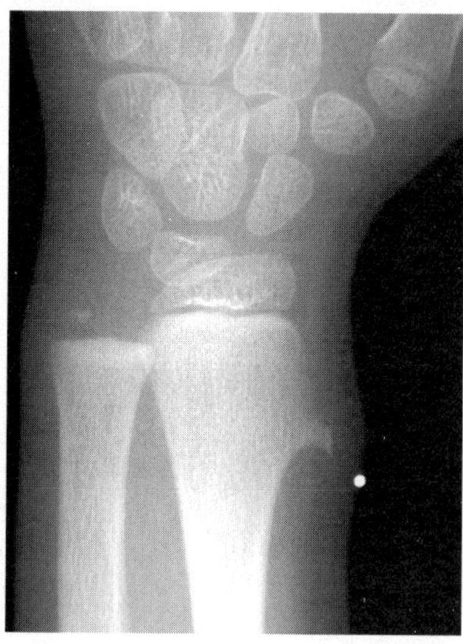

Figure 8-49 Osteochondroma of the distal radius.

and encapsulated and can extend into joints and around tendons. They occur more commonly in adolescents than in young children. Complete excision is curative.

Lipoma

Lipomas manifest as large, soft, painless masses in the palm. They are much less common in children than in adults. Surgery is reserved for symptomatic lipomas; they are encapsulated and usually "shell out" easily. Recurrence is rare.

Benign Bone Tumors

Enchondroma

Enchondroma, the most common primary bone tumor in children, is frequently associated with Ollier disease (multiple enchondromatosis) or Maffucci syndrome (multiple enchondromas and vascular malformations). The proximal phalanges are most frequently involved. Enchondromas usually manifest in adolescence and young adulthood as pathologic fractures. The radiographs show thinning of the cortex and replacement of the cancellous bone by a radiolucent mass containing calcifications. The fracture is reduced and allowed to heal before curettage of the enchondroma and cancellous bone grafting are performed.

Osteochondroma (Exostosis)

Osteochondromas are benign outgrowths from a bone that are capped by cartilage (Fig. 8-49). Most osteochondromas of the hand in pediatric patients are found in those with multiple hereditary exostoses. Osteochondromas are excised only if they cause symptoms such as pain, nerve impingement, restriction of joint motion, and angulation of the underlying bone.

Malignant Hand Tumors

Malignant pediatric hand tumors are exceedingly rare, representing only 2% of the cases in Colon and Upton's[11] series. The most common soft tissue malignancies are sarcoma (Fig. 8-50) and melanoma. The most common skeletal malignancies are osteosarcoma and Ewing sarcoma. The key to treatment of malignancies is tissue diagnosis. Incisional biopsy is preferred for large lesions; small tumors can be excised as long as the incision is oriented so that the biopsy site can be completely excised at the time of definitive resection without compromising the chances for limb salvage. Complete staging of the tumor to define the extent of local invasion and the presence of metastases is mandatory *before*

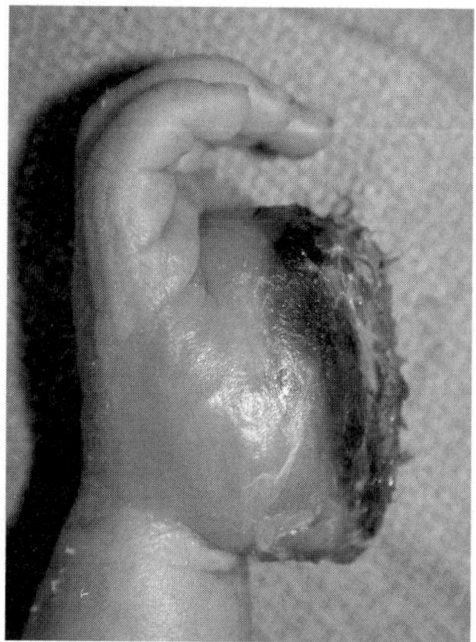

Figure 8-50 Infantile fibrosarcoma in a newborn.

definitive treatment. MRI, CT, and bone scan of the extremity as well as CT of the chest are frequently used for staging. For some tumors, limb-sparing surgery combined with radiation or chemotherapy produces survival rates comparable to those for amputation alone while preserving hand function.

NEUROMUSCULAR DISORDERS

Cerebral Palsy

Cerebral palsy affects 5 of every 1000 children in the United States.[14] Despite much speculation by plaintiff's attorneys, birth asphyxia probably accounts for only a small fraction of children with cerebral palsy. In most cases, the etiology is unknown. The spastic paralysis of the muscles in cerebral palsy produces the following common pattern of deformities in the upper limb: flexion of the fingers, flexion of the thumb with or without adduction in the palm, flexion of the wrist, pronation of the forearm, flexion of the elbow, and adduction and internal rotation of the shoulder (Fig. 8-51). Early treatment with therapy and splinting is essential to avoid fixed joint contracture. The upper extremity paralysis is often accompanied by some sensory deficit, particularly in proprioception, stereognosis, and light touch. There appears to be a direct relationship between the use of the hand and its sensibility, and in some instances, this sensory loss causes the patient to totally disregard the hand. If the patient uses the paretic hand to play, eat, or assist the opposite hand, the hand probably has good sensibility and may be improved by surgery.

The most useful procedures are tendon transfers for wrist extension and thumb abduction when the patient is 7 or 8 years old. In addition to having adequate sensibility of the hand, patients should meet the following criteria before consideration for tendon transfer surgery: reasonable intelligence, only mild spastic cerebral palsy, and no fixed joint contracture. If the patient has fixed joint contractures or is older, a bony procedure, such as arthrodesis, or release of the joint contracture with lengthening or release of the tendon can improve the appearance of a grotesquely positioned joint but may not dramatically improve function. In severe cases of spastic contracture of the digits, release of joint contractures and tendons may be indicated simply to allow for proper hygiene of the palmar skin.

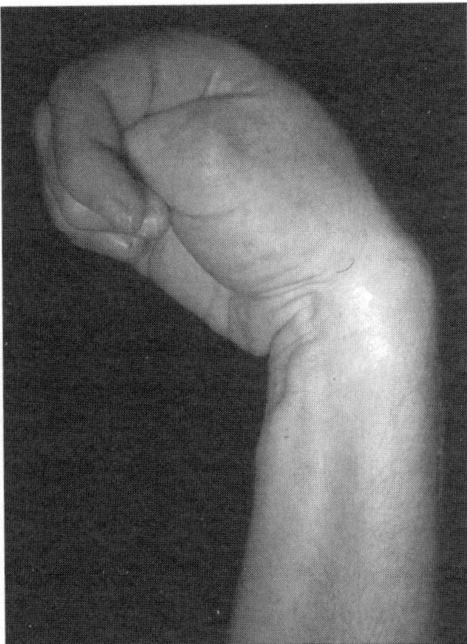

Figure 8-51 Hand flexion deformity in a 14-year-old boy with cerebral palsy.

Obstetrical Brachial Plexus Palsy

In contrast to cerebral palsy, obstetrical brachial plexus palsies are now generally agreed to be caused by an injury at the time of birth—specifically, traction on the brachial plexus. Breech delivery and high birth weight are the two main risk factors. Birch found that of his 512 patients with obstetrical brachial plexus palsy, 90% weighed more than 4 kg at birth.[15] As expected, the incidence has risen over the past few decades as average birth weights continue to rise. The prognosis for spontaneous recovery varies widely in published reports, possibly because the severity of the initial injury is the most important determinant of ultimate recovery but is hard to assess accurately in the newborn. A useful classification for obstetrical brachial plexus palsies is summarized in Table 8-8.[15]

Diagnosis is usually made shortly after birth, when medical staff or the parents notice a significant disparity in the tone and spontaneous motion in the two arms. Physical examination and radiographs should exclude other causes of decreased motion, such as humeral or clavicular fractures, cerebral palsy, arthrogryposis, and stroke. At birth, physical findings can range from a subtle weakness in the shoulder and elbow to complete flaccid paralysis of the arm. Patients with group 2 disease (C5, C6, C7 palsy) exhibit the classic "waiter's tip" posture: shoulder adducted and internally rotated, elbow extended, and wrist flexed. The presence of Horner syndrome (group 4) is a poor prognostic sign.

The main difficulty in treating a patient with obstetrical brachial plexus palsy is in determining whether the patient will recover spontaneously or will be left with a significant impairment without intervention. The trick is to be able to accurately predict the ultimate extent of recovery within the first few months of life, when nerve repair is most likely to be successful. The classification shown in Table 8-8 generally correlates levels of nerve injury with prognosis; patients with only upper root injuries usually do better than those with injuries to many roots. However, for an individual patient, this

Table 8-8 Classification of Obstetrical Brachial Plexus Palsy

Group	Nerves	Paretic Muscles	Clinical Recovery	Rate of Full Recovery (%)
1	C5, C6	Deltoid, biceps	Begins by 3 months	90%
2	C5, C6, C7	Deltoid, biceps Wrist and digit extensors	Deltoid and biceps by 3-6 months	65%
3	C5-T1	All weak, except some finger flexors	25% of patients never recover wrist/finger extension	<50%
4	C5-T1 sympathetics	All atonic, Horner syndrome	20% have limb length discrepancy	None

classification alone is not accurate enough to determine whether surgery should be performed. Extent of recovery within the first 2 to 3 months of life is a better indicator of prognosis. Patients who recover normal grip by 1 month and some shoulder and elbow flexion by 2 months are likely to achieve full spontaneous recovery. Gilbert and Tassin[16] advocate exploration and nerve repair if there is no biceps function by 3 months of age. Some investigators propose surgery at 2 months if the arm remains completely flaccid. The most difficult decisions are for patients with group 2 and 3 palsy, who recover some function by 3 months but have not progressed to full function by 6 to 9 months of age. Would they have done better with early nerve repair? Adjunctive imaging and neurophysiologic tests have been used to aid in this decision, but serious reservations about their accuracy and utility remain. As with many difficult problems, the ideal treatment may be prevention.

INFECTION

Infections of the hand in children often arise from traumatic wounds contaminated by skin flora or saliva. Diagnosis is evident from swelling, erythema, tenderness, and fluctuation. Infection may involve a variety of tissues and spaces—skin (cellulitis and paronychia), subcutaneous tissues (felon), bone (osteomyelitis), flexor tendon sheath (tenosynovitis), and joint space (septic arthritis). Early diagnosis, adequate drainage of purulent collections, and treatment with appropriate antibiotics are the keys to successful outcome. Undrained collections are the most common reason for failure of antibiotic therapy. Purulent collections can usually be diagnosed from physical examination, but ultrasonography and MRI may be needed for diagnosis of deep collections. Radiographs should be obtained to look for osteomyelitis in all cases of deep infection.

Choice of antibiotic should be based on results of culture and susceptibility testing whenever possible. Material for cultures should be obtained by incision or aspiration before empiric antibiotic therapy is initiated (Table 8-9). Appropriate tetanus prophylaxis should be given.

All animal and human bites of the hand require irrigation and prophylactic antibiotic treatment with amoxicillin-clavulanate (clindamycin and ciprofloxacin for the penicillin-allergic patient). Common infectious organisms are gram-positive cocci, anaerobes, *Pasteurella multocida* (cat), *Eikenella corrodens* (human), and *Pasteurella canis* (dog). In general, bites should be left open for drainage to minimize chance of infection. The patient who experiences a cat, dog, or wild animal bite should receive prophylactic rabies treatment with both antirabies globulin and the vaccine if the animal has not been immunized and cannot be observed for 10 days.

Table 8-9 Empiric Antibiotic Therapy for Hand Infections

Clinical Condition	Empiric Treatment	Duration
Cellulitis, felon, paronychia	Dicloxacillin *or* cephalexin *or* erythromycin	7-14 days
Septic arthritis, tenosynovitis	Nafcillin and 3rd-generation cephalosporin *or* vancomycin and gentamicin	2-4 weeks
Osteomyelitis	Nafcillin and ciprofloxacin *or* ampicillin/sulbactam *or* vancomycin, ciprofloxacin, and clindamycin	6 weeks
Human or animal bite	Ampicillin/sulbactam *or* clindamycin and ciprofloxacin	Depends on location

Patients with cellulitis, felon, and paronychia can usually be treated as outpatients. Exceptions are patients who are immunocompromised, diabetic, or unreliable and those who have signs of systemic infection, such as lymphangitis, leukocytosis, and fever. Patients with septic arthritis, flexor tenosynovitis, osteomyelitis, and human bites of the hand must be hospitalized for adequate wound drainage and at least a few days of intravenous antibiotics until clinical signs show improvement.

Paronychia

An infection of the soft tissues around the nail is called a *paronychia* (Fig. 8-52). The infection may start as a cellulitis and progress to a localized abscess. It may involve the nail fold (eponychial fold) or may dissect under the nail, creating a subungual abscess. Untreated paronychia can evolve into osteomyelitis and septic arthritis. The infection is usually due to *Staphylococcus aureus* but may be caused by oral flora in children who suck their fingers.

Early infections in the cellulitis stage can be treated with oral antibiotics, hand washing, and warm soaks several times a day. Palpable fluctuance signifies the presence of an abscess, which should be drained by incision of the entire diameter of the abscess through the thinnest portion of the abscess wall. If the abscess extends under the nail, the nail should be elevated or partially excised for adequate drainage. All infected bone must be débrided. Wounds are left open and treated with soap-and-water washing and warm soaks several times a day to promote drainage. These procedures can usually be accomplished with the use of digital block anesthesia. Antistaphylococcal antibiotics are used for 7 to 14 days, depending on clinical improvement. Osteomyelitis requires 6 weeks of intravenous antibiotics.

Felon

A *felon* is an infection of the volar subcutaneous tissues of the distal phalanx. The volar pad becomes tense, exquisitely tender, and erythematous. Early infection may respond to antistaphylococcal antibiotics alone. Once an abscess cavity develops, it must be incised and packed open for a few days to promote complete drainage. The incision is best made in the thinnest portion of the abscess wall; any loculations created by the vertical fibrous septa should be drained by division of the septa. All necrotic soft tissues and infected bone must be débrided. A felon can extend into the flexor tendon sheath, causing a suppurative tenosynovitis.

Flexor Tenosynovitis

A sheath extending from the distal palm to the distal phalanx encloses the flexor tendons. The potential space between the tendon and the sheath can become infected through penetrating trauma (Fig. 8-53) or hematogenous or contiguous spread. This is a true hand emergency. Delay in treatment would cause adhesions to form between the tendon and the sheath, impairing tendon gliding and range of motion. Left untreated, the infection would destroy the tendon and could track proximally into the palm and forearm along the bursae that surround the tendons.

The diagnosis of flexor tenosynovitis can usually be made from physical examination (Box 8-4). All of the signs need not be present for the flexor tenosynovitis to be diagnosed. Conversely, a subcutaneous abscess or severe cellulitis can sometimes produce all four signs and masquerade as flexor tenosynovitis. If there is any question as to the diagnosis, the tendon sheath should be explored in the operating room.

The treatment for suppurative flexor tenosynovitis involves prompt incision, drainage, and irrigation of the

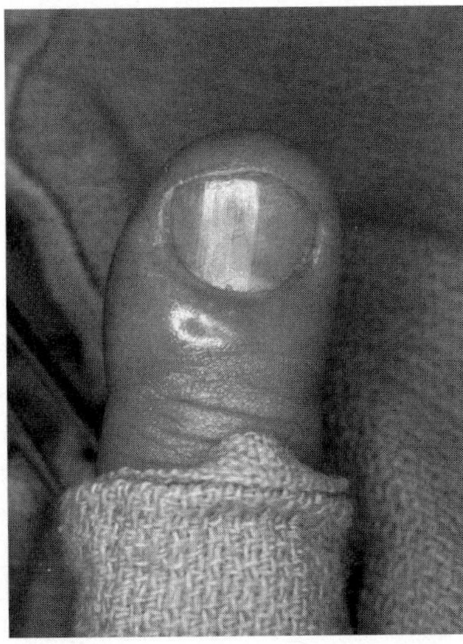

Figure 8-52 Paronychia in a nail-biter.

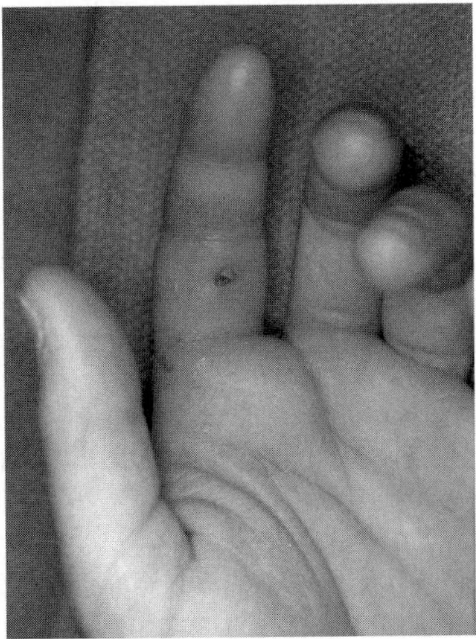

Figure 8-53 Flexor tenosynovitis after cat bite.

Box 8-4 Kanavel's Signs of Flexor Tenosynovitis

Symmetrical swelling along the flexor tendon sheath
Tenderness and erythema over the flexor tendon sheath
Flexed position of the finger
Severe pain on passive extension

flexor tendon sheath. Broad-spectrum antibiotic therapy should commence immediately after culture specimens are obtained. With the patient on the operating table, the tendon sheath is opened proximally in the palm, and an 18-gauge intravenous catheter is inserted into the flexor tendon sheath for postoperative irrigation. A counter-incision is made in the distal sheath at the distal interphalangeal flexion crease for egress of the irrigation fluid. The sheath is then irrigated until the fluid runs clear. The hand is placed in a bulky gauze dressing and waterproof splint. After surgery, the catheter is left in place for 48 hours, and the sheath irrigated with saline solution at 10 mL/hr by means of an intravenous pump. The catheter is then removed, and active range-of-motion exercises are begun under the supervision of a hand therapist. The most common complication of this infection is stiffness of the finger. The wounds are left open to heal by secondary intention. Hand washing and twice-daily soaks in warm water help keep the wounds clean and promote drainage.

Septic Arthritis

Infection of a joint usually arises from penetrating trauma. Delayed diagnosis and treatment can lead to devastating joint destruction, osteomyelitis, and ascending, limb-threatening infection. One should suspect any laceration to the dorsum of the hand over a joint to be a human bite from a clenched fist striking an opponent's tooth. The MP joint is most commonly injured by this mechanism. A radiograph should be obtained to look for fracture and foreign body (Fig. 8-54). The wound should be anesthetized, irrigated, and explored with the joint in flexion and extension to check for penetration into the joint. If the extensor tendon mechanism is punctured, the joint space has probably been violated, and the patient should be taken to the operating room for exploration and irrigation of the joint. If the wound was indeed a human bite, it should be left open, and amoxicillin-clavulanate therapy, to "cover" the common infective organisms (*S. aureus,* streptococci, *E. corrodens,* and anaerobes) should be started.

More commonly, the patient does not present for treatment until there are signs and symptoms of established infection in the joint, such as swelling, erythema, pain on passive motion, lymphangitis, and frank purulence. Such a patient should be taken to the operating room for arthrotomy and placement of an irrigation catheter in the joint. The wound is left open, and the joint is continuously irrigated for 48 hours with saline at 10 mL/hour. The tendon is not repaired primarily; the wound is allowed to heal by secondary intention, with early active motion to prevent joint stiffness. Intravenous ampicillin-sulbactam is given empirically until bacterial culture results are available. Antibiotic therapy is continued for 2 to 4 weeks, depending on clinical response.

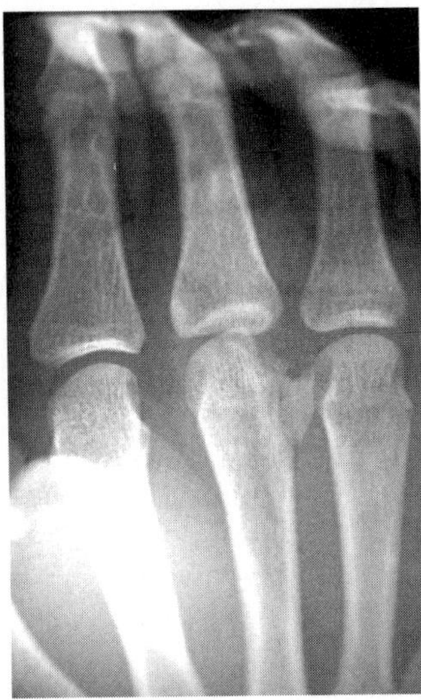

Figure 8-54 Metacarpal head fracture and septic arthritis after punching an opponent in the mouth.

Septic arthritis not associated with penetrating trauma can arise from hematogenous spread (e.g., gonococcus) or contiguous spread from paronychia, felon, or local abscess. Treatment consists of aspiration or incision and drainage of the joint, followed by empiric antibiotic treatment with nafcillin and a third-generation cephalosporin (or vancomycin and gentamicin for penicillin-allergic patients) until culture results are available. Rheumatoid arthritis, gout, and pseudogout should be considered in the differential diagnosis of septic arthritis.

SUMMARY

The hand is important for mechanical interaction with the environment in both adults and children. In children, it also plays a critical role in brain development and sensory input. When treating children with upper extremity disorders, one must pay particular attention to their functional requirements and growth potential. Conditions that interfere with function or are made worse by growth should be corrected early. Diagnosis may be made more difficult by the young patient's inability to report symptoms or cooperate with examination. However, children generally have better recovery potential than adults because of superior wound healing and adaptability.

MAJOR POINTS

Examine the injured hand from distal to proximal.
Plain radiographs should be obtained on all bony tumors and all injured hands.
To control bleeding, elevate the extremity and apply direct pressure to the bleeding vessel with a gloved finger.
Suspect skeletal injury when swelling and bruising accompany point tenderness.
Suspect a tendon injury if there is pain on resisted motion or if there is evidence of nerve or arterial injury.
Pain in a muscle compartment out of proportion to injury is usually the first symptom of compartment syndrome. Pain on passive stretch of those muscles is pathognomonic.
All animal and human bites to the hand require irrigation and prophylactic antibiotic coverage.
A single layer closure with absorbable suture is preferable in the fingers and palm.

REFERENCES

1. Seiler JG (ed): Essentials of Hand Surgery. Philadelphia, Lippincott Williams & Wilkins, 2002.
2. Smith P: Lister's the Hand, 4th ed. London, Churchill Livingstone, 2002.
3. Martin DS, Collins ED (eds): Manual of Acute Hand Injuries. St. Louis, Mosby, 1998.
4. Doyle JR: Extensor tendons—acute injuries. In Green DP, Hotchkiss RN, Pederson WC (eds): Green's Operative Hand Surgery. 4th ed. Philadelphia, Churchill Livingstone, 1999.
5. Abouzahr MK: Compartment syndromes of the upper limb. In Aston SJ, Beasley RW, Thorne CHM (eds): Grabb and Smith's Plastic Surgery, 5th ed. Philadelphia, Lippincott-Raven, 1997.
6. Flatt AE: The care of Congenital Hand Anomalies. St. Louis, Quality Medical, 1994.
7. Knight SL, Kay SPJ: Classification of congenital anomalies. In Gupta A, Kay SPK, Scheker LR (ed): The Growing Hand: Diagnosis and Management of the Upper Extremity in Children. London, Mosby, 2000.
8. Carroll RE: Congenital absence of ulna. In Buck-Gramcko D (ed): Congenital Malformations of the Hand and Forearm. London, Churchill Livingstone, 1998.
9. Kay SPJ, Lees VC: Anomalies of the tendons. In Gupta A, Kay SPK, Scheker LR (eds): The Growing Hand: Diagnosis and Management of the Upper Extremity in Children. London, Mosby, 2000.
10. Wassel, HD: The results of surgery for polydactyly of the thumb. Clin Orthop 64:175-193, 1969.
11. Colon F, Upton J: Pediatric hand tumors: A review of 349 cases. Hand Clin 11:223-244, 1995.
12. Fleming ANM, Smith PJ: Vascular cell tumors of the hand in children. Hand Clin 16:609-624, 2000.
13. Upton J, Coombs C: Vascular tumors in children. Hand Clin 11:307-336, 1995.
14. Tonkin M: The upper limb in cerebral palsy. In Gupta A, Kay SPK, Scheker LR (eds): The Growing Hand: Diagnosis and Management of the Upper Extremity in Children. London, Mosby, 2000.
15. Birch R: Obstetric brachial plexus palsy. In Gupta A, Kay SPK, Scheker LR (eds): The Growing Hand: Diagnosis and Management of the Upper Extremity in Children. London, Mosby, 2000.
16. Gilbert A, Tassin JL: Obstetrical palsy: a clinical, pathologic, and surgical review. In Terzis JK (ed): Microreconstruction of Nerve Injuries. Philadelphia, WB Saunders, 1987, pp. 529-53.

CHAPTER 9

Pediatric Lower Limb Disorders

DAVID M. WALLACH

RICHARD S. DAVIDSON

Pediatricians are commonly asked to evaluate the alignment and function of the pediatric lower extremity. Understanding normal limb development and being able to recognize pathologic conditions are essential in the care of children and adolescents. In the first part of this chapter, we address issues of axial (i.e., in-toeing) and coronal (i.e., bowing) alignment. Then we discuss conditions of the foot—specifically, metatarsus adductus, clubfoot, the causes of a flat foot and a high arch, and abnormalities of the toes.

ROTATIONAL ABNORMALITIES

A parental complaint that a child's foot or leg turns "in" (internal or medial rotation) or "out" (external or lateral rotation) during gait is one of the most common reasons for orthopaedic referral. Limb position is determined by the sum of dynamic forces (muscle function and ligamentous laxity) and static forces (from bones). During normal gait, muscles contract concentrically (shorten) or eccentrically (lengthen) in a well-defined sequence. When muscle pull is absent, weak, too vigorous, or prolonged, an abnormal gait results. In neuromuscular conditions such as cerebral palsy, there may be persistent activity of the medial hamstrings and adductors, causing the limb to rotate internally. Children with excessive ligamentous laxity (i.e., Ehlers-Danlos syndrome) have excessive rotation. Dynamic factors, although important to limb rotation, do not play as great a role as static factors in "normal children." Static forces are discussed later.

The hip joint forms by the eleventh gestational week, although the proximal femur and acetabulum continue to develop until physeal closure in adolescence. At birth, the femoral neck is rotated forward an average of 40 degrees. Hip orientation is referred to as *femoral anteversion* when the femora face forward and *femoral retroversion* when the femora face backward. During gait, the limb is automatically positioned to ensure full and concentric seating of the femoral head within the acetabulum. Therefore, anteversion of the hip encourages internal rotation of the leg, and retroversion, external rotation. In the absence of a neuromuscular abnormality, femoral version decreases to 15 to 20 degrees by the time a child is 8 to 10 years old (Fig. 9-1). In the first year of life, the effect of femoral anteversion is masked by an external hip rotation contracture that resolves soon after the child begins walking.

A second osseous source of limb rotation can be found in the tibia. Infants may have as much as 30 degrees of internal rotation of the tibia. Although spontaneous external reorientation of the tibia can occur in the medially rotated tibia, medial rotation of a

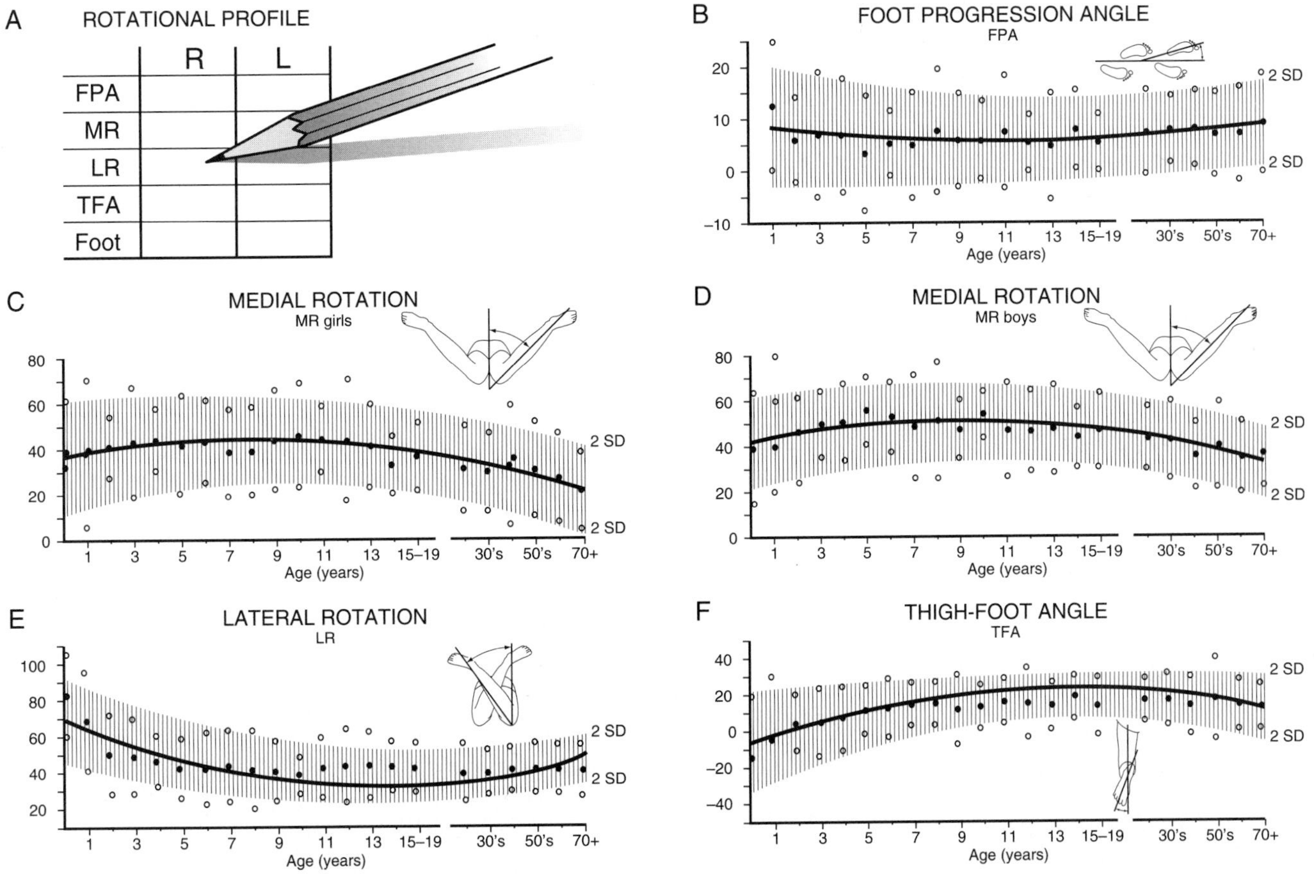

Figure 9-1 The rotational profile from birth to maturity is depicted graphically. All graphs include 2 standard deviations from the mean for foot progression angle, femoral medial and lateral rotation (for boy and girls), and the thigh-foot angle. (Redrawn from Morrissy RT (ed): Lovell and Winter's Pediatric Orthopaedics, 3rd ed, vol 2. Philadelphia, Lippincott Williams & Wilkins, p 742, 1990).

laterally rotated limb may not correct. By 4 years of age, the tibia assumes its permanent alignment. At maturity, the normal range of tibial alignment is from 5 degrees medial to 15 degrees of lateral rotation. Excessive medial rotation is referred to as *medial* (or internal) *tibial torsion* (MTT). *Rotational abnormality* is defined as two standard deviations outside the normal range. External rotational abnormalities can occur. Either MTT or external rotational abnormalities can be unilateral.

Limb rotation may also be found in the foot. The foot may be adducted (i.e., metatarsus adductus, metatarsus primus varus, clubfoot and skew foot) or abducted (i.e., planovalgus). These conditions are addressed in further detail later; however, we describe the method of recognizing the foot as the source of rotation here.

The position of the limb during gait is expressed as the *foot progression angle* (FPA). The examiner determines the FPA by observing the longitudinal axis of the foot during single leg stance in relation to the direction the child is walking.

The FPA is a summation of femur, tibia, and foot rotations. Rotation at each level must be assessed separately. Children with femoral anteversion are able to sit in the "W" position (Fig. 9-2). When the child runs, internal rotation of the hips causes the heels to drift outward, and

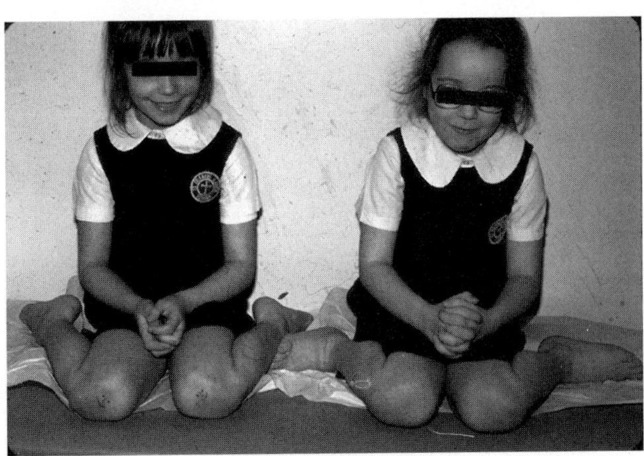

Figure 9-2 Photo of children sitting in "W" position.

the child appears to be kicking the feet out to the sides. On physical examination, the patellae face medially during gait ("squinting patellae" sign).

The standard method of measuring hip rotation is with the child prone. The hips are adducted and in neutral extension-flexion, and the knees are flexed to 90 degrees (Fig. 9-3). By convention, *zero rotation* is present when the tibia is perpendicular to the table. Rotation of the leg toward the ipsilateral side of the body is *medial rotation*. Rotation of the leg toward the contralateral side of the body is *lateral rotation*.

Tibial rotation is measured by the transmalleolar angle (TMA). The TMA is the angle formed by an imaginary line drawn along the axis of the thigh and a second line perpendicular to the axis of the medial and lateral malleoli. In the absence of a foot deformity, the thigh-foot angle (TFA) is easier to use. The TFA is also measured with the child lying prone. It is the angle formed between the longitudinal axis of the thigh and the longitudinal axis of the foot. Any difference between the TMA and TFA is produced by an adduction or abduction deformity of the foot. Staheli and colleagues have collected age adjusted normative values for hip and tibial rotation.[1]

Foot adduction and abduction can also be evaluated with the heel bisector line (HBL). The HBL is formed by a line that divides the plantar heel in half along its longitudinal axis and is then extended to the toes. The normal HBL goes across the second toe. When the heel bisector line points medial to the second toe, the forefoot is abducted, and when the HBL is lateral to the second toe, the forefoot is adducted (Fig. 9-4).[2] Radiographs are not needed during screening of tibial and foot rotation. It is reasonable to obtain an anteroposterior (AP) pelvis radiograph, however, to rule out hip dysplasia.

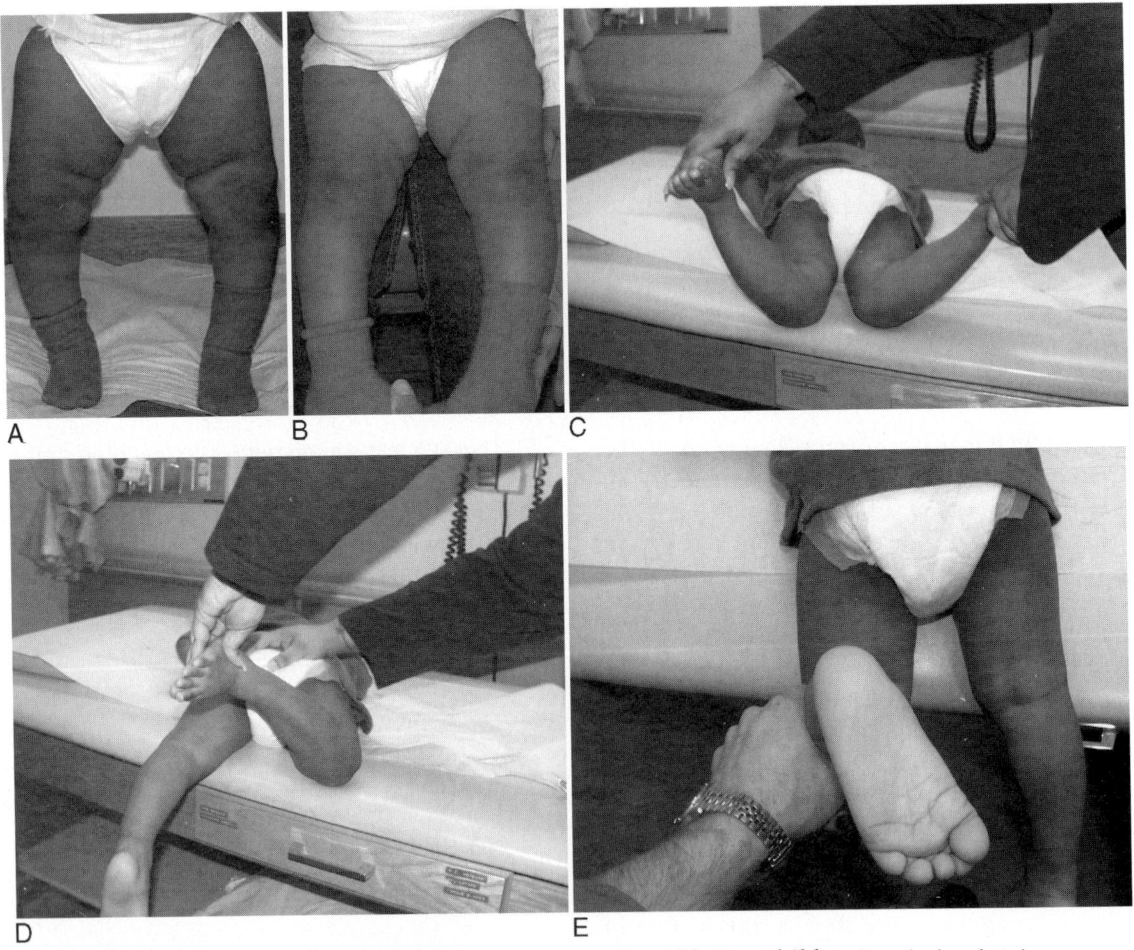

Figure 9-3 Clinical method of static rotational profile in a child. A, Pseudo-bowlegs in child with tibial torsion. Note that feet are forward and patellae are lateral and flexed. **B,** Same child with legs turned so the patellae are forward, knees extended, and feet crossed. Note that legs are now straight. Radiographs must be taken with the legs in the same position. **C,** Measurement of medial rotation of the hip. **D,** Measurement of lateral rotation. Note that the pelvis is maintained in neutral. **E,** The tight-foot angle is seen. The medial rotation of the tibia in this child accounts for the appearance of the patellae in **A** and **B**.

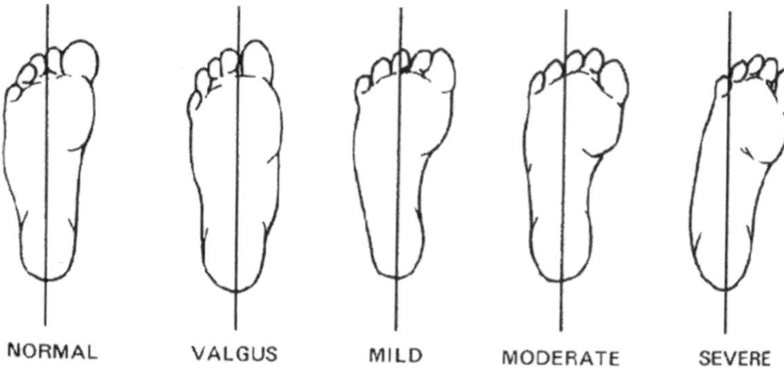

Figure 9-4 The heel-bisector line is demonstrated schematically. Lateral deviation of the foot is abduction, and medial deviation is adduction. (From Bleck EE: Developmental orthopaedics: Chapter III: Toddlers. Dev Med Child Neurol 24:533-555, 1982.)

The natural history of femoral and tibia torsional abnormalities is benign. There is no evidence that these conditions lead to arthritis of the hip, knee, or ankle. In the absence of a neurologic disorder, children with either medially or laterally rotated limbs are not at increased risk for falling. The initial treatment for rotational abnormalities consists of observation and reassurance. Although the parents of many children with such abnormalities were themselves treated with physical therapy, braces, or custom shoes, none of these measures has proved to alter limb alignment.[3] Frequently, parents bring their child to the pediatrician at the insistence of grandparents. It may at times seem easier to prescribe one or all of these modalities. However, time spent on patient education reduces the family's frustration, concerns, and monetary expense. Only surgery consisting of corrective osteotomies is effective in altering limb alignment. For many families, cosmesis is the central issue. Most families decline surgery once they learn of its risks, which include infection, hematoma, non-union, malunion, neurovascular injury, and scar formation.

Coronal Limb Abnormalities (Frontal Prone)

Genu varum (bowed legs) and genu valgum (knock knees) are the two most common deformities found in the coronal plane. The infant is born with knees in varus. Varus persists until 2 years of age, when the legs straighten. The limbs then overcorrect and become maximally valgus between 3 and 4 years of age. In a child 6 to 7 years old, a mature knee alignment is achieved, with 5 to 7 degrees of valgus (Fig. 9-5).[4] Physiologic genu varus and genu valgus, which are characterized by spontaneous resolution, must be distinguished from pathologic conditions that will persist without treatment.

The differential diagnosis of pathologic genu varum includes traumatic genu varum, skeletal dysplasia (e.g., achondroplasia), rickets, fibrous dysplasia, and Blount disease. Many of these conditions can be identified on the basis of information obtained from the history, as exemplified by post-traumatic genu varum. Trauma can cause deformities of the lower extremity in multiple planes.

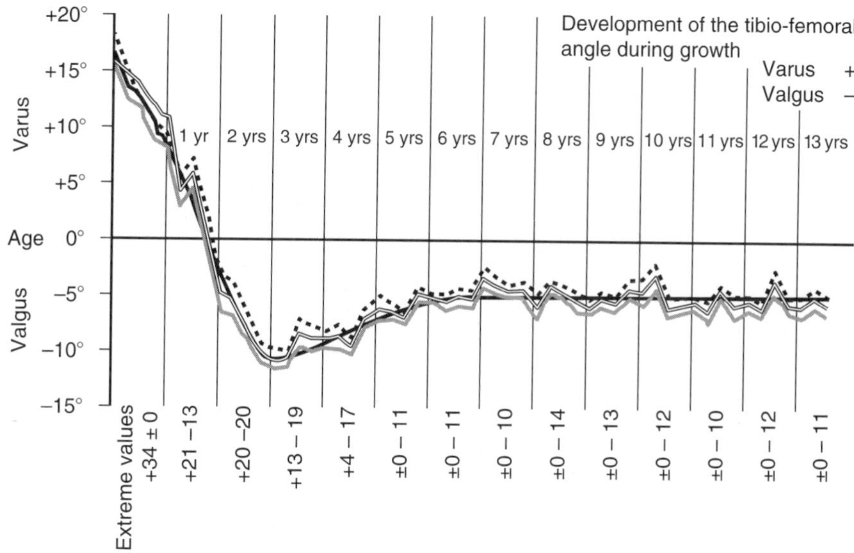

Figure 9-5 The normal coronal alignment of the knee plotted for age. (From Salenius P, Vankka E: The development of the tibiofemoral angle in children. J Bone Joint Surg 57:259-261, 1975.)

Limb deformity can result from angulation produced through a bone at the time of injury, or from partial growth arrest after physeal injury. The distal femoral physis is especially prone to growth arrest. A complete or partial arrest occurs in 50% of cases of physeal fracture of the proximal tibia. The exact location of an angular deformity is not always obvious on radiographs. A helpful sign is the Harris growth arrest line, a radiographic sign of abnormal longitudinal bone growth after illness or trauma.[5] When there is diminished growth in a portion of the physis, the arrest line develops nonparallel to the physis. The line is nearer the portion of the physis where growth is diminished and farther from a region of relative normal growth. Deformities that are expected to lead to mechanical dysfunction are treated surgically. Factors to consider during surgical planning include the location of physeal arrest, percentage of physeal involvement, amount of angular deformity, and amount of growth remaining. Surgical options are physeal bar excision, physeal closure, redirection osteotomy, and limb equalization procedures.

Genu varum from skeletal dysplasias is associated with short stature. The height of affected children is usually below the fifth percentile. Many skeletal dysplasias cause a characteristic facial appearance and body habitus. For example, achondroplasia is associated with frontal bossing, trident hand, and rhizomelic dwarfism. Developmental delay is also common. Most lower limb deformities seen with skeletal dysplasias are treated with observation. The indication for surgical correction of limb malalignment is based on the presence of symptoms (i.e., ankle or knee pain).

Rickets, like the skeletal dysplasias, is associated with short stature. Children with severe rickets may have limb deformities in multiple planes. The physeal regions are enlarged secondary to a deficiency in mineralization in the zone of provisional calcification. Clinically, this enlargement is seen as swollen wrists and "rosary ribs" (Fig. 9-6A). Widened physeal regions are readily apparent on a plain radiograph (Fig. 9-6B). Treatment of limb deformity in rickets begins with the medical control of the disease. Spontaneous resolution may occur once the metabolic abnormality is addressed. Surgical intervention is considered in patients once there a plateau in limb correction has been reached after medical stabilization of the disease.

Blount Disease

Blount disease is an idiopathic, nonphysiologic form of genu varum. Classification is based on age at presentation. The infantile (presentation from birth to 4 years) and juvenile (5 to 10 years) forms of Blount disease are grouped together as early onset, and the adolescent form (presentation from11 years to maturity) is categorized as late onset. Risk factors for infantile Blount disease are early ambulation and weight more than the 95% for age. It should be remembered, however, that Blount disease does occur in thin people.

Distinguishing physiologic genu varum from Blount disease is a difficult task in patients younger than 2 years. Making the correct diagnosis is more challenging in patients who also have MTT. As discussed previously, MTT may persist until a child is 4 years old. MTT

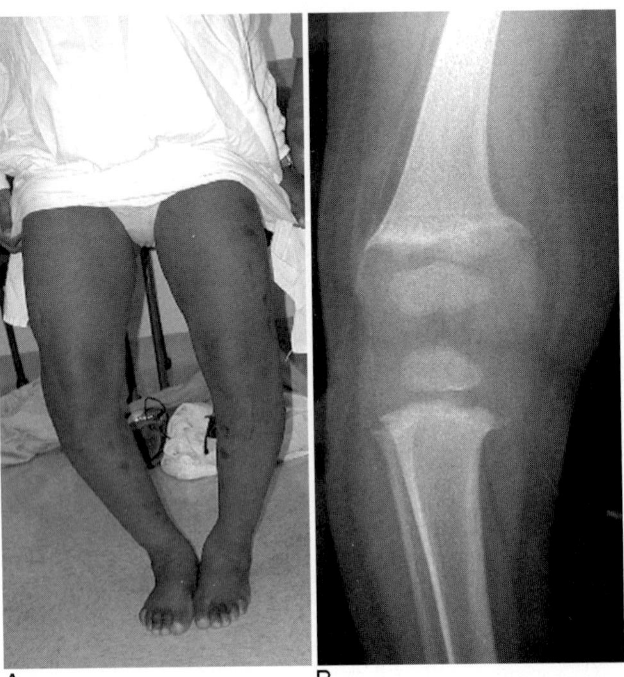

Figure 9-6 **A,** Clinical appearance of child with bowlegs secondary to rickets, a deformity recurring 6 years after surgical correction. **B,** Radiograph of infant with rickets. Note the thickened physis, widened and cupped metaphysis.

increases the appearance of genu varum. Knee angulation is measured both clinically and radiographically by means of the femoral-tibial angle (FTA). The FTA is formed by the longitudinal axes of the femoral and tibial shafts. It should be measured with the patellae facing forward to eliminate the apparent increase in genu varum secondary to axial rotation. In the child with MTT, the patellae face laterally when the feet face forward. Physical findings associated with physiologic genu varum include a smooth angular deformity with contributions from both the femur and tibia. A lateral thrust—a sudden and visible outward excursion of the knee during the weight acceptance phase of gait—is also absent. In contrast, the child with infantile Blount disease has an angular deformity isolated to the proximal tibia (no femoral involvement), and a lateral thrust is typically present (Fig. 9-7).

Blount disease is confirmed with a patellae-forward AP radiograph. The radiographic changes associated with infantile Blount disease were described and divided into six stages by Langenskiöld[6] (Fig. 9-8). These stages are characterized by progressive medial physeal inclination of the proximal tibia. In the most severe stage, a medial physeal bar is present. The changes described by Langenskiöld may not appear before a child is 2 years old. Levine and Drennan[7] proposed use of the metaphyseal-diaphyseal angle (MDA), a radiographic measurement technique that predicts the likelihood of development of infantile Blount's disease in a given limb (Fig. 9-9). The MDA is measured on an AP knee radiograph. An angle larger than 11 degrees is predictive of the development of infantile Blount disease. Feldman and Schoenecker[8] have challenged the 11-degree threshold for too small a confidence interval. They advocate thresholds of 9 degrees for absence of disease and 16 degrees for presence of disease so as to obtain a 95% confidence interval.

Observation is the mainstay of treatment for infantile Blount disease in children younger than 3 years. A brace is prescribed before 3 years of age for a child with a lateral thrust. In the absence of spontaneous correction, a valgus-producing knee-ankle-foot orthosis (KAFO) is worn. Surgery is recommended after brace failure or once a child is older than 4 years. Surgery consists of a proximal tibial realignment osteotomy. Recurrence is common in procedures performed after 4.5 years of age.[9]

Late-onset Blount disease, although different entity from early-onset Blount disease, shares its pathophysiology. The prevailing theory, known as the *Heuter-Volkmann theory*, holds that excessive loads produced by the patient's body weight and preexisting genu varum inhibit proximal medial physeal growth. A lateral thrust may be seen on physical examination, as in early-onset Blount disease, but the distal femur may also be angulated. Late-onset Blount disease is more commonly unilateral and has less tibial torsion than early-onset disease. Medial physeal and epiphyseal hypoplasias with proximal tibial angulation are evident on AP radiographs. The treatment for late-onset Blount disease is surgical, consisting of proximal tibial osteotomies, or lateral physeal hemiepiphysiodesis (selective closure of half of the growth plate to allow the contralateral portion of the physis to correct with growth), or both.

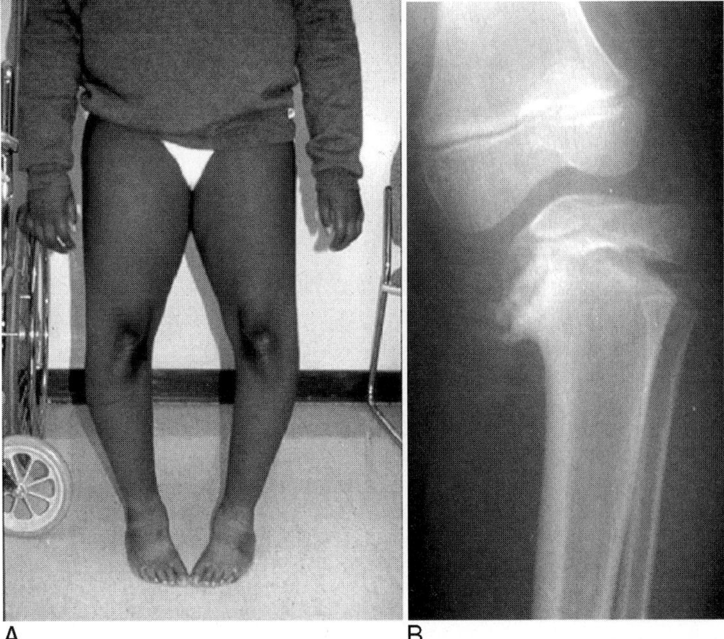

Figure 9-7 **A,** Child with infantile Blount disease. The patellae are forward, and the legs are in varus rotation. **B,** Radiograph of infantile Blount disease. Note the medial epiphyseal deficit, which is not seen in adolescent Blount disease.

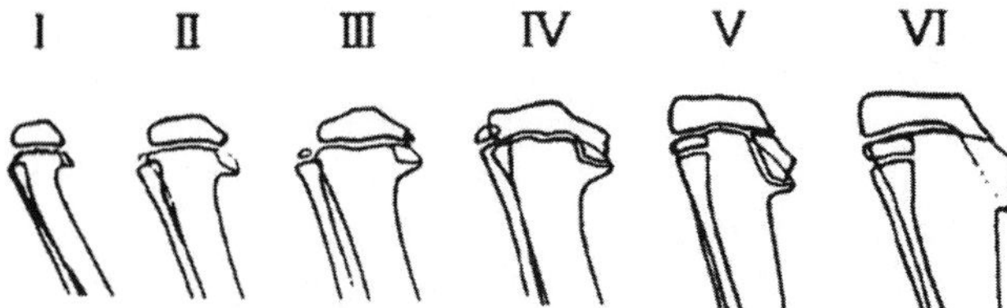

Figure 9-8 Depiction of the stages of infantile Blount disease. (From Langenskiöld A: Tibia vara [osteochondrosis deformans tibiae]: A survey of 23 cases. Acta Chir Scand 103:1, 1952.)

Genu Valgum

The causes of genu valgum are similar to those of genu varum. Trauma, skeletal dysplasia, and metabolic disorders are all possible causes.

Multiple hereditary exostosis (MHE), or osteochondromatosis, is a skeletal dysplasia that warrants discussion. MHE is inherited in an autosomal dominant manner. Patients present to the physician with multiple firm subcutaneous masses, most of which are painless. Causes of pain are external compression (contusion of prominent mass), neurovascular compression, and malignant transformation. The incidence of malignant transformation in MHE is unknown but is believed to be less than 1%. Malignant transformation is very uncommon in the growing child. Indications for treatment of MHE are intractable pain, restriction of motion, neurovascular compression, limb length discrepancy, and progressive limb deformity. Ankle valgus and knee valgus are the two most common deformities of the lower extremity in MHE. Treatment of the angular deformity is based on its severity as well as the expected growth of the limb. Removal of the osteochondromas may be combined with metaphyseal osteotomies, epiphysiodesis, or both (Fig. 9-10).

The diagnosis of idiopathic genu valgum is one of exclusion. When the disorder is severe, patients complain of knee instability or pain. The angular deformity is apparent on physical examination. The degree of knee deformity is measured on plain radiographs. Computed tomography (CT) may be needed to rule out a physeal bar. Treatment is surgical, and a medial hemiepiphysiodesis is performed if adequate growth remains for the lateral physis to catch up. On average, 7 degrees of deformity can be corrected by a hemiepiphysiodesis performed in

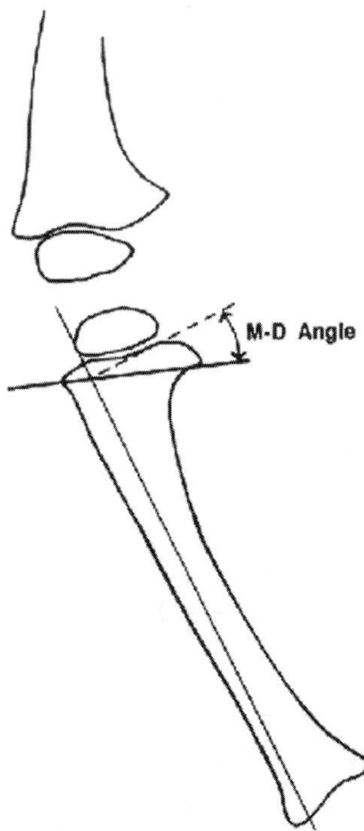

Figure 9-9 Drawing showing the metaphyseal-diaphyseal angle used to diagnose Blount disease. Draw a line through the proximal tibial physis. Draw a second line along the lateral tibial cortex. Then drawn a third line perpendicular to the shaft line at the level of the physeal line. If the angle is smaller than 11 degrees, the patient is unlikely to have Blount disease. An angle greater than 16 degrees is likely to indicate Blount disease. (From Morrissy RT [ed]: Lovell and Winter's Pediatric Orthopaedics, 3rd ed, vol 2. Philadelphia, Lippincott Williams & Wilkins, p 749, 1990).

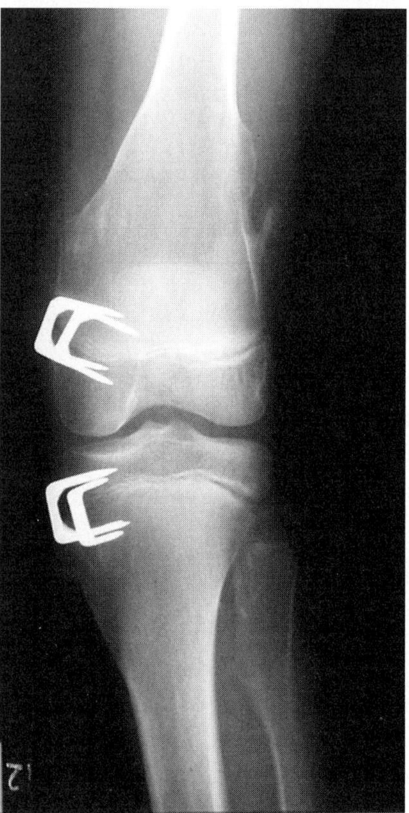

Figure 9-10 Radiograph of knee with genu valgum secondary to multiple hereditary exostosis. Staples placed medially are correcting the deformity.

the distal femur, and 5 degrees in the proximal tibia.[10] In the mature patient or the child in whom inadequate growth remains in the lateral physis for correction, a realignment osteotomy is performed.

Tibial Bowing

Lower extremity bowing can occur in oblique plains. The apex of the deformity defines the direction of bowing. Posterior medial bowing is associated with a calcaneovalgus foot deformity and is discussed along with that deformity (see later). Other directions of bowing are anterior and anterolateral. Anterolateral deformity is associated with congenital pseudoarthrosis of the tibia, whereas anterior bowing is associated with fibula hemimelia.

Congenital pseudoarthrosis of the tibia is a structural defect within the tibia that is susceptible to fracture and resistant to healing. A pseudoarthrosis can occur in any bone, although the tibia is most commonly affected. Typically, the lesion is diaphyseal, located at the junction of the middle and distal thirds. Neurofibromatosis is the most common associated condition, accounting for almost 50% of cases. Other associated conditions are Ehlers-Danlos and amniotic band syndromes. With rare exception, the natural history of congenital pseudoarthrosis is that of limb angulation, repeated fracture, and limb length discrepancy. Radiographs show a narrowing and sclerosis of the diaphysis. The medullary cavity may have cysts at the apex of the deformity or may be completely ablated. Early treatment, before the occurrence of fracture and significant angular deformity, consists of a full-contact clamshell ankle-foot orthosis (AFO) or knee-ankle-foot orthosis and regular visits to an orthopaedist. Fracture or progressive bowing is an indication for surgical intervention. The best surgical procedure is a matter of debate. Placement of an intramedullary nail that crosses the ankle joint is the procedure most often recommended in North America.[11] Three unsuccessful attempts to maintain limb alignment constitute a relative indication for a Syme or Boyd amputation.[12] Although neither amputation heals the pseudoarthrosis, they both allow for better prosthetic application to facilitate ambulation.

Fibula hemimelia is a longitudinal deficiency in the lateral portion of the lower limb in which part or all of fibula may be missing. The foot commonly is missing its lateral rays and may be in severe valgus. Ankle instability and ankle equinus are common. The knee lacks supportive ligaments. Fibula hemimelia can occur in isolation or along with a longitudinally and structurally deficient femur, acetabulum, or both. Treatment is directed at producing a sound limb for ambulation. This goal may be accomplished with limb equalization procedures, provided that the limb is not shortened by more than 30%. Large limb length discrepancies can be addressed with lengthening procedures using the Ilizarov method. However, it is prudent to exercise restraint when considering multiple lengthening procedures. The patient so treated may reach maturity with legs of equal length; however, the cost is a lost childhood, because he or she will have spent years in an external fixator. Substantial leg lengthening procedures yield stiff limbs that may be less functional than limbs with prostheses.[13]

Toe Walking

Physical development occurs in a predictable and orderly fashion. Children gain head control, followed by sitting balance, cruising, and, finally, ambulation. Ninety-five percent of children begin ambulation between 10 and 17 months of age. A toddler's gait has a short stride length, rapid cadence, and is broad-based. The gait lacks both side-to-side symmetry and a consistent cadence. An adult gait pattern occurs by 7 years of age.[14] Toe walking, or equinus gait, can be a normal gait pattern in children until the third year of life. After 3 years, "toe walking" is considered abnormal. The term "equinus" comes from the Latin *equus* ("horse"). These children, like horses, walk on their toes.

The list of conditions that cause pathologic toe walking is extensive. To narrow down the differential diagnosis, it is helpful to separate patients into acute and chronic toe walkers. Acute toe walkers have previously walked with a plantigrade gait, whereas chronic toe walkers have not. Acute toe walking can be further classified as painful or painless. Acute painful toe walking can be the result of a recent trauma (calcaneal fracture) or the presence of a foreign body (i.e., glass, splinter, or thorn) in the plantar aspect of the foot. Acute painless toe walking suggests a neuromuscular differential diagnosis consisting of muscular dystrophy and spinal cord disorders (i.e., tumor, syringomyelia, tethered cord). The typical child with Duchenne muscular dystrophy is a boy with calf pseudohypertrophy, presence of Gower sign, and, in 65% of cases, a positive family history for the condition. Spinal cord disease may be associated with upper motor neuron lesions (i.e., hyperreflexia—clonus, Babinski sign), sensory abnormalities, and dysfunction of the bowel and/or bladder.

Chronic toe walking is seen with limb length discrepancy, congenital limb anomalies (e.g., proximal femoral focal deficiency, fibula hemimelia) and neuromuscular conditions such as cerebral palsy. The diagnosis of limb length discrepancy or congenital anomaly is easily made with physical examination and standard radiographs and so is not discussed further here.

In contrast, although the topic of cerebral palsy is discussed in Chapter 13, some points deserve mention here. *Cerebral palsy* is a collection of neurologic conditions, the common denominator of which is an insult to the brain about the time of birth. The injury occurs during a brief period in the development of the immature brain. The motor dysfunction types seen with cerebral palsy are spastic, athetoid, ataxic, hypotonic, and mixed. Some or all of the limbs can be involved, depending on the portion of the brain affected. Hemiplegia affects the arm and leg on one side of the body; diplegia affects predominantly the lower extremities; and quadriplegia affects all four limbs. A history of prematurity is common among children with cerebral palsy. Toe walking is seen most commonly in patients with spastic hemiplegic. The presence of hand dominance before 1 year of age is suggestive of hemiplegia, because children are normally ambidextrous during the first year of life. The affected lower extremity of a child with hemiplegia is in equinus with a footdrop (absence of active ankle dorsiflexors). The heel may be in varus secondary to overactivity of one or both of the tibial tendons.

The diagnosis of idiopathic (also known as "habitual") toe walking (ITW) is one of exclusion. There may be a family history of this condition. Physical examination begins by distinguishing between fixed equinus deformity and dynamic toe walking (foot can be placed in a plantigrade position). The technique of examining an ankle with an equinus deformity involves inversion of the subtalar joint before ankle dorsiflexion. Inversion locks the subtalar joint, preventing dorsiflexion through the midfoot. Midfoot dorsiflexion gives a false impression of normal ankle motion. The angle is measured from the shaft of the tibia to the lateral border of the foot. The ankle should dorsiflex 10 to 15 degrees.

A fixed ankle contracture is treated initially with physical therapy to stretch the gastrocnemius-soleus muscle complex. If therapy does not correct the contracture, either serial casting or botulinum toxin injections should be prescribed. The failure of conservative measures is the indication for surgical lengthening of the Achilles tendon. The same conservative measures are recommended for dynamic toe walking. However, surgical correction should be used more cautiously because it may lead to overlengthening of the Achilles tendon, with a resultant crouch gait.

FOOT DEFORMITIES

Patients present to their pediatricians with a host of painful or painless foot conditions. During analysis of a foot deformity, it is helpful to identify the location and plane of the abnormal rotation or translation. In general terms, the regions of the foot can be divided into the *forefoot* (metatarsals and phalanges), *midfoot* (cuneiforms, cuboid, and navicular) and *hindfoot* (talus and calcaneus). In the hindfoot, coronal rotation is heel varus (medial) and valgus (lateral). Axial rotation of the hindfoot is coupled with varus (internal) and valgus (external) rotation of the subtalar joint. Sagittal plane rotation of the hindfoot (equinus and calcaneus) primarily occurs at the ankle joint; however, it may be present between the talus and calcaneus. In the midfoot and the forefoot, coronal rotation is described as adduction or abduction as it relates to medial or lateral deviation of the foot. Pronation and supination are axial rotations through the midfoot and the midfoot-forefoot articulation. *Pronation* is a plantar-flexion, and *supination* a dorsiflexion, of the medial column of the foot as it relates to the position of the hindfoot. Lastly, the toes may rotate through the sagittal plane (flexion and extension). The next few sections use these terms to describe specific pediatric foot conditions.

Metatarsus Adductus

As mentioned in the discussion of rotational abnormalities, in addition to the femur and tibia, the foot can be a source of an internal foot progression angle. The three conditions to consider are metatarsus adductus and clubfoot, which are common, and skewfoot, which is not. *Metatarsus adductus* is a medial deviation of the forefoot at the level of the midtarsal joints of the foot. In this condition, the hindfoot is in neutral to valgus alignment (never in varus), and the forefoot may be in varying amounts of supination. The patient with clubfoot, in contrast, has ankle equinus, hindfoot varus, midfoot cavus (pronation of midfoot), and adduction. Skewfoot, also known as serpentine or "Z" foot, consists of metatarsus adductus, midfoot abduction (with or without lateral translation), and hindfoot valgus. Clubfoot is discussed in greater detail later in the chapter.

Metatarsus adductus is the most common congenital foot deformity, present in 1 of 1000 live births. The etiology is not completely understood, but the disorder is theorized to result from intrauterine mechanical forces applied to the foot. For example, in twin births or oligohydramnios, there may be insufficient room within the uterus for normal foot development. Conditions such as metatarsus adductus, torticollis, and hip dysplasia, which have a common etiology, are considered "packing abnormalities." During the initial interview with the parents, questions pertaining to prenatal care will reveal the presence or absence of these predisposing conditions.

The musculoskeletal examination should include a thorough and careful examination of the cervical spine and hips to rule out the associated conditions mentioned previously. The purpose of the foot examination is to judge the extent of deformity and the level of flexibility. The foot with metatarsus adductus is described as "bean shaped" (kidney bean). The foot has a deep medial crease along the instep and a convex lateral border

(Fig. 9-11A and B). The heal bisector line is valuable in measuring and documenting the deformity. Documentation of the deformity should state which toe or web space the HBL crosses (Fig. 9-11C). Photocopying the soles of the child's feet, by resting them on the glass of the copier, is an easy pictorial means of recording foot adduction.[15] One must take care not to allow the child's entire weight to rest on the copier screen during the process, so as not to break the glass. Foot flexibility is of equal importance in treatment decisions. Bleck[16] defined a *flexible foot* as one that can be corrected beyond the midline (second web space), a *moderately flexible foot* as correctable to the midline, and a *severe foot* as uncorrectable. Radiographs are usually unnecessary in the initial evaluation of metatarsus adductus.

The treatment for metatarsus adductus is best determined through an appreciation of the natural history (untreated) of the condition. Rushforth[17] published the largest natural history study of this condition. He monitored 179 feet in children as they grew from 3 years to 11 years old. At study completion, 86% of the feet were normal or had a mild deformity, 10% had a moderate deformity, and 4% had a severe deformity. Ponseti and Becker[18] reported that 88% of their patients with metatarsus adductus experienced complete resolution of the deformity without treatment. The remaining 12 percent (44 patients) underwent manipulation and casting. Five percent of the feet treated in plaster had significant residual deformity.

Once the deformity and flexibility of the foot with metatarsus adductus have been documented, the physician must decide whether an intervention is necessary. It has been suggested that a foot that corrects beyond the midline when its lateral border is stroked does not require treatment. This finding has not been substantiated in the literature; however, the personal experience of one of the chapter authors (DW) agrees with this observation. When a foot is flexible but corrects only to the midline, a course of home stretching is reasonable, although there is no proof of its efficacy.

The technique of stretching is as follows: While facing the child, the caregiver cups the heel of the foot (with

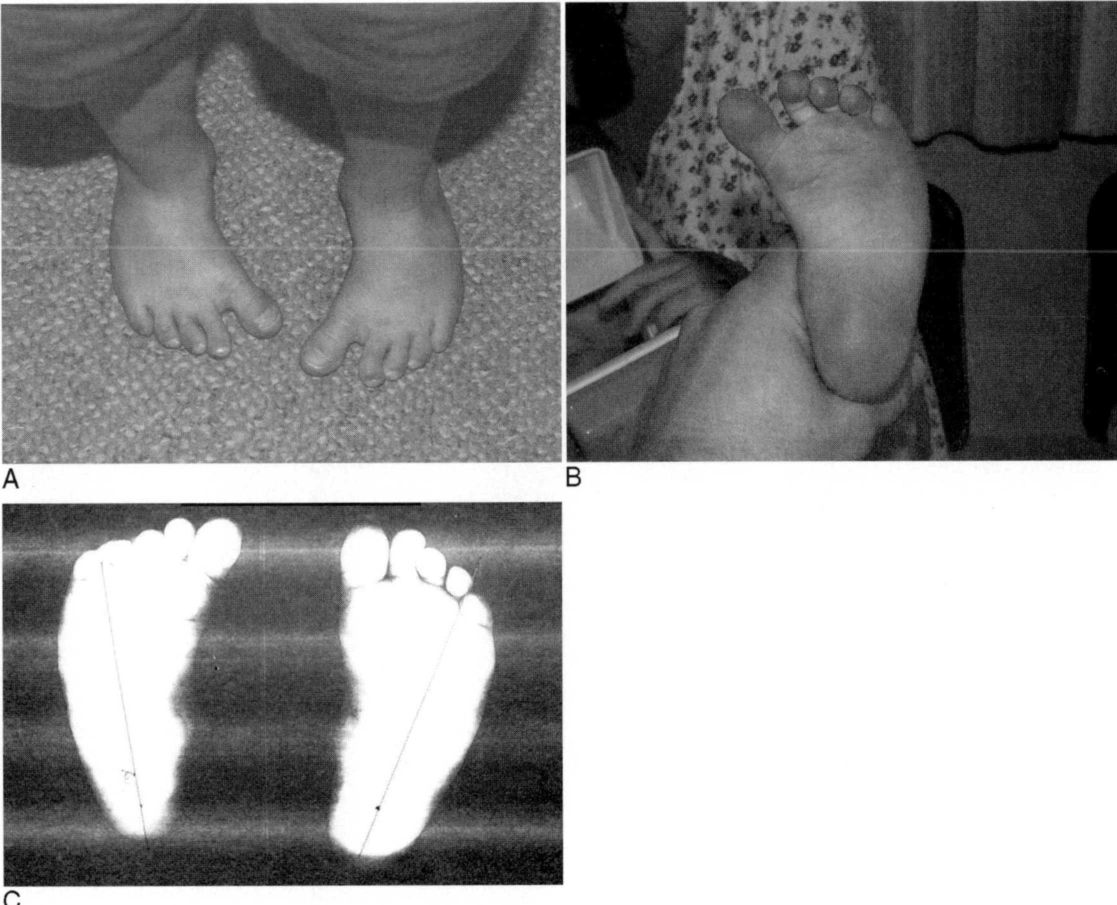

Figure 9-11 **A,** Clinical photograph of the dorsal aspect of the feet of a child with metatarsus adductus. **B,** The same child's feet viewed from the plantar aspect. **C,** A photocopy of the feet of a child with metatarsus adductus for documentation.

the left hand for the right foot, and or the right hand for the left foot). Keeping the heel in varus with that hand, the caregiver abducts the foot with the other hand. Pressure is applied gently enough across the metatarsals so that the infant does not cry. The infant whose foot does not correct to the midline or has not responded to stretching before the patient is 8 months old should be referred to an orthopaedist experienced in the treatment of pediatric foot conditions. Serial casting may then be applied, with a new cast placed every 1 or 2 weeks. The results of casting are best when it is instituted before 8 months of age. An alternative approach is to have the child begin high-top, open-faced, reverse last shoes for 22 hours a day. The high-top style is chosen only to discourage the child from removing them. They are open-toed to prevent damage if the toes are turned under. They are reverse last to stretch out the abductor hallucis.

The indication for surgery is the inability to achieve treatment goals through nonoperative means. Treatment goals for all foot conditions are the attainment of a painless, plantigrade, "shoeable," flexible foot. The foot does not have to look "normal," however; as long as it meets the other criteria, the result is acceptable. In the majority of cases, metatarsus adductus resolves spontaneously by 2 years of age. Surgery is not considered before a child is 4 years old. In the past, a capsulotomy of the metatarsal-tarsal joints was recommended.[19] Because the procedure was associated with an unacceptably high rate of recurrence, it is no longer routinely performed. The use of multiple metatarsal osteotomies through the bases of the metatarsals is a more reasonable operation. However, care must be taken not to damage the first metatarsal's growth plate, which is located near the osteotomy site. An alternative procedure is a cuboid-shortening and medial cuneiform-lengthening osteotomy. This double tarsal osteotomy has yielded excellent results without damage to the first metatarsal physis.

Adduction of the forefoot occurs in both skewfoot and metatarsus adductus. The difference is that skewfoot also involves abduction (with or without lateral translation) of the midfoot and valgus of the hindfoot (Fig. 9-12). Skewfoot occurs idiopathically, from neuromuscular conditions, and iatrogenically after improper casting for metatarsus adductus. Without treatment, skewfoot can lead to pain and problems with the wearing of shoes. Corrective casting is the same as that described for metatarsus adductus. Failure of conservative care along with the inability of the foot to accommodate a standard shoe is a relative indication for surgery. Numerous procedures have been recommended. The concept is to lengthen the medial midfoot with an opening wedge osteotomy and to shorten the lateral midfoot with a cuboid-closing wedge osteotomy. Hindfoot valgus is corrected with a calcaneal osteotomy.[20] Fusions are reserved for the severe foot deformity in the mature patient.

Clubfoot

The term "clubfoot" was initially applied to any deformity of the foot in equinus. The term has come, however, to be applied only to the foot deformed in hindfoot equinus, midfoot varus, and forefoot adductus or talipes equinovarus (Fig. 9-13). The deformity has been further divided into congenital and acquired. Acquired clubfoot is associated with neuromuscular diseases, such as cerebral palsy, myelomeningocele, and polio, or external forces such as amniotic band syndrome. This discussion focuses on the more common congenital clubfoot.

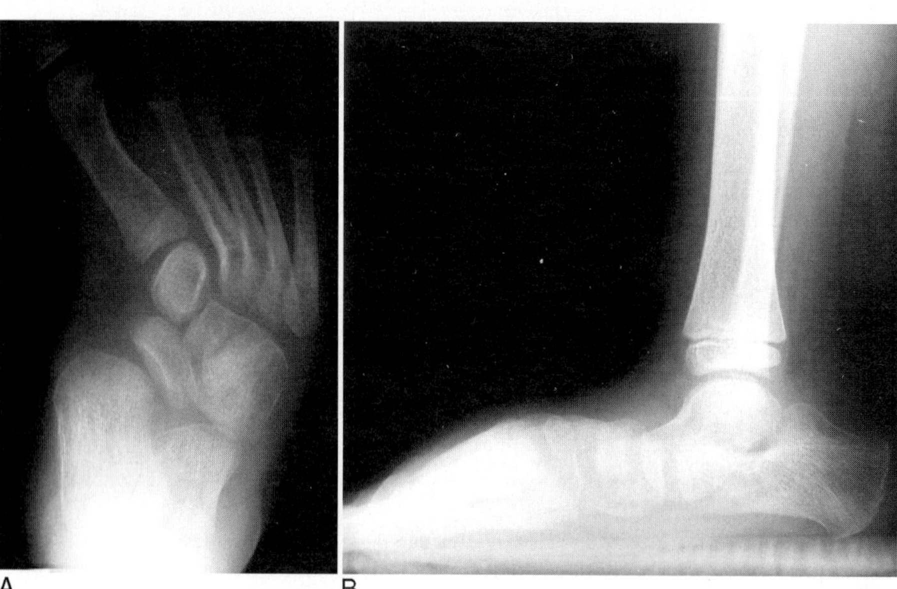

Figure 9-12 Radiographs of a skewfoot. **A,** On an anteroposterior radiograph, note the forefoot adduction, hindfoot abduction, lateral translation, and hindfoot valgus. **B,** Lateral radiograph demonstrates collapse of the arch.

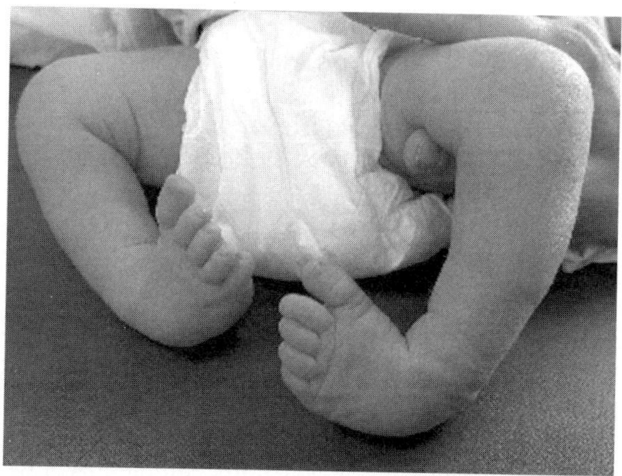

Figure 9-13 Clubfoot, with the foot in hindfoot varus, hindfoot equinus, and forefoot varus.

In spite of new scientific developments and theories concerning the origins of clubfoot, the etiology remains unknown. The cause is most likely a combination of genetic and environmental factors.

The incidence of clubfoot varies widely with race and sex. It rises with the number of affected relatives of a patient with clubfoot, suggesting genetic influence.[21] Chesney and colleagues[22] observed that, although no gene has as yet been identified, many epidemiologic studies suggest inheritance patterns. Lochmiller and associates[23] identified a 24.4% incidence of clubfoot in high-risk families. The incidence among different races varies from 0.39 per 1000 among Chinese to 1.2 per 1000 among white and to 6.8 per 1000 among Polynesians.[24-26] Males are affected twice as often as females. Lochmiller and associates,[23] working in Texas, reported a 2.5:1 ratio of males to females with clubfoot. Siblings have up to a 30 times increased risk of clubfoot deformity.[25] Clubfoot affects both siblings in 32.5% of monozygotic twins but only 2.9% of dizygotic twins.

Histologic anomalies have been reported, but none has been linked as yet to gene anomalies. Almost every tissue in the clubfoot (muscle, nerve, vessels, tendon insertions, ligaments, fascia, tendon sheaths) has been described as being abnormal.[27] Ultrastructural muscle abnormalities were identified by Isaacs and coworkers.[28] Handelsman and Badalamente[29] demonstrated a higher ratio of type I to type II muscle fibers (7:1, compared with 1:2 in normal feet), suggesting a possible link to a primary nerve abnormality.[30]

A primary germ plasm defect of bone resulting in deformity of the talus and navicular was suggested by Irani and Sherman[31] in 1963. Defects in the cartilage of clubfeet were demonstrated by Shapiro and Glimcher.[32] Ionasescu and colleagues[33] identified increased collagen synthesis in clubfeet. In an anatomic study, Ippolito and coworkers[34] demonstrated deformity of the talus with medial neck angulation, medial tilting and rotation of the body of the talus. Together with the medial tilting and rotation of the calcaneus, these deformities accounted for the varus deformity of the hindfoot, which in turn accounted for the supination of the forefoot. Using MRI, Davidson and associates[35] have demonstrated plantar-flexion and varus angular deformity of the talus, os calcis, and cuboid in the infant clubfoot. Their findings suggest growth disturbance secondary to abnormal mechanical forces.

Dietz and coworkers[36] identified reductions in cell number and cytoplasm in the posterior tibial tendon sheath compared with the anterior tibial tendon sheath, indicating a regional growth disturbance. These investigators suggested that there is evidence that localized soft tissue contraction is involved in the pathogenesis of clubfoot. Carroll[37,38] and Shimizu and associates[24] speculated on the possibility of a neuromuscular dysfunction with intrauterine partial loss of innervation and reinnervation as an underlying cause of the clubfoot deformity.

Hootnick and coworkers[39] and Muir and associates[40] found a significantly greater prevalence of the absence of the dorsalis pedis pulse in the parents of children with clubfeet. Muir and associates theorized that the vascular deformity might be primary and the resultant anatomic deformity secondary, occurring through one of the following three possible mechanisms: (1) a poorly vascularized anterior compartment, which would lead to muscle imbalance, (2) ischemic fibrosis in the medial aspect of the foot, and (3) abnormal talar development, secondary to poor vascular supply to the talus from the abnormal anterior tibialis artery.

Turco[26] identified anomalous muscles in about 15% of clubfeet. Porter[41] described an anomalous calf flexor muscle in five children with clubfoot. He also observed that patients with this anomalous muscle had a greater frequency of first-degree relatives with clubfoot.

Turco[26] credits Hippocrates with first proposing the mechanical theory of the cause of clubfoot. This theory holds that the foot is held in a position of equinovarus by external uterine compression and oligohydramnios. Turco[26] finds it unlikely that such increased pressure would produce the same deformity repeatedly, especially when there is plenty of room in the uterus at the time a clubfoot forms (first trimester).

Bohm,[42] in 1929, described the following four stages of fetal development of the foot: (1) marked equinus and severe adduction of the hindfoot and forefoot, (2) rotation into supination, 90 degrees of plantar-flexion, and forefoot adduction, (3) decreased plantar-flexion, and (4) development toward the adult position. He considered the possibility that clubfoot represents an interruption in the development of the normal foot. However, the medial displacement of the navicular bone so common in clubfoot is not seen at any stage in the normal developing foot, and there is no distortion of the bones in the early stages of normal fetal development, even though these changes could occur later. Kawashima and Uhthoff[43] studied the anatomy of the human foot from the 8th to the 21st intrauterine week in 147 specimens. Their findings showed that the normal foot looks similar to a clubfoot during the 9th week of gestation. They posited an interruption in development as responsible for the deformity.

Studies of the complications of amniocentesis have observed the association of clubfoot with early amniocentesis (before the 11th week). Farrell and coworkers[44] reported a rate for clubfoot of 1.1% after amniocentesis, about ten times greater than the risk of live birth (0.1%). The risk of bilateral deformity was noted to be about the same as in the general clubfoot population. Birth weight, gestational age at delivery, chromosome results, and sex were the same as in a group of infants whose mothers underwent amniocentesis later in pregnancy and who did not demonstrate the increased risk of clubfoot. When early amniocentesis was associated with an amniotic fluid leak, the risk of clubfoot deformity increased to 15%, compared with 1.1% for amniocentesis without leakage. Farrell and coworkers[44] postulated that some event during early amniocentesis with fluid leakage interrupted the normal development of the foot, stopping development at a time when the foot was in the clubfoot position. Although the link with early amniocentesis and fluid leakage was clear, these investigators could not conclude that mechanical factors were to blame. They observed that persistent oligohydramnios was not present in subsequent ultrasonography examinations. They also postulated that altered pressure from the leak could change the developmental process. The CEMAT (Canadian Early and Mid-Trimester Amniocentesis Trial) Group[44] did not find the same association with clubfoot; they proposed that the amount of fluid removed at the time of amniocentesis might be responsible for the difference seen in results of their study and that of Farrell and coworkers.

Another, later study may have theoretical correlation. Robertson and Corbett[45] retrospectively reviewed the medical records of 330 children who were born with uncomplicated clubfoot deformities, to determine the month of conception for each. These researchers found that the mean month of conception for children born with clubfoot deformity was June, a finding at variance from the peak months of conception for the overall population of the United States for the same period. They then theorized that an intrauterine enterovirus infection, whose summer and fall peak infection rates could cause anterior horn cell lesions at the appropriate stage of fetal development, might lead to a deformity such as congenital clubfoot. If the mechanism for association between early amniocentesis and clubfoot is not related to mechanical factors and pressure changes, as suggested by Farrell and coworkers,[44] perhaps infection is to blame. Greater leakage of amniotic fluid, associated with a greater risk of clubfoot, could be associated with a higher infection rate.

Evidence for a neuromuscular cause of clubfoot can be found in a variety of published studies. White and Blasier[46] identified intrauterine peroneal nerve lesions in clubfeet. Isaacs and Handelsmanl[28] showed evidence of neurogenic disease in most clubfeet by means of histochemical and electron-microscopic studies. As already described, Handelsman and Badalamente[29] demonstrated higher content of type I muscle fibers in clubfeet, suggesting a primary nerve abnormality. Arthrogryposis, spina bifida, and sacral agenesis have all been associated with congenital clubfoot deformity, implicating a neuromuscular cause.[25,47]

At this time, our knowledge cannot distinguish which of these observations represent primary changes and which represent secondary changes of the developing clubfoot. The more we explore, with increasingly sophisticated technology, the more likely we are to discover new abnormalities. Clearly, there is a complex interrelationship between genetics and environment on a primary level that manifests as an even more complex physiologic interplay among the different tissues of the foot. This results in the collection of deformities that we call clubfoot.

Congenital talipes equinovarus feet are positioned in hindfoot equinus, hindfoot varus, midfoot adduction and, often, cavus. However, they vary greatly in stiffness, bone deformity, muscle involvement, and response to treatment. Although often subjective and difficult to quantify, the physical and radiographic findings can be useful to understanding the individual clubfoot. A standardized examination of the clubfoot should be performed at first encounter and after each manipulative casting to assess progress of treatment and, eventually, to help determine the need for surgery. Physical and radiographic examinations, although not accurate or reproducible, can provide significant information about severity, improvement with treatment, and the need for surgery.

It is important to examine the whole patient with a clubfoot. Associated anomalies of the upper extremities, back, legs, abnormal reflexes, and so on, can provide information about etiology as well as the likelihood of successful treatment.

The knee, flexed to 90 degrees, can serve as a reference point for measurement. Torsional alignment, varus and valgus, and the overall size and shape of the leg, ankle, and foot should be assessed. Transverse plantar crease or clefts at the midfoot and at the posterior ankle should be noted.[38] Calf atrophy is an expected component of clubfoot, particularly in the older child with severe or residual deformity.

Equinus should be assessed with the knee in extension and in flexion. Contracture of the gastrocnemius muscle is indicated by the equinus measured with the knee extended. The difference between the equinus measured with the knee flexed and extended indicates the amount of ankle joint stiffness and isolated soleus muscle contracture. The posterior os calcis must be palpated carefully during measurement of the equinus of clubfoot, because the bone may be pulled proximally away from the heel pad (Fig. 9-14).

The varus or valgus position of the heel at rest and in the position of best correction should be measured. Flexibility of the subtalar joint is difficult to quantify but may give an indication about stiffness.

The talar head should be palpated dorsolaterally at the midfoot. The talar head usually is lined up with the patella, although plantarflexed. Manipulation to reduce the forefoot onto the talar head demonstrates the amount of midfoot stiffness. This type of examination helps distinguish the clubfoot from metatarsus adductus (in which the foot lacks the hindfoot varus and equinus) and vertical talus (in which there is hindfoot equinus but also hindfoot and forefoot valgus).

In the older child, an abnormal plantar callus pattern may indicate persistent deformity. Increased callus over the plantar-lateral aspect of the forefoot indicates hindfoot equinus and supination. Lack of callus over the heel usually signifies equinus of the forefoot in the presence of a stiff ankle or ankle equinus. Medial calluses over the talar head usually indicate over correction of the hindfoot (valgus). Thick calluses over the metatarsal heads and the heel can suggest a cavus deformity.

Radiographic examination has been used to demonstrate the deformities of the tarsal bones of clubfeet; however, the images are hard to reproduce, evaluate, and measure, for several reasons. First, it is difficult to position the feet in a standard fashion in the x-ray beam, particularly those that are very stiff and deformed. Second, the ossific nuclei do not represent the true shape of the mostly cartilaginous tarsal bones.[35] Third, in the first year of life, only the talus, os calcis, and metatarsals may be ossified. In normal feet, the cuboid is ossified at 6 months, the cuneiforms after 1 year, the navicular bone 3 years; ossification occurs even later in clubfeet.[48] Fourth, rotation distorts the measured angles and makes the talar dome look flattened. Last, the feet are not held in the position of best correction, the radiograph will make them look worse than they are.

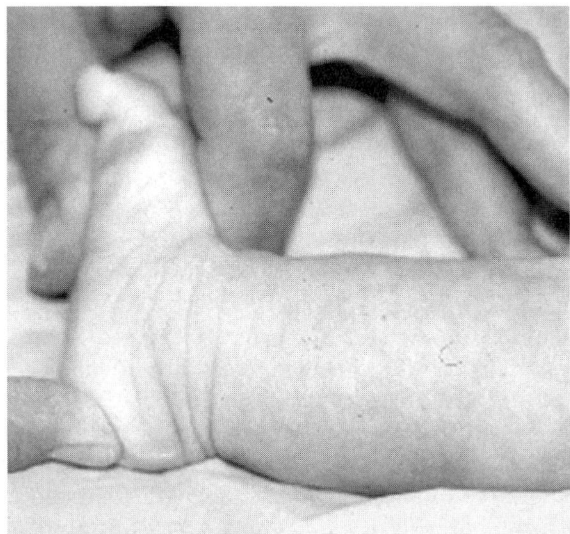

Figure 9-14 In this casted clubfoot, the foot appears to be corrected to neutral, but the heel pad is empty, and the calcaneus is in equinus. The foot should dorsiflex at least 20 degrees.

Radiographic evaluation is useful in documenting the deformity just before surgical correction or to confirm adequate correction by any method. In the older patient with clubfoot, radiographic evaluation can help identify deformity, degenerative changes, and stress changes and fractures.

To optimize the radiographic studies, the feet should be held in the position of best correction, in weight bearing or, for the infant, simulated weight bearing. Because the AP and lateral talocalcaneal angles are the most commonly measured angles (Kite angles[49]), the x-ray beam should be focused on the hindfoot (about 30 degrees from the vertical for the AP angle; the lateral view should be transmalleolar with the fibula overlapping the posterior half of the tibia, to avoid rotational distortion.).

In the older child, it may be useful to focus the x-ray beam on the midfoot. This view assesses dorsolateral subluxation and narrowing of the talonavicular joint. Lateral dorsiflexion and plantar-flexion views may be useful to assess ankle motion (as with flat-top talus), abutting of the anterior tibia against the talar neck, and hypermobility in the midfoot.

The following are common radiographic measurements for the clubfoot.[49,50] On the AP view, the following three observations should be made:

- *The AP talocalcaneal angle:* Lines are drawn through the long axes of the talus and the os calcis (when it is difficult to outline the os calcis, a line can be drawn parallel to the lateral border). The AP talocalcaneal angle typical for clubfoot is less than 20 degrees (Fig. 9-15).
- *The talar to first metatarsal angle:* Lines are drawn through the long axes of the talus and the first metatarsal. In the normal foot, this angle is mild valgus to about 30 degrees; in the clubfoot, it is mild to severe varus (see Fig. 9-18).
- *Medial displacement of the cuboid ossific center on the os calcis axis:*[50,51] This apparent displacement may represent angular deformity of the calcaneus or medial subluxation of the cuboid on the calcaneus.

For the lateral view, the foot should be held in maximum dorsiflexion with the foot laterally rotated but

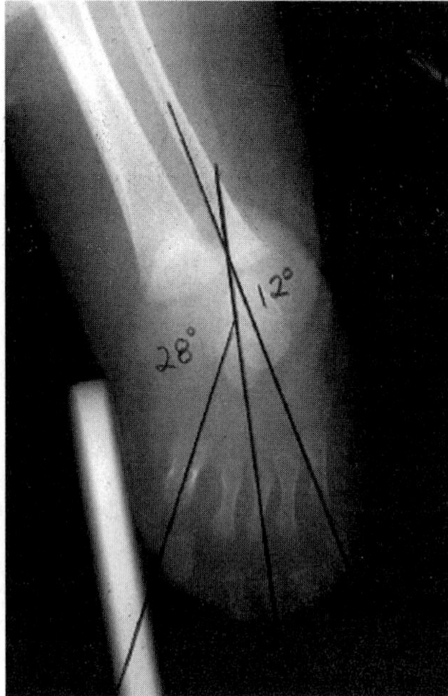

Figure 9-15 Anteroposterior radiograph of a clubfoot. The talocalcaneal angle is reduced to 12 degrees (normal is 30 to 55 degrees). The talar first metatarsal angle is varus (normal is valgus).

without pronation. The x-ray beam should be focused on the hindfoot. The foot should be positioned with the plate held laterally against the posterior half of the foot. The foot is bean shaped, and medial placement of the x-plate would force the foot to be laterally rotated in the x-ray beam. The following two observations should be made on the lateral view:

- *The talocalcaneal angle:* Lines are drawn through the long axis of the talus and the inferior margin of the os classes. The resulting angle for clubfoot demonstrates hindfoot equinus and is typically less than 25 degrees (Fig. 9-16).
- *The talar to first metatarsal angle:* Lines are drawn through the long axes of the talus and the first metatarsal. Plantar-flexion of the forefoot on the hind foot indicates contracted plantar soft tissues or midtarsal bone deformity (triangular navicular bone).

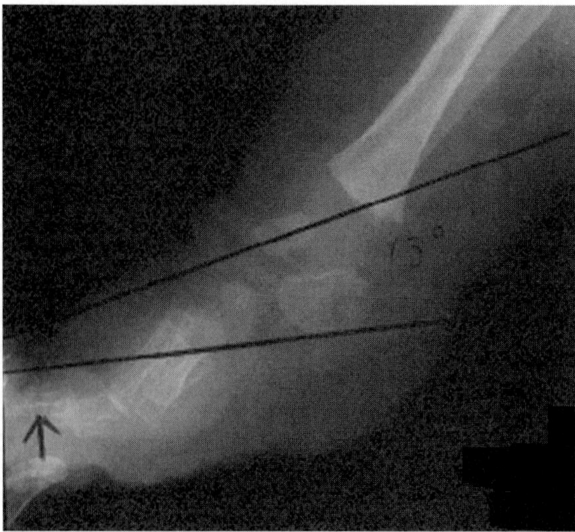

Figure 9-16 Lateral radiograph of clubfoot. The talocalcaneal angle is reduced (normal is 25 to 55 degrees).

As the natural history of clubfoot shows, the patient with an untreated or incompletely treated clubfoot can walk and run surprisingly well throughout childhood in spite of the deformity. However, as the child gets older and larger, the reduced weight-bearing surface (lateral forefoot) develops a thickened callus, which becomes painful. Wearing of ordinary shoes becomes difficult. The stigma of the deformity may cause the child to be shunned in some societies. Because treatment is relatively easy in the infant, it should be started as early as is reasonable.

Hippocrates described the earliest known treatment of clubfoot around 400 B.C.E. He described a manipulation of the deformed foot and wrapping with bandages to maintain the correction. He reported that when the correction was begun in infancy and the deformity was not too severe, treatment was successful and surgery was not necessary.

With the development of mechanical devices in the 17th through 19th centuries, many physicians designed gradual correcting turnbuckle devices to stretch clubfeet over years. Plaster-of-Paris bandages, developed in 1838, soon supplanted these devices because of their ease of use.

Inadequate patient compliance with treatment leads to many failures. With continued failure, tenotomy of the Achilles tendon became popular in the first quarter of the 19th century. Pain and gangrene were dreaded complications until the development of anesthesia in 1846 and of antisepsis in 1865, after which surgeons designed increasingly complex surgical treatments. Throughout the 20th century, physicians offering surgical treatment vied with physicians promoting nonsurgical treatments to develop the ultimate management of clubfoot.

During the last decade, the Ponseti method of combined manipulation and Achilles tenotomy has become very popular.[27] The Ponseti method dramatically reduced the need for extensive surgery while successfully treating up to 90% of clubfeet. Treatment, begun as soon as is practical after birth, consists of weekly casting for 4 to 8 weeks or until the foot has been abducted 60 degrees (Fig. 9-17). Achilles tenotomy is then performed with the use of local or general anesthesia, followed by continued casting for 1 month. The Ponseti manipulation and casting technique differs in many subtle ways from previous techniques that had failure rates as high as 90% and should be performed by specially trained and experienced orthopaedic surgeons. After Ponseti manipulation

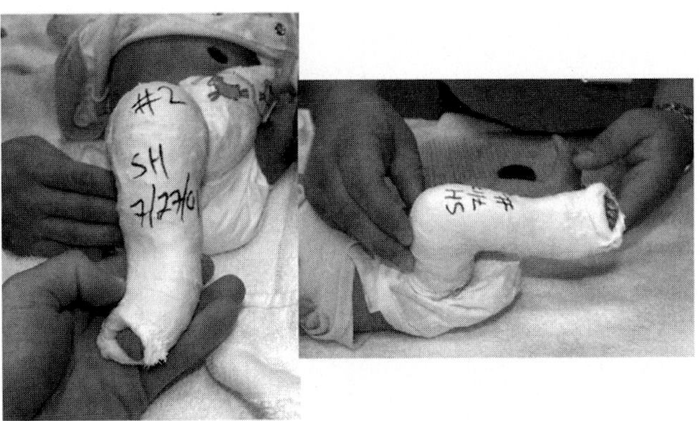

Figure 9-17 Ponseti-type casting of clubfoot. The foot is spun laterally around the talus with pressure applied to the talar head. The long-leg cast with the knee flexed at 90 degrees helps control rotation. The forefoot is supinated slightly.

and tenotomy, the child must wear a Denis Browne–style bar-and-shoes set with the feet externally rotated 70 degrees for the clubfoot. The bar is worn 23 hours per day for 3 months after tenotomy, and then nightly for 2 to 4 years to avoid recurrence.

Ponseti holds that about 30% of patients treated with his technique will need lateral transfer of the anterior tibialis tendon to better balance the foot.[27] Failure of this technique may require additional surgery.

Flat Foot (Planovalgus)

Flat or planovalgus foot is a common deformity consisting of hindfoot valgus with compensatory midfoot supination and abduction. Staheli and colleagues[52] plotted the development of the arch in growing children. They found that the arch increases in height with maturity as the fatty tissue along the sole of the foot decreases. The true incidence of planovalgus feet is unknown. Depending on the criteria used to define the condition, it may be present in as many as 23%[30] of the adult population, and most cases are asymptomatic. Therefore, the fact that a foot is "flat" does not make it an abnormal foot in need of treatment.

Foot flexibility and pain are the central issues to consider when one is evaluating the child with planovalgus feet. Flexible flat feet without pain require no treatment. Conversely, stiff feet even in the absence of pain are cause for concern and require investigation. Stiff feet frequently become painful with maturity and increased body weight. Although flexible flat feet are usually normal, stiff or painful feet are never normal. The differential diagnosis for planovalgus foot consists of flexible flat foot, calcaneovalgus foot, accessory navicular bone, tarsal coalition, congenital vertical talus, and flat foot due to neuromuscular disease.

These conditions are differentiated through information gathered from the history and physical examination. The history also serves to better clarify parental concerns. The role of radiographs is to confirm a diagnosis and aid in treatment planning. Pain, when present, should be localized and characterized. Inciting, aggravating, or alleviating activities or modalities are identified during the interview. Birth and developmental history are helpful in uncovering a neuromuscular origin for the foot deformity (i.e., spastic diplegic cerebral palsy). A family history of flat or painful feet may be reported.

Physical examination begins with observation of the standing child. When the examiner looks at the child with flat foot from the rear, the heel is in significant valgus and the "too many toes" sign may be present, resulting from significant midfoot abductus. The arch (instep) is reduced. With the patella facing forward, knee alignment is examined. Valgus knee alignment causes the patient to stand on the medial aspect of the foot. The child should be asked to rise up on the balls of the feet. A flexible foot with a functioning posterior tibial tendon inverts the heel and reconstitutes the arch (Fig. 9-18).

The flexibility of the arch can also be demonstrated with the Jack test,[53] which consists of dorsiflexion of the first metatarsophalangeal joint. With this maneuver, the plantar fascia raises the arch by shortening the distance between the metatarsal heads and the calcaneal insertion for the fascia, the so-called windlass mechanism, if the foot is flexible. The feet are palpated for tenderness. Free and unrestricted motion should be obtained while the heel is moved into varus and valgus and the midfoot is everted and inverted. The ankle should be examined for a contracted gastrocnemius-soleus muscle complex, as described for idiopathic toe walking.

Flexible Planovalgus Foot

Flexible painless flat foot, in the absence of a tight Achilles tendon, requires reassurance only. There is no evidence that a flat foot is either a disorder or a condition that predisposes to foot pain in adulthood. The wearing of orthotics with a custom instep does not affect arch development.[54] Orthotics are expensive and must be replaced periodically; this is not to say that there is no role for orthotics. Occasionally, a child with a flexible flat foot experiences pain in the instep as a teenager or young adult. The pain is described as achy and usually follows prolonged periods of standing, walking, or running. Pain is alleviated with rest. In these patients, a shoe or sneaker with arch support is recommended. When the patient continues to have pain despite improved shoe wear, an orthotic is appropriate.

A small subgroup of patients with flexible flat foot has tight Achilles tendons. Contracture of the gastrocnemius-soleus muscle complex limits ankle dorsiflexion. The foot compensates by shifting the heel into valgus. Increased dorsiflexion stress is thus dissipated through

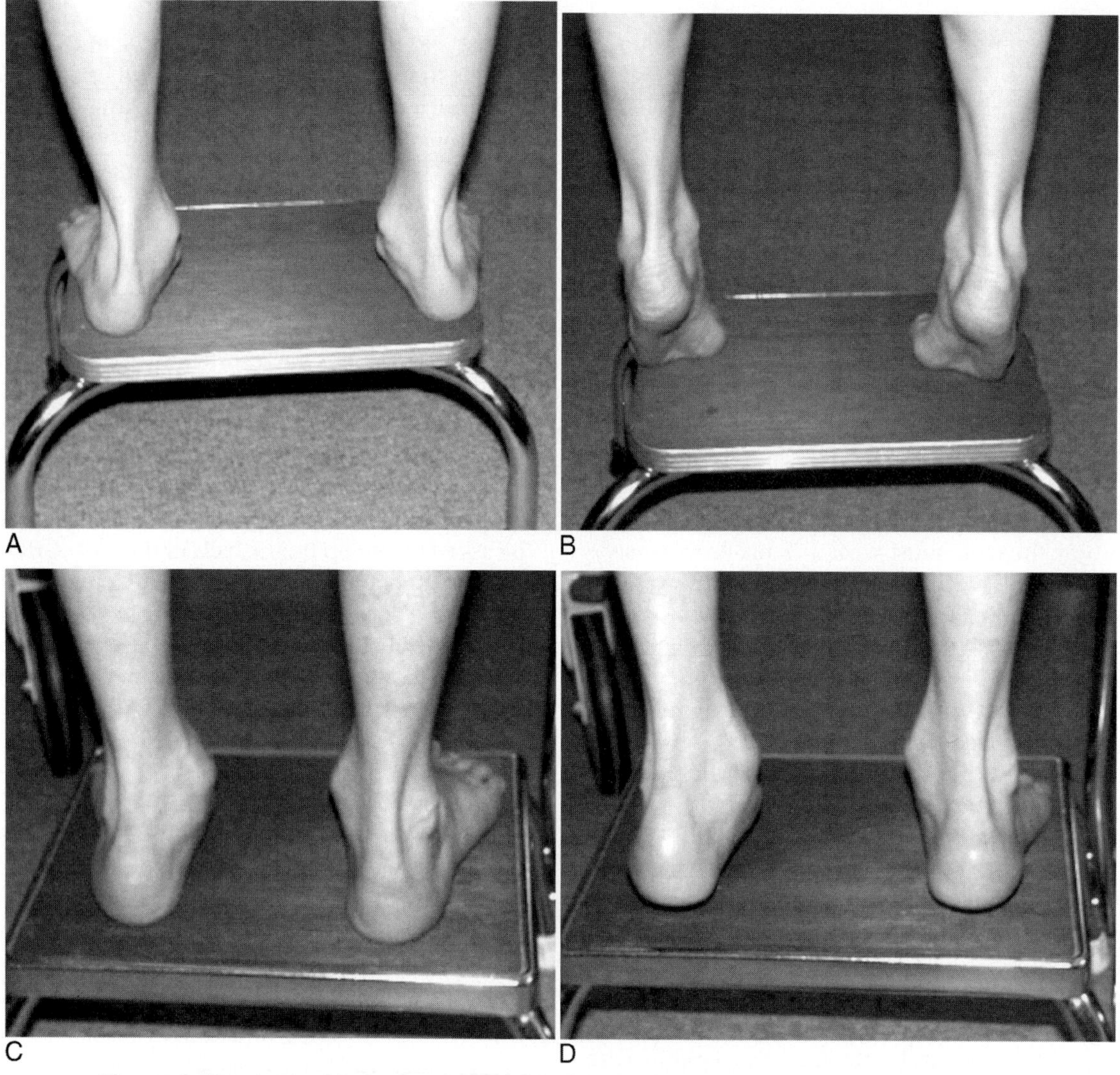

Figure 9-18 A, Flexible flat feet. **B,** Hindfoot inversion of same feet with ankle plantarflexion. **C,** Photograph of another child with a stiff flat foot secondary to a tarsal coalition in which the hindfoot remains in valgus. **D,** The patient rises up on the toes, but hindfoot doesn't invert.

the subtalar joint during the second half of the stance. With time, the foot becomes painful. A course of physical therapy with an emphasis on Achilles tendon stretching is prescribed. Serial casting and botulinum toxin injections are useful as well. Surgery is reserved for patients with persistent Achilles tendon contracture or persistent pain. Several procedures have been advocated. The Achilles tendon is lengthened if involved. Procedures that reconstitute the arch are medial displacement osteotomy, lateral column lengthening, arthrorisis of the subtalar joint, and subtalar arthrodesis.

Calcaneovalgus Foot

Calcaneovalgus foot deformity is included in the differential diagnoses of a congenital rocker-bottom foot. The condition is another example of the fetal "packing abnormalities" discussed previously. The fetus's foot is maintained in extreme dorsiflexion against the uterine wall. The dorsal aspect of the foot comes to rest against pretibial skin after birth. The site of deformity therefore is the ankle joint. In severe cases, the tibia is also bowed with a posteromedial apex.

The natural history of a calcaneovalgus foot is spontaneous correction with some loss of ankle plantar-flexion. Stretching is of debatable efficacy, but it appears to do no harm and gives the family a feeling of empowerment. Ankle motion improves over several weeks. Tibial bowing, however, takes several years to resolve and may be incomplete. With unilateral involvement, the affected leg may be 1 to 5 centimeters shorter than the normal leg.[55] Monitoring limb length at yearly physical examinations identifies children with significant discrepancy and allows a timely referral to an orthopaedist for treatment.

Congenital Vertical Talus

Congenital vertical talus (CVT) is an anomaly characterized by a stiff rocker-bottom foot (Fig. 9-19A).[56] The appearance is secondary to a dorsal dislocation of the navicular bone onto the head of the talus. CVT may occur without a predisposing condition (idiopathic), although more commonly it is associated with another condition. Examples of conditions seen with CVT are arthrogryposis multiplex congenital (AMC), myelomeningocele, congenital myopathy, and intraspinal lesion (i.e., syringomyelia).

History and physical examination are directed at seeking evidence of an associated condition and identifying the deformity. For example, children with AMC have decreased fetal motion, stiff limbs, and an absence of flexion creases in affected limbs. Examination of the foot reveals an equinus hindfoot and a dorsiflexed and abducted midfoot. The talar head is palpable along the plantar surface of the foot. The talar head is not normally a weight-bearing structure and, with time, it becomes callused and painful. The deformity is rigid, and the talonavicular dislocation is not reducible.

Diagnosis of CVT is confirmed with radiographs. The navicular bone does not ossify before 4 years of age; therefore, a dorsal dislocation cannot be directly observed on a radiograph. The position of the navicular bone can be inferred, however, because it is in line with the first metatarsal on a lateral radiograph. When the talonavicular joint is normal, a line can be drawn through the talus and shaft of the first metatarsal on a lateral forced plantarflexion radiograph of the foot. Because the talonavicular dislocation in CVT is irreducible, the talus never comes to lie in the plane of the first metatarsal on such a radiograph in a foot with this deformity (Fig. 9-19B to E).

Without treatment, CVT leads to progressive foot pain in ambulators. Non-ambulators may therefore be treated with shoes that accommodate their deformity. However, the ability to walk is not always predicable in early infancy (e.g., in AMC or myelomeningocele). Manipulation and casting techniques stretch the skin, making wound closure easier at the time of surgery, but cannot reduce the dislocation. The only corrective treatment for CVT is surgery, with best results in children who undergo an operative intervention before they are 2 years old. As with clubfoot surgery, numerous surgical techniques have been described. Few studies are available with adequate patient numbers and duration of follow-up to prove the superiority of any given technique.

Tarsal Coalition

A tarsal coalition is a failure of segmentation between adjoining tarsal bones so that a normal mobile joint does not form. The coalitions are composed of fibrous tissue *(syndesmosis)*, cartilaginous tissue *(synchondrosis)*, or osseous tissue *(synostosis)*. Persistent motion between the tarsal bones despite the coalition produces pain in some patients. The subtalar joint is typically maintained in valgus, although a varus deformity has been described. Subtalar motion is important in negotiation of uneven terrain. Therefore, a history of frequent ankle sprains or fractures is common in patients with this disorder.

Coalitions may exist between any two of the tarsal bones, but talocalcaneal (TCC) and calcaneonavicular (CNC) coalitions are the most common. Pain from a talocalcaneal coalition is located in the medial hindfoot by the sustentaculum tali, a prominence just distal and anterior to the medial malleolus. Patients with CNC have pain in the sinus tarsi, a depression anterior to the tip of the fibula. With both TCC and CNC, lateral heel pain, from fibula impingement on the valgus calcaneus, is common. Subtalar motion is limited or absent. Normal active subtalar motion can be confirmed through observation of the inversion, where the calcaneus moves into varus, of the hindfoot in patients who are standing on the balls of their feet. In the presence of a coalition, the hindfoot stays in valgus and does not shift into varus with equinus (Fig. 9-20). Passive subtalar motion may also be assessed with the patient lying prone with the ankles plantigrade and the knees flexed to 90 degrees. This position affords an excellent view of the hindfoot during the application of inversion and eversion forces by the examining physician.

The presence of a tarsal coalition is confirmed on standing weight-bearing AP, lateral, Harris, and oblique radiographs (Fig. 9-21). Evidence of a TCC is seen on the lateral radiograph with the C sign. If there is any question, a Harris-Beath radiograph should be obtained. On a lateral radiograph, the "anteater's nose" is a sign of a CNC. CNC is best appreciated, however, on the oblique view of the foot. CT is helpful in assessing the location and percentage of joint surface occupied by the coalition. A CT scan can also detect coalitions between other articular surfaces.

Initial treatment consists of 1 month of immobilization in a short-leg walking cast. Once symptoms subside, the patient is placed in a University of California Berkley Laboratories (UCBL) custom orthosis. This orthosis decreases subtalar motion and may provide lasting pain relief. There are two types of surgical procedures for patients in whom conservative measures fail. Patients with a small TCC (less than 50% of the subtalar joint) or CNC undergo coalition resection with fat, muscle, or tendon interposition. Extensive or multiple coalitions are treated with an arthrodesis.

Accessory Navicular Bone

As the word implies, an accessory bone or ossicle is an "extra" one. It may be a located within a tendon, as

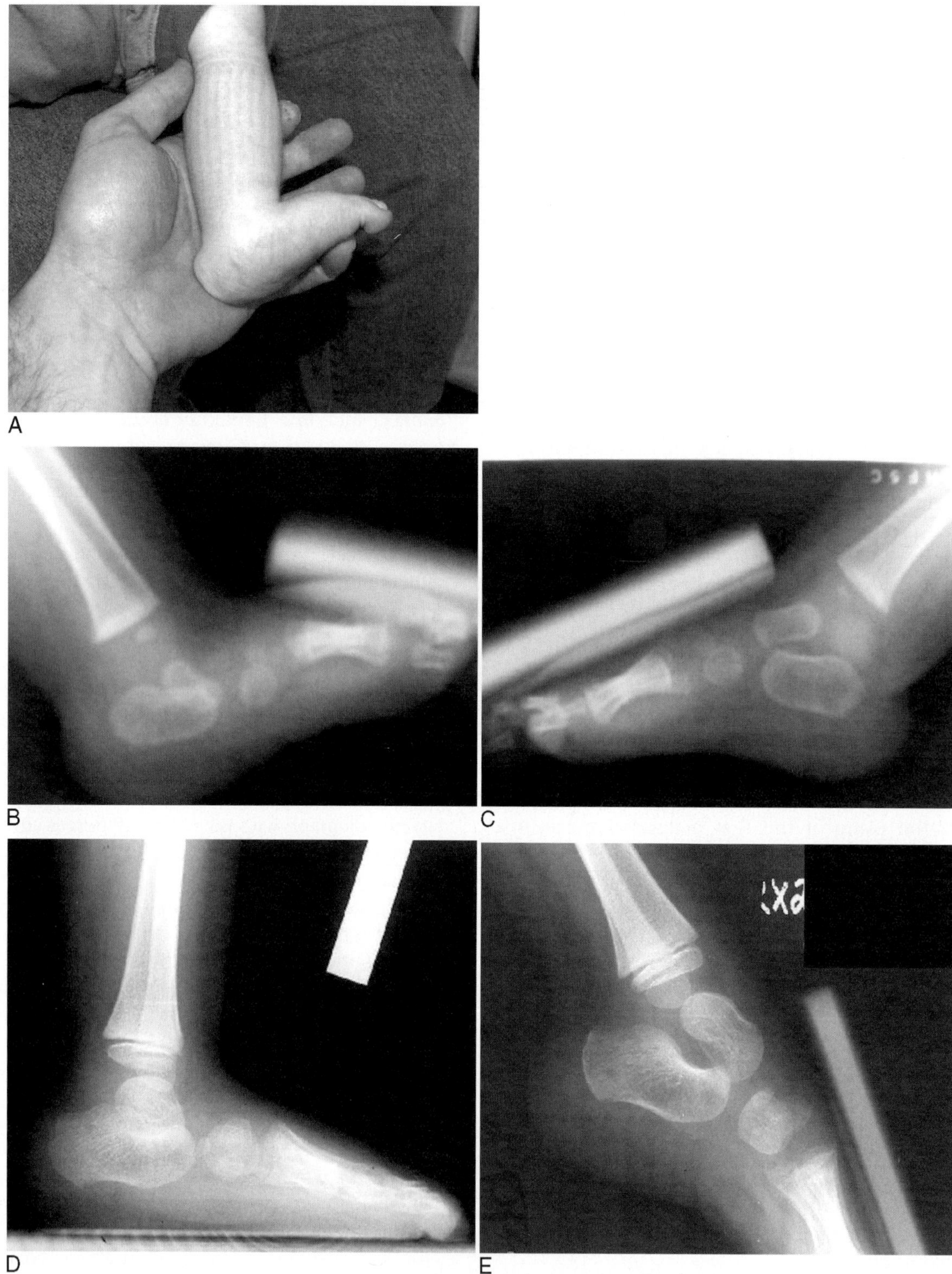

Figure 9-19 **A,** Congenital vertical talus with a rocker-bottom foot. **B,** Plantar-flexion lateral radiograph demonstrating the inability to reduce the navicular on the talus. **C,** A normal foot with the hindfoot, midfoot, and forefoot well aligned. **D,** An "oblique talus" with apparent plantar-flexion of the talus. **E,** Reduction of the "oblique talus" with the plantar-flexion view distinguishing the condition from congenital vertical talus.

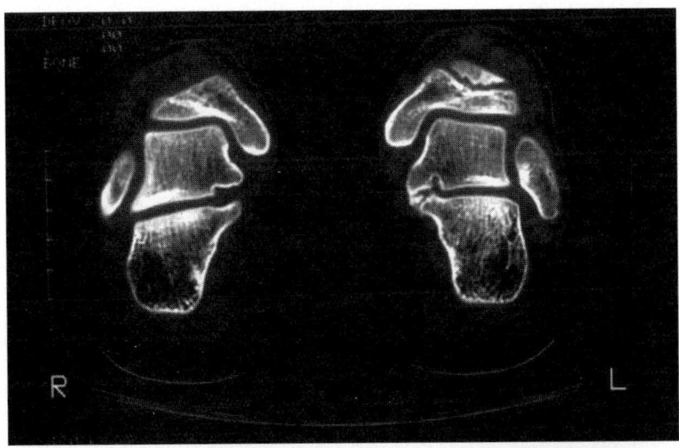

A

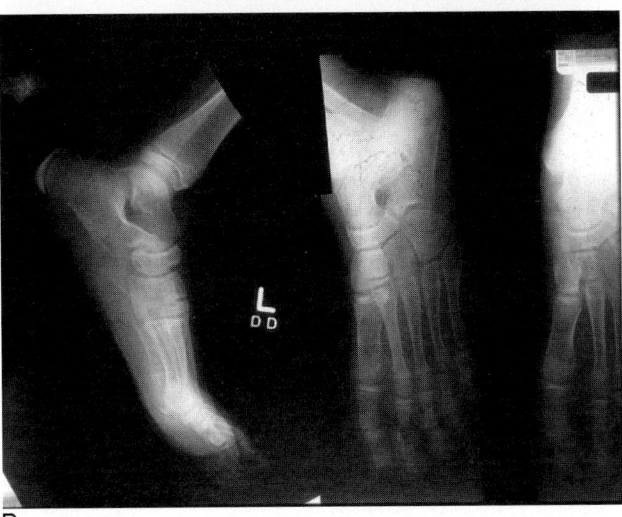

B

Figure 9-20 **A,** Computed tomography scan of normal joint (right) and a talocalcaneal coalition (left). **B,** Lateral oblique and anteroposterior radiographs of calcaneal navicular coalition. Note the prominence of anterior calcaneal process.

is the case with os peroneum, or as a separate bone, such as the os trigonum. These ossicles are common and usually asymptomatic. An accessory navicular bone, present in 12% of the population, is located within the tibialis posterior tendon (TPT). The TPT is important in maintaining the arch. Contraction of the TPT, which occurs when one rises up onto the balls of the feet, causes the hindfoot to invert. An accessory navicular bone is one of the causes of a painful planovalgus foot.

Pain, when present, is located along the medial-plantar aspect of the navicular bone. The diagnosis is confirmed with standing AP and oblique radiographs of the foot. There are three morphologic types of accessory navicular bone.[57] Type 1 is a small, oval to round ossicle within the tendon of the TPT'; type 2 is a larger lateral projection from the medial aspect of the navicular with a clear separation from the base of the navicular; and type 3 is a connected horn-shaped prominence. Pain is most common with type 2 lesions. The causes of pain are midfoot dorsiflexion stress in a planovalgus foot, direct pressure on the prominence, and motion through the navicular-accessory navicular pseudoarthrosis.

Treatment is directed toward pain relief. A short-leg cast is applied for 4 weeks with weight-bearing as tolerated. After successful cast treatment, a custom orthosis is prescribed. A relief is molded into the orthotic to reduce pressure on the prominent navicular bone. Persistent pain is an indication for surgery, which involves removal of the accessory navicular bone through a split in the TPT. There is no demonstrable benefit to plicating the TPT.

Foot Cavus

The deformity in a cavovarus foot is the opposite of that in a planovalgus foot. A cavus foot has a "high arch" with no contact between the floor and the instep (Fig. 9-22). Elevation of the arch is due to plantar-flexion of the medial metatarsals. The forefoot is thus pronated in relation to the hindfoot. For purpose of discussion, one must regard the foot as a stable tripod with a base composed of the first and fifth metatarsal heads and the calcaneal tuberosity.[58] Depression (plantar-flexion) of the first ray causes the calcaneus to assume a varus position to maintain tripod stability. As plantar-flexion of the first ray increases, the patient puts more weight on the lateral aspect of the foot. Ambulation on the lateral border of the foot leads to fifth metatarsal pain and predisposes to inversion injuries (ankle sprains and fractures). The subtalar joint is initially mobile and passively correctable; with time, however, heel varus becomes fixed. Foot rigidity is a function of contractures of the plantar fascia, and tibialis anterior and posterior muscles and osseous adaptations.

Cavus is the result of a peripheral neuropathy that affects intrinsic foot muscles and peroneal muscles, especially the peroneal longus. Intrinsic weakness can also lead to clawing of the toes. Conditions that lead to a Cavus foot may be idiopathic or due to Charcot-Marie-Tooth (CMT) disease, myelomeningocele, Friedreich ataxia, or a spinal cord lesion (i.e., syringomyelia and tumors).

During the history taking and physical examination, evidence of one of the preceding conditions is sought. Examination of the shoes demonstrates lateral tread wear. The barefoot patient, as viewed from behind, has heel varus. The arch is elevated with a plantar-flexed first ray. Mobility of the hindfoot is assessed with the Coleman block test (Fig. 9-23).[59] The test is performed with the patient standing and the lateral border of the foot on an elevated surface. In this position, the unsupported first metatarsal drops below the sole of the foot. The heel assumes a neutral to valgus alignment when the hindfoot is still flexible. A rigid hindfoot, in contrast, stays in varus.

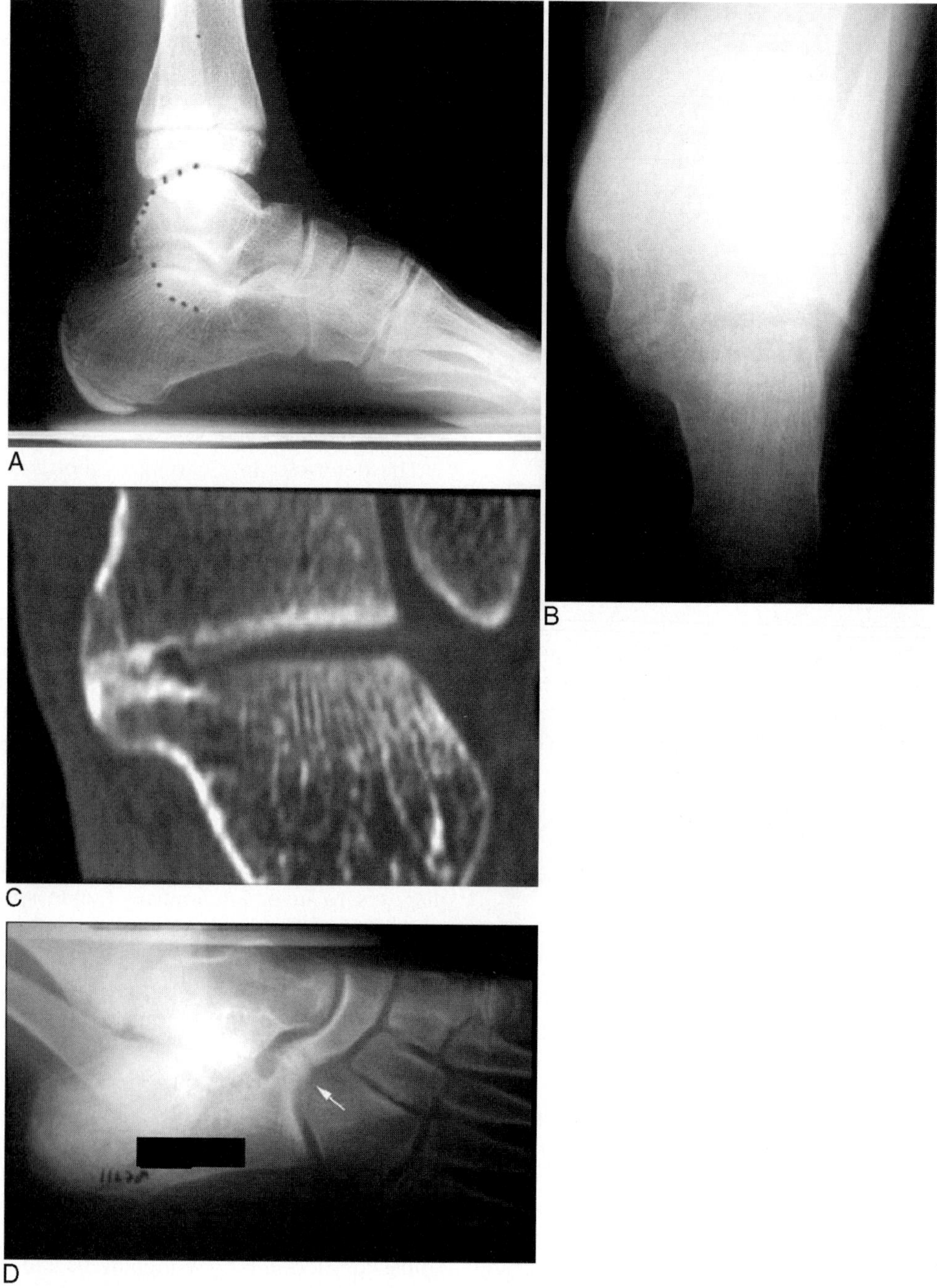

Figure 9-21 **A,** Lateral radiograph of foot with talocalcaneal coalition. The C sign is outlined. **B,** Harris view demonstrating narrowing of the subtalar joint. **C,** Computed tomography scan demonstrating an osseus coalition of the talocalcaneal joint. **D,** An oblique radiograph of the foot with a calcaneal-navicular coalition.

Treatment begins with appropriate tests and referrals to confirm and manage any underlying disease. Patient with diminished plantar sensation must be instructed about appropriate foot care and encouraged to perform frequent self-examination. An orthosis is prescribed for patients with footdrop and ankle instability. An orthosis, however, does not retard disease progression. All patients with cavus foot should be referred to an orthopaedist who can treat the foot as well as associated conditions, such as scoliosis and hip dysplasia, that occur with some of the diseases listed previously. Foot surgery is indicated in progressive or painful deformities. Tendon transfers, plantar releases, and first metatarsal dorsiflexion osteotomies are reserved for the flexible

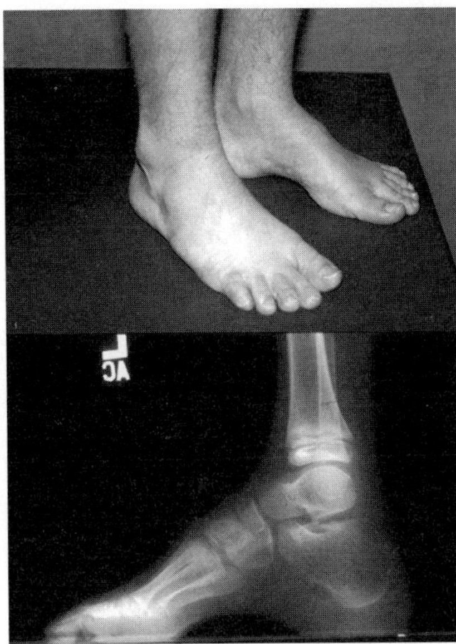

Figure 9-22 Clinical picture and radiograph of cavus foot with the pathognomonic elevated arch.

foot. Calcaneal osteotomies are performed in patients with fixed hindfoot deformity. Arthritis and recurrent deformity are treated with realignment and arthrodesis.

Foot Pain

Several conditions cause foot pain in the absence of a deformity (i.e., cavus and planovalgus). The causes of nonmechanical foot pain are divided into inflammatory, infectious, vascular, neoplastic, and traumatic. Systemic symptoms, multiple joint involvement, morning stiffness, a positive family history, and presence of serum markers are evidence of an inflammatory arthropathy such as juvenile rheumatoid arthritis. Fever, chills, and malaise are seen with an infectious cause, although at times, differentiating infectious from inflammatory arthritis can be challenging. Neoplasm in the foot may or may not cause pain. The lesion itself may be discovered as an incidental finding after trauma or may be the locus of a pathologic fracture. Three other conditions that do not fit into the groupings previously listed that deserve discussion. They are Köhler disease, Freiberg infraction, and Sever disease.[60-62]

Köhler disease, Freiberg infraction, and Sever disease are examples of osteochondrosis of unknown etiology. Köhler disease involves the navicular bone, Freiberg infraction the metatarsal head, and Sever disease the calcaneal apophysis. The etiology has been theorized to be vascular embarrassment after repetitive microtrauma on the young foot.

Patients with Köhler disease are typically younger than 6 years and present with a sudden onset of foot pain. Pain is worse with activities and improves with rest and oral analgesics. Radiographs show fragmentation of the navicular bone. Eight weeks of immobilization in a short-leg cast constitute the initial treatment.[63] Ultimately, the condition resolves. No long-term problems have been reported in children after resolution of Köhler's disease.

In contrast, the outcome of patients with Freiberg infraction is not always favorable. The condition occurs in adolescents and frequently in running athletes. The

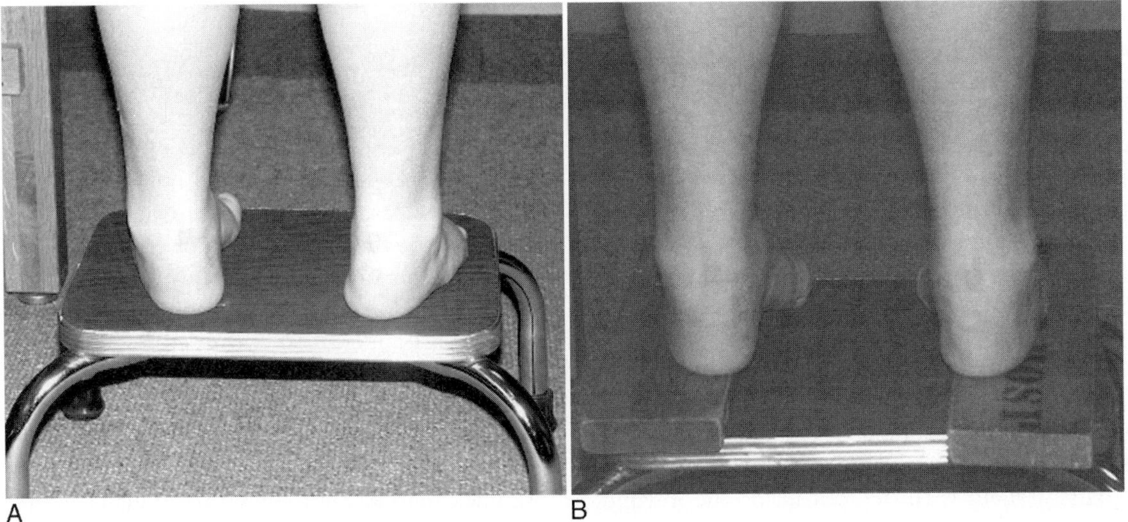

Figure 9-23 Demonstration of the Coleman block test. A, Hindfoot in varus with weight-bearing upon a flat surface. **B,** The hindfoot is now in neutral once the first ray is allowed to hang free. This foot thus has a flexible hindfoot.

patients complain of pain under a metatarsal head, most commonly of the second metatarsal. On physical examination, gait is antalgic and the metatarsal is tender. Radiographs taken early in the disease demonstrate increased density of the metatarsal head. With disease progression, the subchondral bone collapses, producing a crescent sign. After collapse of the articular surface, a period of fragmentation ensues, followed by reformation. Treatment consists of no weight-bearing until symptoms resolve. Metatarsal pads reduce weight-bearing forces on the involved metatarsal and provide some relief. Pain that persists is addressed with decompression and bone grafting. Metatarsal resection and arthrodesis are salvage procedures reserved for severely involved bones.

Sever disease is an enthesopathy of the calcaneus etiologically related to Osgood-Schlatter disease. Sever disease occurs in children with tight Achilles tendons. It can also be part of an inflammatory arthropathy such as spondyloarthropathy. On examination, the child has pain involving the plantar calcaneus and reduced ankle dorsiflexion. Treatment consists of rest, anti-inflammatory medication, the use of heel pads, and Achilles tendon stretching. Sever disease resolves over weeks to months with conservative care and rarely needs surgical intervention.

Juvenile Bunion

Hallux valgus is a deformity of the first ray characterized by abduction of the first metatarsal, with adduction and pronation of the great toe (Fig. 9-24). The prominence formed by the medial aspect of the first metatarsal is known as a *bunion*. Both extrinsic and intrinsic factors lead to the development of hallux valgus. Extrinsic factors include shoes with a narrow toe box, an elevated heel, or both. Improper shoes may not be the culprit in most pediatric case of bunions, but in some cases, adolescents, like their adult counterparts, have become victims of western shoe fashion. Intrinsic factors include hereditary tendency and planovalgus foot. Patients with valgus hindfoot walk on the medial border of the first ray during toe-off. The laterally deviating stress promotes the formation of bunions.

The history begins with a discussion of the chief complaint. Although bunions can be painful, most are not. Some patients are merely unhappy with their foot's aesthetic but do not have functional problems. Inquiry as to the type of shoes worn is helpful in identifying extrinsic causes of the bunion. The examiner should trace the patient's shoe onto a piece of paper, and then have the patient stand with the foot inside the tracing. The toe box is too small if the forefoot extends beyond the tracing. This maneuver is a helpful tool in patient education. Bunion tenderness, swelling, redness, and blistering occur from shoe irritation on the prominence. Pain with dorsiflexion of the metatarsophalangeal joint is consistent with arthrosis, incongruence, or both, of the first metatarsophalangeal joint. Hindfoot valgus and Achilles tendon contracture are predisposing conditions that must be identified and treated in order to prevent recurrence of a bunion.

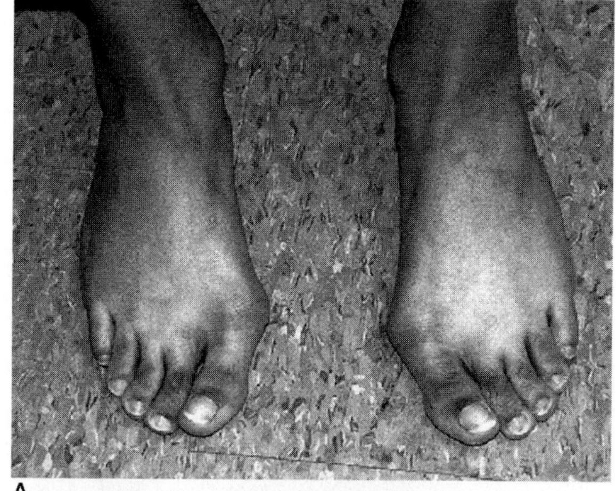

A

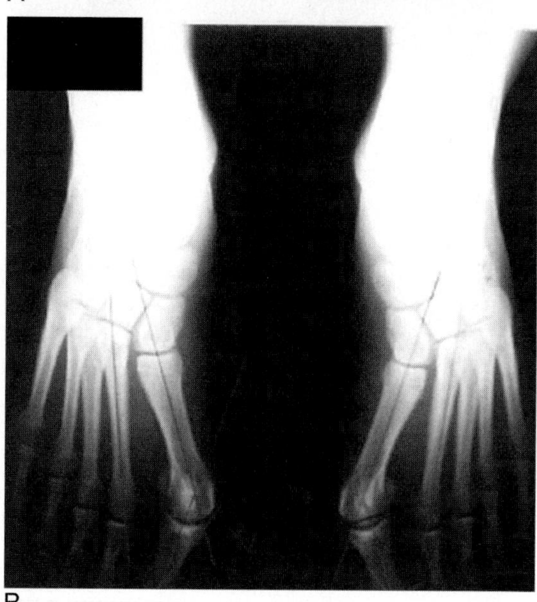

B

Figure 9-24 Clinical **(A)** and radiographic **(B)** appearances of feet with hallux valgus.

Treatment begins with shoe modifications. Patients should wear a shoe with a wide toe box. In the summer, sandals are particularly comfortable. Hindfoot valgus and Achilles tendon contracture are initially treated with a medial arch support (orthosis) and physical therapy. Fixed hindfoot deformity or an Achilles tendon that remains "tight" should be addressed surgically. The goal of surgery is a painless, shoeable foot. Most patients are not able to wear "fashionable" shoes after surgery and should be informed of that fact beforehand. The surgical treatment of juvenile bunions has a high recurrence rate. Patient education includes information about the possibility of chronic pain after surgery secondary to avascular necrosis, infection, neuroma, and arthrosis. In light of the potential risks of surgery, a painless bunion should never be treated operatively.

Deformities of the Lesser Toes

Deformities of the lesser toes make wearing of shoes challenging and may be the cause of a painful gait. *Curly toes* is a nonprogressive flexion deformity of a lesser toe. Most cases are idiopathic. Curly toe is to be distinguished from *claw toe*, or dorsiflexed metatarsophalangeal joint with plantarflexed interphalangeal joints. Claw toe is a progressive deformity associated with spinal cord disease (e.g., myelomeningocele, syringomyelia) or a hereditary motor sensory neuropathy such as Charcot-Marie-Tooth disease.

Curly toes occur most frequently to the fourth and fifth toes. The deformity is initially flexible and painless. Pain does not appear until the child begins to wear shoes. Shoes with a low toe box rub the elevated toe, leading to a painful callosity. Taping and stretching are not effective.[64] Observation is the initial treatment. For most children, the condition either resolves spontaneously or remains asymptomatic. Persistent pain and difficulty with shoe wear are the indications for surgery. Surgical correction consists of lengthening the toe flexors.

Syndactyly is a failure of segmentation of digits. Toe syndactyly can be either partial (a portion of the toe) or complete (entire toe) and either simple (skin only) or complex (involves osseous connections). Syndactyly is usually of no clinical significance because few humans need their feet for fine motor function (i.e., writing). There are thus few indications for separation of the toes without a coexisting condition such as polydactyly.

Polydactyly is an error of duplication, resulting in an extra digit. The extra digit can be pre-axial (medial to the first toe), postaxial (lateral to the fifth toe) or central. Patients with foot polydactyly may have extra digits on their hands as well. The extra toe may be rudimentary (lacking osseous structures) or may be a complete digit with its own metatarsal. Isolated polydactyly is more commonly postaxial, and is seen more often in children with a positive family history and among African Americans. The indications for amputation are cosmesis, difficulties with shoe wear, and foot pain. A rudimentary digit can be "tied off" in the newborn nursery; the digit will "fall off" several weeks after the ligature is placed. More complete digits need surgical excision, especially when they are syndactylized to neighboring digits.

Macrodactyly is digital enlargement. During the history and physical examination, evidence of associated conditions is sought. The causes of macrodactyly include Proteus syndrome, neurofibromatosis, vascular anomalies (Klippel-Trenaunay-Weber syndrome), and lymphangioma. Difficulty with shoe wear is found more commonly with macrodactyly than with any of the other toe conditions and therefore is the primary indication for surgery. The foot or toe can be debulked by excision of associated fat, or débridement of the vascular structures. The length of the digit can be reduced by a timely epiphysiodesis; however, this procedure reduces the toe only longitudinally and does not affect transverse growth. In severe cases, partial toe or foot amputation may be required to allow normal shoe wear.

Ingrown Toenail

Ingrown toenail is largely a preventable condition. The causes are improper nail trimming and tight shoes or socks that rub the ends of the toes. Dancers who perform "en pointe" are a population particularly at risk for this condition. The toenail should be cut squarely and not too short. When too much nail is removed, the nail grows into or under the paronychia, the medial and lateral nail fold. Irritation from the toenail under the paronychia causes the toe to become painful, swollen, and red. With time, the toe may become secondarily infected, most commonly with *Staphylococcus aureus*.

The treatment of an ingrown toenail begins with cleaning and soaking of the foot to address the infection and soften the nail plate. On a daily basis, the skin should be pushed off the edge of the nail with a clean cotton-tipped applicator. A small piece of cotton is then left under the corner of the nail to keep the skin from falling back over the edge of the nail. Treatment continues until the nail "grows out." The process is time consuming and sometimes painful.

Failure of conservative treatment may require partial or complete ablation of the nail. The patient must be clearly informed that procedures that remove portions of the nail, including the germinal matrix, are not always successful. They may have to be revised and can leave the patient with an ugly, distorted nail. Therefore, every effort should be made to allow the nail to grow out naturally. Infected ingrown toenails are best treated with antibiotics and drainage. Hospital admission with administration of intravenous antibiotics is indicated for a patient with systemic symptoms, lymphangitic streaking, or lymphadenopathy.

MAJOR POINTS

Rotational deformities of the lower extremity can occur at the hip (femoral anteversion), tibia (tibial torsion) and/or the foot (metatarsus adductus).

Spontaneous correction is possible until 4 years of age for tibial torsion and 8 years of age for femoral anteversion.

Surgery is reserved for limbs with severe persistent rotational deformity.

Rigid feet with metatarsus adductus should be treated with manipulation and casting. Severe resistant cases are treated surgically.

Children normally have varus knees prior to their 2nd birthday and have maximum knee valgus by their 4th birthday.

Clubfeet are best treated with early manipulation and casting.

Failure of conservative care is the indication for surgical correction of clubfeet.

Flexible painless flat feet (planovalgus) do not require treatment.

Orthotics and an achilles tendon stretching program are appropriate for the painful flexible flat foot.

A thorough physical and radiographic examination are required for patients with rigid flat feet.

A neurologic work-up is required in all patients with cavus feet to rule out spinal cord lesions and peripheral neuropathies.

Juvenile bunions should be treated with shoe modifications unless they are progressive or pain persists despite large toe box shoes.

REFERENCES

1. Staheli LT, Corbett M, Wyss C, et al: Lower-extremity rotational problems in children: Normal values to guide management, J Bone Joint Surg Am 67:39-47, 1985.
2. Bleck EE: Developmental orthopaedics. III: Toddlers. Dev Med Child Neurol 24:533-555, 1982.
3. Knittel G, Staheli LT: The effectiveness of shoe modifications for in-toeing. Orthop Clin North Am 7:1019-1025, 1976.
4. Salenius P, Vankka E: The development of the tibiofemoral angle in children. J Bone Joint Surg Am 57:259-261, 1975.
5. Hynes D, O'Brien T: Growth disturbance lines after injury of the distal tibial physis: Their significance in prognosis. J Bone Joint Surg Br 70:231-233, 1988.
6. Langenskiöld A: Tibia vara [osteochondrosis deformans tibiae]: A survey of 23 cases. Acta Chir Scand 103:1, 1952.
7. Levine AM, Drennan JC: Physiological bowing and tibia vara: The metaphyseal-diaphyseal angle in the measurement of bowleg deformities. J Bone Joint Surg Am 64:1158-1163, 1982.
8. Feldman MD, Schoenecker PL: Use of the metaphyseal-diaphyseal angle in the evaluation of bowed legs. J Bone Joint Surg Am 75:1602-1609, 1993.
9. Ferriter P, Shapiro F: Infantile tibia vara: Factors affecting outcome following proximal tibial osteotomy. J Pediatr Orthop 7:1-7, 1987.
10. Bowen JR, Torres RR, Forlin E: Partial epiphysiodesis to address genu varum or genu valgum. J Pediatr Orthop 12:359-364, 1992.
11. Anderson DJ, Schoenecker PL, Sheridan JJ, et al: Use of an intramedullary rod for the treatment of congenital pseudarthrosis of the tibia. J Bone Joint Surg Am 74:161-168, 1992.
12. Jacobsen ST, Crawford AH, Millar EA, et al: The Syme amputation in patients with congenital pseudarthrosis of the tibia. J Bone Joint Surg Am 65:533-537, 1983.
13. Herring JA: Syme's amputation for fibular hemimelia: A second look in the Ilizarov era. Instr Course Lect 41:435-436, 1992.
14. Sutherland D, Olsen RA, Cooper L, et al: The development of mature gait. J Bone Joint Surg Am 62:336-353, 1980.
15. Smith J, Bleck E, Gamble J, et al: Simple method of documenting metatarsus adductus. J Pediatr Orthop 11:679-680, 1991.
16. Bleck EE: Metatarsus adductus: classification and relationship to outcomes of treatment. J Pediatr Orthop 3:2-9, 1983.
17. Rushforth GF: The natural history of hooked forefoot. J Bone Joint Surg Br 60:530-532, 1978.
18. Ponseti I, Becker J: Congenital metatarsus adductus: results of treatment. J Bone Joint Surg Am 48:702-711, 1966.
19. Heyman C, Herndon C, Strong J: Mobilization of the tarsometatarsal and intermetatarsal joints for the correction of resistant adduction of the fore part of the foot in congenital club-foot and metatarsus varus. J Bone Joint Surg Am 40:299-310, 1958.
20. Moses W, Allen BL Jr, Pugh LI, et al: Predictive value of intraoperative clubfoot radiographs on revision rates. J Pediatr Orthop 20:529-532, 2000.
21. Wynne-Davies R: Family studies and the cause of congenital clubfoot, talipes equinovarus, talipes calcaneo-valgus, and metatarsus varus. J Bone Joint Surg Br 46:445-463, 1964.
22. Chesney D, Barker S, Miedzybrodzka Z, et al: Epidemiology and genetic theories in the etiology of congenital talipes equinovarus. Bull Hosp Jt Dis 58:59-64, 1999.

23. Lochmiller C, Johnston D, Scott A, et al: Genetic epidemiology study of idiopathic talipes equinovarus. Am J Med Genet 79:90-96, 1998.

24. Shimizu N, Hamada S, Mitta M, et al: Etiological considerations of congenital clubfoot deformity. In Simons G (ed): The Clubfoot: The present and a view of the future. New York, Springer-Verlag, 1994, pp 31-38.

25. Tachdjian M: The foot and leg. In Pediatric Orthopedics: The foot and leg. Philadelphia, WB Saunders, 1990, pp 2612-2626.

26. Turco V: Surgical correction of the resistant clubfoot. One-stage posteromedial release with internal fixation: A preliminary report. J Bone Joint Surg Am 53:477-497, 1971.

27. Ippolito E, Ponseti IV: Congenital club foot in the human fetus: A histological study. J Bone Joint Surg Am 62:8-22, 1980.

28. Isaacs H, Handelsman JE, Badenhorst M, et al: The muscles in club foot—a histological histochemical and electron microscopic study. J Bone Joint Surg Br 59:465-472, 1977.

29. Handelsman JE, Badalamente MA: Neuromuscular studies in clubfoot. J Pediatr Orthop 1:23-32, 1981.

30. Harris R, Beath T: Army foot survey: An investigation of foot ailments in Canadian soldiers. Vol 1, Ottawa, National Research Council of Canada, 1947.

31. Irani RN, Sherman MS: The pathological anatomy of idiopathic clubfoot. Clin Orthop 84:14-20, 1972.

32. Shapiro F, Glimcher MJ: Gross and histological abnormalities of the talus in congenital club foot. J Bone Joint Surg Am 6:522-530, 1979.

33. Ionasescu V, Maynard J, Poseti I, et al: The role of collagen in the pathogenesis of idiopathic clubfoot: Biochemical and electron microscopic correlations. Helv Paediatr Acta 29:305-314, 1974.

34. Ippolito E, Ricciardi-Pollini PT, Tudisco C, et al: The treatment of relapsing clubfoot by tibialis anterior transfer underneath the extensor retinaculum. Ital J Orthop Traumatol 11:171-177, 1985.

35. Davidson R, Hahn M, Hubbard A: MRI of talipes equinovarus under the age of twelve months. Amsterdam, Netherlands, 1996.

36. Dietz FR, Ponseti IV, Buckwalter JA: Morphometric study of clubfoot tendon sheaths. J Pediatr Orthop 3:311-318, 1983.

37. Carroll NC: Clubfoot: What have we learned in the last quarter century? J Pediatr Orthop 17:1-2, 1997.

38. Carroll NC: Pathoanatomy and surgical treatment of the resistant clubfoot. Instr Course Lect 37:93-106, 1988.

39. Hootnick DR, Levinsohn EM, Crider RJ, et al: Congenital arterial malformations associated with clubfoot. A report of two cases. Clin Orthop 167:160-163, 1982.

40. Muir L, Laliotis N, Kutty S, et al: Absence of the dorsalis pedis pulse in the parents of children with club foot. J Bone Joint Surg Br 77:114-116, 1995.

41. Porter RW: Clubfoot: Congenital talipes equinovarus. J R Coll Surg Edinb 40:66-71, 1995.

42. Bohm M: The embryonic origin of clubfoot. J Bone Joint Surg Am 11:229, 1929.

43. Kawashima T, Uhthoff HK: Development of the foot in prenatal life in relation to idiopathic club foot. J Pediatr Orthop 10:232-237, 1990.

44. Farrell SA, Summers AM, Dallaire L, et al: Club foot, an adverse outcome of early amniocentesis: Disruption or deformation? CEMAT. Canadian Early and Mid-Trimester Amniocentesis Trial. J Med Genet 36(11): 843-846, 1999.

45. Robertson WW Jr, Corbett D: Congenital clubfoot: Month of conception. Clin Orthop 338:14-18, 1997.

46. White R, Blasier R: Clubfoot: nature and treatment. Todays OR Nurse 16:29-35, 1994.

47. Jones K: Smith's Recognizable Patterns of Human Malformation, 4th ed. Philadelphia, WB Saunders, 1988.

48. Howard CB, Benson MK: The ossific nuclei and the cartilage anlage of the talus and calcaneum. J Bone Joint Surg Br 74:620-623, 1992.

49. Kite JH: Nonoperative treatment of congenital clubfoot. Clin Orthop 84:29-38, 1972.

50. Simons G: The Clubfoot. New York, Springer-Verlag, 1994.

51. McKay DW: New concept of and approach to clubfoot treatment: Section III—Evaluation and results. J Pediatr Orthop 3:141-148, 1983.

52. Staheli LT, Chew DE, Corbett M: The longitudinal arch: A survey of eight hundred and eighty-two feet in normal children and adults. J Bone Joint Surg Am 69:426-428, 1987.

53. Jack E: Naviculo-cuneiform fusion in the treatment of flat foot. J None Joint Surg Am 65:533-537, 1983.

54. Gould N, Moreland M, Alvarez R, et al: Development of the child's arch. Foot Ankle 9:241-245, 1989.

55. Hey C, Herdon C, Heiple K: Congenital posterior angulation of the tibia with talipes calcaneus: A long-term report of eleven patients. J Bone Joint Surg Am 41:476-488, 1959.

56. Drennan JC: Congenital vertical talus. Instr Course Lect 45:315-322, 1996.

57. Grogan DP, Gasser SI, Ogden JA: The painful accessory navicular: A clinical and histopathological study. Foot Ankle 10:164-169, 1989.

58. Paulos L, Coleman SS, Samuelson KM: Pes cavovarus: Review of a surgical approach using selective soft-tissue procedures. J Bone Joint Surg Am 62:942-953, 1980.

59. Coleman SS, Chesnut WJ: A simple test for hindfoot flexibility in the cavovarus foot. Clin Orthop 12:60-62, 1977.

60. Freiberg A: Infraction of the second metatarsal bone: A typical injury. Surg Gynecol Obstet 19:191, 1914.

61. Ippolito E, Ricciardi-Pollini P, Falez F: Köhler's disease of the tarsal navicular: Long-term follow-up of 12 cases. J Pediatr Orthop 4:416-417, 1984.

62. Sever J: Apophysitis of the os calcis. N Y Med J 95:1025, 1912.

63. Williams G, Cowell H: Köhler's disease of the tarsal navicular. Clin Orthop 158:53-58, 1981.

64. Sweetnam R: Congenital curly toes: An investigation into the value of treatment. Lancet 2:398, 1958.

CHAPTER 10

Sports Medicine

THEODORE J. GANLEY
JULIA E. LOU
KRISTEN PRYOR
JOHN R. GREGG

Childhood and adolescence are periods of rapid development, growth, and maturation. These features as well as an interest in many and varied physical activities make young athletes uniquely susceptible to injury. Sports injuries account for nearly a quarter of all injuries in children and adolescents. Those caring for young athletes must be aware of the special characteristics of injuries incurred on the field of play. The treating physician is in a unique position to counsel patients and families about prevention and to alleviate anxiety by offering prognosis and appropriate rehabilitation for return to activity after an injury. These traits can enable young athletes to enjoy the camaraderie and teamwork that may inspire lifelong habits of exercise.

INJURY PREVENTION

Responsibilities of Coaches, Parents, and Treating Physicians

Coaches and parents as well as physicians have a responsibility for the safety and well-being of young athletes in their care. Physicians are in a position to counsel parents and coaches in an effort to prevent injuries. A team representative for children involved in organized sports, especially contact sports, should have a basic first aid kit, a mobile telephone, and medical sheets listing the special medical needs of each athlete on the team (Box 10-1). Parents and coaches should be aware of activity limitations prescribed for players by a physician during the preseason evaluation. At the start of the season, coaches and caregivers should be familiar not only with team plays but also with the individual needs of each athlete.

Caregivers at the field of play can be reminded that some risks to players come from the environment such as weather and field conditions. Those responsible should inspect playing areas, being mindful of unevenness as well as rocks, holes, glass, and obstacles in or close to the playing field that may increase injury risk. Fields and playing areas should be briefly inspected daily so that necessary safety changes can be made. In outdoor arenas, weather conditions such as extreme heat, high humidity, lightning, and cold can increase risk of injury, and these issues must be addressed before play begins.

Box 10-1 Basic Elements of a First-Aid Kit

First aid manual—a quick reference illustrating basic first aid techniques
Medical sheets for each participant should contain the following information:
- Emergency contact numbers of parents/guardians, local hospitals, and paramedics
- List of allergies and medications, any activity modifications, and special considerations for each participant

Sterile bandages:
- 3 × 3-inch gauze
- 5 × 9-inch individually packaged pads
- Nonstick dressings (at least three of each)

Adhesive tape and scissors:
- ½-inch-width roll of tape
- 1-inch-width roll of tape

Adhesive bandage assortment:
- Small (¾-inch width)
- Medium (1-inch width)
- Large (2-inch width)

Antiseptic Ointment—antibacterial ointment for covering small cuts and abrasions
Antiseptic Solution—hydrogen peroxide for cleaning wounds
Screwdriver or bolt cutter (to remove a face mask if necessary)
Ice bags (large plastic bags with crushed ice)
Towels (to place on skin under ice bags, or to sponge an athlete with heat illness)
Mobile phone (readily available for emergency calls to paramedics and/or parents)
Water (should always be available regardless of temperature and time of day)

REMEMBER: ANYTIME AN ITEM IN THE FIRST-AID KIT IS USED, IT SHOULD BE REPLACED BEFORE THE NEXT PRACTICE OR GAME.

Adapted from Ganley TJ, Pill SG, Gregg J, et al: Pop Warner Football & Cheerleading Injury Prevention: A Guide to Common Injuries. Rosemont, IL, The American Orthopaedic Society for Sports Medicine, 2000.

Strength Training

Many youth athletes undergo strength training, which is beneficial for development and maintenance of muscular strength and for enhancement of endurance, flexibility, and prevention of injury. Adolescents participating in such activities should practice resistance training as well as endurance training as part of a well-balanced fitness program. Light weights with high repetitions focusing on single- and multiple-joint exercises are most beneficial and safest for athletes of this age group. Because the joints of children are not fully developed, ballistic or maximal lifting should be avoided. Likewise, it is not advised that adolescents use supplements, other than a multivitamin, to enhance performance. Although steroids and other supplements may enhance strength, some have been associated with serious or potentially life-threatening side effects. Additionally, no conclusive studies have been performed to assess the long-term effects of supplements. Thus, adolescents concentrating on becoming physically fit should practice safe fitness programs and healthy eating habits to achieve optimal physical condition.

THE KINETIC CHAIN OF FUNCTION

The upper and lower extremities are linked in a kinetic chain of function to the trunk, which acts as a core stabilizing structure. Elements and portions of the upper and lower extremities as well as the trunk may serve in different circumstances to support the more distal and proximal structures. The periosteum, a connective tissue membrane that closely invests all bones except at articular surfaces, is considered the strongest link in the skeletal structure of growing bones, as demonstrated by biomechanical testing. Periosteum frequently remains intact even when significant trauma is imparted, resulting in displaced or angulated fractures. The joint capsule and ligaments act as extensions to the periosteal sleeve and can, in many instances, transfer stress beyond the weaker elements of the chain, mainly the epiphysis and physis. The adjacent soft tissue structures and articular cartilage absorb shock to protect the epiphysis.

Nevertheless, the weakest link in this kinetic chain is the physis. The physis is increasingly vulnerable during later periods of growth and development as the perichondral ring at the physeal periphery narrows. Also, bone, although stronger than the physis, is weaker in skeletally immature patients than in adults because of greater porosity due to a larger number of haversian canals per unit area of cortical bone. Therefore, in the young athlete with open physes, there is a greater propensity for fracture of the bone to extend into the physis; in contrast, adult patients more frequently sprain ligaments or dislocate joints.

SOFT TISSUE INJURY

Contusions

Soft tissue injuries or contusions involve direct impact to soft tissues, which causes associated bleeding and crushing of the tissues without breaking the skin. The muscles of young patients are susceptible to severe contusion and hematoma formation because of their greater vasculature. Parents, coaches, and other caregivers should be counseled that blows to certain locations can cause more severe damage, most notably the kidneys, spleen, and testicles. Athletes in contact sports, such as football, can be instructed to wear extra padding at these locations, especially around the ribs and abdomen. Protection of these areas should be stressed for quarterbacks and other players who are at high risk. Caregivers should be advised to watch for intense pain in the flank with bruising and other signs, such as blood in the urine and left-sided abdominal pain.

Sprain

Sprains occur when forces placed on a ligament or joint capsule cause them to stretch or, in some cases, rupture. The extent of injury depends on the amount of force applied as well as the rate of application of this force in accordance with the viscoelastic properties of these structures. In grade I sprains (Table 10-1), the integrity of the ligament is intact, although tearing of some fibers occurs. There is no pathologic laxity and generally no restriction of the range of motion in this injury. Grade II sprains involve damage to the ligament with tearing of fibers as well as pathologic laxity and loss of motion. Some resistance occurs when ligamentous stress testing is performed. In grade III sprains, complete rupture is noted, and instability is evident on ligamentous stress testing. Complete rupture of a muscle of grade III severity is uncommon but possible in children and adolescents.

Strain

Strains involve injuries to the muscle-tendon unit as a result of muscle contraction. Specifically, eccentric contraction, which stretches a preloaded muscle, appears to play a substantial role in causing strains. The myotendinous junction is most often the site of muscle strains, although there is evidence that muscle strain can occur in the muscle fibers.[1] Muscles with a high content of fast-twitch muscle fibers (type II fibers) and muscles that cross two joints are most susceptible to strain. The hamstrings are at high risk for strain because of these two factors and the eccentric contractions that occur with running and deceleration in athletics. Strains are classified much like sprains (see Table 10-1). A first-degree strain results in mild tenderness and pain with stretching. Second-degree strains involve muscle spasms. Third-degree strains result when complete tearing of the musculotendinous junction occurs, at which point a palpable defect can be found on physical examination. With

Table 10-1 Classification of Sprain or Strain Injury with Corresponding Symptoms

Sprain	Strain
Grade I: Integrity of ligament is intact although some tearing occurs, no pathologic laxity, normal ROM	*First-degree:* Mild tenderness and pain with stretching
Grade II: Ligamentous damage with tearing of fibers, pathologic laxity, motion loss, some resistance to ligamentous stress testing	*Second-degree:* Muscle spasms
Grade III: Complete rupture, instability to ligamentous stress testing	*Third-degree:* Complete tearing of musculotendinous junction, palpable defect

proper treatment, rapid recovery is expected, and morbidity in young athletes is minimal.

Management

Management of soft tissue injury involves rest, ice, compression, and elevation (RICE). This first line of treatment should be given within the first 48 to 72 hours after the injury, as it minimizes swelling and increases rate of recovery. Resting protects the soft tissue structures from re-injury and minimizes swelling. Ice minimizes swelling and discomfort; it should be applied for periods of 20 minutes six to eight times throughout the day. Icing causes constriction, which diminishes bleeding and inflammation, helping to reduce edema and relieve pain.

Compression controls edema by limiting compartment volume, increasing interstitial pressure, and reducing transduction of fluid from the capillary bed. To achieve compression, an elastic wrap or bandage is applied from the end of the limb to well past the injured area. Family members and coaches should be counseled that the fit should be snug enough to reduce swelling, but not too tight so as to cause swelling below the wrapped area. During wrapping, attempts should be made to avoid leaving gaps in which skin is exposed. Ideally, the compression should be most snug at the distal end of the limb and slightly less snug above the injury, to enhance circulation. Elevation assists in controlling edema by improving lymphatic and venous return from the injury site. The injured extremity should be elevated above the level of the heart, if possible, until swelling resolves.

Once soft tissues have responded to initial rest, ice, compression, and elevation, the rehabilitation phase of treatment is emphasized. Parents and coaches are counseled that although range of motion (ROM) and strength are restored, the use of brief intervals of the RICE principles should be continued judiciously. Contact or full-intensity activities are inappropriate until pain has resolved and strength and motion have returned. Reassurance of young patients and their families that no single competition is worth the price of re-injury as a result of playing with an injury can ease pressures on the players, family members, and therapists. After range of motion and strength have returned, endurance, proprioceptive, and agility training are encouraged and should be practiced before the patient returns to competition.

CHRONIC AND OVERUSE INJURIES UNIQUE TO SPORTS MEDICINE

Sports can provide young athletes with fulfillment, enjoyment, and camaraderie. The number of children participating in organized athletic activities in the United States is currently at 30 million, and nearly a quarter of all injuries in children and adolescents are attributable to sports.[2] As sports specialization and competition has become more prevalent, training regimens have increased in intensity and duration, with shorter rest periods during and between seasons. Although stress is normal for connective tissue development, excessive stress without intervening periods of rest can cause soft tissue as well as chondral and bone injuries. Sports injuries can occur not only in the unconditioned athlete with poor biomechanics of body alignment or technique but also in the more highly conditioned athlete whose training regimen exceeds the limits of the musculoskeletal system.

The diagnosis of stress injuries entails identifying the factors leading to the development of symptoms, such as training levels, environmental factors, and anatomic factors. The patient's history of symptoms is essential in determining the cause of the injury. Patients may describe pain with intensive activity, with lower levels of activity and training, or with activities of daily living. Marked changes in the intensity, duration, or frequency of workouts may produce overuse syndromes. Environmental factors such as equipment and playing surfaces should also be considered.

Thrower's Shoulder

The proximal humeral physis is susceptible to overstress that may result in a fatigue fracture causing widening of the physis. Although symptoms are frequently nonspecific, pain and aching with throwing are common.

Imaging

Radiographs are useful for imaging widening of the physis in the shoulder with a fatigue fracture (Fig. 10-1). Using comparison views of the other shoulder can prevent physicians from misreading the appearance of physeal widening in a normal shoulder as a result of projection.

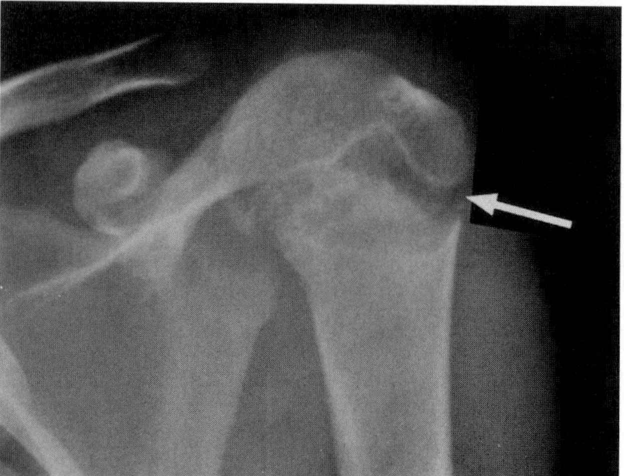

Figure 10-1 Radiograph showing physeal widening *(arrow)* in a patient with thrower's shoulder.

Management

Patients with tenderness at the proximal humeral physis but no physeal widening may be treated with 4 weeks of rest followed by a program of strengthening and gradual return to activity. Those for whom physeal widening is evident on plain radiographs (see Fig. 10-1) are recommended to refrain from throwing for a period of 3 months. A program of progressive strengthening and interval throwing is then instituted. One study of thrower's shoulder demonstrated that 21 of 23 patients treated with an average rest of 3 months were subsequently asymptomatic.[3]

Rehabilitation of thrower's shoulder has the following components: (1) teaching of proper throwing mechanics, (2) helping the athlete understand the injury in order to prevent further injury, (3) education as to the early recognition of discomfort, and (4) education as to limitations for pitches thrown. Although some investigators advocate limiting pitchers to no more than 6 innings per week with 3 days of rest between outings, others have advocated specifically counting pitches during games and practice and limiting players to 60 to 80 pitches per game and 30 to 40 pitches per practice. Coaches and parents should not simply limit patients who pitch to a specific quantitative number; rather, caregivers should monitor players closely for changes in throwing mechanics that may suggest fatigue.

Thrower's Elbow

Thrower's elbow encompasses a number of conditions. It most commonly consists of overstress of the medial elbow-stabilizing structures and repetitive compression injury to the lateral radiocapitellar articulation (Fig. 10-2). Overuse problems involving secondary ossification centers of the proximal ulna and distal humerus have been observed in throwing athletes. Microtrauma to the medial chondral osseous structures is caused by repetitive forces on the medial aspect of the elbow from the pull of the medial musculature. Macrotraumatic acute fractures have also been demonstrated in adolescents and athletes; this injury is avulsion of part or all of the medial epicondyle. This complete separation of the medial epicondylar apophysis occurs from repetitive throwing (Fig. 10-3). Repetitive compressive forces on a lateral side of the elbow may result in irregular fragmentation of the ossific nucleus of the capitellum or osteochondral fracture of the capitellum (Fig. 10-4). Physical findings include lateral pain and loss of motion. However loose bodies from fragmentation of the capitellum may cause elbow joint locking.

The forces experienced at the elbow during pitching have been described throughout each phase of the throwing motion (Box 10-2). A number of different forces are at work throughout the throwing motion, but it has been observed that during the cocking phase, significant tension is placed on the medial structures with lateral compression. Although forces significantly neutralize during the acceleration phase, forearm pronation during a follow-through exerts both compression and shearing forces laterally with tension at the olecranon.

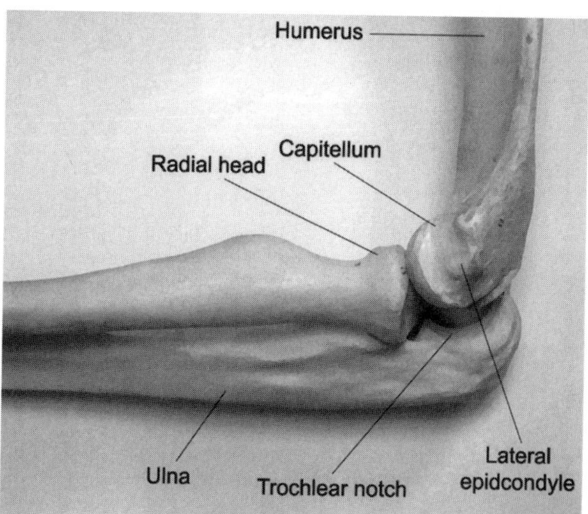

Figure 10-2 Skeletal anatomy of the radiocapitellar articulation.

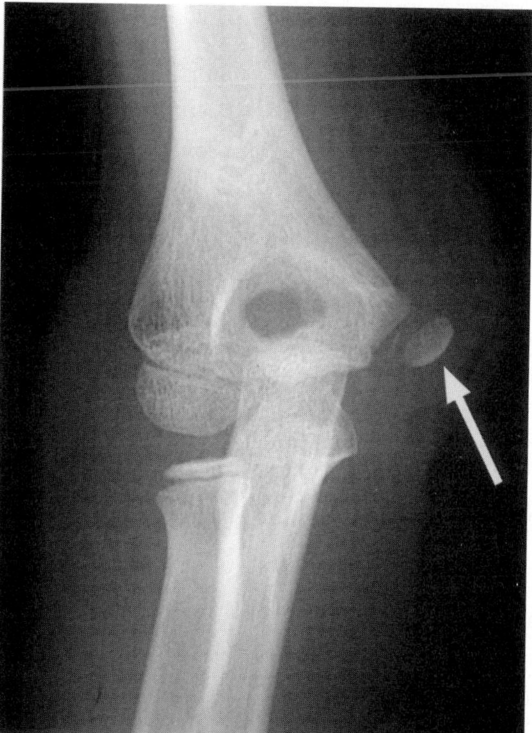

Figure 10-3 Radiograph showing complete separation of the medial epicondylar apophysis *(arrow)* in a repetitive thrower with an acute injury.

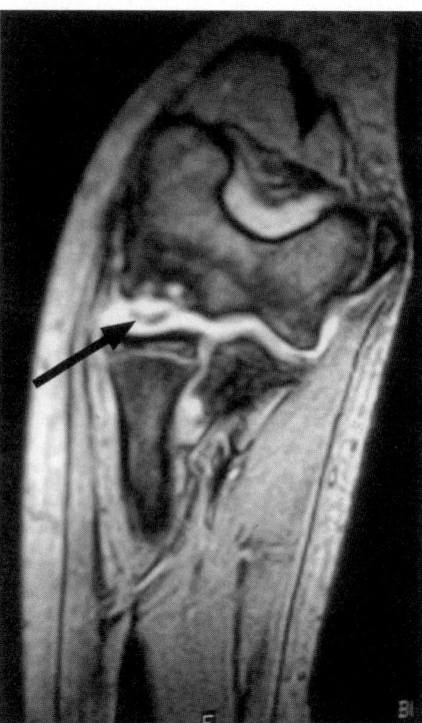

Figure 10-4 Magnetic resonance image demonstrating elbow osteochondritis dissecans lesion with a loose body *(arrow)* from the capitellum within the radiocapitellar joint.

Box 10-2 Phases of Throwing

Arms move apart, front leg steps forward.

COCKING

Front foot touches ground.
Arms are abducted.
Throwing arm is flexed at elbow, continues to rotate externally at shoulder.
Hips, shoulder rotate forward.
Arm reaches maximal external rotation.
Scapular muscles position glenoid under humeral head.
Rotator cuff muscles control glenohumeral distraction.
Internal rotators act to decelerate external rotation.

ACCELERATING PHASE

Arm extends, internally rotates at shoulder.
Internal rotators contract concentrically.
Rotator cuff muscles and scapular muscles are active.
Ball is released.

DECELERATING PHASE

Arm continues to extend and internally rotate; hand appears to pronate.
External rotator muscles act to decelerate internal rotation and prevent glenohumeral join distraction.
Arm reaches point of maximal internal rotation.

The repetitive force on the medial apophysis at the muscle insertion leads to inflammation.

Management

Nonoperative measures, including use of a splint and rest, are recommended. Treatment of medial elbow apophysitis initially consists of rest in the form of activity modification by refraining from throwing and heavy lifting. Three to 4 weeks of activity modification are followed by a graduated rehabilitation program and then, after strength and flexibility have been restored, a throwing program.

The most appropriate treatment for thrower's elbow and other overuse injuries in young athletes is prevention, which consists of monitoring the number of pitches thrown and limiting the number of innings pitched. Caregivers should also ensure that the principle of several days of rest between outings is adhered to by pitchers and catchers.

Gymnast's Wrist

Chronic repetitive mechanical overload of the distal radius has been described in competitive gymnasts. The specific disorder ranges from discomfort without radiographic changes to disabling pain and mechanical symptoms secondary to alteration in anatomy and subsequent biomechanical changes at the wrist. Physeal damage may lead to permanent asymmetric deformity of the wrist. Because approximately 80% of the compressive load across the wrist is transmitted through the radius, early recognition of this problem can allow for treatment to decrease mechanical loads and thereby prevent physeal damage and deformity. Wrist pain and physeal damage correlate with the hours of training per week as well as the number of years of competition and the level of competition. As competition intensifies and level of training increases, competitive gymnasts more frequently use their upper extremities for weight-bearing. Physeal injury at the distal radius may cause progressive radiographic changes, including widening of the physes with irregularity of metaphyseal margins as well as haziness of the physis.

Management

Treatment of gymnast's wrist consists of early recognition followed by modification of activity to permit healing. Patients without radiographic changes have been noted to heal after 4 weeks, whereas those with radiographic changes need 3 months of rest to become asymptomatic.[4]

Osgood-Schlatter Disease

Children are susceptible to overuse injuries at the muscle-tendon, tendon-cartilage, and cartilage-bone interfaces. The most common overuse injury, which occurs at the knee of young athletes, is Osgood-Schlatter disease, an apophysitis at the anterior tibial tubercle. Although adults experience inflammation at the tendon, such as patellar tendonitis at the knee and lateral epicondylitis at the elbow, preteen and teenage athletes more commonly have inflammation at the tendon-bone interface, such as the anterior tibial tubercle. Osgood-Schlatter disease commonly affects rapidly growing preteen girls and young teenage boys during periods of growth and can be noted bilaterally in some patients. Because 70% of the growth of the lower extremities occurs at the physis about the knee, hamstrings and quadriceps can become tight in young athletes. Symptoms include a painful prominence at the anterior proximal tibia and intermittent or constant pain with high-impact running or jumping sports, kneeling, and walking on stairs. Poor flexibility and high-impact sports are contributing factors for this disorder in the growing athlete. Osgood-Schlatter disease may significantly interfere with sports and, in more severe cases, activities of daily living.

Imaging

Radiographs demonstrate fragmentation prominent at the anterior tibial tubercle, which is a consequence of the traction stress at this apophysis (Fig. 10-5).

Management

Patients with Osgood-Schlatter disease are started on a flexibility program to stretch the hamstrings and quadriceps, a straight-leg raising exercise regimen to strengthen the quadriceps muscle, and activity modification to eliminate sports while they are symptomatic. This is not a condition associated with significant long-term problems. Patients are encouraged to follow a home regimen of daily maintenance stretching during their years of growth and development. Patients who are actively involved in sports are counseled that they must interpret pain and limping as nature's signals to discontinue activities for the day. Patients with pain and limping on three successive days are counseled to discontinue their sports participation and follow the stretching regimen for 4 weeks before gradually returning to full sports activity.

This problem is almost universally resolved with closure of the growth plate. There are rare exceptions, such as development of an ossicle at the anterior tibial tubercle that may become symptomatic. In those rare, skeletally mature patients with a persistently symptomatic ossicle at the tibial tubercle that has not responded to nonoperative measures, including activity modification and stretching, this fragment may be excised.

Sinding-Larsen-Johansson Syndrome

Sinding-Larsen-Johansson syndrome is an apophysitis of the inferior pole of the patella. It is caused by chronic repetitive tension and overstress in the form of tension. Fragmentation in a small ossicle may be visualized at the inferior pole on anteroposterior (AP) and lateral radiographs (Fig. 10-6). The treatment of this condition is the same as that for Osgood-Schlatter disease.

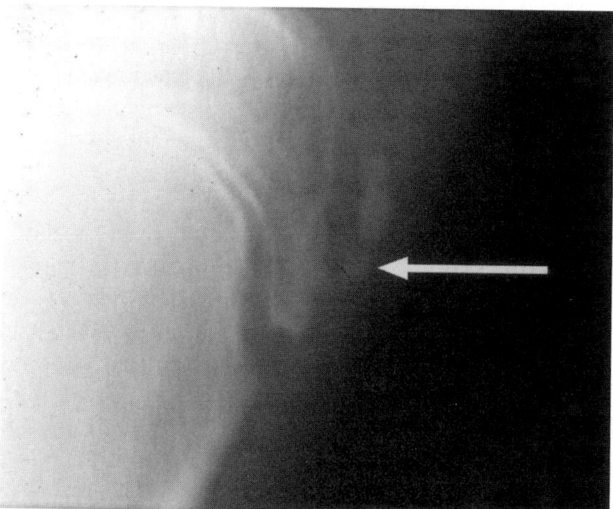

Figure 10-5 Lateral radiograph of a patient with Osgood-Schlatter disease. Note the prominent fragment *(arrow)* at the anterior tibial tubercle.

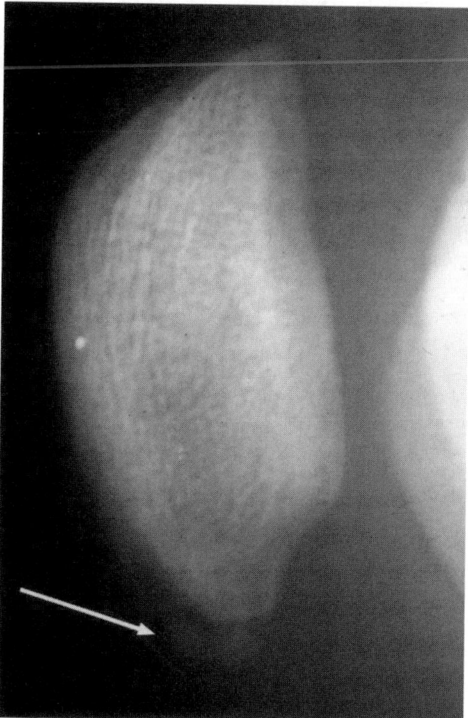

Figure 10-6 Lateral radiograph of a patient with Sinding-Larsen-Johansson syndrome. Note the fragmentation *(arrow)* at the inferior pole of the patella.

Sever Disease

Sever disease is an inflammation of the apophysis at the posterior aspect of the calcaneus (Fig. 10-7). Patients with this condition tend to be younger than children with Osgood-Schlatter disease. The patients are primarily in the early phase of accelerated growth and are most commonly 9 through 12 years old, although they may be younger. Factors contributing to Sever disease are a tight gastrocnemius muscle–soleus muscle–Achilles tendon complex as well as a tight plantar fascia. High-impact running and jumping sports, such as basketball, soccer, and gymnastics, that impart repeated loading on this growth center may cause pain in one or both heels. Symptoms are swelling and tenderness at the insertion of the Achilles tendon into the posterior calcaneus and pain with running and jumping sports. This pain tends to be most prominent during preseason and early season training, especially on hard playing surfaces, in patients with poorly cushioned shoes. Swelling and tenderness are limited to the location at the posterior heel and sometimes the distal aspect of the Achilles tendon, and this finding is not associated with other pathologic findings in the foot or ankle.

Management

Treatment recommendations include education and counseling about the nature and self-limiting condition of this process, activity modification including rest when symptoms appear, appropriate ice application, flexibility exercises, heel cushioning, and the use of a heel lift. Patients are instructed that if they have pain and limping, they are to discontinue their activities for the day. If they have pain and limping on 3 or 4 successive days, they are to discontinue their athletic activities for a month and perform only stretching exercises. Patients are encouraged to change their athletic footwear from cleats to turf shoes if they are playing on dry ground, in an effort to eliminate a component of the shearing forces on the posterior calcaneus. Heel cups and other forms of shock-absorbing insoles may be used to treat this condition as well. Although insoles can secondarily help improve patients' symptoms, activity modification and flexibility training are of primary importance.

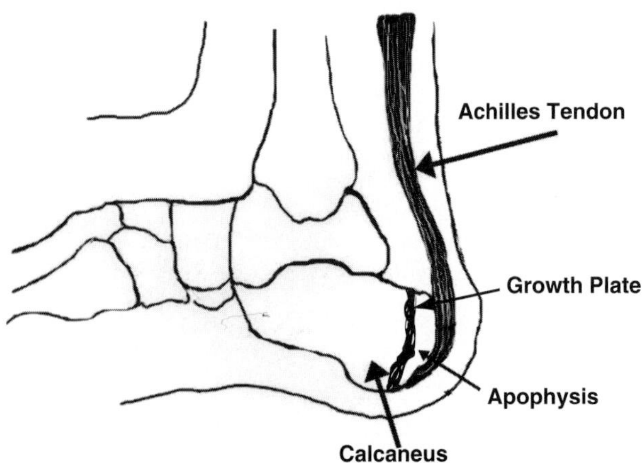

Figure 10-7 Diagram of the ankle. Inflammation of apophysis at posterior aspect of the calcaneus results in Sever apophysitis.

Symptoms usually resolve within a few weeks, or occasionally months, with appropriate treatment without any forms of immobilization. In patients with refractory symptoms, we find that several weeks of immobilization can relieve severe symptoms, after which a formal therapy regimen can be started. Radiographs are not required in routine cases but can be of benefit to rule out other disease, such as tumor, infection, or bone cyst at the ankle or calcaneus in patients with refractory symptoms. Patients are also counseled about appropriate activities that they can continue to perform to maintain their fitness, including swimming, walking, and riding on a stationary bike. Patients are also encouraged to maintain a home baseline stretching program after symptoms resolve in order to prevent recurrences, which are possible during periods of rapid growth.

Osteochondritis Dissecans

Osteochondritis dissecans (OCD) is an osteochondral lesion that affects the subchondral bone and overlying articular cartilage. With OCD, a fragment of bone or cartilage partially or completely separates from the joint surface (Fig. 10-8). In mild cases, the fragment may stay in place in the bone. In more severe cases, however, the fragment completely separates and falls in into the joint. There are four stages of OCD that describe the progression of the condition.[5] The stage 1 lesion is a small area of subchondral compression. The stage 2 lesion is a partially detached fragment. In stage 3, a loose body is present, and by stage 4, the loose body is displaced (Table 10-2). This condition may occur at any time of life but most commonly manifests in teenagers 13 to 17 years old. OCD more commonly affects one joint, usually the knee, although multiple joint involvement has been reported. The elbow and ankle are next most commonly affected, followed by the shoulder, wrist, hand, and hip joints. The etiology of OCD is unknown. Trauma, interruptions in blood supply to bone, uneven or excessive pressure, and genetic factors are all suspected as causes. OCD manifests as generalized pain that worsens with strenuous activity and twisting motions, accompanied by swelling. The joint may become locked, and the patient may complain of a sense of instability in the joint.

Imaging

Radiographs may confirm the presence and location of OCD lesions (Fig. 10-9). Magnetic resonance imaging

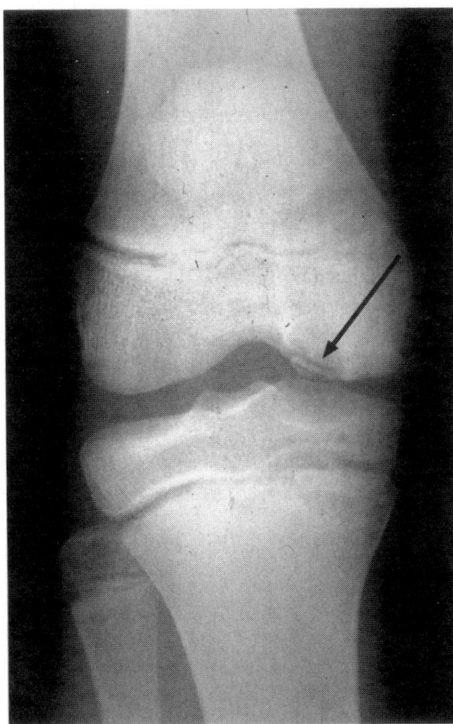

Figure 10-8 Anteroposterior radiograph of osteochondritis dissecans lesion of the lateral aspect medial femoral condyle. Note fragmentation *(arrow)*.

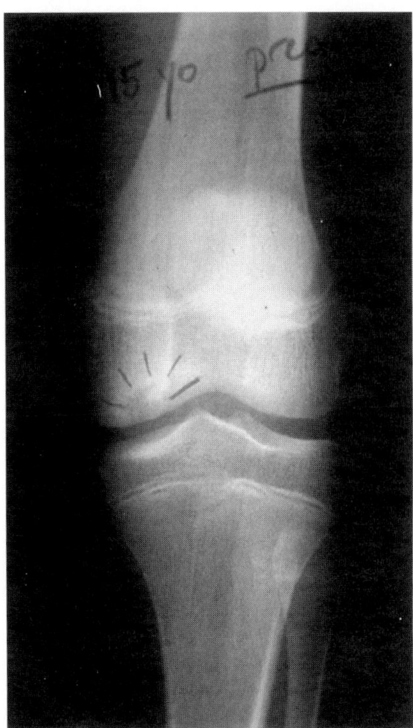

Figure 10-9 Anteroposterior radiograph of 15-year-old patient with osteochondritis dissecans lesion, before drilling.

(MRI) is useful for evaluation of the status of the overlying cartilage and the amount of subchondral edema, features that help the clinician grade lesions and predict clinical outcome.

Management

OCD is usually treated by adjustment of activity levels, which may include changing or stopping the patient's participation in sports. Healing of OCD may be confirmed by follow-up radiographs, at which point the patient can return to normal activity levels. However, older patients with closed growth plates tend to have a worse prognosis. More severe cases may require immobilization with casts or braces. Cases that progress despite nonoperative measures, developing lesion fragmentation and mechanical symptoms that do not improve or that become worse, may require surgical treatment to stimulate increased blood flow to the area or to remove or secure any loose pieces. Bone and cartilage grafting may be necessary in very severe cases with loss of large fragments. After surgery, patients participate in a physical therapy program and may or may not be allowed to return to preoperative activity levels. Treating OCD early and effectively (Fig. 10-10) often prevents recurrent symptoms in adulthood, although some very severe lesions may be symptomatic later in life.

Table 10-2 Berndt and Harty's Four Stages of Osteochondral Lesions

Stage	Description
I	Small area of subchondral compression
II	Partially detached fragment
III	Completely detached fragment remaining in the crater
IV	Fragment loose in the joint

From Berndt AL, Harty M: Transchondral fractures (osteochondritis dissecans) of the talus. J Bone Joint Surg Am 41:988-1020, 1959.

Stress Fractures

Stress fractures after repetitive trauma are well documented in athletes such as runners, football players, gymnasts, and ballet dancers. Stress fractures have been described as spontaneous fractures of normal bone resulting from the summation of stresses, any of which by itself would be harmless.[6] The most common site for stress fracture in children is the proximal tibia, followed by the distal fibula.[7] Sprints, hurdles, and jumps account for a significant number of such injuries. Professional female ballet dancers suffer most commonly from metatarsal fractures,[8] whereas ice skaters often suffer fractures in the distal fibula.

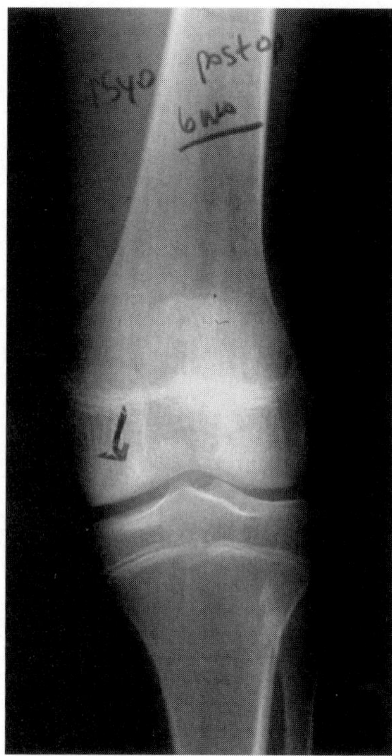

Figure 10-10 Anteroposterior radiograph of the 15-year-old patient with osteochondritis dissecans lesion shown in Figure 10-9, after drilling.

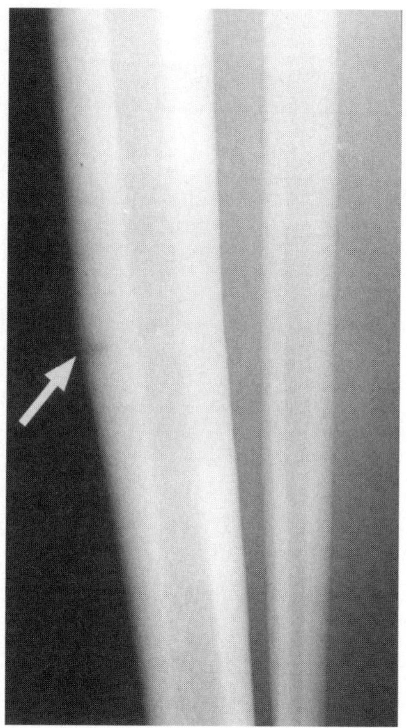

Figure 10-11 Cortical hypertrophy at the mid-anterior tibia with a horizontal radiolucency *(arrow)* indicative of a chronic tibial stress fracture. This radiolucency is called the "dreaded black line," because untreated patients are at risk for development of a complete fracture.

Patients present with localized pain that is related to activity; they may also complain of dull aching discomfort at rest and tenderness to palpation of the affected area. Radiographs are helpful because they may demonstrate a radiolucent line suggestive of a stress fracture (Fig. 10-11). However, a bone scan is most beneficial in confirming a diagnosis.

Patients are typically treated with immobilization in a cast, followed by a progressive return to activity. The goal of treatment is to complete healing, achieved by keeping patients pain free for 2 to 3 months with immobilization followed by activity modification.

Discoid Lateral Meniscus

Discoid lateral meniscus is the cause of "snapping knee" and, when torn, can be a cause of locking and knee pain in children. This is due to an abnormally thick meniscus covering a large percentage of the overall tibial surface. The etiology of this phenomenon is still debated. Some investigators speculate a developmental origin, but others believe the discoid meniscus to be congenital. Its incidence varies from 1.5% to 15.5%, and it occurs almost exclusively in the lateral compartment of the knee.[9,10] On rare occasions, the discoid meniscus may occur on the medial side of the knee.

The Watanabe's system[11] classifies the discoid meniscus into three groups—complete, incomplete, and Wrisberg variant—on the basis of the amount of tibial surface covered by the meniscus and whether the meniscus has normal posterior horn attachments (Fig. 10-12). Both the complete and incomplete types of discoid meniscus have normal posterior horn attachments. However, the complete type covers the entire tibial surface, and the incomplete type covers only a portion.

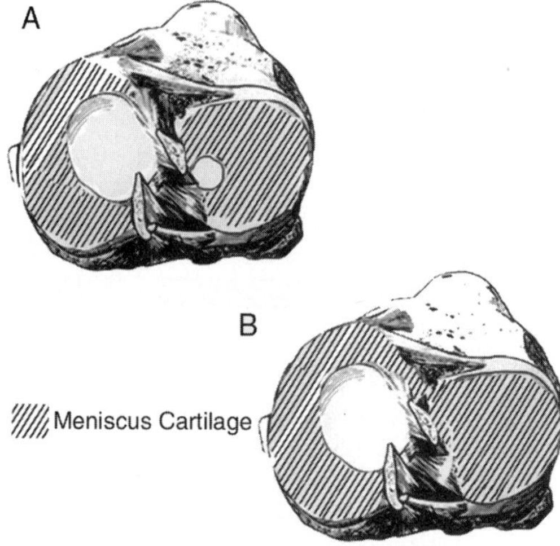

Figure 10-12 Watanabe system for classifying discoid meniscus: **A**, incomplete; **B**, complete.

The Wrisberg variant lacks normal posterior horn attachments and is bonded posteriorly to the medial femoral condyle only by the meniscofemoral ligament, the ligament of Wrisberg.[9,10]

In children and adolescents, the most common symptom of discoid lateral meniscus is pain. The onset of knee pain is associated with a traumatic event or, more often, has an insidious onset. Children may describe mechanical symptoms such as locking, catching, clicking, or the knee "giving way." The classic snapping knee usually manifests in children and is associated with the Wrisberg variant discoid meniscus. Patients with the classic snapping knee describe a painless, audible snap as the knee extends from a flexed position. The symptoms are attributed to reduction of the trapped meniscus with knee extension. On physical examination, the patient has joint line tenderness. Signs include decreased range of motion, quadriceps atrophy, and a knee effusion. Provocative testing may yield a positive McMurray test result and reveal knee instability.

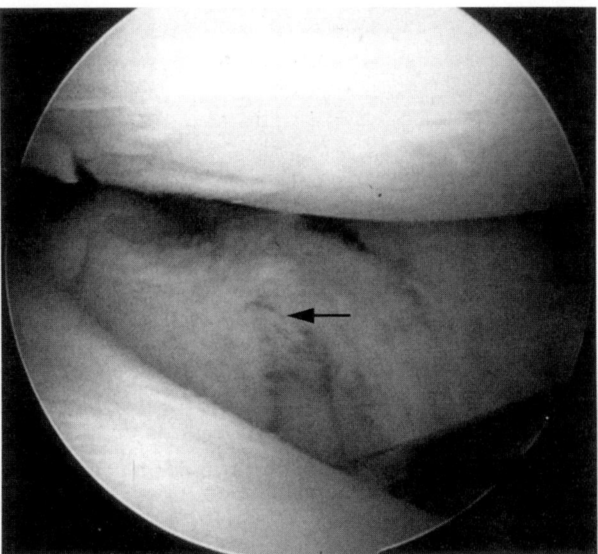

Figure 10-13 Intraoperative photograph of degenerative discoid meniscus with intrasubstance delamination and degenerative tearing.

Imaging

Diagnostic imaging modalities useful in the evaluation of the discoid meniscus are plain radiographs, which are often obtained at the time of initial patient presentation and usually appear normal in cases of discoid meniscus, and MRI. Occasionally, however, radiographs show widening of the lateral joint space and squaring of the lateral femoral condyle.

MRI has become the imaging modality of choice for confirming a diagnosis of discoid meniscus. MRI findings of continuity between the anterior and posterior meniscal horns on three consecutive sagittal images signify a discoid meniscus. Diagnosis of a discoid meniscus also requires demonstration of an abnormally large meniscus with an abnormally large free medial edge. Other MRI findings in discoid meniscus are a transverse diameter greater than 15 mm at the midbody and a difference between medial and lateral meniscal heights of at least 2 mm.[12]

Management

The treatment approach varies according to Wantanabe meniscal type and the presence of any coexisting knee disease. Traditionally, an asymptomatic discoid meniscus requires no intervention as long as there is no clinical evidence suggesting meniscal disease and there are no signs of meniscal hypermobility.

The treatment approach for the discoid meniscus consists initially of rest, activity modification, and quadriceps and hamstrings strengthening. Surgery is required for a complete or incomplete discoid meniscus with evidence of meniscal degeneration, and for meniscal tear (Fig. 10-13) or meniscal hypermobility for which conservative management has failed. Loose fragments of meniscus causing symptoms must undergo removal accompanied by meniscoplasty performed along the remaining meniscal substance to form a more normal meniscal rim. Symptomatic complete and incomplete types are often treated with partial meniscectomy.

The treatment of the symptomatic Wrisberg variant also remains controversial. Total meniscectomy has been advocated for this disorder, and peripheral reattachment for the symptomatic Wrisberg variant is less often performed.

ACUTE UPPER EXTREMITY INJURIES

Shoulder Dislocation

Shoulder joint mobility allows the arm to be moved in the correct direction in space so that the hand can be in a desired location. Many static and dynamic mechanisms contribute to the stability of the glenohumeral joint. The bony constraint is limited to the glenoid fossa, which is somewhat deepened by the labrum. The primary stabilizer is believed to be the capsular-ligamentous complex, and the four rotator cuff muscles serve as the dynamic secondary stabilizer that keeps the humeral head in place as the humerus moves through a full range of motion (Fig. 10-14).

In traumatic shoulder dislocation, the arm and shoulder are forced into an abducted and externally rotated position as the humeral head is levered over the glenoid anteriorly. Posterior dislocations are much less common, probably representing about 2% to 4% of all dislocations. Immediately after the injury, there is pain and swelling around the shoulder. The humeral head can often be palpated anterior to the glenoid. The axillary nerve is most commonly injured, and its examination should be

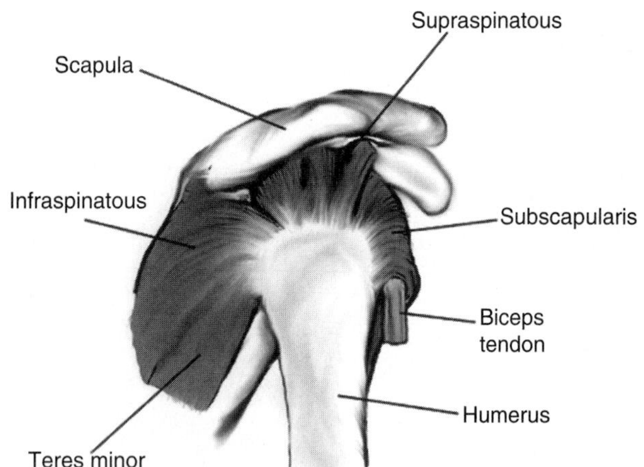

Figure 10-14 **Anatomy of the shoulder.** The rotator cuff forms a "sleeve" around the shoulder.

carefully documented before reduction. The axillary nerve provides sensory innervation to the lateral upper arm and motor function to the deltoid and the teres minor muscles. Generalized ligamentous laxity, if present, should also be noted at clinical examination.

Imaging

Radiographs of shoulder dislocations in skeletally immature patients are similar to those in the adults. Although many different radiographic techniques have been described, the basic series should consist of a true AP view of the glenohumeral joint, the scapular Y view, and an axillary view. An impression fracture at the posterolateral humeral head, commonly known as a Hill-Sachs lesion, can be seen with an internal rotation view of the proximal humerus. If there are mechanical symptoms suggesting an associated intra-articular problem, such as a Hill-Sachs lesion or labral injury with a shoulder dislocation or subluxation, further imaging should be performed. Arthrograms alone were commonly used in the past, but they have been largely used in conjunction with or replaced by CT and MRI performed with "cuts" through the glenohumeral joint.

Management

Acute dislocation of the shoulder should be reduced by one of the standard methods. Adequate sedation is essential for a successful close reduction. Intra-articular injection of local anesthetic can be used as an adjunct, providing added postreduction analgesia.

A commonly used technique involves traction and countertraction (Fig. 10-15). An assistant pulling a sheet wrapped around the trunk of the patient at the level of the scapular body from the contralateral side provides countertraction while the physician applies steady, continuous traction to the affected arm. As the muscle fatigues, spasms that lock the humeral head lessen, allowing reduction of the shoulder joint with gentle manipulation. The Stimson

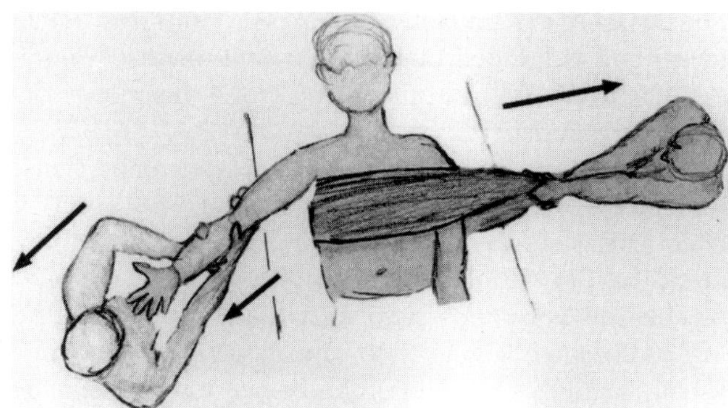

Figure 10-15 Diagram showing glenohumeral traction used for correcting a dislocated shoulder.

maneuver positions the patient prone with the affected arm hanging over the edge of the examination table. Hanging weights from the arm provides traction. Reduction then follows the same principles as described previously. After relocation, a plain radiograph should be obtained to assess the adequacy of reduction. The arm is then placed in a sling for immobilization.

The issue of surgical intervention after an initial dislocation remains a topic of debate. Treatment should be tailored to the individual patient and his or her goals in life. As with the advances in knee surgery a decade ago, a greater understanding of the shoulder and its pathology has led to a refinement of surgical techniques and enthusiasm for minimally invasive operations.

The incidence of recurrent dislocation after the first traumatic event is closely related to the energy of the initial insult, the soft tissue involvement, the age at first dislocation, and the activity level and the overall ligamentous condition of the patient.

Early range-of-motion exercise prevents the formation of adhesions, which would compromise overall function of the arm. Rehabilitation should also focus on scapular stabilization exercises as well as rotator cuff and deltoid strengthening to enhance the dynamic stabilizers of the shoulder joint.

Acromioclavicular Separation

The acromioclavicular (AC) joint is a diarthrodial joint between the lateral clavicle and the acromion of the scapula. The primary stabilizer of the shoulder is the strong coracoclavicular ligament. The acromioclavicular ligament is weaker, serving as a secondary stabilizer.

In sport activities, the acromioclavicular joint can be injured during a violent fall. Typically, the scapula, and therefore the acromion, is driven inferiorly as the top of the shoulder strikes the ground. At the same time, the clavicle stays elevated and extended because the medial end remains attached to the sternoclavicular joint. The classification system for this injury in children and adolescents is similar to that used in adults

(Table 10-3).[13] However, because of the thick periosteal sheath around the clavicle, dislocations in this area tend to split out of the periosteal tube, much like a banana being peeled out of its skin (Fig. 10-16). Type I and type II injuries may have only mild to moderate swelling and tenderness. The gross deformity is usually obvious with type III and type V separations. Type IV injuries are probably the most commonly missed, because the distal end of the clavicle can be buried inside the belly of the trapezius muscle. Type VI injuries are rare, usually causing remarkable restriction in shoulder motion.

Imaging

Plain radiographs are essential to determining correct diagnosis and eliminating associated fractures and dislocations. Stress views are obtained by hanging 5- to 10-lb weights on the injured arm. Traction exaggerates any instability of the acromioclavicular joint on an AP view, and the contralateral side is filmed simultaneously for comparison.

Management

In the pediatric population, type I, II, and III injuries can be expected to heal and remodel without major sequelae. Often, a sling to support the weight of the arm is required. Surgical treatment with internal fixation is reserved for type IV, V, and VI injuries with gross displacement and deformity. In patients older than 16 years, some acromioclavicular separations are true dislocations rather than periosteal splits and therefore may need more aggressive intervention in high-performance athletes.

ACUTE LOWER EXTREMITY INJURIES

Pelvic Avulsion Fractures

With an ever-increasing number of children and adolescents participating in sports activities, pelvic avulsion fractures are becoming more prevalent. These injuries are caused by sudden powerful contractions of a muscle pulling on a developing apophysis. Knowledge of the muscle origins and insertions around the pelvic area aids in the diagnosis (Fig. 10-17). The sartorius muscle originates from the anterior superior iliac spine (ASIS), the direct head of the rectus femoris originates from the anterior inferior iliac spine (AIIS), and the hamstrings and adductors originate from the ischial tuberosity.

ASIS avulsions and ischial avulsions are the most common, each accounting for about 30% of the total number of injuries.[14] Pulling of the sartorius, especially when it is stretched while the hip is extended and the knee flexed, causes ASIS avulsion fractures. Ischial avulsions are produced by contraction of the hamstrings in a similar manner. These injuries are commonly associated with gymnastics, football, and track. The apophysis of the ischium ossifies at the age of 15 years but may not unite until the age of 25 years, making the diagnosis of pelvic avulsion fracture plausible even in young adults.

Physical examination elicits pain and localized swelling around the injured apophysis. Although plain film radiographs may demonstrate gross displacement when present (Fig. 10-18), subtle changes can be detected only with the use of comparison views of the other side. Care should be taken to avoid overtreating a normal anatomic variant.

Management

Usually, the treatment necessary for pelvic avulsion fracture is a period of rest in the form of protected weight-bearing. Positioning of the hip should limit stretching of the muscle involved, thus decreasing the amount of traction on the injured apophysis. Weight-bearing is limited with crutches until appropriate callus is visible on a radiograph. Prognosis is excellent for the patient's return to sports after complete healing and adequate rehabilitation. Occasionally, excessive callus formation that is symptomatic must be excised surgically.

Patellar Dislocations

The patella is a sesamoid bone that increases the mechanical advantage of the extensor mechanism of

Table 10-3 Rockwood Classification of Acromioclavicular (AC) Injuries

Type	Description
I	Mild sprain of the AC ligament without disruption of the periosteal tube
II	Partial disruption of the dorsal periosteal tube with some instability at the distal clavicle
II	Large dorsal, longitudinal split in the periosteal tube with gross instability of the distal clavicle
IV	Similar to Type III separation, but with the distal clavicle displaced posteriorly and buttonholed through the trapezius muscle fiber
V	Complete dorsal periosteal split with superior subcutaneous displacement of the clavicle. There is often an associated deltoid and/or trapezius attachment split
VI	An inferior dislocation of the distal clavicle, which is lodged beneath the coracoid process

From Dameron TB, Rockwood CA: Fractures and dislocations of the shoulder. In Rockwood CA, Wilkins KE, King RE (eds): Fractures in Children. Philadelphia, JB Lippincott, 1984, pp 625-653.

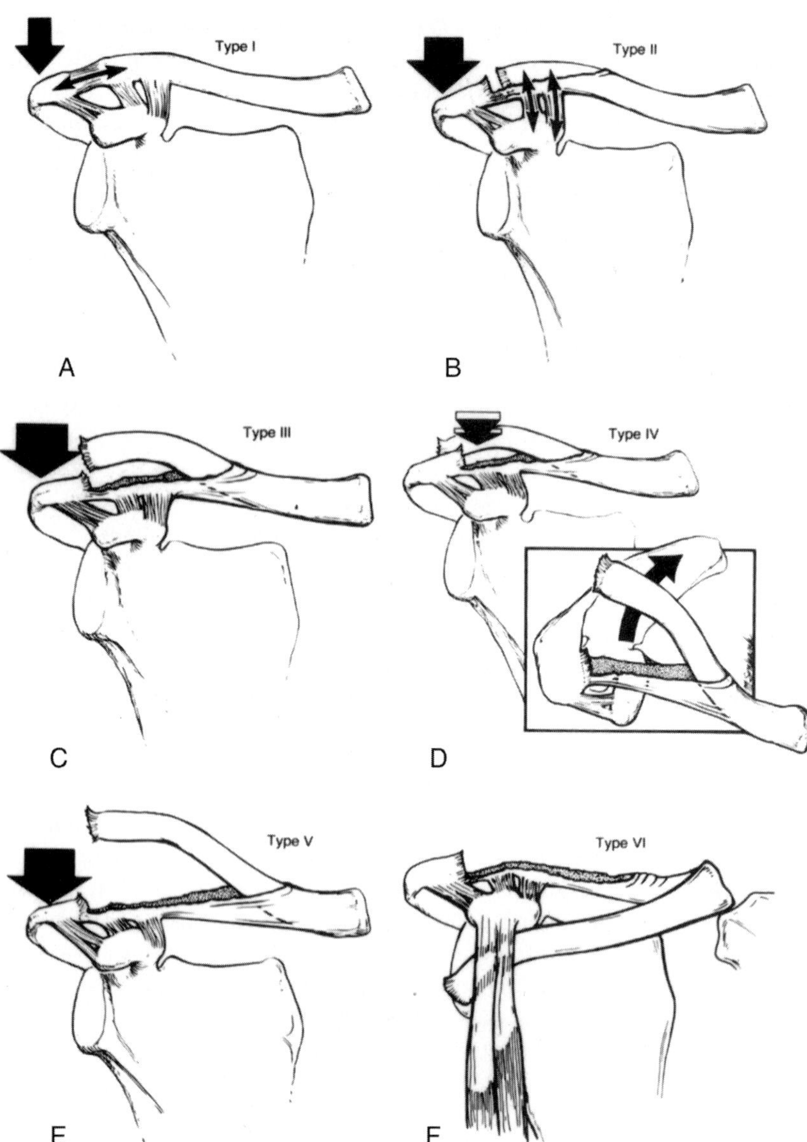

Figure 10-16 Classification of acromioclavicular sprains. (From Rockwood CA Jr, Wilkins KE, Beaty JH: Fractures in Children, 4th ed. Philadelphia, Lippincott-Raven, 1996.)

the knee joint. Because the quadriceps muscle pull is not perfectly in line with the tracking of the patella in the femoral groove, there is a tendency for the patella to be displaced laterally. Patellar dislocation is relatively common in children and more common in girls. Patellar dislocation should be considered in all athletic injuries to the knee, especially if a sizable effusion is present. Pain is diffuse but typically severe at the medial side of the knee. Retinacular tear causes hemarthrosis, which can also be a result of an osteochondral fracture.

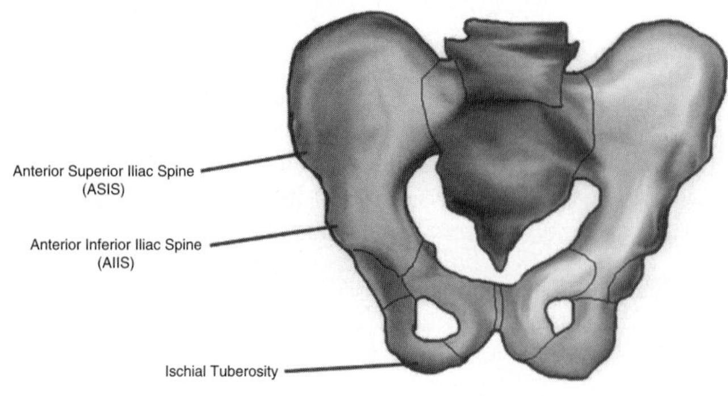

Figure 10-17 Anatomy of the pelvis.

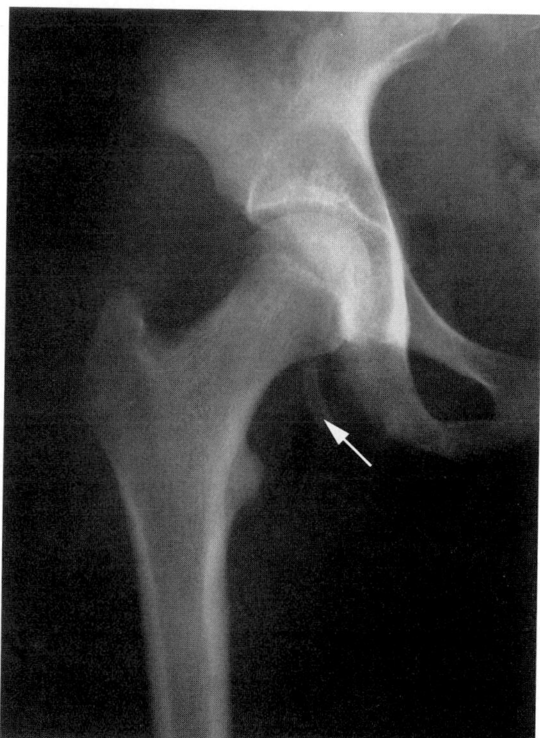

Figure 10-18 Anteroposterior radiograph of an ischial avulsion fracture.

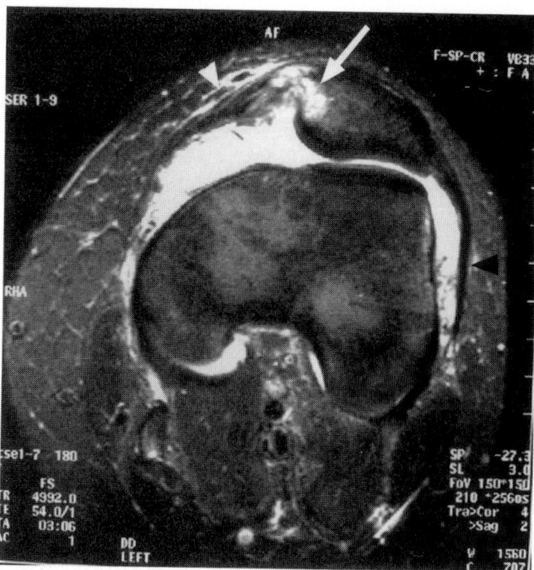

Figure 10-19 Magnetic resonance image demonstrating lateral patellar dislocation of the right knee and subchondral contusion ("bone bruise") *(white arrow).* Notice the torn medial *retinaculum (white arrowhead)* in comparison with the intact retinaculum *(black arrowhead).*

Imaging

Radiographs should be obtained to delineate the exact location of the patella and to rule out osteochondral fracture. A Merchant view shows the position of the patella within the femoral grove when the knee is flexed 30 degrees. MRI can also visualize patellar dislocations (Fig. 10-19).

Management

Rarely seen is the acutely dislocated patella that remains in the displaced position (Fig. 10-20). Usually, the patella reduces spontaneously with knee extension after dislocation. The physician must reduce acute dislocations that do not reduce spontaneously. With the use of adequate sedation and analgesia, the hip is flexed to relax the quadriceps muscle. With the knee gradually extended, the patella can usually be pushed back in place. The knee is then usually immobilized by a cast or a knee immobilizer for 2 to 4 weeks. Surgical management should be reserved for children in whom nonoperative measures fail and who have debilitating subluxations or dislocations. Many procedures have been described for treatment of patellar instability. Most approaches use isolated or combined proximal or distal realignment, lateral releases, and medial reefing.

Rehabilitation after an isolated dislocation or surgery should focus on progressive strengthening of the quadriceps muscles, in particular the vastus medialis oblique, and range-of-motion exercises. About one in six pediatric patellar dislocations develops into recurrent dislocation. The first line of management is aggressive physical therapy after the initial inflammation and swelling subside. Bracing with a neoprene knee sleeve and lateral patellar supports can be helpful. Patients should also be counseled on activity modification. High-risk activities include jumping, pivoting, and twisting sports. More appropriate exercises are walking, biking, swimming, and light jogging.

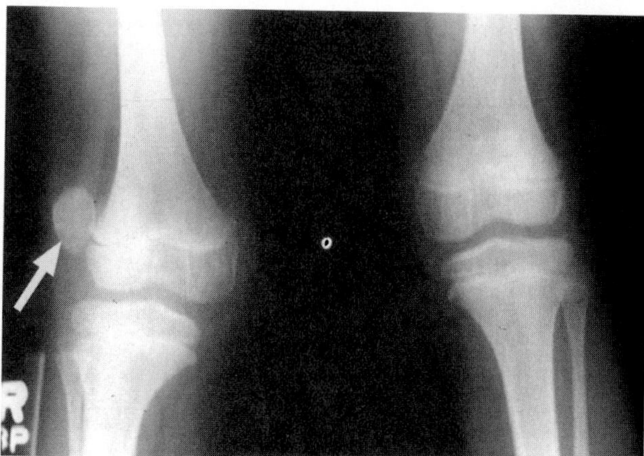

Figure 10-20 Radiographs showing patellar dislocation *(arrow)* of the right knee. The patella of the left knee is in correct anatomical position.

Patellar Fractures

Fracture of the patella after a direct blow to the patella rarely occurs. A variant of patellar fracture is the sleeve fracture, in which the infrapatellar tendon avulses a fragment of bone from the inferior pole of the patella along with articular cartilage. When displacement is minimal and the extensor mechanism still functions, patellar fractures are typically treated nonoperatively with immobilization in extension. Displaced fractures and inability to actively extend the knee are indications for surgical reduction and fixation with a tension-band wire technique.

Meniscal Tears

The menisci arise from the intermediate zone of mesenchyme between the distal femur and proximal tibia. Their semilunar appearance is formed by the tenth week of gestation. As growth continues, the menisci increase in size but retain their shape. They primarily function to transmit and distribute load across the articular surfaces.

Meniscal tears are much less common in children than in adults. The mechanism of injury is typically rotation as the flexed knee is being extended. Pain is present in the majority of patients. Knee effusion is possible, and special maneuvers such as the McMurray and Apley tests can be difficult to perform because of pain. Positive physical findings include a knee effusion, joint line tenderness, and a painful click with knee flexion and circumduction maneuvers such as the McMurray test.

Imaging

Plain radiographs should be obtained to rule out other occult diseases. MRI can be helpful in patients with equivocal radiographic findings.

Management

While many different techniques for meniscal repair have been described, their success is based largely on the blood supply to the area, with peripheral tears having a better prognosis than central tears. The most repairable lesions are vertical tears in the most peripheral third of the meniscus, which are sufficiently vascular to heal after repair.

At present, recommendations for management of meniscal injuries are immobilization for small peripheral tears (<1 cm), repair of large peripheral tears, and limited partial meniscectomy for complex degenerative tears that cannot be repaired, with preservation of as much healthy meniscus as possible (Fig. 10-21). Data suggest the development of degenerative changes after total meniscectomy. Knee motion should be restricted by means of a brace or a cast for 6 weeks after meniscus repair.

Anterior Cruciate Ligament Tear

Anterior cruciate ligament (ACL) tears, like many other sports-related injuries, are seen more and more commonly. This situation is probably the result of a combination of factors such as increased participation of children and adolescents in sports activities, greater participation at a more competitive level, and improved

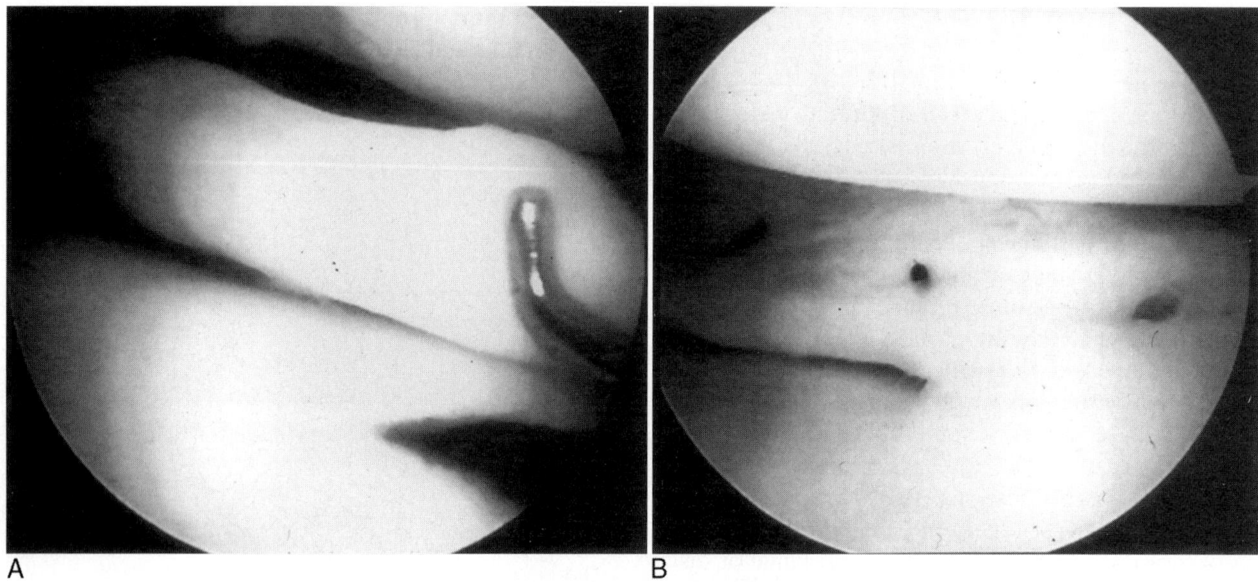

Figure 10-21 **A,** Intraoperative photograph of a peripheral meniscus tear with torn portion interposed within the joint. **B,** Intraoperative photograph of suture repair of meniscus into anatomic position.

diagnostic techniques.[15,16] Children with ACL injuries constitute a unique patient population because of their open growth plates and different ligamentous and bone strength. Damage to a child's open physes potentially causes angular deformity, limb length discrepancy, condylar dysplasia, and subsequent functional limitations. Generalizations should not be made about all ACL injuries in the pediatric population, because children grow at different rates. One patient at a given age may be prepubescent, with significant remaining growth, but another at the same age may be nearing skeletal maturity.

The ACL functions as a primary stabilizer to anterior tibial translation (Fig. 10-22). The mechanisms of ACL injury in children and in adults are similar, resulting from knee twisting, a blow to the knee, or knee hyperextension during which the foot is planted on the ground. Usually, a "pop" is heard or felt by the patient, and a hemarthrosis follows. "Giving way" is a common presenting complaint, as are sudden swelling of the injured knee, knee hemarthroses, a feeling of knee instability, and inability to bear weight on the leg. During physical examination, increased anterior tibial translation can be appreciated by either the Lachman test (with the knee tested at 30 degrees of flexion) or the anterior draw test (with the knee tested at 90 degrees of flexion). It is important to ensure that the thigh muscles, especially the hamstrings, are relaxed during these provocative tests, because false-negative results can be obtained if tensed muscles prevent movement of the tibia relative to the femur.

Some children present with congenital ACL deficiencies, either the absence of the ACL or constitutional laxity. Additionally, physiologic laxity is often seen in the prepubescent knee and can also mislead the clinician. For these reasons, it is essential that the uninvolved knee be examined in all children presenting with knee laxity. The child's account of which motions and positions are responsible for the "giving way" and physical examination of both knees enable the examiner to determine presence or absence of ACL deficiency.

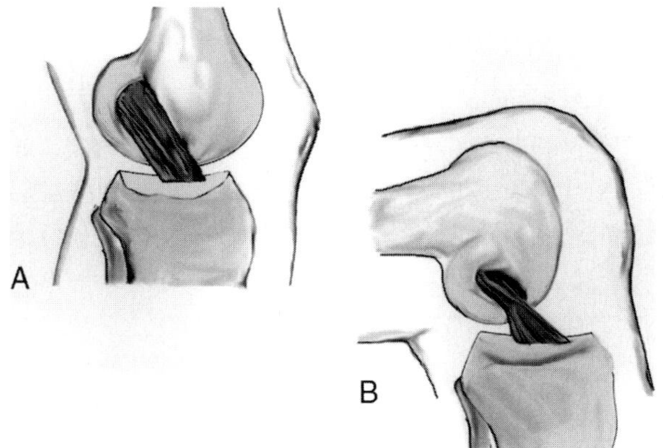

Figure 10-22 Schematic drawing of anterior cruciate ligament in extension **(A)** and flexion **(B)**.

Imaging

Radiographs and MRI determine the diagnosis and extent of the injury while revealing the presence of associated problems in the adjacent cartilage, bone, meniscus, and other ligaments. A plain radiographic study consisting of AP, lateral, tunnel, and patellar radiographs can rule out tibial eminence fractures, osteochondral fractures, and other bony damage. MRI is routinely ordered to establish the diagnosis, to delineate other internal derangement of the knee, such as the presence of occult fractures, and to determine the extent of soft tissue damage to the ACL and other supporting structures, including the menisci (Fig. 10-23).

Management

The treatment of ACL tears in the pediatric population revolves around the issue of skeletal age and how to address the open physis, where approximately 65% of lower extremity growth occurs. In order to select a treatment plan for the pediatric patient, the examiner must accurately evaluate the child's skeletal age and remaining growth to avoid physeal and epiphyseal growth disturbances and subsequent angular deformity, leg length discrepancy, and condylar dysplasia. Several factors are helpful in determining skeletal age, including bone age evaluation on wrist radiographs according to the method of Greulich and Pyle[17] and assessments of secondary sex characteristics, patient and familial height, and recent foot growth. On the basis of these factors, the orthopaedist can make an informed decision about risk to the growth plates.

ACL tears may be partial or complete. Treatment goals for partial ACL tears are to reduce swelling and return full range of motion to the knee. Nonoperative treatments

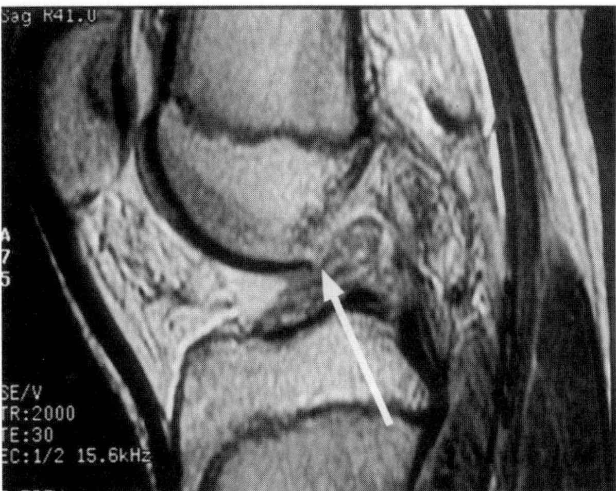

Figure 10-23 Increased signal intensity on a T1-weighted magnetic resonance image at the intercondylar notch consistent with anterior cruciate ligament tear *(arrow)* in a skeletally immature patient.

include muscle strengthening, bracing, activity modification, and counseling. However, nonsurgical treatment of ACL tears in skeletally immature patients has characteristically led to recurrent instability and further meniscal damage, with a poor outlook for returning patients to previous athletic levels.[18-21] Extra-articular and intra-articular surgical options have therefore received more attention. Also, because children may not comply with activity restrictions, or because of a child's lack of understanding of the severity and nature of the injury, nonoperative management is less likely to be successful. Bracing is not sufficient to allow patients to return to sports activities.

Complete ACL tears require surgery for reconstruction of the ligament. The goal of operative reconstruction should be establishment of a stable joint, prevention of the internal soft tissue damages that results from recurrent instability, and return of the patient to sports activities. Primary repair of midsubstance ACL tear has shown limited success, with persistent instability and decreased activity levels being well documented. Intra-articular reconstruction with either an autograft (e.g., part of the patellar tendon or hamstring) or allograft (e.g., Achilles tendon) fixed in bone tunnels in the proximal tibia and distal femur is a common practice for skeletally mature adults (Fig. 10-24). However, in patients with open physis around this area, growth arrest becomes a concern with use of this technique. A debate continues among orthopaedists regarding the age and maturity level at which it is safe to drill across open physes. Extraphyseal procedures aim at working around the open physis to produce knee stability and may have a role in treating skeletally immature patients. These procedures have achieved mixed results. Patients with a nearly closed physis can be treated with an intra-articular soft tissue graft provided that the fixation is not at the level of the physis. Surgery is followed by bracing and physical rehabilitation to regain range of motion and strength. Patients are usually able to return to unrestricted activity in approximately 6 months. Once the clinician determines that the knee is fully rehabilitated and strengthened, the patient may be able to return to sports participation.

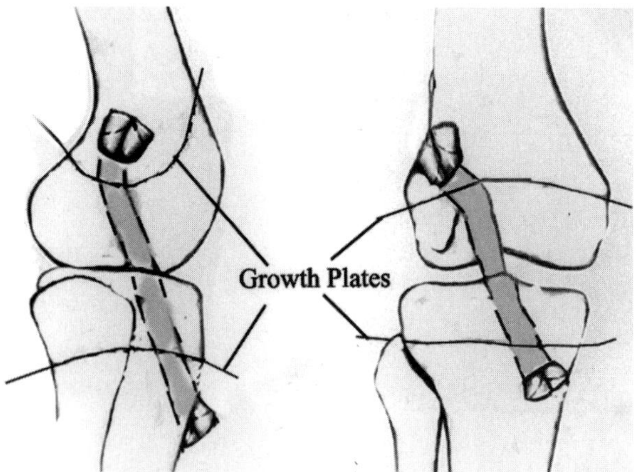

Figure 10-24 Drawing of anterior cruciate ligament reconstruction with soft tissue graft only across physes.

Tibial Spine Fractures

In young children, bone fails before ligaments under tensile or shear stresses. This feature helps explain why ACL injuries in children frequently involve a breach in the bone at the tibial spine, where the ACL inserts, rather than the mid-substance tear seen in older adolescents.[14,15] The association of tibial eminence avulsion with collateral ligament and meniscal damage underscores the importance of a thorough examination and evaluation of all imaging studies. These fractures occur with valgus rotational stress on the knee or hyperflexion occasionally and may cause a large hemarthrosis. The tibial eminence fracture may be nondisplaced, hinged, or displaced. In 1970, Meyers and McKeever[22] classified fractures of the intercondylar eminence into three types (Table 10-4). Zaricznyj[23] later added a fourth type to this classification system. Type I fractures have minimal or no displacement (Fig. 10-25). Type II fractures display a partially attached portion of the tibial eminence, and type III fractures are characterized by complete displacement of a bony fragment, which may be rotated. Type IV fractures are comminuted.

Management

Anatomic reduction should be the goal of treatment. With type I and type II injuries, reduction can usually be achieved with aspiration of the bloody effusion followed by casting of the knee in full extension. Postmanipulation radiographs should be obtained to confirm the adequacy of reduction. Type III and type IV fractures routinely require open reduction and internal fixation with metal pins, wires, or screws, depending on the preferences and level of comfort of the surgeon. Even with perfect reduction and fracture healing, residual

Table 10-4 Classification of Tibial Eminence Fractures

Fracture Type	Description
I	Minimal or no displacement
II	Partial displacement
III	Complete displacement (may have rotational malalignment)
IV	Comminuted fracture

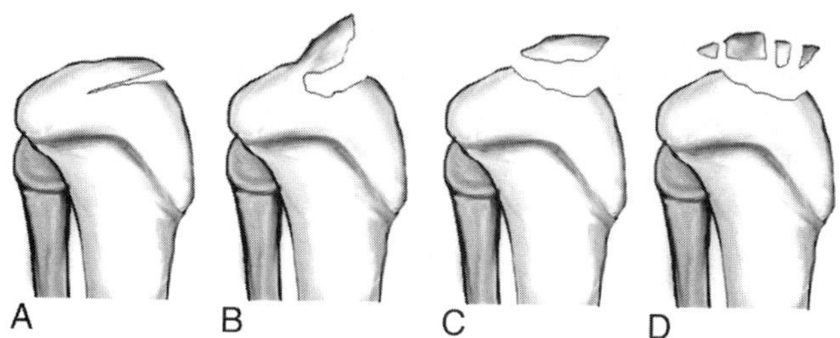

Figure 10-25 Diagram showing the four types of tibial (eminence) spine fractures.

laxity can result, because of plastic deformation or stretching of the ACL under excessive load before fracture actually occurs. Patients and their parents should be warned of this possibility.

Tibial Tubercle Fractures

Avulsion of the tibial tubercle at the attachment of the infrapatellar tendon is found primarily in patients 14 to 16 years old. Open reduction and internal fixation are necessary if the fracture is displaced or occurs at the level of the physis. Nondisplaced or minimally displaced fractures may be treated with a cast holding the leg in extension.

Knee Osteochondral Fractures

Acute osteochondral fractures of the knee typically involved the medial or lateral femoral condyle, or the patella. As with all acute sports injuries, there is an acute onset of symptoms with a well-defined event. According to Kennedy,[24] there are two distinct mechanisms of injury, one exogenous and one endogenous. A direct blow resulting in a shearing force to the femoral condyles is considered exogenous, whereas a flexion-rotation twist of the knee is deemed endogenous.

Most pediatric patients with acute osteochondral fractures present with a history of flexion-rotation injury consistent with patellar dislocation. A bloody effusion is almost always present. Tenderness to palpation can be elicited in the medial or lateral femoral condyle or the medial patella. The knee joint is frequently held in 15 to 20 degrees of flexion, and motion in any direction is restricted.

Imaging

Osteochondral fractures can be difficult to identify on plain radiographs because a significant portion of the lesion is cartilage rather than calcified bone. Often, only a small defect is seen on a regular radiograph. A tunnel projection may be helpful in evaluation of the intercondylar notch. Arthrography, computed tomography (CT), and MRI have also been used (Fig. 10-26).

Management

The treatment of osteochondral fracture is based on the size and origin of the fragment. In general, small fragments (<2 cm) in a non–weight-bearing area of the knee can be removed by an arthroscope. Fragments larger then 2 cm, especially when located in a weight-bearing area, may benefit from internal fixation. Small fragments from non–weight-bearing areas have the best prognosis. Potential complications are adhesions, quadriceps muscle insufficiency, and loose body formation in the case of a fragment which fails to heal.

Ankle Injury in the Young Athlete

The ankle is one of the most frequently damaged structures in adolescents. In fact, the ankle is the most commonly injured body part in athletes of all ages (Fig. 10-27). In adolescents, the ankle is also the most common site of physeal injuries. The effects of these injuries may become more noticeable as sports participation among young athletes increases. Structures important to lateral ankle stability are the peroneal longus and peroneal brevis tendons, which provide stability, and the calcaneofibular (anterior and posterior) ligaments, which provide static support. The primary medial stabilizing structure is the deltoid ligament, with less contribution from the tibialis posterior, flexor digitorum longus, and flexor hallucis longus tendons.

Ankle morphology also contributes to ankle stability. The wider anterior portion of the talus is well seated within the mortise when the foot is in dorsiflexion, providing stability in this position. Inversion injuries occur to the ankle more easily with the foot plantar-flexed, because the talus is narrower posteriorly. The anterior talofibular ligament is taut during plantar-flexion and is therefore more susceptible to injury than the calcaneofibular and posterior talofibular ligaments.

The patient should be asked about the position of the ankle at the time of injury as well as the direction of forces at the time of injury. This history can provide information about the most likely type and location of injury. A history of deformity, swelling, or inability to bear weight immediately after an injury is suggestive of a more severe ligamentous injury or fracture. A history of underlying illnesses, previous ankle injuries, or an underlying disorder of the foot or ankle, such as pes planus, pes cavus, tarsal coalition, or clubfoot, may influence the patient's evaluation and treatment and should, therefore, be noted.

An evaluation of lower extremity pain in skeletally immature patients should involve an evaluation of hip range of motion, so as to avoid missing a slipped capital femoral epiphysis and other disorders. Severely limited and painful hip range of motion, especially if restricted to one side, is an indication for AP and lateral hip

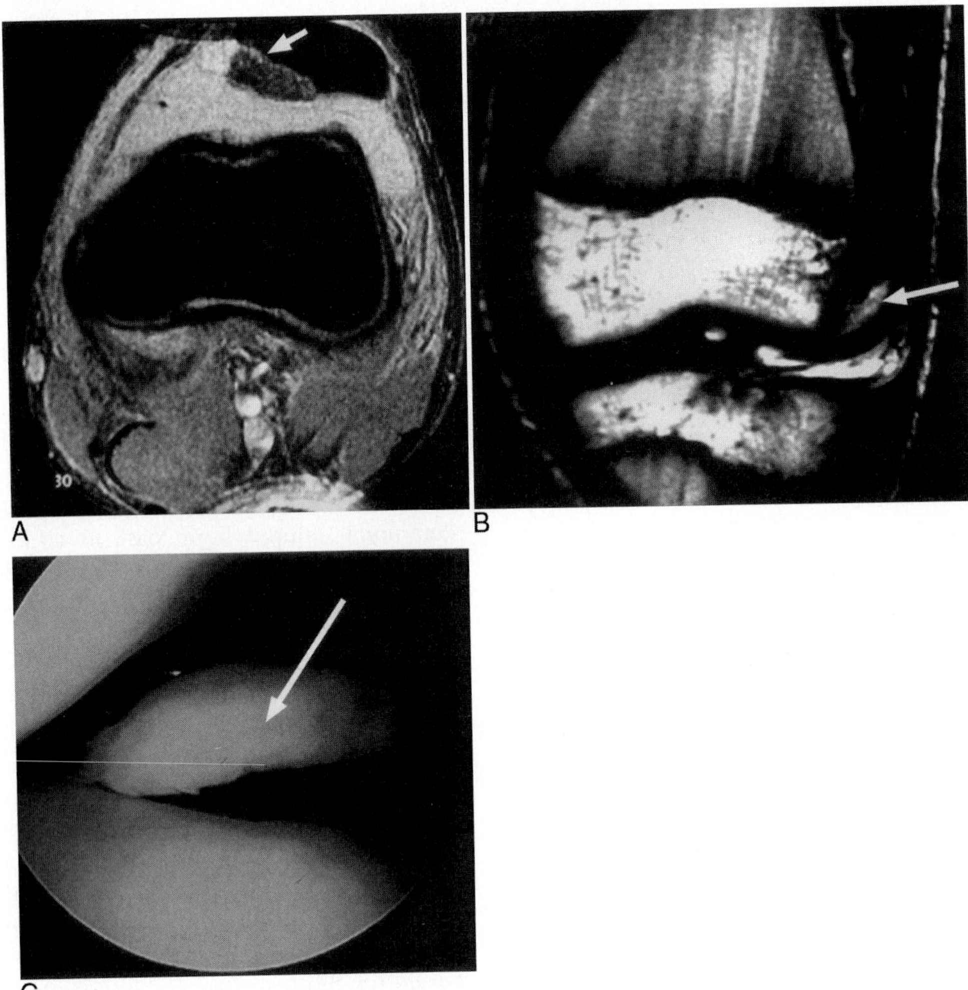

Figure 10-26 Acute osteochondral fracture. A, Patellar fracture *(arrow)* demonstrated on magnetic resonance image. **B,** Chondral loose body *(arrow)* adjacent to femoral condyle demonstrated on magnetic resonance image. **C,** Arthroscopic photograph of chondral loose body *(arrow).*

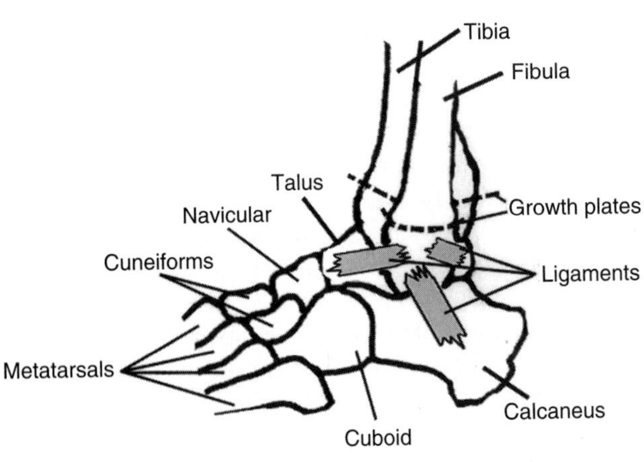

Figure 10-27 Drawing of the anatomy of the skeletally immature ankle.

radiographs. Provided that examination of the hips, knees, and other ankle is unremarkable, the examination can next be focused on the affected ankle and lower leg. Deformity and location of swelling and ecchymosis at the ankle should be noted. The physis, located within 2 cm of the most distal tip of the tibia and fibula, should be palpated as well. An acute inversion injury strongly suggests a growth plate fracture if tenderness and swelling are noted over the physis. Lateral ankle sprain, a less common injury in more immature patients, is found in patients with severe isolated tenderness over the lateral ligamentous complex. Aversion injuries are rare; they occur secondary to the strength of the deltoid ligament as well as the bony configuration of the ankle and orientation of the foot at heel strike. Immediate tenderness and swelling, however, may occur after aversion injuries and can be associated with a fracture. Patients are encouraged to perform active range of motion of the ankle—dorsiflexion, plantar-flexion, inversion, and aversion. Because there is significant variability in motion and laxity in young patients, an evaluation of the other ankle provides a basis for comparison.

A helpful test to assess the status of the ankle's ligamentous structures, the result of which is most commonly positive in adolescents with closed physes, is the anterior drawer test. This test assesses ligamentous stability with the patient's knee in slight flexion and the ankle in 30 degrees of plantar-flexion. To perform the test, the examiner grasps the patient's heel and places a forward pull on the foot while the tibia is maintained in a fixed position. Significant side-to-side difference suggests a tear of the anterior talofibular ligament. Patients experiencing the severe discomfort that tends to appear immediately after or very shortly after an inversion ankle injury may not tolerate passive range-of-motion testing or the anterior drawer test.

Imaging

A number of guidelines, including the Ottawa ankle rules, are used to recommend radiographs if the patient feels pain in specific locations around the foot and ankle. The findings that prompt radiographic evaluation are pain and bone tenderness at the posterior edge of the lateral medial malleolus, midfoot pain with tenderness at the base of the fifth metatarsal, pain in the area of the midfoot, and an inability to bear weight. It should be noted that Ottawa ankle rules do not universally apply to patients with open physes. We recommend obtaining radiographs, including an AP and lateral mortise view, for patients with significant ankle pain and tenderness and inability to bear weight on the ankle and for patients who can bear weight on the ankle but limp.[25]

Management

Type I and II ankle fractures, classified according to the Salter-Harris typing of growth plate injuries, should heal rapidly after simple reduction. The rapid healing is due in part to the thick periosteal sleeve found in patients with open physes. By definition, type III and type IV injuries are intra-articular. Open reduction and internal fixation are often indicated to restore a smooth joint surface for such injuries. Surgery is also recommended to prevent displacement of the growth plate, which could lead to physeal arrest or growth disturbance.

Ankle rehabilitation varies according to the severity of injury. Regardless of severity, a functional rehabilitation program is more efficient than early surgical intervention for restoring comfort, strength, and function. Skeletally immature patients are permitted to progressively bear weight on the ankle with the use of lateral and medial stabilizing supports after 48 to 72 hours of rest, ice, compression, and elevation (RICE). We recommend 2 weeks in a short-leg, weight-bearing cast for children who have severe sprains with marked swelling and limited motion.

Rest and protected weight-bearing with supports or casts is followed by a rehabilitation program focused on restoring ankle range of motion, strength, balance, agility, and endurance. Initially, a general active and pain-free range-of-motion program helps reduce stiffness and pain. In patients with markedly diminished resistance, ankle exercises with elastic tubing and toe raises may be instituted. Balance training can begin with patients standing on the affected leg with eyes open and closed under the supervision of a caregiver or therapist. Aerobic fitness is managed with low-impact aerobic exercises, such as swimming and cycling. A patient with more severe sprains would benefit from formal physical therapy, including the use of balance boards and sport-specific strength and proprioceptive exercises.

Rehabilitation is not complete until strength and proprioception are fully restored and the patient has demonstrated proficiency with sports-specific and functional activities. Patients must be able to jog and then run and should perform straight running before incorporating changes in direction. Efforts may be made to incorporate figure-of-eight running and other activities that involve sharper changes in direction. Sprinting, hopping, jumping, and cutting should be performed before the patient returns to full sports participation. Bracing and taping may make patients feel more comfortable and may provide appropriate proprioceptive feedback; however, these measures are no substitute for appropriate physical rehabilitation.

Rehabilitation should begin within the first few days after an ankle injury, once the most severe initial symptoms have subsided. Rehabilitation promotes rapid return of strength, function, and comfort, reducing the recurrence of sprains. Ultimately, the rehabilitation program should focus on restoring ankle range of motion, strength, balance, agility, and endurance.

Tillaux and Triplane Fractures

Tillaux fractures and triplane fractures are seen in patients with partially closed growth plates. As the distal tibial physis closes from central to medial and then lateral, there is a transitional period during adolescence when the growth plate is fused medially but not laterally, making the lateral part the only one vulnerable to injuries. The Tillaux fracture is a Salter-Harris type III injury involving the unfused anterolateral segment of the distal tibial epiphysis (Fig. 10-28). In this injury pattern, the anterior tibiofibular ligament avulses the epiphyseal segment when the foot is externally rotated. Reduction is therefore achieved by internally rotating the foot relative to the tibia and applying direct pressure over the avulsed epiphyseal fragment. CT is a valuable tool for evaluation of the articular surface after manipulation. If the reduction is deemed adequate, it can be treated with a long-leg

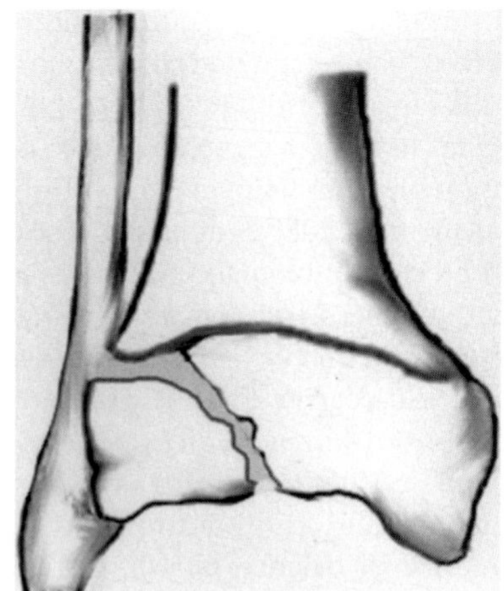

Figure 10-28 Drawing of a Tillaux fracture.

cast for 3 weeks followed by a short-leg walking cast for 3 weeks. Open reduction with internal fixation would be indicated if an intra-articular stepoff persists after closed reduction.

The triplane fracture is so named because the injury has coronal, sagittal, and transverse components (Fig. 10-29). It can be viewed as a Tillaux fracture with a Salter-Harris type II extension to the posterior distal metaphysis of the distal tibia. The typical radiographic hallmark of this injury is the appearance of a Salter-Harris type III injury on the AP view, as seen in Tillaux fractures, with the Salter-Harris type II component visible only on the lateral view. Slightly displaced two-part triplane fractures may be reduced by internally rotating the foot.[13] As with Tillaux fractures, CT should be performed after any closed reduction of a triplane fracture, to delineate the extent of the joint involvement. Surgery should be recommended if CT shows a residual articular stepoff. Otherwise, the reduced injury can be treated with a long-leg, non-weight-bearing cast for 3 to 4 weeks followed by a short-leg cast for 3 to 4 weeks.

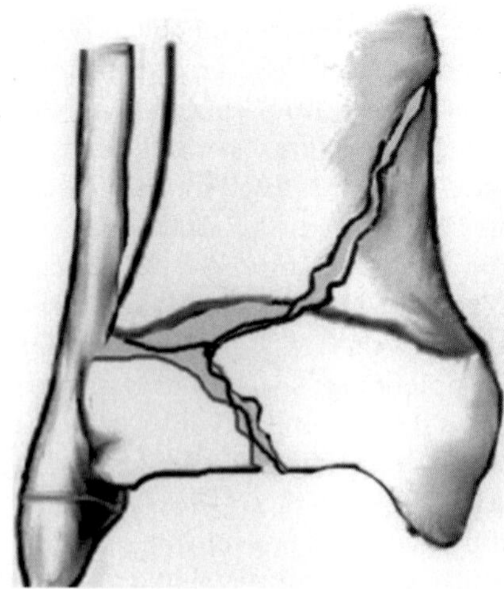

Figure 10-29 Drawing of a triplane fracture.

Fifth Metatarsal Fractures and Midfoot Sprain

Fractures of the fifth metatarsal are common in young athletes. They are categorized according to whether the fracture is located at the tuberosity or within the metatarsal shaft (Fig. 10-30). Older patients tend to suffer tuberosity fractures more commonly than younger patients, who are more likely to present with shaft fractures. Overall, these injuries generally occur in patients 15 years or older. Patients younger that 15 years tend to sustain a proximal apophyseal separation rather than a true fracture. It is important to differentiate between a stress reaction due to trauma and an acute metatarsal fracture. Nonoperative treatment is standard for most patients with a fifth metatarsal fracture. In most cases, the foot and leg are immobilized in a short-leg cast with no weight-bearing. If there is no evidence of healing after 3 months, surgical treatment by percutaneous compression screw insertion is considered. Complications associated with fifth metatarsal fracture are delayed union, non-union, and, rarely, refracture after nonunion.[26]

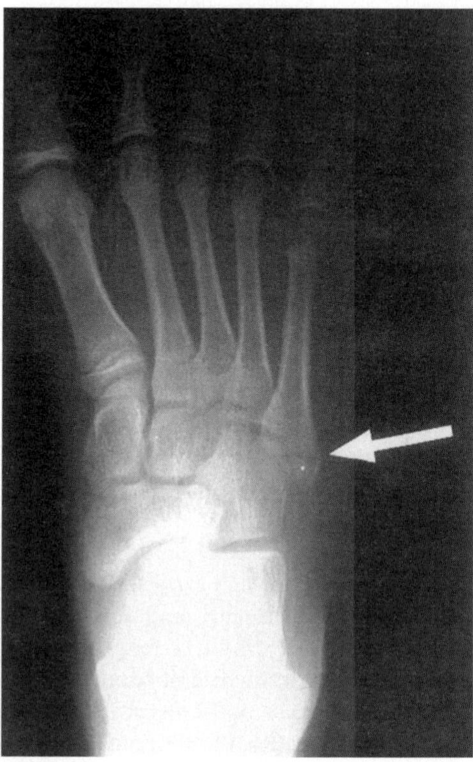

Figure 10-30 Radiograph of a fifth metatarsal fracture *(arrow)* at the tuberosity of the left foot.

SPLINTING

A wide variety of splinting techniques is available for temporary immobilization and for treatment of extremity injuries. Frequently, initial care of a sports injury necessitates immobilization for pain relief, protection, and reduction of swelling. A simple splint may be fashioned with three to four layers of cast padding, 10 to 12 layers of plaster bandage, and a stretch gauze roll or elastic bandage; however, care should be taken not to apply the last too tightly. Various prepared splint materials in both fiber-glass and plaster are also readily available and simple to apply. Children's skin is sensitive and burns easily. Thus, because plaster splints set with an exothermic reaction, cold water should be used, and care should be taken to avoid skin contact. When a splint is applied, the position of the splint and extremity must be maintained until the material has set completely.

Helpful splints for the arm are (1) the volar forearm splint (Fig. 10-31) for wrist and hand injuries, (2) the posterior elbow splint (Fig. 10-32) for elbow and forearm injuries, and (3) radial as well as ulnar gutter splints (Fig. 10-33) for the thumb or small finger aspects of the hand. Sugar-tong splints are extremely useful for the humerus and forearm (Fig. 10-34). The arm may be positioned with the elbow flexed 90 degrees, the forearm in neutral rotation, the wrist in slight dorsiflexion, and the hand with the thumb slightly opposed and the metacarpophalangeal and interphalangeal joints slightly flexed. However, positioning of the extremity plays a secondary role to neurovascular status, which should not be comprised.

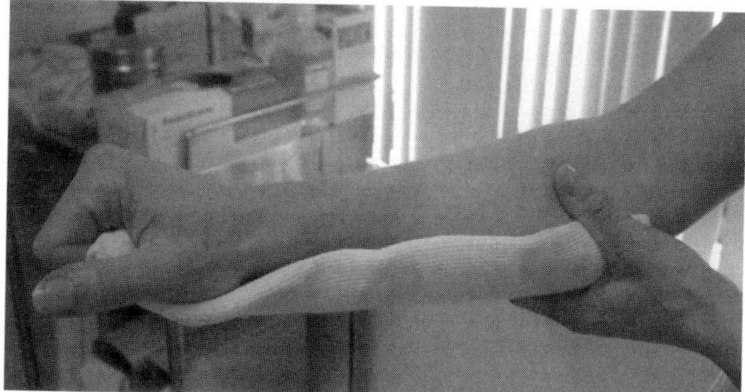

Figure 10-31 Patient wearing a volar forearm splint.

Splints for the leg are (1) the long posterior or long U-splint, which is placed medially and laterally on the leg for femoral and tibial fractures, (2) the medial and lateral coaptation or Jones splints for injuries about the knee, and (3) the short-leg posterior (Fig. 10-35) and short U-splint for ankle and foot injuries. The leg may be positioned with the knee extended and the ankle in neutral dorsiflexion.

SUMMARY

Exercise and athletic activity are beneficial to every child and adolescent. These activities facilitate weight control, help strengthen bones, and can improve cardiovascular risk factors. Mental health may also benefit from athletic activity. An active childhood lays the groundwork for a lifetime of fitness. Athletic involvement is a sound and largely risk-free investment in the present and

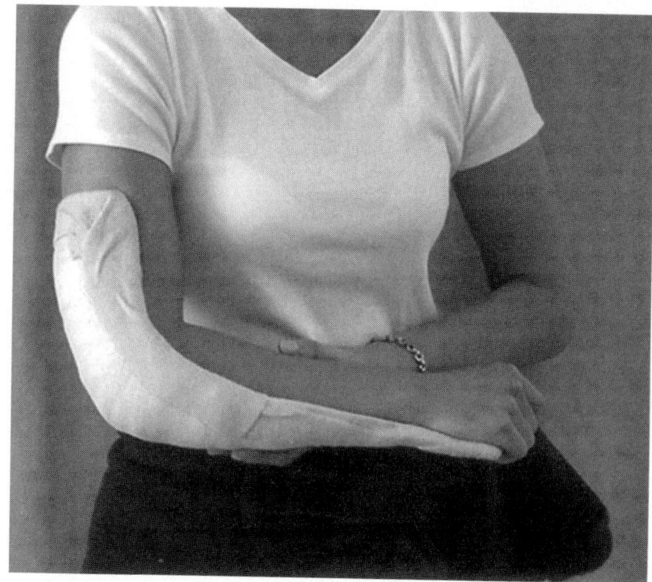

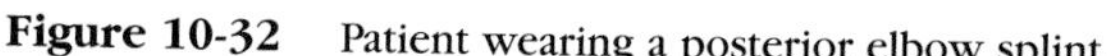

Figure 10-32 Patient wearing a posterior elbow splint.

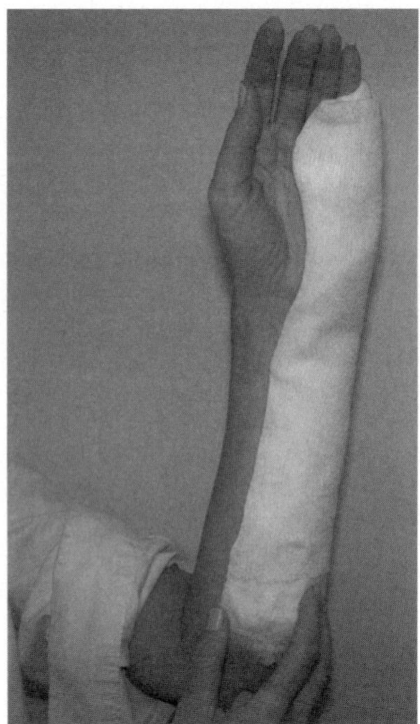

Figure 10-33 Patient wearing an ulnar gutter splint.

future health of children and adolescents. Sports instill the values of teamwork as well as lifelong habits of exercising.

Physicians who care for young patients should take an active role in helping them choose and maintain activities appropriate to their age, physical condition, stage of development, and interests. Physicians are in an important position to assess children's weight status and activity levels during a routine physical examination. With simple recommendations to children and parents, physicians can play a key role in helping young patients find and maintain activities they enjoy while keeping the risk of injury to a minimum. Physicians must be aware of the injuries and injury patterns that often occur in the child athlete. They must also recognize that various childhood sequelae may become manifest as exertion and agility demands increase in conjunction with the higher levels of competition encountered in the adolescent years. This knowledge enables the physician to appropriately diagnose, counsel, and rehabilitate these athletes for a safe and timely return to their activities. Ultimately, the goal of practicing safe, enjoyable activities to promote a lifelong habit of good health and fitness is readily attainable by virtually all youngsters.

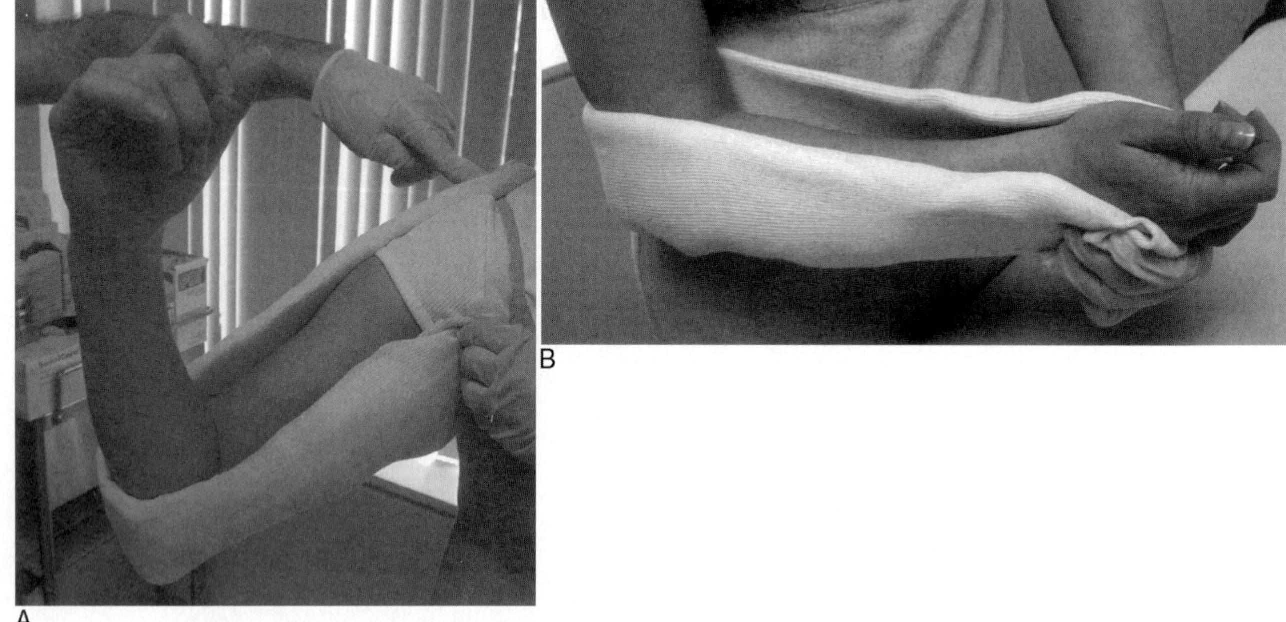

Figure 10-34 Patients wearing a sugar-tong splint for the humerus **(A)** and short-arm sugar-tong splint for the forearm **(B)**.

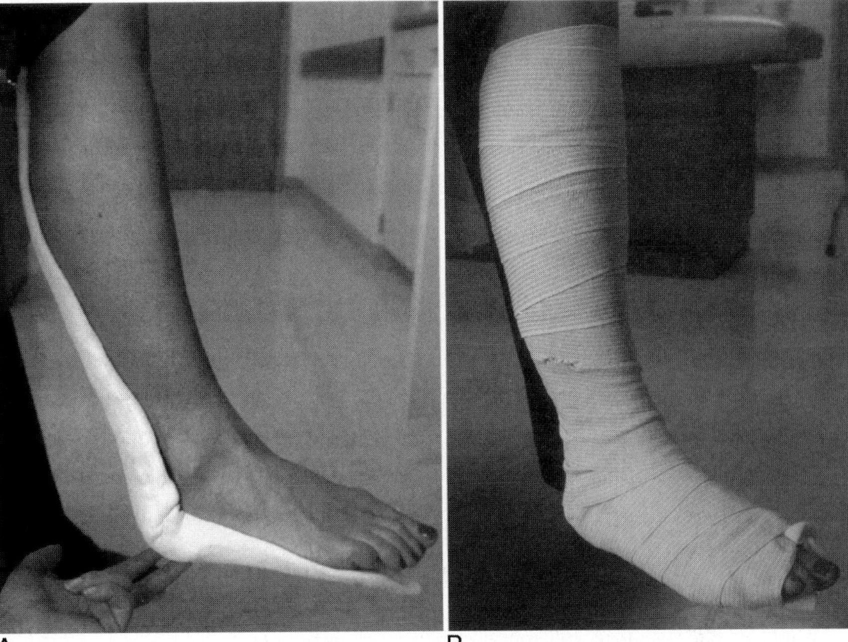

Figure 10-35 A and B, Patient wearing a short-leg posterior splint.

MAJOR POINTS

Rapid development, growth, and maturation as well as participation in many and varied physical activities make many young athletes uniquely susceptible to injury.

Those caring for young athletes must be aware of their unique anatomic and physiologic features, which affect the type of injuries encountered.

Adolescents undergoing supervised strength training should practice resistance as well as endurance training as part of a well-balanced fitness program.

In the young athlete with open physes, there is a greater propensity for fracture of the bone to extend into or through the physis.

The muscles of young patients are more vascular than those of adults and may be susceptible to contusion and hematoma formation.

Management of soft tissue injury includes rest, ice, compression, and elevation (RICE).

Sports injuries can occur in the unconditioned athlete with poor biomechanics of body alignment and/or technique. Injuries can also occur in the more highly conditioned athlete with appropriate biomechanical alignment whose training regimen exceeds the limits of the musculoskeletal system.

The diagnosis of stress injuries entails identification of the factors leading to the development of symptoms, including training levels, environmental factors, and anatomic factors.

Children are susceptible to overuse injuries at the muscle-tendon, tendon-cartilage, and cartilage-bone interfaces.

The most common overuse injury, which occurs at the knee of young athletes, is Osgood-Schlatter disease, an apophysitis at the anterior tibial tubercle.

Osgood-Schlatter disease is almost universally resolved with closure of the growth plates.

The most common site for stress fractures in children is the proximal tibia followed by the distal fibula.

Children with ACL injuries constitute a unique patient population because of their open growth plates and differing ligamentous and bone strength.

To select a treatment plan for the pediatric patient with an anterior cruciate ligament tear, the physician must consider the child's skeletal age and remaining growth, in order to avoid physeal and epiphyseal growth disturbances and subsequent angular deformity, leg length discrepancy, and condylar dysplasia.

In young children, bone usually fails before ligaments under tensile or shear stress.

The ankle is the most commonly injured body part in athletes of all ages; in adolescents, the ankle is the most common site of physeal injury.

(Continued)

MAJOR POINTS—cont'd

Frequently, a sports injury initially must be immobilized via splinting for pain relief, protection, and reduction of swelling.

Exercise is beneficial to every child and adolescent.

Physicians who care for young patients should take an active role in helping them choose and maintain activities appropriate to their age, physical condition, stage of development, and interests.

With simple recommendations to children and parents, physicians can play a key role in helping young patients find and maintain activities they enjoy while keeping the risk of injury to a minimum.

REFERENCES

1. Tidball JG, Chan M: Adhesive strength of single muscle cells to basement membrane at myotendinous junction. J Appl Physiol 67:1063-1069, 1989.
2. Ganley TJ, Pill SG, Gregg J, et al: Pop Warner Football & Cheerleading Injury Prevention: A Guide to Common Injuries. Rosemont, IL, The American Orthopaedic Society for Sports Medicine, 2000.
3. Brighton CT: Structure and function of the growth plate. Clin Orthop 136:22-32, 1978.
4. Roy S, Caine D, Singer KM: Stress changes of the distal radial epiphysis in young gymnasts: A report of twenty-one cases and a review of the literature. Am J Sports Med 13:301-308, 1985.
5. Berndt AL, Harty M: Transchondral fractures (osteochondritis dissecans) of the talus. J Bone Joint Surg Am 41:988-1020, 1959.
6. DeLee JC, Evans JP, Julian J: Stress fracture of the fifth metatarsal. Am J Sports Med 11:349-353, 1983.
7. Devas MB: Stress fractures in children. J Bone Joint Surg Br 45:528-541, 1963.
8. Kadel NJ, Teitz CC, Kronmal RA: Stress fractures in ballet dancers. Am J Sports Med 20:445-449, 1992.
9. Dickhaut SC, DeLee JC: The discoid lateral meniscus syndrome. J Bone Joint Surg Am 64:1068-1073, 1982.
10. Washington ER, Root L, Liener UC: Discoid lateral meniscus in children. J Bone Joint Surg Am 77:1357-1361, 1995.
11. Watanabe M, Takeda S, Kieuchi H: Atlas of arthroscopy, 3rd ed. Tokyo: Igaku-Shoin, 1979.
12. Silverman JM, Mink JH, Deutsch AL: Discoid menisci of the knee: MRI imaging appearance. Radiology 173:351-354, 1989.
13. Dameron TB, Rockwood CA: Fractures and dislocations of the shoulder. In Rockwood CA, Wilkins KE, King RE (eds): Fractures in Children. Philadelphia, JB Lippincott, 1984, pp 625-653.
14. Waters PM, Millis MB: Hip and pelvic injuries in the young athlete. In Stanitski, CL, DeLee JC, Drez D (eds): Pediatric and Adolescent Sports Medicine. Philadelphia, WB Saunders, 1994, pp 279-293.
15. Aronowitz ER, Ganley TJ, Goode JR, et al: Anterior cruciate ligament reconstruction in adolescents with open physes. Am J Sports Med 28:168-175, 2000.
16. Lo IK, Bell DM, Fowler PJ: Anterior cruciate ligament injuries in the skeletally immature patient. Instr Course Lect 47:351-359, 1998.
17. Greulich WW, Pyle SI: Radiographic atlas of skeletal development of the hand and wrist. Stanford, CT, Stanford University Press, 1950.
18. Andrews M, Noyes FR, Barber-Westin SD: Anterior cruciate ligament allograft reconstruction in the skeletally immature athlete. Am J Sports Med 22:478-484, 1994.
19. Graf BK, Lange RH, Fujisake CK, et al: Anterior cruciate ligament tears in skeletally immature patients: Meniscal pathology at presentation and after attempted conservative treatment. Arthroscopy 8:229-233, 1992.
20. Mizuta H, Kubota K, Shiraishi M, et al: The conservative treatment of complete tears of the anterior cruciate ligament in skeletally immature patients. J Bone Joint Surg Br 77:890-894, 1995.
21. Parker AW, Drez D, Cooper JL: Anterior cruciate ligament injuries in patients with open physes. Am J Sports Med 22:44-47, 1994.
22. Meyers MH, McKeever FM: Fracture of the intercondylar eminence of the tibia. J Bone Joint Surg Am 52:1677-1684, 1970.
23. Zaricznyj B: Avulsion fracture of the tibial eminence: Treatment by open reduction and pinning. J Bone Joint Surg Am 59:1111-1114, 1977.
24. Kennedy JC: The Injured Adolescent Knee. Baltimore, Williams & Wilkins, 1979.
25. Canale ST, Belding RH: Osteochondral lesions of the talus. J Bone Joint Surg Am 62:97-102, 1980.
26. Ganley TJ, Flynn JM, Gregg JR: Sports medicine of the adolescent foot and ankle. Foot Ankle Clin 3:767-785, 1998.

CHAPTER 11

Musculoskeletal Tumors in Children

BULENT EROL
LISA STATES
BRUCE R. PAWEL
JUNICHI TAMAI
JOHN P. DORMANS

Pediatric musculoskeletal tumors are uncommon and, when they occur, usually benign. They often are overlooked as the cause of a child's complaints. As a result, diagnosis of these tumors is often delayed. Therefore, the physician must remain alert and aware of the presentation of childhood musculoskeletal tumors. Early detection of a malignant musculoskeletal tumor may make the difference not only between life and death but also between saving and amputating a limb. The bone and soft tissue tumors of childhood can be classified on the basis of their tissue origin (Box 11-1).

EVALUATION

Children with a musculoskeletal tumor usually present with pain, mass, pathologic fracture, or incidental findings on radiographs (Box 11-2). Pain is the most common presenting symptom. Pain from a musculoskeletal malignancy is usually a dull, continuous pain that is characteristically worse at night and typically is not related to physical activity. If pain has been present for an extended time, it is usually from a benign process. The presence of a mass is the second most common symptom. Children with an aggressive neoplastic process usually have a painless mass that grows slowly over a period of weeks or months. A child or adolescent can also present with a bony neoplasm after a pathologic fracture. Most aggressive benign tumors and malignant tumors produce pain before the bone is weakened enough to fracture. A patient without prefracture pain, however, normally has an inactive benign process. Finally, asymptomatic bone tumors can be detected incidentally on radiographs obtained for other reasons.

Most musculoskeletal tumors occur more commonly in boys than in girls. The gender of the patient, however, usually does not play a significant role in formulating the differential diagnosis. Ewing sarcoma is unusual because it shows a race association; it is very prevalent in white persons and rarely seen in African Americans. The age of the patient is important in establishing a differential diagnosis, because certain tumors tend to occur in certain age groups (Table 11-1).

The patient with a suspected musculoskeletal tumor should be given a complete physical examination. The gait pattern of the patient, neurovascular examination of the affected extremity, and range of motion of the adjacent joint should be noted. The size, consistency, and mobility of the mass should be evaluated (see Box 11-2). Small (<5 cm), soft, movable, nontender masses, especially those in the superficial tissues, are usually benign. Large (>5 cm), firm, fixed, tender, and deep masses raise suspicion of malignancy and are rarely benign.

Box 11-1 Classification of Pediatric Musculoskeletal Tumors Based on Tissue of Origin

- Bone tumors
  - Bone origin: osteoid osteoma, osteoblastoma, osteosarcoma
  - Cartilaginous origin: osteochondroma, chondroblastoma, chondromyxoid fibroma, enchondroma, periosteal chondroma
  - Fibrous origin: fibrous dysplasia, ossifying fibroma, nonossifying fibroma, desmoplastic fibroma
  - Miscellaneous: unicameral bone cyst, aneurysmal bone cyst, giant cell tumor, Langerhans cell histiocytosis, Ewing sarcoma
  - Musculoskeletal manifestations of leukemia
  - Bone lymphomas
  - Metastatic tumors: neuroblastoma, retinoblastoma, hepatoblastoma
- Soft tissue tumors
  - Vascular tumors: hemangioma, vascular malformations
  - Nerve origin: neurolemmoma, neurofibroma, malignant peripheral nerve sheath tumor
  - Fibrous origin: fibromatosis, fibrosarcoma
  - Muscular origin: rhabdomyosarcoma
  - Miscellaneous: synovial sarcoma
  - Primitive neuroectodermal tumors (PNETs)
  - Ganglion and synovial cyst

Box 11-2 Clinical Presentations of Pediatric Musculoskeletal Tumors

- Pain
  - Duration
  - Localization
  - Severity
  - Character
  - Relief and how obtained
- Mass
  - Duration
  - Size
  - Consistency
  - Mobility
- Pathologic fracture (spectrum from microfractures to displaced fractures)
  - Prior symptoms and signs
  - Mechanism of fracture
  - Characteristics of fracture
- Incidental radiographic findings
  - Prior symptoms and signs
  - Why radiograph obtained

Table 11-1 Peak Age Ranges for Common Pediatric Musculoskeletal Tumors

Age (years)	Benign	Malignant
0-5	Langerhans cell histiocytosis	Fibrosarcoma
		Metastatic tumors
	Osteomyelitis	Leukemia
	Osteofibrous dysplasia	Ewing sarcoma
5-10	Unicameral bone cyst	Osteosarcoma
	Aneurysmal bone cyst	Rhabdomyosarcoma
	Nonossifying fibroma	
	Fibrous dysplasia	
	Osteoid osteoma	
	Langerhans cell histiocytosis	
10-20	Fibrous dysplasia	Osteosarcoma
	Osteoid osteoma	Ewing sarcoma
	Fibroma	Chondrosarcoma
	Aneurysmal bone cyst	Rhabdomyosarcoma
	Chondroblastoma	Synovial cell sarcoma
	Osteofibrous dysplasia	

After careful history and physical examination, viewing the radiographic imaging studies of the lesion is the next step in the evaluation. Plain radiographs give the most detailed information about skeletal lesions. Good-quality plain radiographs, at least two views (anteroposterior [AP] and lateral), that show the entire lesion are necessary. Thirty percent to 40% of a bone must be destroyed before changes can be seen in plain radiographs. It is difficult to see soft tissue tumors and soft tissue extension from bony neoplasms with plain radiographs. When evaluating plain radiographs of bony lesions, the physician may find it useful to ask the following questions: Where is the lesion located in the bone? What is the lesion doing to the bone? What is the bone doing to the lesion? What is the periosteal response?[1]

Some bony lesions have a tendency to occur in certain long bones (e.g., humerus, tibia) or flat bones (e.g., pelvis). The anatomic location of the lesion (in the long bone) should also be identified as epiphyseal, metaphyseal, or diaphyseal, and central or eccentric (Table 11-2). The lesion may be destroying or replacing the existing bone. Bone destruction as seen on radiographs can be described as geographic, "moth-eaten," or permeative (Fig. 11-1). Although none of these features is pathognomonic for any specific neoplasm, the type of destruction may suggest a benign or a malignant process. *Geographic* bone destruction is characterized by a uniformly destroyed area usually within sharply defined borders. It typifies slow-growing, benign lesions, such as simple bone cyst, enchondroma, and giant cell tumor. *Moth-eaten* bone destruction (i.e., characterized by multiple, small, often clustered lytic areas) and *permeative* bone destruction (i.e., characterized by ill-defined, very small oval radiolucencies or lucent streaks) mark rapidly growing, infiltrating tumors, such as Ewing sarcoma, osteosarcoma, and lymphoma.[2]

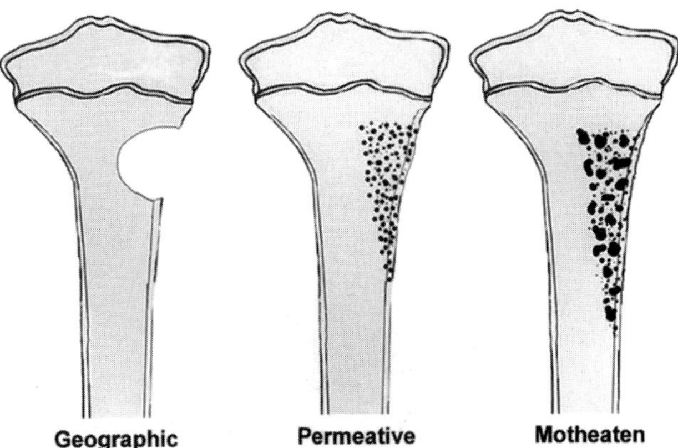

Figure 11-1 Different patterns of bone destruction. (Modified from Madewell JE, Ragsdale BD, Sweet DE: Radiologic and pathologic analysis of solitary bone lesions. Part I: Internal margins. Radiol Clin North Am 19:715, 1981.)

Table 11-2 Common Locations of Pediatric Bone Tumors

Location	Tumors
Epiphysis	Chondroblastoma Brodie abscess of the epiphyses Giant cell tumor Fibrous dysplasia
Metaphysis	Any tumor
Diaphysis (FAHEL)	Fibrous dysplasia Osteofibrous dysplasia Langerhans cell histiocytosis Ewing sarcoma Leukemia, lymphoma
Pelvis	Ewing sarcoma Osteosarcoma Osteochondroma Metastasis Fibrous dysplasia
Anterior elements of spine	Langerhans cell histiocytosis Leukemia Metastatic Giant cell tumor
Posterior elements of spine	Aneurysmal bone cyst Osteoblastoma Osteoid osteoma
Rib	Fibrous dysplasia Langerhans cell histiocytosis Ewing sarcoma Metastasis
Multiple locations	Leukemia (metastasis) Multiple hereditary exostoses Langerhans cell histiocytosis Polyostotic fibrous dysplasia Enchondromatosis

The response of the bone to the neoplastic process involves the response of the adjacent cortex and periosteum.[3] The lesion may be contained by the cortex or "walled off" by dense sclerotic bone, implying a very slow-growing or static lesion, or it may destroy the cortex and form a soft tissue mass, usually indicating an aggressive neoplastic process. Like the pattern of bone destruction, the pattern of periosteal reaction is an indicator of the biologic activity of a lesion. Bone neoplasms elicit periosteal reactions that can be categorized as uninterrupted (*continuous*) or interrupted (*discontinuous*) (Fig. 11-2). Any widening and irregularity of bone contour may represent periosteal activity. Although no single periosteal response is unique for a given lesion, a continuous periosteal reaction indicates a longstanding (slow-growing) benign process, such as osteoid osteoma, osteoblastoma, osteomyelitis, or stress fracture. A discontinuous periosteal reaction, on the other hand, is commonly seen in malignant tumors; in these tumors, the periosteal reaction may appear in a sunburst ("hair-on-end") or onionskin (lamellated) pattern. A reactive periosteal cuff at the periphery of the tumor, a *Codman's triangle*, also may form.

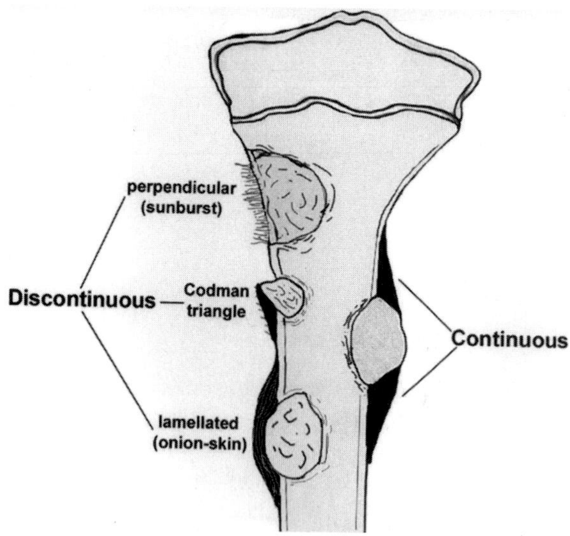

Figure 11-2 Different patterns of periosteal reaction. (Modified from Greenspan A, Wolfgang R: Radiologic and pathologic approach to bone tumors. In Greenspan A, Wolfgang R [eds]: Differential Diagnosis of Tumors and Tumor-Like Lesions of Bones and Joints. Philadelphia, Lippincott-Raven Publishers, 1998, pp 1-24.)

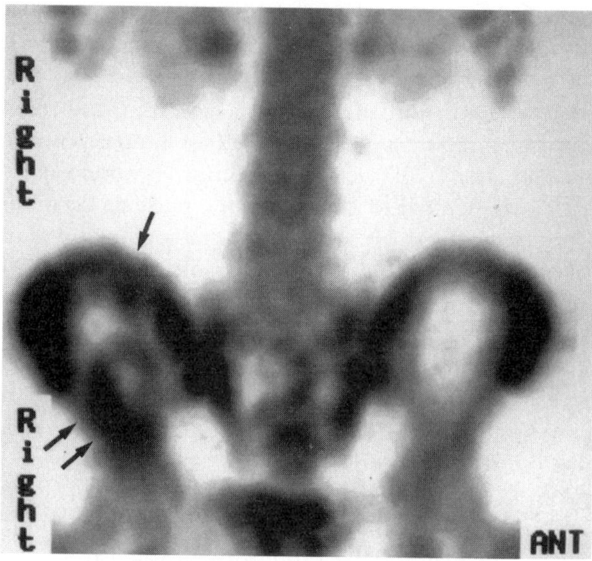

Figure 11-3 Radionuclide bone scan. Radionuclide bone scan of the pelvis shows focal photopenic areas with a hyperintense rim *(double arrows)*. An additional focus of increased activity is present in the right iliac wing *(single arrow)*.

Most bone tumors can be diagnosed correctly after the history taking, physical examination, and examination of plain radiographs. Additional studies are requested only if the specific diagnosis cannot be made or they are necessary for treatment. Conventional radiographs often cannot adequately evaluate sites such as the pelvis, sacrum, and vertebrae; in these locations, computed tomography (CT) or magnetic resonance imaging (MRI) is particularly helpful. Radioisotope bone scanning, CT, and MRI can also show early bone lesions in patients whose conventional radiographs appear normal.

Radionuclide bone scanning is the most practical method to survey the entire skeleton. A lesion that is associated with an increase in bone production increases the local uptake of technetium Tc^{99m} and produces a "hot spot" on a bone scan. Radionuclide bone scanning can be used to evaluate the activity of a primary bone lesion, determine its local extent, and search for other bone lesions (Fig. 11-3).

CT has two features that make it useful for musculoskeletal imaging, particularly of the axial skeleton; it can show cross-sectional anatomy and detect the exact anatomic extent of a tumor (Fig. 11-4). The cortical and medullary bone involvement, periosteal new bone formation, soft tissue component of a bone tumor, and soft tissue tumors can be demonstrated with CT. This modality can also detect calcifications and bone formation within the tumor. CT cannot show the soft tissue and bone marrow as well as MRI, however, and is also unable to screen a large anatomic area effectively.

MRI is a valuable diagnostic method for evaluating the axial skeleton, bone marrow, soft tissue masses (soft tissue extension of bone tumors and soft tissue tumors), and relationship of tumor to neurovascular structures. Its ability to produce images of the body in all three planes (axial, sagittal, and coronal) offers a significant advantage in defining the extent of many tumors.[4] The coronal and sagittal planes show a long axis view and can determine both the location and extent of a lesion (Fig. 11-5A). This modality can also identify skip lesions in the bone marrow. The axial plane can best define the anatomic relationships among tumor, bone, soft tissue, nerves, and vessels (Fig. 11-5B). MRI can also detect cortical destruction and periosteal new bone formation. MRI remains the modality of choice for staging, for evaluating response to preoperative chemotherapy, and for long-term follow-up of bone and soft tissue sarcomas.

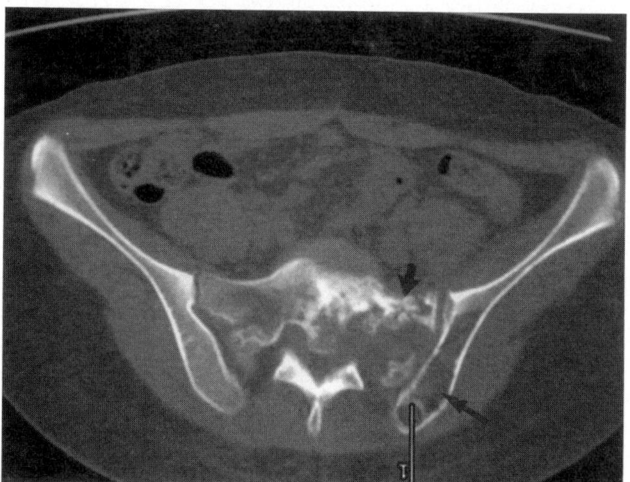

Figure 11-4 Computed tomography. Axial computed tomography image of the pelvis shows several areas of bone destruction *(arrow* and *arrowhead)*.

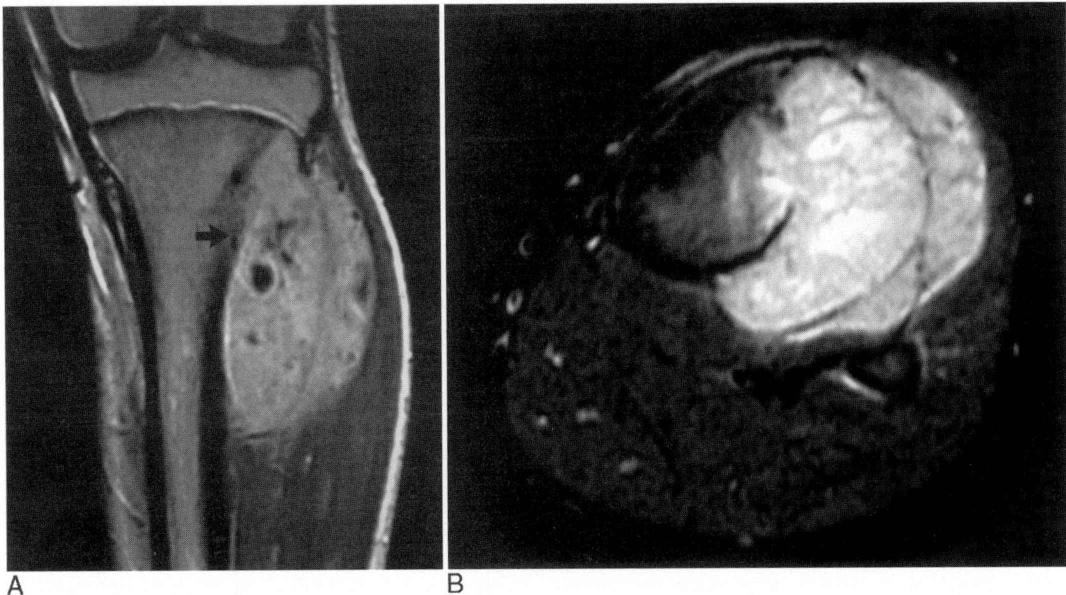

Figure 11-5 Magnetic resonance imaging. A, On coronal T1-weighted image of the proximal leg, an enhancing mass can be seen arising from the proximal tibial metaphysis. The site where the mass breaks through the cortex *(arrow)* is easily visualized. This view clearly shows the mass abutting the growth plate. The epiphysis is spared. **B,** The axial T2-weighted image is most useful in showing the extension of the mass into the soft tissues. Extension of the mass through the cortex is well demonstrated.

Staging of lesions that appear to be malignant is required before biopsy. Staging involves (1) a whole-body bone scan (or skeletal survey, particularly in very young children) to look for bone metastasis and diagnose skip lesions, (2) a CT scan of the chest to search for lung metastasis, and (3) MRI of the primary lesion. MRI should cover the involved portion of the extremity, including the joint above and the joint below. On the basis of these studies, a biopsy can be planned to confirm the diagnosis. Bone marrow sampling (aspirates and biopsy specimens from two sites) should be performed at the time of the biopsy, particularly for suspected Ewing sarcoma.

Biopsy should be the last step in the evaluation of a patient with a bone or soft tissue tumor and should be performed only after careful planning. A well-planned biopsy provides an accurate diagnosis and facilitates treatment. However, a poorly performed biopsy fails to provide a diagnosis and, more important, may have a negative effect on survival and treatment options. Needle aspiration may yield adequate tissue for a histologic diagnosis; however, most oncologic surgeons prefer an incisional technique, which also provides additional tissue for molecular diagnostics. Incisional biopsy involves removal of only a portion of the tumor without contaminating the surrounding soft tissue structures. A biopsy is best accomplished at the institution that would perform the definitive operation if surgery becomes necessary.[5]

ETIOLOGY AND MOLECULAR GENETICS

The discovery of oncogenes has caused an explosion of knowledge of the biology of cancer within the past decade. In general, oncogenes are normal cellular genes *(proto-oncogenes)* that, when normally expressed, are necessary for the normal development and function of the organism. When they become mutated, however, they act through a variety of mechanisms to deregulate cell growth, resulting in a neoplasm. There are two categories of oncogenes, dominant oncogenes and tumor-suppressor genes. The dominant oncogenes encode proteins that are involved in signal transduction. By transmitting an external stimulus from outside the cell, these proteins keep the cell permanently "turned on" so that it keeps dividing. Tumor-suppressor genes encode proteins whose normal role is to restrict cell proliferation and thereby regulate the cell cycle and keep it in check. Proto-oncogenes may become mutated by a variety of mechanisms leading to the ability to transform cells, such as small point mutations (insertion, deletion, or substitution of a base) in DNA coding sequence, gene amplification, and juxtaposition of one gene with another (chromosome rearrangement).

Bone Tumors

Much has been learned over the past several years about the genetic changes that accompany malignant bone tumors. However, the actual cause of these cancers is still unknown, with the exception of ionizing radiation, the only known environmental cause of osteosarcoma. Osteosarcomas generally have complex karyotypic abnormalities without chromosomal translocations. Several nonrandom deletions have been identified, however. The two most obvious gene deletions in osteosarcomas are located on chromosomes 13 and 17, the chromosomes containing the retinoblastoma gene (RB1) and transformation-related protein 53 (p53), respectively.[6] Both of these genes are tumor-supressor genes, and their gene products are important regulators of the cell cycle.

A translocation between chromosomes 11 and 22 has been identified in approximately 95% of all Ewing sarcomas (Table 11-3). The same translocation has been identified in primitive neuroectodermal tumors (PNETs), suggesting that they are members of the same family of sarcoma. This translocation brings a portion of two genes, EWS gene from chromosome 22 and Fli-1 from chromosome 11, into juxtaposition, resulting in a "fusion" gene *(EWS/Fli-1)*. The protein product of this fusion gene acts to regulate DNA transcription (i.e., it is a transcription factor) of other genes presumably responsible for the development of these tumors.[6]

Soft Tissue Tumors

Genetic alterations have been found in many, but not at all, soft tissue sarcomas. They include clonal karyotype abnormalities such as translocations of parts of one chromosome to another. The role of environmental exposures in the development of soft tissue sarcomas remains controversial. There is a causal relationship between therapeutic irradiation and soft tissue sarcomas in some patients, but because of the prolonged latency (10 to 15 years) between exposure and the development of secondary sarcoma, this relationship typically is recognized as a problem in older patients.

Well-defined familial syndromes with an increased risk for the development of soft tissue sarcomas are neurofibromatosis type 1 (NF1 or von Recklinghausen disease), Li-Fraumeni cancer syndrome, and familial pleuropulmonary blastoma.[7] Children with the relatively common, autosomal dominant disorder NF1 have a higher incidence of malignant peripheral nerve sheath tumor (neurofibrosarcoma) and other soft tissue sarcomas, such as rhabdomyosarcoma. Homozygous gene deletions in both the short and long arms of chromosome 17 have been noted in neurofibrosarcomas arising in patients with NF1. This finding suggested that p53 (17p13) and possibly another tumor-suppressor gene are responsible for the NF1-associated malignancies. The candidate tumor-suppressor gene has been cloned (17q11.2) and shown to code for a protein named *neurofibromin*.

The Li-Fraumeni cancer syndrome is an autosomal dominant disorder characterized by germline mutations in the p53 gene and an excess of carcinomas of the breast and adrenal glands, glial neoplasms, leukemias, and childhood sarcomas. Rhabdomyosarcoma is the most commonly diagnosed pediatric soft tissue sarcoma in patients with the syndrome. Spontaneous point mutations of p53 are found in approximately one third to one half of soft tissue sarcomas, and overexpression of the p53 protein is associated with higher tumor grade and poorer overall and disease-free survival.

Familial pleuropulmonary blastoma syndrome is a rare neoplasm of the lung and thoracic cavity that manifests in young children and is frequently associated with soft tissue sarcomas of childhood, including rhabdomyosarcoma and synovial sarcoma. A germ-line mutation has yet to be identified in the familial pleuropulmonary blastoma syndrome.

Embryonal rhabdomyosarcoma does not display any consistent cytogenetic abnormality, but there is evidence that loss of heterozygosity of at least one putative tumor-suppressor gene on chromosome 11 is implicated in the genesis of this neoplasm. Unlike with embryonal rhabdomyosarcoma, a translocation involving chromosomes 2 and 13 [t(2;13)] is documented in a high proportion of alveolar rhabdomyosarcomas (see Table 11-3).[7] In addition, a variant translocation involving chromosomes 1 and 13 [t(1;13)] has been identified in a small subgroup of alveolar rhabdomyosarcomas. At least 90% of synovial sarcomas display the translocation t(X;18)(p11;q11), and many of the remainder have variant translocations involving either chromosome X or chromosome 18 and a different partner (see Table 11-3).

Table 11-3 Pediatric Musculoskeletal Tumors with Nonrandom or Specific Translocations

Tumor	Translocation
Ewing sarcoma/primitive neuroectodermal tumors (PNETs)	t(11;22); t(21;22)
Alveolar rhabdomyosarcoma	t(2;13); t(1;13)
Synovial sarcoma	t(X;18)
Myxoid liposarcoma	t(12;16)

SPECIFIC BONE TUMORS

Bone-Forming Tumors

Osteoid Osteoma

Osteoid osteoma usually affects children between the ages of 5 and 20 years. The male-to-female ratio has been reported as approximately 2:1. Between 70% and 80% of osteoid osteomas are located in long bones, most commonly in the femur, tibia, and humerus.[8,9] The posterior elements of the spine may also be involved. Patients with osteoid osteoma usually present with pain that is characteristically worse at night and is relieved with salicylates. The process may cause growth disturbances, such as limb length discrepancy and bowing of an extremity, or scoliosis.

Osteoid osteoma usually involves the metaphyseal or diaphyseal regions of the long bones. In most cases, the lesion is intracortical and appears on a conventional radiograph as a small (<1 cm in diameter), round to elliptical, radiolucent area within the cortex, termed a *nidus* (Fig. 11-6A). The lesion is surrounded by a dense region of reactive sclerotic bone that may extend for several centimeters from the central nidus. The nidus is best demonstrated with CT; to delineate the lesion, thin (preferably 1- to 1.5-mm) contiguous sections are most appropriate (Fig. 11-6B).[10] The radiographic differential diagnosis of osteoid osteoma most often includes osteoblastoma, Brodie abscess, and stress fracture.

On gross examination, osteoid osteoma is a small, round or oval, reddish brown tumor 1 cm or less in diameter. Histologic examination shows a distinct demarcation between the nidus and the surrounding reactive bone. The nidus consists of an interlacing network of immature, woven bone and bony trabeculae, with focal areas of osteoblastic and osteoclastic activity (Fig. 11-6C).

Osteoid osteoma "burns out" with time. Treatment usually involves complete surgical removal of the nidus; this can be accomplished by en bloc excision (removal of the lesion with a reactive bone around the lesion) or extended curettage and bone grafting (intralesional excision; Fig. 11-7).[11] Surgery is extremely effective, bringing immediate and complete relief of symptoms. Newer techniques for the treatment of osteoid osteoma are percutaneous core removal and thermal ablation of the lesion under CT guidance. Medical management with long-term salicylates may, occasionally, be useful for lesions that are difficult to remove (e.g., in the acetabulum) but is associated with complications, such as gastrointestinal bleeding.

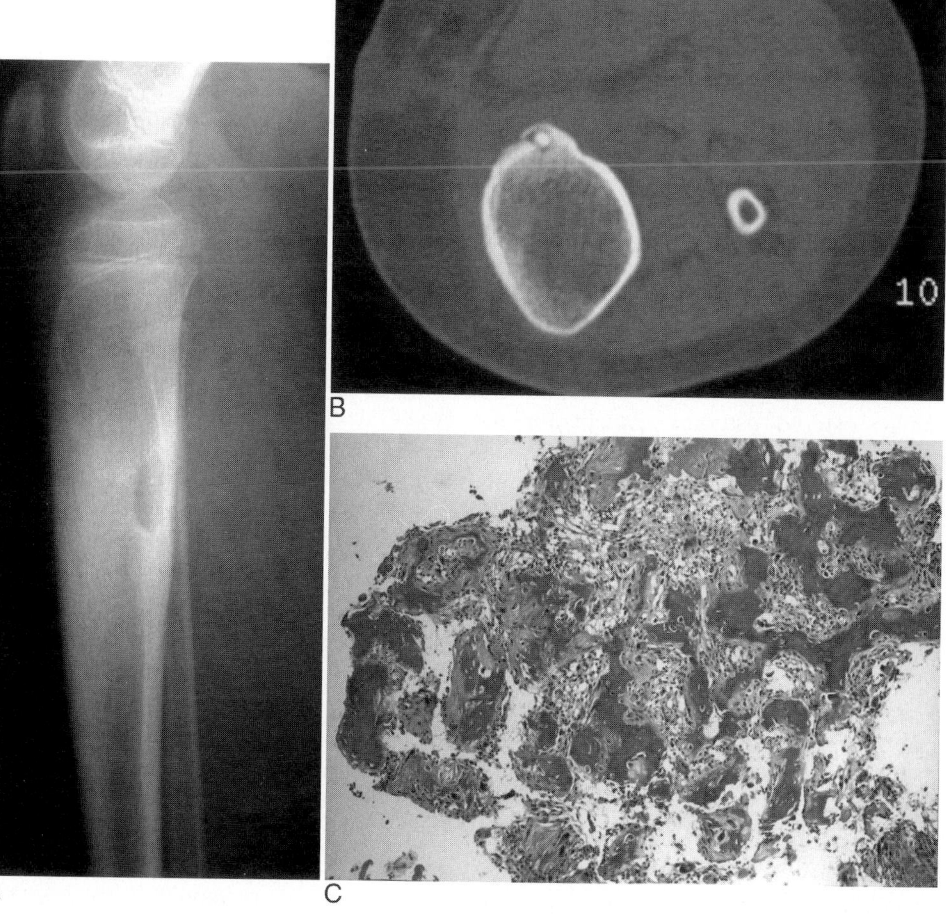

Figure 11-6 Osteoid osteoma. A, Lateral radiograph of the proximal leg shows a well-circumscribed lytic lesion in the posterior cortex of the proximal tibia. Significant cortical thickening surrounds the lesion. The cortical thickening has caused widening of the tibia. **B,** Axial computed tomography scan demonstrates the cortical location of the lesion. A dense, central nidus is surrounded by a lucent rim. Note the extensive cortical thickening. **C,** Photomicrograph of the lesion shows a nidus, with interlacing trabeculae of woven bone dispersed in a vascularized fibrous stroma.

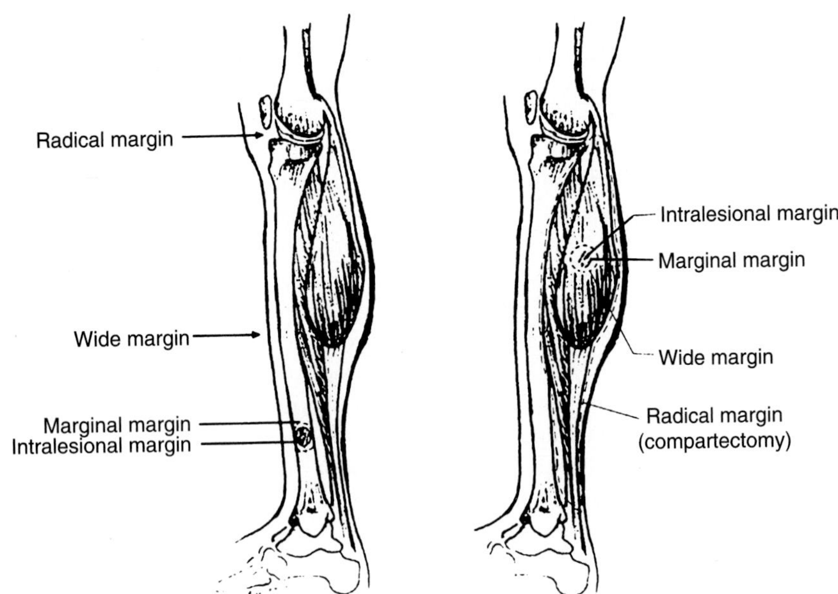

Figure 11-7 Surgical margins for bone (left) and soft tissue (right) lesions. Intralesional margin is within the lesion; marginal margin is through the reactive zone of the lesion; wide margin is beyond the reactive zone, through normal tissue within compartment; and radical margin encompasses normal tissue (extracompartmental). (From Himelstein BP, Dormans JP: Malignant bone tumors of childhood. Pediatr Clin North Am 43:967, 1996.)

Osteoblastoma

Osteoblastoma occurs in patients between 10 and 25 years of age. The male-to-female ratio is between 1.5:1 and 3:1. The area most commonly affected is the posterior elements of the vertebral column.[9,12] Other common sites of involvement are the long bones, especially the femur and the tibia. Patients usually present with pain that is less responsive to nonsteroidal anti-inflammatory drugs (NSAIDs) than osteoid osteoma. Osteoblastoma may cause scoliosis.

Radiographically, osteoblastomas appear as rounded or ovoid osteolytic areas between 2 and 10 cm in diameter and surrounded by a moderate amount of reactive sclerotic bone (Fig. 11-8A). The reactive bone formation is usually less intense, and the margins of the lesion are often less defined, than those in osteoid osteoma.

Gross examination shows osteoblastoma to be similar to osteoid osteoma, except for the larger size. Histologically, osteoblastoma is composed of interlacing trabecular or woven bone lined with variable numbers of osteoblasts within a fibrovascular stroma (Fig. 11-8B). Histologic differentiation among osteoid osteoma, osteoblastoma, and osteosarcoma may be difficult.

Osteoblastoma is a benign, but locally aggressive lesion (Box 11-3). Unless excised surgically, it continues to enlarge and damage the bone and adjacent structures. Marginal excision of the lesion is preferred when practical, but extended curettage is sufficient for most cases (see Fig. 11-7).[13] Most osteoblastomas are controlled by the extended curettage, but recurrence is common. A variant of osteoblastoma, known as *aggressive osteoblastoma* with aggressive behavior and, rarely, metastasis has been described.

Osteosarcoma and its Variants

Osteosarcoma is the most common malignant bone tumor of childhood, with 600 to 800 new cases occurring per year in the United States. It can occur at any age, but more than 75% appear in patients between 12 and 25 years old. Males are affected slightly more often than females. Osteosarcoma is commonly subclassified according to whether it is primary or secondary as well as its site of origin, either within the bone (intramedullary) or on the surface (juxtacortical). Primary osteosarcoma occurs with no evidence of a preexisting lesion or prior treatment of the bone, such as radiation therapy. More than 95% of osteosarcomas in children and young adults are primary. Two major types of primary osteosarcoma have significantly different clinical presentations and prognoses, classic high-grade intramedullary (HG-IM) osteosarcoma and juxtacortical osteosarcoma.

High-Grade Intramedullary Osteosarcoma (Conventional Osteosarcoma)

HG-IM osteosarcoma is the most common type of osteosarcoma, constituting approximately 85% of all forms of osteosarcoma. HG-IM osteosarcoma usually occurs at the metaphyseal ends of the long bones that have the greatest growth potential. The knee (distal femur and proximal tibia) is the most commonly affected site, followed by the proximal humerus.[8,9] Involvement of the axial skeleton (spine or pelvis) is uncommon in children. Pain and swelling are the most common presenting symptoms. Approximately 15% of patients with HG-IM osteosarcoma present with clinically evident metastases, most commonly in the lungs. The presence of metastases at diagnosis indicates poor prognosis.

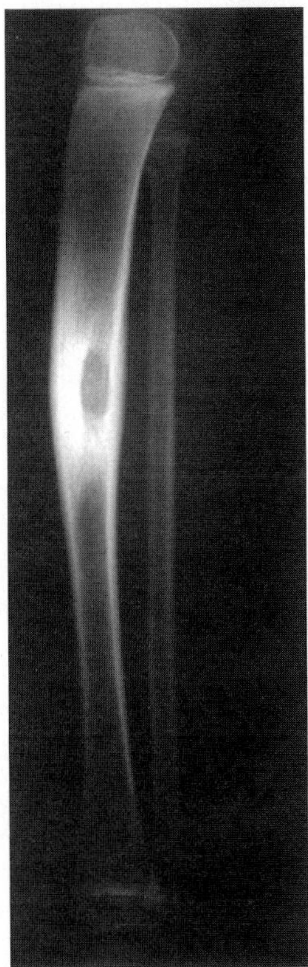

A

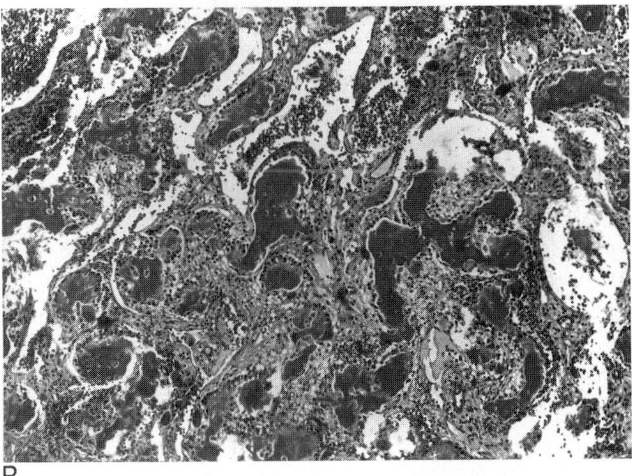

B

Figure 11-8 Osteoblastoma. A, Lateral radiograph of the leg shows an ovoid, well-circumscribed, lytic lesion in the diaphysis of the tibia with extensive reactive sclerosis and cortical thickening. **B,** Photomicrograph of the lesion demonstrates haphazard trabeculae of woven immature bone in a fibrovascular stroma, histologically similar to osteoid osteoma.

Radiographs show that the tumor is typically located in the metaphysis, involves the medullary canal, and consists of lytic (or destructive) or blastic (sclerotic) lesions, or a combination of the two (Fig. 11-9A). Extensive periosteal reaction may be seen. The presence of a soft tissue mass with sclerotic foci (tumoral bone formation), is a common finding. MRI can effectively demonstrate the extent of the lesion, including intraosseous component, soft tissue extension, and the peritumoral edema (Fig. 11-9B and C). Radiographic staging, consisting of an MRI of the primary lesion, a whole-body bone scan, and a CT scan of the chest, is an essential step in the treatment planning.[14]

Box 11-3 Benign But Locally Aggressive Bone Tumors in Children

- Chondroblastoma
- Aneurysmal bone cyst
- Osteofibrous dysplasia-adamantinoma
- Giant cell tumor
- Osteoblastoma
- Chondromyxoid fibroma

HG-IM osteosarcoma has been divided into several histologic subtypes on the basis of the predominant cell type of the tumor—osteoblastic, chondroblastic, or fibroblastic. The osteoblastic subtype is the most common, accounting for about half of HG-IM osteosarcomas.[9] Each of these subtypes is characterized by the formation of osteoid tissue or new bone by the neoplastic cells. Histologic analysis of the lesion usually reveals highly pleomorphic, spindle-shaped and polyhedral tumor cells, producing different forms of osteoid (Fig. 11-9D). These tumor cells have obvious features of malignancy, such as nuclear hyperchromasia and abundant mitotic activity, with atypical mitotic figures.

Twenty to 30 years ago, more than 80 % of patients with an osteosarcoma died, and more than 80% of patients with an extremity osteosarcoma were treated with primary amputation. The current overall survival rate for patients with nonmetastatic osteosarcoma is between 70% and 80%. Currently, more than 80% of patients undergo resection of local disease with limb-preserving operations.[14]

Major advances have been made in the treatment of osteosarcoma in the past two decades. Before the advent of systemic chemotherapy, most patients with localized osteosarcoma of the extremities were treated surgically. Treatment with surgery alone was followed by a long-term survival of less than 25%. These results suggested the presence of a "micrometastatic disease," foci of tumor that are established but too small to be seen macroscopically in the lung. Without systemic chemotherapy to kill these tumor cell rests, they proliferate. Osteosarcoma is therefore treated with a multimodal approach to achieve local control, to eradicate established micrometastases, and to prevent systemic spread. Chemotherapy and surgery are the main components of the treatment, and good results are achieved with application of both modalities.

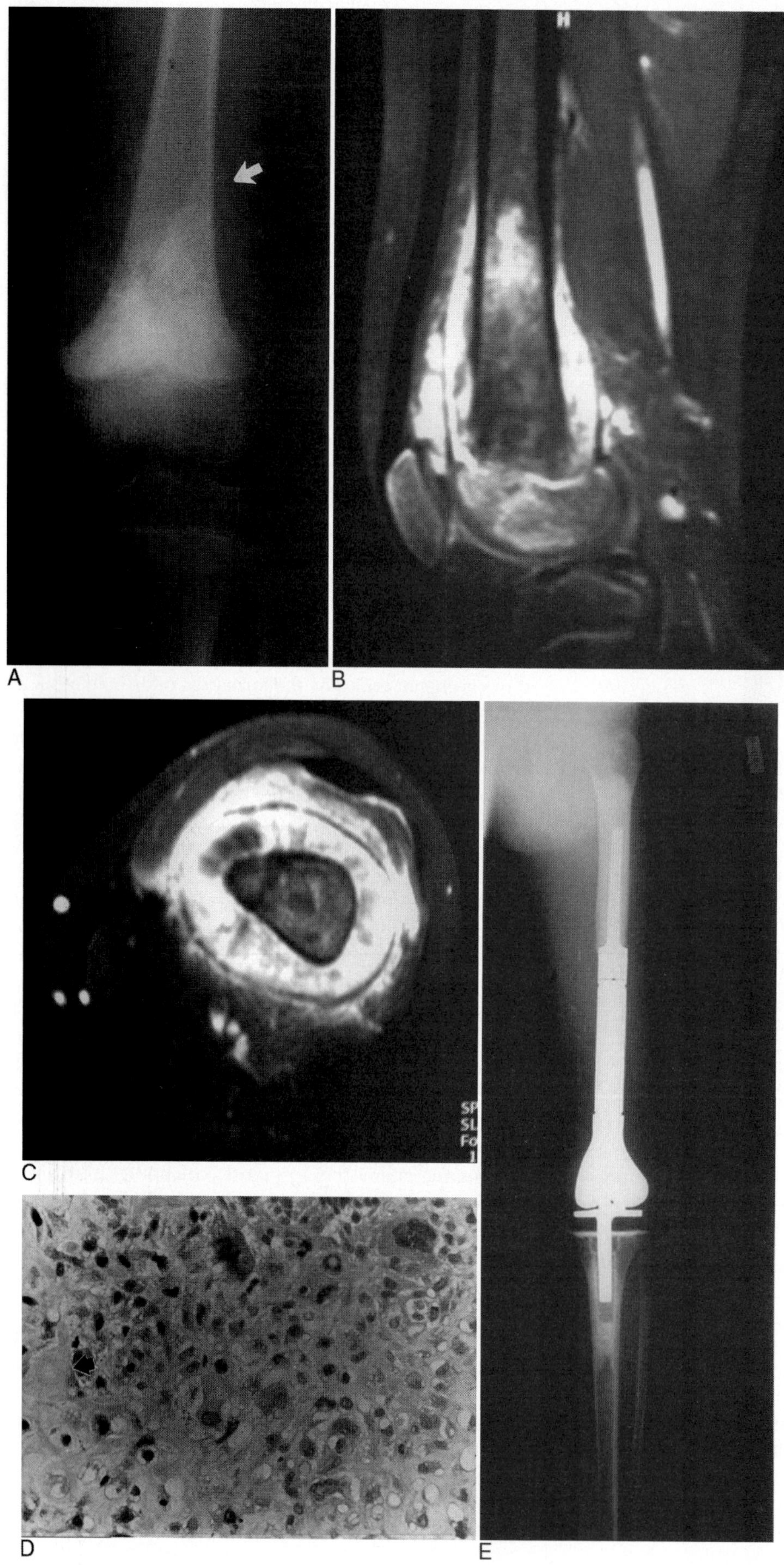

Figure 11-9 High-grade intramedullary osteosarcoma. A, Anteroposterior radiograph of the knee shows sclerosis of the distal femoral metaphysis. A Codman triangle pattern of periosteal elevation *(arrow)* is shown at the superior margin of the mass. **B,** Sagittal T2-weighted magnetic resonance image demonstrates high-signal-intensity tumor in the marrow of the distal femoral metaphysis and epiphysis. The high signal outside the bone represents subperiosteal tumor. There is edema, also high in signal intensity, along the periosteum. **C,** An axial T2-weighted magnetic resonance image shows heterogeneous infiltration of the marrow. A high-signal mass encases the bone. Hazy ill-defined, high signal at the border of the mass represents edema. The neurovascular bundle is clearly separate from the mass. **D,** High-power photomicrograph of the lesion shows scattered pleomorphic, frankly malignant cells in an osteoid matrix (*arrow* points to osteoid). **E,** Radiograph of the leg of a patient who underwent limb salvage surgery with endoprosthetic reconstruction.

Preoperative multiagent chemotherapy (neoadjuvant chemotherapy) is given to most patients with osteosarcoma to treat the micrometastatic disease present at diagnosis, to induce necrosis of the tumor, and, in some instances, to decrease the primary tumor size in order to facilitate limb salvage procedures (see later). The majority of current protocols incorporate doxorubicin, cisplatin, and high-dose methotrexate. The combination of bleomycin, cyclophosphamide, and actinomycin D is also used. Additional maintenance chemotherapy (adjuvant chemotherapy) is given after local tumor control is achieved through surgery, to eliminate any micrometastases still present. The most significant prognostic factor for patients with osteosarcoma is the extent of chemotherapy-induced necrosis in the resection specimen.[15] A good response, usually defined as more than 90% necrosis of the tumor, is associated with higher survival rates.

Osteosarcoma responds poorly to radiation therapy, so surgery is the mainstay of local control of the primary tumor. Excision of the tumor with wide surgical margins is the goal of the operation (see Fig. 11-7). It can be achieved through amputation or through resection leaving uninvolved distal parts, also called *limb salvage surgery*. The success of chemotherapeutic agents in improving local control of the tumor and advances made in surgical techniques have made limb salvage surgery possible in most patients. There is no survival disadvantage for patients treated with limb salvage surgery compared with those treated with amputation, as long as wide surgical margins are achieved.[16] Limb salvage reconstruction involves various surgical techniques, such as endoprosthetic reconstruction (Fig. 11-9E), allograft reconstruction, and rotationplasty reconstruction. The indications for amputation in a patient with osteosarcoma are a grossly displaced pathologic fracture, inability of surgery to achieve wide surgical margins, and a tumor that enlarges during preoperative chemotherapy and is adjacent to the neurovascular bundle.

Tumors Of Cartilaginous Origin

Osteochondroma

Osteochondroma, also known as *exostosis*, is very common, accounting for approximately 50% of benign bone tumors. It is usually diagnosed in patients younger than 20 years. There appears to be a slight preponderance in male patients. Osteochondroma most commonly involves the metaphyses of long bones, particularly around the knee and the proximal humerus. The most common symptom is a hard swelling, usually of long duration, adjacent to a joint. Pain may result from irritation of overlying soft tissues.

The characteristic roentgenographic appearance is a projection composed of a cortex continuous with that of the underlying bone and a spongiosa, similarly continuous. The base may be broad (sessile osteochondroma) or narrow (pedunculated osteochondroma) (Fig. 11-10). Irregular zones of calcification may be present, especially in the cartilaginous cap. Osteochondromas usually point away from the adjacent joint. CT can demonstrate the continuity of cancellous portions of the lesion and the host bone as well as the thickness of the noncalcified cap (usually <3 mm), knowledge of which may occasionally be required to differentiate osteochondromas from malignant lesions such as juxtacortical osteosarcoma and chondrosarcoma.[10]

On gross inspection, an osteochondroma looks like a cauliflower. Histologic examination reveals that the lesion is composed of a cartilaginous cap (usually 2 to 3 mm thick) with a pedunculated or sessile base of bone. A thicker cartilaginous cap may imply the possibility of transformation to chondrosarcoma.[9] Deep to the cartilaginous cap, there is a variable amount of calcification, enchondral ossification, and a normal bone with a cortex and cancellous marrow cavity (Fig. 11-11).

Malignant transformation to chondrosarcoma is extremely rare, occurring in less than 1% of solitary lesions. A growing lesion after the patient has reached skeletal maturity, with a thick cartilaginous cap, is highly suspicious for this complication. The treatment usually consists of alerting the patient and family about signs of malignant transformation. Surgical excision should be reserved for lesions that cause pain or discomfort or are cosmetically unappealing.

Hereditary multiple exostoses is an autosomal dominant disorder often associated with skeletal deformities, short stature, and a significant frequency of malignant transformation (Fig. 11-12). It has been associated with tumor-suppressor genes, termed *exostosin* (EXT) genes (see Chapter 5). Secondary chondrosarcoma in pediatric patients is very rare. However, patients older than 30 years with this disorder have an increased risk of development of a secondary chondrosarcoma. Excision of one or more exostoses is often necessary in patients with osteochondroma because of discomfort or mechanical symptoms.

Dysplasia epiphysealis hemimelica, also known as *Trevor disease*, is a condition that manifests as an intra-articular osteochondroma with pain, deformity, and restricted motion in the affected joint (Fig. 11-13). This disorder is characterized by asymmetric cartilaginous overgrowth of one or more epiphyses in the lower and, occasionally, upper extremities. Histologic appearance of the lesion is almost identical with that of osteochondroma.

Chondroblastoma

Chondroblastoma is a rare tumor usually occurring in patients between 10 and 20 years old. Males are almost twice as frequently affected as females. The most

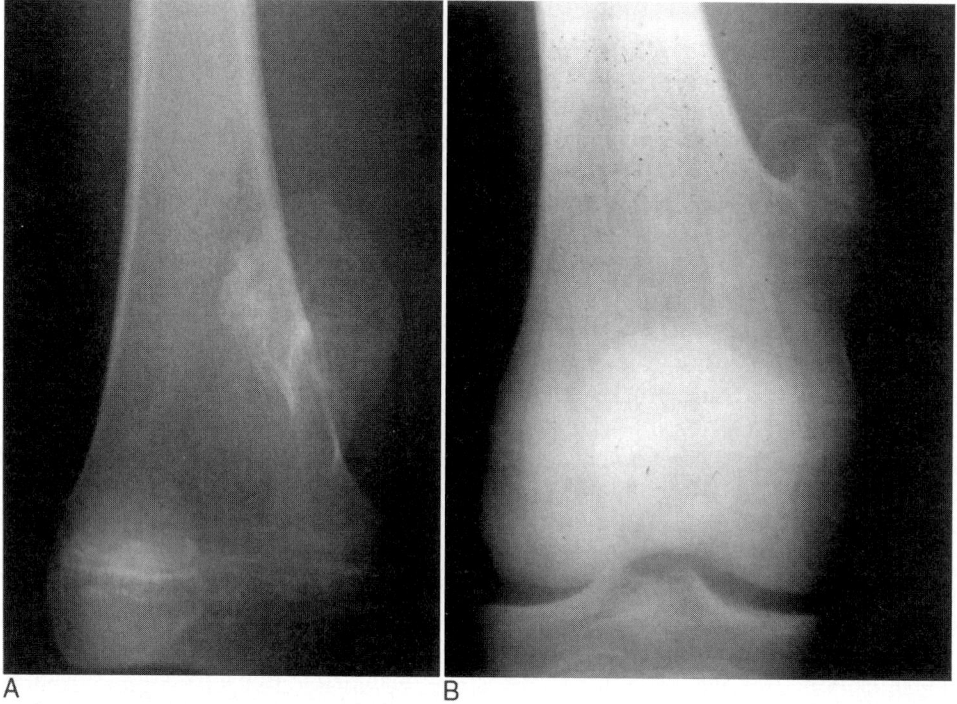

Figure 11-10 Osteochondroma. A, Anteroposterior radiograph of the distal femur shows a bony mass arising from the metaphysis. The trabeculae within the mass and the cortex are continuous with the bone. The broad base is characteristic of a sessile osteochondroma. **B,** Radiograph in a different patient with a pedunculated osteochondroma. Note the narrow pedicle.

common sites of occurrence are the proximal humerus, distal femur, and proximal tibia.[8,10] Presenting symptoms, including pain and swelling, are usually localized to the adjacent joint.

Radiographs show an epiphyseal, sharply marginated lytic destruction, usually with a sclerotic rim of bone (Fig. 11-14A). Only 25% of chondroblastomas have the calcifications that can be characteristic of cartilaginous tumors. The lesions show increased uptake on bone scans and are well defined with MRI. The radiographic differential diagnosis of chondroblastoma may include giant cell tumor of bone, chondrosarcoma, and, sometimes, osteosarcoma.

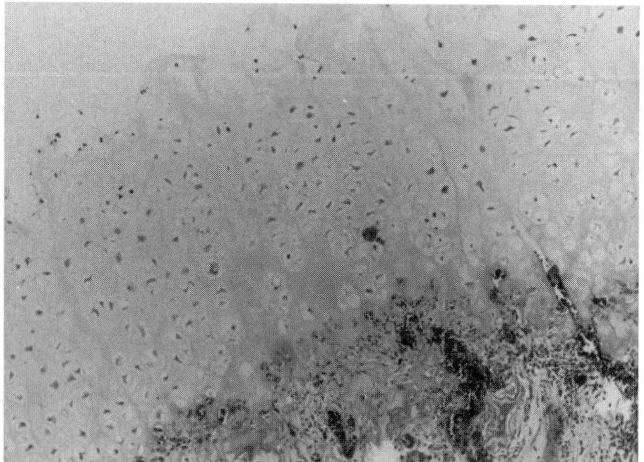

Figure 11-11 Histopathology of osteochondroma. Photomicrograph demonstrates a cartilaginous cap overlying cancellous bone.

Histologically, chondroblastomas are distinguished by the presence of immature chondroblasts, usually with multinucleated giant cells and areas of thin collections of ("chicken-wire") calcification.[9] Chondroblasts are identified from their eccentric nuclei, prominent cytoplasm, and surrounding immature cartilage matrix (Fig. 11-14B).

Chondroblastomas are benign but locally aggressive lesions (see Box 11-3). They may progress and invade the joint and, occasionally, metastasize. They should be treated when detected. Treatment usually consists of extended curettage and bone grafting, but recurrence rates of up to 15% to 20 % have been reported. With recurrence, en bloc resection may be considered. Large lesions that compromise the neighboring joint with a pathologic fracture may require wide resection and reconstruction with allograft, prosthesis, or arthrodesis.

Chondromyxoid Fibroma

Chondromyxoid fibroma is the least common of the benign cartilage tumors seen in children, occurring between the ages of 10 and 30 years. Males are more frequently affected than females at a ratio of 2:1. More than

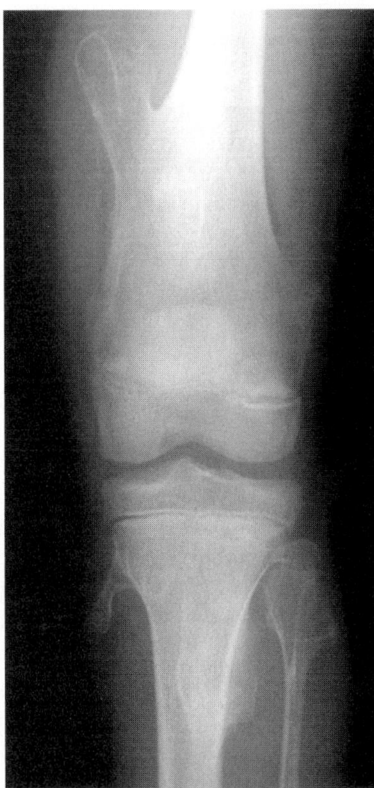

Figure 11-12 Hereditary multiple exostoses. Anteroposterior radiograph of the knee shows multiple lesions extending from the metaphyses of all the bones. All the lesions contain trabeculae and blend imperceptibly with the bone. Note that the lesions point away from the joint. Widening of the distal femoral metaphysis is caused by osteochondromas with a broad base.

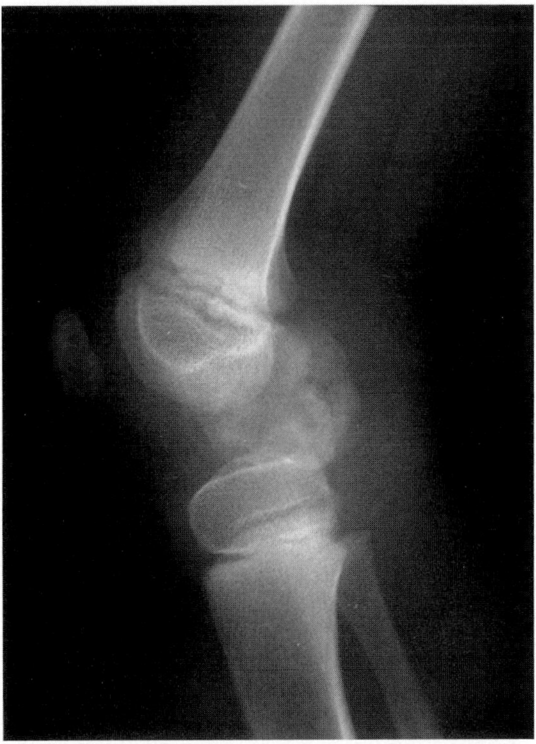

Figure 11-13 Dysplasia epiphysealis hemimelica (Trevor disease). Lateral radiograph of the knee shows marked enlargement of posterior aspect of the medial femoral condyle. Multiple, rounded, ossific densities representing osteochondromas blend with the trabeculae. Note the loss of the cortex.

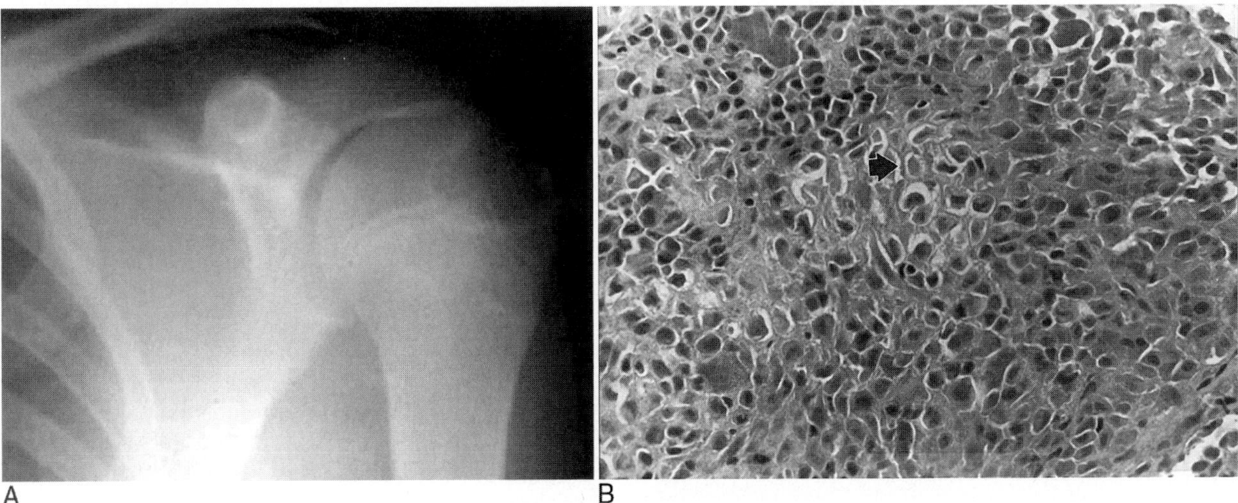

Figure 11-14 Chondroblastoma. A, Anteroposterior radiograph of the shoulder shows a well-circumscribed, lytic lesion in the lateral epiphysis of the humerus. The lesion does not cross the physis. **B,** High-power photomicrograph of the lesion demonstrates closely packed polyhedral cells surrounded by a lacelike, lightly calcified matrix *(arrow)*.

75% of these tumors occur in the lower extremities, the proximal tibial metaphysis being the most common location. Patients complain of a dull, steady pain that is usually worse at night.

Radiographically, chondromyxoid fibromas are metaphyseal, eccentric, sharply circumscribed lytic lesions. Cortical erosion and expansion may occur, giving a "soap-bubble" appearance. The radiographic differential diagnosis includes nonossifying fibroma, aneurysmal bone cyst, and chondroblastoma. On histologic examination the lesions are often lobular, with areas of distinct fibromyxoid cartilage (Fig. 11-15). Because chondromyxoid fibroma commonly has significant cytologic atypia, clinical and radiographic correlation is essential to prevent misdiagnosis of the tumor as chondrosarcoma. Extended curettage and bone grafting constitute the treatment of choice for the children with chondromyxoid fibroma. Local recurrence is rare and can usually be treated with curettage or en bloc excision.

Enchondroma

Enchondromas are benign tumors of mature hyaline cartilage. The peak age of occurrence is in the second decade, but the tumors are found in all age groups with no sex predilection. They usually manifest as solitary lesions. The short, tubular bones of the hand and foot (i.e., phalanges, metacarpals, metatarsals) are preferred sites, followed in frequency by the femur, humerus, tibia, and ribs.[8,9] The lesions are often asymptomatic unless a pathologic fracture occurs.

Radiographs show a sharply circumscribed lytic defect with a central region of rarefaction within the metaphysis or diaphysis of the involved bone (Fig. 11-16A). Calcification may be present and usually is stippled. As an enchondroma becomes more mature, the lobules of cartilage may undergo peripheral enchondral ossification, which is apparent on plain radiographs and CT scans as "popcorn" ossification.[9,10] Expansion of the cortex is common.

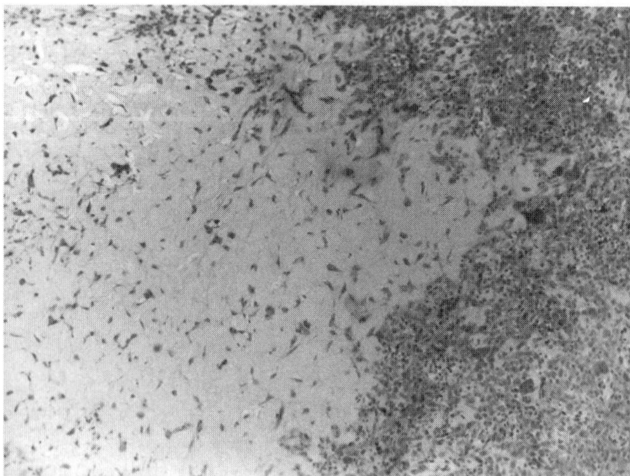

Figure 11-15 Histopathology of chondromyxoid fibroma. Photomicrograph demonstrates the variegated appearance of relatively hypocellular chondromyxoid tissue juxtaposed with a cellular, fibrous component.

On gross examination, enchondromas are lobular and bluish. Histologic preparations show lobules of hyaline cartilage with varying cellularity which are recognized from their blue matrix (Fig. 11-16B). The chondrocytes are located in rounded spaces called *lacunae*. The nuclei are uniformly small, regular, and darkly stained. The differential diagnosis includes bone infarction and chondrosarcoma.

Malignant transformation of enchondromas occurs infrequently (<1%) and is rare in the skeletally immature.[9,10] Patients experiencing pain in a previously asymptomatic lesion without evidence of a pathologic fracture should be evaluated for malignant transformation. In a solitary enchondroma, malignant transformation occurs predominantly in a long or flat bone, never in a short tubular bone.

Asymptomatic solitary enchondromas do not require any treatment other than a periodic follow-up evaluation. Symptomatic or large lesions in the short tubular bones of the hand without pathologic fracture can be managed with curettage and bone grafting. If a pathologic fracture occurs through an enchondroma, the fracture should be allowed to heal before curettage and bone grafting are performed.[11] Recurrence after curettage and bone grafting is rare. Biopsy should be performed for suspicious lesions.

Multiple enchondromatosis, also known as *Ollier disease*, is an inherited condition with widespread enchondromas that are often unilateral (Fig. 11-17). The small tubular bones of the hands and feet and the flat bones are most commonly affected. Unlike solitary enchondroma, enchondromatosis can cause symptoms at an early age. Shortening of the involved bone, angular deformity, and pathologic fracture are common presenting symptoms. Histologically, the lesions closely resemble solitary enchondromas. Malignant transformation has been reported to occur in about 25% of patients with Ollier disease.[17] Multiple enchondromatosis with vascular anomalies of the skin or soft tissues, known as *Maffucci syndrome*, is associated with an extremely high rate of malignant degeneration.

Periosteal Chondroma

Periosteal chondromas, also known as *juxtacortical chondromas*, are extremely rare benign cartilaginous tumors forming beneath the periosteum and external to the cortex of bone. They are discovered mainly in patients in their 20s and 30s. The male-to-female ratio is 2:1. The proximal humerus is the classical location, followed by small bones of the hands or feet. Radiographs show a cup-shaped or saucer-shaped erosion of the cortex with surrounding sclerotic bone (Fig. 11-18).

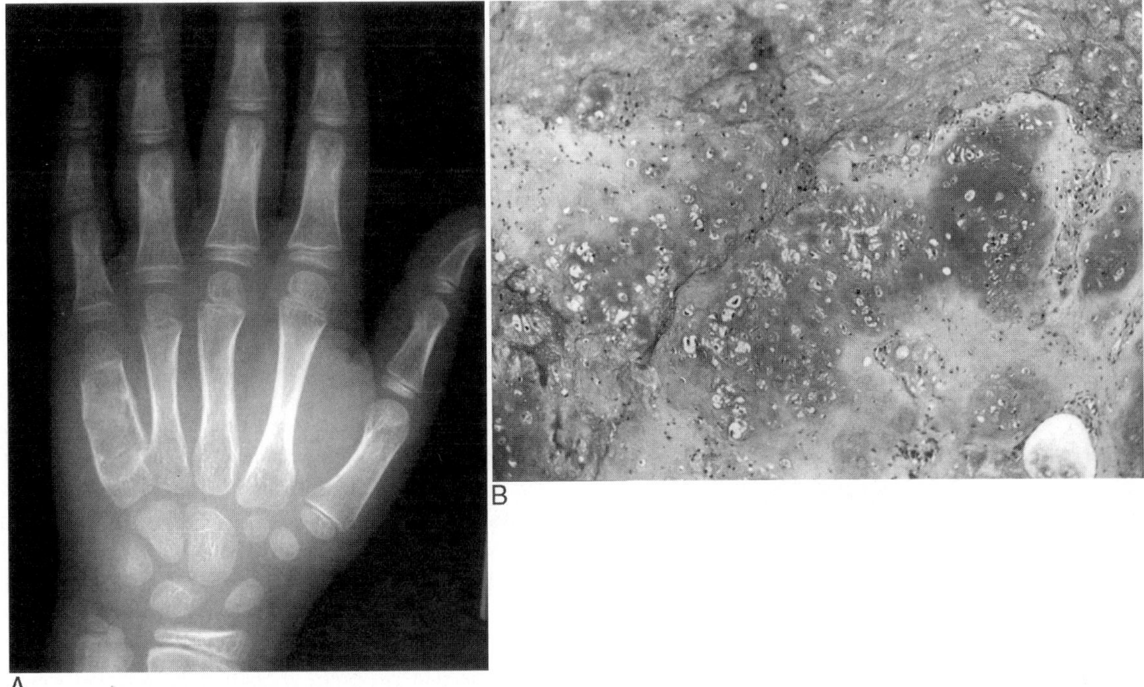

Figure 11-16 Enchondroma. **A,** Anteroposterior radiograph of the hand shows an expansile, lytic lesion involving the diaphysis of the fifth metacarpal with extension into the distal metaphysis. There is saucerization (scalloping) of the inner cortex. **B,** Photomicrograph demonstrates the lobular nature of this cartilaginous lesion.

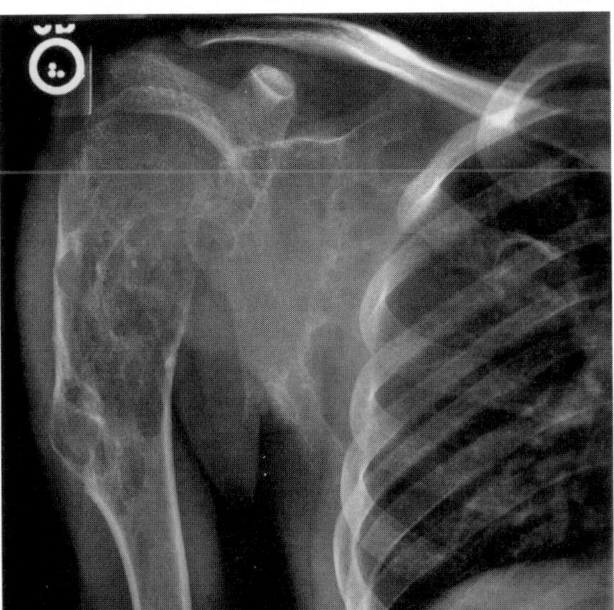

Figure 11-17 Multiple enchondromatosis (Ollier disease). Anteroposterior radiograph of the shoulder shows an expansile process in the proximal humeral metaphysis composed of multiple, lytic lesions with well-defined borders. Note the scalloping of the inner cortex, a characteristic of cartilaginous lesions. The angular deformity is the result of a healed pathologic fracture. Lytic lesions are also scattered along the edges of the scapula and in the glenoid region. In addition, there is a lesion at the anterior rib end of the second rib.

Histologically, these tumors are composed of lobules of hypercellular, immature cartilage; double nuclei; faintly staining matrix; little, if any, calcification; and hypercellularity with some cellular atypia.[9] Malignant transformation of periosteal chondromas has not been reported. Treatment is usually extended curettage or en bloc excision. Depending on the size of the lesion, bone grafting may be indicated.

Lesions of Fibrous Origin

Fibrous Dysplasia

Fibrous dysplasia is a fibro-osseous lesion characterized by the replacement of normal lamellar cancellous bone by an abnormal fibrous tissue. The lesions appear early in childhood and remain active during growth. After the cessation of growth, the disease subsides to a static phase; however, it may be reactivated with pregnancy. Fibrous dysplasia may affect one bone (monostotic form, 80% of cases) or several bones (polyostotic form, 20%). The most common locations for monostotic fibrous dysplasia are the ribs, proximal femur, tibia, and base of the skull. Fibrous dysplasia is usually asymptomatic, being discovered incidentally on radiographs obtained for other reasons. Occasionally, pain accompanied by swelling is present. Pathologic fracture, the most common complication, may occur repeatedly and lead to deformity ("shepherd's crook" deformity) (Fig. 11-19A).

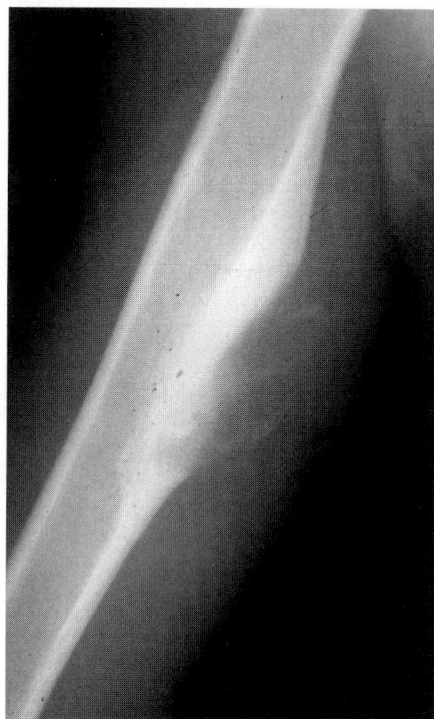

Figure 11-18 Periosteal chondroma. Anteroposterior radiograph of the humerus shows spicules of bone formation within a lucent mass. Note the fusiform area of cortical thickening with a central pattern of erosion, referred to as *saucerization*. The axis of the mass is parallel with the bone, and the cortex at each end of the lesion has a triangle configuration, these features are keys to the origin of the lesion.

Radiographically, fibrous dysplasia usually is shown to involve the full width of the bone, appearing as a radiolucent lesion with slight expansion and thinning of the cortex, and partial loss of trabecular pattern in the cancellous bone, giving the characteristic "ground-glass" appearance (Figs.11-19A and 11-20).[10] The lesions are usually diaphyseal, and the differential diagnosis may include other common diaphyseal lesions of bone.

Histologically, fibrous dysplasia, both the monostotic and polyostotic forms, is composed of trabeculae of woven bone in a background of moderately cellular fibrous tissue (Fig. 11-19B).[8,9] There are few if any osteoblasts, and the osteoid and bone seem to arise directly from the background fibrous stroma. The trabeculae often obtain a variety of shapes (Cs and Os) and are sometimes referred to as "Chinese letters."

Asymptomatic, monostotic lesions do not require any treatment other than observation. Symptomatic lesions may be treated by curettage and bone grafting, although there is a high recurrence rate.[11] Cortical allografts are usually preferred to cancellous bone grafts. With polyostotic disease, problem areas usually require straightening and strengthening procedures. Extensive involvement of long bones may be successfully treated with long-term intramedullary stabilization and corrective osteotomies.

Polyostotic fibrous dysplasia may occur as a part of a condition known as *McCune-Albright syndrome*, which is characterized by the classic triad polyostotic fibrous dysplasia, café au lait skin lesions, and precocious puberty (Fig. 11-21). Activating missense mutations of the guanine nucleotide-binding protein gene (GNAS), encoding the alpha subunit of the stimulatory G protein, have been

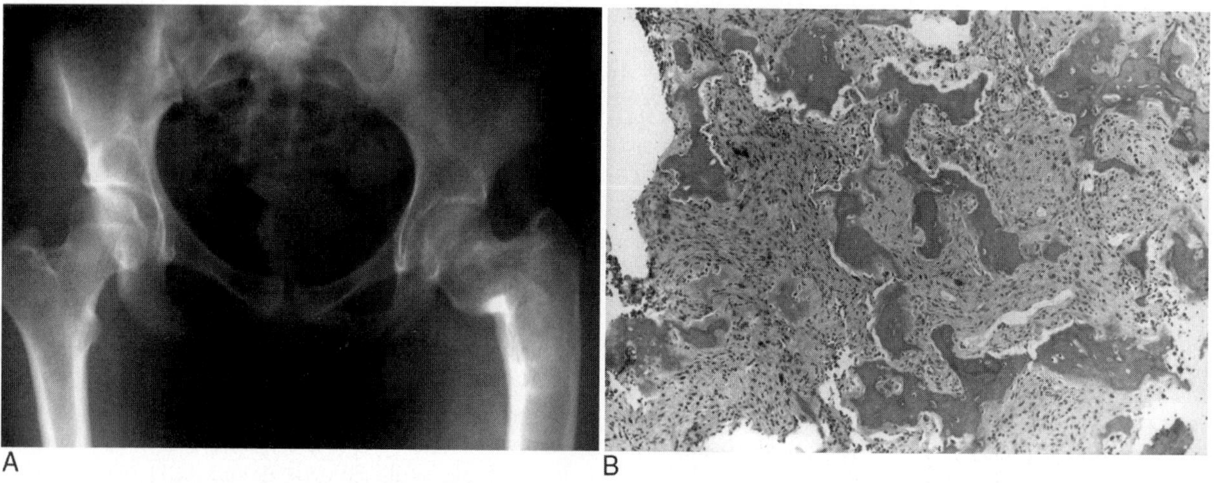

Figure 11-19 Monostotic fibrous dysplasia. A, Anteroposterior radiograph of the pelvis shows widening of the left femoral neck and proximal diaphysis with a diffuse, ground-glass density and scattered lucencies. Note the "shepherd's crook" deformity of the femoral neck. **B,** Photomicrograph of the lesion demonstrates characteristic curvilinear and irregularly shaped trabeculae of woven bone dispersed in a matrix of fibrous tissue. Osteoblastic rimming is largely absent.

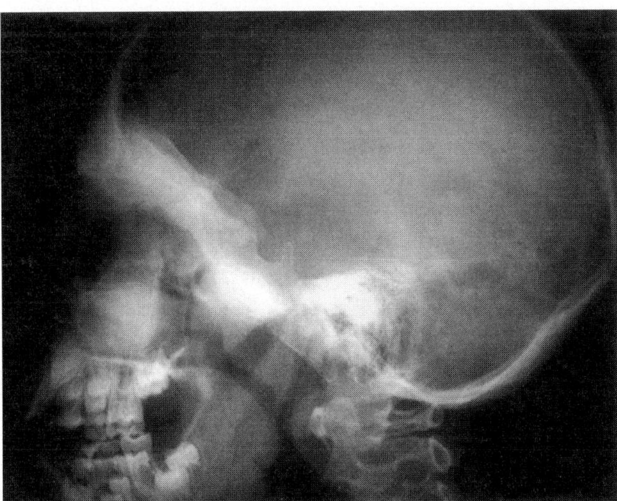

Figure 11-20 Monostotic fibrous dysplasia. Lateral radiograph of the skull shows expansion of the sphenoid bone, adjacent frontal bone, clivus, and maxilla with ground-glass density.

identified in patients with this syndrome. These G proteins play a role in regulation of the activity of hormone-sensitive adenylate cyclase and transduce extracellular signals received by transmembrane receptors to effector proteins. The occurrence of GNAS mutations has been shown in individual cases of fibrous dysplasia.

Osteofibrous Dysplasia

Osteofibrous dysplasia, or *Kempson-Campanacci lesion* (formerly called *ossifying fibroma*), is a rare disorder of childhood. More than 60% of affected patients are younger than 5 years. Boys are slightly more commonly affected. The process originates intracortically, in contrast to fibrous dysplasia, which has an intramedullary origin. Approximately 90% of lesions occur in the tibia, followed by the fibula and ulna. Osteofibrous dysplasia is usually asymptomatic, but occasionally, it may be revealed clinically by the enlargement and bowing of the tibia. There is a growing association of this tumor with adamantinoma of bone. Transition from osteofibrous dysplasia to adamantinoma has been documented.[18]

Radiographically, osteofibrous dysplasia appears as a diaphyseal, intracortical lytic lesion associated with expansion and thinning of the cortex and lobulated sclerotic margins (Fig. 11-22). Larger lesions may destroy the cortical bone and invade the medullary cavity. The lesion rarely involves the entire circumference of the shaft in the tibia but may do so in the fibula.

Histologically, osteofibrous dysplasia is similar to fibrous dysplasia, but with osteoblasts lining the trabeculae.[8,9] A fibrous tissue background is present with numerous fibrous-bony trabeculae. The trabeculae are rimmed by plump normal-appearing osteoblasts. The

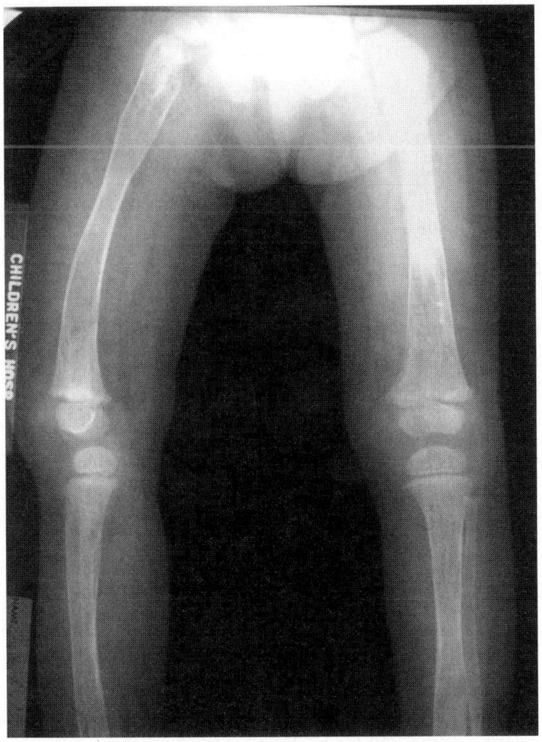

Figure 11-21 Polyostotic fibrous dysplasia (McCune-Albright syndrome). Anteroposterior radiograph of the lower extremities reveals expansion of the diaphyses of all the bones with ground-glass opacity.

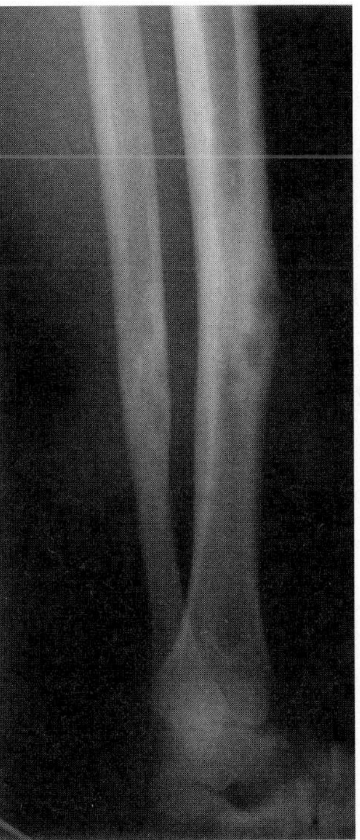

Figure 11-22 Osteofibrous dysplasia. Lateral radiograph of the leg shows cortical thickening of the diaphyses of both the tibia and fibula. Small, focal lytic lesions expand the cortical bone and can be seen centrally as well.

differential diagnosis often includes lesions such as fibrous dysplasia and adamantinoma.

Osteofibrous dysplasia is benign but may be locally aggressive (see Box 11-3). Treatment depends on the age of the child, the radiographic characteristics of the lesion, the presence or absence of progression, and results of biopsy, if performed.[11] Observation is recommended for children younger than 10 years with asymptomatic and nonprogressive lesions. Bracing may be indicated for a child with progressive bowing of the tibia. If the lesion progresses, curettage and bone grafting, or even resection, are suggested. If the patient presents after the age of 10 years, especially if the lesion is large or has aggressive features on the plane radiographs, a biopsy is suggested to rule out an adamantinoma. An adamantinoma requires a wider resection than an enlarging osteofibrous dysplasia. En bloc removal of the lesion with reconstruction is the treatment of choice.

Nonossifying Fibroma

Nonossifying fibroma, *fibrous cortical defect*, *metaphyseal fibrous defect*, and *fibroma* all refer to the same histopathologic process in bone. Fibrous cortical defect is a small, asymptomatic lesion that occurs in 30% of the normal population during the first and second decades of life (Fig. 11-23). The term *nonossifying fibroma* is applied to this lesion if it enlarges and encroaches on the medullary portion of the bone.[10] The lesions are not true neoplasms but, rather, a developmental defect in which areas that normally ossify are occupied by fibrous connective tissue. Nonossifying fibroma occurs more commonly in boys, in a ratio of 2:1. There is a predilection for the long bones, particularly the femur and tibia. Most nonossifying fibromas are asymptomatic. The clinical significance is that these lesions may contribute to pathologic fracture by nature of their size and location.

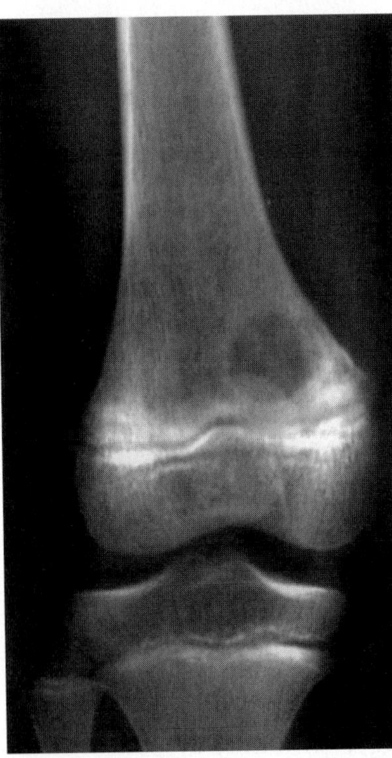

Figure 11-23 Fibrous cortical defect. Anteroposterior radiograph of the knee shows a small, round, well-defined lytic lesion in the medial distal femoral metaphysis.

Radiographically, nonossifying fibromas appear as metaphyseal, eccentric, elongated lesions with sclerotic scalloped borders (Fig. 11-24A and B). They range in size from 0.5 to 7 cm, with their long axes aligned with the long axis of the affected bone. Nonossifying fibromas may scallop the outer cortex of the bone, making them radiographically similar to chondromyxoid fibroma.

Histologically, the lesions characteristically show a spindle cell proliferation with a loose storiform arrangement of the cells (Fig. 11-24C). Hemosiderin pigment is present within the spindle cells. Clusters of giant cells and foam cells containing lipid are almost always found in nonossifying fibroma. Typically, the lesions do not contain bone.

Most of nonossifying fibromas can be observed if they are asymptomatic. They may undergo spontaneous healing by the remodeling process of the tubular bone. Large lesions (occupying more than 50% of the cross-sectional area of the bone involved) with a risk of pathologic fracture should be treated. Treatment consists of curettage and bone grafting and, occasionally, prophylactic internal fixation.[19]

Desmoplastic Fibroma

Desmoplastic fibroma, also known as *periosteal desmoid*, is a fibrous cortical defect occurring typically on the posteromedial aspect of the distal femur. It usually occurs between the ages of 12 and 20 years, mainly in boys. The lesion is usually asymptomatic, being detected incidentally on radiographs taken for some other reason. Radiographically, desmoplastic fibroma appears as shallow erosion of the cortex with a sclerotic base. If the lesion is removed for some reason, histologic evaluation shows fibrous replacement of a portion of the cortex. Desmoplastic fibroma is a benign lesion to be left alone, without biopsy.

Miscellaneous Tumors and Tumor-Like Lesions

Unicameral Bone Cyst (Simple Bone Cyst)

Unicameral bone cyst (UBC) is a tumor-like lesion of unknown cause that has been attributed to a local disturbance of bone growth. Although the pathogenesis is still unknown, the lesion appears to be reactive or developmental rather than to represent a true neoplasm. UBCs

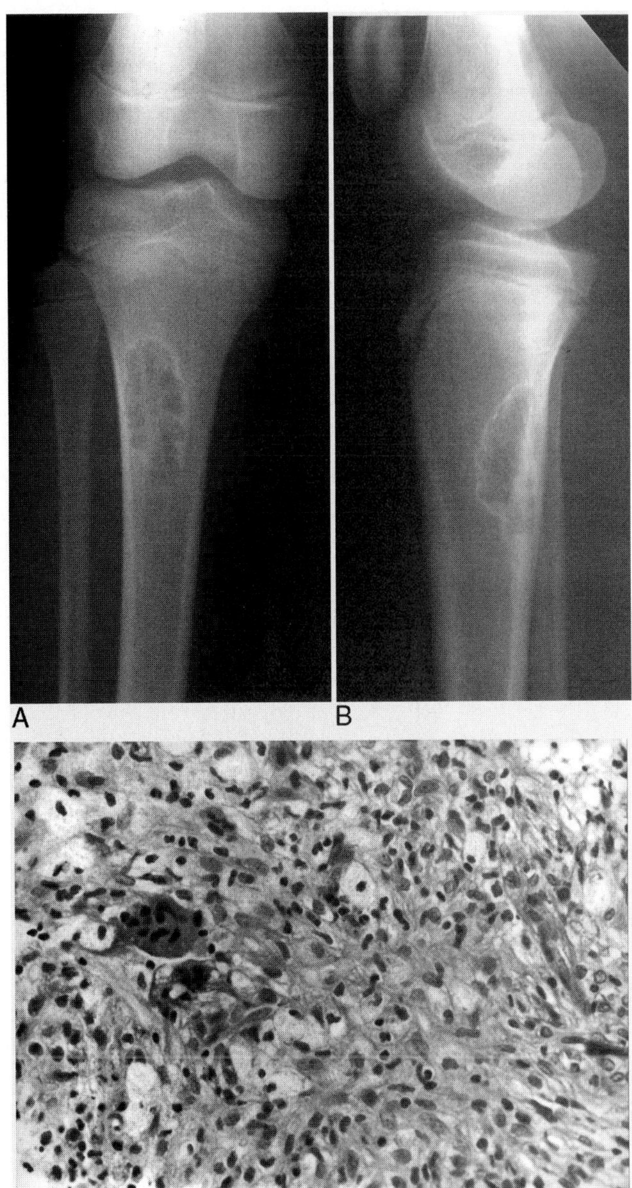

Figure 11-24 Nonossifying fibroma. Anteroposterior (**A**) and lateral (**B**) radiographs of the knee show a large, cortically based, lobulated, lytic lesion with a sclerotic border in the metadiaphysis of the tibia. **C**, High-power photomicrograph demonstrates a spindle cell stroma that is populated by foamy histiocytes, a sparse lymphocytic inflammatory infiltrate, and scattered giant cells.

are frequently seen in childhood, with a high incidence in patients between 5 and 15 years old. Boys are more frequently affected than girls at a ratio of 2:1. The most common locations are the proximal humerus and femur, followed by the calcaneus. The lesions are commonly asymptomatic, coming to attention in most patients only after pathologic fracture has occurred. Occasionally in these situations, the callus formation induces cystic healing as well as fracture consolidation.

Radiographically, UBCs are metaphyseal, centrally located, well-circumscribed, radiolucent lesions with sclerotic margins (Fig. 11-25A).[9] When a UBC is with a pathologic fracture, the characteristic "fallen leaf" sign may be observed. This sign consists of a fragment of thinned cortex fractured and displaced into the cyst, confirming the cystic nature of the lesion.

The cystic cavity is usually filled with a clear or yellowish fluid of low viscosity. If a pathologic fracture has taken place, the fluid is stained by hemorrhage. Histologically, a cyst lining is present, usually consisting of a single layer of mesothelial cells with underlying connective tissue or bone (Fig. 11-25B).

Traditional treatment options for UBC are observation, steroid injections, and open curettage with bone grafting, all of which are associated with high rates of complications and recurrence. Newer techniques include injection with demineralized bone matrix and percutaneous curettage and grafting with bone graft substitutes (calcium sulfate); these techniques have high healing and low complication rates.[19]

Aneurysmal Bone Cyst

Aneurysmal bone cysts (ABCs) are vascular lesions consisting of widely dilated vascular channels that are not lined by identifiable endothelium. Many are believed to be secondary to or related to other benign lesions. They are frequently seen in the second decade with no sex predilection. ABCs can be observed in almost every skeletal site, but the most common areas of occurrence are the long bones and the posterior elements of the spine. The presenting symptom in 70% of the patients is pain. Pathologic fracture is a common complication (Fig. 11-26).

Radiographically, ABCs are expansile, lytic, and sharply circumscribed lesions that usually involve the metaphyseal regions of the long bones (Fig. 11-27A). The lesion may start in an eccentric location and can expand to involve the entire width of the bone. An ABC can destroy the cortex but grows slowly enough that there is usually a rim of overlying calcified periosteum, which stimulates a thinned but intact bony cortex. ABCs frequently have internal septations and fluid-fluid levels that are well shown on MRI (Fig. 11-27B).[20]

The essential histologic features of ABCs are cavernous spaces, the walls of which lack the normal features of blood vessels (Fig. 11-27C). Thin strands of immature woven bone are often present in the fibrous tissue of these walls. The septa almost invariably contain scattered osteoclast-like giant cells and hemosiderin-laden macrophages.

Although they have a well-differentiated benign histology, ABCs can show aggressive local behavior (see Box 11-3). They usually require surgical treatment. En bloc resection is recommended for lesions located

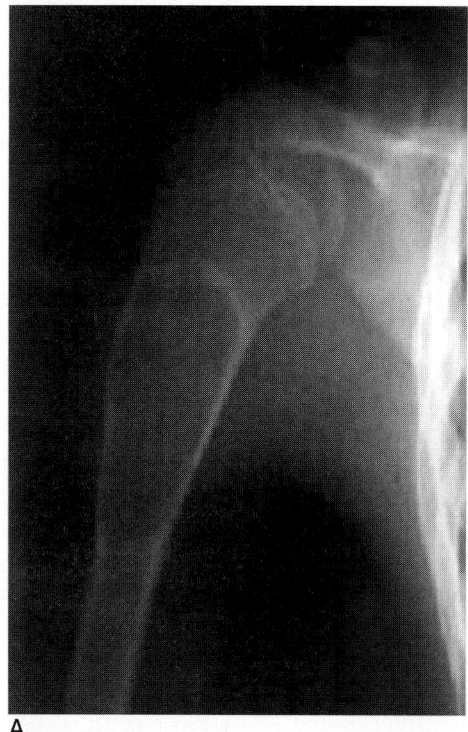

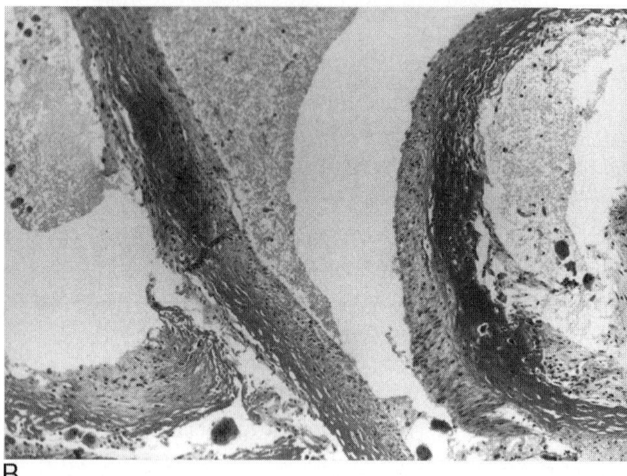

Figure 11-25 Unicameral bone cyst. A, Anteroposterior radiograph of the humerus shows a lytic lesion with sclerotic borders filling the entire medullary canal. **B,** Photomicrograph of the lesion demonstrates cyst membranes lined by loose connective tissue with underlying bands of osteoid. Amorphous debris partially fills the cyst cavities.

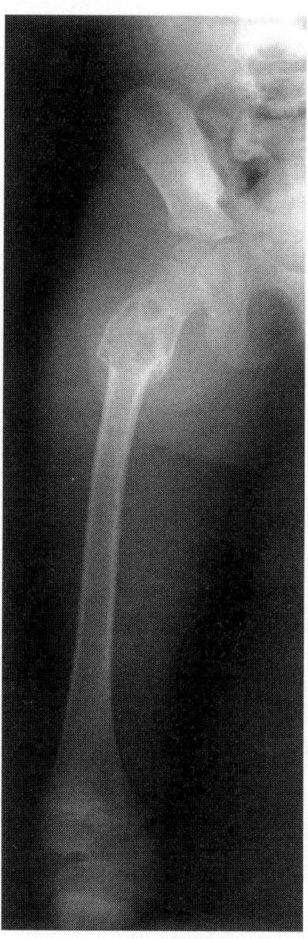

Figure 11-26 Aneurysmal bone cyst. Anteroposterior radiograph of the femur shows a pathologic fracture through an aneurysmal bone cyst.

in expandable bones (e.g., fibula, ribs, metacarpals, metatarsals). In other locations, extended curettage with bone grafting is the treatment of choice.[19]

Giant Cell Tumor

Giant cell tumors (GCTs) commonly occur in patients between the ages of 20 and 40 years, usually after physeal closure. There is a female preponderance, with a female-to-male ratio of 2:1. Most of the lesions arise in long bones, most commonly the femur, tibia, radius, and proximal humerus. In the spine, giant cell tumor usually involves the anterior elements.[12] The most common presenting symptoms are pain, swelling, and tenderness of the affected area. Limited motion of the adjacent joint may also be seen.

Radiographically, a GCT is a radiolucent lesion with sharply circumscribed margins that involves the epiphysis and metaphysis of a long bone (Fig. 11-28A). The lesion may invade articular cartilage. Neither calcification nor ossification is present within the lesion. No periosteal reaction occurs.

Histologically, the lesion consists of stromal cells and multinucleated giant cells that are usually distributed uniformly throughout the tumor (Fig. 11-28B).[8,9] Although these giant cells bear some resemblance to osteoclasts, they do not appear to participate in bone resorption. Mitoses are common, but they are normal in appearance. Areas of spontaneous necrosis may be seen.

GCT is a benign but locally aggressive lesion (see Box 11-3). Treatment usually involves extended curettage and bone grafting or methyl methacrylate cementation of the lesion. If bone cement is used, it should be removed later and replaced with bone graft.

Langerhans Cell Histiocytosis

Langerhans cell histiocytosis (LCH) is a rare group of disorders with a wide spectrum of clinical presentations. Although etiology and pathogenesis remain unsettled,

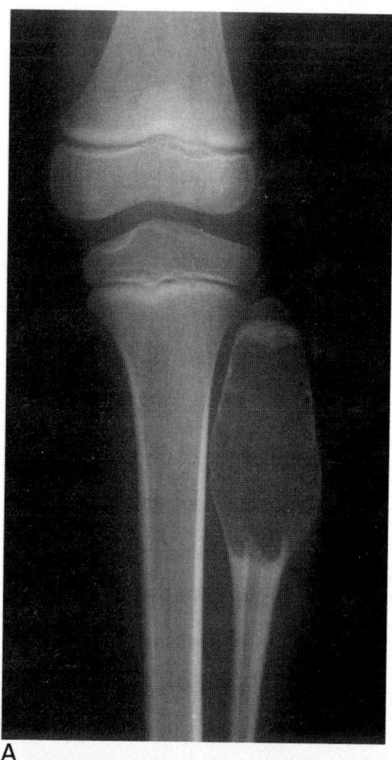

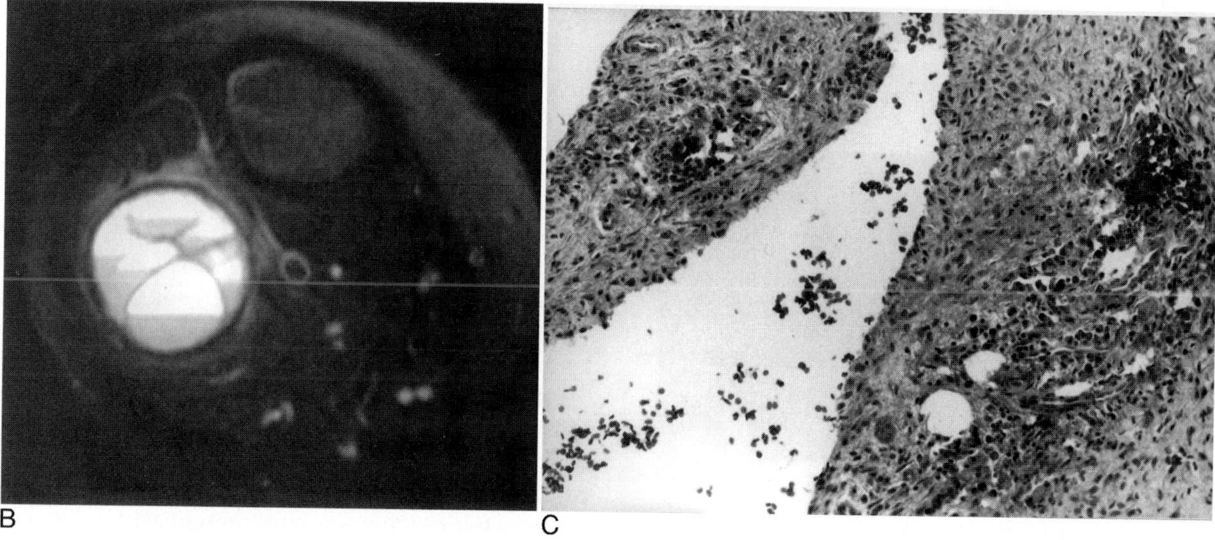

Figure 11-27 Aneurysmal bone cyst. **A,** Anteroposterior radiograph of the knee shows an expansile, lytic lesion with a well-circumscribed border and multiple bony septations throughout the lesion. Note the absence of periosteal new bone formation. **B,** Axial T2-weighted magnetic resonance image shows fluid-fluid levels in this multiloculated lesion. A thin, encapsulating rind of low signal intensity surrounds the lesion. **C,** Photomicrograph demonstrates a cavernous, nonendothelialized space containing red blood cells, with inflammatory cells and rare giant cells in the underlying stroma.

LCH is now considered a disorder of immune regulation rather than a neoplastic process.[10] Some molecular studies of clonality and the role of viruses initiating this disease are nevertheless under study. LCH can manifest at any age, from the neonatal period to old age. The peak incidence is in children 1 to 3 years old, and males are more often affected than females at a radio of 2:1. LCH most often occurs in the flat bones, with a predilection for the skull. Long bone involvement is usually limited to the femur, tibia, and humerus. The process is represented by a spectrum of overlapping syndromes ranging from the more serious and life-threatening Letterer-Siwe disease to Hand-Schüller-Christian variants to the solitary eosinophilic granuloma of bone. Pain is the most common

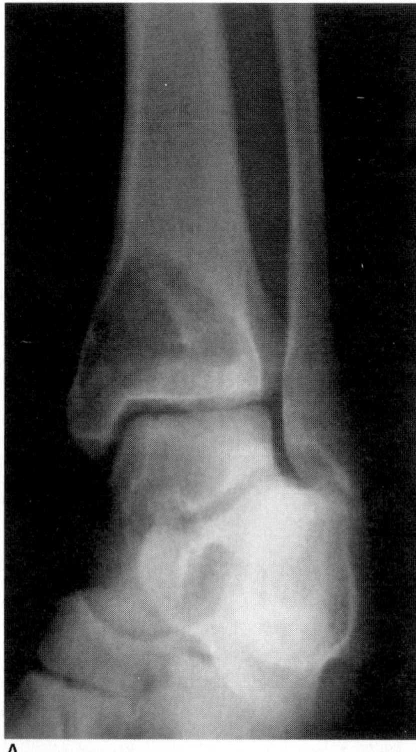

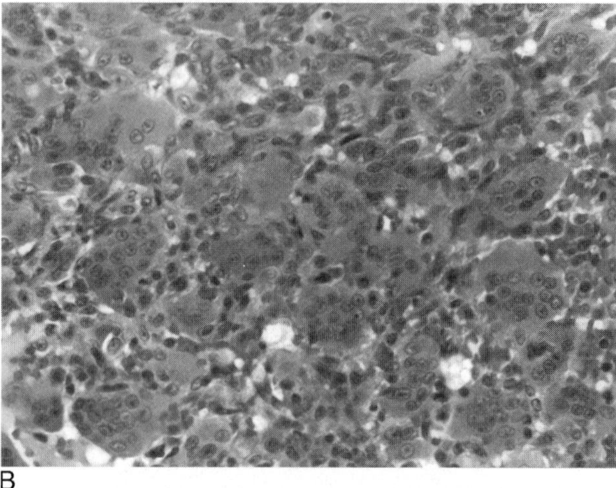

Figure 11-28 Giant cell tumor. A, Oblique radiograph of the ankle shows a lytic lesion in the distal tibia involving the metaphysis and epiphysis. The borders are well defined. Scalloping of the inner cortex is seen. **B,** High-power photomicrograph of the lesion demonstrates the diffuse distribution of multinucleated giant cells in a cellular stroma of mononuclear cells.

presenting complaint and may be accompanied by a tender mass detected on physical examination.

The radiographic appearance is highly variable. Initially, lesions may be either solitary or multiple. They are typically lytic with well-defined margins (Fig. 11-29A). Expansion of the overlying cortex, solid periosteal new bone formation, and surrounding sclerosis may occur with time. A soft tissue mass may be associated. In LCH, the progression and disappearance of the bony lesions are very rapid.[8] Spinal involvement usually results in variable compression of the vertebral body ("vertebra plana" when complete) (Fig. 11-30).[10,12]

Histologically, the lesion is characterized by a proliferation of Langerhans cells in an inflammatory background (Box 11-4) (see Fig. 11-29B). These cells commonly have ill-defined cytoplasmic boundaries and characteristically contain an oval or indented nucleus. Multinucleated giant cells, eosinophils, lymphocytes, plasma cells, and neutrophils are also commonly seen. Langerhans cells can be specifically identified on electron microscopy from the presence of racquet-shaped cytoplasmic organelles, known as Birbeck granules.[9,10] Immunohistochemical phenotyping shows that Langerhans cells react positively for S100, CD1a, CD11, and CD14 (see Fig. 11-29C).

The clinical course of LCH in patients with localized or single-system disease, usually of bone, lymph nodes, or skin, is generally benign. Patients have a good chance of spontaneous remission and a favorable outcome over a period of months to years. A single osseous lesion usually does not require treatment other than biopsy to confirm diagnosis. For LCH in the spine, no treatment is recommended, unless a neurologic deficit is present.

Ewing Sarcoma

Ewing sarcoma is the second most common primary malignant bone tumor in children. It most commonly affects individuals between the ages of 10 and 20 years but may occur at any age. The disease shows a distinct predilection for males. Ewing sarcoma occurs most frequently in the long bones (predominantly the femur, tibia, and humerus) and pelvis. It may also involve the spine. Pain and local swelling are the most common presenting symptoms. Some patients may have generalized symptoms such as, fever, weight loss, and malaise. These symptoms, together with common laboratory evidence such as a high white cell count and elevated erythrocyte sedimentation rate, may suggest osteomyelitis as a differential diagnosis. Approximately 25% of patients with Ewing sarcoma present with overt metastases, typically in the lungs, bone marrow, or bone.[14]

Box 11-4 Round Cell Lesions

Benign
- Langerhans cell histiocytosis

Malignant
- Ewing sarcoma/primitive neuroectodermal tumors (PNETs)
- Bone lymphomas (non-Hodgkin lymphoma and Hodgkin lymphoma)
- Multiple myeloma (plasmocytoma)

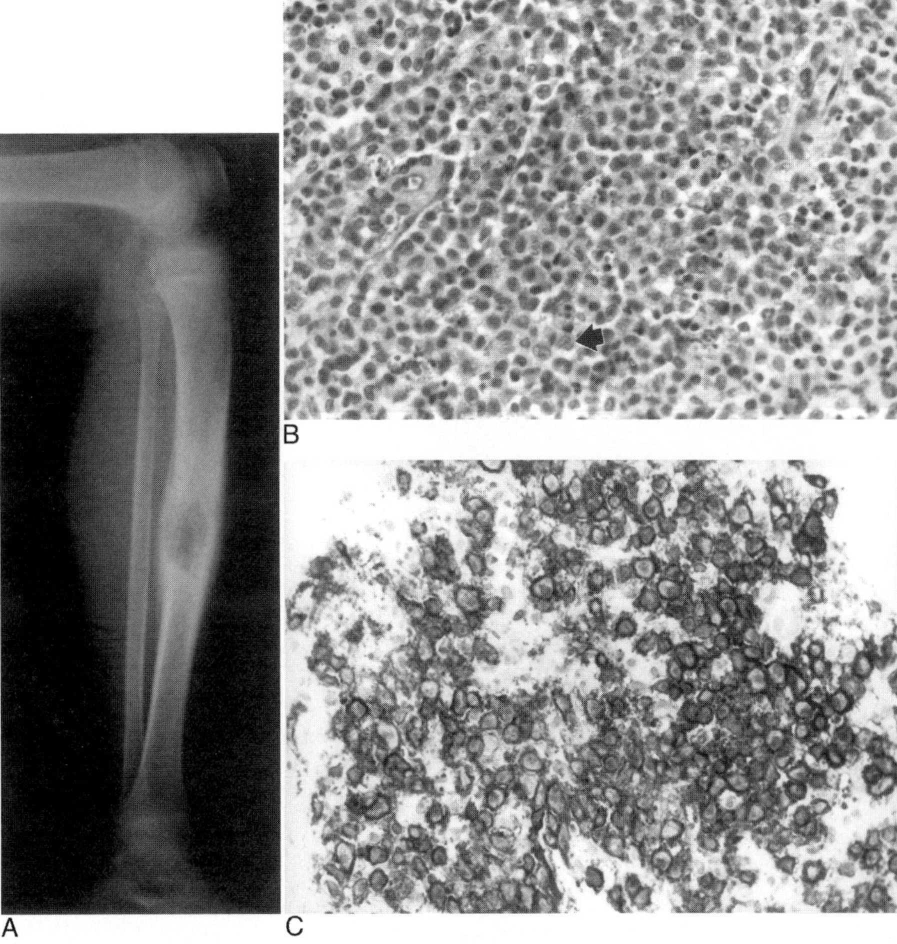

Figure 11-29 Langerhans cell histiocytosis. A, Lateral radiograph of the leg shows a cluster of lytic lesions in the diaphysis of the tibia associated with extensive sclerosis. The lesions have sharply defined borders. There is, however, destruction of the cortex, both anteriorly and posteriorly. Thick periosteal new bone formation bridges the areas of destruction and extends along the diaphysis. **B,** Photomicrograph of the lesion shows sheets of Langerhans cells, many with characteristic deep nuclear clefts (*arrow*) and nuclear grooves. Smaller, darkly staining cells are eosinophils. **C,** Photomicrograph of a CD1a immunohistochemical preparation demonstrates crisp cell membrane positivity.

Radiographically, Ewing sarcoma demonstrates diffuse permeative, destructive bone lesions, usually developing in the diaphyseal regions of long bones or in flat bones of the axial skeleton (Fig. 11-31A).[8-10] The lesion usually is associated with a lamellated periosteal new bone formation that has an onion-skin appearance or, less commonly, a sunburst type of periosteal reaction, and a large soft tissue mass. On radionuclide bone scan, Ewing sarcoma shows a highly increased uptake (Fig. 11-31B); this modality provides reliable information about the presence or absence of skeletal metastases. MRI is essential for definite demonstration of the extent of the bone marrow spread and soft tissue involvement by the tumor (Fig. 11-31C and D). Radiographic staging of the local and metastatic disease should be performed before biopsy. In addition, bone marrow sampling (aspirates and biopsy specimens from two sites) should be performed at the time of biopsy for suspected Ewing sarcomas.

Histologically, Ewing sarcoma consists of small, uniformly sized cells characterized by an almost clear cytoplasm and nuclei that are round and slightly hyperchromatic (see Box 11-4; Fig. 11-31E).[9,10] Prominent septa composed of fibrous connective tissue divide the tumor tissue into strands and lobules. Areas of necrosis and hemorrhage are often observed. There are glycogen granules in the cytoplasm, and these are usually present in enough abundance to produce a positive periodic acid–Schiff (PAS) diastase sensitive stain on routine histology. With immunohistochemistry, Ewing sarcomas typically have a strong perimembranous staining pattern with MIC-2 (CD99).

Ewing sarcoma is typically sensitive to both chemotherapy and radiotherapy.[14] Multiagent chemotherapy has made a significant difference in the prognosis of Ewing sarcoma, improving the 5-year survival rate from 5% to 10% to more than 70%. The chemotherapeutic agents most widely used are vincristine, cyclophosphamide, doxorubicin, ifosfamide, and etoposide. As long-term survival has increased, the importance of local control has become better appreciated. Radiation therapy is still an important modality in treating Ewing sarcoma locally. Unfortunately, the modality is associated with a number of complications, such as radiation-induced malignancies, especially in children given higher doses. For nonmetastatic Ewing sarcoma, surgical excision and chemotherapy constitute the mainstay of local control.

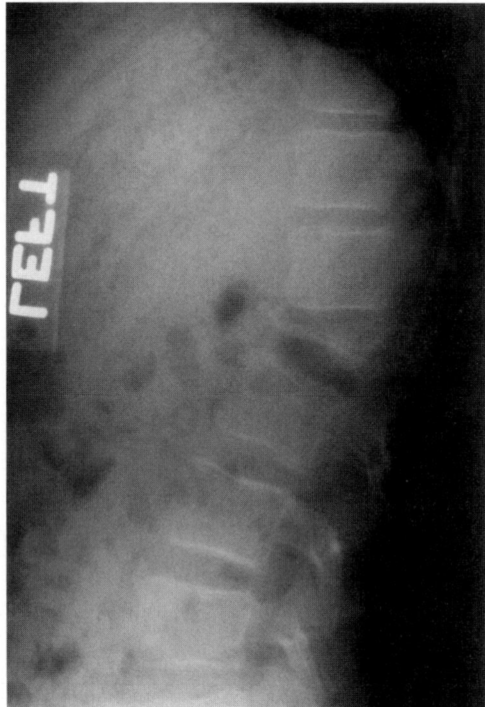

Figure 11-30 Langerhans cell histiocytosis. Lateral radiograph of the spine shows complete collapse of the first lumbar vertebral body that results in kyphosis. Note the preservation of the disk spaces.

After the diagnosis is confirmed with biopsy, a patient with Ewing sarcoma should first receive neoadjuvant chemotherapy, which will reduce the soft tissue component of the lesion dramatically in most cases. After neoadjuvant chemotherapy, surgical excision should be considered when possible. Surgical excision involves removal of the tumor with wide surgical margins. Limb salvage surgery is possible in majority of patients. If the margins are close and viable tumor is present in the resected specimen, postoperative irradiation is recommended. The prognosis is still poor for patients with metastatic Ewing sarcoma.

Musculoskeletal Manifestations of Leukemia

Acute leukemia is the most common cancer in childhood. Acute lymphoblastic leukemia represents 80% of cases and has a peak incidence at 2 to 5 years, with a male preponderance (Table 11-4). Leukemic involvement of bones and joints is common in patients with acute lymphoblastic leukemia. Bone or joint pain is the most common presenting symptom in majority of patients (Box 11-5). Leukemic involvement of bone should be suspected in a child with bone pain who also has cytopenia, fever, bleeding manifestations, hepatosplenomegaly, or lymphadenopathy. A diffuse osteopenia of the skeleton is frequently detected in children with acute leukemia. Common radiographic changes include lytic lesions in the medullary cavity or cortex, radiolucent metaphyseal bands ("leukemia lines"), and periosteal new bone formation (see Box 11-5; Fig. 11-32A).[21] The diagnosis should be made if typical leukemic blasts are found in an aspiration specimen of bone marrow (Fig. 11-32B). Treatment involves prolonged multiagent chemotherapy, with overall survival rates approaching 70% for children with acute lymphoblastic leukemia.

Table 11-4 Types and Distribution (%) of Acute Pediatric Leukemia

Type	%
Acute lymphoblastic leukemia (ALL)	80%
Acute myelogenous leukemia (AML)	18%
Chronic myelogenous leukemia (CML)	2%

Box 11-5 Musculoskeletal Manifestations of Leukemia

Clinical
- Musculoskeletal pain
  - Bone pain: intermittent, localized, sharp, severe, and sudden in onset
  - Joint pain: migratory

Radiographic
- Diffuse osteopenia: alterations in protein and mineral metabolism
- Radiolucent metaphyseal bands (generally is the first radiographic abnormality): diminished osteogenesis of the epiphyseal growth plate
- Periosteal bone formation: leukemic infiltrate lifts the periosteum from the cortex of the bone
- Osteolytic lesions: leukemic infiltration of the bone marrow, local hemorrhage, and osteonecrosis of adjacent trabecular bone
- Osteosclerosis: late manifestation
- Mixed lesions: simultaneous production of bone by osteoblasts at one site and increased osteoclastic activity at another site
- Permeative pattern: indicates an aggressive lesion with rapid growth
- Pathologic fracture: most commonly associated with osteoporosis of the spine; also occurs at other locations after minor trauma

Lymphoma of Bone

Bone lymphomas are typically non-Hodgkin large cell lymphomas or, occasionally, lymphoblastic lymphomas.

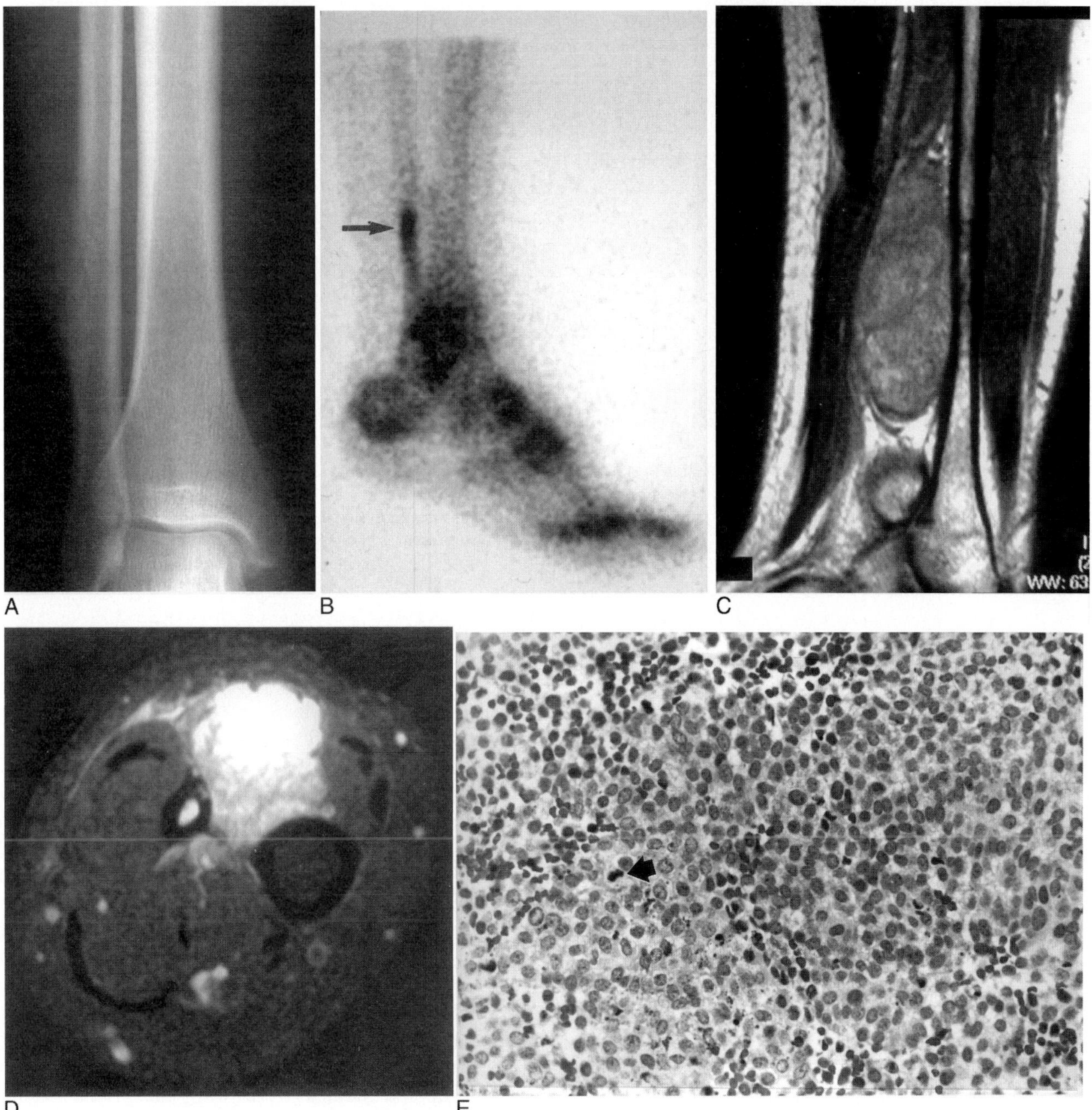

Figure 11-31 Ewing sarcoma. A, Anteroposterior radiograph of the lower leg shows a "moth-eaten" pattern of bone destruction within a fusiform area of cortical thickening in the distal fibular diaphysis. An ill-defined layer of new bone formation is present. **B,** Radionuclide bone scan shows the increased uptake localized to the site of the lesion *(arrow)*. **C,** On a coronal T1-weighted magnetic resonance image, heterogenous signal can be seen within the marrow of the distal fibula. The extraosseous component of the lesion has well-circumscribed borders. **D,** An axial T2-weighted image shows a high-signal-intensity mass in the anterior compartment of the leg. The tumor extends across the interosseous membrane into the posterior compartment and laterally along the fascia. Note the high signal in the medullary cavity of the fibula and the cortex. **E,** Photomicrograph of the lesion demonstrates monotonous sheets of small round cells with scattered mitoses *(arrow)* and ill-defined cytoplasm.

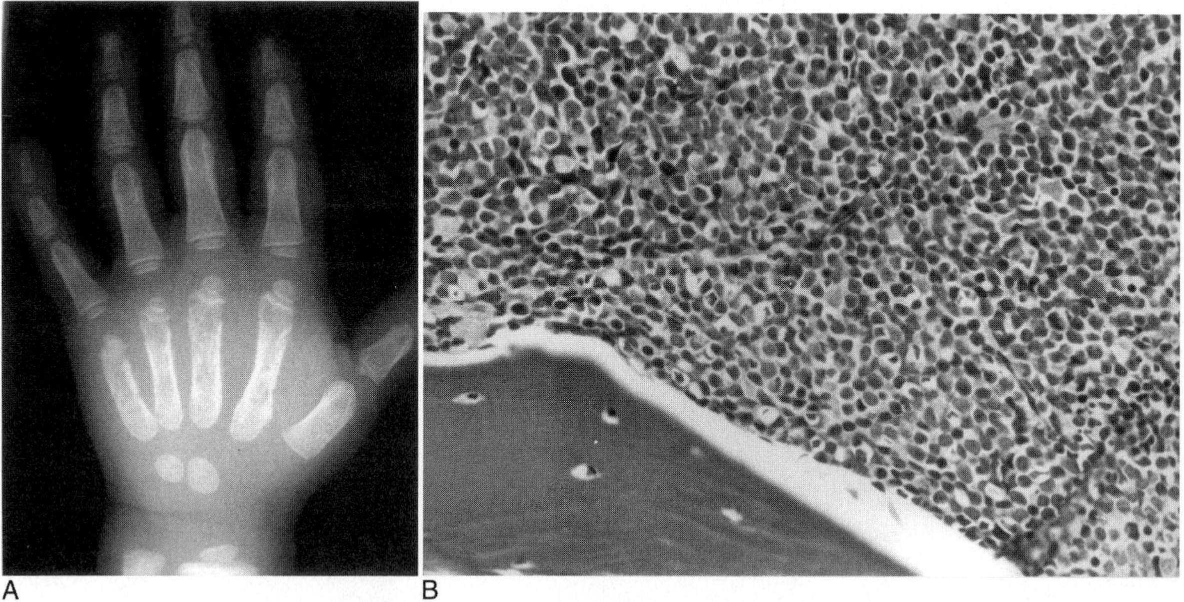

Figure 11-32 Musculoskeletal manifestations of leukemia. A, Anteroposterior radiograph of the hand shows a "moth-eaten" pattern of bone destruction and a single layer of periosteal new bone formation in all the metacarpals except the first. Also note the lucent metaphyseal bands in the distal radius and ulna. **B,** Photomicrograph demonstrates features of high cellularity and inconspicuous cytoplasmic borders.

They manifest most commonly in adults, but bone lymphomas have been reported as occurring in the second decade of life. Bone lymphomas usually occur in femur and pelvis, and manifest as pain and swelling.[9,10] Systemic signs and symptoms, such as fever, weight loss, anemia, and elevated erythrocyte sedimentation rate, may be present. Radiographically, the lesions commonly are extensive, involving a large portion of the affected bone. Bone destruction is a predominant feature and can be shown effectively on CT (Fig. 11-33A). MRI is valuable for establishing the soft tissue and bone marrow involvement. Bone lymphomas may be clinically and radiographically indistinguishable from Ewing sarcomas. Histologically, they are composed of large blastic cells that are either round or pleomorphic (see Box 11-4; Fig. 11-33B). An extensive staging evaluation should be performed at the initial presentation of the patient. Treatment is primarily determined by the extent of the primary tumor and the presence or absence of metastases to the bone marrow or cerebrospinal fluid. Treatment for bone lymphomas consists of multiagent chemotherapy.

Metastatic Tumors of Bone

Neuroblastoma

Neuroblastoma is the most common extracranial solid tumor of childhood, accounting for 10% to 20% of childhood cancers. It typically affects children younger than 5 years, with a peak incidence around 2 years of age. Neuroblastoma usually manifests as a mass lesion along the sympathetic nervous chain. The most common anatomic site is the abdomen, in the adrenal gland or in a paraspinal ganglion, followed by paraspinal tumors in the chest, neck, and pelvis. Bone metastases, usually multiple, are more common in older children and may be heralded by bone pain, limp, or refusal to put weight on a limb. Children with vertebral compression fractures and spinal cord compression due to paraspinal tumors may present with severe back pain or neurologic symptoms. Metastatic bone lesions of neuroblastoma may be detected on plain films or bone scans (Fig. 11-34). Metastatic neuroblastomas are treated with systemic chemotherapy, surgical excision of the primary tumor, radiation therapy to areas of bulk disease, and very-high-dose ablative chemotherapy with bone marrow rescue. Despite such intense treatment, to which most cases temporarily respond, the prognosis for patients with neuroblastoma is poor.

Retinoblastoma

Retinoblastoma is the most common ocular tumor of childhood. It may spread hematogenously to the bones and bone marrow. Multiple bony metastases may be present and are usually associated with bone pain and local tenderness. Because it is distinctly unusual to find

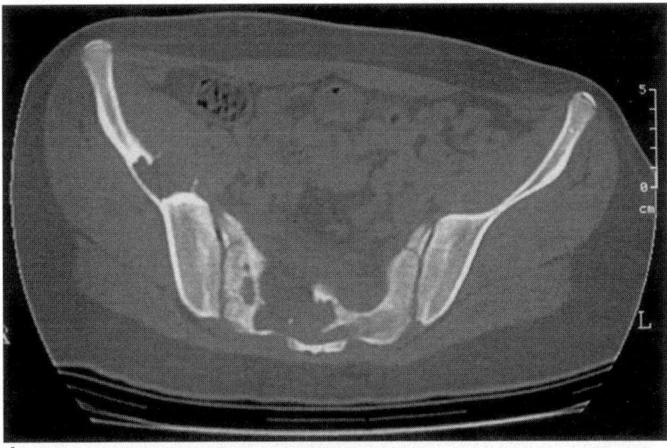

A

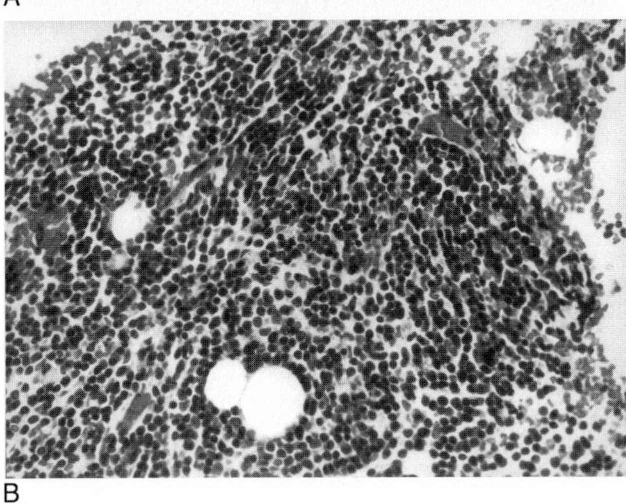

B

Figure 11-33 Lymphoma of bone. A, Axial computed tomography scan of the pelvis (at the third sacral segment) shows the destructive lesions and a mottled appearance of the adjacent bone. **B,** Photomicrograph of the lesion demonstrates densely arranged, large pleomorphic cells with roundish nuclei.

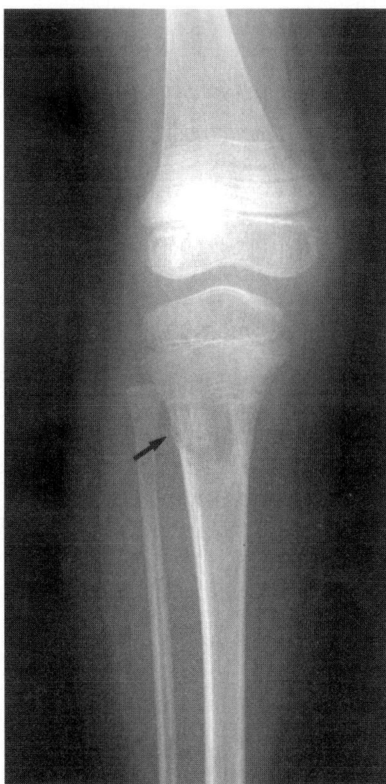

Figure 11-34 Metastatic neuroblastoma. Anteroposterior radiograph of the knee shows a geographic pattern of bone destruction in the proximal tibia. Severe, diffuse osteopenia affects all the bones. A cortical disruption *(arrow)* represents a pathologic fracture. Note the multiple dense bands representing lines of growth recovery during periods of healing.

bone metastases in patients with this disease without concomitant invasion of the bone marrow, bone marrow sampling should be undertaken first in the evaluation of possible metastasis in patients with retinoblastoma. Primary retinoblastoma is chemosensitive and radiosensitive, but the outcome for patients with metastatic disease is poor.

It is notable that osteosarcomas occur very commonly in patients with retinoblastoma. Osteosarcomas in these patients, as well as spontaneous osteosarcomas, carry mutations or deletions of the RB1 gene (see earlier discussion of etiology and molecular genetics).

Hepatoblastoma

Hepatoblastoma, an unusual liver tumor of childhood, typically manifests as an asymptomatic abdominal mass. Occasionally, however, affected children present with severe osteopenia, pathologic fractures in long bones and compression fractures of the vertebrae.

SPECIFIC SOFT TISSUE TUMORS

The majority of soft tissue tumors in children are benign. Soft tissue sarcomas represent only 7% of all malignancies in children younger than 15 years. Over a year, approximately 600 cases of soft tissue sarcomas are newly diagnosed in children younger than 15 years in the United States. Pediatric soft tissue sarcomas are slightly more common than pediatric bone tumors (8.9 versus 7.7 per 1 million population) and occur with a slightly higher incidence in younger patients (younger than 10 years versus older than 10 years) regardless of gender or race. Rhabdomyosarcomas account for 45% to 50% of all soft tissue sarcomas in children. Synovial sarcomas, fibrosarcomas, and malignant peripheric nerve sheath tumors are the other common malignant soft tissue tumors of childhood.

Vascular Tumors

Hemangioma

Hemangiomas are true neoplastic lesions with endothelial hyperplasia. They are the most common benign soft tissue tumors of childhood, occurring in 4% to 10% of all children. Hemangiomas are infrequently present at birth but grow rapidly during the first 2 to 3 weeks after birth.[7] They occur more commonly in males, at a ratio between 3:1 and 5:1. Hemangiomas may be located in the superficial or deep dermis, subcutaneous tissue, musculature, bone, or viscera. The head and neck are the most commonly involved sites. Superficial hemangioma manifests as a bright red lesion that can be macular (like a port-wine stain) or raised and bosselated, whereas deep hemangioma may appear as only a soft tissue mass. The natural history of hemangiomas is pathognomonic and has three distinct phases, referred to as proliferation, involution, and involuted.[22]

When physical examination and natural history are not enough, ultrasonography, CT, and MRI are all suitable imaging modalities for assessment of hemangiomas. On T1-weighted magnetic resonance images, hemangiomas have a low to intermediate signal intensity often similar to that of surrounding muscle (Fig. 11-35A). On T2-weighted images, they appear as areas of very high intensity signal (Fig. 11-35B). Histologically, a proliferating hemangioma demonstrates rapidly dividing endothelial cells with hyperchromatic nuclei and abundant cytoplasm, but lacking atypical mitoses. (Fig. 11-36) The long involution phase is characterized by dilation of the vascular lumen and flattened endothelial cells with reduced mitotic activity.

Most clinical studies show that 75% to 95% of hemangiomas resolve by age 7, and improvement is possible until age 10 to 12. Some lesions, however, do require intervention. Treatment involves steroid therapy, which is thought to accelerate the involution, as well as chemotherapy, embolic therapy, radiotherapy; and surgical intervention. Laser treatment to reduce proliferating cutaneous hemangiomas has gained favor.

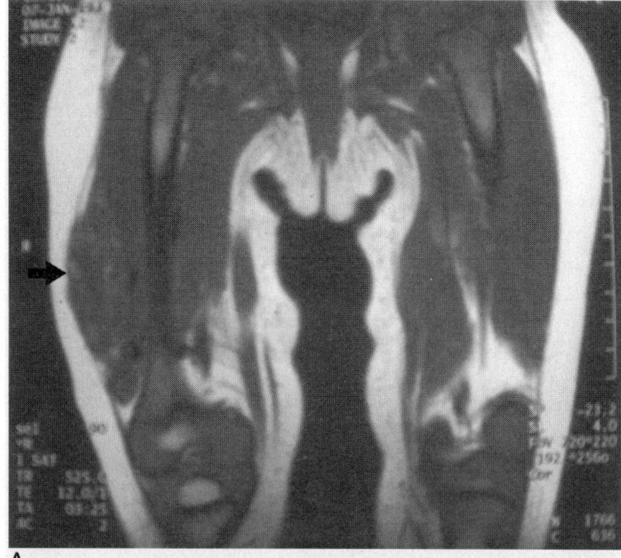
A

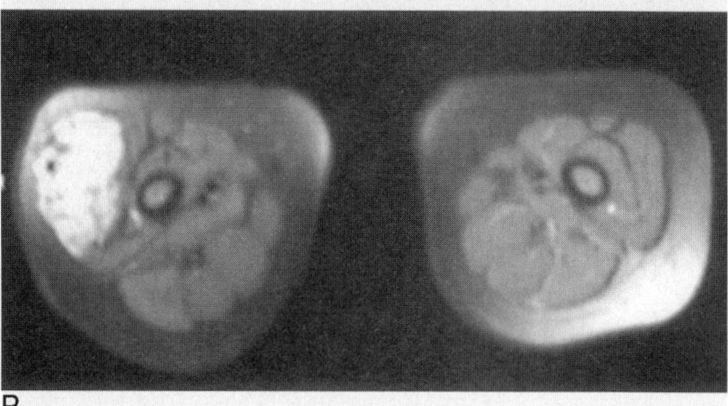
B

Figure 11-35 Hemangioma. A, On a coronal T1-weighted magnetic resonance image of the thighs, a mass is shown in the lateral soft tissues of the right thigh *(arrow)*. It has the same signal intensity as muscle. The slight heterogeneity and bulging of the muscle planes are the only clues to the presence of the mass. **B,** An axial T2-weighted image shows the large, lobulated, high-signal soft tissue mass in the vastus lateralis muscle. Low-signal septations are scattered throughout the mass.

Vascular Malformations

The second category of vascular anomalies is vascular malformations, which are congenital lesions with normal endothelial turnover. Many of the common vascular malformations manifest at birth, but some may appear in adolescence or adulthood. These lesions grow commensurate with the child. Boys and girls are equally affected. The majority of vascular malformations involve the skin and subcutaneous tissue, but extensive involvement of structures such as muscle, joint, bone, abdominal viscera, and central nervous system is not uncommon. The most commonly affected sites are the head and neck. Vascular malformations may be subdivided into several forms—capillary, venous, arterial, and lymphatic[7,23]—but also may be mixtures of those categories.

MRI is an excellent modality for confirming the nature of the vascular malformations and defining their relationship to adjacent structures.[22] MRI findings in vascular malformation vary with the form of the lesion; arteriovenous malformations have low signal intensity on both T1- and T2-weighted images, whereas venous and lymphatic malformations have low signal intensity on T1-weighted images and high signal intensity on T2-weighted images (Fig. 11-37). Ultrasonography or color Doppler ultrasonography may also be used to evaluate vascular malformations. Angiography is still helpful in patients requiring surgical intervention or preoperative embolization.

Vascular malformations do not improve with time like hemangiomas, and they usually require treatment. Use of compression stockings is the mainstay of treatment for venous malformations, and low-dose aspirin may also be used to minimize thrombophlebitis. Asymptomatic arteriovenous malformations are treated conservatively, whereas symptomatic lesions are treated with selective

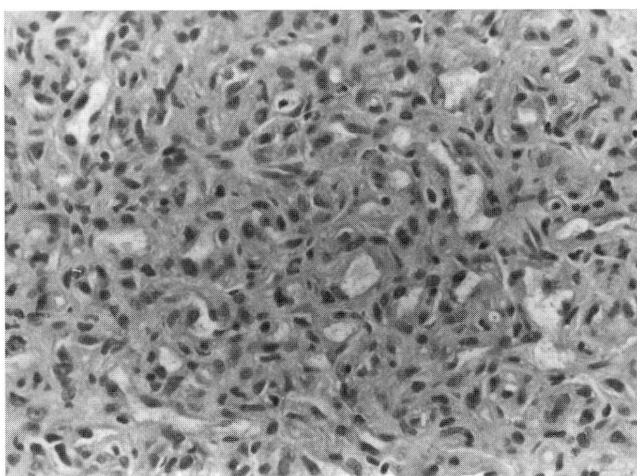

Figure 11-36 Histopathology of hemangioma. Photomicrograph of this juvenile capillary hemangioma shows small capillary channels that are scattered throughout a background of compressed, plump endothelial cells.

embolization followed by surgical resection. Capillary malformations are best treated with pulsed yellow-dye laser therapy under the care of a plastic surgeon or dermatologist.

Associated Syndromes

Vascular malformations may be part of several rare syndromes. Maffucci syndrome is a premalignant condition involving venous vascular malformations and enchondromas. The vascular lesions are often present at birth, and enchondromas develop later. This syndrome often occurs in the subcutaneous tissue and bones of the limbs. The cartilage tumors have a high risk of malignant transformation to chondrosarcomas.

Angiomatosis is a vascular syndrome that usually involves multiple tissue types (e.g., subcutis, muscle, bone). Generally, angiomatomas grow commensurately with the child. The characteristics of angiomatosis are haphazard proliferation of small or medium-sized blood vessels that diffusely infiltrate the skin, muscle, or bone. Treatment options include compression stockings, laser ablation, embolization, electrocautery, irradiation, local or systemic steroids, antiangiogenic therapies, and surgery.

Tumors of Nerve Origin

Neurolemmoma

The neurolemmoma, also referred to as *schwannoma*, is a benign, usually encapsulated neoplasm derived from Schwann cells. Neurofibroma and neurolemmoma are the most common peripheral nerve sheath tumors. Neurolemmoma commonly occurs in early adulthood, with no sex predilection. The tumor has a predilection for the head, neck, and flexor surfaces of the extremities. It usually manifests as a painless, slowly growing, solitary mass in the subcutaneous tissue.

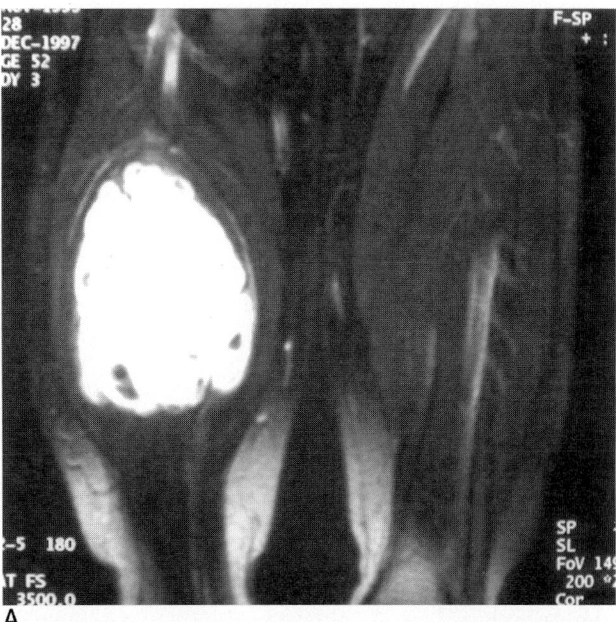

A

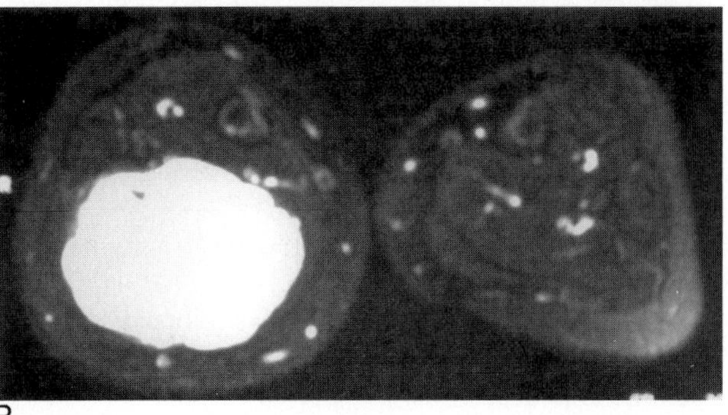

B

Figure 11-37 Vascular malformation (venous malformation). A, A sagittal T2-weighted magnetic resonance image of the lower legs shows a large, lobulated, high-signal mass in the right calf. The areas of low signal intensity represent blood products due to hemorrhage in the mass. **B,** An axial T2-weighted image demonstrates the displacement of the muscles of the posterior compartment by this large soft tissue mass.

Neurologic symptoms are uncommon unless the tumor becomes large. Neurolemmomas are rarely associated with neurofibromatosis, and they do not have a significant malignant potential.

In general, benign neural tumors appear as well-circumscribed, round or ovoid masses on MRI. Neurolemmoma is a mass of low or intermediate signal intensity on T1-weighted images and highly intense signal on T2-weighted images. The lesions are usually located in intramuscular planes, sometimes in association with a large peripheral nerve. Histologically, the neurolemmoma is a nodular mass surrounded by a well-defined fibrous capsule consisting of epineurium and residual nerve fibers. There are two distinct alternating groups of cells within the lesion, termed Antoni A and Antoni B areas. The relative amounts of these two

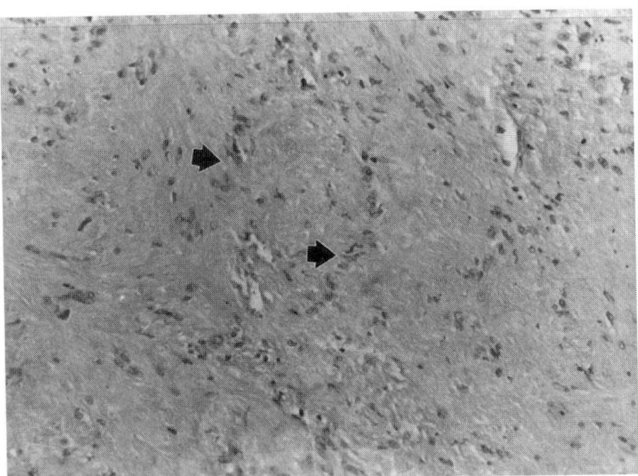

Figure 11-38 Histopathology of neurolemmoma. *Arrows* point to the Antoni A areas with compact spindle cells. The nuclei are stacked, giving the palisaded appearance with formation of Verocay bodies.

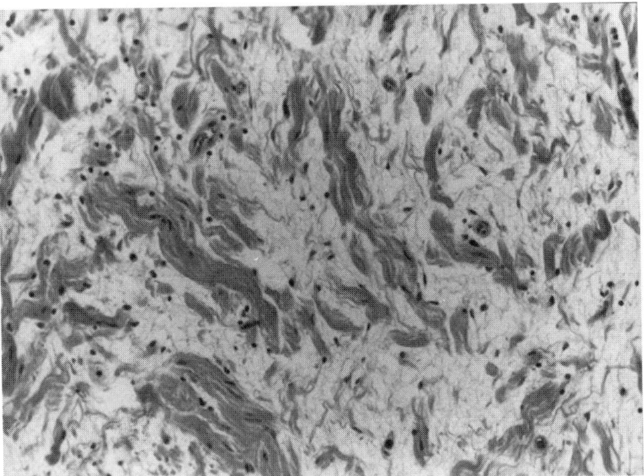

Figure 11-39 Histopathology of neurofibroma. High-power photomicrograph of the lesion demonstrates elongated, wavy spindle cells and bundled collagen fibers (so-called shredded carrot appearance). Smaller, dark-staining cells are mast cells.

components vary. The Antoni A area is highly cellular and composed of compact spindle cells (Fig. 11-38); the nuclei are stacked, giving the lesion a palisaded appearance with formation of numerous Verocay bodies. The Antoni B area is composed of myxomatous tissue with less cellularity.[23]

Symptomatic lesions are treated with marginal excision without sacrifice of the affected nerve. The tumor can be separated from the nerve easily, because it does not invade the nerve itself. Recurrence after surgical excision is unusual.

Neurofibroma

Neurofibroma may arise as a solitary lesion or multiple lesions. Solitary lesions account about 90% of neurofibromas. Most solitary neurofibromas develop in patients between 20 and 30 years old, and the tumor affects the sexes equally. Neurofibroma grows slowly as a painless mass in the skin, subcutaneous tissue, or the distribution of a peripheral nerve. Solitary neurofibromas are not associated with neurofibromatosis, and they have little malignant potential.

Like other benign peripheral nerve sheath tumors, neurofibromas typically manifest as lesions of low to intermediate signal on T1-weighted magnetic resonance images. A characteristic "target" appearance on T2-weighted images has been described, consisting of a peripheral area of high signal intensity surrounding a central core of low signal intensity. This appearance has also been described for neurolemmomas, to a lesser degree. The malignant nerve sheath tumors almost never demonstrate this target sign. Histologically, unlike neurolemmomas, neurofibromas are not encapsulated and they do invade the nerve fibers. They contain interlacing bundles of elongated cells with wavy, dark-staining nuclei (Fig. 11-39). Neurites are usually seen within the lesion. Surgical excision is recommended for symptomatic solitary neurofibromas involving a peripheral nerve. Those arising from a major nerve can be resected, but with caution.[7,24]

Neurofibromatosis

Neurofibromatosis is a multisystem disease that primarily affects cellular growth of neural tissue. The disease is usually evident within the first few years of life. Multiple neurofibromas typically occur in the majority of patients with neurofibromatosis type I. These patients have a significant potential for morbidity and mortality because of the possibility (5% to 10%) of development of sarcomatous degeneration in a neurofibroma. Therefore, patients and parents should be very careful in following the changes in size of lesions. Surgery is reserved for lesions that demonstrate significant enlargement or suspected sarcomatous degeneration or cause pain. If sarcomatous degeneration occurs, the prognosis for long-term survival is poor.

Malignant Peripheral Nerve Sheath Tumors

Malignant peripheral nerve sheath tumors, or *neurofibrosarcomas*, are uncommon in children and adolescents. They account about 5% of pediatric soft tissue sarcomas. The majority occurs after the age of 10 years, with an equal sex distribution. Neurofibrosarcomas may arise in a preexisting neurofibroma or de novo in the subcutaneous or deep soft tissues of the extremities or trunk. An enlarging soft tissue mass with pain or dysesthesia is the most common presentation in children.

CT scans demonstrate a bulky soft tissue mass that may have areas of necrosis or calcification. Although MRI findings in malignant and benign peripheral nerve sheath tumors are usually similar, neurofibrosarcomas may show variable intensities on both T1- and T2-weighted images, depending on the extent of intratumoral necrosis (Fig. 11-40A). The extent and aggressiveness of the tumor can be evaluated well with MRI.

Histologically, a nerve of origin and an associated neurofibroma can be identified in most cases. Focal hemorrhage, necrosis, and cystic changes are usually seen. The tumor displays interlacing fascicles of spindle cells, with pale, indistinct cytoplasm and elongated nuclei (Fig. 11-40B).[7,23] The differential diagnosis includes fibrosarcoma, leiomyosarcoma, malignant fibrous histiocytoma, synovial sarcoma, rhabdomyosarcoma, and malignant melanoma.

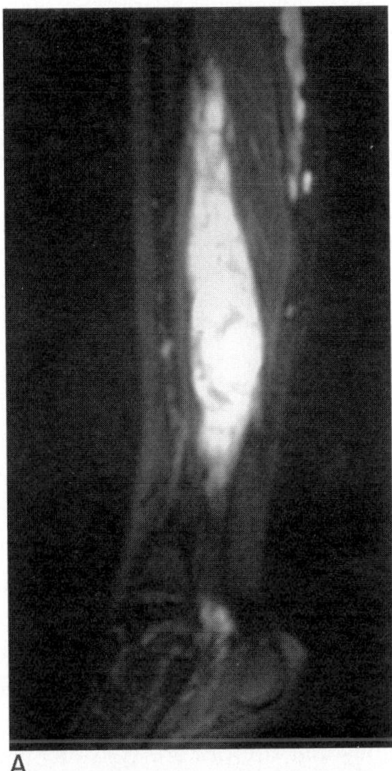

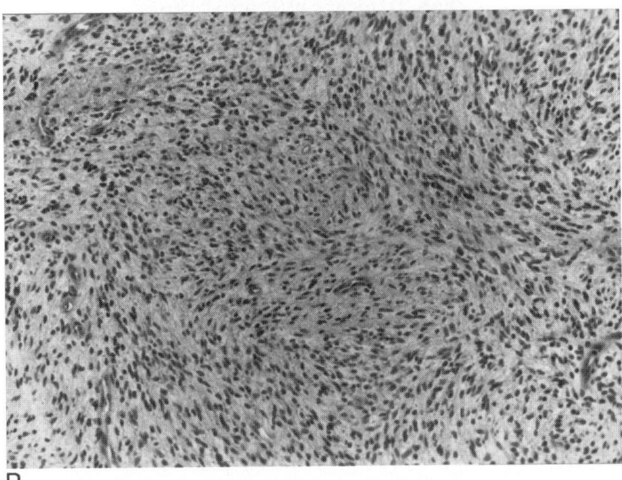

Figure 11-40 Malignant peripheral nerve sheath tumor. A, A sagittal T2-weighted magnetic resonance image of the leg shows fusiform, lobulated, elongated masses of high signal following the neurovascular bundles. **B,** Photomicrograph demonstrates a lesion composed of interlacing cellular spindle cell fascicles.

Wide excision with resection of the entire tumor bed is the mainstay of the treatment for neurofibrosarcomas.[7,13] Adjuvant radiation therapy is recommended regardless of the status of the surgical margins and appears to improve survival. The efficacy of adjuvant chemotherapy remains unproven.

Tumors of Fibrous Tissue Origin

Fibromatosis

The term *fibromatosis* refers a variety of benign fibrous lesions with different manifestations. Benign fibrous lesions, which are relatively common in children, are divided into two groups.[23] The first group consists of *aggressive fibromatosis* or *extra-abdominal desmoid*, which commonly affects children. The second, less common, group is that of fibrous lesions (e.g., fibrous hamartoma of infancy, infantile myofibromatosis) peculiar to infancy and childhood. Aggressive fibromatosis is the most common benign fibrous tumor seen in patients between puberty and 40 years of age. Males and females are affected with equal frequency. The principal location of the tumor is the musculature of the shoulder, followed by the chest wall, back, thigh, and mesentery. The most common presenting symptoms are mild pain and a slowly enlarging mass. The mass usually is deep, firm, and slightly tender.

On radionuclide bone scan, aggressive fibromatosis usually shows an increased uptake. The mass has a density similar to that of muscle on CT but is usually more vascular and can be distinguished best from the surrounding tissue by contrast-enhanced CT. The classic description of the MRI signal characteristics of aggressive fibromatosis is low signal intensity on both T1- and T2-weighted images. However, because the cellularity varies, fibromatosis may have an MRI appearance similar to that of any soft tissue neoplasia (Fig. 11-41A).

Histologically, aggressive fibromatosis looks like scar tissue. The tumor is poorly circumscribed and infiltrates the surrounding normal tissue. It consists of elongated spindle-shaped cells of uniform appearance within dense bundles of collagen (Fig. 11-41B). The nuclei are small, palely staining, and sharply defined.

Malignant transformation of the tumor is extremely rare, but the lesion may behave in a locally aggressive manner.[25] Wide resection should be the initial treatment of aggressive fibromatosis. However, complete local excision of the tumor is difficult because of its infiltrative nature. The local recurrence rate after surgical excision is high. A second wide resection is indicated for a recurrent lesion.

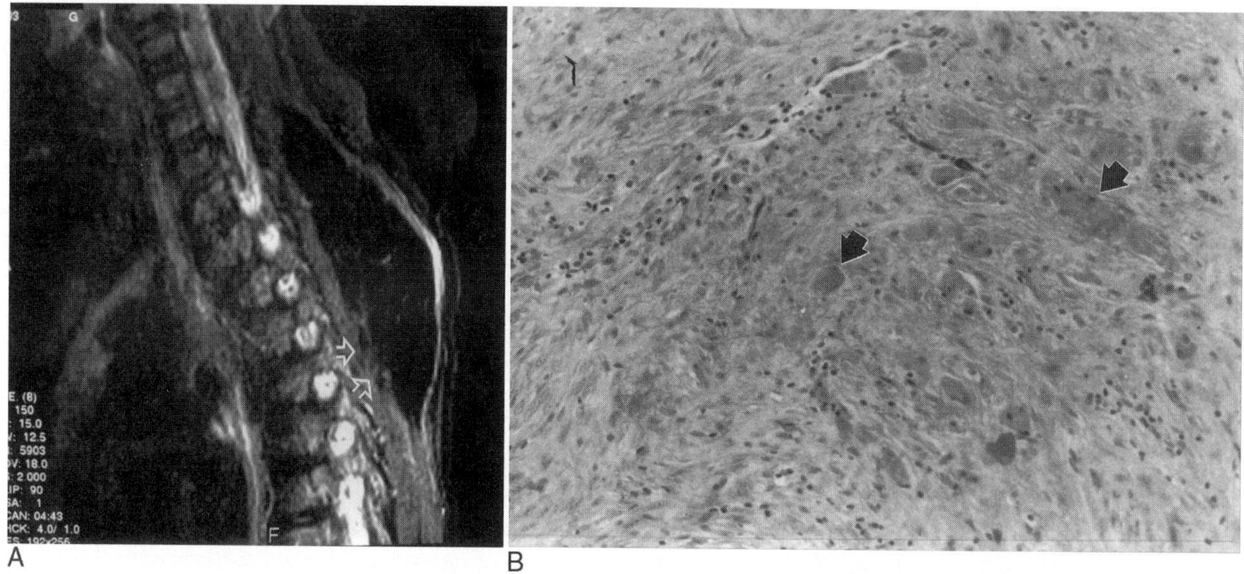

Figure 11-41 Aggressive fibromatosis. A, A sagittal T2-weighted magnetic resonance image of the base of the neck shows a large, fusiform, hypointense mass in the subcutaneous tissues. It is difficult to separate the inferior margin of the mass from the adjacent, higher-signal-intensity, paraspinal muscles *(arrows)*. **B,** Photomicrograph of the lesion demonstrates envelopment of normal skeletal muscle fibers *(arrows)* by fibroblasts and dense collagen.

Fibrosarcoma

Although most common in adults, fibrosarcoma does occur in children and adolescents. It represents approximately 10% of all pediatric soft tissue sarcomas. Twenty-five to 40% of fibrosarcomas in children are diagnosed during the first 5 years of life; they are referred to as "congenital-infantile fibrosarcoma."[7,23] A male preponderance has been noted in most series. The tumor may occur anywhere in the body where fibrous tissue is found. The distal portions of the extremities and the head and neck region are the most commonly involved sites. The lesion usually manifests as a solitary palpable mass that rarely measures more than 10 cm in greatest diameter. In general, the mass is slowly growing and may reach a large size before causing pain. The overlying skin is tense, shiny, and red and may be ulcerated.

Findings on CT and MRI are nonspecific, showing nonhomogenous masses varying from well-defined to very invasive. MRI is best for delineating the extent of the tumor. Fibrosarcomas usually exhibit low signal intensity on both T1- and T2-weighted images (Fig. 11-42A). Grossly, the tumor is lobulated and poorly circumscribed; compression of adjacent tissue gives the appearance of a pseudocapsule. Histologically, the lesion demonstrates a solid pattern of growth of spindle cells, with dense cellularity, prominent mitotic activity, and variable collagen formation (Fig. 11-42B). Although fibrosarcoma rarely metastasizes, its local behavior may be aggressive. The treatment of choice for fibrosarcoma is excision of the tumor with wide surgical margins.[7,13]

Tumor of Muscular Origin

Rhabdomyosarcoma

Rhabdomyosarcoma is the most common pediatric soft tissue sarcoma, with a peak incidence in children younger than 10 years. There are four histologic patterns—embryonal, botryoid, alveolar, and pleomorphic (Box 11-6).[23] Embryonal and alveolar types are more common. Embryonal tumors are typically found in children younger than 10 years and most often in the head and neck or the genitourinary tract. Alveolar rhabdomyosarcomas are more commonly found in teenagers, most often in the extremities and trunk. An extremity lesion usually manifests as a painless mass, whereas paravertebral tumors may cause back pain.

On MRI, rhabdomyosarcomas are often heterogenous masses, indicating the presence of blood or necrosis (Fig. 11-43A and B). Tumor margins are variable; they can be well-circumscribed or poorly defined and infiltrative. MRI provides important information about tumor extent,

Box 11-6 Histologic Subtypes of Rhabdomyosarcoma

Embryonal rhabdomyosarcoma
Botryoid-type rhabdomyosarcoma
Alveolar rhabdomyosarcoma
Pleomorphic rhabdomyosarcoma

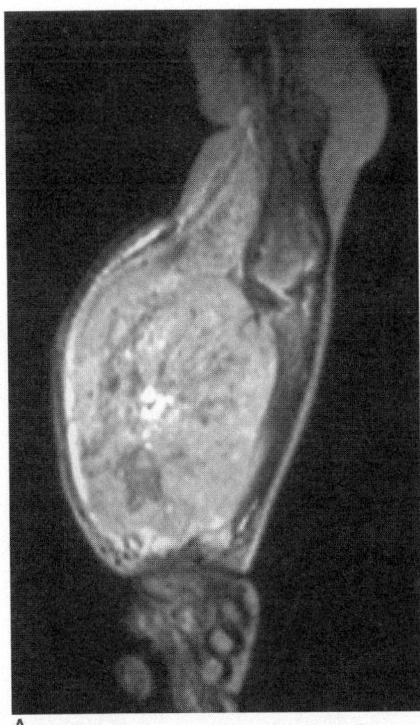

A

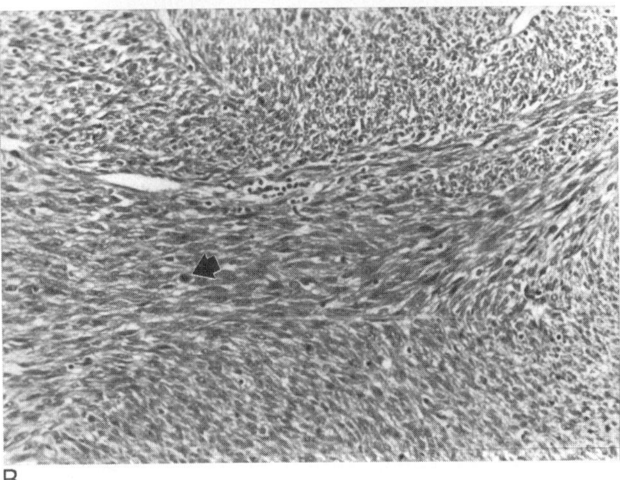

B

Figure 11-42 Infantile fibrosarcoma. A, A sagittal T2-weighted magnetic resonance image of the forearm shows a large, high-signal mass with central, radiating, linear areas of low signal, which represent fibrous tissue. **B,** Photomicrograph of this lesion demonstrates the characteristic "herringbone" pattern imposed by fascicles of malignant spindle cells. Mitotic activity *(arrow)* is brisk.

particularly the relationship of the tumor to bone and neurovascular structures, which is needed for treatment planning. After tumor resection, MRI is useful for monitoring recurrence of tumor and complications of treatment.

The histologic appearance of embryonal rhabdomyosarcoma can vary. It consists of poorly differentiated rhabdomyoblasts with a limited collagen matrix. The rhabdomyoblasts are small, round to oval cells with darkly staining nuclei and limited amounts of eosinophilic cytoplasm. Histologically, alveolar rhabdomyosarcoma is composed of poorly differentiated small, round to oval tumor cells that show central loss of cellular cohesion and formation of irregular alveolar spaces (Fig. 11-43C). The individual cellular aggregates are separated and surrounded by irregularly shaped fibrous trabeculae.

Prognostic variables for rhabdomyosarcomas include histologic subtype, size of the tumor, site of the tumor, and age of the patient. Alveolar subtype, larger tumors, patients older than 10 years, and location in an extremity are associated with a poorer prognosis. Alveolar rhabdomyosarcoma, like the other subtypes, is treated with a combination of chemotherapy and surgery. Irradiation can be used if total surgical resection cannot be achieved without excessive morbidity. Unlike for rhabdomyosarcomas at other sites, preoperative chemotherapy should be considered, because it often makes total resection of an extremity lesion possible. A wide surgical margin is recommended. The overall survival for a patient with extremity rhabdomyosarcoma is approximately 65%.[7,13]

Miscellaneous Lesions

Synovial Sarcoma

Synovial sarcoma is a well-known adult soft tissue sarcoma that occurs in teenagers and occasionally in younger children. Most patients are between 15 and 35 years old, and males are slightly more affected than females. Synovial sarcoma tends to occur in the lower extremities, especially around the knee and ankle joints. It occurs primarily in the para-articular regions, usually in close association with tendon sheaths, bursae, and joint capsules, but rarely within a joint.[7,23] The most common presentation is a palpable deep-seated swelling or mass that is associated with pain and tenderness. The lymph nodes should be examined carefully, because up to 25% of patients have metastases to regional lymph nodes.

Synovial sarcomas may have calcifications or ossifications within the tumor, which are often seen on plain radiographs. The CT scan shows a soft tissue mass, the calcified densities deep within it. Although the small foci of calcifications or ossifications are not seen as well with MRI as with CT, MRI is preferred over CT as the staging modality, as is true for all soft tissue sarcomas.

Grossly, the tumor appears to be well-encapsulated, with white areas of calcification on the cut surface. The classic histologic pattern is biphasic, consisting of epithelial cells and spindle cells (Fig. 11-44). Usually the spindle cell component predominates. The epithelioid foci contain glands with a central lumen lined by cuboidal or tall columnar cells in a spindle cell background.

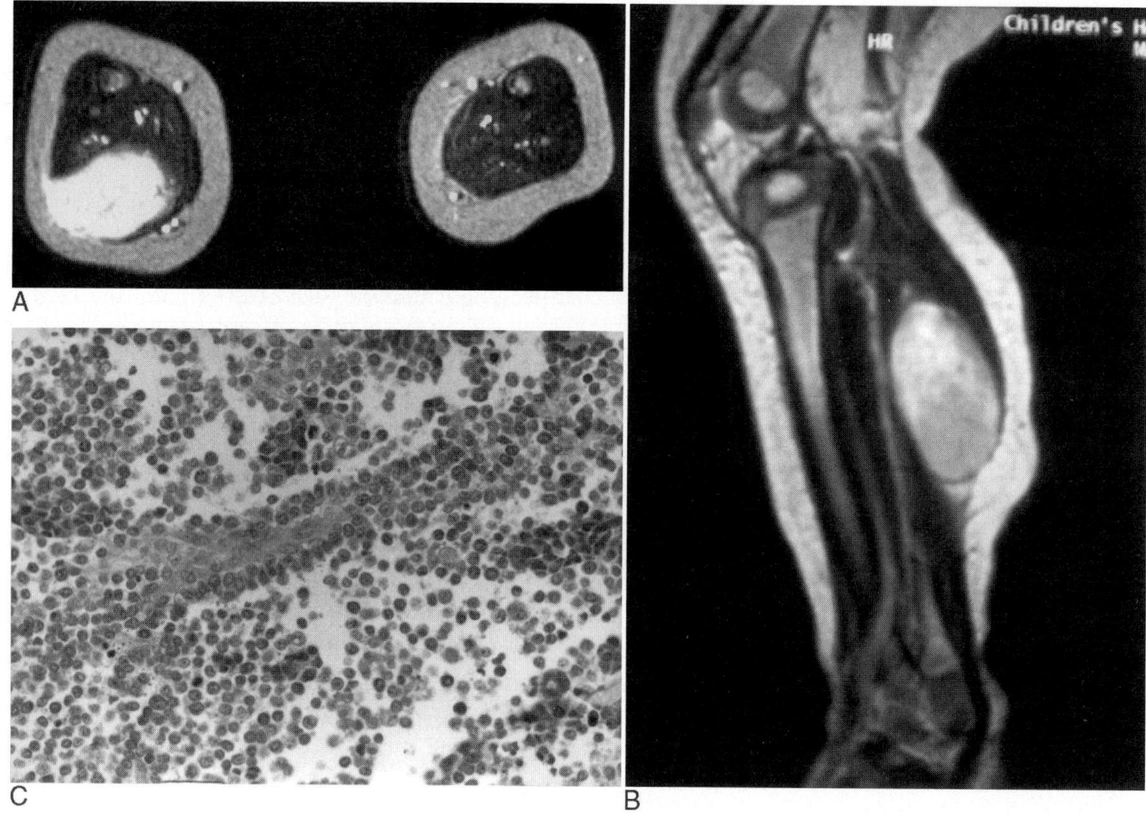

Figure 11-43 Alveolar rhabdomyosarcoma. **A,** An axial T2-weighted magnetic resonance image of the calf shows a high-signal mass replacing the lateral gastrocnemius muscle. The neurovascular bundles are well visualized separate from the mass. **B,** After the administration of intravenous contrast agent, enhancement of the mass is seen on the sagittal image. **C,** Photomicrograph of the lesion demonstrates undifferentiated small round cells with inconspicuous cytoplasm, which are discohesive and line fibrous septa.

The initial treatment of synovial sarcoma is wide local excision with limb salvage if possible, followed by adjuvant chemotherapy and irradiation.[7,13] In adults and older children with synovial sarcoma, as in those with other soft tissue sarcomas, preoperative radiotherapy is used in conjunction with nonradical surgery in an attempt to salvage more extremities.

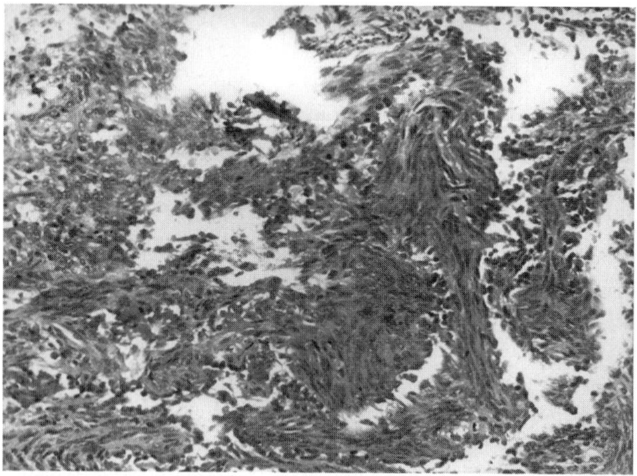

Figure 11-44 Histopathology of synovial sarcoma. Photomicrograph of this monophasic synovial sarcoma shows dense fascicles of atypical spindle cells. An epithelial component is not present in this field.

Primitive Neuroectodermal Tumors

Primitive neuroectodermal tumors (PNETs) refer to a family of soft tissue sarcomas with shared cytogenetic abnormalities involving chromosome 22 (see Table 11-3). PNETs are closely related to Ewing sarcoma; both have the same chromosomal translocation between chromosomes 11 and 22, similar presentations, identical treatments, and almost identical histologic characteristics.[13] PNETs and Ewing sarcoma are thought to arise from the neural crest. PNETs represent approximately 20% of all pediatric soft tissue sarcomas. They most commonly occur in the second decade with 70% to 80% of cases presenting at or before 20 years of age. There is a slight male predominance. The anatomic distribution of PNETs

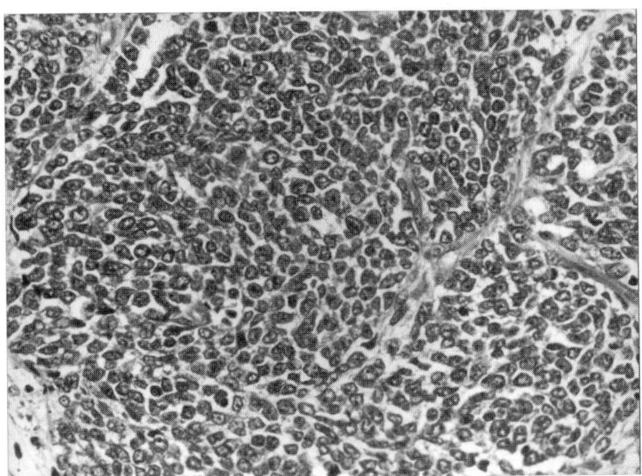

Figure 11-45 Histopathology of primitive neuroectodermal tumor (PNET). Photomicrograph of the lesion demonstrates sheets of small round cells with minimal cytoplasm and no discernible architecture.

shows a predilection for the trunk, especially the chest wall and paraspinal regions, followed by extremities, and head and neck. The lesions usually present as a painful mass. In addition to pain, nerve involvement may be accompanied by paraesthesia, weakness, or loss of function.

PNETs may become quite large, with a median diameter of 8.5 cm, and 40% of cases in excess of 10 cm. Grossly, PNETs may be circumscribed or infiltrative; they present as a multinodular or lobulated mass with alternating solid white areas and soft, partially hemorrhagic, cystic, and necrotic foci. Histologically, the tumors are composed of sheets or lobules of small rounded cells containing darkly staining, round or oval nuclei and minimal cytoplasm (Fig. 11-45; see Box 11-4). Immunohistochemically they demonstrate a strong perimembranous pattern with CD99 (MIC-2).

The clinical course of PNETs is highly aggressive. Tumors occurring along the central axis (head and neck, spine, pelvis) represent the greatest challenge for local control and overall survival. Some studies have indicated that the most effective treatment is surgery with combination chemotherapy and high-dose radiation therapy. As a general rule, PNETs receive chemotherapy protocols similar to those used for Ewing sarcoma.[13] Surgical excision should be performed with wide surgical margins. PNETs have a higher risk of local recurrences and bony metastases than other sarcomas.

Ganglion and Synovial Cysts

Ganglion

Ganglion, the most common soft tissue mass of the hand, is not uncommon in children. It is a superficially located, small (1 to 1.5 cm in diameter) cystic lesion that commonly appears on the dorsal surface of the wrist in young persons, especially women. Ganglion usually manifests as a firm, fluctuant mass associated with mild pain and tenderness. It is usually located adjacent to or attached to the joint capsule and tendon sheath, but the precise origins are not clear. Ultrasonography is helpful to demonstrate the cystic nature of the lesion. Grossly, ganglion is a firm, well-defined nodule composed of one or more mucoid cysts surrounded by a fibrous capsule. Histologically, the cyst typically has no cellular lining (Fig. 11-46). The peripheral zone consists of reactive fibroblasts and mucoid stroma. Treatment is indicated for symptomatic lesions. Various treatment methods are applied, including compression and bursting, aspiration and steroid injection, and surgical excision. Surgical excision is more effective, although up to 35% of ganglia recur after removal.

Synovial Cysts

The synovial cyst usually arises in the popliteal fossa; in this site it is called *popliteal cyst* or *Baker's cyst*. The lesion is more common in boys than girls and has a peak occurrence in children between 2 and 14 years old. The clinical presentation is a soft tissue swelling in the popliteal space (Fig. 11-47A). The cyst is firm to palpation. The diagnosis can be confirmed with transillumination, ultrasonography, or aspiration of gelatinous fluid from the cyst (Fig. 11-47B). MRI is helpful for diagnosis and differentiation of popliteal cyst from popliteal aneurysm, lipoma, pigmented villonodular synovitis, infection, and synovial sarcoma. Grossly, the cysts are 1.5 to 6.5 cm in diameter and filled with clear or white mucoid fluid. Histologic examination shows a single layer of flattened synovial cells lining the cystic space. A thick, densely fibrous capsule or more cellular connective tissue surrounds the cyst. Popliteal cysts may

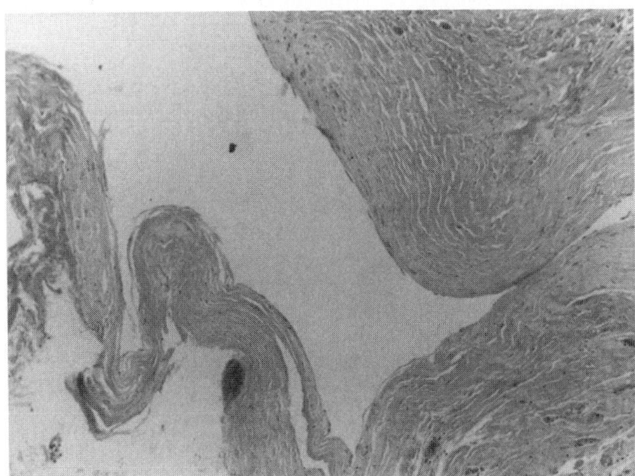

Figure 11-46 Histopathology of ganglion cyst. Photomicrograph demonstrates cystic spaces separated by fibrous stroma without lining epithelium.

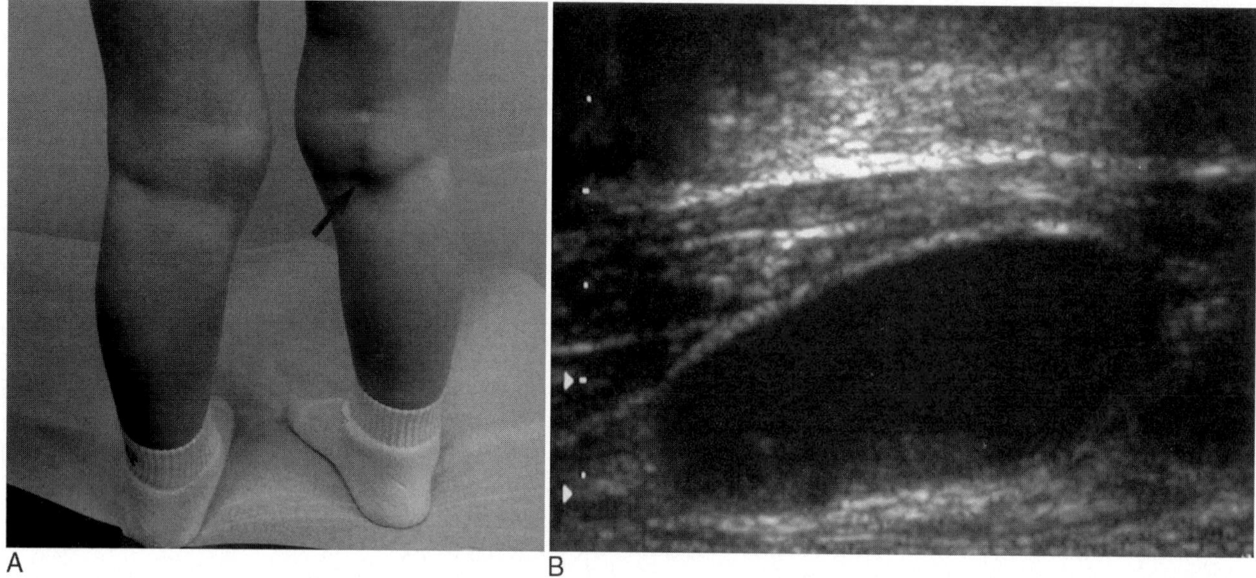

Figure 11-47 **Synovial cyst. A,** Photography of the legs of a 3-year-old boy with a synovial cyst in the right popliteal space (popliteal cyst) *(arrow)*. **B,** Ultrasonography of the region confirms the cystic nature of the lesion.

regress spontaneously. Surgical excision is indicated only for persistent and symptomatic lesions.[11]

SUMMARY

A wide range of musculoskeletal tumors occurs in the pediatric population. Physicians should be aware of the clinical and radiographic manifestations of these tumors in order to provide timely specialist referrals so that early diagnosis and treatment can be achieved. Improvements in diagnosis and treatment have increased survival for many children with malignant musculoskeletal tumors. New molecular genetic discoveries are providing insights into the mechanisms of tumorigenesis and may engender novel therapeutic modalities based on interference with aberrant transcriptional activation by hybrid transcripts.

MAJOR POINTS

The physician must remain alert because a malignant tumor of the musculoskeletal system is an unexpected event in children, and its frequency can result in improper or delayed initital management.

Good quality plain radiographs showing the entire lesion give the most detailed information in the evaluation of children with skeletal lesions.

It is useful to ask specific questions when evaluating plain radiographs of bony lesions: Where is the lesion located in the bone? What is the lesion doing to the bone? What is the bone doing to the lesion? What is the periosteal response?

The extent of many tumors can be best defined by MRI. MRI is the modality of choice for staging, for evaluating response to preoperative chemotherapy, and for long-term followup of bone and soft tissue sarcomas.

Staging of lesions that appear to be malignant is required prior to biopsy. Staging includes a whole body bone scan (or skeletal survey, particularly in very young children), a CT scan of the chest, and a MRI of the primary lesion.

A biopsy is best accomplished by the surgeon who would perform the definitive surgery if it becomes necessary.

The nidus of osteoid osteoma is best demonstrated with thin section (1-1.5 mm) computed tomography.

A growing osteochondroma after the patient has reached skeletal maturity, with a thick cartilaginous cap requires high suspicion for malignant transformation to chondrosarcoma.

Malignant transformation of enchondromas occurs predominantly in long or flat bones, and never in short tubular bones.

Large nonossifying fibromas (occupying more than 50% of the cross-sectional area of the bone involved) with a risk of pathologic fracture should be treated with curettage and grafting and, occasionally, with prophylactic internal fixation.

MAJOR POINTS—cont'd

- The presence of fluid-fluid levels and internal septations on MRI strongly suggests the diagnosis of aneurysmal bone cyst in children.
- Langerhans cell histiocytosis presenting as a single osseous lesion usually does not require treatment other than biopsy to confirm diagnosis. In the spine, no treatment is recommended unless a neurologic deficit is present.
- Children with Ewing sarcoma may present with generalized symptoms (e.g., fever, weight loss, malaise) and common laboratory findings (e.g., high white cell counts, elevated sedimentation rate), suggesting osteomyelitis as a differential diagnosis.
- Bone marrow sampling (aspirates and biopsies from two sites) should be performed at the time of biopsy for children with small round blue cell tumors, including suspected Ewing sarcoma.
- The essential component to the treatment of children with osteosarcoma and Ewing sarcoma is appropriate chemotherapy, including neoadjuvant chemotherapy, and surgical excision of the tumor with wide surgical margins.
- Leukemic involvement of bone should be suspected in a child with bone pain who also has cytopenia, fever, bleeding manifestations, hepatosplenomegaly, or lymphadenopathy.
- The majority of hemangiomas resolve by increasing age, however, vascular malformations do not get better with time and usually require treatment.
- Patients with neurofibromatosis type 1 are at risk of developing sarcomatous degeneration in one of their neurofibromas. Therefore, patients and parents should be very careful in following the changes in the size of lesions.
- Prognostic variables for rhabdomyosarcomas include histologic subtype, size of the tumor, site of the tumor, and age of the patient.
- PNETs are closely related to Ewing sarcoma; both have the same chromosomal translocation between chromosomes 11 and 22, similar presentations, similar treatments, and almost identical histologic characteristics.

REFERENCES

1. Enneking WF: Musculoskeletal tumor surgery. New York, Churchill Livingstone, 1983.
2. Madewell JE, Ragsdale BD, Sweet DE: Radiologic and pathologic analysis of solitary bone lesions. Part I: Internal margins. Radiol Clin North Am 19:715, 1981.
3. Ragsdale BD, Madewell JE, Sweet DE: Radiologic and pathologic analysis of solitary bone lesions. Part II: Periosteal reactions. Radiol Clin North Am 19:749, 1981.
4. Gillespy T III, Manfrini M, Ruggieri P, et al: Staging of intraosseous extent of osteosarcoma: Correlation of preoperative CT and MR imaging with pathologic macroslides. Radiology 167:765, 1988.
5. Simon MA, Biermann JS: Biopsy of bone and soft tissue lesions. J Bone Joint Surg Am 75:616, 1993.
6. Gebhardt MC: Molecular biology of sarcomas. Orthop Clin North Am 27:421, 1996.
7. Coffin CM, Dehner LP, O'Shea PA: Pediatric Soft Tissue Tumors: A Clinical, Pathological, and Therapeutic Approach Baltimore, Williams & Wilkins, 1997.
8. Huvos AG: Bone tumors: Diagnosis, Treatment and Prognosis, 2nd ed. Philadelphia, WB Saunders, 1991.
9. Unni KK: Dahlin's Bone Tumors: General Aspects and Data on 11,087 Cases, 5th ed. Philadelphia, Lippincott-Raven, 1996.
10. Greenspan A, Remagen W: Differential Diagnosis of Tumors and Tumor-Like Lesions of Bones And Joints. Philadelphia, Lippincott-Raven, 1998.
11. Copley L, Dormans JP: Benign pediatric bone tumors. Pediatr Clin North Am 43:949, 1996.
12. Dormans JP, Pill SG: Benign and malignant tumors of the spine in children. In Drummond DS (ed): Spine: State of the Art Reviews. Philadelphia, Hanley & Belfus, 2000.
13. Conrad III EU, Bradford L, Chansky HA: Pediatric soft-tissue sarcomas. Orthop Clin North Am 27:655, 1996.
14. Himelstein BP, Dormans JP: Malignant bone tumors of childhood. Pediatr Clin North Am 43:967, 1996.
15. Picci P, Sangiorgi L, Rougraff B, et al: Relationship of chemotherapy-induced necrosis and surgical margins to local recurrence in osteosarcoma. J Clin Oncol 12:2699, 1994.
16. Rougraff B, Simon M, Kneisl J, et al: Limb salvage compared with amputation for osteosarcoma of the distal end of the femur: A long term oncological, functional, and quality-of-life study. J Bone Joint Surg Am 76:649, 1994.
17. Schwartz HS, Zimmerman NB, Simon MA, et al: The malignant potential of enchondromatosis. J Bone Joint Surg Am 69:269, 1987.
18. Springfield DS, Rosenberg AE, Mankin HJ, et al: Relationship between osteofibrous dysplasia and adamantinoma. Clin Orthop 309:234, 1994.
19. Dormans JP, Flynn JM: Pathologic fractures associated with tumors and unique conditions of the musculoskeletal system. In Beaty JH, Kasser JR (eds): Rockwood and Wilkins' Fractures in Children, 5th ed. Philadelphia, Lippincott Williams & Wilkins, 2001.
20. Sullivan RJ, Meyer JS, Dormans JP, et al: Diagnosing aneurysmal and unicameral bone cysts with magnetic resonance imaging. Clin Orthop 366:186, 1999.

21. Gallagher DJ, Phillips DJ, Heinrich SD: Orthopaedic manifestations of acute pediatric leukemia. Orthop Clin North Am 27:635, 1996.

22. McCarron JA, Johnston DR, Hanna BG: Evaluation and treatment of musculoskeletal vascular anomalies in children: An update and summary for orthopaedic surgeons. The University of Pennsylvania Orthopaedic Journal 14:15, 2001.

23. Enzinger FM, Weiss SW: Soft Tissue Tumors, 3rd ed. St Louis, Mosby, 1995.

24. Smith JT, Yandow SM: Benign soft-tissue lesions in children. Orthop Clin North Am 27:645, 1996.

25. Spiegel DA, Dormans JP, Meyer JS, et al: Aggressive fibromatosis from infancy to adolescence. J Pediatr Orthop 19:776, 1999.

CHAPTER 12

Synovial Disorders

LISABETH V. SCALZI
JULIA E. LOU
RANDY Q. CRON

In the evaluation of synovitis, the physician must be able to compartmentalize in his or her own mind the various categories of presentations. Is the symptomatology acute or chronic? Does it occur after an infection or is it concurrent with an infection? Is it associated with another rheumatologic illness such as vasculitis, or is it consistent with the patient's previously known diagnoses (such as cystic fibrosis or glycogen storage disease)?

Chronic synovitis (duration equal to or greater than 6 weeks) is one of the criteria, according to the American College of Rheumatology, required to make the diagnosis of juvenile rheumatoid arthritis (JRA). Figure 12-1 summarizes the approach to the child with chronic arthritis. In this chapter, *acute synovitis* refers to any arthritis of less than 6 weeks' duration.

When gathering historical information from the patient and parents, the physician should direct questioning to elicit history that will aid in differentiating the acute causes of synovitis. Is there evidence of an active infectious synovitis? Are there fevers, sweats, chills, or a red-hot joint? Was there a preceding streptococcal throat infection? Could the illness be consistent with that of rheumatic fever or post-streptococcal synovitis? Did a viral illness precede the onset of a painful large-joint arthritis consistent with toxic synovitis? Does the patient have a history of a tick bite or live in an area endemic for Lyme disease? Are there other signs or symptoms that indicate Kawasaki syndrome or Henoch-Schönlein purpura? Are there systemic signs of vasculitis, such as severe abdominal pain and cutaneous lesions, that suggest polyarteritis nodosa? A few of the most common acute causes of synovitis, such as post-infectious and rheumatic fever, are discussed in this chapter, but there are many more not reviewed because of our limited scope.

Juvenile rheumatoid arthritis and juvenile spondyloarthropathies are the principal causes of chronic synovial disorders that rheumatologists see in the outpatient clinic setting. Thus, these disorders are the major topics of discussion in this chapter. Other common autoimmune diseases that may cause chronic arthritis, such as systemic lupus erythematosus (SLE) and juvenile dermatomyositis (JDM), are also discussed. The differential diagnosis of chronic and acute synovitis, or the diseases mimicking synovitis, is more completely shown in Box 12-1.

PHYSICAL EXAMINATION OF THE CHILD WITH ARTHRITIS

Whether the child is suspected or known to have synovitis, the physical examination is similar. Aspects unique to the physical examination of individual arthritides are discussed in the sections on those disorders.

The first step of the examination is observation of the joint in comparison with its symmetrical counterpart. Is the joint erythematous? Is it warm to touch? The normal intra-articular temperature is less than 37° C. Knees are approximately 32° C, and ankles are approximately 29° C; therefore, a knee that is the same temperature as the rest of the leg should raise suspicion of inflammation.[1,2]

Palpation includes ballottement, the bulge maneuver, and range of motion. *Ballottement* is a technique performed on the knee. The examiner stabilizes the joint with his or her nondominant hand and then, using either the thumb or the forefinger of the dominant hand, gently pushes the knee cap downward to see whether it "bounces" off the femur because of excessive joint fluid. Some joints are much larger than other joints, and fluid may "hide" in the surrounding soft tissues. In the case of the knee, synovial fluid frequently communicates with the suprapatellar sac. To elicit a *bulge sign*, the examiner "milks" the fluid into the suprapatellar sac, and then on the lateral side, slides one finger from the superior aspect of the knee joint to the inferior pole. Careful observation may demonstrate a bulge along the medial aspect as the fluid is pushed medially. The examiner may notice that the bulge occurs slowly; this is due to the viscosity of the joint fluid.

Chronic synovitis frequently causes localized growth disturbances. Limb length discrepancies are common in children with JRA. Arthritis in the lower extremity causes accelerated growth in the ossification centers of the bone. The level of bony maturation is likely responsible for whether inflammation will cause a limb to be longer or shorter than its unaffected counterpart. In a young child with greater potential for growth, the limb will probably become longer. Mild to moderate limb length discrepancies may resolve spontaneously in young children. In the older child, there may be premature closure of the growth plate, and subsequently, the limb is shortened. Limb length discrepancy can be grossly observed in the supine child by bending both legs at the knees and comparing the height of the two

Text continued on page 341

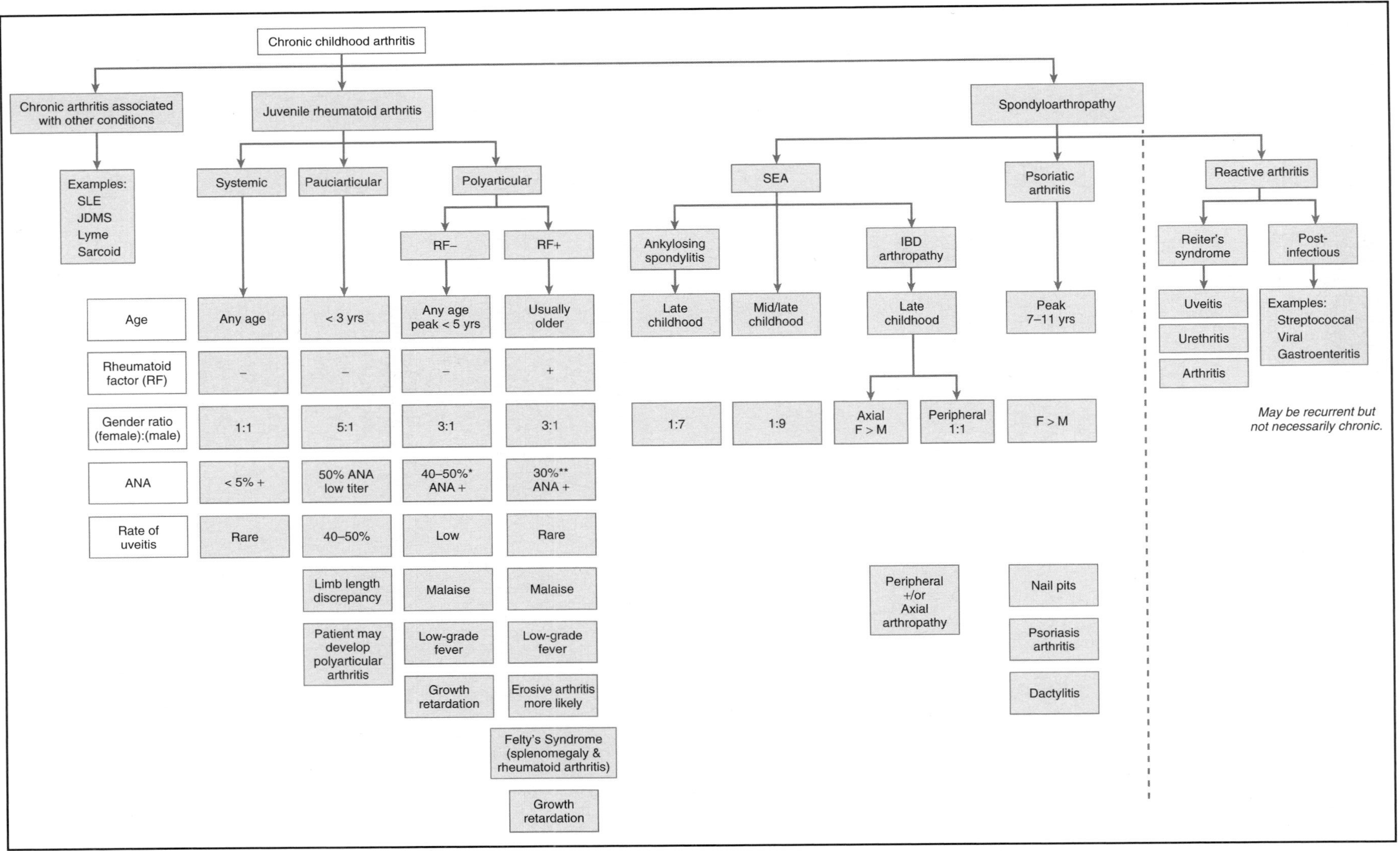

Figure 12-1 Algorithm showing the approach to the child with chronic arthritis. ANA, antinuclear antibody; F, female(s); IBD, inflammatory bowel disease; JDMS, juvenile dermatomyositis; Lyme, Lyme disease; M, male(s); RF, rheumatoid factor; SEA, syndrome of seronegativity, enthesopathy, and arthropathy; SLE, system lupus erythematosus; *, data from Cassidy and Petty[3]; **, data from Chandrasekaran AN, Rajendran CP, Madhavan R: Juvenile rheumatoid arthritis—Madras experience. Indian J Pediatr 63:501-510, 1996.

Box 12-1 Causes of Synovial Disorders in Children

- Juvenile rheumatoid arthritis
  - Pauciarticular
  - Polyarticular
  - Systemic
- Spondyloarthropathies
  - Psoriatic arthritis
  - Reiter syndrome
  - Inflammatory bowel arthropathy
  - Seronegative enthesopathy and arthropathy (SEA) syndrome
  - Juvenile ankylosing spondylitis
- Systemic lupus erythematosus
- Mixed connective tissue disease
- Juvenile dermatomyositis
- Systemic sclerosis
- Eosinophilic fasciitis
- Vasculitic syndromes
  - Leukocytoclastic vasculitis
    - Henoch-Schönlein purpura
    - Hypersensitivity angiitis
    - Hypocomplementemic urticarial vasculitis
    - Mixed cryoglobulinemia
  - Polyarteritis
    - Polyarteritis nodosa
    - Kawasaki disease
    - Cutaneous polyarteritis
  - Granulomatous vasculitis
    - Wegener granulomatosis
  - Giant cell arteritis
    - Takayasu arteritis
  - Behçet disease
  - Mucha-Habermann disease
- Sarcoidosis
- Relapsing polychondritis
- Sweet syndrome
- Septic arthritis (bacterial)
- Arthritis caused by viruses
  - Parvovirus
  - Rubella
  - Hepatitis B and hepatitis C
  - Alpha viruses
  - Mumps
  - Human immunodeficiency virus
  - Human T-lymphotropic virus type1
  - Herpes viruses
- Arthritis caused by other infections
  - Fungal
  - Mycobacteria
  - Spirochetes
    - Lyme disease
    - Leptospirosis
    - Syphilis
  - Sporotrichosis
  - Infective endocarditis
- Rheumatic fever
- Serum sickness
  - Secondary to drugs
  - Secondary to infections
- Reactive arthritis
  - Post-streptococcal arthritis
  - Postdysenteric arthritis
  - Mycoplasmal
- Immunodeficiencies with arthritis
  - Chronic granulomatous disease
  - Familial lipochrome histiocytosis
  - Complement deficiencies
  - Combined immunodeficiency
    - Severe combined immunodeficiency
    - Wiskott-Aldrich syndrome
  - T-cell deficiencies
    - DiGeorge syndrome
  - Hypogammaglobulin syndromes
    - Selective immunoglobulin A deficiency
    - X-linked agammaglobulinemia
    - Common variable immune deficiency
- Mucopolysaccharidoses
- Sphingolipidoses
- Metabolic deficiencies
  - Gout (just a few causes list)
    - Lesch-Nyhan syndrome
    - Becker syndrome
    - Gaucher disease
    - Renal disease with decreased urate excretion
    - Glycogen storage disease type 1
  - Pseudogout (calcium pyrophosphate deposition disease)
  - Ochronosis
  - Hyperlipoproteinemia
- Hematologic disorders
  - Sickle cell disease
  - Thalassemia
  - Hemophilia
- Hemochromatosis
- Multicentric histiocytosis
- Cystic fibrosis
- Familial Mediterranean fever
- Hypothyroidism
- Plant thorn synovitis

knees. At The Children's Hospital of Philadelphia, a shoe insert or orthotic is not recommended until the discrepancy is greater than 1 cm. The difference that is usually compensated for is approximately half of the defect. Other joints may have premature fusion of the physis or destruction of the joint. Micrognathia, resulting from arthritis of the temporomandibular joint, is one example.

In patients who have had arthritis in a particular joint, there may be muscle wasting surrounding that joint. If it is unclear whether a patient has had swelling in the past, a discrepancy in the circumference of the nearby muscle groups may be telling. For example, the patient who has had synovitis of the knee for weeks at a time may have quadriceps wasting on the ipsilateral side.

The clinician should have a consistent and systematic approach to the child with arthritis. An organized examination allows for specific physical diagnostic skills when appropriate, such as measurement of quadriceps circumference and potential leg length discrepancy.

JUVENILE RHEUMATOID ARTHRITIS

Juvenile rheumatoid arthritis is a term that encompasses a number of chronic synovial disorders in children. This identification causes some confusion and has been abandoned in Europe for the more general term *juvenile idiopathic arthritis*. JRA should not be confused with adult-onset arthritides. The adult presentation of rheumatoid arthritis is quite uncommon in children. Likewise, the systemic presentation of juvenile arthritis (Still disease) and seronegative polyarticular arthritis is uncommon in adults. Seronegative pauciarticular arthritis is not seen in adults, whereas the later onset of seronegative spondyloarthropathy is diagnosed in older children and adults.

Although Cornil documented an inflammatory arthropathy in childhood in 1864, it was not until 1890 that Diamantberger presented a review of published cases. The latter noted that the disease process was of an acute onset, involved exacerbations and remissions, affected large joints, and was often accompanied by growth retardation. George Frederick Still, an English pediatrician and pathologist, described systemic onset of JRA in detail in 1897.

JRA is one of the most common diagnoses seen and treated by pediatric rheumatologists. The subtypes of JRA are systemic-onset, polyarticular, and pauciarticular.

Incidence and Epidemiology

Published reports suggest the incidence of JRA is approximately 6 to 20 cases per 100,000 children at risk per year. These data include information from both the United States and Finland.[3]

Etiology

The causes of JRA are unknown. The disease may occur in a genetically predisposed host after initiation by some stimulus. Inciting agents include infection, physical trauma to the joint, emotional stress to the host, and an allergic reaction to environmental agents.

The genetic predisposition to JRA is of great interest. There appear to be different HLA associations with the different subtypes of disease (Table 12-1).

Systemic Juvenile Rheumatoid Arthritis

Presentation

The systemic form of JRA can manifest at any age but is more common in younger age groups. It affects 10% to 20% of all patients with JRA and has no gender bias. Onset of disease may be heralded by polyarticular joint inflammation, weight loss, and an evanescent salmon-colored rash that is usually worse with fevers. Systemic signs may precede arthritis by months and, rarely, even years. The fever curve in systemic JRA is referred to as quotidian or biquotidian. Classically, the *quotidian fever* spikes (up to 40.5° C), and then drops to, or below, the baseline normal temperature once per day (in a *biquotidian* fever, this happens twice a day) without anti-inflammatory agents or antipyretics. The fever may occur at any time during the day but is more common late in the afternoon or in the evening. Joint pain is frequently worse with fever spikes and involves small and large joints in a symmetrical manner. Approximately 20% of patients go on to have chronic arthritis that continues for months or years after their initial systemic symptoms. The common symptoms of all forms of JRA, morning stiffness and "gelling" after

Table 12-1 HLA Associations with Different Subtypes of Juvenile Rheumatoid Arthritis (JRA) and Spondyloarthropathy

Disease Type or Subtype	Associated Angiten(s)
Pauciarticular	
Onset at young age	HAL-A2, HLA-DR5, HLA-DR6, HLA-DR8, HLA-DPw2, HLA-DR4
Spondyloarthropathies	HLA-B27
Polyarticular	
Rheumatoid factor–positive	HLA-DR4, HLA-DR7
Rheumatoid factor–negative	HLA-DR8, HLA-DPw3, HLA-DQw4
Systemic	HLA-DR4, HLA-DR5, HLA-DR8
Spondyloarthropathy	HLA-B27

Adapted from Cassidy JT, Petty RE (eds): Textbook of Pediatric Rheumatology, 4th ed. Philadelphia, WB Saunders, 2001.

inactivity, are also common in inflammatory arthritis. The young child may not complain of these symptoms, so the physician should inquire about a limp or disuse of a limb that improves as the day wears on. Pain is often described as an aching. On physical examination, discomfort may be elicited only with extremes of range of motion.

One of the dangerous complications of systemic JRA is *macrophage activation syndrome* (MAS), otherwise known as *hemophagocytic syndrome*. MAS is caused by the overactivation and proliferation of well-differentiated macrophages. Clinically, patients appear acutely ill with one or all of the following findings: fever, hepatosplenomegaly, lymphadenopathy, depression of leukocytes, erythrocytes, and platelets, low erythrocyte sedimentation rate (ESR), elevated liver enzyme values, prolonged prothrombin and partial thromboplastin times, and hypofibrinogenemia. Bone marrow aspirate reveals well-differentiated macrophages engulfing hematopoietic elements.[4] MAS is associated with significant morbidity and mortality; therefore, the clinician should maintain a heightened vigilance for this complication. In patients with JRA, MAS has been associated with medications as well as with poorly controlled disease activity. MAS can also occur in diagnoses other than JRA, including adult Still disease, malignancies, and infections.

Laboratory Studies

Abnormal laboratory findings in JRA include leukocytosis, anemia, thrombocytosis, elevations of inflammatory markers (such as ESR and serum C-reactive protein), presence of D-dimers, mild hyperbilirubinemia, and elevations of aldolase and transaminases. Only 10% of patients with systemic JRA have an antinuclear antibody (ANA). Uveitis is more common in children with an ANA, but uveitis is rare in the systemic presentation of JRA. More information regarding uveitis is presented in the discussion of pauciarticular JRA.

Laboratory values are monitored on a regular basis in patients with systemic JRA who are taking medications. All of the pharmaceuticals used have toxicities, most of which are reversible. Nonsteroidal anti-inflammatory drugs (NSAIDs) may cause microcytic blood loss from the gastrointestinal tract, interstitial nephritis, thrombocytopenia, agranulocytosis, elevated transaminases, and renal compromise; but typically, these agents cause only stomach upset in a minority of children. Methotrexate may cause hepatotoxicity, leukopenia, anemia, and nephrotoxicity. Corticosteroids may cause gastritis with microscopic blood loss, hyperglycemia, adrenal insufficiency, and other problems. Combination therapy, especially with medications that may have combined renal toxicity and hepatotoxicity, requires special attention.

Physical Examination

Physical findings in the patient with systemic JRA may vary widely between patients and at different times in the same patient. The rash is evanescent and, as previously mentioned, is more remarkable and erythematous during periods of fever. The rash is classically described as salmon colored but is frequently erythematous, especially early in the disease course and with high fevers. The macules are often small (usually <5 mm) but may coalesce; they are found on the proximal extremities and trunk. The rash may also be seen on the hands, soles, and face. There may be a surrounding area of pallor. The lesions leave no scarring and may last hours at a time in a migratory and evanescent fashion (Fig. 12-2). Other physical findings that may be seen in the systemically ill child are pericardial or pleural fluid (which is frequently asymptomatic), hepatosplenomegaly, and lymphadenopathy.

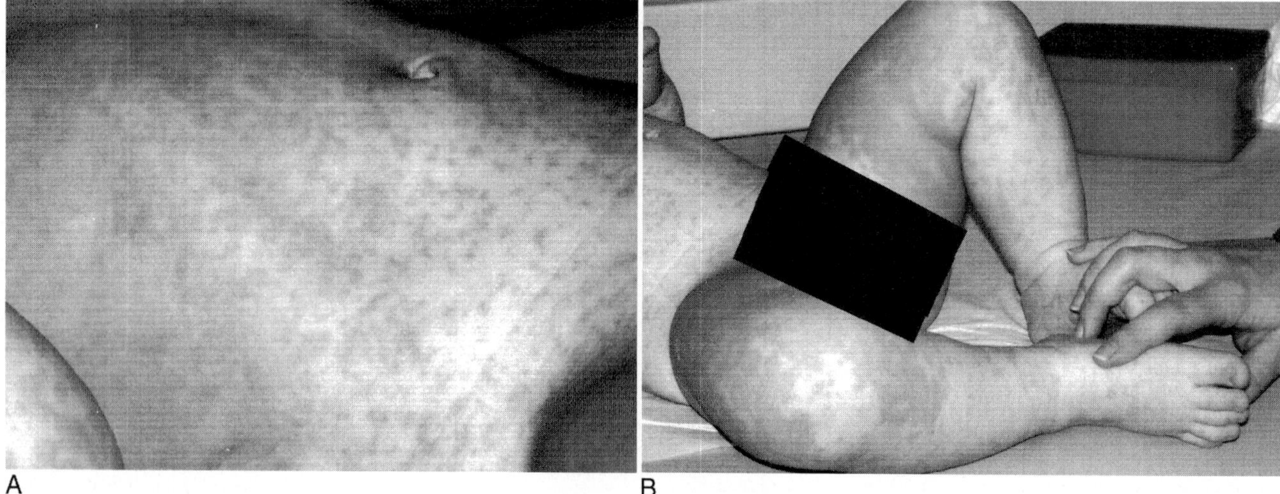

Figure 12-2 The rash of systemic juvenile rheumatoid arthritis on the abdomen **(A)** and perineum and legs **(B)** of an infant.

Imaging

Plain films can show several characteristics of systemic JRA, including osteopenia, bony erosions, effusions, overgrowth, swelling, and enlargement of joints (Figs. 12-3 and 12-4).

Treatment

Treatment of the systemically ill patient with JRA consists of steroids (usually starting at 2mg/kg/day divided twice daily) with or without initial pulse methylprednisolone for 3 consecutive days, weekly methotrexate (up to 1 mg/kg/week), and NSAIDs, typically indomethacin.[5] At our institution, we prefer subcutaneous administration of methotrexate, which avoids the first-pass effect on the liver that occurs with oral administration; also, the absorption of oral methotrexate is highly variable and has a greater incidence of gastrointestinal upset.[6] Newer agents, such as the tumor necrosis factor (TNF) inhibitors, etanercept and infliximab, are used as secondary disease-modifying medications. Steroid dosage is slowly tapered, and the disease-modifying agents, such as methotrexate and TNF inhibitors, are used as primary therapy. A pediatric rheumatologist must monitor laboratory values and disease course very closely.

Physical therapy and occupational therapy are mainstays of therapy for reducing pain, increasing mobility to restore function, and preventing disability in all forms of JRA. Splints, such as the cock-up splint, can be used to maintain a functional position of the wrist. Other splints, such as ring splints, may help prevent joint contractures of the digits. Dynamic splints are helpful for the elbows and knees.

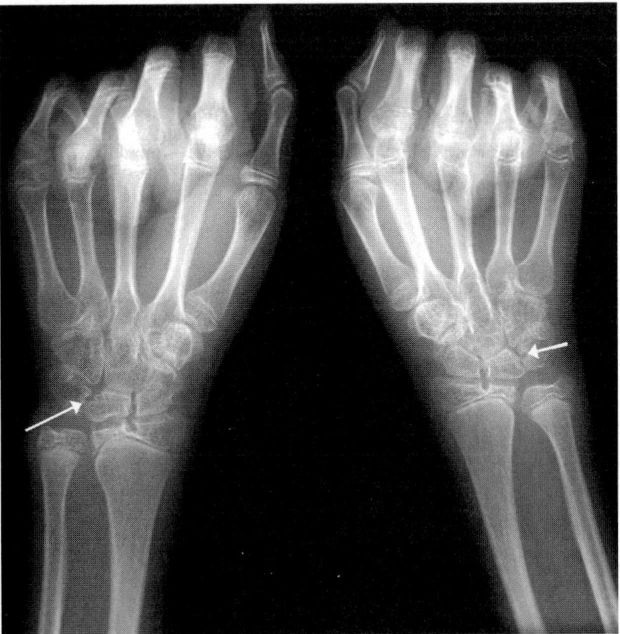

Figure 12-3 Plain radiographs of the hands of an 11-year-old girl with rheumatoid factor–negative system juvenile rheumatoid arthritis, showing osteoporosis of both wrists as well as narrowing of intercarpal spaces. Several bony erosions *(arrows)*, including subchondral cysts, radial epiphyseal erosion, and carpal erosion, are shown.

A great deal of time and effort are devoted to the education of the patient with systemic JRA, the family, and the school. Frequently, children who have limitations secondary to their arthritis are provided with letters of necessity for the use of elevators at school, extended periods of time

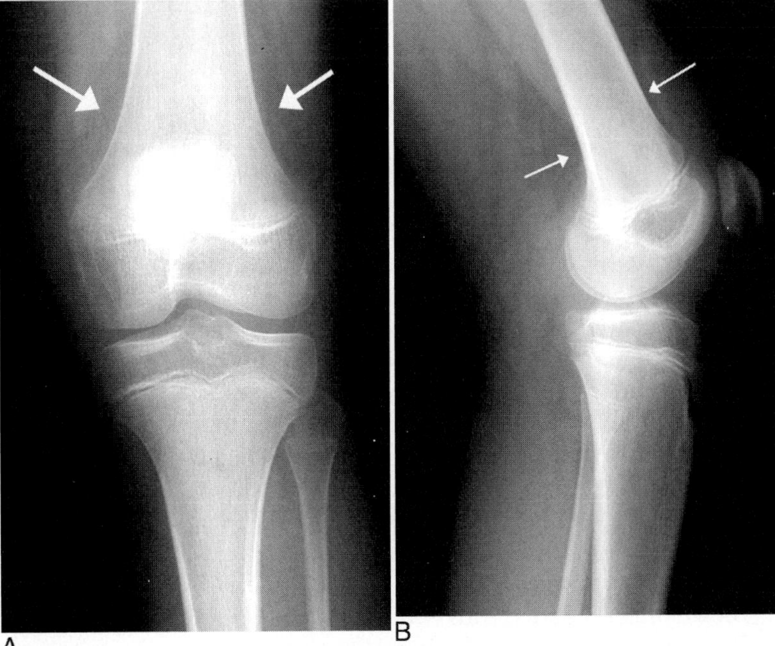

Figure 12-4 **A** and **B,** Plain radiographs of the knee of a 12-year-old girl with systemic juvenile rheumatoid arthritis showing effusions *(arrows)* and diffuse osteopenia.

to get to classes or to take written tests, and a second set of books at home. Teachers and school nurses need to be educated regarding the disease and any special needs the child may have so that adaptations can be made, if necessary, to promote the child's success. In general, children are encouraged to set their own limits on activities.

Disease Course

The disease course of systemic JRA varies. A subset of patients recover completely, another have recurrent systemic signs and symptoms, and still others have continued joint involvement and subsequent disability. The advent of newer medications may change these trends for the better.

An attempt has been made in the literature to identify patients at risk for poorer outcomes. Some of the risk factors are disease onset before the age of 5 years, persistent disease of more than 5 years' duration, and presence of cardiac disease. Poor prognosis has also been shown to be associated with fever, thrombocytosis, and need for corticosteroids 6 months after initial diagnosis.[7]

Differential Diagnosis

The differential diagnosis of systemic JRA includes infections, Kawasaki disease, malignancies, and other connective tissue diseases, such as rheumatic fever, SLE, and the vasculitides. There are no diagnostic laboratory tests for JRA. The diagnosis of this disease is one of exclusion. The fever in a patient with sepsis usually does not return to baseline, or less than baseline, as the quotidian fever of systemic-onset JRA does. In sepsis, the spikes in temperature are often more erratic, and the patient continues to look systemically ill even between spikes. Excluding malignancies such as leukemia and neuroblastoma may be difficult, and bone marrow aspiration may be helpful. A manual differential leukocyte count of the complete blood count is necessary, with examination of the peripheral smear for blasts. Patients with JRA may have significant lymphadenopathy, so differentiating it from lymphoma may be difficult without a lymph node biopsy. Other diseases included in the differential diagnosis for JRA are rheumatic fever, polyarteritis nodosa, dermatomyositis, and SLE. The arthritis of rheumatic fever, although migratory, is exceptionally painful compared with the physical findings. Appropriate screening for recent streptococcal infection should be performed, including an anti-streptolysin O test. The use of other markers such as anti-deoxyribonuclease B, antihyaluronidase, and antistreptokinase, increases the sensitivity of identifying streptococcal illnesses. Any evidence of myocarditis or valvular disease should raise suspicion for acute rheumatic fever (ARF). One of the vasculitides that may manifest as fever of unknown origin is polyarteritis nodosa. This disease does not have the classic JRA rash; rather, it may have a painful purpuric rash. Hypertension and renal bruits are signs that should prompt the suspicion of polyarteritis nodosa.

Polyarticular Juvenile Rheumatoid Arthritis

Presentation

Polyarticular juvenile rheumatoid arthritis is defined as involvement of five or more joints during the first 6 months of disease. Forty percent of cases of JRA are of polyarticular onset. Females outnumber males by approximately three to one. Onset may occur any time during childhood, but there is a peak in toddlers (1 to 3 years). Joint involvement is usually symmetrical and affects the large joints, including knees, ankles, hips, wrists, and elbows; however, small joints may be involved. The cervical spine and temporomandibular joints are often involved in polyarticular disease (Fig. 12-5). Systemic symptoms may be present but are usually much milder than in the systemic presentation. Patients may have a low-grade fever, mild hepatosplenomegaly, and pericardial effusions. Chronic uveitis occurs in approximately 5% of these patients, most of whom test positive for ANA.

There are two distinct subcategories of polyarticular JRA. The first is rheumatoid factor (RF)–positive disease, and the second is RF-negative disease. Patients with RF usually present later in childhood or adolescence, and their disease more closely resembles adult-onset rheumatoid arthritis. They may have early erosive disease, rheumatoid nodules, and a more chronic disease that waxes and wanes over time. Patients with RF-negative

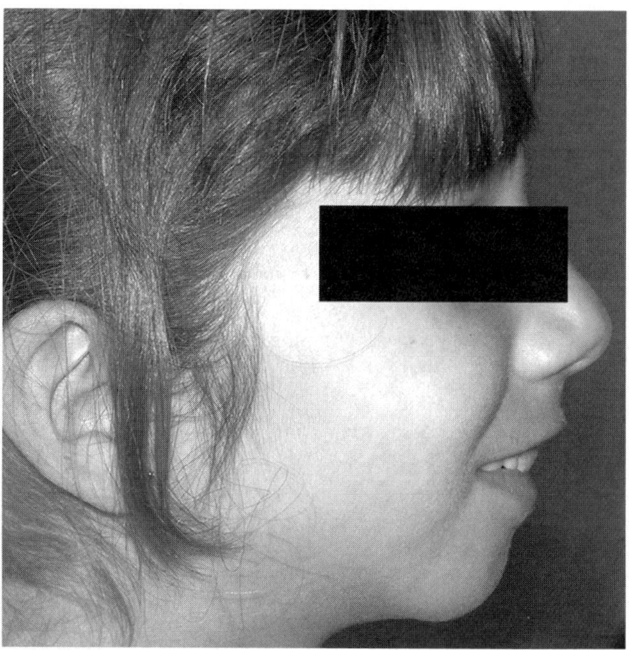

Figure 12-5 A patient with polyarticular juvenile rheumatoid arthritis with involvement of the temporomandibular joint resulting in micrognathia.

disease are likely to have involvement of fewer joints, do not have rheumatoid nodules, and have a better prognosis for regression of disease.

Laboratory Studies

There are no diagnostic laboratory tests for any of the subtypes of JRA. Some patients with polyarticular disease have ANA, and they must be monitored more closely for uveitis than patients without an ANA. (This issue is discussed in more length in the pauciarticular JRA section.) The rate of seropositivity for ANA is 40% to 50% in patients with polyarticular JRA. The rate of uveitis is lower than in patients with early onset of pauciarticular JRA. Inflammatory markers such as ESR and C-reactive protein may be mildly elevated. Children frequently have a normocytic anemia of chronic disease.

Ten percent of patients with polyarticular JRA, or approximately 4% of all patients with JRA, test positive for RF. If a patient has RF-positive disease or the disease process does not seem to be responding to standard therapy, radiographs should be considered. If there is concern that pain in a joint is atypical or could represent another disease process, such as avascular necrosis, magnetic resonance imaging (MRI) should be considered.

Physical Examination

Patients with polyarticular disease have synovitis, as described earlier (Figs. 12-6 through 12-9). They may also have mild hepatosplenomegaly, mild lymphadenopathy, pericardial effusions (usually asymptomatic), and leg length discrepancies. Checking for a leg length discrepancy should be a routine part of the examination in a patient with JRA.

A funduscopic examination should always be performed in every patient, but a slit-lamp examination by an ophthalmologist is crucial for ruling out the "silent" uveitis of JRA. The plan of care should remind the families of patients with JRA when they are due for ophthalmologic evaluation.

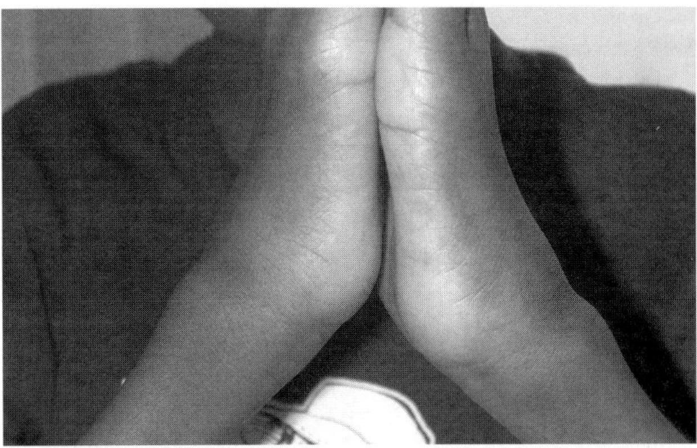

Figure 12-7 Patient with polyarticular juvenile rheumatoid arthritis in whom active arthritis in the wrists prevents complete dorsiflexion, known as a "prayer sign."

Imaging

Plain films can show several characteristics of polyarticular JRA, such as osteopenia, cortical irregularities, joint space narrowing and collapse, sclerosis, and erosions (Figs. 12-10 and 12-11).

Treatment

Initial management of the patient with polyarticular disease depends on the severity of synovitis and whether there are any other signs or symptoms, such as pericarditis. If the patient has significant synovitis or organ involvement, treatment is usually initiated at our institution with corticosteroids and methotrexate.

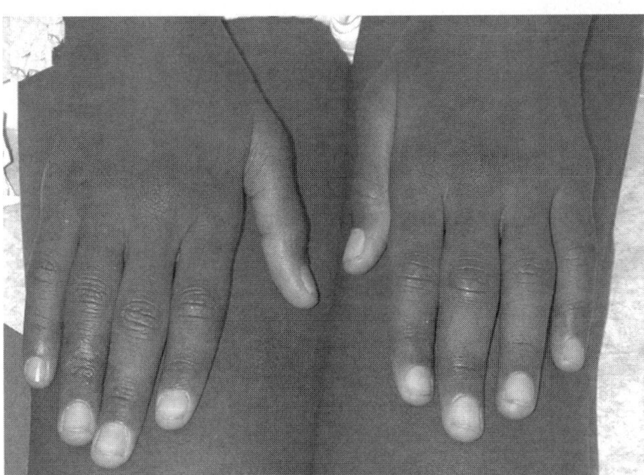

Figure 12-6 Hands of a patient with polyarticular juvenile rheumatoid arthritis with symmetrical inflammation of the proximal interphalangeal joints, greater on the left than the right.

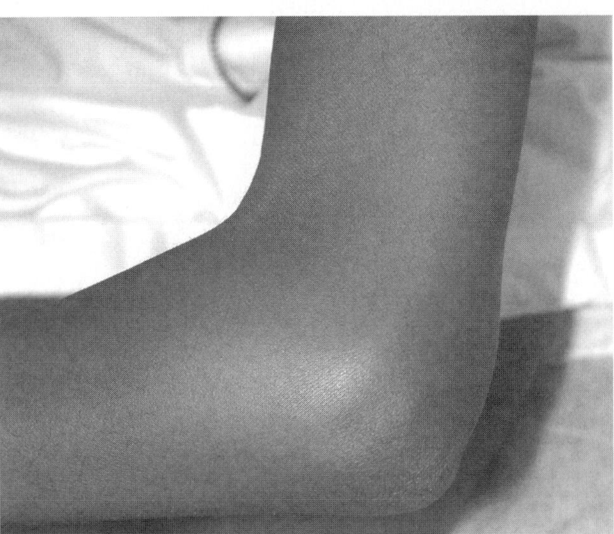

Figure 12-8 Elbow arthritis in a patient with juvenile rheumatoid arthritis.

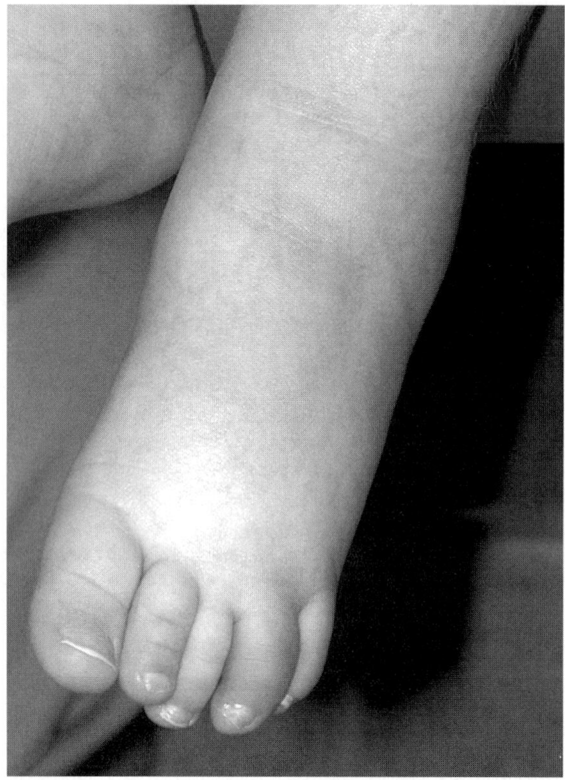

Figure 12-9 Evidence of arthritis in the fourth toe and ankle.

NSAIDs are often used along with methotrexate for long-term therapy. The goal of management for any patient with arthritis is to taper and discontinue steroid use as soon as possible. Other disease-modifying agents, such as parenteral gold and penicillamine, are no longer used, but occasionally, hydroxychloroquine and sulfasalazine are used as adjunctive therapy.[5] TNF inhibitors have also proved to be effective in refractory cases of polyarticular JRA. Frequent physical and laboratory examinations should guide treatment.

Intra-articular injection of glucocorticoids is a useful method to reduce and, in some cases, resolve synovitis. This treatment modality can reduce joint contractures and may prevent leg length discrepancies by minimizing or eradicating synovitis.[8] The uncommon side effects of intra-articular injections with glucocorticoids include subcutaneous atrophy and hypopigmentation at the site of injection, infection (1 in 100,000), chemical synovitis from the injection (usually of short duration), intra-articular calcification, and subchondral bone resorption. Although this list seems formidable, the inflammation of a joint is probably more dangerous than the minimal risk of the injection.[9]

Disease Course

Disease course is difficult to predict in polyarticular JRA. Generally, the poorest outcome is in the older

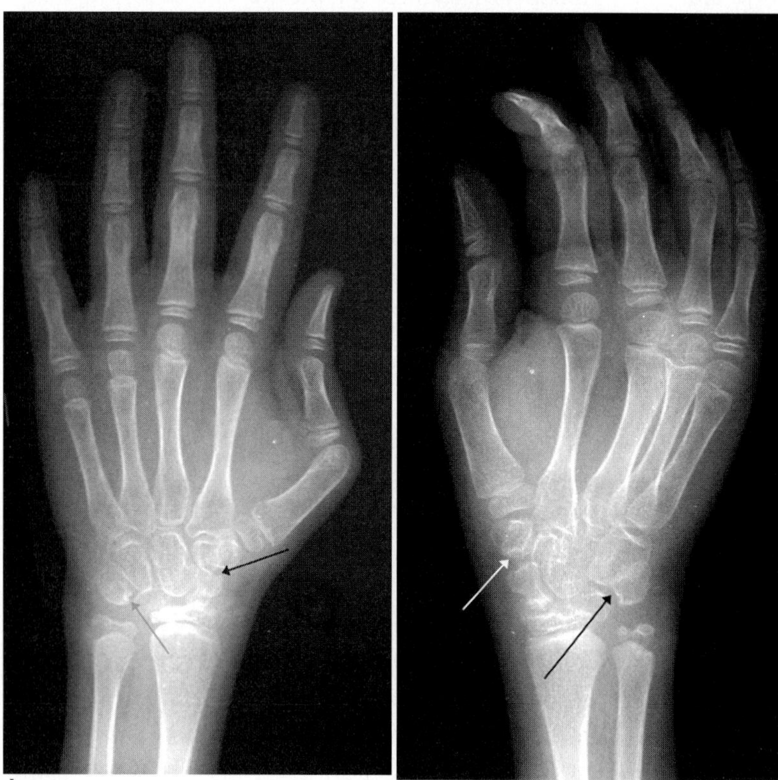

Figure 12-10 Plain radiographs of the hands of a 10-year-old girl with rheumatoid factor–positive polyarticular juvenile rheumatoid arthritis. A, Osteopenia of the left hand is noted, with irregularity of the distal radial epiphysis. Cortical irregularities of the carpal bones with erosions of the triquetrum *(gray arrow)* and navicular bone *(black arrow)* as well as radiolunate joint space narrowing are apparent. **B,** The right hand also has osteoporosis, cortical irregularities, and erosions of the carpal bones *(arrows).*

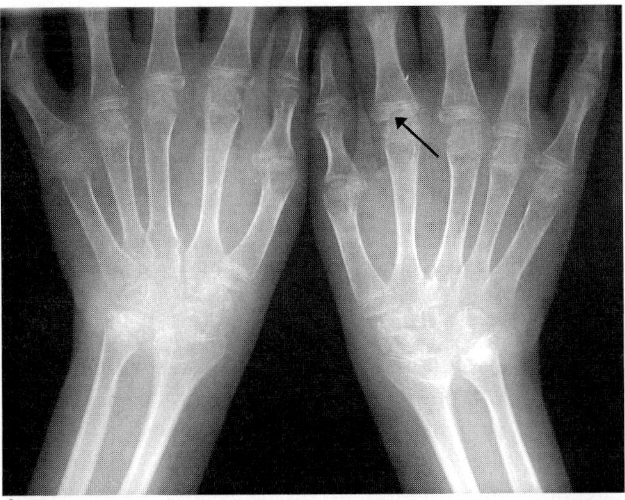

A

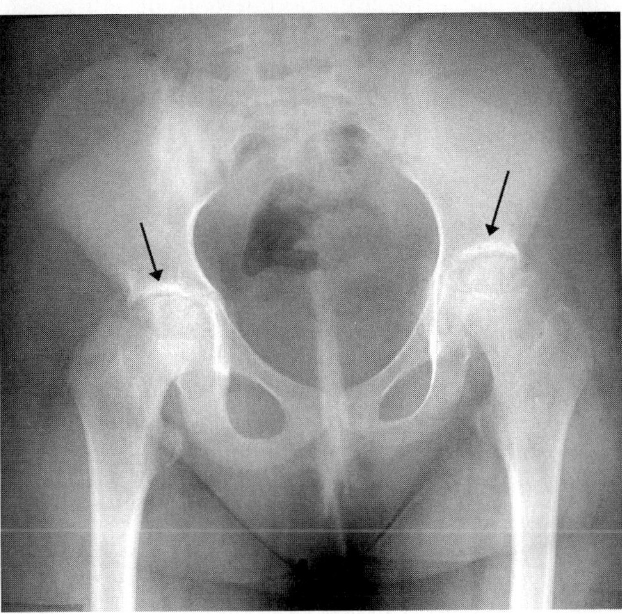

B

Figure 12-11 Plain radiographs of a 14-year-old girl with rheumatoid factor–positive polyarticular juvenile rheumatoid arthritis. A, Radiographs of the wrists show diffuse osteopenia, poorly defined articular surfaces, fusion of the second *(arrow)* and third metacarpal joints, and multiple erosions and deformities throughout the carpal bones. **B,** Joint space narrowing of the hips with sclerosis *(arrows)* as well as collapse and bony irregularities of the left femoral head are visible on a pelvic radiograph.

female patient who has RF-positive disease, early and progressive erosions, nodules, and prolonged duration of disease before initiation of therapy. Younger patients with a RF-negative disease have a better prognosis. Hip involvement can occur with any of the JRA subtypes, but it can lead to significant disability if inflammation interferes with femoral head and acetabular development. Severe hip involvement may be a harbinger of a poorer prognosis.[3]

Differential Diagnosis

The differential diagnosis for polyarticular JRA includes spondyloarthropathy, SLE, Lyme disease, reactive arthritis, sarcoidosis, and the mucopolysaccharidoses (which can mimic arthritis).[3]

Pauciarticular Juvenile Rheumatoid Arthritis

Presentation

Pauci is derived from the Latin word meaning "few," and *pauciarticular* implies that four or fewer joints are involved. Thirty percent to 40% of all patients with JRA have pauciarticular disease. Age of presentation is usually in toddlerhood, with the peak between 1 and 2 years. There is a female preponderance, with a female-to-male ratio of 5:1. In half of all patients with pauciarticular JRA, only one joint is involved (monoarthritis), most commonly the knee, followed by the ankle and the joints of the fingers.[10] The patient may present with a limp or morning stiffness. The pain from pauciarticular JRA is usually much less severe than that felt in systemic JRA or reported by adult patients with rheumatoid arthritis. A significant proportion of children with pauciarticular JRA have painless arthritis.[11]

Uveitis may be the first manifestation of the disease. Twenty percent of patients with pauciarticular JRA have uveitis. Patients who present at an early age, are ANA positive and female, and have the HLA-DR5 allele are at highest risk. Guillaume and associates[12] report that ANA positivity is not as predictive as previously thought for the development of uveitis. This extra-articular complication is often insidious, with most affected patients having no symptoms. Nonetheless, the physician should inquire about photophobia, pain, redness, and any changes in vision. Uveitis usually develops within 5 to 7 years of onset of the arthritis, and 65% of cases of disease are bilateral. The vast majority of cases of uveitis develop within 6 weeks of onset of the JRA.[13]

Signs of disease that may be apparent to the pediatrician or rheumatologist are inflammatory cells within the anterior chamber (seen without slit lamp only if disease is very inflammatory) and synechiae, which make the shape of the iris appear irregular or cause a poorly reactive pupil. Poor and late outcomes include band keratopathy, glaucoma, and cataracts. Management by the ophthalmologist consists of the use of glucocorticoid eye drops, mydriatics, and, in resistant cases, intraocular injections of glucocorticoids. Treatment given in collaboration with the rheumatologist may be necessary, as systemic therapy can reduce the need for topical steroids. Systemic medications used successfully for uveitis include corticosteroids, methotrexate, cyclosporin, chlorambucil, and, most recently, etanercept (Table 12-2).[14]

Laboratory Studies

As mentioned, there is no diagnostic laboratory test to diagnose JRA. ANA is present in 68% of patients with a pauciarticular presentation.[10] The ANA titer allows the physician to identify patients at highest risk for uveitis. Patients must be screened for uveitis by an ophthalmologist every 3 months for the first 2 years of disease if they are ANA positive, and every 6 months if they are ANA negative.

It is of utmost importance that the pediatrician realizes that an ANA titer is not used for diagnostic purposes. This test is used for prognostication about uveitis in a patient who has already been diagnosed with JRA. Approximately 1 in 10 healthy females have an ANA, which is likely inherited and does not indicate a predilection to develop a connective tissue disorder. Children with JRA may have a chronic normocytic anemia and mild elevations in ESR or C-reactive protein value. In our experience, these inflammatory markers are not as sensitive for disease activity as the physical examination.

Physical Examination

The maneuvers to detect synovitis on physical examination are the same in all of the JRA subtypes. The joints should be visualized and compared bilaterally, examined for warmth, ballotted, inspected for a bulge sign. The legs should be checked for length discrepancy. We observe the child's gait at every visit to determine whether orthotics are indicated and whether the child should be referred for a gait analysis at physical therapy.

As mentioned, a funduscopic examination should be performed at every visit, and the care plan should include the patient's follow-up with the ophthalmologist.

Treatment

Treatment modalities are similar for JRA of both pauciarticular and polyarticular onset. There is usually no systemic involvement with pauciarticular onset, so administration of systemic steroids is usually not indicated. The mainstays of therapy are intra-articular corticosteroids, NSAIDs, and methotrexate.[5] Some institutions may use other disease-modifying antirheumatic agents, such as sulfasalazine and hydroxychloroquine, more frequently. In general, early aggressive management with intra-articular steroids and subcutaneous methotrexate yields excellent results.

Intra-articular corticosteroid injections may yield the best results in pauciarticular JRA. In one series, such injections in pauciarticular JRA, resulted in full remission in 82% of patients and discontinuation of all oral medications in 74% of patients.[15] In a series published from Germany, patients with early-onset pauciarticular JRA had the longest duration of relief after intra-articular injections of triamcinolone hexacetonide, a long-acting corticosteroid. The average duration of efficacy in this group was 121 weeks, followed by 105 weeks in patients with RF-negative pauciarticular JRA, 63 weeks in patients with RF-positive pauciarticular JRA, and 36 weeks in patients with systemic-onset JRA.[16]

Table 12-2 Schedule of Ophthalmologic Screening in Juvenile Rheumatic Arthritis

Patient Features	Schedule for First 2 Years of Arthritis	Schedule More than 2 Years After Diagnosis
Pauciarticular disease		
ANA+	Every 3 months	Every 6 months
ANA–	Every 6 months	Every 6 months
Polyarticular disease		
ANA+	Every 3 months	Every 3 months
ANA–	Every 6 months	Every 6 months
Systemic disease	Every year	Every year

ANA, result of antinuclear antibody titer.

Disease Course

The disease course in the patient who presents with pauciarticular onset is variable. The child may present with monoarticular disease, continue with pauciarticular disease, or progress to polyarticular disease.

Patients with monoarticular disease usually have a good functional outcome. Some may experience a remission of disease within a couple of years. Other patients with pauciarticular involvement may have a waxing and waning of disease. In one group of patients, the pauciarticular disease extends to involve multiple joints.

In the group of patients who progress to a polyarticular type of disease, the disease course is similar to that in patients with polyarticular JRA. These children have a higher risk of joint erosions. A group of French investigators attempted to define risk factors in patients with pauciarticular JRA that were markers of future progression to a polyarticular disease. They demonstrated that patients with pauciarticular disease who presented with involvement of more than one joint and at least one upper limb joint or with a high ESR were at an increased risk for development of polyarticular disease.[12] These children should be aggressively treated, and every attempt should be made to minimize functional limitations.

Differential Diagnosis

The differential diagnosis for pauciarticular JRA includes infection, reactive arthritis, rheumatic fever, toxic synovitis, Lyme disease, sarcoidosis, and malignancy. If there is any question that a joint may be infected, an arthrocentesis should be performed, and the synovial fluid should be sent for cell count with a differential count, Gram stain, and cultures. The history is the most helpful diagnostic tool available to the clinician. Questions about a preceding upper respiratory infection, a preceding streptococcal infection, recent antibiotic use, tick bite, diarrheal illness, progressive weight loss with debilitation, night pain, and fevers should all be included in the proper review of symptoms.

SPONDYLOARTHROPATHIES

The *spondyloarthropathies* are a group of HLA-B27–associated inflammatory disorders that involve arthritis, enthesitis, bursitis, and tendonitis. ***Enthesitis***, or inflammation where tendons and ligaments insert into bone (usually around the knees and feet), distinguishes the spondyloarthropathies from JRA. Some of these illnesses may have cutaneous manifestations. Serologic analysis usually shows that a rheumatoid factor is absent, and an ANA is typically absent but may be present. The subgroups of the spondyloarthropathies are the syndrome of seronegativity, enthesopathy, and arthropathy (SEA syndrome), psoriatic arthritis, arthritis associated with inflammatory bowel disease (IBD), Reiter syndrome and reactive arthritis, and juvenile ankylosing spondylitis (JAS).

Epidemiology and Pathogenesis

The incidence of juvenile spondyloarthropathy in the United States is not clear. Many children with these diseases may be misdiagnosed with JRA, and thus, the incidence of juvenile spondyloarthropathy may have a prevalence approximating that of JRA. In our experience, careful examination for enthesitis, nail pitting and psoriatic patches (associated with psoriatic arthritis), and poor lower back flexibility as well as evaluation for HLA-B27 status identifies a significant percentage of children with juvenile spondyloarthropathy who may otherwise have been misdiagnosed as having JRA.

Multiple pathogenic triggers have been investigated in adult patients with spondyloarthropathy. Peptides bound within the groove of the HLA-B27 molecule, bacterial infections, gastrointestinal inflammation, and differences in immune responses have all been associated with these illnesses. Sixty percent to 90% of patients with spondyloarthropathy are HLA-B27 positive. HLA-B27*05 is the most common subtype found in both the general population and in patients with spondyloarthropathy. Associations with *Salmonella*, *Shigella*, *Yersinia*, *Campylobacter*, *Chlamydia*, and *Klebsiella* have been suggested as possible inciting triggers, especially in reactive arthritis. Inflammatory changes in the terminal ileum or colon have been demonstrated in up to 70% of patients with spondyloarthropathy. Inflammation may allow increased permeability to bacterial antigens that can act as triggers of disease. Studies have demonstrated subclinical inflammatory bowel disease in 81% of patients with juvenile spondyloarthropathy.

Clinical Manifestations

Patients with either undifferentiated or a defined subtype of spondyloarthropathy may have a combination of arthritis, enthesitis, and bursitis or tendonitis. As mentioned, enthesitis is inflammation at the site of insertion of a tendon or ligament into bone. Enthesitis most frequently affects the lower extremities, and enthesitis of the feet may be one of the most disabling features of spondyloarthropathy in a child. On examination, there is tenderness to palpation at the insertion of tendons, ligaments, or joint capsules into bone. Some of the more common locations are the insertion site of the Achilles tendon, the insertion sites on the calcaneus and the metatarsal heads on the plantar fascia, and the insertion site of the patellar ligament onto the anterior tibia. There may or may not be demonstrable swelling, but these sites are tender to palpation. High-definition ultrasound analysis may help define an enthesitis more objectively. The clinician must be careful to recognize that tenderness at an enthesis may represent a noninflammatory disorder such as Osgood-Schlatter or Sever disease.

SEA Syndrome

Patients with the syndrome of seronegativity, enthesopathy, and arthropathy do not have a rheumatoid factor or an ANA. SEA syndrome may be a form of spondyloarthropathy or it may be a harbinger of a separate subtype of spondyloarthropathy that develops in the future. In one study, with SEA syndrome had evolved into a different subtype of spondyloarthropathy at 9-year follow-up in 70% of patients.[17] There may be two forms of SEA syndrome, one in children who are HLA-B27 negative and in whom a separate subtype of spondyloarthropathy does not develop, and the other in children who are HLA-B27 positive and may progress to have JAS.[18] Arthritis in the latter group often involves the small and large joints of the leg Approximately 72% of patients with SEA syndrome are HLA-B27 positive.[3]

Management of SEA syndrome usually consists of NSAIDs and intra-articular corticosteroids.[5] If the arthritis is refractory to treatment, other disease-modifying agents, such as sulfasalazine and methotrexate, may have to be used.

Psoriatic Arthritis

Juvenile-onset psoriatic arthritis is defined as arthritis occurring at 16 years of age or earlier with a typical psoriatic rash. The alternative categorization is arthritis with three of the four minor criteria (dactylitis, nail pitting or onycholysis, psoriasis-like rash, and family history of a first or second-degree relative with psoriasis). This form of arthritis is more common in girls, and the peak age at onset is between 7 and 13 years. There is less of an association with HLA-B27 in psoriatic arthritis than in other spondyloarthropathies. Arthritis is the initial presentation in 50% of patients, and psoriasis in 40%. In 10% of patients, the skin and joint manifestations occur simultaneously.

Oligoarticular involvement is the most common presentation of the arthritis. The joints most commonly involved are the knees, ankles, proximal interphalangeal (PIP) joints of the feet and hands, and distal interphalangeal (DIP) joints of the feet. Dactylitis, or "sausage digit," is also seen in psoriatic arthritis. As the disease progresses over time, polyarticular involvement of the elbows, DIP joints of the fingers, wrists, temporomandibular joints, and cervical spine may become more prevalent. Findings on radiographs of involved joints include periarticular osteopenia, joint space narrowing, and erosions. An aggressive form of psoriatic arthritis is called *arthritis mutilans* for its severely erosive nature.

Cutaneous manifestations of psoriatic arthritis may be mild in children, so the clinician must have a high index of suspicion for the disease. Locations of skin involvement include the umbilicus, scalp, anal area, and extensor surfaces of the limbs. Careful examination of the nails must include an investigation for pits and striae.

Arthropathy Associated with Inflammatory Bowel Disease

Joint disease in patients with IBDs may be divided into peripheral disease and axial (sacroiliac or spinal) disease. Peripheral joint involvement is usually of the lower extremity. Peripheral joint involvement is usually not associated with HLA-B27 and coincides with bowel symptoms only 50% of the time.[19] Half of patients may only have one episode of arthritis that is self-limited. The remaining patients with peripheral joint involvement may have oligoarthritis or monoarthritis that lasts for less than 1 month. Erosions may be evident on radiographic examination, but it is rare for such a patient to have permanent functional limitation.

Axial involvement tends to follow intestinal flares of the IBD, and children with this type of disease are more frequently HLA-B27 positive.[20] Some patients with spondylitis also have peripheral joint disease. A disease course resembling that of JAS may evolve in some patients whose IBD becomes quiescent.

Reactive Arthritis and Reiter Syndrome

Reactive arthritis and Reiter syndrome are linked by their association of arthritis preceded by an infection. Infections (e.g., those mentioned previously in the epidemiology of spondyloarthropathy) usually antedate arthritis by approximately 2 to 4 weeks. The organisms implicated in these arthritides in children are usually of an enteric origin. In adolescents, sexually transmitted *Chlamydia trachomatis* is a common trigger. Reiter syndrome consists of a triad of arthritis, conjunctivitis, and urethritis (or cervicitis).

The arthritis in children with reactive arthritis or Reiter syndrome is often acute. It is frequently asymmetric and usually involves few joints, and dactylitis is not uncommon. Knees and ankles are the most commonly affected. Enthesitis, especially at the patella and calcaneus, can be extremely painful.

Urethritis is present in 30% of children at the onset of disease and may manifest as dysuria, a sterile pyuria, or inflammation at the meatus or may be completely asymptomatic. If symptoms are mild, or the physician suspects Reiter syndrome in a patient with conjunctivitis and arthritis, the urinary sediment should be centrifuged to look for white blood cells (WBCs).[3]

Conjunctivitis is present in two thirds of patients with Reiter syndrome and is usually bilateral. Symptoms include photophobia, erythema of the bulbar or palpebral conjunctiva or both, or a scratchy sensation in the eye. More severe complications can be seen, although less frequently, such as mucopurulent discharge, iritis, keratitis, optic neuritis, and corneal ulcerations.[3]

Occasionally, Reiter syndrome may be confused with Kawasaki disease.[21] Kawasaki disease has some of the same features, including conjunctivitis, urethritis, and arthritis. The other signs and symptoms seen in Kawasaki disease are fever, lymphadenopathy, rash, and changes of the oral mucosa (dry fissured lips, "strawberry tongue," and erythema of the oropharynx). Rashes are unusual in Reiter syndrome, but keratoderma blennorrhagicum and balanitis circinata are occasionally seen. Mucocutaneous lesions, if present, tend to be short-lived.[18]

Laboratory abnormalities include an elevated ESR (average equaling 50 to 60 mm/hr), an elevated WBC count (up to 20,000 cells/mm^3) with a left shift, and pyuria (with 5 to 1000 WBCs per high-power field). Results of microbiologic cultures have been positive for organisms in some cases but are usually negative. Examples of isolated organisms are *Chlamydia* in conjunctival and urethral swabs, and *Shigella* and *Salmonella* in stool samples. Radiographic changes that may be seen include periarticular osteoporosis, erosions at ligamentous insertions, and asymmetric changes in the sacroiliac joints.[3]

The prognosis for children with reactive arthritis or Reiter syndrome tends to be good. A large proportion of cases undergo remission, and some patients may have waxing and waning disease. In one series of 26 patients with Reiter syndrome, two thirds of the patients were HLA-B27 positive.[22] It is possible that Reiter syndrome and reactive arthritis may be the initial presentation of a seronegative arthropathy.

Juvenile Ankylosing Spondylitis

Juvenile ankylosing spondylitis is a chronic inflammatory arthritis that begins in children younger than 16 years. The arthritis affects the peripheral and axial skeleton and may also involve inflammation of the entheses. The male-to-female ratio is approximately 7:1, and the disease has a strong association with the presence of HLA-B27. True JAS is rare in childhood, whereas SEA syndrome is relatively common.

At presentation, involvement of peripheral joints of the lower extremities is more common than axial symptoms. The majority of patients present with involvement of four or fewer joints but often progress to have polyarticular disease within a year. When axial disease occurs, it usually appears in the lumbar and thoracic regions. Stiffening of the spine is a result of inflammation within the vertebral joints. Spinal and sacroiliac joint pain, stiffness, and decreased anterior flexion of the spine or decreased chest expansion usually worsen after disease has been present for 2½ years and reach a peak 5 to 10 years after onset. In adult patients, there is marked spinal stiffness in the morning that gradually improves with movement and time. The pattern is just the opposite in children; pain often worsens with activity and time and decreases with rest. Enthesitis can be quite disabling in JAS and is frequently an early manifestation of the disease.

Radiographic findings include periarticular osteopenia, joint space narrowing, spur formation, erosion at ligamentous insertions, and ankylosis of tarsal, hip, and axial joints.[18] Changes seen in the vertebral column in patients with ankylosing spondylitis, such as epiphysitis, anterior vertebral squaring, anterior ligament calcification, and "bamboo spine," are uncommon in childhood.[3]

JAS has a number of extra-articular manifestations. Acute iritis may occur, characterized by a red, photophobic, painful eye. It usually does not cause long-term sequelae or precede the onset of the arthritis. Aortic insufficiency is less common in children than adults. Decreased vital capacity, secondary to impairment of chest wall expansion because of arthritis, is possible. Atlantoaxial subluxation has been reported in only a few children with JAS.

Treatment of patients with JAS involves medications and physical therapy. NSAIDs can be helpful for the pain of JAS but likely do not alter disease progression. Indomethacin and tolmetin sodium have both been shown to be beneficial. Studies are under way to confirm initial reports that TNF inhibitors are effective in the management of ankylosing spondylitis.[23] Physical therapy is vital to limit functional disabilities and contractures as much as possible; it consists of range-of-motion exercises and splints. Insoles can be made to relieve the discomfort of painful enthesitis.[3]

RHEUMATIC FEVER AND POSTSTREPTOCOCCAL ARTHRITIS

Rheumatic Fever

Incidence and Epidemiology

Acute rheumatic fever appears to be growing in frequency, having begun to do so in the 1980s. Zanguill and associates[24] initially published a report documenting the higher incidence of ARF in western Pennsylvania between 1985 and 1987. Their study was then extended, and they were able to demonstrate that the number of cases continued to rise between 1987 and 1990.[24] The change in incidence of rheumatic fever may be secondary to an alteration in the subtype of streptococci bacteria.

Rheumatic fever occurs equally in boys and girls with a peak age at onset between 5 and 15 years; the disease is uncommon in children younger than 4 years.[3] It occurs more frequently in highly populated areas with crowding and poverty.

Etiology

Rheumatic fever is precipitated by a pharyngeal infection with group A β-hemolytic streptococci (GABS). The pathogenesis of rheumatic fever is probably multifactorial. Investigations have demonstrated that the mechanisms responsible include cross-reactivity between GABS and host molecules, GABS virulence factors, and host susceptibility. A number of GABS antigens have been shown to be cross-reactive with human tissue. One example is the M protein. Human antibodies directed against myosin also react against M protein. Antigens found within human synovium have been shown to be cross-reactive with streptococcal antigens. M protein can also function as a superantigen, eliciting a cascade of inflammation.

A variety of GABS virulence factors have been elucidated. Besides M protein, GABS may also be heavily encapsulated with hyaluronic acid, which may increase its resistance to being encapsulated by macrophages. Host factors include a B-cell marker, identified by the monoclonal antibody D8/17, which most patients with ARF carry; this marker is inherited in an autosomal recessive fashion.[25] HLA-DR*B*1*01 has also been associated with rheumatic fever.[26]

Clinical Manifestations

Clinical manifestations of rheumatic fever commonly begin 2 weeks after a streptococcal pharyngitis. Patients usually have high fevers, which frequently subside after 3 weeks. Patients may not have a known history of streptococcal infection, so the clinician's index of suspicion for the disease must be high. The modified Jones criteria aid the physician in diagnosing ARF, which, like that of most other rheumatic illnesses, is still a diagnosis of exclusion (Table 12-3).

Arthritis

The arthritis of ARF is the most common symptom. It usually affects the large joints of the lower extremity, is asymmetric, and is migratory, and the severity of pain is commonly out of proportion to the swelling. Pain may be so great that the patient cannot even bear passive range of motion of the joint. One of the identifying features of the arthritis seen in ARF is its migratory nature: The clinician may see significant erythema and pain on motion in one joint; a few hours later, the joint is fine but a new joint has acquired the same symptomatology. The arthritis is remarkably sensitive to salicylates. If the arthritis is resistant to this medication and there are no other major criteria, the diagnosis of ARF should be reevaluated. Arthritis usually lasts a few days to a couple of weeks.[27] Erosive arthritis does not occur.

Carditis

Carditis is the most serious manifestation of ARF. It may appear as a new murmur, tachycardia, electrocardiographic abnormalities, chest pain, or overt signs of congestive heart failure. Congestive heart failure is a poor prognostic sign. Carditis is more commonly seen in younger patients. The frequency of rheumatic fever carditis in the United States is approximately 40%.[3]

Sydenham's Chorea

The onset of chorea in ARF is usually later than that of arthritis or carditis, often occurring up to 3 months after the streptococcal infection. It is more common in girls than boys and in younger children. The choreiform movements most commonly involve the face, tongue, and hands. It usually does not occur during sleep. The patient may have difficulty controlling the movements fully, and it may be exacerbated by stress. The chorea may last weeks to months.[3]

Erythema Marginatum

This is an unusual manifestation of ARF, occurring in only 10% of patients. The rash may be transient in nature. It usually manifests on the trunk and is erythematous in quality with central clearing (Fig. 12-12). Erythema marginatum is associated with those patients who develop carditis.[3]

Subcutaneous Nodules

Subcutaneous nodules are usually small (<1 cm), appear on bony prominences, and are painless. These lesions are uncommon, occurring in less than 10% of patients, and are usually found in sick patients with carditis or in children with recurrent ARF. Histologically, the nodules seen in JRA cannot be distinguished from those seen in ARF.

Table 12-3 Revised Jones Criteria for Rheumatic Fever

Major criteria	Carditis
	Polyarthritis
	Chorea
	Erythema marginatum
	Subcutaneous nodules
Minor criteria	Clinical
	Fever
	Arthralgia
	Laboratory
	High erythrocyte sedimentation rate OR high C-reactive protein level
PLUS:	
Evidence of preceding streptococcal infection:	Elevated antistreptococcal antibody value and/or throat culture or rapid streptococcal antigen test result positive for streptococci

*The presence of two major or of one major and two minor criteria indicates a high probability of acute rheumatic fever; if supported by evidence of preceding streptococcal infection.

Laboratory Studies

Laboratory studies to document a streptococcal infection are paramount. If a throat culture is not positive for GABS then tests for anti-streptolysin O (ASO) antibodies, anti-deoxyribonuclease B, antihyaluronidase, antistreptokinase, or a combination of these markers, should be completed. A fourfold rise or fall in titers of such markers should be sought over time. The specificity of the diagnosis is higher if more than one titer is documented as being elevated. A rise in the acute-phase reactants (ESR and C-reactive protein values) remains elevated for prolonged periods. If these levels are checked while the patient still has arthritis or carditis, they are usually still quite high. These markers may not be elevated if a

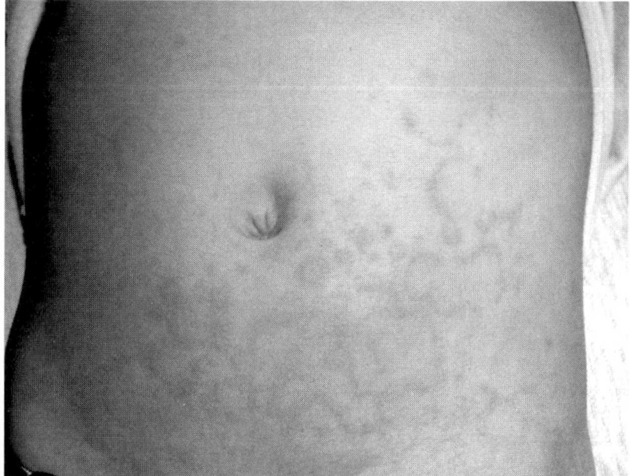

Figure 12-12 Example of erythema marginatum in a patient with rheumatic fever.

patient presents only with chorea. Patients may also have leukocytosis and mild anemia.

Cardiac evaluation should include both electrocardiogram (EKG) and echocardiogram. Abnormalities that can be seen on EKG include PR prolongation and, much less frequently, second-degree or complete heart block. S-T elevations across all leads may be indicative of pericarditis. Chest radiographs may demonstrate cardiomegaly if carditis occurs.

Treatment

Treatment of ARF consists of eradication of the GABS infection, general management of disease manifestations, and prophylaxis of rheumatic heart disease, and prophylaxis of endocarditis. Treatment of the acute GABS should involve a 10-day course of penicillin or an intramuscular injection of benzathine penicillin. If the patient is allergic to penicillin, erythromycin can be used.[3]

General management principles include bed rest for approximately 3 weeks or until the acute phase reactant values are returning to normal. If carditis has been severe, the cardiologist may order a more prolonged period of rest. Aspirin, 75 to 100 mg/kg/day, should be used for fever and arthritis. As mentioned previously, the arthritis responds dramatically to salicylates. Aspirin is usually used for 6 to 12 weeks; however, naproxen has also been shown to be effective.[28] Some physicians may choose to use glucocorticoids for initial management in patients with carditis. Dosages of 1 to 2 mg/kg/day are used initially and tapered after 2 to 3 weeks. Aspirin therapy, initiated after glucocorticoids are tapered, is continued for 3 weeks longer. Treatment of chorea is directed at the symptomatology.[3]

Prophylaxis is administered to prevent future cardiac manifestations of GABS infections. Benzathine penicillin, given intramuscularly every 3 weeks, or oral penicillin V can be used. Prophylaxis is suggested until age 21 years, or throughout life if the patient is at high risk for GABS infection.[3]

Endocarditis prophylaxis for patients with rheumatic heart disease is suggested before dental or surgical procedures. Doses and administration schedules depend on the nature and invasiveness of the procedure to be performed.

Disease Course and Prognosis

Arthritis and carditis are the most common manifestations of ARF, occurring within the first 2 to 6 weeks. Erythema marginatum, subcutaneous nodules, and chorea are less common and may occur later in the disease process (Fig. 12-13). Prognosis is determined by the severity of the carditis. ARF can recur, and the risk of cardiac involvement grows with subsequent attacks. The course of rheumatic fever can be prolonged (e.g., longer than 6 months), but rarely.

Differential Diagnosis

The differential diagnosis of ARF depends on the clinical manifestations. Arthritis and fever may be mistaken for Kawasaki disease, serum sickness, systemic JRA, or infectious arthritis. Confusion may occur in the differentiation of rheumatic fever without carditis, rash, or nodules from post-streptococcal arthritis.

Post-Streptococcal Reactive Arthritis

There are differing opinions as to whether post-streptococcal reactive arthritis (PSRA) is its own entity or, rather, is on a continuum with rheumatic fever. Differences between the two conditions appear to exist but may be based on circular arguments or definitions of the disease.

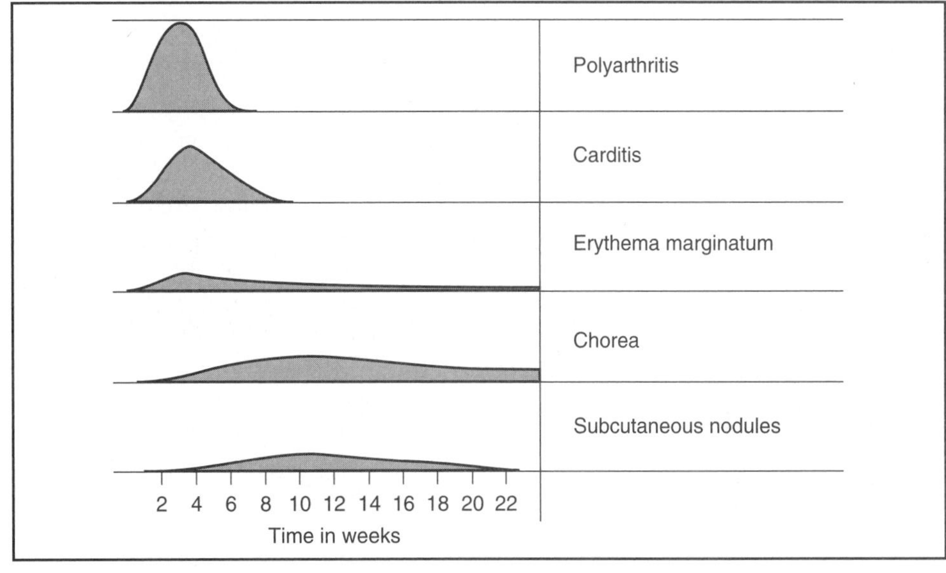

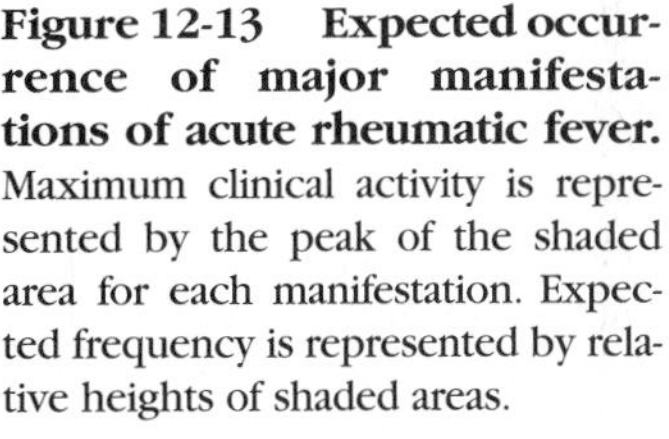
Figure 12-13 Expected occurrence of major manifestations of acute rheumatic fever. Maximum clinical activity is represented by the peak of the shaded area for each manifestation. Expected frequency is represented by relative heights of shaded areas.

Arthritis

The joint symptoms of PSRA typically manifest sooner than those of rheumatic fever. For the majority of patients with PSRA, onset of arthritis occurs within 10 days of the preceding streptococcal pharyngeal infection. The arthritis of PSRA primarily affects large joints, but also involves small joints in 10% to 30% of cases. Small joint involvement is very rare in ARF. Axial skeletal involvement, rare in ARF, has been reported in almost a quarter of patients with PSRA.[27] The arthritis differs from that in rheumatic fever because it is not migratory; rather, it is additive and not as responsive to salicylates or NSAIDs. Symptoms may last months after initiation of NSAID therapy.[27] In contrast to the association of ARF with HLA-DR*B*1*01, PSRA is associated with HLA-DR*B*1*16.[26]

Carditis

Approximately 6% of patients diagnosed with PSRA do have carditis; however, patients who have PSRA and are treated with antimicrobial prophylaxis do not experience carditis.[26] The carditis seen in PSRA tends to be "silent."[29] No patients with PSRA have Sydenham chorea or erythema marginatum; a patient with either of these symptoms most likely has ARF.

Treatment

Although the incidence of carditis is lower in PSRA than in ARF, it is prudent to give prophylactic antibiotics to patients with PSRA. Opinions may differ as to the duration of therapy, but given the dire complications of carditis, one might consider therapy at least until the patient is 21 years old.

LYME DISEASE

Incidence and Epidemiology

Lyme disease is a vector-borne systemic disease that manifests as symptoms mimicking those of many rheumatic, neurologic, and cardiovascular disorders. The disease was originally recognized in 1975 from the geographic clustering of children diagnosed with JRA in Lyme, Connecticut.[30] Lyme disease has become the most prevalent vector-borne disease in the United States (accounting for 90% of cases).[31,32] Almost 92% of reported cases of Lyme disease occur in the northeastern and mid-Atlantic states of the U.S., and most outbreaks appear between April and October (Table 12-4). However, forested regions of Europe and Asia have reported cases as well.[31]

Children between 5 and 9 years old represent the highest population reported with the disease annually.[33] The incidence of the disease continues to rise. In 2000, 13,309 cases were reported to the U.S. Centers for Disease Control and Prevention (CDC), and between 1993 and 2003, approximately 158,448 cases were reported.

Table 12-4 Distribution of Lyme Disease by State, 1992-1998

State	Cases, n (% of Total)	Cases/100,000 Persons
New York	29,172 (32.8)	23.3
Connecticut	15,523 (17.4)	67.9
Pennsylvania	13,020 (14.6)	15.4
New Jersey	10,852 (12.2)	19.9
Wisconsin	3,237 (3.6)	9.5
Rhode Island	3,128 (3.5)	44.8
Maryland	2,758 (3.1)	8.3
Massachusetts	2,118 (2.4)	5.1
Delaware	883 (1.0)	18.5
Minnesota	1,522 (1.7)	5.0

Adapted from Van Solingen RM, Evans J: Lyme disease. Curr Opin Rheumatol 13:293-299, 2001.

However, some studies estimate that the number of reported cases accounts for only 50% to 60% of the actual occurrences of Lyme disease, whereas others argue that the disease is overdiagnosed. Those who believe that Lyme disease is underdiagnosed attribute this state to the strict regulations imposed by the CDC for actual diagnosis coupled with the inaccuracy of laboratory results and overall complexity of the disease. The controversy over the diagnostic accuracy of Lyme disease is just one of the debates surrounding this highly publicized disease. Diagnostic methodology, treatment protocols, and preventive measures are also strongly debated among various members of the medical community.

Etiology

Lyme disease is caused by the spirochete *Borrelia burgdorferi,* which thrives in the gut of the deer tick species *Ixodes scapularis* (East coast strain) and *Ixodes pacificus* (along the Western seaboard). The deer tick undergoes three stages of development: larval, nymph, and adult. The *Ixodes* nymph, which is smaller than its adult counterpart and more abundant, causes the largest number of infections. The *Ixodes* larvae infect mice, deer, birds, and other small animals. The *Ixodes* nymph then feeds on these infected animals, thereby acquiring the disease and passing it on to its hosts and offspring. A small proportion of *I. pacificus* ticks (1% to 3%) are infected with *B. burgdorferi*, most likely because of the feeding habits of the tick in its nymph stage.[31] *I. pacificus* nymphs feed primarily on lizards, which are not susceptible to the spirochete and therefore do not aid in its transmission.

Unfortunately, the *Ixodes* species are capable of transmitting more than one pathogen to their hosts, a feature that appears to increase the severity of symptoms.

Patients suffering from multiple infections often have Lyme disease as well as babesiosis or human granulocytic ehrlichiosis (HGE); fortunately, all of these disorders are responsive to appropriate antibiotic therapy.

Presentation

Lyme disease gives rise to a variety in symptoms, including flu-like symptoms, fever, headaches, Bell palsy, and erythema chronicum migrans (ECM) in more than 60% of patients (Box 12-2). It is estimated that two of every three patients with Lyme disease present with nonspecific systemic features,[31] whereas others experience fevers, diffuse myalgias, arthralgias, headaches, fatigue, malaise, adenopathy, hepatosplenomegaly (rare), and conjunctivitis.

Early Disease

ECM occurs within in 1 month of infection in 50% to 70% of patients with Lyme disease. ECM is an erythematous macule or papule usually found in the groin, thigh, or axilla areas. Approximately one of every four patients has secondary lesions, although these usually fade over time and are thought to result from an immunologic response to the pathogen.[31] The skin lesion is usually painless, but some patients complain of tingling or burning sensations around the area. The rash expands concentrically, giving the appearance of a bull's eye. It is possible to culture organisms from specimens collected at the expanding edge of a lesion.[31] Early disseminated disease may result in satellite ECM lesions (Fig. 12-14). Spirochetes are not found in the margins of these secondary rashes.

Lyme disease commonly affects the joints. The patient may experience brief and recurrent attacks of asymmetric swelling and pain in large joints, especially the knee.[30] Early neurologic manifestations of the disease are meningoencephalitis, cranial neuropathy (typically, Bell palsy), radiculoneuropathy, encephalopathy, and encephalomyelitis. Sensorineural hearing loss is a rare occurrence in the European form of the disease. Ocular manifestations of the disease have also been reported, including a wide range of neuro-ophthalmologic disorders.[33]

Box 12-2 Symptoms of Lyme Disease

EARLY DISEASE: STAGE I (1-4 WEEKS)
- Erythema chronicum migrans (ECM)
- Muscle and joint aches
- Headache
- Fever
- Fatigue

EARLY DISSEMINATED DISEASE: STAGE II (MONTHS)
- Multiple ECM lesions
- Facial paralysis (Bell palsy)
- Meningitis
- Radiculitis (numbness, tingling, burning)
- Brief episodes of joint pain and swelling

LATE CHRONIC DISEASE: STAGE III (MONTHS TO YEARS)
- Arthritis, intermittent or chronic
- Encephalopathy (mild to moderate confusion)

LESS COMMON SYMPTOMS OF LYME DISEASE
- Heart abnormalities
- Eye problems such as conjunctivitis
- Chronic skin disorders
- Encephalomyelitis (limb weakness, motor coordination)

Adapted from the National Institutes of Health: How Lyme Disease Is Diagnosed, 1999. Available online at http://www.niaid.nih.gov/publications/lyme/diagnosis.htm/

Early Disseminated Disease

Sixty percent of untreated patients experience migratory joint involvement of large joints, most commonly the knee. Synovial fluid counts may range from mild

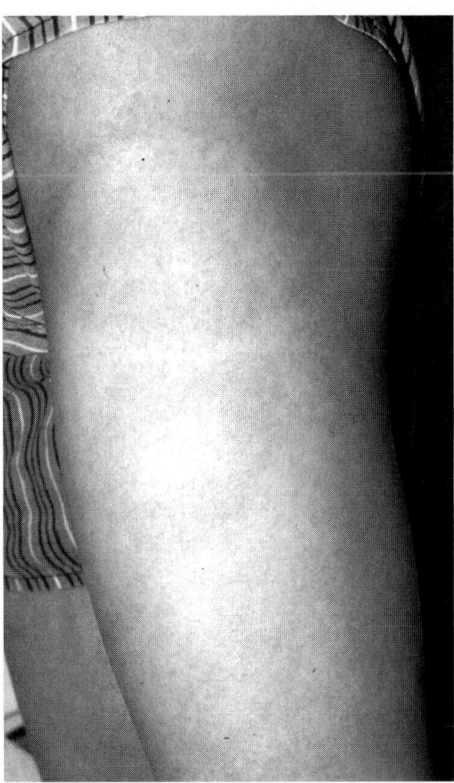

Figure 12-14 Patient with Lyme disease showing erythema chronicum migrans. There are several secondary lesions on the leg. Note the bull's eye pattern.

inflammation to appearing septic. Progressive neurologic manifestations occur in 10% to 15% of untreated patients, resulting in encephalitis, meningitis, cranial or peripheral neuropathy, radiculitis, mild neck stiffness, memory and concentration problems, lymphocytic meningitis, and facial nerve palsy. Only 10% of untreated patients have cardiac symptoms, which include fluctuating degrees of atrioventricular heart block, myopericarditis, and mild congestive heart failure.[31]

Late Chronic Disease

Patients who do not receive treatment may suffer from serious joint and neurologic manifestations months to years after initial infection. These patients may experience acute attacks of arthritis, arthralgia, joint erosion, tendonitis, bursitis, enthesitis affecting the back, neck, and upper body, fibromyalgia resulting in sleep disturbances, and diffuse myalgias. The attacks of arthritis and arthralgia appear to decrease in frequency and duration over time, and only a few large joints tend to be affected. Approximately 1% of untreated patients experience long-term neurologic manifestations such as encephalopathy, polyneuritis, and cognition and psychiatric changes.[31]

Differential Diagnosis

Lyme disease has been called one of the "great imitators" because of its common and sometimes perplexing symptoms. The differential diagnosis for Lyme disease includes JRA, sarcoidosis, SLE, multiple sclerosis, myopathy, ehrlichiosis, Rocky Mountain spotted fever, primary fibromyalgia, rheumatic fever, gonococcal arthritis, temporomandibular joint syndrome, gout, polymyalgia rheumatica, psychogenic rheumatism, Reiter syndrome, seronegative rheumatoid arthritis, and syphilis (Box 12-3).[30,31] The single most common diagnosis to exclude in children in whom Lyme disease is suspected is pauciarticular JRA.[30]

Box 12-3 Differential Diagnosis for Lyme Disease

Juvenile rheumatoid arthritis, specifically pauciarticular
Seronegative rheumatoid arthritis
Gonococcal arthritis
Sarcoidosis
Systemic lupus erythematosus
Multiple sclerosis
Myopathy, ehrlichiosis
Rocky Mountain spotted fever
Primary fibromyalgia
Rheumatic fever
Temporomandibular joint syndrome
Gout
Polymyalgia rheumatica
Psychogenic rheumatism
Reiter syndrome
Syphilis

Physical Examination and Laboratory Studies

Because of the systemic nature of Lyme disease, a careful examination at presentation is essential. Recognizing the history or risk of exposure to infected ticks (i.e., endemic area, outdoor activities) as well as noting symptoms, such as ECM at presentation, provides the physician with a high pretest probability that the result of a blood test for Lyme disease will be positive.

In 1987, the U.S. Food and Drug Administration (FDA) approved a two-step diagnostic protocol for the serologic recognition of Lyme disease in 1987, involving (1) an enzyme-linked immunosorbent assay (ELISA), the results of which would be validated by (2) an immunoglobulin (Ig) G (and/or IgM) Western blot analysis. ELISA is the most effective screening tool because culturing the organism is impractical, and blood cultures produce a low yield. ELISA is an effective test because it can be standardized and automated, and is easily reproducible. The method has a sensitivity of 94% and a specificity of 97%. Sonicated whole *B. burgdorferi* are most often used as an antigen with 41-kDa purified flagellin protein to increase IgM sensitivity. IgM ELISA is most responsive 2 to 4 weeks after infection, whereas IgG response occurs within 6 to 8 weeks.[31] False-positive results may occur from lack of standardization, whereas false-negative results are attributed to attenuation of the antibody response because of antibiotic therapy or testing very early in the course of infection. The accuracy of laboratory diagnosis has been improved by requiring the presence of 5 of 10 bands on Western blot analyses to determine a positive immunoblot result.[32] Nevertheless, serology reports are not 100% consistent. True seronegative Lyme disease is rare in patients with clinical manifestations of disseminated or chronic disease. Furthermore, it is estimated that 8% of people living in areas endemic for *Ixodes* ticks are serologically positive but asymptomatic for the disease.[31]

In 1995, the CDC expanded the diagnostic procedure for Lyme disease by issuing the following criteria: (1) patients must present with ECM, (2) patients must show one or more manifestations of the disease, and (3) these two criteria must be substantiated by positive laboratory findings.[32] However, criterion 1 is often absent in pediatric Lyme disease. Criterion 2 may include the occurrence of arthritis, objective findings of central nervous system (CNS) involvement, encephalopathy in conjunction with a cerebrospinal fluid (CSF) to serum Lyme ELISA titers ratio greater than 1, cardiovascular system involvement, or residence or presence of the patient in an endemic county within 30 days of onset of symptoms. An *endemic county* is defined as a region where two cases have occurred or where infected ticks have been detected.[31] Unfortunately, Lyme disease remains difficult to diagnose.

Although diagnosis based on presence of ECM coupled with characteristic symptoms of articular, neurologic, or cardiac manifestations of Lyme disease with serologic confirmation is standard, new diagnostic techniques are currently being explored. Studies have begun to test the reliability and effectiveness of using recombinant chimeric *Borrelia* proteins with ELISA to gain diagnostic confirmation of the disease.[33]

Treatment and Disease Course

Although much controversy remains as to the proper treatment for Lyme disease, most physicians treat the disease with oral antibiotic therapy (Tables 12-5 and 12-6). Doxycycline, 1 to 2 mg/kg twice daily for children older than 8 years, or amoxicillin, 50 mg/kg/day divided into 2 doses, for 3 to 4 weeks is recommended for early localized or early disseminated Lyme disease in absence of neurologic and cardiovascular involvement. Intravenous ceftriaxone, 75 to 100 mg/kg/day IV in a single dose, or a third-generation cephalosporin should be administered for patients with Lyme disease and neurologic involvement or cardiovascular block. Azithromycin, 10 mg/kg/day, and clarithromycin, 7.5 mg/kg twice daily, have also been found to be effective.

Some reports warn that patients may feel worse at the start of antibiotic therapy, a development that has been regarded as a Jarisch-Herxheimer reaction. It occurs as the antibiotics eradicate *B. burgdorferi* organisms from the circulatory system. Symptoms of this reaction include fever, chills, aches, and fatigue. The reaction occurs in 10% to 14% of patients treated for Lyme disease. Serologic results may remain positive for years after treatment. Therefore, response to treatment must be determined clinically.

Children who are diagnosed and treated for Lyme disease in a timely fashion have an excellent prognosis. If treatment failure occurs, a second treatment with the same antibiotic is recommended. If left untreated, patients may suffer chronic neurologic or articular manifestations. Thus, recognition of the disease and timely treatment are essential for eradicating this disease in the pediatric population.

Table 12-5 Treatment Options for Patients with Lyme disease: Drug Therapy

Drug	Dosage for Children
Preferred oral	
Amoxicillin*	50 mg/kg/day divided into 2 doses (max: 500 mg/dose)
Doxycycline*	Age <8 yr: not recommended Age ≥8 yr: 1-2 mg/kg 2× daily (max: 100 mg/dose)
Alternative oral	
Cefuroxime axetil*	30 mg/kg/day divided into 2 doses (max: 500 mg/dose)
Preferred parenteral	
Ceftriaxone	75-100 mg/kg/day IV in a single dose (max: 2 g)
Alternative parenteral	
Cefotaxime	150-200 mg/kg/day IV divided into 3 or 4 doses (max: 6 g/day)
Penicillin G	200,000-400,000 units/kg/day, divided into doses given every 4 hours (max: 18-24 million units/day)†

*For children intolerant of amoxicillin, doxycycline, and cefuroxime axetil, alternatives are azithromycin, 10 mg/kg/day (max: 500 mg/day); erythromycin, 12.5 mg/kg 4× daily (max: 500 mg/dose); clarithromycin, 7.5 mg/kg 2× daily (max: 500 mg/dose). Patients treated with macrolides should be monitored closely.

†The penicillin dosage should be reduced for patients with impaired renal function.

Adapted from Van Solingen RM, Evans J: Lyme disease. Curr Opin Rheumatol 13:293-299, 2001.

Table 12-6 Treatment Options for Patients with Lyme Disease: Symptom-Based Therapy

Indication	Treatment	Duration (days)
Tick bite	Observe	—
Erythema chronicum migrans	Oral*	14-21
Acute neurologic disease		
Meningitis or radiculopathy	Parenteral*	14-28
Cranial-nerve palsy	Oral*	14-21
Cardiac disease		
1st- or 2nd-degree heart block	Oral*	14-21
3rd-degree heart block	Parenteral*	14-21
Late disease		
Arthritis without neurologic disease	Oral*	28
Recurrent arthritis after oral regimen	Oral or parenteral*	28
Persistent arthritis after two courses of antibiotics	Symptomatic therapy	—
Central nervous system or peripheral nervous system disease	Parenteral*	14-28
Chronic Lyme disease or post–Lyme disease symptoms	Symptomatic therapy	

*See Table 12-5.

Adapted from Van Solingen RM, Evans J: Lyme disease. Curr Opin Rheumatol 13:293-299, 2001.

Additional controversy has arisen over prolonged antibiotic treatment for persistent Lyme disease–related symptoms such as joint pain. Some suggest that such symptoms result from permanent organ damage, slow resolution of the disease, persistence of the organism, or an ongoing immune response.[33] Klempner and associates[34] have reported that patients who were treated with prolonged antibiotic therapy to alleviate persistent symptoms attributed to Lyme disease showed no difference in relief of symptoms from those patients given placebo treatment.[34] Further research continues on this topic.

Research has also provided additional insight to the physiologic implications of Lyme disease. Some studies have indicated that the CD1d gene participates in host defense. Additionally, T cells have been shown to play an active role in the inflammatory response against *B. burgdorferi.* Arthritis-related protein (ARP) appears to be a gene product of the organism that elicits an immune response from the host organism during infection. Studies have also found that *B. burgdorferi* may use surface antigen modulation as a mechanism for evading the host's immune response.[33] Gross and coworkers[35] reported that a peptide from leukocyte function-associated antigen-1 (LFA-1) may act as an autoantigen in treatment-resistant Lyme arthritis.

Prevention

The clear cause of Lyme disease allows for easy methods of prevention. Some authorities suggest wearing light-colored clothing in order to increase visibility of ticks. Children who play outdoors in tick-endemic areas should wear their pants tucked in and long-sleeved shirts. They should be encouraged to walk in the center of paths and to avoid areas of tall grass.

Use of insect repellent is another viable preventive measure. However, it is important to recognize the risks of using insect repellent that contains the chemical *N,N*-diethyl-3-methylbenzamide (DEET). The U.S. Environmental Protection Agency (EPA) currently categorizes DEET with a low-toxicity warning level and allows companies to label insect repellent as "child safe" if the product contains less than 15% of the active ingredient. It is recommended that insect repellent containing DEET not be applied to the hands or around the mouths of children.

Parents should inspect their children after they have been outdoors, remembering that ticks tend to prefer moist, warm locations on the body, such as the groin area, neck, and behind the knees. If a tick is found, tweezers should be used to remove it, grasping the tick's mouth parts as close to the child's skin as possible. The tick should be removed by pulling upward steadily, with care taken not to squeeze. The bitten area should then be cleaned with antiseptic, the child should be observed for signs of the disease, and an ELISA should be performed within 6 to 8 weeks of the bite. If the child demonstrates an ECM rash, treatment for Lyme disease should begin immediately.

It is postulated that a tick must feed for at least 48 hours to infect a host, and some studies have found that transmission is 100% if an infected tick feeds on a host for 72 hours or more.[31] Nevertheless, when infected ticks are removed within 24 to 36 hours, the risk of transmission remains very low. In areas nonendemic for deer ticks and Lyme disease, the risk of acquiring the disease is negligible.

Vaccine

The FDA approved the Lymerix vaccine in December of 1998 for persons 15 to 70 years of age in order to aid in the prevention of Lyme disease.[33] The vaccine, composed of lipidated recombinant OspA protein, works to eliminate or reduce the number of *B. burgdorferi* present within the gut of a tick before entry of the spirochete into the host. The vaccine is given as three doses via intramuscular injection. Side effects have ranged from mild to severe, and its effectiveness is estimated at 78%. Studies have shown that the vaccine for children 2 to 5 years old to be safe and immunogenic,[33] but other studies have found that it may not be cost effective.[36] Nevertheless, controversy remains as to its safety and effectiveness, and further research is necessary to find definitive answers for these concerns.

Summary

Lyme disease is a treatable systemic disease known to mimic the symptoms of a wide range of medical disorders. Although it is the principal vector-borne disease in the United States, the majority of cases arise in the limited geographical area of New England. The etiology of the disease has been traced to the spirochete *B. burgdorferi*, which is transmitted through the feeding habits of infected deer ticks. The symptoms of the disease range from mild skin lesions and moderate joint pain to acute arthritis and cardiovascular or neurologic difficulties. Diagnostic confirmation is based on CDC criteria, although no protocol is 100% accurate. Fortunately, the prognosis for Lyme disease, once treated, is extremely favorable in both children and adults. Further research is needed to alleviate much of the controversy that the diagnostic procedures and treatment protocols for Lyme disease have encountered.

VIRAL ARTHRITIS

A number of viruses have been implicated as causing arthritis and autoimmune disorders in patients. It may be difficult to prove that a virus is the etiologic agent of arthritis. Signs of infection may precede arthritis or an autoimmune syndrome and may be cleared by the immune system, so that testing demonstrates only previous infection by the time the patient presents for medical care. Arthritis and autoimmune processes are not uncommon, so infection with a virus may be coincidental. A few viruses have known clinical features when manifesting as arthritis.

Pathogenesis

Mechanisms of viral arthritis in children are difficult to delineate clearly. Different viruses may cause inflammation in a variety of ways. Certain infections may initiate an immune complex reaction within a joint (e.g., varicella, Coxsackie B, adenovirus), whereas others may cause direct cytopathic changes secondary to viral invasion of the joint (e.g., rubella, mumps).[37]

Rubella Arthritis

Rubella is one of the best-described viral causes of arthritis. The virus is known to cause direct cytopathic changes within the joint, and viral replication has been demonstrated within the joint.[38] The arthritis occurs approximately 1 week after the onset of rash and is typically symmetrical, involving the hands, wrists, ankles, and knees. The pain and morning stiffness are impressive. Most patients experience resolution of symptoms within 1 to 2 weeks, and anti-inflammatory medications are effective for the symptoms. In some patients, a more chronic course reminiscent of rheumatoid arthritis may be initiated. An unusual pediatric presentation of rubella arthritis, called "catcher's crouch," involves acute inflammation and contraction of the knees occurring 1 to 2 weeks after infection.[37] IgM testing is available, but the diagnosis can be made clinically.

Arthritis occurring after rubella immunization is also seen. Its frequency is low, and the course is more benign than that of the wild-type virus infection.

Parvovirus B19 Arthritis

Arthritis initiated by parvovirus B19 should be suspected in a patient presenting with synovitis preceded by a nonspecific viral illness or rash consistent with erythema infectiosum ("slapped cheek" appearance). The clinical course is usually that of acute onset with pain out of proportion to the amount of swelling, and either pauciarticular or polyarticular involvement is seen. Large joints, including knee and hip, are most commonly affected. The course in children is usually benign, with symptoms lasting 2 to 4 weeks. Disease course in adults may be much different, with chronic arthritis and occasionally erosive manifestations. Synovitis may be secondary to the host's immune response or to persistent infection. Parvovirus DNA has been found in the bone marrow, synovial fluid, and synovium, suggesting that failure to clear the organism may be responsible for disease manifestations. Parvovirus IgM should be tested for as soon as possible in any patient suspected of having this postinfectious disease. The presence of IgG antibodies is nondiagnostic because of the high level of seroprevalence in the general population. Cross-reaction with other titers, such as the Lyme ELISA and ANA, can occur.[39] NSAIDs help reduce pain and inflammation until symptoms subside.

Varicella Arthritis

Appearance of arthritis approximately 10 days after varicella infection occurs in a small proportion of children. The arthritis is usually not very painful and presents most commonly as a monoarthritis of the knee. Viral replication is not thought to be a cause of this manifestation; thus, antiviral therapy may not be indicated. Conversely, viral replication may occur with zoster infection when the synovitis occurs in the affected dermatome.[40] NSAIDs should be used for pain; occasionally severe myalgias or arthralgias may require more aggressive pain management.

Epstein-Barr Virus Arthritis

Patients with acute Epstein-Barr virus (EBV) (infectious mononucleosis) may present with a few days of a painful polyarthritis or polyarthralgia. The arthritis tends to be symmetrical, involving the knees and knuckles. The joints may appear dusky in color. Systemic signs of infection, including leukopenia, monocytosis, and thrombocytopenia, should be sought. EBV serologic tests should be obtained, including viral capsid antigen (VCA) IgM as a marker of acute infection. Manifestations of arthritis with EBV are rare and usually respond well to antiinflammatory agents.[39]

Infectious Hepatitis

Both hepatitis B and hepatitis C can cause arthritis. The arthritis seen with hepatitis B is usually of an acute onset, symmetrical, and painful. Other manifestations are rash, lymphadenopathy, palpable purpura, and, in children, acropustulosis palmaris (Gianotti-Crosti syndrome). ANA test results may be positive, and thus, an investigation for SLE may be initiated. A few reports have been published of the rare occurrence of a transient arthritis occurring after immunization against hepatitis B. Any patient with risk factors for hepatitis B who presents with an acute onset of arthritis should be tested.

Hepatitis C virus (HCV) has been associated with a variety of autoimmune symptoms, including arthritis, vasculitis, sicca symptoms (dry eyes and dry mouth), mixed cryoglobulinemia, and positive autoantibody test results, including that for RF. Arthritis is reported in approximately 4% of patients with HCV antibodies.[41] As with hepatitis B, the arthritis is usually symmetrical, painful, and acute in onset. Presence of RF should raise suspicion for HCV in a child with arthritis, given that only 10% of patients with polyarticular JRA are RF positive. This infection should be suspected in patients who have risk factors for hepatitis C or a painful chronic arthritis that is poorly responsive to anti-inflammatory agents.

OTHER CONNECTIVE TISSUE DISEASES WITH CHRONIC ARTHRITIS

Systemic Lupus Erythematosus

SLE is a multisystem autoimmune inflammatory disease involving the blood vessels and connective tissues. Serologic markers (autoantibodies), some of which are highly specific for SLE, characterize it. Disease manifestations are variable from patient to patient, and therefore, so are treatment regimens.

Epidemiology

The incidence of SLE in children younger than 15 years is approximately 1 per 200,000.[42] Ten percent of all patients seen in a pediatric rheumatology clinic have SLE.[43] Disease onset is rare in patients younger than 5 years, but the rate of onset steadily increases until, in adolescence, it is equivalent to that seen in adults. The sex ratio changes with the age at presentation. The ratio of boys to girls with onset from birth to 9 years has been shown to be 3:4; in those 10 to 14 years old, 1:4, and in those 15 to 18 years old, 1:5.[44]

Etiology

The etiology of SLE is unknown, but the disease is presumed to be the manifestation of triggers (environmental, immune dysregulation, hormonal) in a genetically predisposed host. In a study of 107 twin sets, in which one twin fulfilled American College of Rheumatology (ACR) criteria for SLE, the concordance for the disease was 24% in monozygotic twins and 2% in dizygotic twins.[45] There are HLA associations in SLE, some of which are strongly linked with race. A few examples are HLA-DR3 in northern European white persons, and HLA-DR2 in blacks, Chinese, and Japanese persons.[3]

The immune dysregulation in SLE is complex and involves polyclonal immunoglobulin activation by B cells, T-cell dysfunction, and production and deposition of immune complexes. (The immunologic factors involved in the pathogenesis of SLE extend beyond the scope of this text.) An estrogen-mediated effect on SLE has also been suspected. Hormonal abnormalities in children with SLE have been demonstrated, including low levels of testosterone and high levels of follicle-stimulating hormone, luteinizing hormone, and prolactin. Interestingly, patients with Klinefelter syndrome (XXY) have low levels of testosterone and also a higher incidence of SLE than their normal male counterparts. SLE may also be precipitated after infection with viruses or bacteria, medication reactions, and exposure to sunlight.

Presentation

A patient is said to have SLE if 4 of 11 criteria are met. These criteria were revised in 1982,[46] but a later letter suggests that antiphospholipid antibodies should be added, and the LE preparation eliminated from the list (Table 12-7).[1]

Joint Involvement

Arthritis, arthralgia, or both are present in the majority of patients with SLE. The arthritis is often symmetrical and can involve any joint but is most common in the small joints of the hands, wrists, and knees. The arthritis is almost never deforming in nature; it may be of short duration or may become chronic. Significant accumulation of synovial fluid may be asymptomatic (e.g., in the knees), but some patients describe an extremely painful arthritis (e.g., in the hands) with little to no objective findings. Patients with SLE may have ulnar deviation of the hands that is reducible. Swan neck deformities are common and involve extension of the PIP joints and flexion of the DIP joints. No erosions are seen on radiographs, even when subluxation occurs; this finding is called *Jaccoud arthritis*. Tenosynovitis can be an early manifestation of disease and may predispose a patient to development of a tendon rupture. This disorder can be extremely painful, usually is not precipitated by trauma, and is frequently seen in patients who have had prolonged therapy with steroids. Other causes of joint pain must be considered in patients with SLE. Patients are commonly taking steroids and other immunosuppressive medications, so septic arthritis must be considered. Avascular necrosis is not uncommon in this group, especially in patients who have received high doses of or long-term therapy with steroids.

Constitutional Symptoms

Constitutional symptoms are a common presentation for SLE. Patients may have fatigue, malaise, weight loss, and fevers. The clinician must have a high index of suspicion for the diagnosis in a patient with such symptomatology. Children and adolescents may not always present with four criteria for SLE. The disease frequently develops slowly and in stages. Patients may be retrospectively recognized to have had constitutional symptoms for many months before the final diagnosis is made.

Skin Manifestations

Various rashes may be seen in patients with SLE. *Lupus* originates from the Latin word for wolf; it refers to

Table 12-7 1982 American College of Rheumatology Revised Criteria for Classification of Systemic Lupus Erythematosus*

Criterion	Definition
1. Malar rash	1. Erythema over the malar eminences, tending to spare the nasolabial folds
2. Discoid rash	2. Erythematous raised patches with adherent keratotic scaling and follicular plugging; atrophic scarring may occur in older lesions
3. Photosensitivity	3. Rash as a result of unusual reaction to sunlight
4. Oral or nasal ulcers	4. Usually painless, observed by physician
5. Arthritis	5. Nonerosive arthritis involving 2 or more peripheral joints, characterized by tenderness, swelling, or effusion
6. Serositis	6. (a) Pleuritis: pleuritic pain, rub heard by physician, or evidence of pleural effusion
	OR
	(b) Pericarditis: documented by EKG or rub or evidence of pericardial effusion
7. Renal disorder	7. (a) Proteinuria >0.5 grams per day or >3+ if quantitation not performed
	OR
	(b) Cellular casts
8. Neurologic disorder	8. Psychosis in the absence of offending drugs or metabolic derangements
9. Hematologic disorder	9. (a) Hemolytic anemia,
	OR
	(b) Leukopenia (<4000 cells/mm^3 on 2 or more occasions),
	OR
	(c) Thrombocytopenia in the absence of offending drugs
10. Immunologic disorder	10. (a) Anti-double-stranded DNA antibody,
	OR
	(b) Anti-Smith antibody,
	OR
	(c) Positive finding of antiphospholipid antibodies based on (1) an abnormal serum level of IgG or IgM anticardiolipin antibodies, (2) a positive result of test for lupus anticoagulant using a standard method, or (3) a false-positive result of serologic test for syphilis†
11. Antinuclear antibody	11. Abnormal ANA titer not associated with drug

ANA, antinuclear antibody; EKG, electrocardiography; Ig, immunoglobulin; SLE, systemic lupus erythematosus;
*A person is said to have SLE if 4 of the 11 criteria are present.[46]
†Criterion10 adapted from reference 1.
Recreated with permission from American College of Rheumatology. From Tan EM, Cohen AS, Fries JF, et al: The 1982 revised criteria for the classification of systemic lupus erythematosus. Arthritis Rheum 25:1271, 1982.

the facial rash of SLE, which resembles the face of a wolf. The best-recognized rash is the "butterfly" rash, which typically develops over the nasal bridge and along the cheeks (with sparing of the nasolabial fold) secondary to sun exposure (Fig. 12-15). This lesion may last for days, weeks, or longer. Pathologic examination shows immune complexes at the dermal-epidermal junction.

Other SLE rashes may occur in this distribution but are not limited to it. Discoid rashes are chronic cutaneous lesions that begin as erythematous plaques or papules and progress to hypopigmented or hyperpigmented areas; central atrophy may occur. Discoid rashes may appear in a malar distribution, in the ears or on the scalp, torso, or extremities. The areas may have follicular plugging and so may be mistaken for severe acne.

A thorough search must be made to discover subtle lesions. Patients may present with only discoid lesions and no systemic signs or symptoms; these patients are said to have "discoid lupus." Photosensitivity may occur without either a malar or discoid rash. Lymphocytes from patients with SLE appear to be sensitive to ultraviolet light and may trigger a local or systemic inflammatory response. Alopecia, either patchy or diffuse, can manifest as a sign of active SLE secondary to scarring discoid lesions or as a consequence of corticosteroid or cytotoxic therapy.

Oral and Nasal Lesions

Nonpainful oral or nasal lesions are a common manifestation of SLE. Characteristic oral sores are found on the hard palate and are not painful (Fig. 12-16). Nasal lesions may manifest as recurrent epistaxis and are located on the septa. Septal perforations can occur. Similar mucous membrane changes can also be seen on the vagina. The ulcerations are usually shallow and well circumscribed.

Serositis

Serositis may manifest as pleural, pericardial, or peritoneal effusion. Pleuritis is more common than radiographic evidence of pleural effusions, and autopsy evidence of pleuritis is more common than clinical evidence. Pleural effusions are usually small but can be quite large and may also be bilateral.

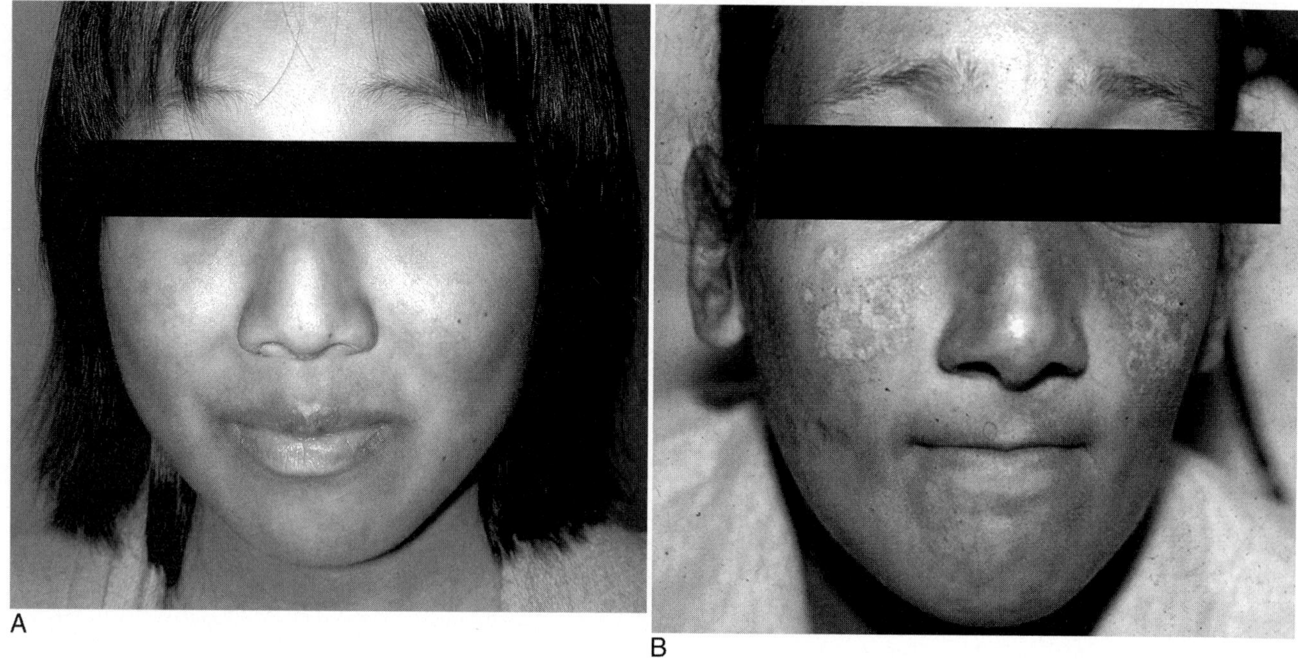

Figure 12-15 **A** and **B**, Patients with systemic lupus erythematosus and malar rashes.

Pericarditis

Pericarditis is the most common manifestation of cardiac involvement in SLE. It is less common than pleuritis, being reported in 20% to 30% of patients but found in up to 60% at autopsy.[47] Pericarditis often manifests as precordial chest pain, pericardial rub, and electrocardiographic changes. Although pericardial effusions are not uncommon, cardiac tamponade is very unusual.

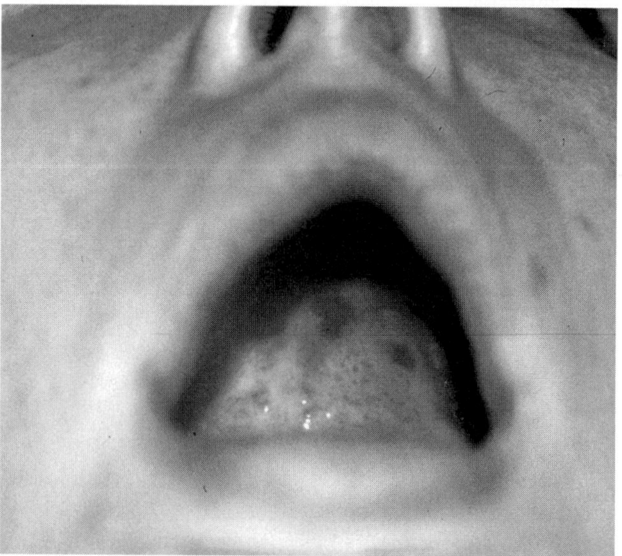

Figure 12-16 Patient with systemic lupus erythematosus with palatal ulcers.

Peritoneal Inflammation

Peritoneal inflammation, although not a formal criterion for SLE, may cause nausea, vomiting, anorexia, and ascites. Autopsy evidence of peritoneal involvement is found in 60% of cases, but clinical evidence is much less common.[48] Lupus ascites may become chronic, is often painless, and may be associated with few other signs or symptoms of active SLE. The differential diagnosis for chronic SLE ascites includes constrictive pericarditis, congestive heart failure, Budd-Chiari syndrome, intraabdominal malignancy, and atypical infections. If infection is a possibility, peritoneal fluid aspiration should be performed as soon as possible.

Cardiopulmonary Involvement

Cardiopulmonary involvement, in addition to serositis, includes pneumonitis, pulmonary hemorrhage, pulmonary hypertension, abnormal pulmonary function values, endocarditis, myocarditis, and coronary artery disease. Coronary artery disease may be vasculitic in nature, but is more commonly atherosclerotic and is much less common in teenage patients.

Renal Involvement

A wide array of renal lesions are involved in SLE. Renal disease, along with CNS disease, accounts for the highest proportion of morbidity and mortality in SLE. The World Health Organization (WHO) has classified these abnormalities (Table 12-8). The WHO classification characterizes renal involvement but does not address the activity or the chronicity of the glomerulonephritis. Commonly, a patient may have a lesion with characteristics that cross classes.

Table 12-8 World Health Organization Classification of Systemic Lupus Erythematosus Nephritis

Class	Description
I	Normal or minimal change in disease
II	Mesangial glomerulonephritis
III	Focal proliferative glomerulonephritis
IV	Diffuse proliferative glomerulonephritis
V	Membranous glomerulonephritis
VI	Advanced sclerosing glomerulonephritis

Common manifestations of glomerulonephritis are asymptomatic hematuria, presence of casts, proteinuria, and pyuria on urine analysis. Patients may present with high serum creatinine level, hypertension, or edema, especially if nephrotic.

Central Nervous System Disease

Nervous system involvement by SLE has neurologic as well as psychiatric manifestations. Signs of neurologic involvement are headaches (most common CNS symptom), strokes, seizures, movement disorders, transverse myelitis, cranial neuropathy, and peripheral neuropathy. Psychiatric involvement may take the form of psychosis, organic brain syndrome, neurocognitive dysfunction, or psychoneurosis.[49] This spectrum of presentations has a variety of pathogenic causes, and in some cases, the pathogenesis is unknown. Some known pathologic findings are thrombotic occlusion of blood vessels, intimal proliferation of small blood vessels, microinfarcts, and, rarely, frank vasculitis. A few antibodies have been associated with neurologic disease in SLE. Antineuronal antibodies have been detected in the CSF and serum of patients with CNS disease, and antiribosomal P protein has been observed in the serum.

Diagnosis of neuropsychiatric disease in SLE is usually clinical. Elevated WBC counts in the CSF along with elevated protein and reduced glucose levels may be present in a third of cases. Elevation of immunoglobulin content in the CSF has been suggested as evidence for CNS disease. Electroencephalographic findings are frequently abnormal in this population but lack specificity. A variety of radiographic imaging modalities have been investigated in SLE, including positron emission tomography (PET), MRI, and phosphorus 32 nuclear magnetic resonance spectroscopy.[49] The utility of these methodologies in screening for CNS involvement by SLE is unclear.

Hematologic Abnormalities

Hematologic abnormalities seen in SLE include anemia, leukopenia, lymphopenia, and thrombocytopenia. Anemia may have many causes, including renal disease, chronic disease, and blood loss, but the hemolytic anemia mediated by autoantibodies is one of the classification criteria for SLE. A Coombs autoantibody test should be performed in all patients with SLE and anemia of unclear etiology. Active SLE frequently causes a leukopenia in the range of 2500 to 4000 WBCs/mm^3. Leukopenia can be complicated by medications known to lower the WBC count. Patients with SLE frequently have antibodies to their own lymphocytes, causing a lymphopenia. Thrombocytopenia of less than 150,000 cells/mm^3 is common in children with SLE. Patients may have antiplatelet antibodies, but sometimes these findings may not be clinically relevant because patients with these antibodies may not be thrombocytopenic. Both immune thrombocytopenic purpura and thrombotic thrombocytopenic purpura may be complications of SLE and must be considered in the appropriate clinical setting.

Immunoserologic Abnormalities

A number of antibodies may be seen in patients with SLE. According to the ACR criteria, anti–double-stranded DNA antibodies (anti-dsDNA), anti-Smith antibodies (anti-Sm), and a false-positive result of the Venereal Disease Research Laboratory test for syphilis, or a combination, constitutes serologic evidence for SLE. In particular, anti-dsDNA and anti-Sm antibodies are very specific for SLE. Approximately 50% to 60% of patients have antibodies to dsDNA, and 25% have anti Sm antibodies. The false-positive VDRL test result suggests antibodies to phospholipid proteins. Antiphospholipid antibodies predispose some patients to having coagulation and thrombotic disorders. In the future, new ACR criteria may be more specific regarding antiphospholipid status as a requirement for diagnosis of SLE.

ANA is present in almost all patients with SLE. A positive ANA response alone, however, is never sufficient evidence to diagnose SLE. Ten percent to 20% of healthy young women have an ANA without any predisposition to an autoimmune process.[50] ANAs may also be present in patients with other autoimmune processes, infections, and malignancies as well as those taking certain medications.

Laboratory Studies

Many possible laboratory abnormalities may be seen in SLE, many of which have been discussed in the presentation section. Other serologic evidence of disease activity includes an elevated ESR and low complement levels (C3 and C4). An elevated ESR may indicate greater disease activity or, in some patients, may remain high for prolonged periods despite disease quiescence. C3 and C4 levels frequently drop during an acute flare, indicating consumption of these substances in an immune complex–mediated process. A number of other autoantibodies can be seen in SLE. Anti-Ro (SS-A) and anti-LA (SS-B) antibodies are seen in SLE and Sjögren's syndrome. These antibodies are associated with neonatal lupus; the presence of SS-A has greater implications for congenital heart block. Antihistone antibodies should be tested in any patient in whom drug-induced SLE is suspected. Drugs that have proved to be associated with drug-induced SLE include minocycline, hydralazine, procainamide, isoniazid, methyldopa, and chlorpromazine.

Physical Examination

Because SLE is a multisystem disease, the physical examination should be a complete one, from head to toe. The hair should be examined for follicular stability. The fundus and eye should be examined for the complications seen with vasculitis, hypertension, corticosteroid therapy, and superimposed infections. The oral and nasal orifices should be checked for lesions. The skin on and around the face should be examined for malar and discoid rashes. The heart should be auscultated for any evidence of new murmurs or rubs, and the lungs for signs of effusion and intrathoracic disease. The abdomen should be examined for hepatosplenomegaly, ascites, and tenderness. If vasculitis is suspected within the abdomen, a rectal examination and stool test for occult blood should be performed.

A thorough examination of the joints should be completed to look for synovitis and limitation of movement. A complete neurologic examination should be done and must test for CNS disease as well as peripheral nerve disease. Deconditioning commonly occurs if a patient is unable to maintain physical activity, so strength should be assessed at each visit. Capillary nail fold loop dilatation is seen less frequently in SLE than in JDM or scleroderma, but its presence may indicate a vasculitic process (Fig. 12-17). Raynaud phenomenon is common in SLE. Affected patients present with the classic color changes to white, blue, and red in the fingertips upon exposure to cold. Occasionally, patients may have ulcerations from ischemia at the tips of the fingers secondary to severe Raynaud phenomenon (Fig. 12-18).

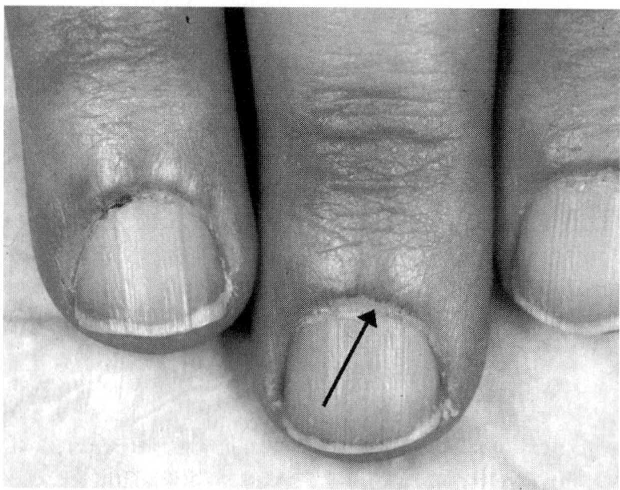

Figure 12-17 Example of grossly visible dilated capillary nail fold loops.

Treatment

A cornerstone of the management of patients with SLE is prevention. SLE activity may wax and wane, and certain measures may prevent a flare. Patients must be reminded to avoid sun exposure. Sun blocks with high level of effective ultraviolet light blockade must be used even in colder weather. Use of long sleeves and hats with brims furthers sun protection. Patients are advised to avoid sulfa-containing antibiotics, which might exacerbate SLE disease activity. Regular follow-up appointments with the pediatrician or rheumatologist are important to monitor urinalysis, blood pressure, laboratory values, and signs of systemic involvement.

Pregnancy often exacerbates disease activity, which can place the mother and fetus at risk if the patient is not closely followed and managed by a high-risk obstetrical specialist; therefore, family planning should be discussed early. If a patient with SLE wishes to become pregnant, it is best to plan the pregnancy at a time when her disease is in remission. Some of the medications used in SLE management are contraindicated in pregnancy (such as cytotoxics). Birth control pills containing estrogen may put patients with SLE at higher risk for thromboembolic disease. A large multicenter trial, the Safety of Estrogen in Lupus Erythematosus–National Assessment (SELENA), is currently under way to evaluate the risk of estrogen-containing birth control pills. Routine immunizations should be given to children with SLE, but live vaccines should not be administered to patients receiving immunosuppressive medications, including corticosteroids.

Medications

NSAIDs are used primarily for the musculoskeletal complaints associated with SLE. This class of medications alleviates the discomfort of arthralgias, myalgias, and arthritis. NSAIDs can also be used for the pain and inflammation

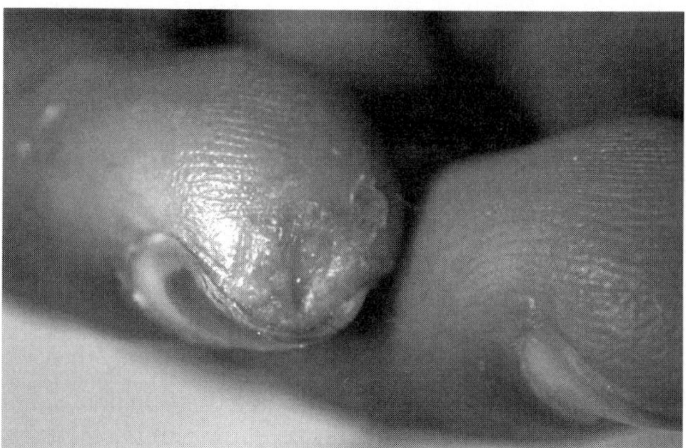

Figure 12-18 Patient with systemic lupus erythematosus and Raynaud phenomena with ulcer.

associated with recurrent pericarditis or pleuritis. Laboratory values must be checked for any alterations in liver function parameters and for any red blood cells or white blood cells in the urine as consequences of these medications. Patients with severe thrombocytopenia should not be given NSAIDs because of their antiplatelet effects.

Antimalarial agents such as hydroxychloroquine (Plaquenil) are used as adjunctive therapy. Hydroxychloroquine is helpful in the management of joint, cutaneous and constitutional symptoms of SLE. It has a very low toxicity profile, but ophthalmology visits every 6 months to 1 year are required to monitor for any retinal damage, including visual field and color testing. Chloroquine, another antimalarial agent, can be used in cases of severe cutaneous disease that is refractory to hydroxychloroquine alone. Liver function parameters must be monitored when this medication is used. Other possible side effects of the antimalarial drugs are dyspepsia, diarrhea, and rash. Hydroxychloroquine has been shown to have a modest lipid-lowering effect.[51] The dose is typically 5 to 6 mg/kg/day, with a maximum dosage of 400 mg per day.

Corticosteroids are widely used in patients with SLE. These agents are effective in quickly decreasing the inflammation that results from active disease. The dose of steroids depends on the complication being treated. Low-dose therapy is typically less than 0.5 mg/kg/day. The arthritis of SLE is usually sensitive to low-dose therapy. Manifestations such as serositis and fever are usually also sensitive to these doses. The dosage is tapered according to the indication for treatment. Higher doses of steroids, 1 to 2 mg/kg/day, usually divided and given twice per day, are used for glomerulonephritis, CNS disease, hemolytic anemia, and vasculitis. Occasionally, pulse-intravenous corticosteroids (30 mg/kg/day, maximum dosage of 1 gram) must be used in a crisis. The side effects of long-term steroid therapy are many, including cataracts, insulin resistance, weight gain with cushingoid features, striae of the skin, and avascular necrosis. The dose should be tapered as is appropriate, and this process should be managed by the rheumatologist, often in conjunction with the nephrologist if glomerulonephritis or hypertension is present.

Cyclophosphamide (Cytoxan) is a nitrogen mustard–alkylating agent used in the management of some glomerulonephritides, some neuropsychiatric diseases, some hematologic manifestations, and some cases of vasculitis. Cyclophosphamide is metabolized by the liver and excreted by the kidney. In patients with either liver or kidney dysfunction, the dose of the medication may have to be altered appropriately. Intravenous cyclophosphamide has been shown to be effective in the management of lupus nephritis and reduces the risk of end-stage renal disease.[52] The possible side effects of cyclophosphamide are substantial. Patients may have nausea and vomiting with administration of the medication and usually require antiemetic medications. Alopecia may result from therapy but is often the result of uncontrolled SLE disease activity. Immune suppression is expected, with the nadir in the WBC count occurring 7 to 14 days after the intravenous dose. Daily oral therapy with cyclophosphamide is occasionally used and requires frequent blood counts. Patients are at greater risk of infection and may need prophylaxis against *Pneumocystis carinii* pneumonia. Bladder damage may result from use of cyclophosphamide, including acute cystitis, hemorrhagic cystitis, fibrosis, and carcinoma. At our institution patients undergoing cyclophosphamide therapy are routinely given mesna (2-mercaptoethanesulfonate), which binds the toxic metabolite known to cause cystitis. Intravenous fluids are also administered before and after the medication to ensure adequate hydration for bladder irrigation.

Purine analogues such as azathioprine and mycophenolate mofetil (MMF) are used in some patients with SLE. MMF, a relatively new medication in the treatment of SLE, has been shown to be effective in membranous nephritis in children and as a steroid-sparing drug.[53] Azathioprine has been used for a longer periods; it is efficacious as an immunosuppressant and a steroid-sparing medication for nonrenal manifestations. In older studies, this agent has been shown to reduce proteinuria, stabilize renal disease, and reduce mortality in patients with diffuse proliferative glomerulonephritis.[54] Side effects include bone marrow suppression; therefore blood counts must be monitored regularly. There are reports of leukemia and non-Hodgkin lymphoma in patients with SLE who were treated with azathioprine.[49]

Other treatments used in SLE, but less frequently, are dapsone, cyclosporine, methotrexate, immune globulin, danazol, and plasmapheresis.

Disease Course

The course of disease in SLE is one of remissions and exacerbations. Some patients may have a benign course marked by constitutional symptoms, positive serologic results, and rash; whereas others have multiorgan involvement and significant morbidity. Morbidity may be a result of the disease or of the treatment. Mortality rates have declined over the years, and surviving patients are now dealing with the long-term consequences of prolonged inflammatory processes and immunosuppressive medications. Complications include the need for dialysis or kidney transplantation, neuropsychiatric alterations, atherosclerosis, osteoporosis, growth delay, infection, malignancy, diabetes, glaucoma, and cataracts.

Prognosis is affected by the patient's socioeconomic status. Non-white race and lower level of education predispose patients to a poorer outcome. Longer disease duration and a higher disease activity also predict a poorer outcome with more extensive organ damage.[55]

Differential Diagnoses

The differential diagnosis for a patient with suspicion of SLE is broad and depends on the symptomatology. Involvement of specialists may play a key role in differentiating the causes of a patient's complaints—for example, psychiatry for CNS symptoms, hematology for cytopenias, and nephrology for declining renal function.

Juvenile Dermatomyositis

JDM is a chronic, systemic vasculopathy that affects the musculature, skin, joints, and, occasionally, visceral organs. An uncommon disease, JDM is nevertheless the most common of the idiopathic myopathies seen in children.

Epidemiology

JDM occurs in approximately 3 per 1 million children. The average age at onset of disease is 7 years. In girls there appears to be two peaks in age of onset, one at 6 years and the other at 10 years. Boys appear to only have one peak, at 6 years. There is some evidence for geographic and seasonal clustering of cases of JDM.

Etiology

The etiology of JDM is unclear. Viral causes have been sought, but no clear evidence has been found; in addition, immunologic factors may play a role. Most studies agree that JDM is an autoimmune condition. Pathogenesis of this disease involves both cell-mediated and immune complex elements. IgG, IgM, and components of C3 have been identified within affected vessel walls in JDM. Genetic predisposition may also predetermine who may be afflicted. There are few familial cases of JDM, but both HLA-B8 and HLA-DR3 occur in a higher proportion of patients with JDM than in the general population.

Presentation

The most common presentation of JDM involves fatigue, proximal muscle weakness, fever, and rash. Fatigue is common in children with JDM, and in young patients, it may represent how parents interpret muscle weakness. Patients may also complain of muscle pain. Muscle disease usually manifests as weakness of the limb-girdle musculature of the lower extremities. Other muscle groups that may be affected are the neck flexors, abdominal musculature, shoulder girdle, facial and extraocular muscles, and, less frequently, distal muscles. Two of the most life-threatening complications are aspiration or choking as a complication of pharyngeal involvement and bowel perforation from vasculitis of the gastrointestinal tract.[3]

Cutaneous disease is pathognomonic in three quarters of patients with JDM. A less characteristic rash is usually seen in the rest of the patients. The most common rashes seen in this disease are heliotrope rash of the eyelids, Gottron papules, and capillary nail fold loop changes. The heliotrope rash is an erythematous to purplish discoloration of the eyelids (Fig. 12-19). There may be marked periorbital edema in patients presenting with JDM. The clinician must be careful to examine along the superior aspect of the eyelid, along the lashes, if JDM is suspected and an obvious heliotrope rash is not present. Gottron papules are erythematous, shiny patches located over the extensor surfaces. The most common location is at the PIP joints and, less commonly, over the metacarpophalangeal (MCP) joints, (DIP) joints, elbows, patellae, and malleoli.

Capillary nail fold loop dilatation, arborization, and dropout are characteristic in JDM. Although this picture is seen also in scleroderma and less frequently in SLE, it is typical of JDM. The nail beds of the fingers can be examined by capillaroscopy. If this diagnostic tool is unavailable, the clinician may use the 40× lens of the ophthalmoscope. We find that petroleum jelly acts as an inexpensive magnifying agent when placed along the nail bed. Dilatation and dropout of capillaries indicates active disease and may denote a disease with a more severe, chronic course.[3]

Arthritis is a common manifestation of JDM. In one series of 80 patients, 61% reported arthritis. Frequently affected joints included the knees, wrists, elbows, and fingers. The arthritis appeared at an average of 4.5 months after the diagnosis of the disease. The initial involvement was oligoarthritis in a third of patients, and polyarticular in two thirds. All cases responded to the therapy instituted for the JDM (41% of patients were taking corticosteroids only), but the arthritis recurred in 39% as the steroid dosages were tapered. In all patients, the arthritis was nonerosive.[56] Arthritis can be a major sequela in JDM, and appropriate measures must be taken to prevent morbidity.

Calcinosis, the accumulation of calcium within the soft tissues, is a cause of long-term morbidity in JDM. Collections frequently appear at sites of trauma, such as the elbows and knees. These areas may exude a milky white fluid when traumatized further. The deposition may cause calcified plaques, nodules, bridging calcification across a joint, clumps in the interfacial planes of muscle (Fig. 12-20), or even exoskeletons in some children. The acute phase of the calcinosis can be inflammatory and painful. Severe calcinosis is thought to occur in patients in whom therapy

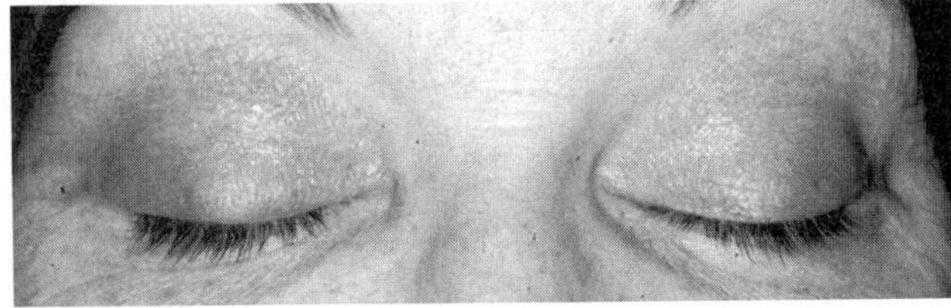

Figure 12-19 Patient with dermatomyositis and heliotrope rash of the eyelids.

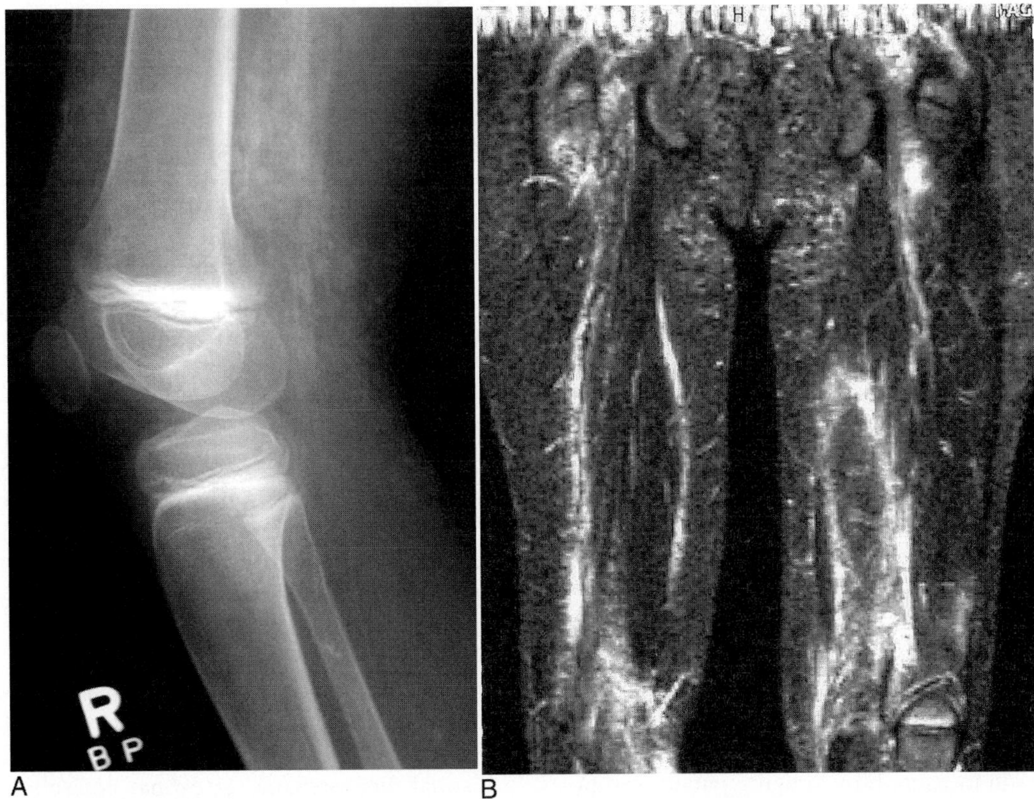

Figure 12-20 Patient with dermatomyositis who presented with diffuse muscle pain of the quadriceps. A, Radiograph shows diffuse soft tissue calcification. **B,** T2-weighted magnetic resonance image of the thighs shows high intensity in soft tissues surrounding muscle groups, a finding consistent with inflammation secondary to calcification, not myositis.

was delayed or whose disease has an aggressive and chronic course. Ulcerated calcium plaques can create a nidus of infection caused by cutaneous microorganisms, and these infections are often exacerbated in children with JDM, who are immunocompromised.

There are other, less common manifestations of disease. *Lipoatrophy,* a localized loss of subcutaneous tissue, frequently occurs in the hands. Pericarditis has been described as well as nonspecific cardiac enlargement and abnormal EKG findings. Subclinical myocarditis may be more common than previously thought, as demonstrated by radioisotope scanning.[57] Vasculitis of the intestines can be life threatening. Affected children present with abdominal pain, melena, and hematemesis. Investigations to rule out intestinal infarction and perforation must be made as quickly as possible. Vasculitis of other visceral organs, such as the urinary bladder, uterus, and testes, can also occur. Respiratory weakness can result in restrictive lung disease, but the interstitial lung disease seen in some adults with myositis is less common in children.

Laboratory Studies

Some of the laboratory abnormalities in JDM are nonspecific markers of inflammation, muscle enzyme elevations, and autoantibodies. Nonspecific markers of inflammation include ESR and C-reactive protein level. These markers can be used to follow disease activity during therapy. The muscle enzymes whose measurements are used include creatine kinase (CK), aldolase, aspartate aminotransferase (AST), and lactic dehydrogenase (LDH). Aldolase and CK are more specific muscle enzymes, and thus, baseline levels of these enzymes should be established to determine how the disease is responding to therapy. CK may be elevated to 20 to 40 times higher than baseline in acute disease. In some children, CK may not be elevated, and other enzymes must be used as markers of disease.

A number of myositis-specific autoantibodies (MSAs) can be seen in myopathies, and a few of these antibodies can be seen in JDM. In adults, identification of a certain MSA may help predict disease course and response to therapy. Approximately 80% of patients with JDM have no identifiable MSA. Anti Mi-2 antibody is one autoantibody detected in some patients with JDM. This autoantibody is associated with disease that responds well to therapy and has a good prognosis.[58]

Muscle biopsy may be a vital procedure in a patient with JDM, to identify the cause of a myopathy if other signs are not prominent. Electromyography (EMG) was formerly used frequently to identify a likely muscle group for biopsy. This practice proved to be problematic for the following reasons: EMG can be painful (especially in a young child), the biopsy cannot be done in the same leg as the EMG because of abnormalities seen on biopsy as a consequence of the EMG, and involvement may be patchy. MRI is now frequently used to identify muscle groups and skin, with inflammation secondary to disease involvement. MRI of the muscles, usually the quadriceps, can aid the surgeon in precisely localizing the proper site for biopsy without the use of EMG. MRI can also be helpful in a patient presenting with acute pain in the proximal musculature in whom it is not clear whether the symptoms are secondary to acute muscle swelling or to inflammation from calcinosis around muscle groups (see Fig. 12-20B).

Physical Examination

The physical examination in a patient in whom JDM is suspected or who has JDM and is being monitored should pay particular attention to skin, joints, and musculature. Muscle strength should be assessed in an organized and reproducible fashion so that the clinician can compare the patient's performances over time. The physician should measure how long the patient can perform certain tasks, such as neck flexion to the chest (the starting position should be with the head extended over the edge of the table) and straight-leg extensions against gravity. Muscle strength, of proximal and distal musculature, should be graded. The child should be asked to perform actions that test proximal muscles, including a complete a sit-up and the Gower maneuver. Gower sign is said to be present if a patient uses the arms to push up the trunk and "climb up the legs" when rising from the floor.

The skin examination should include a thorough search for rash and calcinosis, although calcinosis is usually a late finding. The heliotrope rash may be subtle, especially in dark-skinned children. Gottron papules appear over the knuckles, but other extensor surfaces, such as the knees and elbows, can take on a similar erythematous, shiny appearance. Calcinosis may also be subtle early in the disease. A thorough investigation of the entire body surface area should be completed, and the skin felt for any subcutaneous irregularities. The ophthalmoscope or, if available, capillaroscope should be utilized to examine the nail beds for dilation and dropout of capillary nail fold loops. Interestingly, a careful inspection of the gum line may also show dilated blood vessels.

Treatment

The rarity of JDM prevents the performance of large, controlled, randomized trials of treatment options. Reports of success with treatment regimens are often from single centers and frequently are retrospective. We use 2 mg/kg/day of corticosteroids orally in the initial stages after diagnosis and frequently until laboratory values normalize. If there is any evidence of swallowing difficulty or severe compromise in function, we administer high-dose intravenous prednisolone (Solu-Medrol) promptly. Disease-modifying medications are started almost immediately in order to control disease and allow the tapering of steroids when appropriate. Subcutaneous methotrexate is frequently a first-line therapy.

Hydroxychloroquine is also used in JDM, primarily for skin, arthritis, and constitutional effects. One of the more dangerous total dose–related side effects of hydroxychloroquine is retinal toxicity. Children taking this medication should undergo yearly ophthalmologic examinations, which should include slit-lamp examination as well as testing of color vision, visual acuity, and visual fields. Other drugs that have been used with variable success are intravenous immune globulin, cyclosporine, azathioprine, and cyclophosphamide.

Disease Course

Before the use of steroids, mortality from JDM was near 40%. Mortality in the post-corticosteroid era is down to 3%, and death occurs primarily from gastrointestinal hemorrhage, intestinal infarction, cardiopulmonary complications, and sepsis. The current survival rate is over 90%.

There appear to be four phases involved in the disease course of JDM. The first phase is a prodromal period that lasts weeks to months and involves nonspecific symptoms. In the second phase, the affected child has muscle weakness and rash lasting days to weeks. Continued myositis, weakness, and rash, which can last up to 2 years, marks the third phase. The final phase is the recovery period, in which the child is left with residual weakness, scarring, and calcinosis.

The best prognostic factor in predicting a good outcome is the rapidity with which steroid therapy is initiated. Disease courses may vary greatly, ranging from signs and symptoms lasting less than 1 year to a persistent waxing and waning of symptoms with little resolution. Approximately 20% of children have a more progressive course with poor outcomes. Poor prognosis and mortality are associated with a disease course of rapid onset, cutaneous vasculitis, the finding of severe vascular disease and infarction on muscle biopsy, delay in the institution of therapy, inadequate therapy, and poor response to initial treatment with steroids. Although malignancy is associated with dermatomyositis in adult patients, this is rarely the case in children.[3]

Differential Diagnosis

The list of myopathies and neuromuscular disorders in the differential diagnosis for JDM is a long one; however, most of these are rare. Very few diseases manifest with the classic JDM rash and muscle symptoms. In atypical cases, in which the rash is not classic, other causes of muscle weakness or inflammation should be investigated. Polymyositis is a similar disorder without the typical skin involvement and is more common in African-Americans.

Infectious causes may appear as acute onset of muscle pain. Influenza A and B, Coxsackie B virus, toxoplasmosis, trichinosis, staphylococcal bacteremia, schistosomiasis, and trypanosomiasis have all been implicated in acute myopathies. Infection with *Trichinella spiralis* usually manifests as fever and diarrhea but may be followed by periorbital edema. Swelling of involved muscles, including those of the face, neck, and chest, would be extremely unusual in JDM. Biopsy of the muscles demonstrates the larvae and cysts.

Other connective tissue diseases (CTDs), such as mixed connective tissue disease (MCTD), scleroderma, and SLE, may manifest as myositis and skin involvement. Usually the serologic abnormalities and other systemic complications make differentiation of these diseases from JDM an easy one. The myositis of JDM is usually much more severe and disabling, and involves higher elevations of CK. Vasculopathy is not seen on muscle biopsy in SLE, JRA, or scleroderma. The skin involvement in JDM, if atypical or early, can be mistaken for other entities. Children with JDM may have a malar blush, but it is not usually as intense as that of SLE, and there is not the typical sparing of the nasolabial folds as in SLE. Capillary nail fold changes can be seen in other CTDs that involve vasculitis, such as scleroderma, SLE, and MCTD, but the classic heliotrope rash and Gottron papules are not.

Many neuromuscular diseases and myopathies may have similar signs or symptoms in a patient with an atypical presentation of JDM. Muscular dystrophy is usually a slowly progressive disease that does not evolve as quickly as JDM. There may be similar involvement of the proximal musculature and elevations in CK. Patients with Duchenne muscular dystrophy commonly have calf hypertrophy, a sign not seen in JDM. Myoadenylate deaminase deficiency is an autosomal recessive deficiency of an enzyme that causes muscle fatigue, cramping, and stiffness after exercise; it frequently appears in child hood and may be secondarily associated with a rheumatic disorder. Affected patients may have decreased muscle mass, and usually the elevation of CK is only modest. The diagnostic laboratory test result is a failure to produce increases in plasma ammonia after exercise of the forearm. Lack of the enzyme can be detected on muscle biopsy. Medications may also induce myopathy; some of these are hydroxychloroquine, steroids, alcohol, hMG CoA (3-hydroxy-3-methylglutaryl coenzyme A) reductase inhibitors, and penicillamine. The list of neuromuscular disorders in the differential diagnosis for JDM is a long one, and if indicated, a pediatric neurologist should evaluate the child.

Malignancies Causing Rheumatic Complaints

Musculoskeletal complaint may be one of the initial symptoms in a child with a malignancy. The clinician must have a high index of suspicion and must know what signs and symptoms are consistent with malignancy versus a rheumatologic disorder. In a review of 29 children initially referred for a rheumatic disease and later identified as malignancies, 48% of patients had clinical features atypical for any rheumatic disorder.[59] Signs and symptoms in this series that were considered "worrisome" were monoarticular bone pain and bone tenderness, back pain, severe constitutional symptoms, discordantly high ESR and low platelet count, elevated lactic dehydrogenase (LDH), and abnormal CBC results. The investigators in this study make the point that back pain is a very unusual complaint in pediatric rheumatologic disorders, even JAS and spondyloarthropathy; back pain is usually a late manifestation in these diseases. They also point out that night sweats, a constitutional sign, are extremely unusual in rheumatologic disorders (despite the presence of high spiking fevers) but are not as uncommon in malignancies. Referring diagnoses in this study included JRA, spondyloarthropathy, SLE, Kawasaki disease, mixed connective tissue disorder, Lyme disease, and JDM.

In another study, Ostrov and colleagues compared the cases of 10 children with acute leukemia and 10 children with systemic-onset JRA. Some of their findings are summarized in Table 12-9.[60] They found that certain laboratory findings did not significantly differ in

Table 12-9 Findings at Time of Diagnosis: Acute Leukemia vs. Systemic-Onset Juvenile Rheumatoid Arthritis

	Leukemia	Systemic-Onset JRA
Morning stiffness with high spiking fevers	+	++++
Night-time pain with awakenings	++++	None
Bony pain (not articular)	++++	None
Thrombocytosis	+	++++
WBC differential count	Lymphocytosis	Neutrophilia
^{99m}Tc bone scan findings	Multiple "hot" areas or single "cold" lesions	Arthritis
Arthralgia without arthritis	++++	None
Arthritis	++	++++

JRA, juvenile rheumatoid arthritis; ^{99m}Tc, technetium 99m; WBC, white blood cell; +, <25% of cases; ++, 25% to 50% of cases; +++, 51% to 75% of cases; ++++, >75% of cases.[60]

the two groups, including ANA, RF, uric acid, LDH, and ESR. WBC counts and the differential counts varied between the two groups, depending on time of onset of signs and symptoms versus a delay in time to diagnosis. The total WBC count was not significantly different between the two groups; rather the composition of the total WBC count was different, and only at the time of diagnosis. Specifically, in systemic-onset JRA, there was a neutrophilia, and in leukemia, there was a lymphocytosis.[60]

In a third series examining 10 patients initially complaining of musculoskeletal symptoms who were later determined to have malignancies, the final diagnoses included acute leukemia, non-Hodgkin lymphoma, Ewing sarcoma, and neuroblastoma.[61] The preliminary diagnoses were JRA, PSRA, "post-viral arthralgia," septic arthritis, JDM, and "rheumatic disorder." The researchers in this study found common complaints to be a monoarticular arthritis either of the elbow or knee that was usually transient, pain out of proportion to the extent of swelling, and lack of morning stiffness. Other symptoms were night sweats, hepatosplenomegaly, and lymphadenopathy. Diagnostic procedures were lymph node biopsy and bone marrow aspiration. Interestingly, initial diagnostic aspirates in three of seven patients showed only cellular hypoplasia. Unfortunately, second aspiration procedures were required to make the diagnosis of malignancy.

A misdiagnosis of a rheumatic disease in a patient with a malignancy may delay the time to appropriate treatment. Treatment with corticosteroids could also worsen the prognosis in patients with leukemia.[62] The clinician must maintain a high degree of suspicion and continue to reevaluate the patient who presents with atypical symptomatology.

SUMMARY

There are many causes of acute and chronic synovitis in children. JRA and spondyloarthropathy account for a large majority of chronic arthritides, whereas viral and postinfectious arthritides, Lyme disease, and rheumatic fever are some of the more frequently seen acute causes. SLE and JDM are two of the autoimmune diseases with chronic arthritis that are treated by pediatric rheumatologists. Searching for and discovering specific history and physical findings increase the clinical suspicion for particular diagnoses and improve the pretest probability of certain test results (e.g., HLA-B27 and Lyme ELISA). Worrisome signs and symptoms (such as night-time pain, pain out of proportion to findings, and lymphocytosis) should direct diagnostic testing to rule out malignancies that can be disguised as rheumatic illnesses, with consequent delay in diagnosis. We hope this review has elucidated when appropriate testing should and should not be performed (e.g., ANA and RF). Chronic arthritis in children is not uncommon, but it can be appropriately managed when identified early.

ACKNOWLEDGMENTS

The authors would like to give special thanks for the generous donation of clinical photographs to: Daniel Albert, MD, Jon Burnham, MD, and H. Ralph Schumacher, MD.

MAJOR POINTS

- Childhood chronic arthritis may be painless in up to one third of children.
- Approximately 1 in 1,000 children in the U.S. will develop chronic arthritis.
- A potentially very dangerous complication of systemic JRA is macrophage activation syndrome.
- In endemic regions, Lyme disease should be ruled out when diagnosing chronic arthritis of childhood.
- Children with JRA need frequent ophthalmologic screening to detect silent uveitis.
- Intra-articular corticosteroid injections are often the treatment of choice for children with chronic arthritis.
- Juvenile spondyloarthropathies are a relatively common form of childhood arthritis and can be distinguished from JRA by the presence of enthesitis.
- Chronic arthritis can be associated with underlying connective tissue diseases such as systemic lupus erythematosus and juvenile dermatomyositis.

REFERENCES

1. Hochberg MC: Updating the American College of Rheumatology revised criteria for the classification of systemic lupus erythematosus. Arthritis Rheum 40:1725, 1997.
2. Horvath SM, Hollander JL: Intra-articular temperature as a measure of joint reaction. J Clin Invest 218:543-548, 1949.
3. Cassidy JT, Petty RE (eds): Textbook of Pediatric Rheumatology, 4th ed. Philadelphia, WB Saunders, 2001.
4. Grom AA, Passo M: Macrophage activation syndrome in systemic juvenile arthritis. J Pediatr 129:630-632, 1996.
5. Cron RQ, Sharma S, Sherry DD: Current treatment by United States and Canada pediatric rheumatologists. J Rheumatol 56:2036-2038, 1999.
6. Wallace CA, Sherry DD: A practical approach to avoidance of methotrexate toxicity. J Rheumatol 22:1009-1012, 1995.
7. Spiegel LR, Schneider R, Lang BA, et al: Early predictors of poor functional outcome in systemic-onset juvenile rheumatoid arthritis. Arthritis Rheum 43:2402-2409, 2000.

8. Sherry DD, Stein LD, Reed AM, et al: Prevention of leg length discrepancy in young children with pauciarticular juvenile rheumatoid arthritis by treatment with intraarticular steroids. Arthritis Rheum 42:2330-2334, 1999.

9. Huppertz HI, Tshammler A, Horwitz A, et al: Intraarticular corticosteroids for chronic arthritis in children: Efficacy and effects on cartilage and growth. J Pediatr 127:317-321, 1995.

10. Sharma S, Sherry D: Joint distribution at presentation in children with pauciarticular arthritis. J Pediatr 134:642-643, 1999.

11. Sherry DD, Bohnsack J, Salmonson K, et al: Painless juvenile rheumatoid arthritis. J Pediatr 116:921-923, 1990.

12. Guillaume S, Prieur AM, Coste J, et al: Long-term outcome and prognosis in oligoarticular-onset juvenile idiopathic arthritis. Arthritis Rheum 43:1858-1865, 2000.

13. Kotaniemi K, Kautianen H, Karma A, et al: Occurrence of uveitis in recently diagnosed juvenile chronic arthritis: A prospective study. Ophthalmology 108:2071-2075, 2001.

14. Takei S, Groh D, Bernstein B, et al: Safety and efficacy of high dose etanercept in treatment of juvenile rheumatoid arthritis. J Rheumatol 28:1677-1680, 2001.

15. Padeh S, Passwell JH: Intraarticular corticosteroid injection in the management of children with chronic arthritis. Arthritis Rheum 41:1210-1214, 1998.

16. Breit W, Frosch M, Meyer U, et al: A subgroup-specific evaluation of the efficacy of intraarticular triamcinolone hexacetonide in juvenile chronic arthritis. J Rheumatol 27:2696-2702, 2000.

17. Cabral DA, Oen KG, Petty RE: SEA syndrome revisited: A long-term followup of children with a syndrome of seronegative enthesopathy and arthropathy. J Rheumatol 19:1282-1285, 1992.

18. Burgos-Vargas R, Clark P: Axial involvement in the seronegative enthesopathy and arthropathy syndrome and its progression to ankylosing spondylitis. J Rheumatol 16: 192-197, 1989.

19. Lindsley C, Schaller JG: Arthritis associated with inflammatory bowel disease in children. J Pediatr 84:16-20, 1974.

20. Burgos-Vargas R: Spondyloarthropathies and psoriatic arthritis in children. Curr Opin Rheumatol 5:634-643, 1993.

21. Bauman C, Cron RQ, Sherry DD, et al: Reiter syndrome initially misdiagnosed as Kawasaki disease. J Pediatr 128:366-369, 1996.

22. Cuttica RJ, Scheines EJ, Garay SM, et al: Juvenile onset Reiter's syndrome: A retrospective study of 26 patients. Clin Exp Rheumatol 10:285-288, 1992.

23. Brandt J, Haibel H, Sieper J, et al: Infliximab treatment of severe ankylosing spondylitis: One-year follow-up. Arthritis Rheum 44:2936-2937, 2001.

24. Zanguill KM, Wald ER, Londino AV: Acute rheumatic fever in western Pennsylvania: A persistent problem the 1990's. J Pediatr 118:561-563, 1991.

25. Moreland LW, Koopman WJ: Infection as a cause of reactive arthritis, ankylosing spondylitis, and rheumatic fever. Curr Opin Rheumatol 4:534-542, 1998.

26. Ahmed S, Ayoub EM, Scornick JC, et al: Poststreptococcal reactive arthritis: Clinical characteristics and association with HLA-DR alleles. Arthritis Rheum 41:1096-1102, 1998.

27. Ayoub EM, Majeed HA: Poststreptococcal reactive arthritis. Curr Opin Rheumatol 12:306-310, 2000.

28. Uziel Y, Hashkes PJ, Kassem E, et al: The use of naproxen in the treatment of children with rheumatic fever. J Pediatr 137:269-271, 2000.

29. Schaffer FM, Agarwal R, Helm J, et al: Poststreptococcal reactive arthritis and silent carditis: A case report and review of the literature. Pediatrics 93:837-839, 1994.

30. Steere AC, Schoen RT, Taylor E: The clinical evolution of Lyme arthritis. Ann Intern Med 107:725-731, 1987.

31. Keenan GF: Lyme disease: Diagnosis and management. Compr Ther 24:147-152, 1998.

32. Qureshi MZ, New D, Zulqarni NJ, et al: Overdiagnosis and overtreatment of Lyme disease in children. Pediatr Infect Dis J 21:12-14, 2002.

33. Van Solingen RM, Evans J: Lyme disease. Curr Opin Rheumatol 13:293-299, 2001.

34. Klempner MS, Hu LT, Evans J, et al: Two controlled trials of antibiotic treatment in patients with persistent symptoms and a history of Lyme disease. N Engl J Med 345:85-92, 2001.

35. Gross DM, Forsthuber T, Tary-Lehmann M, et al: Identification of LFA-1 as a candidate autoantigen in treatment-resistant Lyme arthritis. Science 281(5377):703-706, 2001.

36. Kamradt T: Lyme disease and current aspects of immunization. Arthritis Res 4:20-29, 2002.

37. Spruance SL, Metcalf R, Smith CB, et al: Chronic arthropathy associated with rubella vaccination. Arthritis Rheum 20:741-747, 1977.

38. Huppertz HI, Niki JK: Susceptibility of normal joint tissue to viruses. J Rheumatol 18:699-704, 1991.

39. Rose CD, Eppes SC: Infection-related arthritis. Rheum Dis Clin North Am 23:677-695, 1997.

40. Amoura I, Fillet AM, Huraux JM, et al: Isolation of varicella zoster virus from the synovial fluid of a patient with herpes zoster arthritis. Arthritis Rheum 36:1329, 1993.

41. Buskila D, Schnaider A, Neuman L, et al: Musculoskeletal manifestations and autoantibody profile in 90 hepatitis C infected Israeli patients. Semin Arthritis Rheum 28: 107-113, 1998.

42. Hochberg M: The incidence of systemic lupus erythematosus in Baltimore, MD, 1970-1977. Arthritis Rheum 28:80-86, 1985.

43. Bowyer S, Roettcher P: Pediatric rheumatology clinic populations in the United States: Results of a 3 year survey. Pediatric Rheumatology Database Research Group. J Rheumatol 23:1968-1974, 1996.

44. Cassidy JT, Sullivan DB, Petty RE, et al: Lupus nephritis and encephalopathy: Prognosis in 58 children. Arthritis Rheum 20(Suppl 2):315-322, 1977.

45. Deapen D, Escalante A, Weinrib L, et al: A revised estimate of twin concordance in systemic lupus erythematosus. Arthritis Rheum 35:311-318, 1992.

46. Tan EM, Cohen AS, Fries JF, et al: The 1982 revised criteria for the classification of systemic lupus erythematosus. Arthritis Rheum 25:1271-1277, 1982.

47. Bulkley BH, Roberts WC: The heart in systemic lupus erythematosus and the changes induced in it by corticosteroid therapy: A study of 36 necropsy patients. Am J Med 58:243-264, 1975.

48. Schoshoe JT, Koch AE, Clang RW: Chronic lupus peritonitis with ascites: Review of the literature with a case report. Semin Arthritis Rheum 18:121-126, 1988.

49. Gladman DD, Urowitz MB: Systemic lupus erythematous. In Klippel JH, Dieppe PA (eds): Rheumatology. St. Louis, Mosby, 1994.

50. Tan EM, Feltkamp TE, Smolen JS, et al: Range of antinuclear antibodies in "healthy" individuals. Arthritis Rheum 40:1601-1611, 1997.

51. Rahman P, Gladman DD, Urowitz MB, et al: The cholesterol lowering effect of antimalarial drugs is enhanced in patients with lupus taking corticosteroid drugs. J Rheumatol 26:325-330, 1999.

52. Austin HA, Klippel JH, Balow JE, et al: Therapy of lupus nephritis: Controlled trial of prednisone and cytotoxic drugs. N Engl J Med 314:614-619, 1986.

53. Buratti S, Szer IS, Spencer CH, et al: Mycophenolate mofetil treatment of severe renal disease in pediatric onset systemic lupus erythematosus. J Rheumatol 28:2103-2108, 2001.

54. Felson DT, Anderson J: Evidence for the superiority of immunosuppressive drugs and prednisone over prednisone alone in lupus nephritis: Results of pooled analysis. N Engl J Med 311:1528-1533, 1984.

55. Sutcliffe N, Clarke AE, Gordon C, et al: The association of socio-economic status, race, psychosocial factors and outcome in patients with systemic lupus erythematosus. Rheumatology (Oxford) 38:1130-1137, 1999.

56. Tse S, Lubelsky S, Gordon M, et al: The arthritis of inflammatory childhood myositis syndromes. J Rheumatol 28:192-197, 2001.

57. Buchpiguel CA, Roizenblatt S, Lucen-Fernandes MF, et al: Radioisotope assessment of peripheral and cardiac muscle involvement and dysfunction in polymyositis/dermatomyositis. J Rheumatol 18:1359-1363, 1991.

58. Rider LG, Miller FW: Classification and treatment of the juvenile idiopathic inflammatory myopathies. Rheum Dis Clin North Am 23:619-649, 1997.

59. Cabral DA, Tucker LB: Malignancies in children who initially present with rheumatic complaints. J Pediatr 134:53-57, 1999.

60. Ostrov BE, Goldsmith DP, Athreya BH: Differentiation of systemic juvenile rheumatoid arthritis from acute leukemia near the onset of disease. J Pediatr 122:595-598, 1993.

61. Trapani S, Griolia F, Simonini G, et al: Incidence of occult cancer in children presenting with musculoskeletal symptoms: A 10 year survey in pediatric rheumatology unit. Semin Arthritis Rheum 29:348-359, 2000.

62. Revsz T, Kordos G, Kajtar P, et al: The adverse effect of prolonged prednisolone pretreatment in children with ALL. Cancer 55:1637-1640, 1985.

CHAPTER 13

Cerebral Palsy

DAVID A. SPIEGEL

Cerebral palsy is a complex disorder of motion and posture resulting from damage to the immature central nervous system (CNS). Although the CNS lesion is nonprogressive, secondary changes in the musculoskeletal system may be progressive throughout growth and development. The needs and functional capabilities of each child evolve as he or she matures into adulthood. Cerebral palsy may also be viewed as a developmental disability, and coexisting problems within the CNS and other viscera must also be addressed in order to achieve the best overall outcome for the individual patient. The spectrum of clinical findings is large, varying from the patient with normal intelligence and an isolated contracture at the ankle to the totally dependent, nonambulatory patient with multiple contractures and mental retardation who needs a gastrostomy tube for nutritional support. Thus, the treatment plan must be comprehensive and realistic.

Optimal care is provided through a multidisciplinary approach, requiring input from orthopaedic surgeons, neurosurgeons, pediatricians, physiatrists, physical therapists, occupational therapists, and orthotists. Global priorities for care are enhancing communications skills, improving activities of daily living, and enhancing mobility. The overall goal is to facilitate the patient's integration into society and to maximize function in later life.

This chapter focuses on musculoskeletal problems in cerebral palsy. Although several types of motor disturbance are observed in children with cerebral palsy, spasticity is the most common. Both orthopaedic and neurosurgical interventions are directed at spasticity and its secondary effects on growth and development of the musculoskeletal system.

We first attempt to define cerebral palsy, and then we discuss the etiology, epidemiology, pathology, diagnosis, and physical findings. Coexisting medical problems, including the preoperative evaluation in children with greater levels of involvement, are addressed. We emphasize a comprehensive management approach, discussing the role of physical and occupational therapy and orthotics. Neurosurgical approaches to spasticity have evolved, and this chapter discusses both selective dorsal rhizotomy and intrathecal baclofen. Finally, we cover the indications and strategies for orthopaedic surgical intervention in the management of deformities of the spine and extremities.

DEFINITION

The diagnosis of cerebral palsy is based on the presence of the following three components: (1) patients must have a disorder of movement and posture; (2) the disorder must result from damage to the immature CNS; and (3) the damage must be nonprogressive. Although abnormalities within the CNS remain static, the effect of the motor impairment on the musculoskeletal system and functional skills may change with time.

In a more global context, cerebral palsy may be viewed as a developmental disability in which there are abnormalities of both behavior and function (Fig. 13-1).[1] The overall developmental sequence may be divided into physiological-psychological and integrated functional processes. The former may be further subdivided into sensory function, cognitive function, and motor function. The latter may be subdivided into communication and socialization skills, daily living skills, and mobility. Whereas deficits in basic processes are termed *impairments*, abnormalities in integrated processes are referred to as *disabilities*. CNS damage creates impairments, which subsequently affect integrated processes. Orthopaedic interventions treat only a subset of the problems faced by children with cerebral palsy, and coexisting impairments and disabilities may further affect the treatment of musculoskeletal problems.

Priorities for care are directed to the integrated processes to maximize function in adult life. Communication skills are most important, followed by daily living skills, and then functional mobility.

EPIDEMIOLOGY[1,2]

The prevalence of cerebral palsy is approximately 2 to 3 per 1000 and has risen slightly in recent years because of enhanced survival of premature babies with low birth weight. Approximately 50% of patients with cerebral palsy have a history of low birth weight, approximately one in three having weighed less than 1500 g at birth. A host of risk factors have been implicated, including factors related to the pregnancy as well as maternal health issues and problems with previous children. Maternal hyperthyroidism, epilepsy, and mental retardation may increase the risk. There is a higher risk in multiple births, which increases in magnitude from twin to quadruplet births. For a twin pregnancy, the risk is especially high if one twin dies in utero.

ETIOLOGY[1-5]

A definitive cause is present in only about 10% of cases of cerebral palsy, although many patients have one or more of the risk factors cited previously. Most cases are secondary not to birth asphyxia but, rather, to

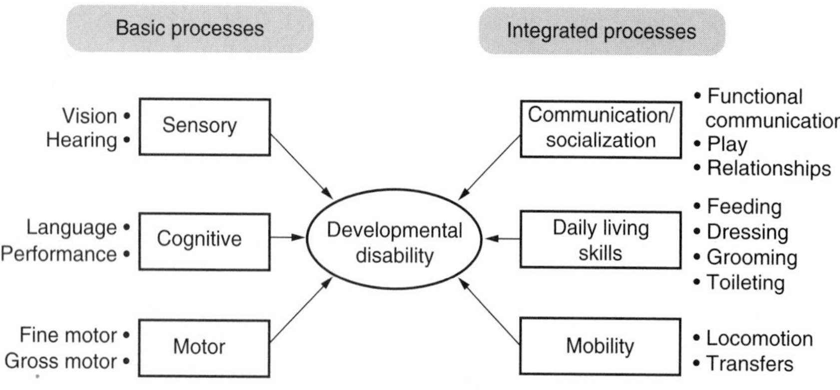

Figure 13-1 Cerebral Palsy as a Developmental Disability. From a global perspective, abnormalities in both basic processes and integrated processes ultimately shape features of the disability in each patient. Orthopaedic management focuses upon improving mobility in order to enhance overall function. (From Pellegrino L, Dormans JP: Definitions, etiology, and epidemiology. In Dormans JP, Pellegrino L [eds]: Caring for Children with Cerebral Palsy: A Team Approach. Baltimore, Brookes Publishing, 1998, p 33.)

prenatal events. Prematurity has been associated with approximately 50% of new cases. Cerebral palsy may result from abnormalities in the structural development of the CNS, for example metabolic disorders or neuronal migration disorders, or from an insult to the developing CNS, such as trauma, ischemia, or infection.

Risk factors associated with the development of cerebral palsy may be chronologically divided into prenatal (from conception through the onset of labor), perinatal (from onset of labor to first few days after birth), and postnatal (the first few years after birth). Although the upper limit for postnatal causes is nebulous, most investigators put it at about 2 years.

Prenatal factors associated with the development of cerebral palsy include developmental abnormalities, exposure to toxins, infections, genetic syndromes, and chromosomal abnormalities. Insults during early embryonic life may result in structural abnormalities in the developing brain. Fetal infections, including toxoplasmosis, rubella, cytomegalovirus, herpes, and syphilis (TORCHES diseases), may be important factors, as may maternal infections such as chorioamnionitis. Maternal use of drugs (marijuana, tobacco, cocaine, others) and alcohol (fetal alcohol syndrome) is also influential. Rhesus incompatibility, which may result in kernicterus, is much less common with the availability of Rh_0D immune globulin (RhoGAM).

Perinatal factors occur around the time of delivery, and hypoxia or ischemia may be secondary to a tight nuchal cord, placental abruption, or other events. Birth trauma, which may result in cephalohematoma, subgaleal hemorrhage, or intracerebral hemorrhage, is becoming uncommon with improvements in obstetric care. Vacuum extraction is performed infrequently today; in the past it has occasionally been associated with intracerebral hemorrhage from tears in either the tentorial membrane or the subdural veins.

In the postnatal period, infectious, hypoxic, and traumatic causes predominate. Infectious causes include neonatal sepsis such as meningitis and encephalitis. Profound hypoxia may occur in traumatic cases of cardiac arrest, respiratory failure, or near-drowning injuries. Traumatic brain injuries may be accidental or nonaccidental (shaken baby syndrome). Neonates requiring extracorporeal membrane oxygenation (ECMO) for physiologic support, as well as those undergoing open-heart surgery within the first month of life, there is a significant chance of having cerebral palsy.

PATHOLOGY[1,6]

Morphologic changes in the developing CNS occur as early as the first 12 weeks of embryonic life, when the various structures of the brain are formed. Neurons are formed during the second trimester of pregnancy, and at the time of birth, a normal number of neurons are typically present. The process of myelination begins at about the sixth month in utero and continues until adolescence. Events culminating in CNS damage may occur early in the embryonic period through the first several years of life.

The mechanisms involved in neuronal damage vary, and in most cases, the final common pathway is hypoxic-ischemic cellular damage. Global asphyxia, hypoperfusion from cardiac arrest, intracerebral hemorrhage, and focal ischemia from vascular occlusion predominate. The cascade of events leading to cell injury and death begins with the primary insult, followed by secondary changes including edema, loss of autoregulation, and diminished blood flow.

Pathologic specimens demonstrate several consistent patterns of injury. Hypoxia produces a diffuse pattern of involvement with scattered areas of necrosis in the cerebral cortex, cerebellum, and subcortical nuclei. This widespread damage often results in spastic quadriplegia. Ischemia typically affects the watershed regions of the brain, in which collateral flow is not well established. Watershed infarcts may be seen in the cerebral cortex but are much more common in the deep periventricular white matter adjacent to the ventricles, causing periventricular leukomalacia. Periventricular leukomalacia is most common in preterm infants and may be associated with intraventricular hemorrhage in more than 50% of cases. This pattern of injury has been most commonly associated with spastic diplegia.

Intraventricular hemorrhage is also associated with hypoxia and may be encountered in up to 50% of preterm infants with birth weights less than 1500 g. A significant risk of intraventricular hemorrhage is seen in patients with asphyxia, respiratory distress, low Apgar scores, and the need for mechanical ventilation. The classification system most commonly used for intraventricular hemorrhage has four grades. In grade 1, the bleeding is confined to the germinal matrix, which is adjacent to the ventricular wall. In grade 2, the hemorrhage extends into the ventricles. Dilatation of the ventricles is seen in grade 3, and extension into the parenchyma occurs in grade 4. Uncommon varieties of intracerebral hemorrhage are subdural, subarachnoid, and intracerebral, which are most often traumatic in origin. Both intraventricular hemorrhage and periventricular leukomalacia may be identified on ultrasonography, computed tomography (CT), and magnetic resonance imaging (MRI).

CLASSIFICATION[1,3,7]

The two schemes commonly used to classify cerebral palsy are the physiologic and geographic classifications. The physiologic classification describes the predominant type of motor disorder, whereas the geographic classification focuses on the anatomic distribution of involvement. Patients may also be classified according to whether they have pyramidal or extrapyramidal involvement. Pyramidal damage affects the motor tracts, and extrapyramidal involvement is caused by damage to the basal ganglia and cerebellum. Figure13-2 integrates all three of these schemes into a comprehensive classification.

Physiologic Classification

- *Spasticity*, the most common motor disorder found in patients with cerebral palsy (approximately 80% of cases), results from damage to the pyramidal tracts. There is an increase in muscle tone that is velocity dependent; the level of muscle tone varies with the rate at which the muscle is stretched. Neurosurgical treatment methods focus on decreasing spasticity (primary problem), whereas orthopaedic surgery is aimed at caring for secondary deformities of the spine and extremities.
- *Athetosis* involves involuntary, writhing movements that develop as a consequence of damage to the basal ganglia. This type of movement disorder was much more common before treatment for Rh incompatibility.
- *Chorea* represents involuntary, random movements of the extremities that are increased when the muscles are resting. These movements typically improve with voluntary use of the extremity. Chorea is secondary to damage in the basal ganglia.
- *Ataxic* cerebral palsy results from lesions in the cerebellum, and patients exhibit difficulties with balance and positioning of the trunk and limbs.
- *Dystonia* consists of involuntary, sustained muscle contractions (simultaneous contraction of agonists and antagonists) that result in abnormal posturing of the head, trunk, and extremities. In contrast to spasticity, the muscle tone fluctuates in dystonia and does not vary with the rate of stretch. Tone often increases with effort and emotion. Primitive reflexes are preserved, and the abnormal tone may cause pain.
- *Mixed* cerebral palsy involves the presence of more than one physiologic subtype. Patients are most often classified according to the predominant physiologic type. For example, a quadriplegic patient with severe spasticity may also have a mild athetoid component.

Geographic Classification

Patients with cerebral palsy may be assigned to any of six categories based on the distribution of involvement. Most have hemiplegia, diplegia, or quadriplegia.

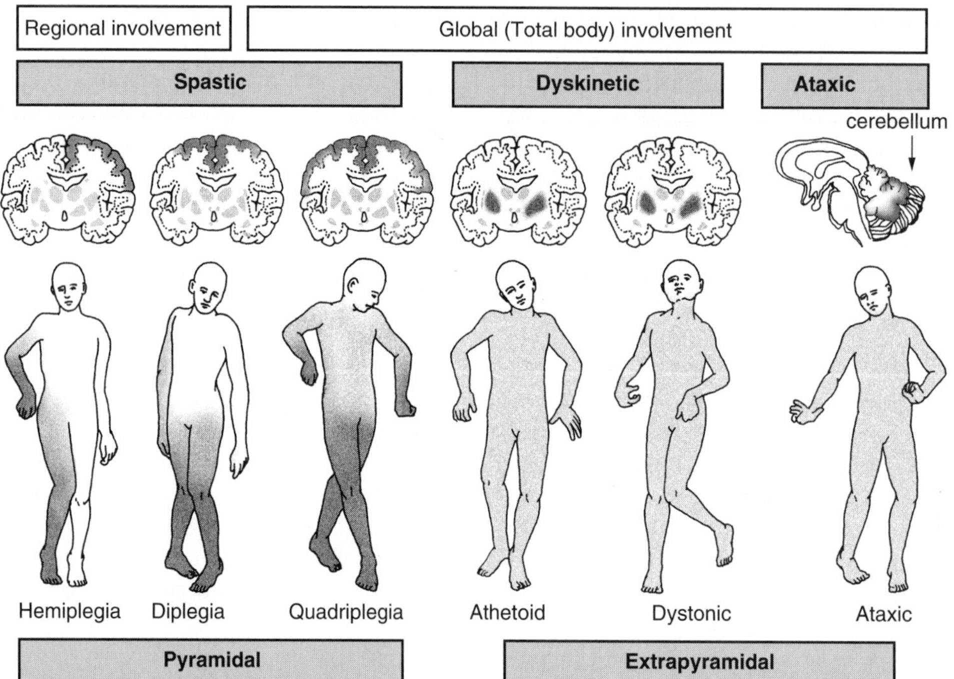

Figure 13-2 Classification of Cerebral Palsy. This figure integrates the three classification schemes for cerebral palsy—physiologic, geographic, and pyramidal versus extrapyramidal—and provides an excellent perspective from which to view each patient. (From Pellegrino L: Cerebral palsy. In Batshaw ML [ed]: Children with Disabilities, 4th ed. Baltimore, Brookes Publishing, 1998, p 502.)

- *Monoplegia* involves a single extremity and is very uncommon. A spinal cord or peripheral nerve problem is more likely the cause than damage to the CNS.
- *Hemiplegia* consists of involvement on one side of the body, and in most cases, the upper extremity is more affected than the lower extremity.
- *Diplegia* is defined as involvement of both sides of the body, with the lower extremities affected more than the upper extremities; this pattern is seen in most premature infants with cerebral palsy.
- *Triplegia* less common; it is similar to diplegia with more pronounced involvement in one of the upper extremities.
- *Quadriplegia* is global involvement of increased severity in both the upper and lower extremities; only about 20% of patients with quadriplegia can ambulate. Coexisting medical problems are very common. Most cases are due to severe anoxia.
- *Double hemiplegia* is an uncommon pattern involving the two sides asymmetrically, with the upper extremities more affected than the lower extremities.

DIAGNOSIS[1,3,7]

The diagnosis of cerebral palsy is made by documenting the three basic features associated with the definition—that there is a disorder of movement and posture, that it results from damage to the immature brain, and that the CNS lesion is nonprogressive. A stepwise approach to diagnosis is presented in Figure 13-3. The history and physical examination will identify a delay in neurologic maturation and should document abnormalities in upper motor neuron function and characterize abnormalities in movement and posture. The examination, with or without the support of imaging studies (ultrasonography, computed tomography, magnetic resonance imaging), should correlate these findings with damage to the immature brain. Finally, any progressive conditions, including neurodegenerative disorders, genetic syndromes, and metabolic diseases, should be ruled out. Rare metabolic conditions that give rise to findings similar to those in cerebral palsy are arginase deficiency, Lesch-Nyhan syndrome, Pelizaeus-Merzbacher disease, metachromatic leukodystrophy, and congenital hypothyroidism. Syndromes with ataxia include Dandy-Walker deformity, Joubert syndrome, and Angelman syndrome. Familial spastic paraparesis and congenital ataxia are genetic disorders that may resemble cerebral palsy. The prognosis for other conditions may differ from that for cerebral palsy, and treatment for the primary processes may be available.

Making a diagnosis of cerebral palsy in a child younger than 2 years may be difficult, because a sufficient level of myelination must be present for some of the physical findings to evolve. A subset of patients who are followed for developmental delay may never meet the criteria for a diagnosis of cerebral palsy, and it is important to keep false-positive diagnoses to a minimum. The diagnosis is usually first suspected by the pediatrician or family physician, and patients are often referred to a neurologist to complete the evaluation. Surgical consultants usually become involved after the diagnosis is made, and physiatrists take part in the medical management of the musculoskeletal system in communities where trained personnel are available. Orthopaedic surgeons, however, may on occasion be first to suspect the diagnosis and must always be prepared to initiate the evaluation.

CLINICAL EVALUATION

The clinical evaluation focuses on both the neurologic system and the musculoskeletal system. After a detailed history is obtained, the physical examination is used to determine the patient's level of neurologic maturation, the presence of increased or decreased muscle tone and any abnormal motions, the patient's posture, and the alignment and range of motion of the spine and extremities. Finally, an assessment of the patient's overall level of function can be made. In those who ambulate, the integrated function of both systems is evaluated through observational gait analysis, which is discussed later. The examination is tailored to the age of the patient. Infants and toddlers are often best examined initially while sitting in a parent's lap, and observation of the patient at play or interacting with family provides many important clues. The examination in older children is similar to that in adults.

History

A detailed history of significant prenatal, perinatal, and postnatal events should be sought. A review of developmental milestones is important, and the presence of any associated medical problems, including seizures, poor feeding or weight gain, gastroesophageal reflux, and respiratory difficulties, should be noted. Normal developmental milestones include achieving head control by 3 to 6 months, independent sitting by 6 to 9 months, crawling by 8 months, pulling up to stand by 8 to 12 months, and ambulating independently by 12 to 18 months. Handedness normally develops around 18 months of age, and an infant demonstrating an early hand preference may ultimately be diagnosed with hemiplegia. By 2 years, toddlers can usually jump. Children should be able to stand on one foot for 10 seconds by 5 years of age, and hop on one foot by 6 years. The level of prematurity must be taken into account when comparing the chronologic age of each infant with these accepted ranges of normal.

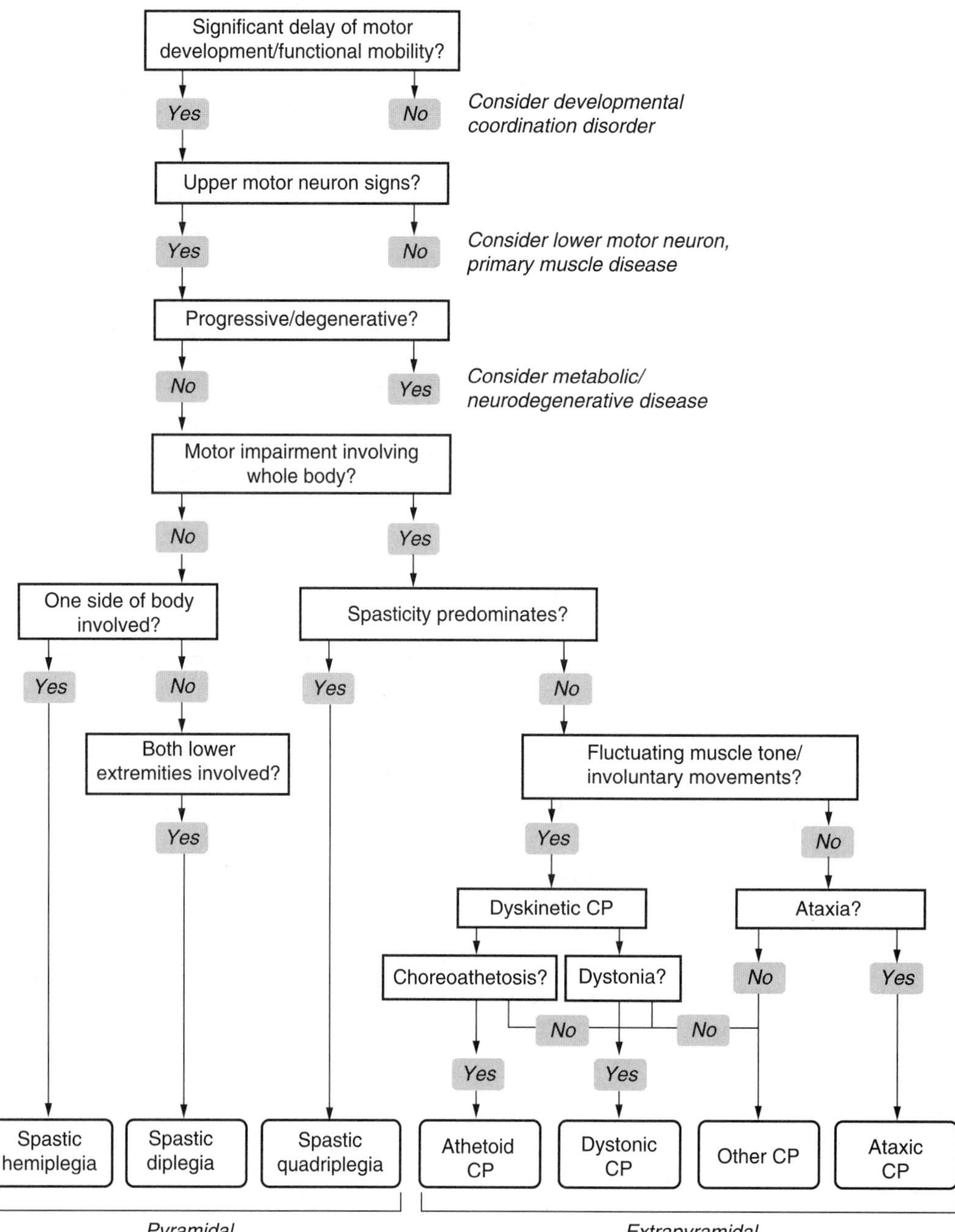

Figure 13-3 A sequential approach to the diagnosis and classification of patients with cerebral palsy (CP). A delay in neurologic maturation is first identified, and then abnormalities in upper motor neuron function must be documented. Progressive conditions are ruled out. Patients may then be characterized according to the distribution and extent of involvement and the type of motor disorder present. (From Pellegrino L, Dormans JP: Definitions, etiology, and epidemiology. In Dormans JP, Pellegrino L (eds): Caring for Children with Cerebral Palsy: A Team Approach. Baltimore, Brookes Publishing, 1998, p 49.)

Neurologic Examination[1,7]

The goal of the neurologic examination is to identify upper motor neuron dysfunction. The evaluation examines the cranial nerves, reflexes (including primitive), muscle strength and tone, selective muscle control, sensation, balance, and posture. The earliest abnormal findings usually involve the primitive reflexes (see later). Other deficits may not become apparent until later, when sufficient myelination has occurred.

In infants as well as some toddlers, the examination focuses on identification of a delay in motor development.

Resting posture should be noted, and the joints should be examined for resting tone (the head should be kept straight). During the first few months of life, mild hypertonia in the flexor muscles of the elbow, hip, and knee may be normal. However, tone should decrease by the third month of life. From 8 to 12 months, it may be normal to find an increase in extensor tone. The scarf sign, which may help identify hypotonia, is elicited with the patient supine. The examiner grasps the infant's hand and gently pulls the upper extremity toward the midline. If the elbow crosses the midline, the scarf sign is present.

Deep tendon reflexes are difficult to test in infants and may be asymmetrical in a subset of normal patients. The plantar reflex (Babinski) is tested by stroking of the plantar surface of the foot (or the lateral border of the foot). A positive response involves immediate dorsiflexion of the great toe with fanning of the lesser toes. Care should be taken to distinguish this from a withdrawal response. In toddlers and older children, a positive plantar reflex and the presence of clonus and hyperactive deep tendon reflexes are suggestive of a lack of cortical inhibition consistent with upper motor neuron dysfunction.

Testing of cerebellar function evaluates balance and coordination. Equilibrium reactions should be tested, gait should be observed if possible, and in older patients, the Romberg test and other standard tests should be performed. Equilibrium (tilting) reactions may be tested with the patient seated or standing. The patient's center of gravity is displaced (gentle push in one of four directions), and protective reflexes should result in righting or maintenance of balance. While seated, the patient should respond to displacement of the center of gravity by reactive changes in head and neck posture, and the arm on the lower side should become extended for protection. This reflex usually appears between 7 and 9 months of age. If the patient is displaced while standing, changing foot placement and hopping are normal responses to maintain balance. Patients with significant deficiency are unsteady and may even fall over. The standing reaction should appear between 12 and 18 months.

Infantile Reflexes

Infantile (primitive) reflexes, also termed *infantile automatisms*, represent complex patterns of movement generated by sensory stimulation (cutaneous, labyrinthine, proprioceptive, multimodal). These patterns originate in the brainstem and spinal cord and disappear with neurologic maturation as a result of inhibitory influences from higher cortical centers. The persistence of these reflexes suggests a delay in neurologic maturation. Whereas the primitive reflexes should disappear during the first months of life, postural (head and neck) and protective (extremities) reactions should emerge during infancy. Postural reflexes facilitate positioning of body segments. The absence of postural and protective reactions at their appropriate time suggests a delay in neurologic maturation. A subset of these reflexes is depicted in Figure 13-4.

Primitive Reflexes

Primitive reflexes are present at birth and normally disappear with time. They are categorized, according to the method of sensory stimulation, as cutaneous (palmar and plantar grasp reflex, Gallant reflex), labyrinthine (prone and supine tonic labyrinthine reflexes), proprioceptive (tonic and asymmetrical tonic neck reflexes), and multimodal (Moro reflex).

The hand *grasp reflex* involves flexion of the fingers after tactile stimulation across the palm of the infant's hand. This reflex normally disappears by 2 to 4 months of age. The plantar grasp reflex is similar and usually disappears by 1 year of age.

The *Gallant reflex* is tested by stroking of the infant's back on one side; the reflex is present if the back curves toward the side being stroked.

For the *prone tonic labyrinthine reflex*, the patient is placed prone, and flexion of the neck results in flexion of the arms, legs, and trunk associated with inward movement of the shoulders. The supine version involves extending the neck with the infant supine. This maneuver should cause extension of the trunk and legs with outward movement of the shoulders.

In the *asymmetrical tonic neck reflex*, the patient is supine, and the examiner turns the head to one side. A positive result consists of extension of the extremities on the side to which the face is turned, with flexion on the contralateral side. The symmetrical tonic neck reflex is tested with the patient sitting; when the head is flexed, flexion of the arms and extension of the legs should occur. The opposite pattern occurs with extension of the neck.

The *Moro reflex* is tested with the infant supine. The head and neck are extended (some prefer to use a loud noise). A positive response involves abduction and extension of all four limbs with extension of the spine and spreading of the digits. This is followed by flexion and adduction of the upper extremities.

Postural and Protective Reactions

Both *postural and protective reactions* are absent at birth and normally appear with time. Postural reactions include segmental rolling reaction, head and trunk righting reaction, and Landau reaction. The *segmental rolling reaction* is tested with the infant supine. When the head is slowly rotated to one side, sequential rolling of the shoulders, trunk and pelvis should follow. The *head and trunk righting reaction* is tested with the infant supine. When the upper body is tilted to one side, the head should also tilt to maintain a vertical position. In the *Landau reaction*, the infant is lifted in the prone

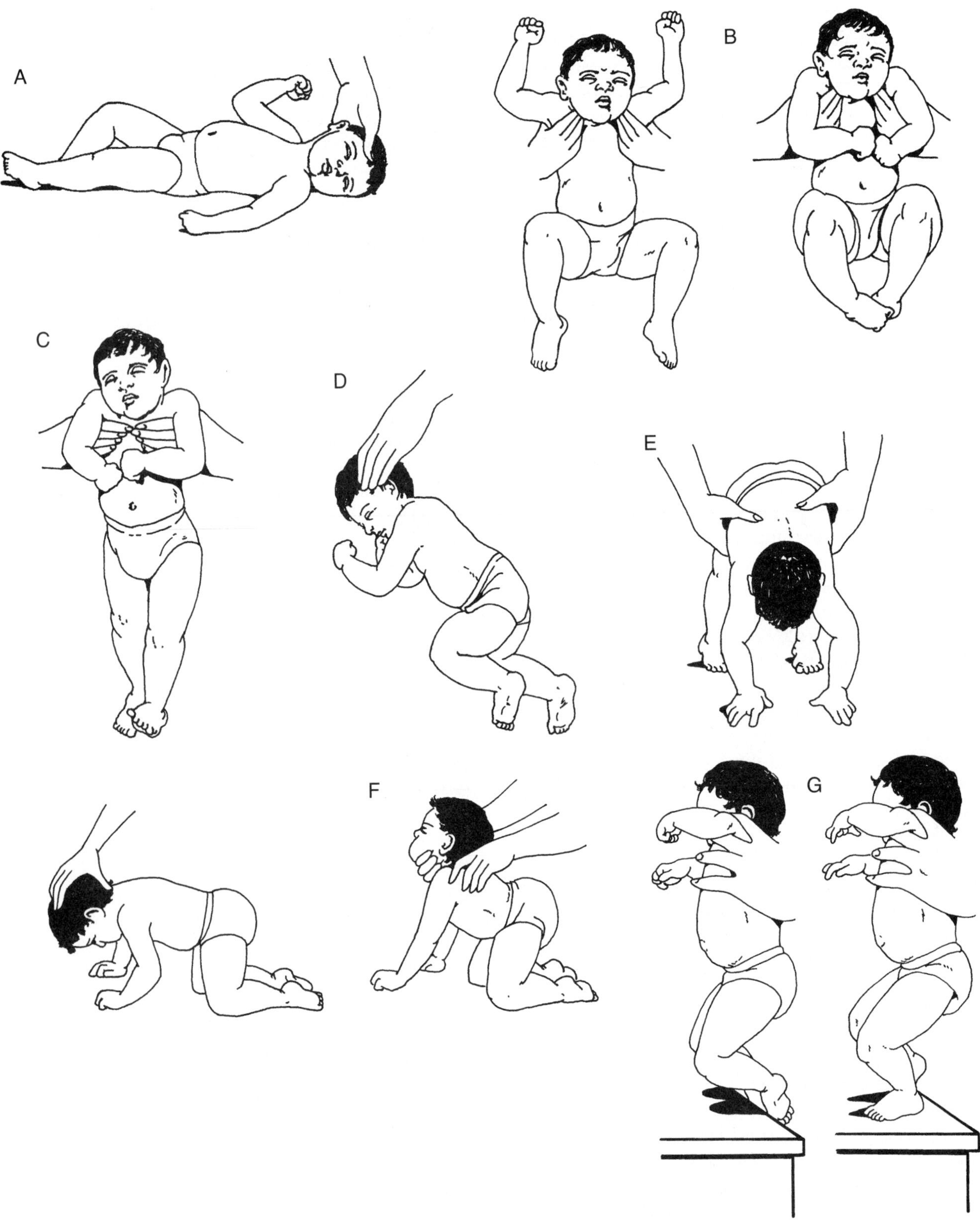

Figure 13-4 Infantile Reflexes and Postural Reactions. This figure illustrates a subset of the infantile reflexes that can be tested: **A,** Symmetrical tonic neck reflex; **B,** Moro reflex; **C,** extensor thrust; **D,** neck-righting reflex; **E,** parachute reaction; **F,** symmetrical tonic neck reflex; **G,** foot placement reaction. (From Dutkowski JP: Cerebral Palsy. In Canale ST [ed]: Campbell's Operative Orthopaedics, 9th ed, vol. 4. St. Louis, Mosby-Year Book, 1998, p 3903.)

position, which causes extension of the arms, trunk, and neck, and flexion of the legs.

Protective reactions include the parachute response, the lateral prop reaction, the foot placement reaction, and the extensor thrust. In the *lateral prop reaction*, the sitting patient is tilted to one side. The appropriate response is to extend the arm on that side for support and balance. In the *parachute reaction*, the patient is suspended vertically and tilted forward. The arms and legs should extend. The *foot placement reaction* is tested with the patient suspended upright; the feet are gently swung into contact with the edge of a table. The normal response is for the infant to place the feet up on the surface. *Extensor thrust* is also tested with the infant suspended vertically; the feet are touched down onto a surface. The limbs should flex, and an abnormal response involves progressive extension of the legs and trunk.

Testing of Reflexes and Motor Strength

Standard reflexes should also be tested, including biceps, triceps, brachioradialis, patellar and ankle jerk. The crossed adductor reflex involves adduction of the contralateral hip when testing the patellar reflex and is abnormal in patients older than 8 months.

Formal muscle testing is impossible in infants and difficult in toddlers. In older children who are able to cooperate, muscle testing is an important component of the examination. A common system uses five grades. Grade 0 represents a complete lack of activity, whereas in grade 1 the muscle contraction is palpable but does not result in any motion at the involved joint. In grade 2, there is sufficient contraction to create motion at the joint, but strength is not sufficient to counteract gravity. In grade 3, there is antigravity strength, but the patient cannot function against any resistance. Grade 4 muscles are active against some resistance, whereas grade 5 muscles offer full resistance (normal strength). In children who ambulate, it is best to gauge strength by observing them play. An overall assessment of balance, posture, and coordination can be made. The presence of any involuntary movements should also be noted.

Musculoskeletal Examination

The musculoskeletal examination identifies and quantifies deformities of the spine and extremities and evaluates ambulation or mobility. The examiner should start by watching the child walk. Ambulatory function should be classified for all patients, in order to maintain realistic goals for their management. *Community ambulators* can walk for extended distances with or without support, and stand to gain the most from reconstructive surgery. *Household ambulators* walk for short distances with support, whereas *nonfunctional ambulators* walk for only limited distances in a therapeutic program. *Nonambulators* are wheelchair bound but may be able to perform transfers. Observational gait analysis is discussed in greater detail in the section on gait.

A systematic evaluation of the range of motion of all joints identifies and quantifies any loss of motion *(contracture)*. When a contracture is diagnosed, the examiner must determine whether it is related solely to spasticity *(dynamic)* or occurs from actual shortening of the muscle tendon unit *(myostatic)*. Many patients have components of both. For the remainder of this chapter, *contracture* is used to describe a decreased range of motion, whether it be dynamic, myostatic, or a combination. Spasticity is difficult to quantify on physical examination, and the degree may vary between examinations. The patient should be relaxed if possible, and gentle but sustained pressure may be required to overcome the spastic component and gain an appreciation of the myostatic component. Myostatic contracture is best quantified during an examination with the patient under anesthesia (which relieves spasticity); patients undergoing surgery are examined under anesthesia to confirm findings of previous examinations.

Spine

Deformities of the spine may be seen in any patient but are most common in those with a high level of involvement. Patients with spastic quadriplegia may have poor trunk control, and spasticity of the paraspinal muscles may lead to asymmetrical muscle action on the spine. These factors may result in a slow collapse or buckling of the spinal column. The examination may be performed with the patient standing (if possible) or sitting. The observer should view the patient from the front and back (coronal plane) and from the side (sagittal plane). Scoliosis is a deformity of the coronal (frontal) plane, whereas kyphosis and lordosis are sagittal plane deformities. Patients with poor trunk control and balance are difficult to examine and are best evaluated in the sitting position. For those who can comply with a standing examination, any limb length discrepancy should be noted, as it may be associated with asymmetry on the forward-bending examination.

With the patient viewed from behind, any asymmetry in the shoulders, scapulae, or back should be noted. The relationship between the patient's head and pelvis should be noted, and the center of the occiput should be in line with the center of the pelvis. Similarly, the trunk should be centered over the pelvis. The Adams forward-bending test is performed by having the patient bend forward while keeping the palms together. A thoracic or lumbar prominence may become evident as the spine flexes. Figure 13-5 illustrates some of the typical findings. From the front, an asymmetry in the chest wall may be suggestive of a scoliosis. Spinal motion is coupled, and

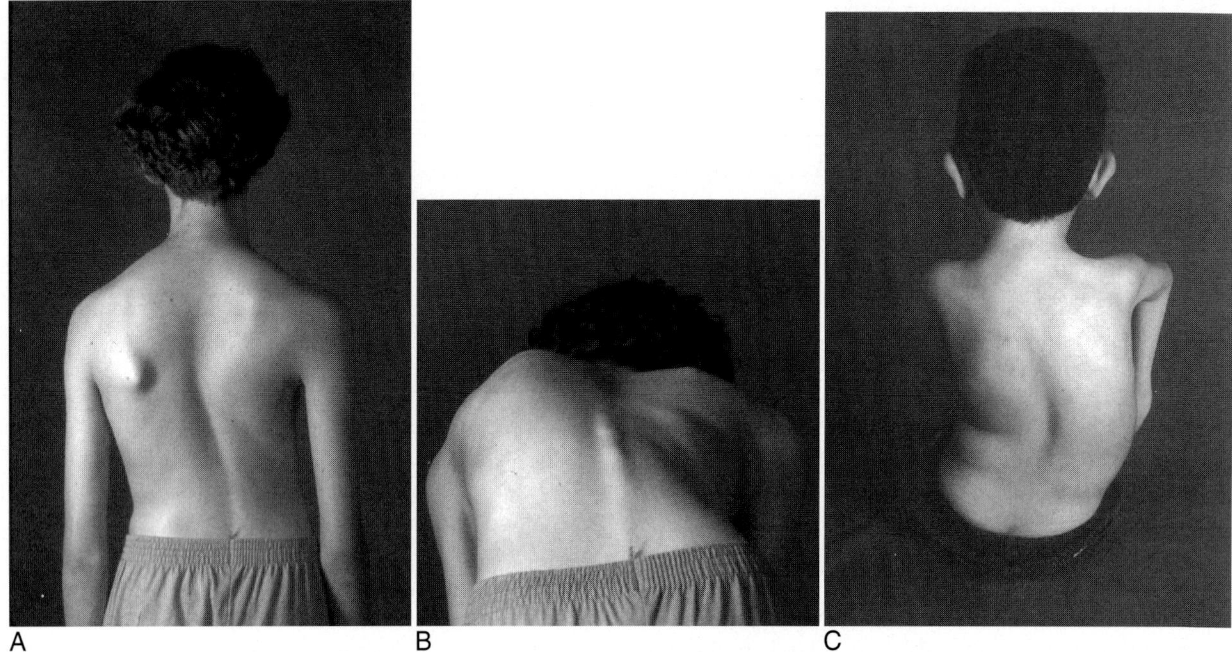

Figure 13-5 Frontal plane examination of the spine. A, With the patient standing, assess the relationship between the head and the center of the pelvis, between the trunk and the pelvis, and between the shoulders. Any asymmetry in the chest wall should be noted, such as prominence of the right scapula and a shift of the trunk to the right in this case. **B,** On forward bending, a rotational prominence, or increase in chest wall asymmetry, may better demonstrate a scoliotic curvature. **C,** The same general assessment is made in nonambulators with the patient seated. This patient has a right thoracolumbar curvature with a shift of the trunk to the right.

movement of a spinal motion segment in one plane is associated with motion in another plane. Flexion of the spinal units is coupled with rotation, a relationship that explains why curvatures are clinically more apparent when the patient bends forward. In the thoracic region, the ribs are attached to the vertebrae, and the greater rotation associated with flexion makes the ribs more prominent. In the lumbar spine, rotation creates a prominence in the paraspinal region on one side.

From the side, the thoracic region should normally be kyphotic, although some patients exhibit an increase in kyphosis (round back). The lumbar region should normally be lordotic.

Findings from an examination in the frontal and sagittal planes must be evaluated within the context of the entire examination, as spinal curvatures may compensate for lower extremity contractures. In the frontal plane, scoliosis may be associated with pelvic obliquity from a unilateral hip dislocation. In the sagittal plane, a flexion contracture of the hip (pelvis tilts anteriorly) is compensated for by an increase in lumbar lordosis, and an extension contracture of the hip (pelvis tilts posteriorly) is compensated for by a loss of lumbar lordosis and an increase in thoracic kyphosis. In these cases, treating the lower extremity deformity may improve the change in alignment of the spine.

The examiner should also evaluate the flexibility of each deformity. For a scoliotic curve, the patient may be asked to bend toward the convexity of the curvature or may be passively positioned to assess the flexibility of the deformity. For patients who are unable to stand, holding the child in the axillary region and gently lifting him or her up off the examining table allows an assessment of flexibility. Alternatively, the patient can be placed laterally with the apex of the curvature on the examiner's thigh. To evaluate an increase in thoracic kyphosis, the examiner may ask the patient to bend backwards, or may passively hyperextend the spine to assess the degree of correction.

Hip

The hip examination documents range of motion, and serial examinations help identify patients at risk for neuromuscular hip dysplasia. In contrast to developmental dysplasia of the hip, which occasionally is seen in patients subsequently diagnosed with cerebral palsy, neuromuscular hip dysplasia evolves slowly, relates to the degree of spasticity of muscles around the hip, and is usually diagnosed from a progressive loss of abduction. In the infant, standard tests for instability should be performed, including the Ortolani and Barlow maneuvers. In older infants and children, a decrease in abduction and presence of the Galeazzi sign are the most common findings. The Galeazzi sign is assessed for with both of the patients' hips flexed to ninety degrees, and the knees maximally flexed. A positive test occurs when one knee appears lower, which indicates shortening of that femoral segment from either subluxation or dislocation of the hip. False-positive results in the neuromuscular patient can occur from asymmetrical muscle contracture.

Sagittal plane deformities involve loss of flexion or extension. The most common finding is a flexion contracture (loss of extension) from spasticity or contracture of the hip flexors (mainly iliopsoas). Loss of extension from hamstring contracture may also be seen, particularly in nonambulatory patients.

There are two well-described techniques for identifying the extent of flexion contracture. The Thomas test, performed with the patient supine, involves flexing the contralateral hip maximally in order to flatten out the lumbar lordosis (Fig. 13-6A). The angle between the affected thigh and the examining table represents the extent of flexion contracture. The Staheli test is performed from the prone position, with the child's pelvis at the edge of the table (Fig. 13-6B). The contralateral hip and knee are flexed, and the affected side is extended maximally. The angle between the thigh and the surface of the examining table represents the loss of flexion on that side.

It is very important to monitor spasticity and contracture of the adductors, especially in nonambulatory patients, who are at the greatest risk for neuromuscular hip dysplasia. Sequential assessment of the extent of hip abduction is essential. The degree of abduction should be measured with the hip in extension and the patient supine. A higher clinical risk is identified in patients with less than 45 degrees of abduction on either side (Fig. 13-7). The rotational examination is described later.

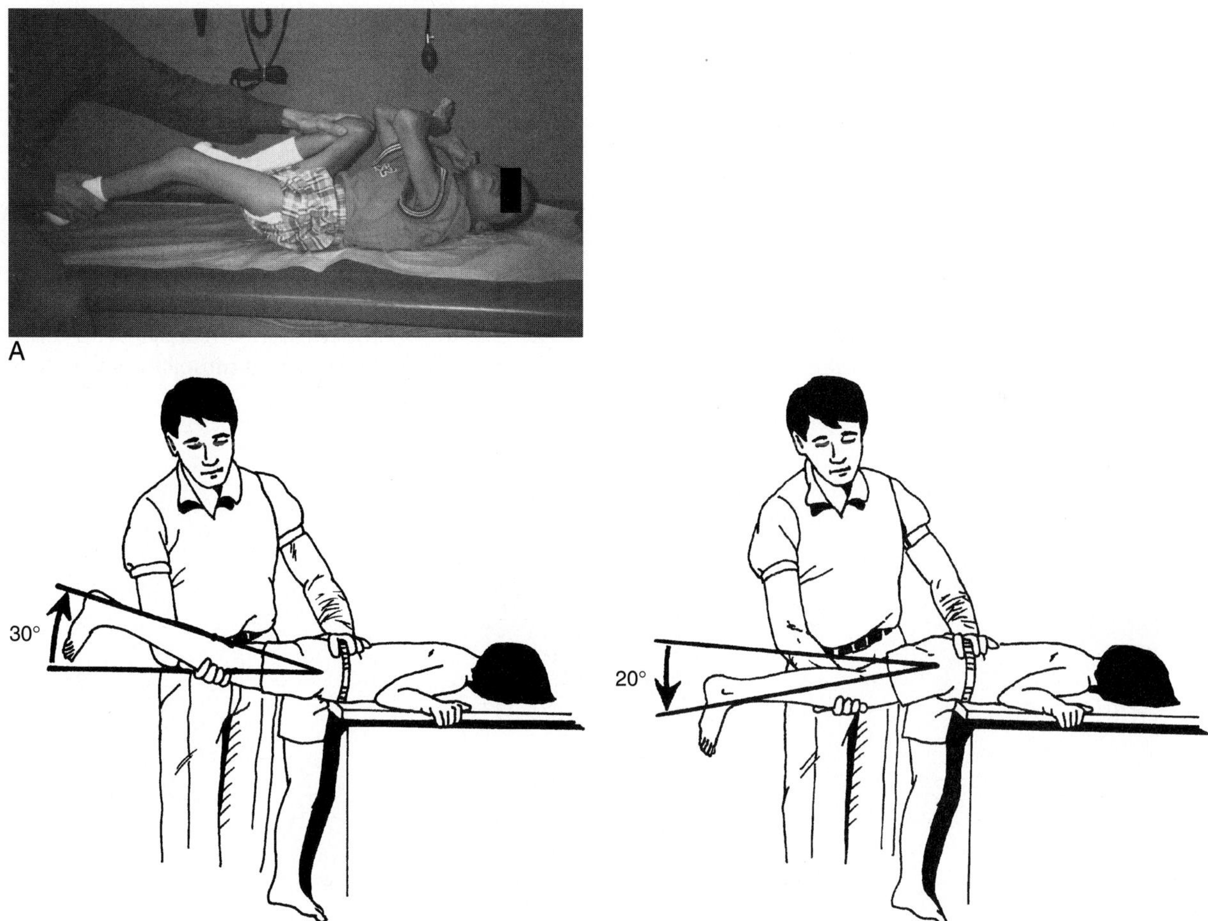

Figure 13-6 Tests for hip flexion contracture. A, The Thomas test is performed with the patient supine, and the lumbar spine is flattened by fully flexing the contralateral hip. The angle between the thigh and the table represents the degree of flexion deformity. **B,** The Staheli test is performed with the patient prone, with the contralateral hip flexed and the pelvis at the edge of the table. The angle between the thigh and the horizontal represents the degree of hip flexion deformity (loss of extension). (**B** from Herring JA [ed]: Tachdjian's Pediatric Orthopaedics, 3rd ed, vol. 2. Philadelphia, WB Saunders, 2001, p 1179.)

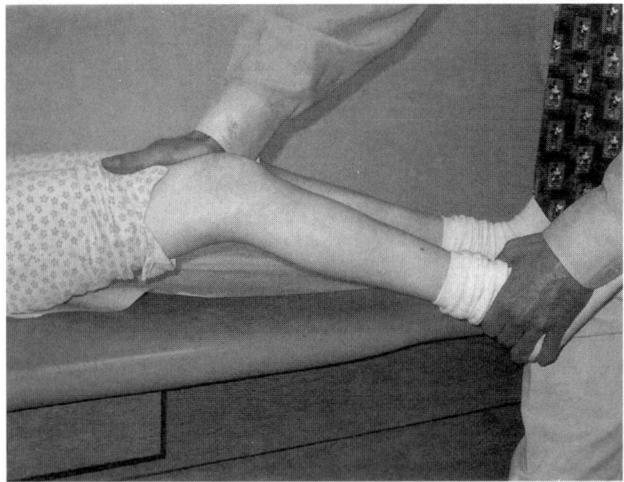

Figure 13-7 The extent of hip abduction is measured with the patient supine and the hips extended. Patients with a combined arc of less than 90 degrees, or with less than 45 degrees on one side, are clinically at risk for progressive hip subluxation and dislocation.

Knee

Range of motion in the sagittal plane is most important, as many patients have contracture of the hamstrings. The popliteal angle is measured with the patient supine, and the contralateral leg fully extended (Fig. 13-8). The affected limb is flexed 90 degrees at the hip, and the knee is brought into extension. The angle between the lower leg segment and the thigh (vertical) is the popliteal angle, and a normal value is 20 degrees or less.

Spasticity of the quadriceps, specifically the rectus femoris, is evaluated with the prone rectus stretch test (Duncan-Ely). With the patient prone and the hip extended, the knee is gradually flexed. A rise in the ipsilateral hemipelvis is abnormal and suggests rectus spasticity (Fig. 13-9). A significant hip flexion contracture on the same side may result in a false-positive result.

Ankle

A plantar-flexion (equinus) contracture at the ankle is very common and involves the gastrocnemius muscle–soleus muscle complex. The gastrocnemius crosses both the knee joint and the ankle joint, while the soleus crosses just the ankle joint. The gastrocnemius muscle originates at the distal femoral condyles, while the soleus originates on the posterior surface of the tibia. The two muscles terminate in a conjoined tendon that inserts into the calcaneus (Achilles tendon). The examiner not only needs to determine the degree of contracture, but also must determine whether there is an isolated gastrocnemius contracture or a contracture of both muscles. The Silverskold test evaluates the degree of dorsiflexion at the ankle with the knee flexed and then maximally extended, a position that allows an assessment of the relative contributions of the gastrocnemius and soleus muscles to the contracture (Fig. 13-10). The foot must be inverted to lock the subtalar joint and prevent spurious dorsiflexion from the midfoot. If dorsiflexion is normal with the knee flexed but limited with the knee extended, the gastrocnemius is contracted. If the degree of dorsiflexion is similar with the knee both flexed and extended, both muscles contribute to the contracture.

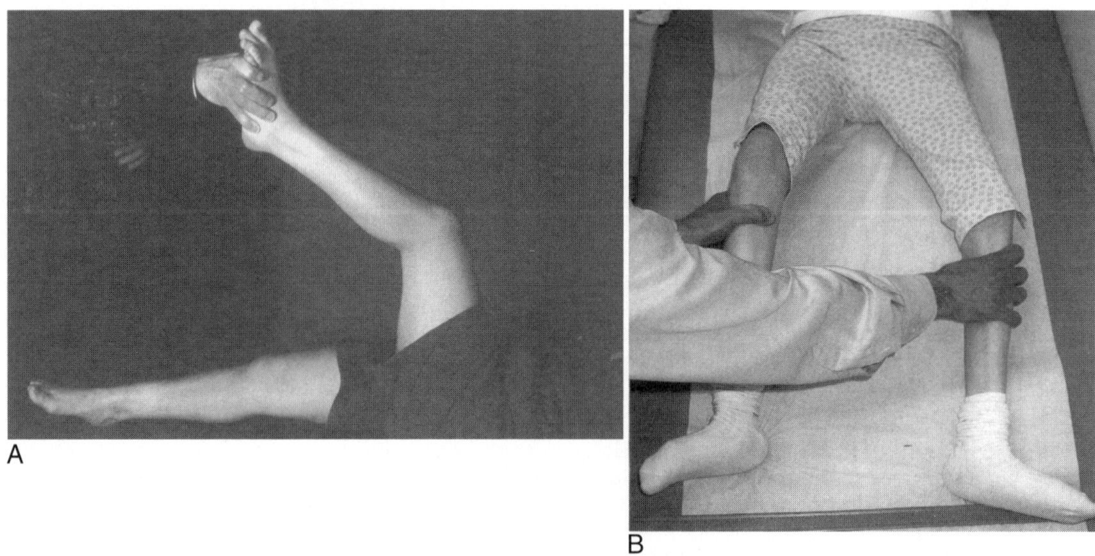

Figure 13-8 Assessments of knee flexion contracture. A, The popliteal angle, measured with the hip flexed, evaluates contracture of the hamstring muscles. **B,** The degree of knee extension with the hip extended demonstrates the contribution from the posterior capsule of the knee (hamstrings are relaxed by extending the hip).

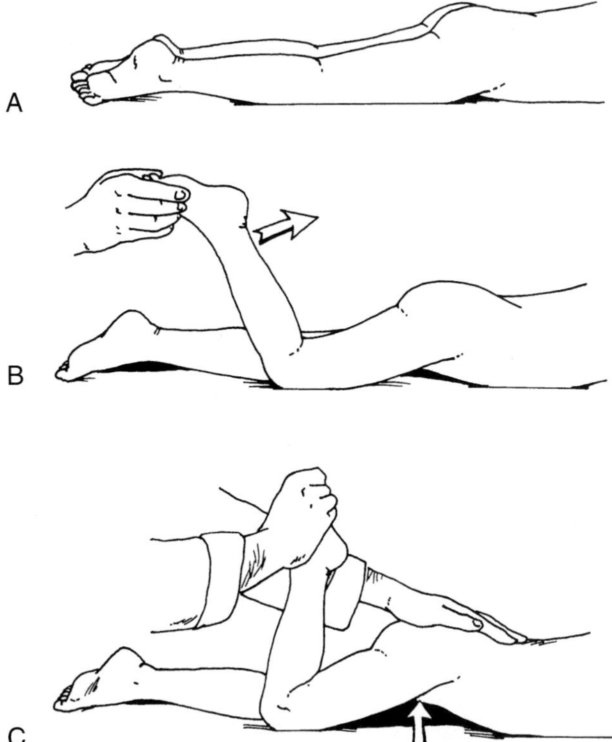

Figure 13-9 The Duncan-Ely test for spasticity of the rectus femoris. With the patient prone, the knee is flexed. Rectus spasticity results in an upward rise of the ipsilateral pelvis. (From Herring JA [ed]: Tachdjian's Pediatric Orthopaedics, 3rd ed, vol. 2. Philadelphia, WB Saunders, 2001, p 1172).

Foot

The foot should be inspected while hanging free to enable the examiner to assess resting position, evaluate the skin for any areas of irritation or callus formation, and test voluntary muscle function. Although deformity, with or without muscle imbalance, may be identified, the weight-bearing examination is most important. Standing alignment can be evaluated starting with the most distal aspect of the foot. The relationship between the forefoot and the hindfoot should be noted, as should the alignment of the hindfoot while the patient is standing. The position and alignment of the foot should also be evaluated during ambulation if possible.

Common deformities include equinus, equinovarus, and equinovalgus (Fig. 13-11). Patients with equinus commonly walk on their toes and may find it difficult to keep their heels down in braces. Patients with equinovarus tend to roll onto the outer border of the foot while walking, and calluses or thickening may develop along this border. Equinovalgus feet resemble flatfeet; the hindfoot is in equinus (tight Achilles tendon), and the forefoot is everted relative to the hindfoot. One may observe overactivity of the peroneal muscles. Patients with equinovalgus feet roll onto the medial aspect of the hindfoot, so callosities and discomfort may develop over the head of the talus medially, making orthotic fitting difficult. Patients with equinovalgus feet may also have hallux valgus (bunion deformities) from mechanical forces during weight-bearing.

Rotational Examination

Torsional deformities occur within the axial plane. Torsional malalignment in the lower extremities contributes to pathologic gait in ambulatory patients. The

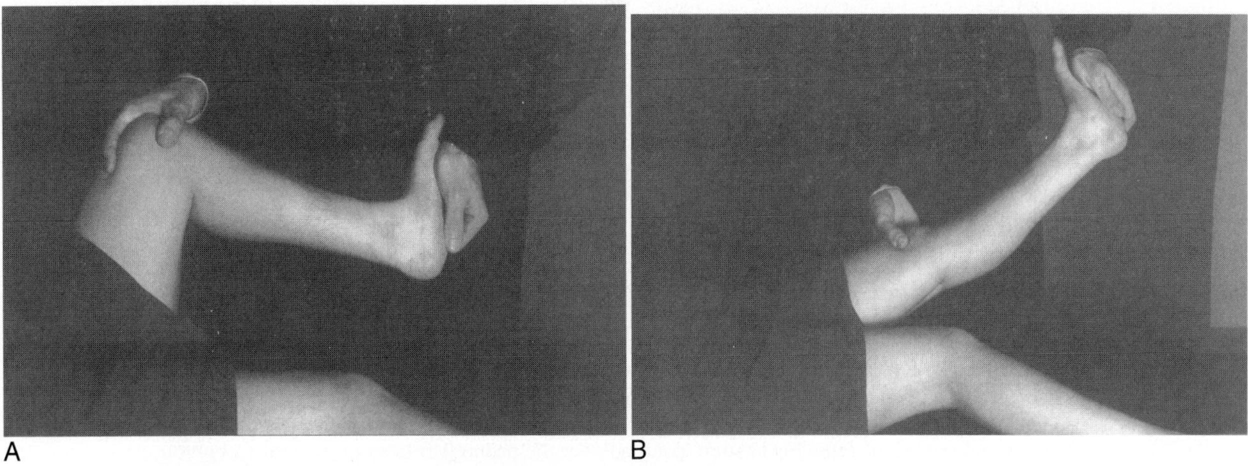

Figure 13-10 The Silverskold test for equinus (flexion) contracture at the ankle. The degree of ankle dorsiflexion is tested with the knee both flexed **(A)** and extended **(B).** The foot should be inverted to avoid any spurious dorsiflexion through the midfoot. If dorsiflexion is limited only with the knee extended, an isolated contracture of the gastrocnemius muscle is present. If dorsiflexion is also limited with the knee flexed, there is an associated contracture of the soleus muscle.

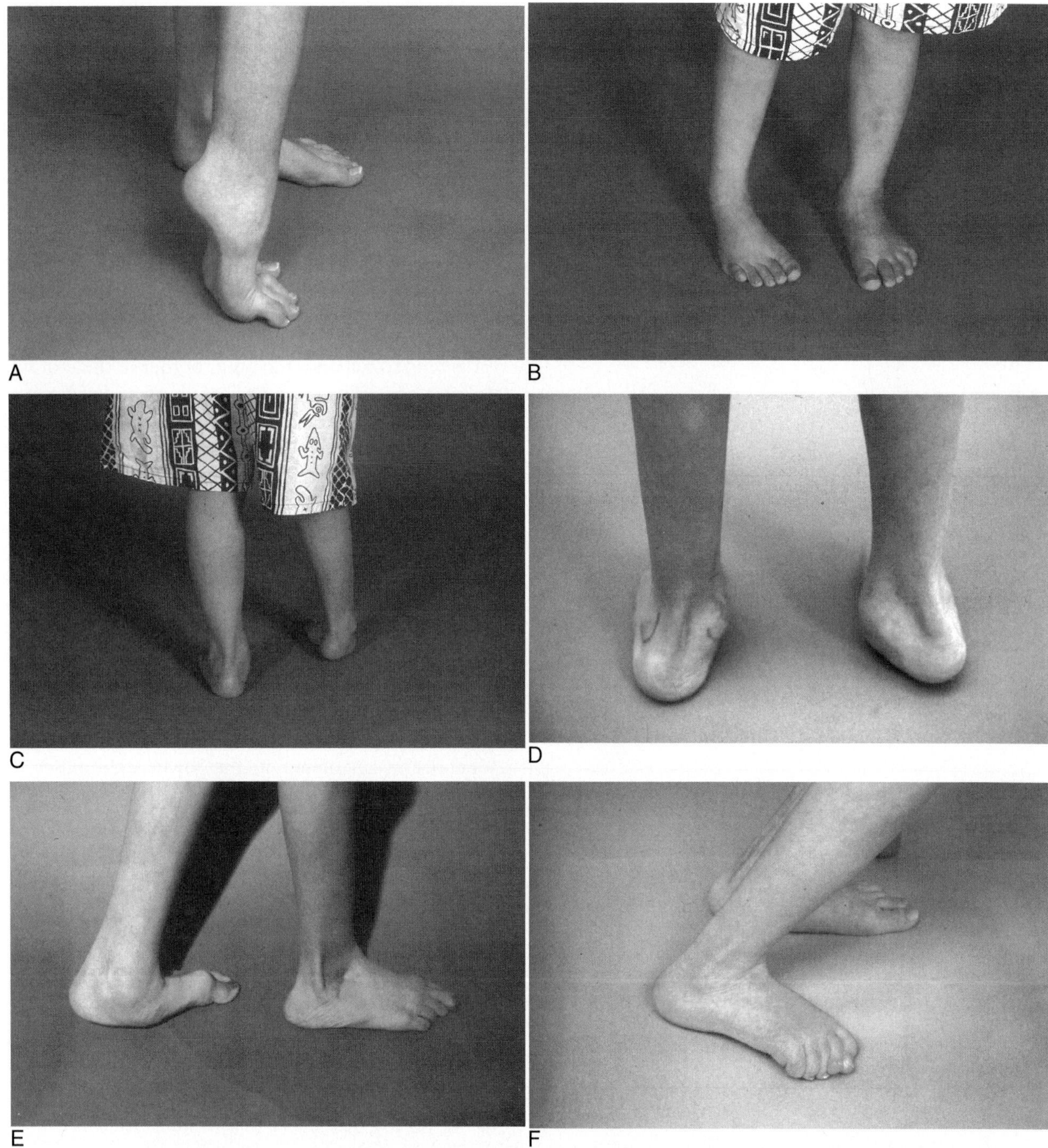

Figure 13-11 **A,** An equinus deformity involves a loss of dorsiflexion at the ankle, and the heel is in neutral alignment. **B,** Equinovarus feet have both equinus and varus of the hindfoot. **C,** In equinovalgus, there is hindfoot valgus in addition to hindfoot equinus. This gives the appearance of a flatfoot, and symptoms often occur from irritation over the prominent head of the talus. A bunion deformity may occur as well from the altered mechanics. **D,** Calcaneus deformity may occur with an overlengthened heel cord, and there is excessive ankle dorsiflexion during stance phase.

terminology surrounding these deformities is often confusing. The term *version* describes rotation about an axis that is within the normal range for a population, whereas *torsion* represents a degree of rotation that lies outside the normal range. Technically, torsion should be defined as two standard deviations from the mean for a population. Torsional limb deformities involve the femur, tibia and fibula, and hindfoot.

At the level of the proximal femur, *anteversion* represents the normal inward rotation of the proximal femur relative to the distal femoral condyles. Newborns normally have approximately 40 degrees of anteversion, and this gradually improves with growth. At maturity, approximately 15 degrees of femoral anteversion is found. Spasticity and muscle imbalance interfere with derotation of the proximal femur during growth in children with cerebral palsy, resulting in a persistence of the fetal anteversion, or excessive femoral anteversion (femoral torsion). Clinically, the upper segment of the limb rotates internally during gait, and patients may have significant in-toeing. Over time, the lower segments (below the knee) may gradually become misaligned to compensate for the femoral torsion. External tibial torsion as well as a planovalgus foot deformity may occur either alone or in combination. In both cases, there is excessive external rotation of the lower limb segment, further decreasing the efficiency of gait. The physical examination, including both the rotational profile and an assessment of ambulation, should identify the relative contributions of the femur, tibia, fibula, and foot to the overall rotational alignment of the extremity.

The rotational examination at the hip quantifies the degree of internal (medial) and external (lateral) rotation and is performed with the hip in extension (Fig. 13-12). The degree of femoral anteversion may be estimated clinically from the degree of medial rotation of the hip. With the patient prone, the knee is flexed to 90 degrees, and each leg is rotated either towards (tests lateral rotation) or away from (tests medial rotation) the midline. The examiner should stabilize the pelvis during the examination. An increase in medial rotation is suggestive of greater femoral anteversion. In general, 60 to 70 degrees of medial rotation is graded as mild, 70 to 90 degrees as moderate, and more than 90 degrees as severe. Femoral anteversion may be measured clinically, also with the patient prone and the knee flexed 90 degrees. The leg is then rotated medially until the greater trochanter is most prominent by palpation. The degree of medial rotation at this point represents the degree of femoral anteversion. The degree of femoral anteversion is usually be less than the degree of medial rotation.

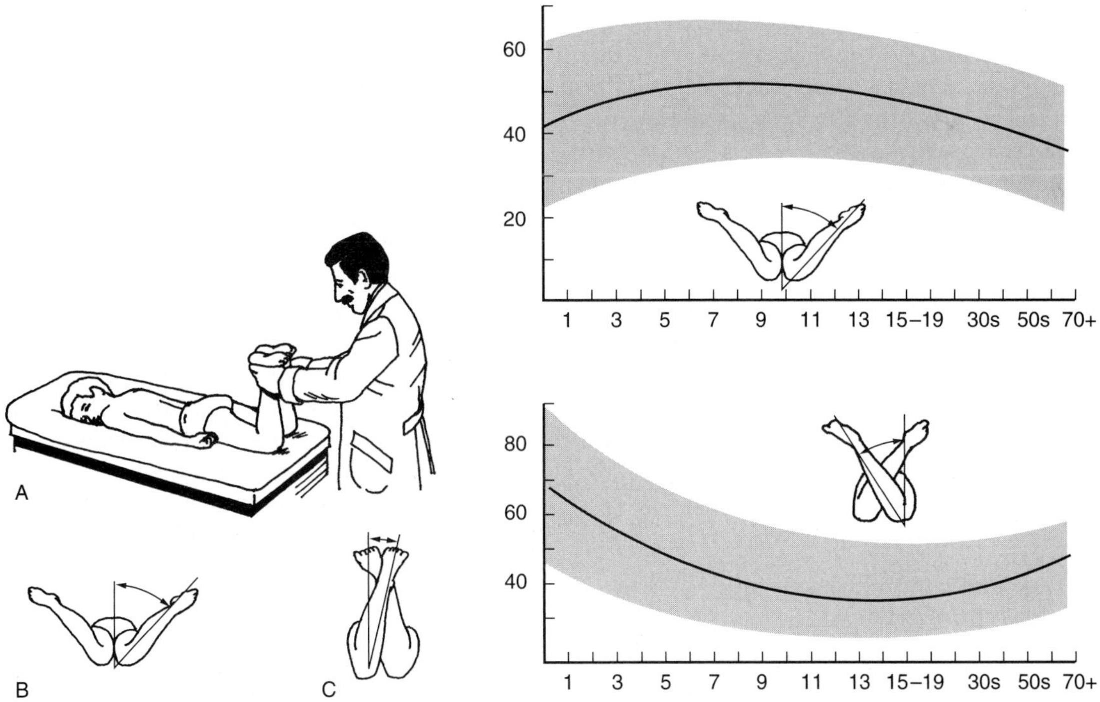

Figure 13-12 Rotational profile at the hip. A, Hip rotation may be tested with the patient prone, the hip in an extended position, and the knee flexed to 90 degrees. **B,** Medial rotation is tested by allowing each leg to rotate outwards; the angle between the vertical and the lower limb segment represents the degree of medial rotation. **C,** Lateral rotation is tested in a similar fashion, but the leg is rotated inwards. The ranges of normal values are shown to the right. (From Staheli LT: Lower limb: Torsion. In Fundamentals of Pediatric Orthopaedics. Philadelphia, Lippincott-Raven, 1998, p 32.)

The rotational alignment from the knee to the foot may be evaluated by two techniques. The *thigh-foot axis* is measured with the patient prone and the knee flexed to ninety degrees (Fig. 13-13). Care must be taken to keep the foot at neutral, because minor degrees of flexion internally rotate the foot and mild degrees of extension have the opposite effect. This measurement represents a composite of the rotation of the tibia-fibula and the alignment of the hindfoot. The *transmalleolar axis* is evaluated with the patient sitting and the legs hanging over the edge of the table. With the knee joint axis made parallel with the edge of the table, the angle between the edge of the table and a line through the malleoli represents the degree of version of the tibia and fibula. The normal transmalleolar axis is 20 degrees external at skeletal maturity.

The *foot progression angle* defines the angle that the foot makes, while in contact with the ground, relative to the line of progression (Fig. 13-14). Normally, this is about 10 degrees external. Patients with increased femoral anteversion, or those with internal tibial torsion, have an internal foot progression angle, and those with isolated external tibial torsion with or without a planovalgus foot deformity have an external progression angle greater than normal.

Upper Extremity

The active and passive range of motion should be tested at the shoulder, elbow, wrist, and hand. Any abnormal movements, such as writhing of the fingers, may suggest extrapyramidal involvement. Grasp can be evaluated by asking the patient to hold a cylindrical object, and fine motor skills can be tested by asking the child to pick up small objects. Sensory changes are very common in patients with upper extremity involvement by cerebral palsy. Testing for *stereognosis*, or shape recognition, is performed by asking the child to identify objects while blindfolded. This is an important sensory test that can help predict the functional level of the extremity and the response to surgical intervention. Older children may be able to cooperate with an examination for two-point discrimination. A paper clip can be modified such that the ends are 5 mm apart, and the patient, with the eyes closed, is asked whether he or she is feeling one or two points.

Coexisting Medical Problems and Preoperative Evaluation[1,7,8]

Coexisting problems are seen in the CNS, the respiratory system, the gastrointestinal system, the genitourinary system, and, less commonly, in other systems. The frequency and severity of these associations increase with greater levels of neurologic involvement, and patients with spastic quadriplegia are most affected. From the surgical standpoint, a comprehensive preoperative evaluation is indicated, particularly when children with diffuse involvement are scheduled for major reconstructive procedures such as spinal fusion and multilevel lower extremity procedures. Close monitoring and support are also required during the perioperative period. Surgical complications are common in patients with spastic quadriplegia but can be minimized through careful patient selection and aggressive medical management during the perioperative period.

Common CNS problems are mental retardation, seizures, visual disturbance (strabismus, cortical blindness) and both behavioral and emotional problems. All of these conditions affect the patient's functional status and are major considerations when surgery on the spine or extremities is being contemplated. Patients are often monitored by a neurologist and should be screened by an ophthalmologist. Use of valproic acid (Depakote, Depakene) may result in a prolonged bleeding time owing to a rise in von Willebrand factor; if possible, an alternate antiseizure medication should be administered during the perioperative period to reduce the risk of bleeding complications. In addition, several of the antiseizure medications may reduce bone mineral density, further raising the risk of fractures in this population. Bone mineral density is already decreased in many patients from poor nutrition and inadequate mechanical loading.

Respiratory problems in cerebral palsy include abnormal hypopharyngeal tone, recurrent aspiration with or without pneumonia, and reactive airway disease. Recurrent episodes of inflammation may create fibrotic changes within the lung parenchyma, further compromising pulmonary function. The ability to clear secretions is also important, and evaluating the patient's cough may be helpful. Although formal pulmonary testing may not be possible in many younger patients or in patients with cognitive deficits, a chest radiograph and arterial blood gas sampling should provide ample information when combined with the history and physical examination. Respiratory function may occasionally be affected by the magnitude of spinal deformity. The decision to proceed with surgery depends in part on this evaluation, and many patients require pulmonary therapy both preoperatively and during the postoperative period. For those with severe aspiration, a gastrostomy tube may be required.

Poor nutritional status relates both to insufficient intake and to the higher metabolic demands imposed by spasticity. Abnormalities in gastrointestinal motility are common, including gastroesophageal reflux, delayed gastric emptying, and constipation. Bulbar involvement may result in dysphagia. Abnormal control of the oropharynx predisposes patients to feeding difficulties, aspiration, and malnutrition. Recurrent infections, such as aspiration pneumonia, further increase metabolic demands and

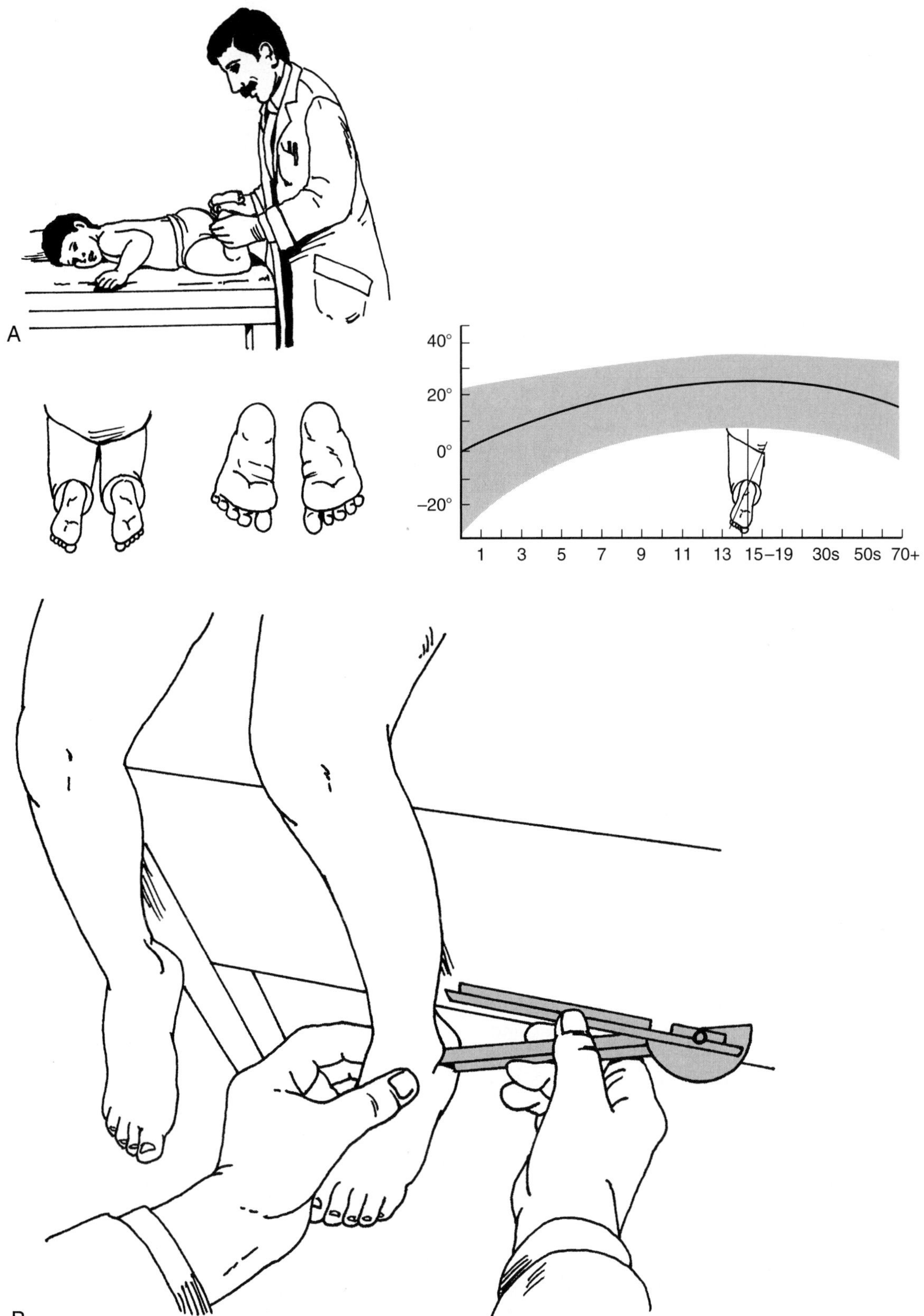

Figure 13-13 Rotational profile of the lower leg. The thigh-foot axis and the transmalleolar axis test rotation below the knee. **A,** For assessment of the thigh-foot axis, the patient is prone, and the knee is flexed 90 degrees. The angle of the foot (held in neutral dorsiflexion/plantar-flexion) relative to the thigh is measured. The normal range of values is shown at the right. This index includes the degree of rotation of both the tibia/fibula and the hindfoot. **B,** The transmalleolar axis is measured with the patient sitting at the edge of the examining table and the distal femoral condyles aligned with the side of the table. The angle between a line through the medial and lateral malleoli and the edge of the table should be approximately 30 degrees external. (**A,** from Staheli LT: Lower limb: Torsion. In Fundamentals of Pediatric Orthopaedics. Philadelphia, Lippincott-Raven, 1998, p 32; **B,** from Bleck EE: Orthopaedic Management in Cerebral Palsy. London, Mac Keith Press, 1987, p 55.)

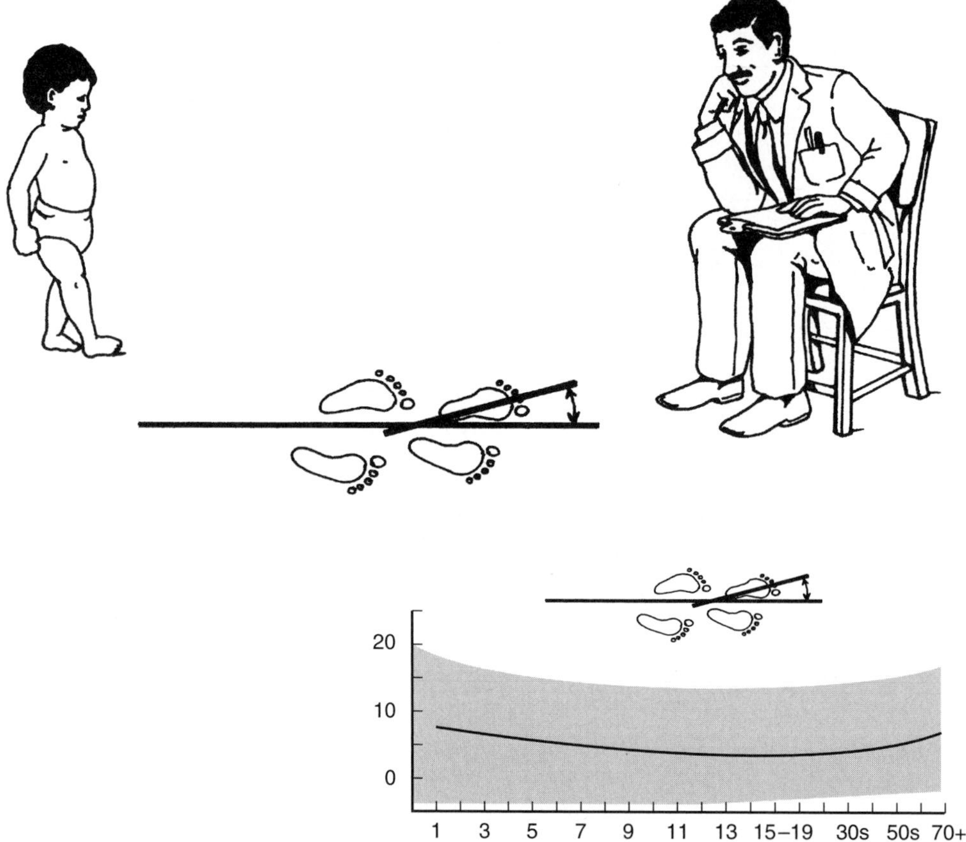

Figure 13-14 The foot progression angle represents the angle of the foot relative to the direction of progression, and may be either internal or external. (From Staheli LT: Lower limb: Torsion. In Fundamentals of Pediatric Orthopaedics. Philadelphia, Lippincott-Raven, 1998, p. 32.)

contribute to malnutrition. Review of the growth chart is helpful, and patients whose height and weight are below the fifth percentile at a high risk for postoperative complications. Laboratory studies to evaluate nutritional status include total lymphocyte count and serum protein measurements (albumin, prealbumin, total protein, and transferrin). Reflux may be treated by Nissen fundoplication, and malnutrition may be reversed by enhancing intake via either a jejunostomy tube or a gastrostomy tube. Elective surgery should be delayed until nutritional status is optimized; this is especially important for children with severe involvement who need major surgery, in whom the infection risk is higher.

PHYSICAL AND OCCUPATIONAL THERAPY[1]

Both physical therapy and occupational therapy play an important role in the overall management of children with cerebral palsy. Goals for physical therapy are to promote a normal neurodevelopmental sequence, to improve functional mobility and activities of daily living, to provide appropriate adaptive equipment, and to improve range of motion and strength during the postoperative period. Occupational therapists focus on improving function in the upper extremities through splinting and adaptive aids, in addition to exercises for gaining and maintaining range of motion and developing better patterns of use.

Therapeutic interventions are determined by the child's functional status and needs, which change throughout the course of growth and development. Strategies for a 3-year-old who is learning to walk are necessarily different from those for a 15-year-old who participates in limited recreational activities. During infancy and early childhood, goals are to facilitate sensorineural development, improve alignment and posture, teach and supervise a home program for stretching and strengthening, and educate the family. As the child grows, emphasis is placed on maximizing ambulatory skills or promoting mobility through the use of a wheelchair. During adolescence, the same principles apply but must be modified. For example, many ambulators suffer a decline in function from factors such as weight gain, and providing a wheelchair for part-time use may be helpful. Therapeutic recreation has also been especially helpful in this age group.

A variety of devices may help patients improve mobility, including standers (prone, supine, parapodium), wheelchairs (manual, electric), walkers (anterior, posterior), and canes and crutches (quad cane, axillary or forearm crutches). The appropriate device for a given patient depends on the severity of involvement. Patients with hemiplegia typically do not need assistance, whereas most diplegics (and the small number of ambulatory quadriplegic patients) may benefit from either a walker or crutches. Most quadriplegics rely on a wheelchair, which may be customized to accommodate the specific deformities and needs of each patient.

Standers help those who are unable to ambulate achieve an upright posture, which helps with social interaction and may provide some mechanical loading to the skeleton (promoting maintenance of bone mineral density). These devices also facilitate therapeutic efforts to improve neuromuscular control and range of motion. Whereas prone standers support the anterior surface of the body, supine standers support the back. A variety of modifications may enhance positioning and support. A parapodium, which supports the patient up to the waist, is of little benefit in patients with poor upper body control.

Both walkers and crutches help support ambulation and are usually prescribed for patients who have difficulties with balance and proprioception rather than weakness. Posterior walkers, in which the frame is behind the body, are recommended most often because they promote extension of the legs and trunk (Fig. 13-15). The device may be outfitted with either two or four wheels. Anterior walkers allow patients to flex forward at the hips, a position that is undesirable in a population predisposed to hip flexion contractures and a crouched pattern of ambulation. For patients with better trunk control and balance, standard or forearm (Lofstrand) crutches may be helpful (Fig. 13-16).

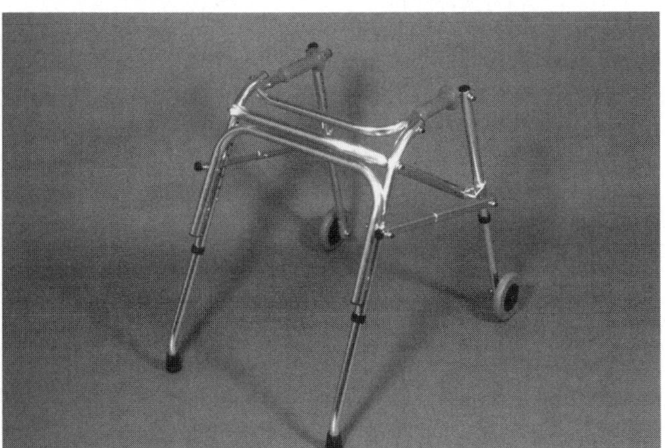

Figure 13-15 A posterior walker promotes extension of the trunk and lower extremities, and either two or four wheels may be added to increase speed in patients with adequate stability. In this example, two front wheels are used.

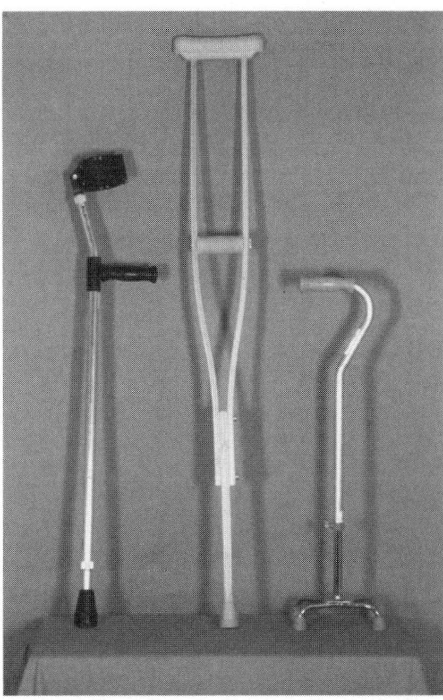

Figure 13-16 Many patients will benefit from the support afforded by assistive devices such as canes or crutches. A quad cane *(left)* is held in one hand and offers more stability than a regular cane because it has four points of contact with the ground. Standard or axillary crutches provide the greatest stability *(center)*. Lofstrand crutches, which transmit forces to the forearm instead of the axilla, require better overall balance than axillary crutches *(right)*. For those who need greater support, a walker may be appropriate.

Nonambulators rely on a wheelchair for mobility, and those with functional use of the upper extremities may have the strength and endurance to propel a manual device. Patients who lack upper extremity strength but have sufficient intelligence may benefit from a motorized design (Fig. 13-17). The totally involved child with severe contractures or mental retardation relies on a caregiver to push the wheelchair. In addition to the basic frame, the wheelchair has an adaptive seating system. The seating system must provide comfort and relief of pressure, and may include a foam- or gel-based cushion. For more difficult cases, an air-based system or thermoplastic urethane may be required. The more sophisticated cushioning systems sacrifice stability to achieve a softer seating surface. Additionally, positional components may be required to support the head, trunk, or pelvis.

ORTHOTIC MANAGEMENT

Orthoses are external devices that support the spine and extremities. Goals for orthotic management include

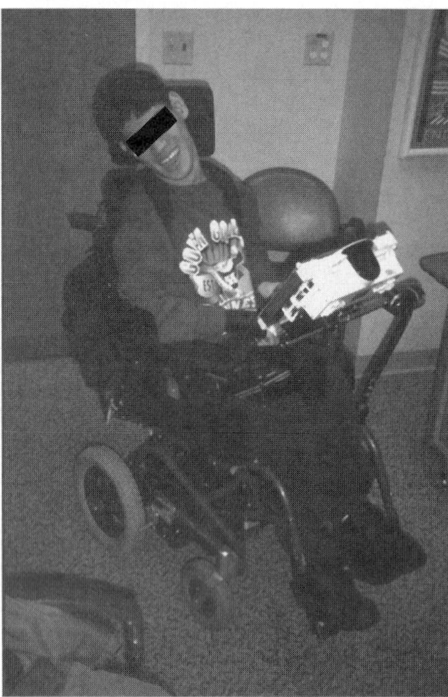

Figure 13-17 A wheelchair is essential for nonambulatory patients and may be required for trips of greater distance by those who ambulate. Each device is customized to the needs of the individual, and modifications are made to accommodate deformities. The electric design is ideal for those who cannot propel themselves yet possess the cognitive ability to operate the controls.

prevention of deformity, provision of support for weakness and spasticity, and improvement of the mechanical efficiency of ambulation.

Foot orthoses stabilize the forefoot, midfoot, hindfoot, or a combination. A variety of designs are available, including a medial arch support, heel cup, University of California Biomechanics Laboratory (UCBL) orthosis, and supramalleolar orthosis (Fig. 13-18). A heel cup supports the calcaneus, whereas the UCBL provides greater control of the hindfoot and extends out onto the forefoot. The supramalleolar orthosis provides even greater support by extension over the malleoli but still allows flexion and extension at the ankle.

An *ankle-foot-orthosis* (AFO), which supports both the foot and the ankle joint, may be employed to improve the mechanics of gait or as a splint (at night) to help maintain range of motion and prevent contractures. Several different designs are available, depending on the clinical scenario (see Fig. 13-18). A solid AFO restricts motion at the ankle and, by blocking dorsiflexion, increases the extension moment at the knee. The solid AFO facilitates clearance during swing phase and helps preposition the foot for initial contact. Patients with a spastic gastrocnemius-soleus muscle (gastrocsoleus) complex and an equinus gait may benefit from such a device, as may those with a very mild crouch.

A ground reaction AFO (GRAFO; also called floor reaction AFO) is constructed with the ankle at neutral or several degrees of plantar-flexion. It has a solid anterior shell over the region of the proximal tibia and transmits the ground reaction force to produce an extension moment at the knee. The GRAFO was originally designed to prevent the crouched gait caused by weak quadriceps muscles in patients with polio. Patients who ambulate in a crouched pattern may benefit from a GRAFO, as long as they have less than 10 degrees of fixed flexion contracture at the knee.

An articulating AFO has a hinge at the ankle and allows varying degrees of plantar-flexion and dorsiflexion. A plantar-flexion stop at neutral (prevents any plantar-flexion) improves clearance during the swing phase of gait in those with a drop-foot pattern while permitting dorsiflexion to enable the tibia to advance over the foot during stance phase. The degree of dorsiflexion may also adjusted. For example, dorsiflexion may be restricted to a specific angle to fine-tune knee motion during the gait cycle. Patients must have at least 5 to 10 degrees of passive dorsiflexion on examination to benefit from an articulating AFO. Patients with a significant hamstring contracture or weakness of the muscles of plantar-flexion may be better served by an AFO with a solid ankle. A leafspring AFO (variant of a solid AFO) provides some sagittal motion by using a more flexible material and decreasing the thickness above the ankle. A dynamic ankle foot orthosis (DAFO) is a total-contact device made of more flexible materials.

A *knee immobilizer* is a removable splint that keeps the knee in an extended position. Patients tend to sleep with their knees flexed, a position that may accelerate the development of hamstring contracture. In addition to stretching, patients may benefit from nighttime use of this device.

A *thoracolumbosacral orthosis* (TLSO) provides support to the trunk and is used to treat progressive spinal deformities (Fig. 13-19). The typical device is made of rigid polypropylene, but soft spinal orthoses made of more flexible materials are also available. The rigid brace, although biomechanically superior, is poorly tolerated in children with cerebral palsy, in whom it has been ineffective in arresting the progression of scoliosis. A soft spinal orthosis, which is more comfortable and much better tolerated, is commonly used to improve sitting balance and may delay surgical intervention in a subset of patients.

Splinting is commonly employed in the management of upper extremity involvement (Fig. 13-20). A dynamic finger splint allows the patient to flex the finger freely but provides a constant extension force at the proximal interphalangeal joint to prevent or improve flexion contracture. A neoprene splint, often used during the daytime, helps keep the wrist extended and the thumb abducted. A more rigid splint, with the same function, may be used at night, when function is not required.

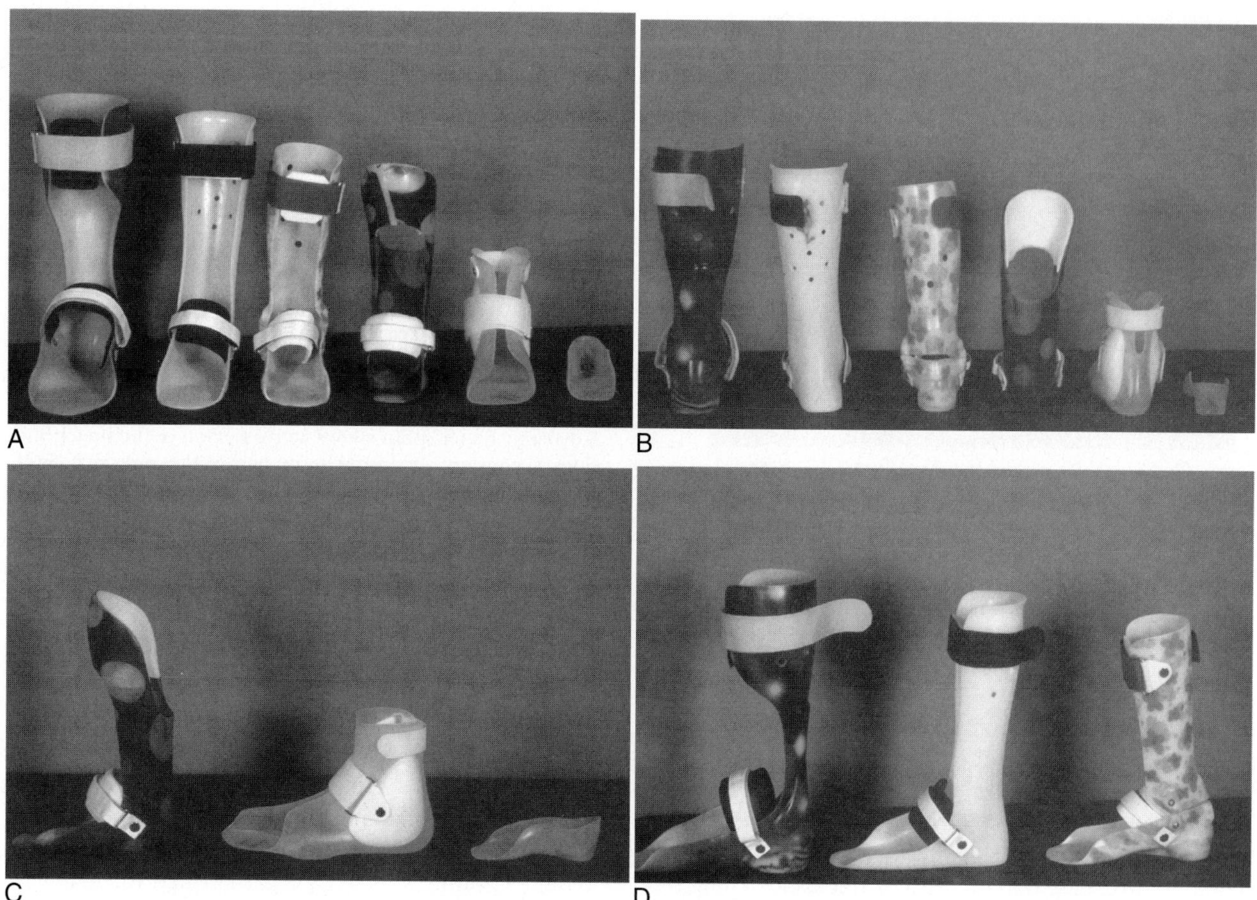

Figure 13-18 Common foot and ankle orthoses viewed from the front **(A)**, the back **(B)**, and the side **(C** and **D)**. From *left* to *right*, these are a University of California Biomechanics Laboratory orthosis (UCBL), supramalleolar-type orthosis, ground reaction ankle-foot orthosis (GRAFO), articulating ankle-foot orthosis (AFO), solid AFO, and leafspring AFO. Ankle orthoses control the alignment of both the foot and the ankle joint, and specific design features may be varied according to the patient's pattern of ambulation. A solid AFO allows no motion at the ankle, whereas an articulating AFO has a hinge at the ankle that can be modified to adjust the range of plantar-flexion and dorsiflexion. Typically, plantar-flexion is blocked past the neutral position. A ground reaction (or floor reaction) AFO transmits a posteriorly directed force to the proximal tibia, which may help prevent crouch during ambulation. A leafspring AFO uses more flexible materials and is thinner posteriorly across the ankle. It affords greater flexibility may improve plantar-flexion during pushoff. However, leafspring AFOs are more prone to failure with higher levels of activity because of their flexible design.

Finally, a dynamic, turnbuckle elbow splint may help with a flexion contracture at the elbow.

SPASTICITY[1,7,9-15]

Spasticity results from damage to upper motor neurons within the pyramidal system. The principle pathophysiologic finding is a loss of supraspinal inhibition, with a resultant hyperexcitability of the stretch reflex. Although the level of spasticity will not change over time, secondary effects on the growth within the musculoskeletal system (end organ) require ongoing evaluation and treatment. Clinically, *spasticity* is defined as a velocity-dependent increase in muscle tone. On physical examination there are a resistance to passive motion that varies with the rate of stretch, an increase in deep tendon reflexes, and clonus. Spasticity may be graded according to the Ashworth Scale. A score of 1 represents no increase in tone, and 2 reflects a slight increase with a palpable "catch" during stretching of the muscle. Scores of 3 and 4 signify a progressive increase in tone, and passive motion becomes more and more difficult. Rigidity is observed with a score of 5.

Spasticity directly affects patient function and ease of care but also has indirect effects on the growth and development of the musculoskeletal system. During normal growth, muscles add on sarcomeres at the

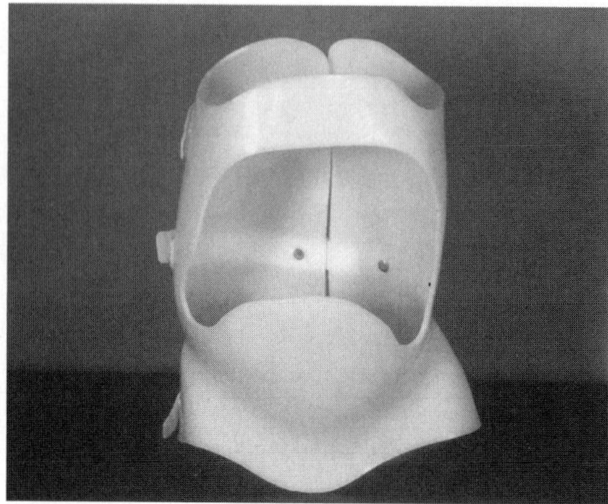

Figure 13-19 A thoracolumbosacral orthosis (TLSO) is the standard device used to manage scoliosis and kyphosis in the thoracic and lumbar spine. Although the standard rigid polypropylene material is generally not well tolerated by patients with cerebral palsy, the soft spinal orthosis, made of more flexible materials, may stabilize the trunk, improve sitting posture, and potentially delay the timing of surgery in those with progressive deformities.

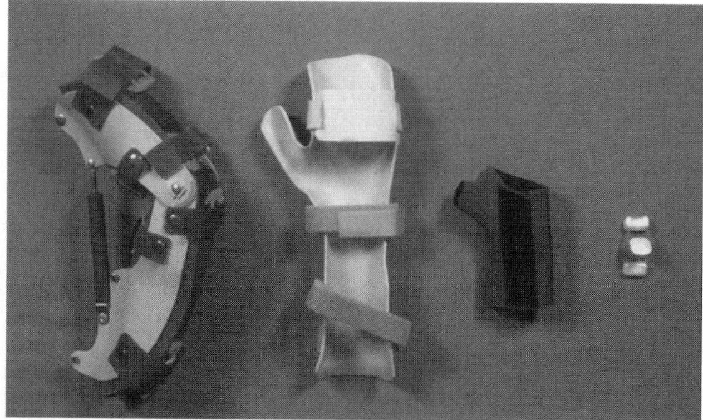

Figure 13-20 Upper Extremity orthotics. *Far left*, A dynamic finger splint allows active flexion of the finger but provides a constant extension force across the proximal interphalangeal joint to help improve or prevent flexion deformity. *Center left*, A soft, neoprene hand and wrist splint is comfortable and is ideal for use during the daytime. The thumb is maintained in abduction, and the wrist in minimal dorsiflexion. *Center right*, A more rigid resting splint, which also promotes wrist extension and thumb abduction, is better suited for use at night. *Far right*, A dynamic elbow extension orthosis may be employed as a night splint to promote elbow extension.

musculotendinous junction in response to the tensile forces exerted through repetitive stretching. Spasticity decreases muscle excursion, thereby reducing the range of motion of the involved joints. Dynamic muscle contractures caused purely by spasticity may ultimately progress to myostatic contractures or fixed shortening of the muscle-tendon unit. Permanent shortening may tether growth, resulting in angular and rotational deformities in the extremities. These secondary deformities further reduce the efficiency of function and gait. Functional capabilities, including ambulation, may be limited by both dynamic and myostatic muscle contracture in addition to angular and rotational bony deformities.

Thus, we may view spasticity as the primary disorder and structural abnormalities in the musculoskeletal system as secondary. The majority of orthopaedic and neurosurgical interventions are directed to managing spasticity and the sequelae of increased muscle tone. Neurosurgical interventions address spasticity directly; they include selective dorsal rhizotomy and the implantation of pumps for intrathecal administration of baclofen. Orthopaedic care focuses on the prevention and treatment of soft tissue contractures, angular and rotational deformities, hip dysplasia, and deformities of the spine.

The evaluation and treatment of spasticity is best performed by a multidisciplinary team consisting of orthopaedic surgeons, neurosurgeons, physiatrists, pediatricians, physical therapists, occupational therapists, and orthotists. Both medical and surgical therapies are available, the goals of which are to improve function, promote the ease of care, relieve muscle spasms and pain, and potentially prevent the development of secondary deformities in the musculoskeletal system. Treatment decisions are often based on whether the spasticity is focal, such as an isolated dynamic contracture of the gastrocsoleus complex in a patient with hemiplegia, or generalized with involvement in both the upper and the lower extremities, as in diplegia or quadriplegia.

In addition to physical therapy and splinting, options for the management of spasticity include oral antispasmodic agents, intramuscular injections with phenol, alcohol, or botulinum toxin A (Botox or Dysport), selective dorsal rhizotomy, and the intrathecal administration of baclofen. Patient selection is critical to the success of each of these modalities, and although each may have the same goal, their indications are different. Even when spasticity is decreased, other components of a patient's motor disorder, such as problems with selective motor control, deficiencies in balance and proprioception, and the underlying weakness that is often uncovered by successful treatment, persist.

Oral Medications[3,9]

A number of oral antispasmodics—baclofen (Lioresal), dantrolene sodium, tizanidine (Zanaflex), and the benzodiazepines, such as diazepam (Valium), clonazepam (Klonopin), and clorazepate (Tranxene)—have been prescribed in patients with cerebral spasticity.

Both the benzodiazepines and baclofen modulate γ-aminobutyric acid (GABA), an inhibitory neurotransmitter. Most of the literature on these oral agents describes their use in adults, although a limited number of studies in children with cerebral palsy have been published. Some reduction in spasticity is seen; however, the dosages required for a more effective response are limited by side effects, the most common of which is sedation.

The benzodiazepines achieve their effect through increased binding of GABA at both spinal and supraspinal levels. Valium has been used most often and may be very helpful in managing postoperative muscle spasm after orthopaedic procedures.

Baclofen binds to GABA receptors, causing hyperpolarization. It is the most commonly prescribed oral agent, and dosage is limited by sedation effects. Other undesirable effects experienced by a limited number of patients are confusion, memory loss, deficits in attention, dizziness, weakness, and ataxia. Symptoms of withdrawal include increased spasticity, hallucinations, and confusion. When withdrawal occurs patients, must be weaned off the agent. Patients with moderate to severe spasticity who are too young for consideration of tone-reducing procedures may be candidates for oral baclofen therapy.

Dantrolene sodium acts at the level of skeletal muscle by inhibiting the release of calcium at the sarcoplasmic reticulum, which decreases or inhibits the response to excitatory stimuli. Increased muscle weakness is common, and hepatotoxicity is observed on occasion. Further studies are necessary to define the precise role of these agents.

Tizanidine acts at central α_2-adrenergic receptor sites (spinal and supraspinal) to prevent the release of excitatory neurotransmitters (glutamate and aspartate). Side effects include somnolence, dizziness, hallucinations, possible hypotension, and hepatotoxicity. There is limited published material on the use of tizanidine in cerebral palsy, although the agent has been effective in spasticity associated with multiple sclerosis and spinal cord injury.

Intramuscular Injections[10,11]

There has been considerable interest in the use of intramuscular botulinum toxin A to achieve a temporary reduction of spasticity in isolated muscle groups. The indications for botulinum toxin are evolving.

Botulinum toxin type A is an exotoxin, produced by *Clostridium botulinum*, which acts upon cholinergic neurons to block release of acetylcholine at the neuromuscular junction (reversible chemical denervation). The substance is injected directly into the target muscle. Some physicians employ electromyography (EMG) to help guide the injections. Reinnervation occurs by sprouting at the neuromuscular junction. Two forms of this drug are currently available (Botox and Dysport). Most injections are completed with the use of topical anesthesia and on an outpatient basis; some patients may require conscious sedation. Patients needing injections at multiple sites, as well as those requiring electrical stimulation to identify the sites of injection, must be given a general anesthetic. An example of such a case is the patient requiring injections in smaller muscle groups of the upper extremity. Side effects of this agent include pain at the site of injection and excessive weakening of the involved muscle group.

Although the indications for injection of botulinum toxin A are evolving, candidates typically have a limited number of muscles involved (<4), and ideally have a purely dynamic muscle contracture. The results are less reliable in those with myostatic contracture. Because the effects of botulinum toxin A are short lived, the goal of treatment is usually to delay surgical intervention. The temporary reduction in spasticity facilitates an aggressive stretching program, and therapy may also focus on motor training. Most patients with a predominantly dynamic contracture have some level of fixed shortening. Therefore, the program may be supplemented by a series of stretching casts to help gain muscle length.

In the lower extremities, the most commonly injected muscle is the gastrocnemius (with or without the soleus), in patients between 1 and 5 years old. Patients who have difficulty keep their feet down in their ankle foot orthoses may benefit, as well as those with an equinus gait without crouch. Other injection sites are the hamstrings, adductors, and tibialis posterior. Upper extremity muscles include the biceps, flexor carpi ulnaris, pronator teres, and thumb adductor.

The maximum dosage is 12 U/kg or 400 U. The typical dose for large muscles is 3 to 6 U/kg, and for small muscles, 1 to 2 U/kg. The maximum dose at a single injection site is 50 U. Re-injection can be considered after a minimum of 3 months.

Phenol blocks are performed less commonly and require general anesthesia because electrical stimulation is used to localize the motor end plates. Risks of phenol block include dysesthesias (15%) and paresthesias. Therapeutic effects last 9 to 12 months.

Dorsal Rhizotomy[12,13]

Dorsal rhizotomy is an operative neurosurgical procedure that permanently decreases spasticity by sectioning a subset of sensory rootlets at the level of the cauda equina. The procedure is most commonly employed in ambulatory patients with diplegia. However a limited number of centers have used the technique in quadriplegics to improve positioning and ease of care as well as to alleviate pain from muscle spasms. In contrast to intrathecal baclofen, the reduction in spasticity is permanent and cannot be adjusted. Spasticity reduction unmasks weakness in the lower extremity musculature, and it is critical to perform the procedure only in patients who have sufficient underlying strength so that function, including the ability to ambulate, is not lost. The ideal candidate for dorsal rhizotomy is a diplegic child (3 to 7 years) who ambulates independently and has "pure" spasticity, no fixed contractures, and good voluntary muscle control. The use of rhizotomy has not been studied in hemiplegics and has not achieved widespread acceptance for quadriplegics.

After a laminectomy from L1 or L2 to S1, the rootlets are gently dissected free, and 25% to 50% of the sensory rootlets are cut. In selective dorsal rhizotomy, each rootlet is stimulated electrically, and the response is gauged both by EMG and by physical examination. Only the rootlets with an abnormal response are sectioned. An abnormal response may be defined by EMG criteria or by physical evidence of contraction of multiple muscle groups with stimulation of a single rootlet *(spread)*. Some centers practice nonselective sectioning.

Compliance with an extensive postoperative rehabilitation program is essential for the patient to enjoy the maximum benefits, which may not be realized until 1 year after the procedure. Overall, complications are rare; they include temporary dysesthesias (common and usually resolve within several days), permanent sensory changes in the lower extremities, and neurogenic bladder.

The results of several studies have documented a significant improvement in spasticity, and minor improvements have been observed in upper extremity function, bladder function, speech, and swallowing *(supraspinal effects)*. Selective dorsal rhizotomy does not seem to alter the need for orthopaedic surgical procedures, and several specific musculoskeletal problems have been observed after rhizotomy. A rapidly progressive unilateral hip subluxation, presumably due to altered muscle balance, has been reported. Heterotopic ossification is more common after reconstructive procedures about the hip in those who have undergone rhizotomy, and patients should receive prophylaxis against it. Spinal deformities have also been reported, including scoliosis, lumbar hyperlordosis, spondylolysis, and spondylolisthesis.

Overall, the literature suggests that selective dorsal rhizotomy may provide significant benefits for a subset of children with cerebral palsy, and the best results are seen with adherence to strict criteria for patient selection.

Intrathecal Baclofen[14,15]

The limited success with oral agents has led to the development of localized delivery of baclofen at the level of the spinal cord. Intrathecal infusion of baclofen has been successful in alleviating spasticity from spinal cord injuries and multiple sclerosis, and studies have demonstrated efficacy of this approach in spasticity of cerebral origin. Baclofen acts in the superficial layers of the spinal cord to increase inhibitory impulses. The indications include moderate to severe spasticity that decreases function, creates difficulties with care, and causes progressive contractures. Intrathecal baclofen may be indicated for tone reduction in ambulatory patients with poor underlying muscle strength, in whom a rhizotomy would be expected to cause excessive postoperative weakness. The technique has become popular in diplegics and in a small subset of quadripegics. Unlike rhizotomy and orthopaedic surgery, intrathecal baclofen has shown some benefit for dystonia.

Patient response is assessed by a test dose (lumbar puncture), and if a sufficient reduction in spasticity is seen, a pump is implanted at a later date with the patient under general anesthesia. The catheter is inserted into the spinal canal within the lumbar region and is advanced to the desired level (C4-C5 for dystonia, T1-T4 for spastic quadriparesis, mid- to lower thoracic spine for spastic diplegia). Placement of the catheter tip is important because the concentration of the agent varies in different regions of the spinal canal. The reservoir is placed subfascially in the abdomen and requires refilling (percutaneously) every 3 weeks to 5 months, depending on the daily dosage required. Most centers use patient weight, rather than age or size, as a cutoff for pump implantation. The dosage is titrated, and the pump may be programmed to deliver higher dosages at certain times of the day, when spasticity may be greater. Because a reduction in spasticity may unmask weakness, the dose may be increased gradually as greater strength is gained through physical therapy. Constipation is a common side effect.

Complications are becoming less frequent with additional experience in the procedure as well as modifications in pump design. Infection occurs in 10% to 20% of patients and requires pump removal followed by a course of antibiotics. The pump may be reinserted once the infection has cleared. Catheter-related problems, seen in approximately 25% of patients, include migration and breakage, and cerebrospinal fluid may leak around the catheter. Baclofen overdose is uncommon and is treated by stopping the infusion, draining off cerebrospinal fluid to decrease the concentration of the drug, and supporting respiratory function if necessary until the agent is metabolized.

Intrathecal baclofen reliably reduces muscle tone and appears to improve patient function and ease of care. Complications are becoming less common, and future studies will likely address the effects of this modality on a variety of associated functions in children with cerebral palsy. The effect of this strategy on the need for orthopaedic procedures remains to be determined, and whether deformities of the spine or extremities may be prevented by its use is unclear.

ORTHOPAEDIC SURGERY

Orthopaedic surgeons employ a host of procedures in the treatment of children with cerebral palsy. The surgical treatment plan is individualized, and goals for the lower extremities are based on the ambulatory potential of the child. For nonambulators, the goals are to relieve pain (usually from spasticity or hip subluxation-dislocation), to improve sitting balance and upper extremity use, and to facilitate positioning and ease of care. For patients who ambulate, the goal is to correct limb deformities that adversely affect gait in order to decrease energy expenditure. For the upper extremity, goals are to improve function and, in some cases, cosmesis, as well as to facilitate care. Patients with progressive spinal deformities may need stabilization to maintain an upright or seating posture. All extremity procedures result in postoperative weakness, and physical therapy is essential to restore muscle strength and provide gait training in those who ambulate as well as to implement a stretching program to maintain range of motion. Orthoses remain an important component of the treatment plan, and surgery rarely eliminates the need for them.

Expectations for the procedure should be realistic, and the family should be educated in detail. Orthopaedic procedures do not affect coexisting abnormalities in the CNS, such as spasticity, loss of selective motor control, problems with balance, abnormalities in cognition or vision, and underlying weakness.

After a discussion of general principles, we address the spectrum of orthopaedic procedures on the spine and extremities according to patient function, in both ambulatory patients (lower extremity procedures) and nonambulatory patients (procedures in the spine and lower extremities); Table 13-1 offers an overview of the host of common procedures for the lower extremities. We then discuss upper extremity procedures in both ambulatory and nonambulatory patients. Although both spinal deformities and hip dysplasia may be found in any patient with cerebral palsy, their prevalence is by far the highest in nonambulators; and these issues are addressed in the section on nonambulators. Many patients, particularly ambulators with spastic diplegia, will benefit from multiple interventions to both lower extremities in the same sitting. Although the procedures are described in this section individually, they are typically employed in combination. The last section of the chapter, on gait in hemiplegics and diplegics, deals with the rationale for and orchestration of these multiple interventions.

General Principles

Procedures on soft tissue and bone are available to treat the range of deformities seen in patients with cerebral palsy. Soft tissue procedures involve muscle lengthening and muscle transfer. Osteotomies are used to correct angular and rotational bony deformities and to realign joints. Joints may be permanently stabilized by arthrodesis (fusion), which relieves pain in joints with significant degenerative changes.

The goal of muscle lengthening is to treat contractures by restoring the length of the muscle-tendon unit. Techniques are release, recession, and lengthening (Fig. 13-21). Complete release of a muscle at its site of origin or insertion creates significant weakness and is rarely indicated in children who ambulate. Given the underlying muscle weakness in patients with cerebral palsy, either muscle release (or overlengthening) may decrease efficiency and endurance. Muscle release may be indicated in nonambulators to improve range of motion, enhance function, or promote the ease of care. Muscle recession is rarely performed; it involves releasing a tendon at the site of insertion and resuturing it more proximally. Most procedures lengthen the tendon either by Z-plasty or by releasing the fascia at the muscle-tendon junction. The latter technique, aponeurotic or musculotendinous lengthening, preserves muscle power and is preferable in patients who ambulate if sufficient length can be gained. This procedure is commonly performed for lengthening of the iliopsoas, hamstrings, and gastrocsoleus complex. Although the rate of recurrence of contracture is higher with this technique, there is less chance of overlengthening the muscle, which would lead to a decrease in function.

The main goal of muscle (tendon) transfers is to balance the muscular forces across a joint. Two types of

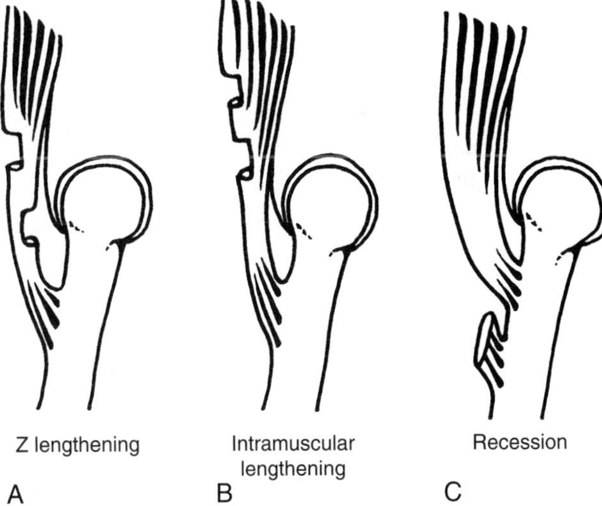

Figure 13-21 There are three general techniques for lengthening muscles. A, In a Z lengthening, the tendon is longitudinally divided, and the two ends are sutured together after the desired amount of lengthening is achieved. **B,** An intramuscular, or aponeurotic, lengthening releases the tendinous portion at the musculotendinous junction. Repair is not necessary, and the chances of overlengthening the muscle are minimized; however, the chance of recurrence is higher. **C,** A recession involves release of the tendon at its insertion, with resuturing to proximal soft tissues (joint capsule) or bone. (From Dormans JP, Copely LA: Orthopaedic approaches to treatment. In Dormans JP, Pellegrino L [eds.]: Caring for Children with Cerebral Palsy: A Team Approach. Baltimore, Brookes Publishing, 1998, p 149.)

Table 13-1 Common Orthopaedic Procedures in Ambulatory and Nonambulatory Patients

Ambulation Status	Hip Problem	Clinical Findings	Procedures	Knee/Leg Problem	Clinical Findings	Procedures
Ambulatory	Flexion contracture	Crouch Lumbar hyperlordosis	Iliopsoas lengthening (intramuscular)	Flexion contracture	Crouch gait	Hamstring lengthening
	Adduction contracture	Scissoring	Adductor myotomy	Rectus femoris spasticity	Stiff-knee gait	Rectus femoris transfer
	Excessive femoral anteversion	In-toeing	Femoral derotational osteotomy	Internal or external tibial torsion	In-toeing, out-toeing	Tibial derotational osteotomy
Nonambulatory	Flexion contracture	Lumbar hyperlordosis	Iliopsoas release or lengthening	Extension contracture	Loss of lumbar lordosis Problems with seating balance	Hamstring release (proximal or distal)
	Mild subluxation	Decreased abduction	Adductor/psoas release			
	Moderate/severe subluxation	Decreased abduction ? problems with perineal care ? Pain	VDRO ± pelvic osteotomy			
	Dislocation (reconstructive)	Chronic pain Problems with perineal care	VDRO ± pelvic osteotomy ± open reduction			
	Dislocation (salvage)	Chronic pain Problems with perineal care	Resection Arthroplasty Valgus osteotomy Arthrodesis Prosthesis			

VDRO, varus derotational osteotomy of the proximal femur.

tendon transfer are performed, a complete transfer and a split-tendon transfer. The entire tendon may be transplanted to a different site of insertion to remove a deforming force, to augment a weaker muscle, or both. However, spastic muscles often act either inappropriately (out of phase) or continuously throughout the gait cycle, and the results of complete transfers are less predictable, often causing the opposite deformity. A split muscle transfer reroutes half of the tendon to a different site of insertion. Transfers are usually employed for deformities around the foot and ankle and in the upper extremity.

Procedures in bone aim to correct angular and rotational abnormalities and to realign or fuse joints. An osteotomy involves division of a bone at a particular location. After the fragments are realigned to correct an angular or rotational deformity, fixation is usually achieved with a metal plate and screws, although other means may be employed. In joint arthrodesis or fusion, the cartilaginous surfaces are denuded down to fresh cancellous bone, and the joint surfaces are then brought together in the appropriate alignment and secured by fixation.

Lower Extremity Procedures in Ambulators[1,3,7,16-22]

All patients with hemiplegia will walk, as will most patients with spastic diplegia. Orthopaedic procedures are recommended to maintain adequate range of motion, restore muscle balance, and improve angular and rotational deformities. These interventions should decrease the energy expended on ambulation and also improve function and cosmesis.

Hip[1,3,7,16,17,22]

A flexion contracture at the hip results from contracture of the iliopsoas muscle associated with weakness of the hip extensors (gluteal muscles). It may be treated with intramuscular release of the iliopsoas tendon at the level of the pelvic brim, which preserves hip flexion power.[17] Complete release of the iliopsoas tendon at the lesser trochanter may be performed in nonambulators. An imbalance between the strong adductors and the weaker abductors may contribute to adduction at the hip during gait (femoral anteversion and overpull by the anterior fibers of the gluteus medius may also be involved), which may be treated by adductor lengthening. The adductor longus and gracilis are typically released, and the adductor brevis is preserved. Care is taken to avoid injury to the anterior branch of the obturator nerve, which might lead to excessive weakness and produce a wide-based gait.

In addition to dysplasia of the proximal femur and acetabulum (discussed in the section on surgery in nonambulators), the most common bony abnormality is increased femoral anteversion, which results in in-toeing. The treatment is derotational osteotomy of the proximal femur, which is usually performed at the subtrochanteric level but may also be performed at the level of the distal femur.

Knee[1,3,7,16,18,20-22]

Flexion contracture of the knee due to hamstring contracture and weakness of the knee extensors (quadriceps) is treated by hamstring lengthening, which may include the semimembranosus, semitendinosus, gracilis, and biceps femoris muscles (Fig 13-22). The medial hamstrings are approached first, and the biceps is addressed only if additional length is necessary. The semitendinosus may be either lengthened at the musculotendinous junction or Z-lengthened, and the semimembranosus, gracilis, and biceps femoris are all lengthened with a musculotendinous technique. If both the medial and lateral hamstrings are lengthened, the patient should be monitored closely during the early postoperative period for any signs of stretch of the neurovascular bundle, which include decreased perfusion and any neurologic symptoms (dysesthesias) or findings. Patients may be immobilized in either a long-leg cast or a knee immobilizer postoperatively; occasionally, serial casting may be required to maximize range of motion.

In addition to contracture of the hamstring muscles, there may be an associated contracture of the posterior capsule of the knee. When the patient is examined with the hip in extension, the hamstrings are relaxed, and the loss of extension at the knee represents the severity of capsular contracture. For significant capsular contractures, either a posterior capsulotomy (release of the joint capsule), or an extension osteotomy of the distal femur may be required to achieve adequate knee extension.

Spasticity of the rectus femoris muscle may lead to a stiff-knee gait with insufficient flexion. The muscle fires inappropriately during swing phases (see discussion of gait). This problem is treated by transfer of the tendon of the rectus femoris to one of the medial hamstrings (sartorius or gracilis), in order to remove the deforming force and augment knee flexion during swing phase.[18,20,21] The procedure is usually combined with a distal hamstring lengthening as part of a lower extremity reconstruction.

Ankle and Foot[1,3,7,19,22,23]

Common procedures are listed in Table 13-2. An equinus contracture is most common, and lengthening of the gastrocsoleus complex may be required if less invasive approaches fail to maintain the range of motion. Options include an open Z lengthening, a percutaneous lengthening, and a musculotendinous lengthening by recession (at the musculotendinous junction) of the tendon of the gastrocnemius, the fascia overlying the soleus, or both (Fig. 13-23).[22] For patients with a tight Achilles tendon with the knee extended but not flexed, a musculotendinous

Table 13-2 Common Orthopaedic Procedures for the Foot and Ankle

Foot	Clinical Findings	Procedures
Equinus	Plantar-flexion contracture Limited dorsiflexion Toe walking Difficulty tolerating orthoses	Gastrocsoleus muscle complex lengthening
Equinovarus	Hindfoot in equinus and varus In-toeing Toe walking Tripping Difficulty tolerating orthoses	Gastrocsoleus muscle complex lengthening Tibialis posterior intramuscular lengthening Split-tendon transfer (tibialis posterior and/or tibialis anterior)
Equinovalgus	Flatfoot Hindfoot equinus and valgus, forefoot abduction Irritation or pain over prominent talar head medially Difficulty tolerating orthoses	Calcaneal osteotomy (lateral column lengthening) Extra-articular subtalar arthrodesis Triple arthrodesis

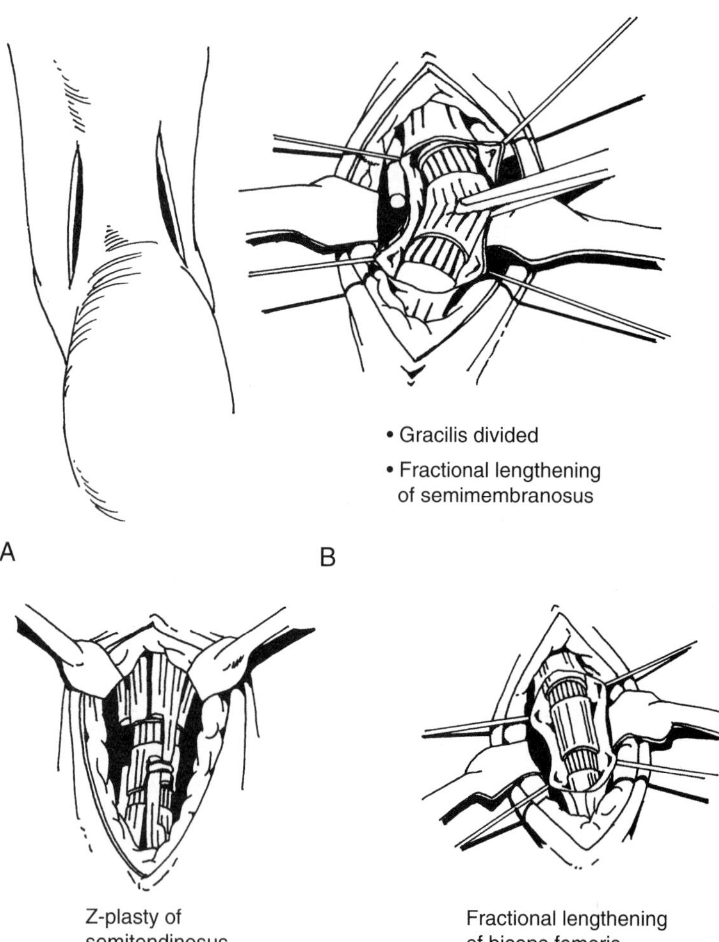

Figure 13-22 The hamstring muscles include the gracilis, semitendinosus, semimembranosus, and the biceps femoris. Surgical lengthening of the medial hamstrings typically involves release or musculotendinous lengthening of the gracilis, Z lengthening of the semitendinosus, and a musculotendinous lengthening of the semimembranosus. With persistent contracture after medial surgery, the biceps femoris may also be lengthened with a musculotendinous technique. Either a long-leg cast or a knee immobilizer is usually applied for 5 to 6 weeks after the procedure. (From Herring JA [ed]: Tachdjian's Pediatric Orthopaedics, 3rd ed, vol 2, Philadelphia, WB Saunders, 2001, p1171.)

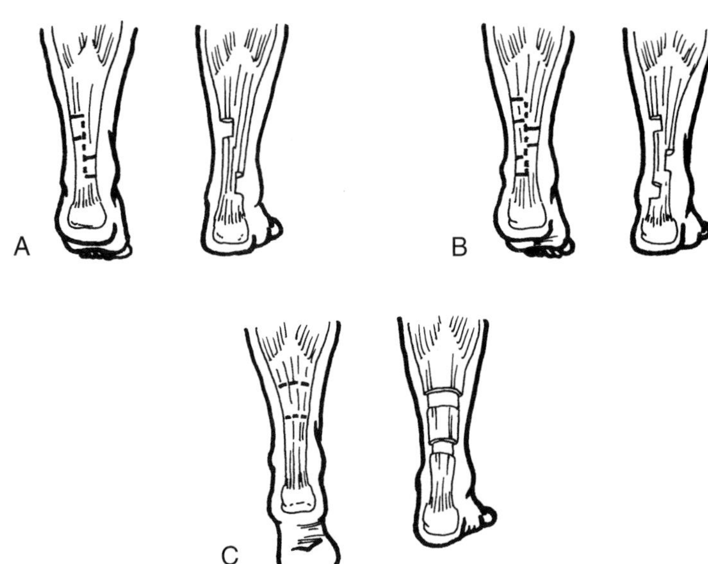

Figure 13-23 Techniques used for an equinus contracture at the ankle, **(A)** and **(B).** In a sliding lengthening, two or three incomplete cuts are made in the tendon, and the foot is dorsiflexed to achieve correction. **C,** In a musculotendinous recession, the tendon is divided at the musculotendinous junction. The underlying muscle fibers are stretched to achieve the desired correction. (From Dormans JP, Copely LA: Orthopaedic approaches to treatment. In Dormans JP, Pellegrino L [eds]: Caring for Children with Cerebral Palsy. A Team Approach. Baltimore, Brookes Publishing, 1998, p 160.)

lengthening of the gastrocnemius may be sufficient, and several techniques have been employed. Limited dorsiflexion with the knee both flexed and extended signifies contracture of both the gastrocnemius and soleus muscles. Musculotendinous recession of both muscles may be sufficient in milder cases. Greater degrees of deformity require a lengthening of the Achilles tendon distally. Care must be taken to avoid overlengthening in ambulators, which would create a calcaneus gait (excessive foot dorsiflexion during stance, which leads to crouch at the knee and hip).

An equinovarus deformity is common in hemiplegics. There is an Achilles tendon contracture, and the foot is pulled into inversion by either the tibialis posterior (most common) or the tibialis anterior. In addition to lengthening of the Achilles tendon, muscle balance must be achieved. If the varus component is mild, an intramuscular lengthening of the tibialis posterior may be sufficient. In most cases, a transfer of the spastic inverter must be performed to remove the deforming force and augment eversion. A split-tendon transfer of the tibialis posterior is commonly performed, in which half of the tendon is rerouted laterally and woven into the tendon of the peroneus brevis (Fig. 13-24).[19] If the tibialis anterior is producing the deformity, a split-tendon transfer to the cuboid may be beneficial. Some surgeons have performed a combined transfer of both the tibialis anterior and the tibialis posterior with acceptable results. Many patients have been able to discontinue the use of an orthosis after undergoing these procedures.

An equinovalgus (flatfoot) deformity is common and may interfere with wearing of braces and shoes (see Fig. 13-11). The head of the talus is prominent at the level of the medial midfoot, and chronic irritation and

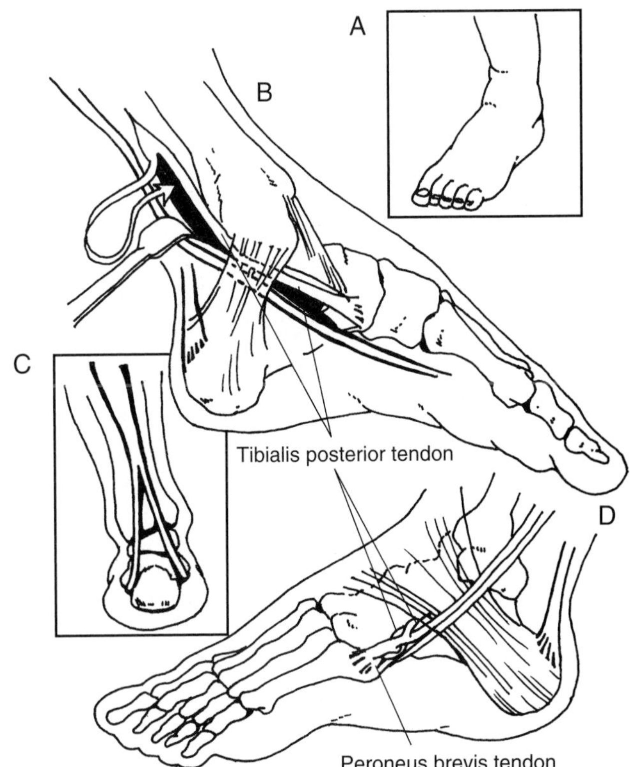

Figure 13-24 **A,** The equinovarus foot. **B,** One half of the tibialis posterior tendon is detached from the navicular and split proximally. **C** and **D,** One half of the tendon is routed laterally and sewn into the peroneus brevis tendon. For a dynamic equinovarus deformity in which the foot is pulled into inversion during the swing phase of gait, a split tibialis posterior tendon transfer achieves better balance by removing some of the deforming force (inversion) and supplementing eversion by rerouting one half of the tendon to the peroneus brevis. (From Dutkowski JP: Cerebral Palsy. In Canale ST [ed]: Campbell's Operative Orthopaedics, 9th ed, vol 4. St. Louis, Mosby-Year Book, 1998, p 3919.)

pain may impede wearing of braces or shoes. There is equinus at the ankle from a tight Achilles tendon, in conjunction with valgus of the hindfoot from the tight Achilles tendon with or without overpull by the peroneal muscles. Lengthening of the peroneal muscles has not been successful as an isolated procedure. Several techniques have been employed to realign the hindfoot, including extra-articular subtalar joint fusion, calcaneal osteotomy, and triple arthrodesis.

Calcaneal osteotomy has become a popular solution to this problem.[23] The procedure corrects the deformity without sacrificing any joints. An osteotomy of the anterior calcaneus is performed, and a trapezoidal bone graft is inserted to lengthen the bone (Fig, 13-25). Correction can also be achieved with arthrodesis of the subtalar joint. The extra-articular technique involves placing a bone graft (usually a bone peg) between the talus and the calcaneus in the sinus tarsi. An alternative is the

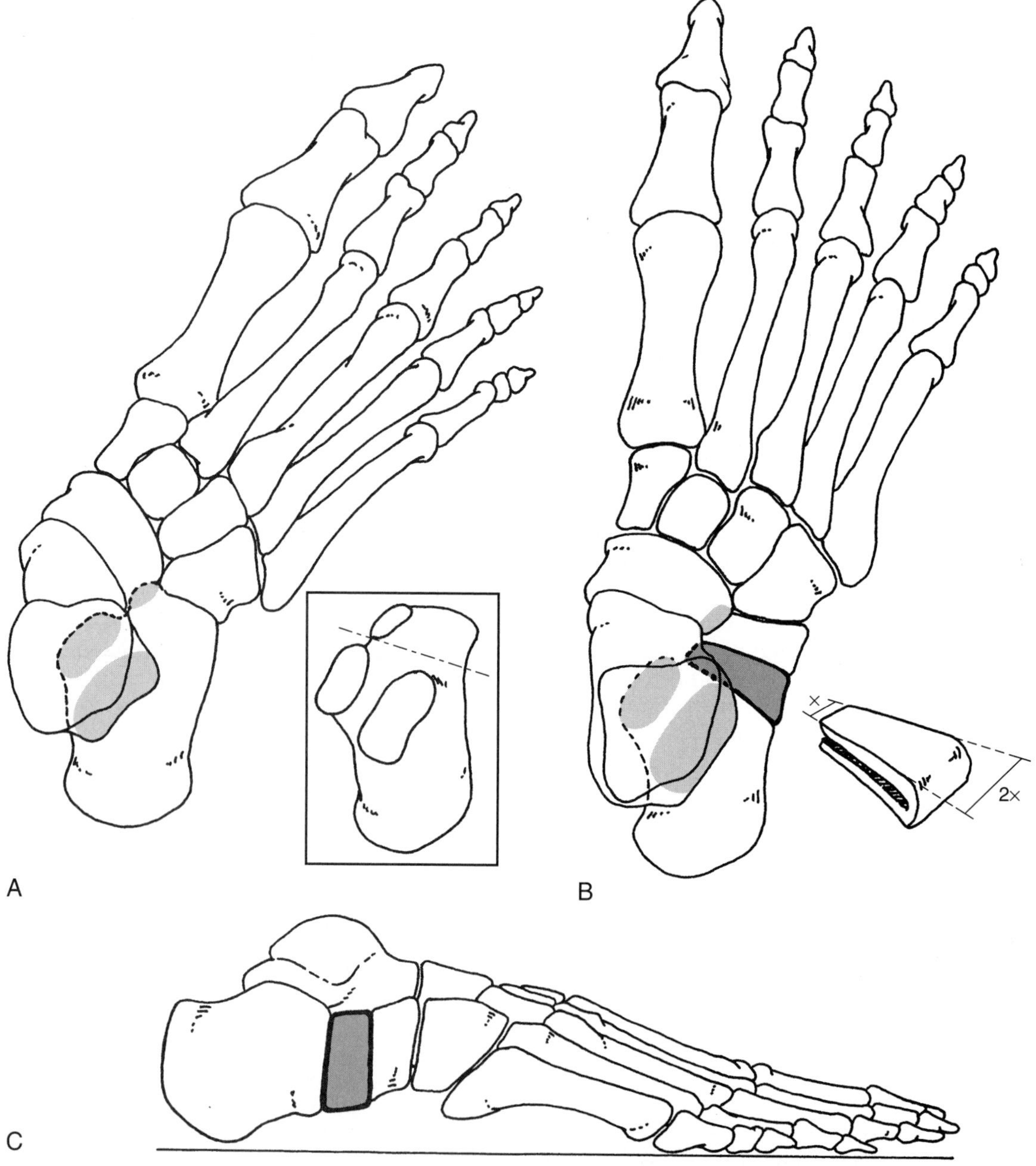

Figure 13-25 One option for managing an equinovalgus deformity of the foot is by lengthening the lateral column of the foot by an osteotomy of the anterior portion of the calcaneus (calcaneal osteotomy). **A**, An osteotomy of the anterior portion of the calcaneus is performed, in between the anterior and middle facets. **B** and **C**, A trapezoidal bone graft is inserted into the osteotomy site, which results in a three-dimensional realignment of the bones of the hindfoot. (From Mosca VS: Calcaneal lengthening for valgus deformity of the hindfoot. J Bone Joint Surg Am 77:502-503, 1995.)

Dennyson-Fulford technique, in which cancellous graft is placed between the two bones, and alignment is secured with a screw (Fig. 13-26). Although arthrodesis permanently corrects the deformity, it results in permanent loss of motion of the joint. The loss alters the stress distribution in neighboring joints, which then may be subjected to greater stresses that may in turn accelerate degenerative changes. Triple arthrodesis may be the best option for salvage in an older child or adolescent with a rigid deformity; it involves fusion of the subtalar, talonavicular, and calcaneocuboid joints. Hallux valgus (bunion) may be painful, may interfere with brace or shoe wear, and may create skin breakdown. If the deformity is flexible, a soft tissue rebalancing procedure may help. For stiffer, severe deformities or in patients with recurrence, an arthrodesis of the first metatarsophalangeal joint is the treatment of choice.

Lower Extremity and Spine Procedures in Nonambulators

Only about 20% of patients with spastic quadriplegia will ambulate, and the goals for mobility in this population differ from those in patients with hemiplegia or diplegia. Treatment strategies focus on achieving a stable sitting posture, preventing deformities, facilitating wheelchair use, and improving the ease of care. Patients ideally will have a straight spine, a level pelvis, painless and mobile hips without significant subluxation (or dislocation), and plantigrade feet for wearing shoes.

Neuromuscular Hip Dysplasia[1,3,7,24-28]

Dysplasia of the hip is common, and both spasticity and muscle imbalance may result in progressive subluxation or dislocation in up to 40% of patients. The risk of spastic hip disease relates to the child's level of function; independent community ambulators have the lowest risk, whereas nonambulatory patients with spastic quadriplegia have a much higher risk. A spectrum from mild subluxation, in which the femoral head is partially displaced from the acetabulum, to frank dislocation, is seen (Fig. 13-27).

The pathophysiology of hip dysplasia relates to imbalance between the spastic adductors-flexors and the weak abductors-extensors. A fixed contracture in adduction and flexion may develop, and the femoral head may gradually migrate superiorly and laterally. Secondary changes develop in the acetabulum over time, with flattening (deficiency) of the posterior and lateral margins. Acetabular dysplasia further compromises the bony coverage of the femoral head. In longer-standing cases of subluxation or dislocation, the femoral head may become deformed by asymmetrical pressure on the acetabulum, resulting in degenerative changes. Hip subluxation-dislocation may compromise perineal care, create difficulties in sitting, and, in some patients, cause pain with time.[3,7,27,28] Patients with unilateral dislocation may experience pelvic obliquity, and an associated scoliosis may further affect patient function, symptoms, and ease of care. The preferred approach is to identify and treat neuromuscular hip dysplasia before dislocation to maintain mobile, located hips.

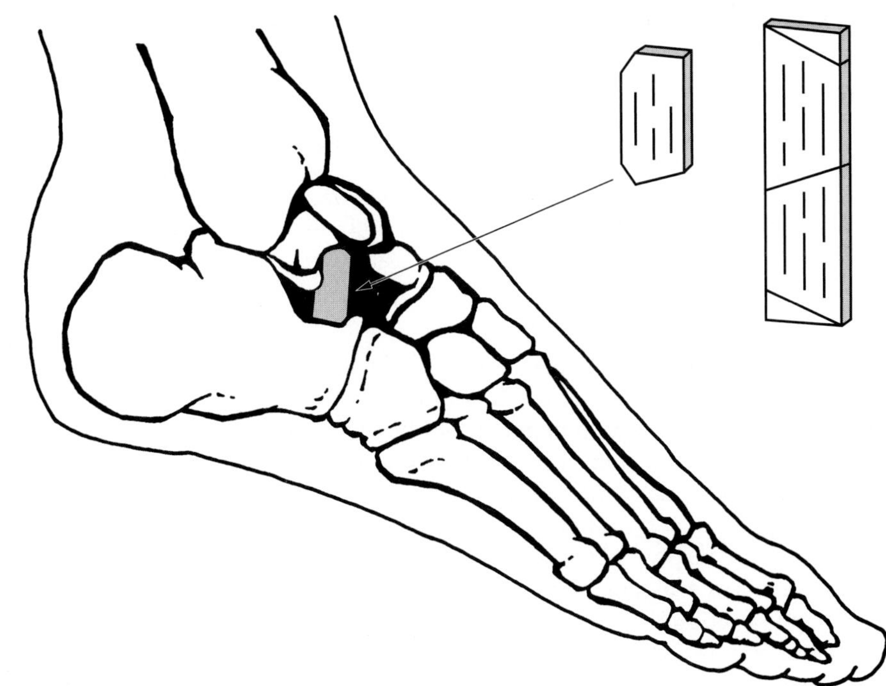

Figure 13-26 Another technique to realign the foot in equinovalgus deformities is arthrodesis (fusion) of the subtalar joint in the corrected position. In the extraarticular technique, a corticocancellous graft B placed between the talus and the calcaneus, at a right angle to the axis of motion. (From Grice DS: An extra-articular arthrodesis of the subastragalar joint for correction of paralytic flat feet in children. J Bone Joint Surg 34A:927-40, 1952.)

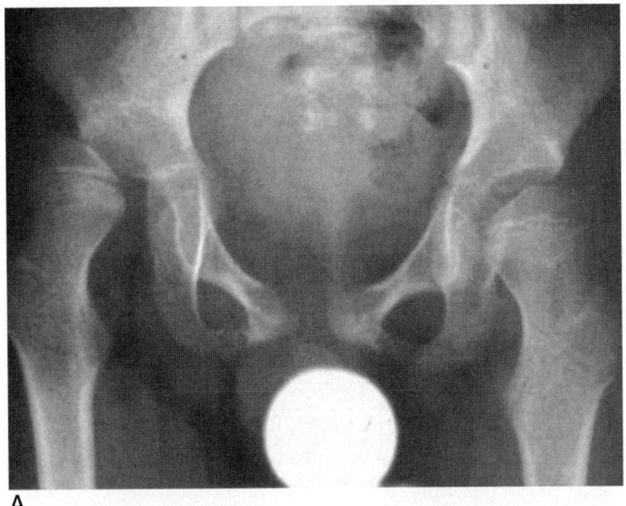

A

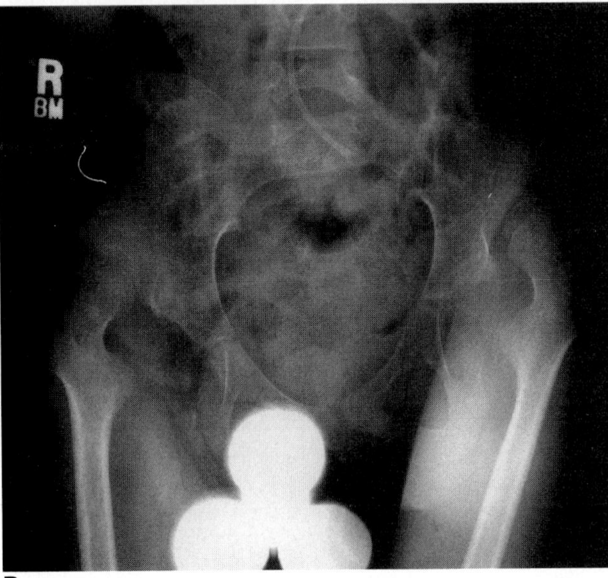

B

Figure 13-27 Progressive hip subluxation leading to dislocation is relatively common in children with spastic quadriplegia and may also be seen in those with lesser involvement (diplegia or hemiplegia). **A,** Subluxation represents incomplete migration of the femoral head from the acetabulum. **B,** In a complete dislocation, there is no contact between the femoral head and the acetabulum.

Neuromuscular hip dysplasia develops gradually, and close follow-up throughout growth is essential to identify patients at risk and to monitor those showing signs of progressive subluxation. Patients with moderate to severe spasticity have the greatest risk. Those with greater degrees of subluxation have a higher risk of progression to dislocation. Although hips that are normal at skeletal maturity will remain stable, subluxated hips may progress to dislocation even after growth is completed.

Clinical risk factors for hip dysplasia include progressive loss of abduction with or without a progressive flexion contracture. Patients should be examined with the hip in full extension, and those with less than 45 degrees of abduction should be monitored closely. In addition to the physical findings, radiographic parameters are measured to monitor progression. The migration index (described by Reimer), has been found to be most reliable. Sequential measurements may be used to monitor a patient for progression of subluxation (Fig. 13-28). A normal migration percentage is less than 30% in children with cerebral palsy; those whose migration index remains within this range are at low risk for progressive instability. An intermediate risk is seen in those with 30% to 60% migration, and all hips with more than 60% migration eventually progress to dislocation. Age is also a relative risk factor, because younger patients are more likely than patients who are older or skeletally mature to experience progression to hip dysplasia.

Nonoperative treatment focuses on preventing contractures, and involves stretching of the psoas, hamstrings, and adductors. Splinting in abduction has also been employed and may be supplemented with injections of botulinum toxin A into the spastic adductors (investigational). In those patients who have progression despite a nonoperative program, and in those who present with advanced deformity, surgical intervention may be indicated.

For the hip at risk with mild subluxation (migration percentage in the range of 30% to 50%) despite adequate stretching and splinting, the goal of surgery is to release the contracture and rebalance the muscular forces about the hip. Surgical release or lengthening of the adductors and the psoas muscle (Fig. 13-29), followed by splinting and a program of physical therapy, may prevent further subluxation.[26] Some surgeons have also sectioned the anterior branch of the obturator nerve (obturator neurectomy) with the goal of preventing recurrence. In a subset of patients, however, a disabling abduction and extension contracture that impairs positioning may develop. The current trend is to avoid obturator neurectomy. For those with greater degrees of subluxation (>50% to 60%), hip reconstruction with both soft tissue and bony procedures is performed.[25] In addition to muscle lengthening, a varus derotational osteotomy of the proximal femur, with or without an acetabular procedure to increase the coverage of the femoral head, may be indicated (Fig. 13-30). The femoral derotation corrects excessive femoral anteversion (femoral torsion), and placing the proximal femur in greater varus corrects valgus malalignment and redirects forces around the hip to promote greater stability. This approach may also be useful in recently established dislocations in which deformity of the femoral head has not yet occurred, and an open reduction of the hip may also be needed. Open reduction involves opening the hip capsule, clearing out any structures that may impede placement of the femoral head in

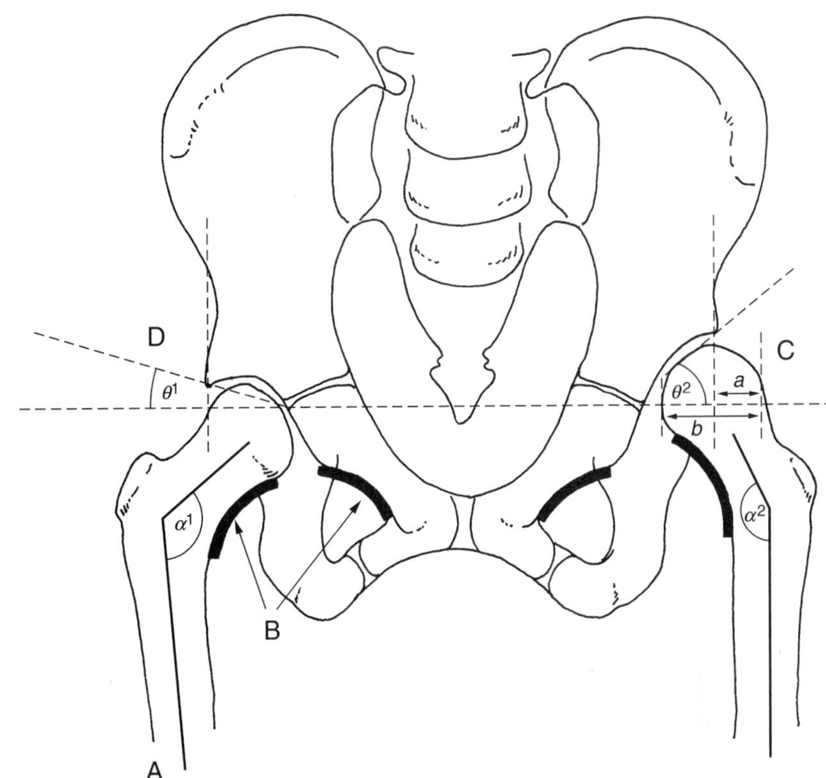

Figure 13-28 The four major radiographic parameters used to evaluate the spastic hip are the femoral neck-shaft angle **(A)**, the Shenton line **(B)**, the Reimer migration index **(C)**, and the acetabular index **(D)**. In this diagram, the right hip is normal and the left is subluxated. In patients with cerebral palsy, the femoral neck shaft angle (α^2) is increased (normal is approximately 135 degrees). The Shenton line is drawn along the medial portion of the femoral neck and should form a smooth arc with a line drawn on the inferior portion of the superior pubic ramus. This arc is typically broken in the presence of subluxation. The migration percentage measures the percentage of the capital femoral epiphysis that lies outside the lateral margin of the acetabulum and may be used to sequentially follow progressive lateral migration of the femoral head. The migration percentage is distance $a/b \times 100$, and hips with greater than 50% to 60% of migration nearly always progress to dislocation. The acetabular index (θ) is one way to assess the morphology of the acetabulum; and if this measurement is greater than 25 degrees (normal is typically less than 20 degrees), the acetabulum is dysplastic. (From Herring JA [ed]: Tachdjian's Pediatric Orthopaedics, 3rd ed, vol 2. Philadelphia, WB Saunders, 2001, p 1189.)

the acetabulum, and then resuturing the capsule after the femoral head is reduced. Direct inspection of the femoral head enables an assessment of the cartilaginous joint surface to identify degenerative changes. In the presence of significant degenerative changes or deformity in the femoral head, a salvage procedure may be preferable to relocating the hip.

For those with a symptomatic, chronic dislocation with deformity of the femoral head or degenerative changes, several options for salvage are available (Fig. 13-31). Resection of the proximal femur, usually at the subtrochanteric level, is one. The abductor muscles and capsule are interposed between the acetabulum and the proximal femoral remnant. Patients must undergo prophylaxis against heterotopic bone formation, and maximal relief of pain may not be achieved for up to a year after the procedure. Traction is commonly employed for several weeks during the postoperative period to allow for a sufficient scar to form, in order to prevent symptomatic bony impingement of the femoral segment on the acetabulum. An alternative is to perform a valgus osteotomy at the subtrochanteric level, which realigns the proximal femur and reorients the femoral head away from the acetabulum. This procedure may be combined with a resection of the femoral head and neck with interposition of the muscle and capsule. Fusion of the hip joint reliably relieves pain but has a limited role in this patient population. Replacement of the proximal femur with a prosthesis, or total hip arthroplasty, in which both sides of the joint are replaced, may be an option in a limited number of patients.

Hips, Knees, Feet

The orthopaedic goals for the lower extremities are modified for nonambulatory patients. Flexion or extension contractures at the hip may interfere with sitting. The hamstrings typically become contracted because nonambulatory patients spend most of their time in a wheelchair with the knees flexed 90 degrees. Hamstring contracture causes the pelvis to rotate posteriorly, and the lumbar spine compensates by flexing (loss of lumbar lordosis) to balance the center of gravity. The inability to compensate causes seating difficulties because patients tend to slide forward in the wheelchair. Lengthening of the hamstrings may be appropriate in this situation, and a proximal release of the origin from the ischial tuberosity may be considered as an alternative to distal release of the muscles at the level of the knee. Hip flexion contractures result in a compensatory increase in lumbar lordosis; if the lordosis becomes severe, a release of the iliopsoas tendon off the lesser trochanter may be required. Maintaining plantigrade feet is important for retaining their ability to fit into standard shoes as well as allowing them to be accurately positioned on the footrests of a wheelchair. Bracing and stretching may help maintain alignment, and in some cases, a soft

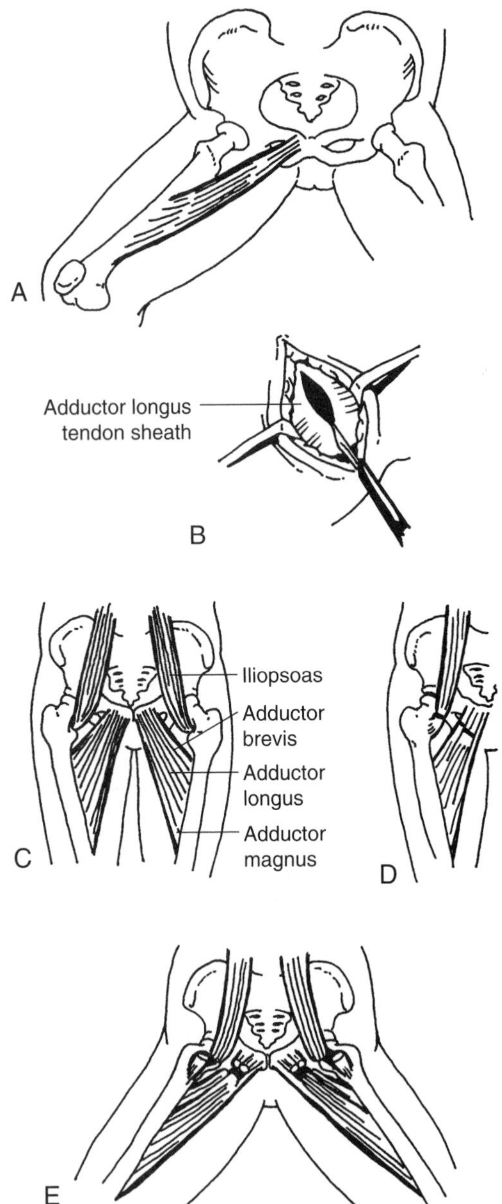

Figure 13-29 For children with early subluxation who have significant spasticity and contracture in adduction and flexion, a soft tissue release of the adductor muscles and the iliopsoas tendon may prevent the progression of subluxation. Typically, the adductor longus, adductor gracilis, and a portion of the adductor brevis are released, in addition to the iliopsoas tendon. Release of the iliopsoas tendon should be performed only in nonambulators. In ambulatory patients, a musculotendinous lengthening of the iliopsoas muscle preserves hip flexor power. (From Dormans JP, Copely LA: Orthopaedic approaches to treatment. In Dormans JP, Pellegrino L [eds]: Caring for Children with Cerebral Palsy: A Team Approach. Baltimore, Brookes Publishing, 1998, p 151.)

tissue release, osteotomy, or triple arthrodesis (in older patients with stiff deformities) may be needed to restore alignment.

Spine[1,3,7,29]

Spinal deformities are scoliosis, kyphosis, and lordosis. A radiograph in the frontal plane should show a straight spine, and on the lateral view (sagittal plane), there should be 20 to 40 degrees of kyphosis in the thoracic spine, and lordosis in the lumbar spine. Most spinal deformities in patients with cerebral palsy involve scoliosis. The patient with scoliosis may have a coexisting kyphotic or lordotic deformity in the thoracic or lumbar spine. Primary deformities in the sagittal plane are uncommon, and more often, an accentuation of thoracic kyphosis or lumbar lordosis represents compensation for contracture about the hips. Scoliosis is often seen in association with pelvic obliquity and unilateral hip dislocation.

Scoliosis occurs in 25% to 68% of patients, usually in nonambulators with spastic quadriplegia. The management of the spinal deformity is often complicated by coexisting pelvic obliquity, hip subluxation or dislocation, and lower extremity contractures. Coexisting medical problems, including malnutrition, seizures, gastroesophageal reflux, and pulmonary difficulties, often make management decisions more difficult. The etiology of neuromuscular curvatures involves asymmetrical paraspinal spasticity, and mechanical factors become important with larger curves. The typical pattern in neuromuscular patients is a long, sweeping, C-shaped curvature that extends from the thoracic region down to the pelvis (Fig. 13-32). Decisions about treatment are often difficult in this complex situation and must be individualized. Each patient should be assessed with respect to the magnitude of the deformity, the effect it has on functional status and ease of care, the overall medical status, the presence of any symptoms, and the desires of the family and caregivers.

Symptoms often depend on the level of patient function. Progressive curves may interfere with sitting balance and the use of the upper extremities by nonambulators, and ischial pressure sores may occasionally develop from the altered pressure distribution in the buttock area. Severe deformities may result in the loss of upright posture. Pain does not appear to be a significant problem in most patients.

Options for treatment of scoliosis include observation, nonoperative measures such as wheelchair modifications and orthoses, and operative treatment, which involves spinal fusion with instrumentation. The presence of associated soft tissue contractures and bony deformities also influences treatment decisions for the spine.

The more rigid braces (typically used in patients with idiopathic scoliosis) have not been shown to arrest progression of spinal curvatures and are often poorly tolerated. There has been some enthusiasm for the use of a soft spinal orthosis to support the trunk and

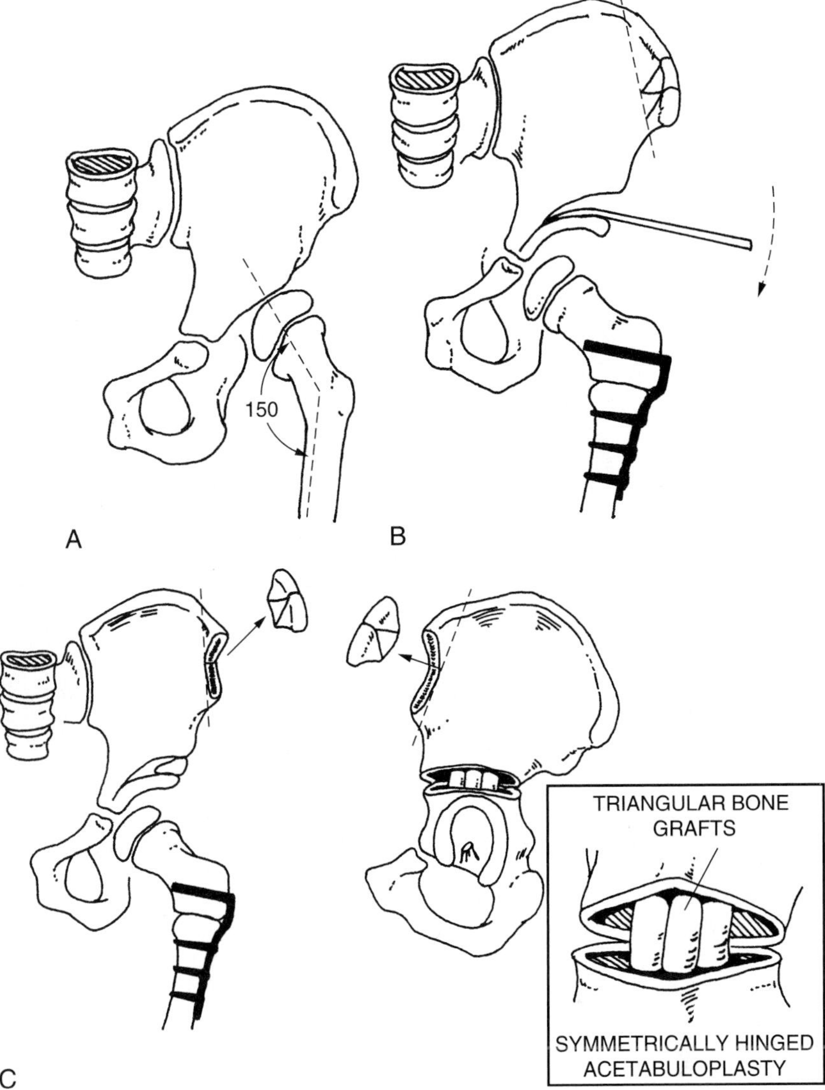

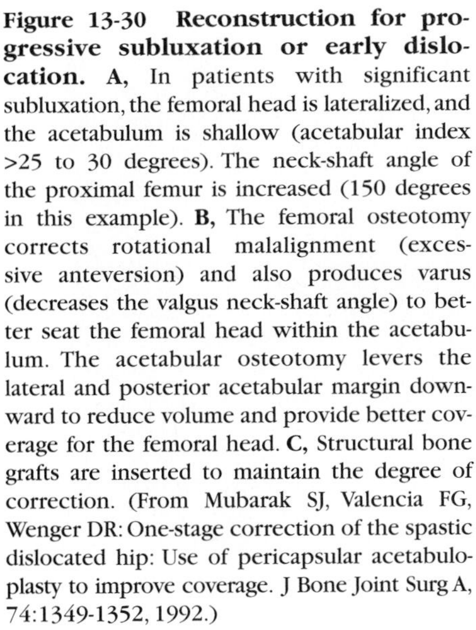
Figure 13-30 Reconstruction for progressive subluxation or early dislocation. A, In patients with significant subluxation, the femoral head is lateralized, and the acetabulum is shallow (acetabular index >25 to 30 degrees). The neck-shaft angle of the proximal femur is increased (150 degrees in this example). **B,** The femoral osteotomy corrects rotational malalignment (excessive anteversion) and also produces varus (decreases the valgus neck-shaft angle) to better seat the femoral head within the acetabulum. The acetabular osteotomy levers the lateral and posterior acetabular margin downward to reduce volume and provide better coverage for the femoral head. **C,** Structural bone grafts are inserted to maintain the degree of correction. (From Mubarak SJ, Valencia FG, Wenger DR: One-stage correction of the spastic dislocated hip: Use of pericapsular acetabuloplasty to improve coverage. J Bone Joint Surg A, 74:1349-1352, 1992.)

improve sitting balance, potentially to delay the need for surgical intervention in patients for whom surgery is medically or nutritionally unsuitable or for whom stabilization would ideally be performed at a later time.

The goals of surgical intervention are to arrest progression of the deformity, to achieve sufficient correction to restore or improve sitting balance and upper extremity function, and to avoid the potential complications associated with a severe spinal deformity. The patient and family should be educated about the natural history and should be given a frank description of the anticipated benefits and risks of the procedures. In comparison with idiopathic scoliosis, neuromuscular curves in patients with cerebral palsy have a greater propensity to progress after skeletal maturity. Although each case should be viewed individually, the general indications for spinal instrumentation and fusion include progressive curvatures greater than 40 to 50 degrees (these curves continue to progress). The procedures are often technically challenging, and complications are common. A thorough medical evaluation is necessary before any surgical intervention is considered.

The standard surgical procedure is a posterior spinal fusion with instrumentation. The goals are to straighten the spine and to obtain fusion across all the vertebrae such that the deformity is permanently stabilized. The instrumentation is used to apply corrective forces, which help to achieve realignment, and also to stabilize the spine during healing of the fusion. Without spinal implants, the patient would have to remain immobilized in a body cast for 6 to 12 months. The principle is to achieve segmental fixation (secure each vertebra or motion segment) in order to maximize the rate of fusion and minimize the chance of implant failure and

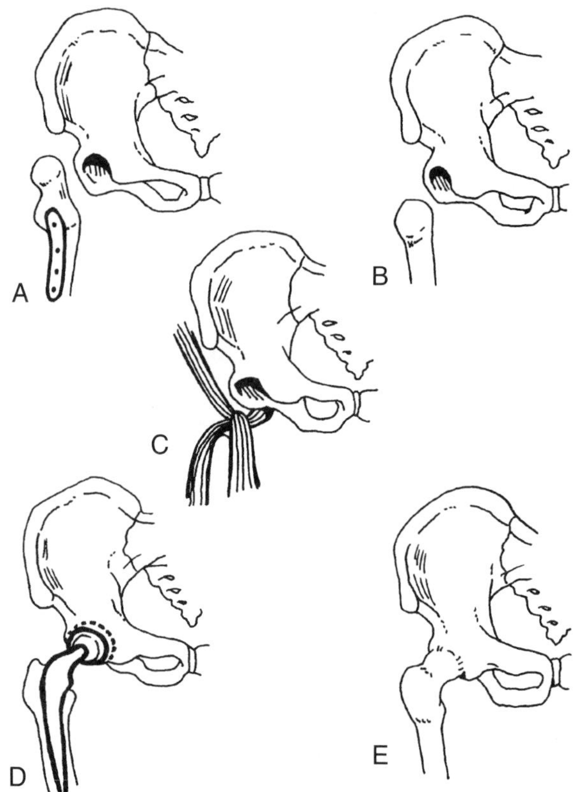

Figure 13-31 Several options are available if the hip dislocation is of long standing, or if femoral head deformity or degenerative changes in the articular cartilage are discovered during an attempted open reduction. **A,** With a valgus osteotomy, the proximal femur is redirected away from the acetabulum; this procedure may also be combined with interposition of soft tissues. **B,** A resection arthroplasty removes the proximal end of the femur, most often at the subtrochanteric level; and interposition of the hip capsule and abductor muscles is usually performed as well **(C). D,** Total joint arthroplasty involves replacement of the joint with prosthetic components. Some surgeons have replaced just the proximal femur, leaving the acetabular side alone. **E,** Arthrodesis, or fusion, involves removal of the cartilaginous surfaces, realignment of the joint in the desired position, and securing of the joint with hardware to promote permanent healing. Joint replacement and hip fusion are rarely performed. (From Dormans JP, Copely LA: Orthopaedic approaches to treatment. In Dormans JP, Pellegrino L [eds]: Caring for Children with Cerebral Palsy: A Team Approach. Baltimore, Brookes Publishing, 1998, p 155.)

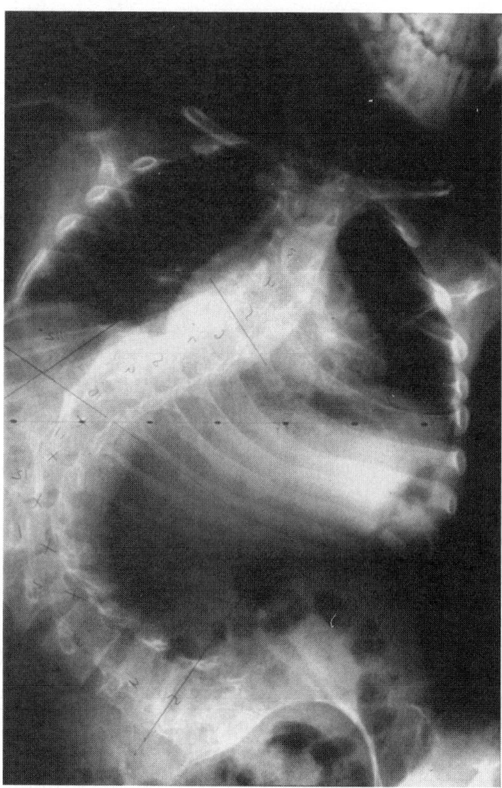

Figure 13-32 Neuromuscular scoliosis. This nonambulatory patient with spastic quadriplegia developed a severe thoracolumbar curvature with the typical C-shaped appearance. Sitting balance is impaired, and there is associated pelvic obliquity with elevation of the hemipelvis on the concave side of the deformity.

non-union. Most patients do not require a brace postoperatively if segmental spinal instrumentation is used.

A basic spinal implant construct consists of two rods, which are attached to points of fixation in the posterior elements of the spine. The rods are then cross-linked to each other to further enhance the rigidity of the construct. Implants used for fixation include hooks (attached to the laminae, pedicles, or transverse processes), wires (placed under the lamina at each involved level), or screws (placed through the pedicles into the vertebral bodies). The instrumentation and fusion is typically performed from the upper thoracic spine to the pelvis, especially in patients with significant pelvic obliquity (Fig. 13-33). For pelvic fixation, the distal portions of the rod on each side may be contoured to fit within the iliac wing (Galveston technique). For patients who ambulate, it may be beneficial to avoid extension of the fusion across the lumbosacral junction. This subset of ambulatory patients with scoliosis are treated like patients with idiopathic scoliosis.

In patients with larger, rigid deformities, it may be advantageous to perform an anterior spinal release before a posterior spinal fusion. This is best accomplished during the same day (less anesthesia time and blood loss, shorter hospital stay, better nutritional status), but the two procedures may have to be performed 10 to 14 days apart in some patients. Greater correction improves spinal balance, decreases pelvic obliquity, and reduces the chance of pseudarthrosis. In the anterior procedure, the spine is approached through the chest or abdomen, and as many disks as possible are excised near the apex of the curvature. This release, particularly of the anulus fibrosus, improves the flexibility of the curve. A greater correction can then be achieved during the

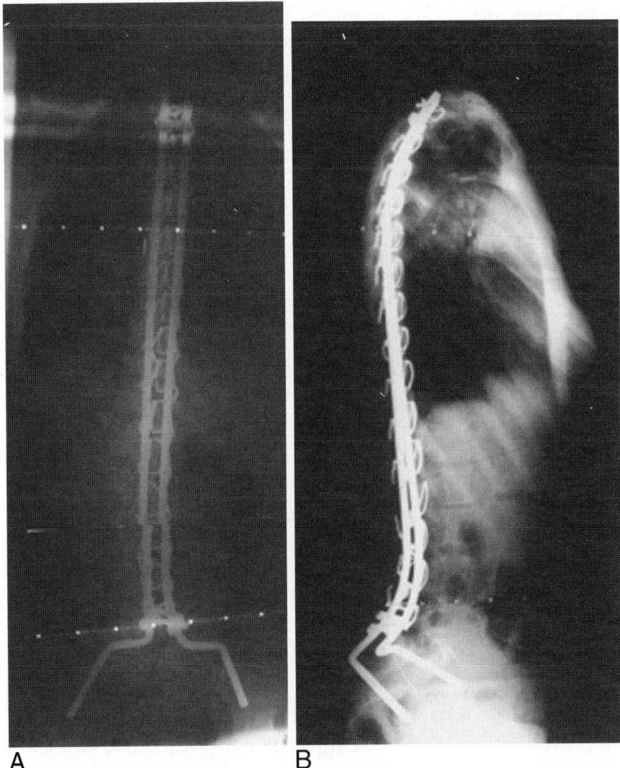

Figure 13-33 Spinal instrumentation for neuromuscular scoliosis. Posteroanterior **(A)** and lateral **(B)** radiographs demonstrate the typical spinal construct used to stabilize long neuromuscular curves with pelvic obliquity. Fixation is achieved at each level with sublaminar wires, which are tightened to the spinal rods. The rods extend down into the pelvis (iliac wing) on each side to stabilize the lumbosacral junction. Metal cross-links stabilize the construct further by locking the rods to one another. Corrective forces are applied gradually during the sequence of instrumentation.

posterior instrumentation and fusion. In addition, bone graft is placed in each interspace, which enhances the surface area for bony fusion and decreases the chance of a pseudarthrosis (non-union).

Upper Extremity Procedures[1,3,7,30]

Upper extremity problems requiring treatment are seen in hemiplegics and a limited number of quadriplegics. Nonoperative measures including range-of-motion exercises and splinting are the mainstay of treatment. Very few (5% to 10%) patients are candidates for surgical intervention, and it is critical to define realistic goals preoperatively. Upper extremity procedures are recommended mainly to improve function and, occasionally, to enhance cosmesis or the ease of care in patients with severe contractures. Function can often be improved by repositioning of the joints. Options include muscle release or lengthening, muscle transfer to rebalance the forces across the joint, and arthrodesis to stabilize the position of the joint in space or promote functions such as grasp, release, and pinch. As for the lower extremities, it is best to perform multiple procedures, if indicated, at the same time, with the goal of treating the entire limb. The ideal candidate for these procedures is intelligent and motivated, has voluntary use of the hand, has spasticity without fixed contractures, and has reasonable sensory function, including stereognosis, proprioception, and light touch. Patients with a significant athetoid component or with dystonia do not benefit from upper extremity surgery.

A comprehensive history focuses on psychosocial development, functional capabilities, and the presence of any symptoms or limitations in activities of daily living. The physical examination, in addition to noting the presence and overall pattern of deformities, documents active and passive range of motion of the joints, motor strength, sensibility, and functional activities. Most patients have spasticity, and a limited number have flaccidity or exhibit athetoid or extrapyramidal movements. Deficiencies in sensibility and in grasp, release, and pinch are very common. The pattern of joint contractures usually involves internal rotation of the shoulder, flexion of the elbow, pronation of the forearm, and flexion and ulnar deviation at the wrist. Hand deformities include thumb-in-palm deformity, swan neck deformities of the fingers, and clenched fist.

Nonoperative treatment consists of occupational therapy to promote bimanual skills and facilitate adaptive skills for daily living. Splinting is also employed. Functional splints, such as a neoprene thumb orthosis (for thumb in palm deformity) and a dorsal ring splint (for wrist flexion deformity) are used during the daytime to better position the wrist and thumb. A dynamic finger splint may help in treating a swan neck deformity. Static splints for thumb abduction or extension of the hand and wrist are used at night to prevent or improve contracture. Botulinum toxin injections may facilitate stretching and may enable strengthening of antagonist muscles. Injections may be performed in the biceps, flexor carpi ulnaris, pronator teres, and thumb adductors.

A host of procedures, and combinations of procedures, may be employed in the management of the upper extremity. At the level of the shoulder, a soft tissue release may rarely be indicated for adduction and internal rotation deformity. Contracture of the biceps, brachialis, and brachioradialis results in flexion deformity at the elbow, and lengthening of the involved muscles may be required. Pronation deformity, which may be complicated by subluxation or dislocation of the radial head, may be treated with release or transfer of the pronator teres or with transfer of the flexor carpi ulnaris to the extensor carpi radialis brevis. For severe deformities, an osteotomy of the radius, coupled with release of the pronator quadratus, may be required. Flexion and ulnar deviation at the wrist are usually treated with lengthening of the flexor carpi radialis or the flexor carpi ulnaris; release of the flexors at their origin on the medial epicondyle serves as an alternative. Transfer of the flexor carpi ulnaris into the extensor carpi radialis brevis may augment extension at the wrist and is often combined with a lengthening of other muscles. Arthrodesis of the wrist in a more functional position may be necessary in patients with severe deformities. The thumb-in-palm deformity is treated with soft tissue release, first metacarpophalangeal joint stabilization (soft tissue tightening or joint fusion), and tendon transfer to augment abduction and extension. Swan neck deformities are generally treated with soft tissue release and rebalancing.

GAIT

A major focus of orthopaedic care in ambulatory children with cerebral palsy is to improve the quality and energy efficiency of ambulation. Treatment decisions are complex, and serial examinations are required. Ultimately, treatment recommendations are based on results of both the bench examination (range of motion, angular and rotational alignment, degree of spasticity) and the observational gait analysis. Instrumented gait analysis may complement the clinical evaluation, especially in patients for whom multilevel interventions are planned. This section presents a basic overview of normal gait, explores some of the common gait deviations in ambulatory children with cerebral palsy, and briefly discusses instrumented gait analysis.

Normal Gait[3,7,31]

In the normal developmental sequence, infants begin to ambulate independently between 12 and 14 months of age. The infants' gait exhibits greater flexion at the hip and knee, and instead of making contact with the ground with the heels, they land with the feet flat. The base (distance between the feet) is wide to improve balance. The lower extremities are often externally rotated. The arms are held in abduction at the shoulder and extension at the elbow; reciprocal arm motions do not develop until about 2 years of age. Infants have a shorter step length and need to take more steps to increase their velocity. Normal children develop a mature pattern by 3 to 5 years of age, although those with cerebral palsy may take 7 years to reach a plateau. The adult pattern is characterized by an increase in velocity, step length, and time in single-limb stance, with a decrease in cadence and a narrower base of support.

Observational gait analysis should be performed from both the front and the side, and children with assistive devices (walker, braces, crutches) should be evaluated both with and without these aids. Each clinician should develop a comfortable sequence for evaluating the head, arms, trunk, hips, knees, and ankles during the different phases of the gait cycle. Watching the child run provides additional information. Ample floor space is required to obtain an accurate impression of a child's gait.

Gait Cycle[31]

The gait cycle may be divided into a *stance phase* (60%), in which the foot is in contact with the ground, and a *swing phase* (40%), in which the foot is off the ground while the limb is propelled forward. The cycle begins as the heel strikes the ground, and both stance phase and swing phase are subdivided into different events (Fig. 13-34). Stance phase consists of initial contact, loading response, midstance, terminal stance, and preswing; swing phase comprises initial swing, midswing, and terminal swing.

Prerequisites for a normal gait are stability during stance phase, clearance during swing phase, appropriate pre-positioning of the foot at the end of swing phase, an adequate step length, and conservation of energy. Individual muscles, or groups of muscles, have specific functions during each event and phase of the gait cycle. There are three types of muscle contraction, and the type of contraction a given muscle performs may vary at different times within the cycle. A muscle may contract concentrically (shorten during contraction), eccentrically (lengthen during contraction), or isometrically (contract without any change in length).

The cycle begins with *initial contact*, as the heel strikes the ground. During the *loading response*, the ankle plantar-reflexes as the heel makes contact with the ground, and the tibialis anterior functions to decelerate the foot as it flexes forward at heel strike. Both the hip and knee are flexed as the limb lands, and the hamstrings and hip flexors contract to help decelerate the limb. During *midstance*, the body advances over the foot, which is now fully in contact with the ground. The foot dorsiflexes as the tibia advances over the foot, while the knee and hip extend. In *terminal stance*, the body continues to advance forward over the foot, and the gastrocsoleus muscle complex contracts to plantarflex the ankle (which is in dorsiflexion) and stimulate the heel to rise in preparation for swing phase. Both the hip and knee remain extended. During *preswing*, the gastrocsoleus complex contracts to push the limb off the ground. Both the hip and the knee flex passively.

During *swing phase*, the goal is to advance the limb forward and achieve clearance of the foot. The hip flexors initiate forward motion of the limb, and during *initial swing*, both the hip and the knee are in flexion. The tibialis anterior dorsiflexes the foot to facilitate clearance. Clearance is achieved at *midswing*, and flexion

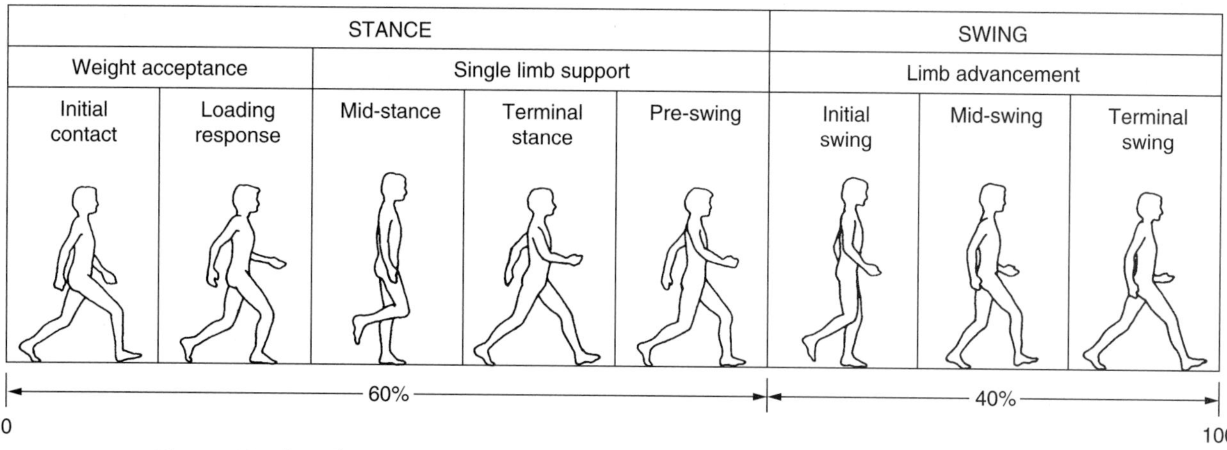

Figure 13-34 The gait cycle has a stance phase, when the lower extremity is in contact with the ground, and a swing phase, in which the limb is off the ground. The cycle begins with heel strike, and the cycle for the right leg is demonstrated here. (From Herring JA [ed]: Tachdjian's Pediatric Orthopaedics, 3rd ed, vol 1. Philadelphia, WB Saunders, 2001, p 76.)

persists at the hip and knee while the ankle remains at neutral. *Terminal swing* involves deceleration of the limb and preparation for contact of the heel. As in midswing, the tibialis anterior contracts to keep the foot at neutral. The knee extends by contraction of the quadriceps, and the hamstring muscles act to decelerate flexion at the hip and extension at the knee. The foot is now prepositioned for initial contact and the start of a new cycle.

Gait in Cerebral Palsy

The etiology of gait deviations in cerebral palsy is multifactorial. The primary abnormalities lie within the CNS, and although spasticity is most important, problems with weakness, selective motor control, balance, proprioception, and vision may also have an impact. Problems associated with spasticity include muscle weakness, imbalance between agonists and antagonists across each joint, and inappropriate muscle activation during different phases of the gait cycle. Structural problems, such as myostatic contractures and both angular and rotational bony deformities, further contribute to pathologic gait. Finally, the ultimate pattern of ambulation depends on both primary abnormalities (summation of the factors previously listed), and the compensatory strategies developed to alter these primary deviations.

All children with hemiplegia will ambulate independently, usually by 21 months of age, and nearly 9 of 10 patients with spastic diplegia will walk by 4 years of age. Figure 13-35 shows a typical patient with diplegia ambulating with a posterior walker. A subset of patients with spastic quadriplegia also possesses some ambulatory potential.

Prognosis for ambulation in children with cerebral palsy depends on the extent of neurologic involvement. A poor prognosis has been suggested for patients with persistent primitive reflexes after 15 months of age, the inability to achieve sitting balance by 2 years, and the inability to achieve head control by 20 months. Bleck studied the presence of four primitive reflexes (asymmetrical tonic neck, neck righting, Moro, symmetrical tonic neck) and the absence of three protective reactions (parachute, foot placement, extensor thrust) in a group of patients older than 12 months.[33] Each persistent primitive reflex, or absence of a protective reflex, received a score of 1. The prognosis for ambulation was good for a score of 0, guarded for a score of 1, and poor for a score of 2 or higher. Most investigators believe that

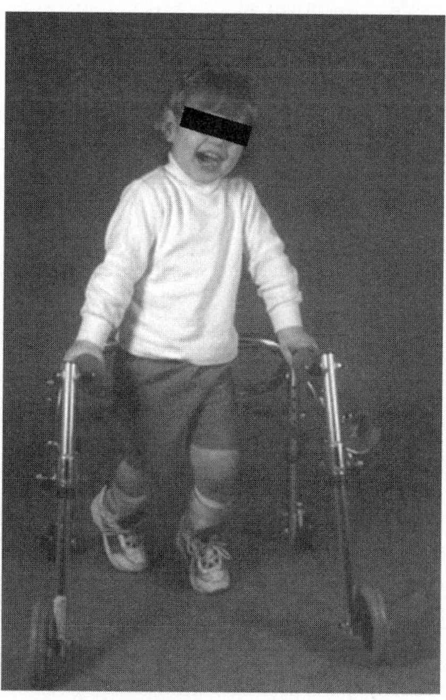

Figure 13-35 Diplegic child.

if a child is not walking by 7 years of age, the potential for ambulation in the future is minimal.

In general, ambulatory patients with cerebral palsy reach a plateau in walking by 7 years of age. The current trend is to avoid orthopaedic intervention until a mature pattern of gait has been achieved, and then to simultaneously correct all deformities at one time. Patients with moderate to severe spasticity may benefit from a tone-reducing procedure (rhizotomy or intrathecal baclofen) before undergoing orthopaedic intervention. Although rhizotomy does not appear to decrease the need for orthopaedic surgical procedures in the future, long-term follow-up data are not yet available for intrathecal baclofen.

Gait Deviations in Cerebral Palsy[7,16,18,20-22,32]

Common gait abnormalities in patients with hemiplegia and diplegia, and the few ambulatory patients with quadriplegia, result from abnormalities at the hip, knee, and ankle. Problems encountered at each joint are discussed separately. We use the term *contracture* to represent a dynamic deformity from spasticity, a fixed shortening of the muscle-tendon unit (myostatic), or a combination of both (most common).

Hip

Excessive flexion and adduction at the hip may be seen alone or in combination with other lower extremity contractures. Flexion contracture causes the trunk to lean forward, and compensatory changes include an increase in lumbar lordosis and an increase in flexion at the knee. If there is an equinus contracture at the ankle, the patient will walk in a crouch ("jump" gait pattern), up on the toes. If the foot is flat during stance (Achilles tendon is normal length or overlengthened) the result is a "crouch" gait pattern. Excessive adduction of the hip is caused by contracture of the adductors, and clinically, patients bring the leg inward during swing phase (scissoring). Coexisting femoral torsion may exacerbate this pattern. Lengthening of the hip flexors (intramuscular iliopsoas tenotomy), adductors, or both may be necessary.

Knee

Excessive flexion at the knee usually results from a hamstring contracture and weakness of the quadriceps but may also be used to compensate for a hip flexion contracture or a weak or overlengthened gastrocsoleus muscle complex. Primary contracture of the hamstrings may often be associated with a hip flexion contracture as well. Patients typically walk in a crouched pattern ("crouch" gait or "jump" gait). Persistent flexion during stance phase increases the demands on the quadriceps mechanism, and patients often complain of anterior knee pain, from both quadriceps muscle overload and increased stresses at the patellofemoral joint. In addition, the patellar tendon may gradually elongate from chronic tension, resulting in proximal migration of the patella, or patella alta. Patients may experience degenerative changes in the patellofemoral joint in adolescence or adulthood. A GRAFO and quadriceps-strengthening exercises may help patients with mild crouch and minimal flexion contracture. Those with greater involvement need hamstring lengthening. Salvage for patella alta, especially with degenerative changes, is difficult. Hamstring lengthening (with or without an extension osteotomy of the distal femur) combined with distal transfer of the tibial tuberosity represents one option for treatment. Alternatively, soft tissue plication of the patellar ligament may also be performed. For advanced cases with arthrosis of the patellofemoral joint, patellectomy may be the only salvage.

An extension contracture, or loss of knee flexion, is usually dynamic and occurs during ambulation. It is caused by spasticity of the rectus femoris muscle, which usually remains active inappropriately during swing phase, resulting in a stiff-knee gait. Normally, approximately 62 degrees of flexion occurs at the knee during swing phase, allowing for adequate clearance. Flexion is usually limited by at least 15 degrees in patients with a stiff-knee gait. Achieving clearance is difficult, and compensatory patterns include circumduction, vaulting, and both upward tilt and external rotation of the pelvis on the ipsilateral side. Transfer of the rectus femoris tendon to the gracilis or sartorius helps to relieve the deforming force and to augment the effect of the hamstrings on knee flexion. This procedure is commonly employed in concert with hamstring lengthening and other lower extremity procedures.

Ankle

Excessive plantar-flexion at the ankle (equinus) may interfere with achieving the normal heel strike during initial contact and may impair clearance during swing phase. Contracture of the gastrocsoleus complex is responsible, and weakness of the tibialis anterior contributes to decreased clearance during swing phase. Equinus contracture results in a loss of active and passive dorsiflexion, and the heel is prevented from making initial contact (toe walker). Residual equinus may cause the knee to hyperextend during stance (back-knee or "recurvatum" gait). An AFO may help, and lengthening of the gastrocsoleus complex may also be required. Weakness or impaired control of the tibialis anterior results in the inability to dorsiflex the foot actively during swing phase, making clearance difficult. The child may drag the toes, and the front of the shoe shows a characteristic pattern of wear. An AFO is needed to block plantar-flexion and keep the foot at neutral.

Instrumented Gait Analysis[32]

Instrumented gait analysis uses sophisticated methodology to objectively document gait parameters in the laboratory setting. The gait laboratory evaluation includes a detailed history and physical examination, and the final recommendations reflect both the clinical findings and the data generated in the instrumented motion analysis. Members of the assessment team generally are an orthopaedic surgeon, a physical therapist, and a biomechanical engineer. The referring physician may then integrate his or her clinical impression with the objective data, as well as with the final recommendations of the motion analysis team, to design a plan for management.

The availability and usage of gait laboratories varies in different regions of the United States. Ambulatory patients with hemiplegia and diplegia are studied most often, and a common indication for a motion study is fine-tuning the preoperative plan in patients about to undergo multilevel soft tissue and bone surgical procedures. Proponents of performing gait analysis for this purpose believe that the surgical plan is altered in a significant number of cases. Efforts to standardize data collection among laboratories are ongoing, and the final recommendations from a particular gait laboratory will necessarily reflect the experiences and biases of the professionals completing the analysis. The ultimate role of instrumented gait analysis in cerebral palsy is evolving.

In addition, instrumented gait analysis has been an excellent research tool, enhancing our insights into pathologic patterns of gait in children with cerebral palsy. Studies have evaluated the benefits of different orthoses, the results of orthopaedic surgical procedures and the results of tone-reducing interventions, including botulinum toxin A injection, selective dorsal rhizotomy, and intrathecal baclofen.

A typical study has several components. *Kinematic* data is collected in order to reconstruct the relationships between limb segments during ambulation. Surface markers are placed in different locations throughout the skeleton, and four to six cameras collect data as the patient walks. The video data are processed through a computer, which facilitates a reconstruction of the relationships between body segments during gait and enables a calculation of the range of motion, velocity, and acceleration of the involved joints. *Kinetic* data is collected through the use of a force plate, which measures forces along different axes of motion. This information can be used to calculate the magnitude and location of forces acting around each joint.

Dynamic surface EMG data assesses muscle activity during the various periods of the gait cycle, and one can determine whether muscles are acting in the appropriate phase, in an inappropriate phase, or throughout the gait cycle. This information is particularly helpful when a muscle transfer procedure is being considered. In patients who ambulate with a stiff-knee gait, documenting inappropriate activity of the rectus femoris during swing phase helps identify those who may benefit from a rectus femoris transfer. In patients with an equinovarus foot, this technique may be used to determine whether the tibialis anterior or the tibialis posterior is responsible for the muscle imbalance across the ankle joint, knowledge that defines the appropriate muscle for transfer. Finally, oxygen consumption can be calculated during instrumented gait analysis.

CASE EXAMPLE

The following hypothetical case describes the evaluation and management of an ambulatory patient with spastic diplegia. Information from the history and physical examination is integrated with data from an instrumented gait analysis to finalize the plan for surgical management.

An 8-year-old child with spastic diplegia presents for a gait evaluation. A community ambulator, he has been wearing bilateral solid AFOs. His chief complaint is that he crouches down and that his feet point inward. He tends to cross his legs over one each other and often trips. His endurance has decreased as the crouch has worsened. He has also been treated with several injections of botulinum toxin A to various muscles in the lower extremity, which achieved temporary improvement.

Observational gait analysis demonstrates that in the sagittal plane, this patient walks with flexion at both the hip and the knee, and is up on his toes. In the frontal plane there is scissoring, and the femoral segment is internally rotated. His foot progression angle is external, and the longitudinal arches of his feet are collapsed when bearing weight.

Physical examination demonstrates muscle contractures at multiple levels. He has a 20-degree hip flexion contracture, and passive hip abduction is 35 degrees bilaterally. His popliteal angle is 60 degrees, and with the hip in extension, he lacks several degrees of extension at the knee (no significant capsular contracture). His foot can be dorsiflexed 5 degrees with the knee flexed, and he lacks 5 degrees of dorsiflexion when his knee is in extension. His rotational profile includes 80 degrees of medial rotation at the hip, and his thigh-foot axis is 30 degrees external bilaterally. He has bilateral equinovalgus deformities of the feet, with callus formation and mild tenderness in the region of the head of the talus.

In summary, clinical examination demonstrates crouch gait and scissoring, with contracture of the psoas, adductors, hamstrings, and Achilles tendon on both sides. The patient has coexisting rotational deformities, including internal femoral torsion, external tibial torsion, and equinovalgus foot deformities. A radiograph of the pelvis shows no significant hip dysplasia. Data from the gait laboratory corroborates the clinical findings.

The surgical strategy for this spectrum of deformities might include both soft tissue and bony procedures, and the specific choices would be at the discretion of the treating surgeon. One possible approach consists of the following procedures: bilateral intramuscular lengthening of the iliopsoas and hamstring muscles and the gastrocsoleus complex; bilateral femoral derotational osteotomies (subtrochanteric level); bilateral tibial derotational osteotomies; and bilateral calcaneal osteotomies. Postoperatively, the patient's legs might be placed in bilateral short-leg casts with knee immobilizers, rather than bilateral long-leg casts. If bone quality is believed to be poor, or fixation of the femoral osteotomies to be inadequate, a hip spica cast (body cast) may be used until healing is sufficient.

MAJOR POINTS

Cerebral palsy is a nonprogressive disorder of motion and posture resulting from injury to the immature brain.

Secondary changes in the musculoskeletal system may be progressive throughout growth and development, and each patient's level of function and needs may change as he or she matures into adulthood.

The global care plan should be directed to maximizing function in adulthood, and a multidisciplinary team is often involved in the management of patients with cerebral palsy.

Priorities for management, in order of importance, are communication skills, activities of daily living, mobility, and ambulation.

A definitive cause of cerebral palsy is identified in only 10% of patients, and the prevalence has remained constant over the past few decades. Approximately 50% of new cases have been associated with prematurity.

The diagnosis involves establishing a delay in development, identifying physical findings of an upper motor neuron disorder, and ruling out congenital or metabolic conditions that are progressive, have a different natural history, and may be amenable to treatment.

Classification schemes include physiologic (spasticity, athetosis, ataxia, dystonia, mixed), geographic (hemiplegia, diplegia, quadriplegia), and pyramidal versus extrapyramidal.

Spasticity results from upper motor neuron damage and represents a velocity-dependent increase in muscle tone. The sequelae of spasticity include muscle contracture and angular and rotational deformities of the extremities.

Neurosurgical procedures to treat spasticity include selective dorsal rhizotomy and intrathecal baclofen pump implantation.

Dorsal rhizotomy, which involves either selective or nonselective sectioning of spinal nerve roots, results in a permanent decrease in spasticity. Strict selection criteria are essential to achieve adequate results.

Intrathecal baclofen allows modulation of spasticity by titrating the dosage directly at the level of the spinal cord; it has been helpful in ambulatory diplegics, in patients with dystonia, and in a subset of quadriplegics.

Orthopaedic procedures target the secondary affects of spasticity on the musculoskeletal system, and goals are based on the patient's level of function.

Nonambulators (usually quadriplegics), in addition to muscle contractures, often have progressive hip subluxation or dislocation and are at a higher risk for progressive scoliosis. Treatment is aimed at maintaining or improving sitting posture, preventing pain, and promoting the ease of care. Common procedures are muscle releases to improve positioning and hip reconstructive surgery to prevent progressive subluxation or to reduce a dislocation. Early diagnosis and treatment may allow goals to be achieved with less extensive surgery. Spinal instrumentation and fusion are necessary to stabilize progressive scoliosis.

Ambulators (hemiplegics and diplegics) often benefit from surgical treatment of contractures, muscle imbalance, and both angular and rotational deformities of the extremities in order to improve the pattern of ambulation and decrease energy expenditure during locomotion. Common procedures are muscle lengthening and transfer and osteotomies to realign bones or joints. These patients usually require lower extremity orthoses to counteract spasticity, provide support, and improve the pattern of ambulation. Orthopaedic procedures rarely eliminate the need for braces.

Orthopaedic and neurosurgical procedures do not treat the primary central nervous system disorder. Coexisting deficits, such as weakness, loss of selective motor control, poor balance, altered cognition, and vision, affect the outcome after these interventions.

Realistic goals are essential, and families should be counseled in detail about the risks and proposed benefits of each procedure.

REFERENCES

1. Dormans JP, Pellegrino L: Caring for Children with Cerebral Palsy: A Team Approach. Baltimore, Brookes Publishing, 1998.
2. Mutch L, Alberman E, Hagburg B, et al: Cerebral palsy epidemiology: Where are we now and where are we going? Dev Med Child Neurol 34:547-551, 1992.
3. Herring JA (ed): Disorders of the brain. In Tachdjian's Pediatric Orthopaedics, 3rd ed, vol 2. Philadelphia, WB Saunders, 2001, pp1121-1248.
4. Nelson KB, Ellenberg JH: Antecedents of cerebral palsy: Multivariate analysis of risks. N Engl J Med 315:81-86, 1986.
5. O'Shea TM, Dammann O: Antecedents of cerebral palsy in very low-birth weight infants. Clin Perinatol 27:285-302, 2000.
6. Menkes JH, Sarnat HB: Perinatal asphyxia and trauma. In Menkes JH, Sarnat HB (eds): Child Neurology, 6th ed. Philadelphia, Lippincott Williams & Wilkins, 1998, pp 401-457.
7. Bleck EE: Orthopaedic Management in Cerebral Palsy. Philadelphia, JB Lippincott, 1987.
8. Winter S: Preoperative assessment of the child with neuromuscular scoliosis. Orthop Clin North Am 2:239-245, 1994.
9. Krach L: Pharmacotherapy of spasticity: Oral medications and intrathecal baclofen. J Child Neurol.16:31-36, 2001.
10. Koman L, Mooney J, Smith B: BOTOX Study Group: Botulinum toxin A neuromuscular blockade in the treatment of lower extremity spasticity in cerebral palsy: A randomized, double-blind, placebo-controlled trial. J Pediatr Orthop 20:108-115, 2000.
11. Graham K, Aoki K, Autti-Ramo I, et al: Recommendations for the use of Botulinum toxin A in the management of cerebral palsy. Gait Posture 11:67-79, 2000.
12. Steinbok P: Outcomes after selective dorsal rhizotomy for spastic cerebral palsy. Childs Nerv Syst 17:1-18, 2001.
13. Peacock WJ, Staudt LA: Functional outcomes following selective posterior rhizotomy in children with cerebral palsy. J Neurosurg 74:380-385, 1991.
14. Albright AL: Intrathecal baclofen in cerebral palsy movement disorders. J Child Neurol 11(Suppl 1): S29-S35, 1996.
15. Gilmartin R, Bruce D, Storrs B, et al: Intrathecal baclofen for management of spastic cerebral palsy: Multicenter trial. J Child Neurol 15:71-77, 2000.
16. Renshaw TS, Green NE, Griffin PP, et al: Cerebral palsy: Orthopaedic management. J Bone Joint Surg Am 77:1590-1606, 1995.
17. Sutherland DH, Zilberfarb JL, Kaufman KR, et al: Psoas release at the pelvic brim in ambulatory patients with cerebral palsy: Operative technique and functional outcome. J Pediatr Orthop 17:563-570, 1997.
18. Sutherland DH, Davids JR: Common gait abnormalities of the knee in cerebral palsy. Clin Orthop Rel Res 288:139-147, 1993.
19. Green NE, Griffin PP, Shiavi R: Split posterior tibial-tendon transfer in spastic cerebral palsy. J Bone Joint Surg Am 65:748, 1983.
20. Gage JR: Surgical treatment of knee dysfunction in cerebral palsy. Clin Orthop Rel Res 253:545-554, 1990.
21. Gage JR, Perry J, Hicks RR, et al: Rectus femoris transfer to improve knee function of children with cerebral palsy. Dev Med Child Neurol 29:159-165, 1987.
22. Winters TF, Gage JR, Hicks R: Gait patterns in spastic hemiplegia in children and young adults. J Bone Joint Surg Am 69:437-441, 1987.
23. Mosca VS: Calcaneal lengthening for valgus deformity of the hindfoot. J Bone Joint Surg Am 78:500-512, 1995.
24. Moreau M, Drummond DS, Rogala EJ, et al: Natural history of dislocated hips in cerebral palsy. Dev Med Child Neurol 21:749-753, 1979.
25. Mubarak SJ, Valencia FG, Wenger DR: One-stage correction of the spastic dislocated hip: Use of pericapsular acetabuloplasty to improve coverage. J Bone Joint Surg Am 74:1347-1357, 1992.
26. Miller F, Cardoso Diaz R, Dabney KW, et al: Soft-tissue release for spastic hip subluxation in cerebral palsy. J Pediatr Orthop 17:571-584, 1997.
27. Bagg MR, Farber J, Miller F: Long-term follow-up of hip subluxation in cerebral palsy patients. J Pediatr Orthop 13:32-36, 1993.
28. Cooperman DR, Bartucci E, Dietrick E, Millar EA: Hip dislocation in spastic cerebral palsy: Long term consequences. J Pediatr Orthop 7:268-276, 1987.
29. Buhlman W, Dormans JP, Ecker M, Drummond DS: Posterior spinal fusion for scoliosis in patients with cerebral palsy: A comparison of Luque rod and unit rod instrumentation. J Pediatr Orthop 16:314-323, 1996.
30. Waters PM, Van Heest A: Spastic hemiplegia of the upper extremity in children. Hand Clin 14:119-134, 1998.
31. Davids JR: Normal gait and assessment of gait disorders. In Morrissy RT, Weinstein SL (eds): Lovell and Winters' Pediatric Orthopaedics, 4th ed. Philadelphia, Lippincott-Raven, 1997, pp131-156.
32. Gage JR, DeLuca PA, Renshaw TS: Gait analysis: Principles and applications: Emphasis on its use in cerebral palsy. J Bone Joint Surg Am 77:1607-1625, 1995.
33. Bleck EE: Locomotor prognosis in cerebral palsy. Dev Med Child Neurol 17:18-25, 1975.

CHAPTER 14

Spina Bifida

BENJAMIN D. ROYE
RICHARD S. DAVIDSON

The spectrum of congenital neural tube defects, referred to as *spina bifida*, produces a wide variety of disabilities, ranging from benign defects in the skin of the back to devastating paralysis and deformity of the lower extremities, urinary and fecal incontinence, hydrocephalus, spasticity and mental retardation. The care of children with spina bifida usually requires a multidisciplinary approach. Early intervention by a team of trained caregivers can significantly improve the disabilities and permit many children to be integrated into normal social environments with high levels of independence. This chapter is describes the overall management of spina bifida (myelomeningocele) with special emphasis on the orthopedic management.

DEFINITIONS

Spina bifida consists of a spectrum of congenital injuries or failures of development of the dorsal spinal column and cord. These can be broadly differentiated into *spina bifida occulta*, in which the spinal cord and meninges remain inside the spinal canal, and *spina bifida cystica*, in which the meninges, spinal cord, or both protrude through the defect in the neural arch. Spina bifida cystica can be further divided into meningocele, myelomeningocele, myeloschisis, and lipomyelomeningocele. Of note, when describing the level of the lesion in a child with a neural tube defect, the level assigned the child is the last level functioning in a *clinically significant manner*. For example, a child with an L4 level myelomeningocele has a functional L4 nerve root that does not merely provide a flicker of muscle contraction to the quadriceps, but is strong enough to enable the limb to at least resist gravity.

Similar problems that are less common are caudal regression syndrome and spinal sacral agenesis. Associated anomalies include hydrocephalus, tethered cord, Arnold-Chiari type II malformation, diastematomyelia, and hydromyelia. These are further described later in the chapter.

ETIOLOGY AND EMBRYOLOGY

In spite of extensive study, two opposing concepts of the etiology of spina bifida have persisted since the early descriptions of the disease. Von Recklinghausen hypothesized that the defect was caused by lack of closure of the spine, whereas Morgagni proposed rupture of a previously closed neural tube. Both events are believed to occur by the third or fourth week of gestation.

The central and peripheral nervous systems, including the spinal cord, develop from the neural plate. Formed from the ectodermal layer of the trilaminate embryo, the neural plate gives rise to neural folds on either side of the midline, with a neural groove running between them. The neural folds fuse dorsally to form a neural tube in a process known as *neurulation*. This process starts cranially around the 24th day of gestation and is complete by the 26th day. The cells of the neural tube begin to differentiate, forming the cord, peripheral nerves, and three layers of coverings—the pia, arachnoid, and dura mater.

Longitudinal ultrasonographic studies of the developing myelomeningocele fetus suggest that there is progressive deformity, including Arnold-Chiari malformation, ventriculomegaly, and clubfeet. Early lower extremity movement has been observed to cease during fetal development. Secondary trauma from direct abrasion of the exposed cord against the uterus and exposure to amniotic fluid may cause late damage to the cord. Erosion, abrasion, and pressure necrosis have been reported in the myelomeningocele fetus.

DIAGNOSIS: PRENATAL EVALUATION

Three modalities (maternal serum screening, ultrasonography, and amniocentesis) are available to evaluate neural tube defects, such as myelomeningocele and its related condition, anencephaly, in the fetus.

Elevations of maternal serum α-fetoprotein between the 15th and 18th weeks of pregnancy are indicative of fetal neural tube defect. The rate of false-negative results is 10% with this measurement, which also carries a risk of false-positive results. Twin pregnancy and other obstetric complications can produce false-positive results. A positive result should be followed by additional tests such as amniocentesis and ultrasonography.

Ultrasonography, when performed by an experienced ultrasonographer between the 10th and 12th weeks of gestation and again at the 18th week, can provide reliable evidence of neural tube defects.

Amniocentesis is performed between the 15th and 16th weeks of gestation to obtain amniotic fluid for evaluation of α-fetoprotein levels. Confirmation of the results by ultrasonography is advised. Chromosomal analysis of cells cultured from amniocentesis can identify additional disorders.

DEMOGRAPHICS AND GENETIC AND ENVIRONMENTAL FACTORS

Traditionally, the incidence of spina bifida has shown significant regional and racial variation. However, later data have shown a leveling of the incidence across both geographic and racial lines. In the United States, the incidence of neural tube defects is about 3 per 10,000 live births; and in 1990 this number was similar for Hispanic, white, and African-American persons.[1] In fact, in 1990, the incidence was lower in white persons than in African Americans, a group with a historically lower incidence. In Europe, studies have reported an incidence of approximately 1 per 10,000 live births.[2] Many later studies have also shown a diminishing incidence of myelomeningocele,[1,2] which has been attributed to voluntary terminations of pregnancy and the more regular use of perinatal folic acid.

The male-to-female ratio for spina bifida is about 3:2. Studies suggest etiologic heterogeneity for the disorder, meaning that there is more than one cause and both genetic and environmental factors probably play a role. A study out of the Netherlands demonstrated a greater risk of high spina bifida than of low lesions in patients with a family history positive for spina bifida.[3]

For a family who has one child with a neural tube defect, the risk that a second child will have a neural tube defect is approximately 2% to 4%,[4] approximately the same as the risk of a major birth defect in the general population.[5] For the parents of two or three children with a neural tube defect, the risk becomes approximately 10% or 25%, respectively.[6]

Environmental factors have also been implicated in the development of neural tube defects. Valproic acid, which is used in the treatment of seizures, is one. Folic acid deficiency has been associated with neural tube defects since the late 1960s.[7,8] In 1987, Yates and colleagues[9] demonstrated that inherent maternal problems with folic acid metabolism are associated with a higher incidence of spina bifida.

PREVENTION

Many studies have shown the benefit of vitamin supplementation in preventing neural tube defects. Adequate levels of folic acid in a woman's diet for at least 1 month before conception and during the first trimester of pregnancy have been estimated to reduce her risk of having a baby with a neural tube defect by 50% or more.[10] In fact, since the U.S. Food and Drug Administration (FDA) approved the enrichment of grain products with folic acid in 1996, the incidence of neural tube defects dropped by at least 19%.[11] The most recent statistics published by the U.S. Centers for Disease Control and Prevention (CDC) show a 25% decrease in live births involving spina bifida between 1996 and 2001, from 25 per 100,000 to 20 per 100,000 live.[12] This decrease translates to avoidance of an absolute value of approximately 920 cases of spina bifida per year, or of approximately 4000 cases of spina bifida since folate enrichment began in 1996 in the United States. The mechanism by which folic acid protects against neural tube defects is not understood.

NATURAL HISTORY

As suggested by Lindseth,[13] the natural history of myelomeningocele has changed since the advent of routine neural tube closure and ventricular shunting and may change again if in utero closure of the neural tube proves to be beneficial. Untreated open neural tube defects have an astronomical mortality rate, with death usually secondary to meningoventriculitis. In the early 1970s, forays into selective neural tube closure as suggested by Lorber[14] were met with great resistance, but routine neural tube closure soon after birth has now become the standard of care. Routine closure and survival are much improved, but the children tend to deteriorate with time; that is to say, the neurologic level of the patient can worsen with time, usually because of hydrocephalous (often from shunt failure), Arnold-Chiari deformity, or tethered cord syndrome. These entities are described in full detail later. To preserve function, the caregivers of the patient with myelomeningocele must be vigilant for signs of neurologic deterioration. If subtle signs are detected and investigated, a problem such as a malfunctioning shunt or tethered cord may be identified and treated before severe and permanent loss of function occurs.

In addition to deterioration in neurologic function, many children experience deterioration in social function as they age. This development is caused by the interplay among the child's physical and intellectual handicaps, factors related to provision of health care, and community attitudes.[15] For children with myelomeningocele, socialization is impaired from birth; most children are at home being properly stimulated during infancy, but children with myelomeningocele are often confined in the hospital, interfering with their normal development. Then, although these children are typically accepted in elementary school, many problems arise in the transition to adolescence. Adolescents normally have body image problems, an issue understandably magnified in the handicapped. Teenagers with myelomeningocele typically have tremendous difficulty finding an accepting peer group. Many issues contribute to this problem, ranging from mobility and continence difficulties to overprotective parents to the fact that wheelchairs, braces, and skeletal deformities simply make children with meningomyelocele look different. These problems culminate in difficulties finding employment and developing romantic relationships.

SPECTRUM OF DISEASE: GENERAL OVERVIEW

A major goal in the treatment of a child involves "preventing complications or further disability and maximizing functional independence and inclusion in society."[15] Many different medical specialists and allied health practitioners are required to achieve this lofty goal.

Role of the Multidisciplinary Clinic

As described in the remainder of this section, children affected by spina bifida need many different services. Taking these mobility-challenged children to ten different doctor visits per month is difficult if not impossible for many families, especially as the children grow. The multidisciplinary clinic evolved to address this issue. It can be thought of as a type of one-stop shopping. All the different services and specialists needed by these children and their families, from social work to urology to orthopaedics, are in one location to provide comprehensive care. The benefits of this model include fewer demands on the family and better communication among caregivers.

Nursing

Nurses play an important role in the care of children with spina bifida in both the hospital and the home. They both care for patients and educate patients and families about skills necessary for daily survival. For instance, nurses instruct patients with bowel and bladder incontinence about bowel regimens and self-catheterization. Nurses teach families how to avoid pressure sores and, when such sores do occur, nurses assist with dressing changes and monitor healing.

Specialty Pediatrics (Developmental Medicine)

Most children with myelomeningocele have cognitive defects ranging from mild to severe. Because of the special needs and delayed intellectual development of such children, developmental pediatricians can be a great resource. These specialists can work with the children and their families to establish a developmentally appropriate education program. Also, they can assist with the many psychosocial issues these children experience, especially as they enter adolescence and lose their "darling of the classroom" status.

Physical and Occupational Therapy

Therapists are central to the development and progress of children with myelomeningocele and probably have more contact with these children than any other single group of specialists. By manipulating joints and placing them in physiologic positions, the physical therapist can accelerate the achievement of gross motor skills and improve overall functioning. As a child with myelomeningocele grows, therapists continually reassess both child and environment in order to set new goals and work with the rest of the team to maximize function and independence. The therapy program may involve transfers, gait training, or wheelchair skills; improvement of strength and flexibility; and development of conditioning and coordination. Also, therapists refer the patient back to the physician when they notice changes that may reflect a deterioration in neurologic status or some other problem. Therapists are in a unique position to perform this function because of their intimate relationship with the child and family.

The occupational therapist (OT) works to develop and improve fine motor skills, activities of daily living (ADLs), and seating or positioning. The aim of occupational therapy is to maximize independence in a wide range of activities, from the basic (dressing, hygiene) to the more complex (shopping, cooking, economic budgeting). Although the primary neurologic lesion of meningomyelocele affects the lower extremities, hydrocephalus can lead to cognitive deficits, ataxia, and problems with upper extremities, making many of these tasks much more difficult for the patient. Much of the benefit of the OT's intervention is attained through early intervention programs. Such programs, when begun at a very early age, have been shown to significantly decrease the number of orthopaedic and urologic operations, improve locomotion, and increase the probability of normal schooling for children with this disorder.[16]

Wheelchair Assessment

Because the spectrum of disability from spina bifida varies widely, not only from child to child but also for the individual child with growth, the decision whether and when to use a wheelchair requires constant monitoring of function. Most children with spina bifida have some ability to ambulate or stand, often with orthotic assistance. However, the functional level of many children deteriorates as they grow older and heavier, so they become increasingly dependent on wheelchairs.

For children who spend the majority of their waking hours in a wheelchair, proper wheelchair selection is critical. The chair must be (1) designed to facilitate transfers according to the function of the child, (2) well padded to prevent pressure sores, (3) and bolstered to improve seating balance and maximize the child's ability to interact with the environment.

Orthotics (General Principles)

For the child with spina bifida, orthotics are ubiquitous, a normal part of life from the time he or she begins trying to stand. Menelaus's classic text lists six major roles of orthotics, an approach that constitutes a convenient framework for thinking about these devices.[17]

The most general and important element is to improve function. This improvement can take many forms. For example, orthotics may aid mobility. An ankle-foot orthotic (AFO) can help place the foot in a more advantageous position for better walking, making gait faster and more efficient. Orthotics can also help improve posture. Children with thoracic level lesions may use a stander to encourage weight-bearing and help prevent the osteopenia associated with no weight-bearing. Protection of sites of recent surgery or of a fracture can also be accomplished by orthotics. They are often preferable to casts, which are heavy and can cause skin problems in insensate areas. A common indication for orthotics is prevention of the development or recurrence of joint contractures. It is important to remember, however, that orthotics cannot correct a rigid deformity. They are static devices that can hold a joint in a certain position, but the joint must be able to be passively manipulated into the position determined by the brace.

Finally, orthoses can facilitate gait in children who would otherwise be completely wheelchair bound. Orthotics for the entire lower extremity from the knee to the foot (a knee-ankle-foot orthosis, or KAFO) or from the hip to the foot (an HKAFO) can provide the necessary support for children with weak legs to ambulate who otherwise could not. Reciprocating-gait orthoses (RGOs) link the hip joints with a mechanism that causes extension in one hip as the other hip is flexed. RGOs can facilitate non-wheelchair ambulation even in children with thoracic level lesions.

Urology

Difficulty with urinary continence is nearly universal in this population. A neurogenic bladder can contribute to recurrent urinary tract infections and even lead to problems with the kidney parenchyma (renal failure or hypertension). To prevent or minimize these complications, most urologists recommend a routine program of clean intermittent catheterization, which is a safe, effective technique.[18] Oral anticholinergic agents can be very helpful, but some patients do not tolerate their side effects. The effectiveness of intravesicular injection of botulinum toxin in this population is being studied. Finally, bladder augmentation can play a role in selected patients. Urinary function must be constantly monitored to preserve renal function through discovery of problems before they cause permanent damage.[19]

Other Issues

Children with myelomeningocele are subject to other secondary problems. Visual disturbances and dental problems are very common issues that require specialty care. Additionally, psychiatrists can help manage the difficult emotional problems that arise when these children reach adolescence.

TYPES OF SPINA BIFIDA

Spina bifida occulta is a defect of the posterior neural arch extrusion of the meninges or spinal cord. Approximately 10% to 15% of the population may have spina bifida occulta, most commonly in the fourth and fifth lumbar and first sacral vertebrae. Although this is usually a benign, incidental diagnosis, spina bifida occulta can rarely be associated with intraspinal lesions (like tethered cord and diastematomyelia) and progressive neurologic symptoms. However, an isolated radiographic finding in the absence of neurologic abnormality should not be an indication for referral to spina bifida specialists.

Meningocele refers to a defect in the posterior vertebral elements associated with a cyst of the meninges or tissue layers surrounding the cord. The underlying cord and nerve roots remain restricted to the spinal canal and are not involved in the cyst. Hydrocephalus is uncommon, and although there may be associated intraspinal lesions, the typical patient is neurologically normal. Treatment is excision of the cyst with repair of the defect.

Myelomeningocele is the most common variant of spina bifida cystica, representing approximately 90% of all cases. In this condition, the spinal cord, spinal nerve roots, or both protrude with the meninges outside the spinal canal through a defect in the posterior vertebral arch (Fig. 14-1). Neurologic deficits are present, and there is a strong association with hydrocephalus, Arnold-Chiari type II malformation (Fig. 14-2), and tethered cord (Fig. 14-3).

In *myelocele*, also called *rachischisis* or *myeloschisis*, the neural tube fails to tubularize, and the unfused neural plate is exposed with no overlying tissue cover. This rare defect is the most severe and debilitating form of spina bifida cystica.

Like meningocele and spina bifida occulta, *lipomyelomeningocele* is a skin-covered deformity with a subcutaneous lipoma connected by a fibro-fatty stalk to an intraspinal lipoma (see Fig. 14-3). These deformities typically occur in the lumbar or sacral spine. They are commonly associated with cord tethering and neurologic symptoms, including motor and sensory deficits and bladder continence problems. Other associated abnormalities are diastematomyelia (Fig. 14-4), dermoid sinus or dimple, and dermoid cyst.

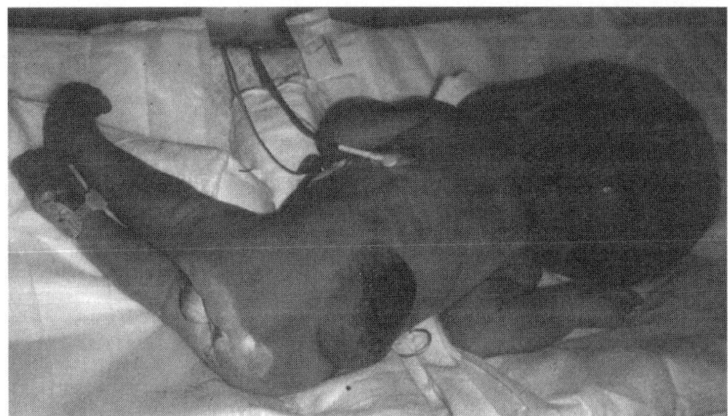

Figure 14-1 Newborn with as yet unrepaired myelomeningocele. Note the clubfeet and the extensile posturing of the knees.

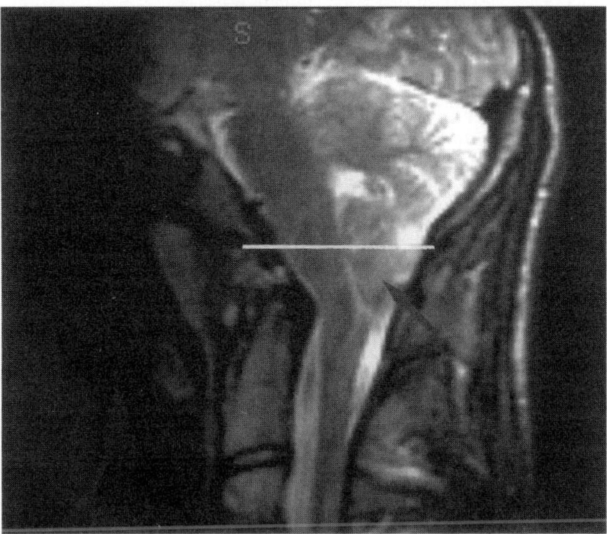

Figure 14-2 In Arnold-Chiari malformation type I, the cerebellar tonsils herniate *(arrow)* below the foramen magnum *(white line)*. In type II lesions, the cerebellar vermis herniates as well, often resulting in disruption of cerebrospinal flow and hydrocephalus.

ASSOCIATED ANOMALIES AND THEIR TREATMENT

In addition to the neuromuscular deficits present at birth, other anomalies may arise and can lead to progressive deformity and disability.

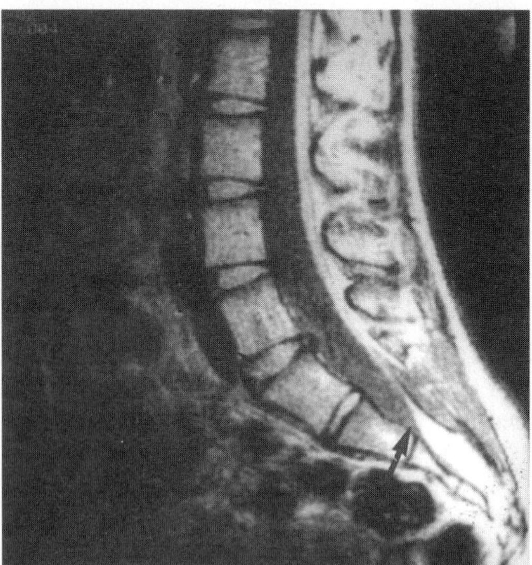

Figure 14-3 Tethered spinal cord. Normally the spinal cord terminates at the L1-L2 level at the conus. In this magnetic resonance image, the conus *(black arrow)* can be seen in the midsacral region, a clear indication of tethering. Magnetic resonance imaging may show evidence of a tether in most children with myelomeningocele, but unless they demonstrate neurologic deterioration, surgical release is usually not indicated. Note that this child also has a fatty lesion near the end of the cord, a lipomeningocele.

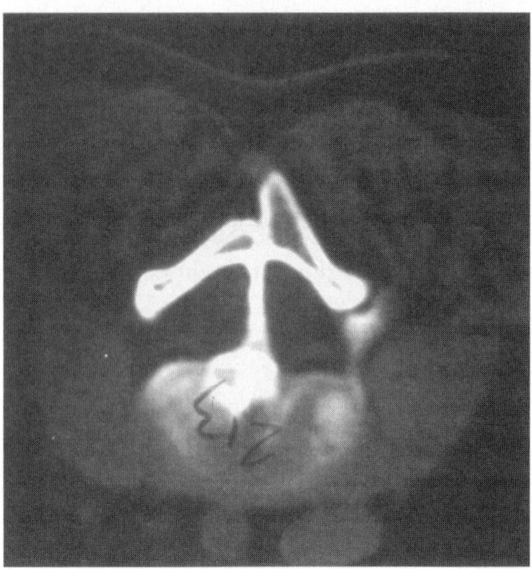

Figure 14-4 An axial computed tomography scan demonstrating a bony septum through the middle of the spinal canal, a condition known as diastematomyelia.

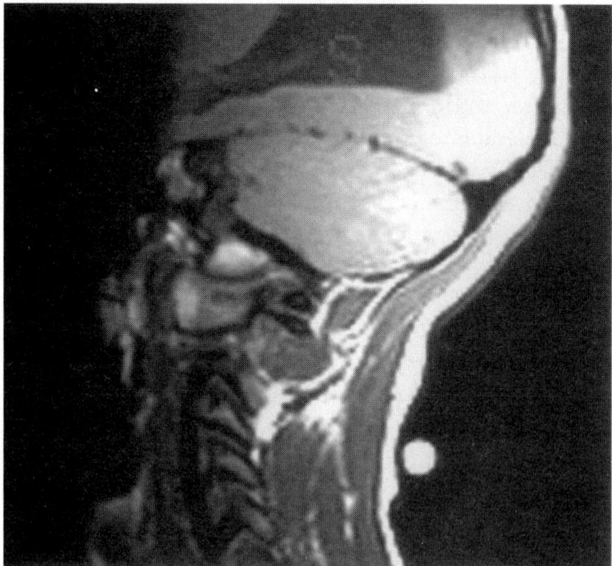

Figure 14-5 Hydrocephalus, or abnormally large cerebral ventricles typically caused by abnormalities in cerebrospinal fluid flow, is commonly seen in children with myelomeningocele. In this magnetic resonance image, the dilated fourth ventricle can be seen as the large, dark structure in the brain.

The accumulation of cerebrospinal fluid (CSF) in the skull with dilation of the cerebral ventricles is known as *hydrocephalus* (Fig. 14-5). This disorder occurs in about 80% of patients with spina bifida cystica and is more common in higher lesions than in lower lesions.[20] If progressive, hydrocephalus can cause neurologic deterioration. Lorber[14] showed that 80% of patients with myelomeningocele had IQs greater than 80, whereas only 50% of those with hydrocephalus did so. Hydrocephalus is usually the result of deranged CSF flow, and in the case of spina bifida, this is commonly the result of an Arnold-Chiari type II malformation (see later).

Most children with myelomeningocele have some element of hydrocephalus that requires decompression in the first few weeks of life, usually in the form of a ventriculoperitoneal (VP) shunt placed by a neurosurgeon. Hydrocephalus that progresses later in life is usually secondary to occlusion of a VP shunt, although occasionally the disorder may arise de novo late in children who do not have a VP shunt and have not experienced problems with CSF flow previously. Nausea, vomiting, and headache classically herald shunt occlusion. Hydrosyringomyelia may result from uncontrolled hydrocephalus, leading to growing paralysis of the lower extremities, spasticity, back pain, scoliosis, and involvement of the upper extremities.

Hydromyelia is an abnormal collection of CSF within the spinal cord itself (Fig. 14-6). The collections can vary greatly in size and amount of dilation. The hydromyelic cavity, or *syrinx*, classically causes lower motor neuron findings in the upper extremities and spasticity in the lower extremities. There can be a variable sensory loss as well. Although common in children with spina bifida, hydromyelia can occur in individuals without vertebral lesions. Treatment in symptomatic patients involves neurosurgical decompression.

Arnold-Chiari malformations occur when the cerebellum herniates through the foramen magnum into the

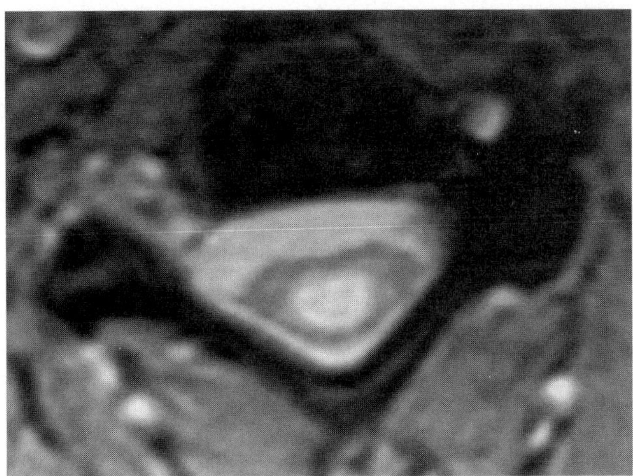

Figure 14-6 Syrinx, or hydromyelia, is an abnormal collection of cerebrospinal fluid within the spinal cord itself. Pressure from this fluid can damage the spinal cord, leading to deterioration of neurologic function.

spinal canal. An Arnold-Chiari type I lesion (see Fig. 14-2) occurs when the cerebellar tonsils herniate, and there are usually no problems with the fourth ventricle or with CSF flow. The much rarer Arnold-Chiari type II lesion is often found in conjunction with spina bifida cystica; it involves a herniation of the cerebellar vermis into the spinal canal. The type II lesion, thought to be caused by in utero loss of CSF through the defect in the meninges, can cause late neurologic deterioration. In essence, the spinal cord and hind brain above it are sucked down as the fluid flows out. This theory is borne out by the observation of spontaneous reduction of Arnold-Chiari malformations when myelomeningoceles are repaired with fetal surgery. In patients in whom the Arnold-Chiari malformation is thought to be causing neurologic deterioration, treatment usually consists of decompression of the foramen magnum. This procedure is usually performed by neurosurgeons, although a concurrent upper cervical fusion is sometimes required by their orthopaedic colleagues.

Tethering of the spinal cord occurs when a fibrous band connects the spinal cord to the bony sacrum, preventing proximal migration of the spinal cord with longitudinal growth of the spinal column (see Fig. 14-2). In children with myelomeningocele, this tethering most commonly occurs at the level of the surgical repair and is likely a consequence of scarring from the procedure. Tethering may also occur via a thickened filum terminale, the usually thin fibrous tissue that connects the conus medullaris to the sacrum and coccyx. Tethering can result in a slow neurologic deterioration, a condition known as *tethered cord syndrome*. However, not all children with myelomeningocele and spinal cord tethering have neurologic sequelae. In fact, nearly 100% of children with myelomeningocele have what appears to be tethering on magnetic resonance imaging (MRI), but because only a portion have neurologic deterioration from tethering, routine surgical untethering is not recommended. Only children with neurologic problems should undergo surgical release of the spinal cord.

Diastematomyelia is a split in the spinal cord, often with a bony or cartilaginous septum (see Fig. 14-4). It should be differentiated from *diplomyelia*, which, as the name implies, is a true duplication of the spinal cord. Treatment consists of resection of the septum by neurosurgery.

A rare condition usually associated with maternal diabetes, *sacral agenesis* consists of failure of development of part or all of the sacrum, including the ventral spinal cord responsible for the motor nerves. The dorsal columns do develop with variable deformity and loss of sensation. *Caudal regression syndrome*, also associated with maternal diabetes, is a more severe condition involving hypoplasia of the lower extremities and associated cardiac malformations, including transposition of the great vessels.

NEUROSURGICAL INTERVENTION

Neurosurgeons are intimately involved in the care of children with spina bifida from the first day of life, and sometimes even earlier (see later). They close the initial defect, usually within the first 2 days of life. Spina bifida is treated as an urgent, not emergency, problem, and infants are no longer whisked from the delivery room to the operating room as in years past. As already stated, neurosurgeons are also instrumental in caring for many of the associated problems discussed previously, including hydrocephalus, hydromyelia, Arnold-Chiari malformation, and tethered cord.

Prenatal Surgery

In 1984, reports of two animal models of myelomeningocele treated with fetal surgery appeared, one from Germany[21] and the other from Italy.[22] In 1996, neurosurgeons at the University of California, San Francisco, documented improved neurologic function after in utero repair of myelomeningocele in their sheep model.[23] The first human studies were reported in 1998.[24] Currently, a multicenter trial funded by the National Institutes of Health is being conducted to determine the safety and efficacy of such surgery. Results so far suggest that there may be an improvement of one or two neurological levels and a significant decrease in the number of Arnold-Chiari malformations and cases of hydrocephalus.[25]

NONNEUROLOGIC ISSUES

Latex Allergy

In the early 1990s, the significance of latex allergies in children with spina bifida came to light. Upwards of 40% of children with spina bifida have serum antibodies to latex, and although many fewer actually have a clinical allergy, fatal reactions have been reported. The allergy, an immunoglobulin E-mediated response,[26] probably develops because of repeated early exposures to latex, especially in the first year of life.[27] With greater awareness of these facts, most institutions undertake latex allergy precautions in all patients with spina bifida. This practice has been demonstrated to dramatically decrease the prevalence of latex sensitivity.[28]

Malignant Hyperthermia

In addition to latex allergies, an association has been reported between malignant hyperthermia and myelomeningocele.[29] Although not been many more cases have been reported since the initial description, this association is something that must be kept in mind every time a child with spina bifida goes to the operating room, because of the potentially devastating consequences of malignant hyperthermia.

Skin Breakdown

Pressure sores and frank ulcers are important issues in any population with sensory deficits, and children with myelomeningocele can have major skin problems. Pressure sores develop in as many as 60% of such children, typically on the feet and over the sacrum, the ischial tuberosities, and the greater trochanter. These lesions can be very difficult to manage, especially if they are infected.

Pressure sores and ulcers are caused by unchecked pressure, usually over a bony prominence or prominent hardware. The pressure may be caused by normal sitting or positioning or by an external brace, orthosis, or cast. Because of their deficient sensation and absence of motor power, children with myelomeningocele are unable to protect their skin. They do not feel ischemic pain, and they are unable to shift regularly the way neurologically intact people do without even thinking about it.

Aside from the obvious neurologic problems, children with myelomeningocele have other issues that contribute to the development and perpetuation of pressure sores and ulcers. The postural and positional problems that develop, including kyphosis, hip dysplasia and dislocation, and joint contractures, all lead to abnormally prominent bones. The bony prominences can tent the skin, placing it at high risk for breakdown. Also, many children have multiple scars from their many operations. The scars can be problematic with respect to initial healing and late breakdown. Finally, for children with fecal incontinence, urinary incontinence, or both, soiling of ulcers in the pelvic region can be a serious problem. When it occurs and infection cannot be controlled, temporary diverting ostomies of the bowel or genitourinary tract provide a means to keep the ulcers clean until they heal.

As with many problems in pediatrics, the proverbial ounce of prevention is worth the well-known pound of cure. The supervising medical staff, family members, and the children themselves must all keep constant vigil about potential areas of pressure. Position must be changed regularly frequently, and proper fitting and padding of all orthoses is a must. When early signs of skin breakdown become apparent, local wound care, possibly including wet to dry dressings, must be instituted. Additionally, the affected area must be relieved of all pressure until healing is complete. This requirement can be a major inconvenience, especially if the sore is in the ischial or sacral area, for which seating must be avoided. However, failure to comply with such a regimen can lead to extension of the ulcer and necessitate operative intervention.

Treatment of established pressure sores has already been touched on. Conservative treatment must precede surgical closure to obtain a clean and relatively sterile bed over which to close or graft skin. Ulcers require frequent dressing changes and débridements. Any cavities should be packed with a moist dressing to eliminate empty space and to gently débride the deep portions of the wound. Ideally, this packing should be changed at least four times a day. Once the bed of the ulcer consists of healthy granulation tissue and quantitative wound cultures show an acceptably low level of bacterial colonization, surgery can proceed.

The obvious goal of surgery is to cover the sore, either with skin around the defect or with skin grafted from a distant site. Plastic surgeons are often involved in this aspect of care. If there is bone or tendon in the ulcer bed, or if the wound is very large, a myocutaneous graft with a vascular pedicle may be required. However, in addition to achieving coverage, the surgeon must evaluate the underlying cause of the ulcer and determine whether anything can be done to prevent recurrence. For example, when skin breakdown occurs over a severe kyphotic deformity, the kyphosis should be corrected or resected to relieve pressure in this area. This type of surgery often must be staged to be successful. A less obvious example is the child with an ulcer over the greater trochanter because of spinopelvic obliquity. Such a child sits on the lateral aspect of the hip because of a scoliotic deformity of the spine. Instead of resection of the offending trochanter to remove the source of pressure, a more elegant solution may be to correct the scoliosis, eliminating the spinopelvic obliquity and thus allowing the child to sit properly. Similarly, it is preferable to correct a deformity that is causing an ulcer than to merely cover the ulcer, because the ulcer is likely to recur if its cause is not removed.

SPECIFIC ORTHOPAEDIC CONCERNS

Upper Extremity Dysfunction

Problems with dexterity of the arms are very common in children with spina bifida.[30] These problems are most likely secondary to hydrocephalus, and children with more shunt problems have been shown to have worse hand function.[31] If upper extremity function appears to be deteriorating, a shunt blockage should be considered. An ascending syrinx is another possible cause. Problems with upper extremity function are typically handled by the occupational therapist.[32]

Lower Extremity Deformity

The following section outlines the basic deformities of the joints of the lower extremities in terms of etiology and treatment. The guiding principle for treatment of these deformities is to create a limb, via therapy or surgery, that can be placed in a functional position and held there with a brace (orthosis). The brace will supplement the dysfunctional muscles to maintain the proper position of the limb to facilitate mobility and activities of daily living.

Foot and Ankle

Interestingly, the development of foot and ankle deformities found in patients with spina bifida have little relation to neurologic level or spontaneous motor activity. Broughton and colleagues[33] showed no correlation between neurologic level (excluding sacral level lesions) and the incidence or morphology of foot and ankle deformities. In fact, they found that nearly 90% of patients with thoracic and high lumbar lesions had foot deformities even though they had no voluntary motor activity in their feet. Deformity present at birth, if symmetric, may be due to intrauterine positioning. In patients in whom deformity develops in childhood, reflex spasticity may play an etiologic role, although spasticity was present in only one out of four patients with deformity and in none of the patients with no deformity.[33]

Equinus and equinovarus deformities are among the most common foot deformities in spina bifida. The typical equinovarus (clubfoot) deformity present at birth is quite rigid and recalcitrant to conservative treatment (Fig. 14-7). Serial casting is still the first treatment to correct deformity. Surgery is almost always required and involves complete release of all involved joint capsules and deforming muscles. The tendons are tenotomized or excised. Lengthening is usually followed by recurrence of deformity because the underlying deficit persists. Tendon transfer usually fails because the transferred tendon is out of phase, is weak owing to the spina bifida, and loses a grade of strength in transfer. Postoperative splinting with orthotics is helpful in maintaining correction (Fig. 14-8), but recurrences and reoperation are common.

Talipes calcaneus, an abnormal dorsiflexion of the foot (as opposed to equinus) commonly associated with ankle valgus, is another common abnormality in this population. A spastic or unopposed tibialis anterior muscle is typically responsible for this problem (note that the tibialis anterior is the only functional tendon crossing the ankle in child with spina bifida at the L4 functional level). Treatment varies with the rigidity of the deformity. Flexible deformities may respond to stretching or casting to obtain a plantigrade foot that can be held with a brace. However, bracing the feet in a child with talipes calcaneus is notoriously difficult, and surgery to release the anterior ankle capsule and ligaments is often required. Some investigators have reported success with tibialis anterior transfers,[34,35] although others have found that the transferred muscle does not fire in phase to assist with ambulation, and bracing needs are not typically changed.[36]

Talipes calcaneus can also be associated with the so-called vertical talus (Fig. 14-9). This condition is typified by a dorsiflexed, everted midfoot on a fixed plantarflexed (vertical) talus.[37] Treatment consists of soft tissue releases combined with tendon transfers, fusion, or navicular excision.

Ankle valgus can also occur independently from a talipes calcaneus. The valgus can be either isolated or associated with a flat foot (planovalgus deformity) (Fig. 14-10). If the deformity is flexible, bracing should be used to hold the foot in a corrected position. The presence of fixed valgus becomes clinically important in the ambulatory child or the child in whom medially based ulcers develops as a result of the abnormal posture of the foot. In these cases, surgical treatment is usually required. Valgus in the subtalar joint can be treated with calcaneal osteotomy or, occasionally, fusion. Valgus in the ankle joint, associated with a wedge-shaped distal tibial epiphysis, can be treated in the skeletally immature by arresting the growth of the medial tibial physis (epiphysiodesis) either by stapling or insertion of a medial malleolar screw. Realignment of the ankle can also be accomplished by an osteotomy of the distal tibia (supramalleolar). Ankle (tibiotalar) fusions have a miserable track record in children with spina bifida and are to be avoided.[38]

Rotational deformities of the tibia can hinder ambulation. Infants and young children tend to have internal

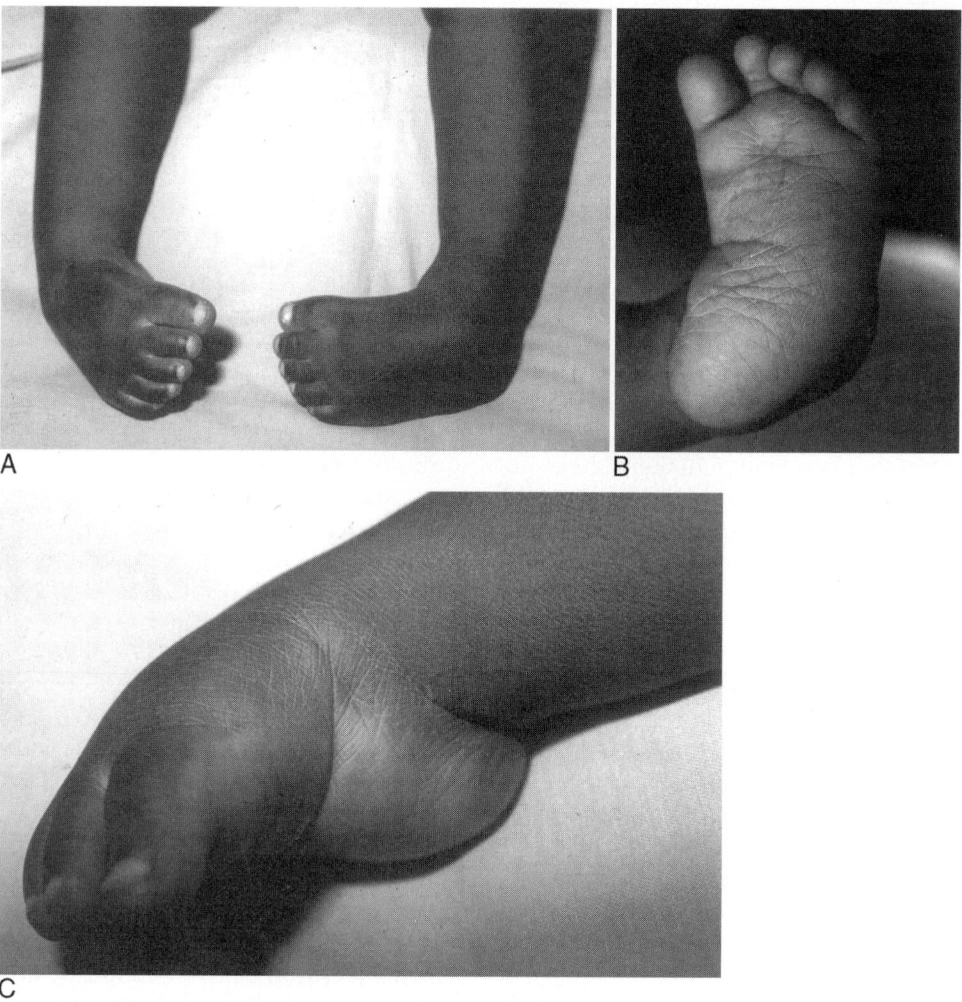

Figure 14-7 The clubfoot deformity is commonly seen in children with myelomeningocele. This deformity is defined by a fixed, rigid equinus and varus of the ankle, associated with forefoot adductus and commonly cavus. **A,** Severe ankle varus. **B,** Forefoot adductus with a medial foot crease. **C,** Medial view showing equinus and deep creases in both the midfoot and heel.

tibial torsion, possibly the result of an imbalance between the medial and lateral hamstrings. In the ambulatory child, this torsion can lead to difficulty in walking and so needs surgical intervention. External tibial torsion usually occurs after the age of 6 years and is commonly associated with a planovalgus foot. As for the valgus ankle, treatment initially consists of orthotics management. When this modality fails, a derotational osteotomy (plus appropriate management of ankle valgus) achieves the necessary correction.[39]

Knee

Although the knee requires less surgery and clinical attention than the hip and foot in children with spinal bifida, the knee can be a significant source of morbidity. Valgus deformity and flexion and extension contractures are the most common deformities seen. Clinically significant knee arthropathy has been demonstrated in ambulatory young adults with spina bifida and is probably secondary to abnormal walking mechanics.[40] Emphasizing the need for forearm crutches to reduce the impact on the knees is important to prevention of this problem.[41]

Knee valgus deformity is unusual and rarely requires orthopaedic intervention. Severe valgus may be seen in cases of renal osteodystrophy, but children with this disorder tend to be quite ill and so not to be candidates for surgery.[42] Rarely, contracture of the iliotibial band is associated with distal femoral valgus deformity, which may progress in spite of release.

Knee flexion contractures are more common, especially in patients with spina bifida at a thoracic or high lumbar level. Deformity greater than 10 degrees can be treated with well-padded serial casts, whereas deformity greater than 30 degrees may require posterior release fol-

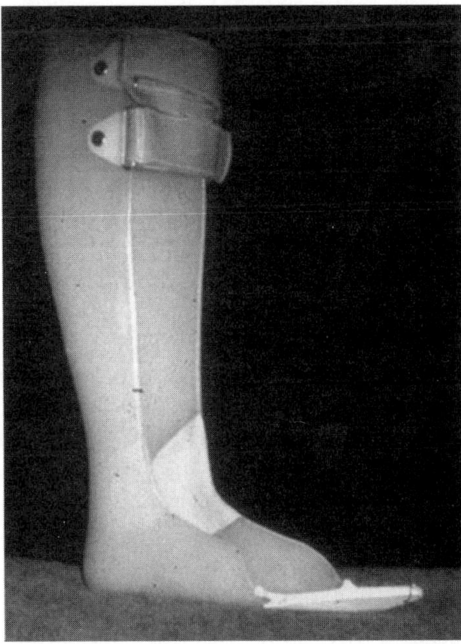

Figure 14-8 This solid ankle-foot orthosis helps control ankle equinus and, with the raised sides, can also help control ankle varus and valgus. Some models have hinged ankles, and most have straps crossing ankle and foot to hold the foot down.

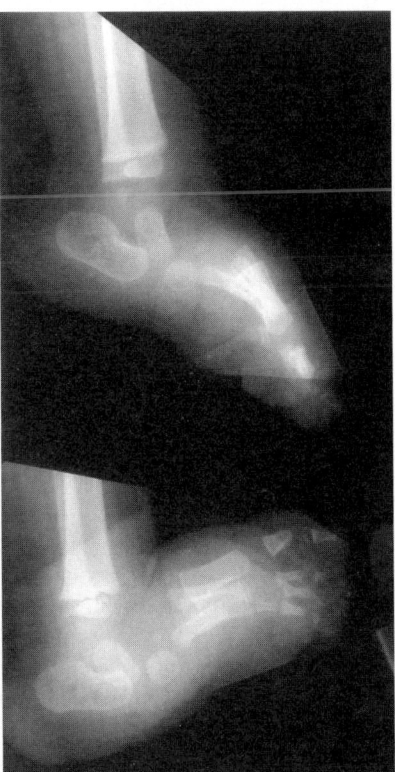

Figure 14-9 Vertical or oblique talus, shown in this radiograph, can be confused with clubfoot. The diagnostic *sine qua non* is the persistence of a plantar-flexed talus relative to the calcaneus when the foot is brought into dorsiflexion.

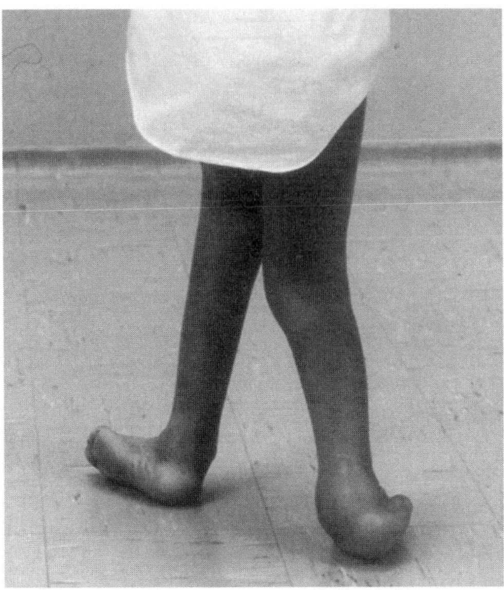

Figure 14-10 Flatfoot (planovalgus foot) is a deformity that can almost be thought of as the opposite of clubfoot. It is characterized by a flat arch and valgus heel. Surgery may be required to correct a planovalgus foot that cannot be passively brought into a neutral position.

lowed by serial casting to attain hyperextension of the knee. Acute hyperextension is usually not possible because of problems with wound closure, shortness of the neurovascular structures. Treatment is not required in patients who are nonambulatory unless the contracture is interfering with standing, sitting, or transfers.[42]

Fixed knee extension is seen to occur in patients with both an active and inactive quadriceps muscles. In infancy, serial casting can be helpful to obtain 90 degrees of flexion.[42] Later in life, ambulatory patients with recurvatum typically do not need treatment, although patients without clinically significant leg power can benefit from a release of the patellar tendon to improve seating.[43]

Hip

Problems about the hip joint, ranging from joint contractures to subluxation to dislocation, are very common in spina bifida (Fig. 14-11). The presence of hip deformity and dislocation is related to the neurologic level of the disorder but not to muscle imbalance, a point stressed by Menelaus.[48] For example, muscle imbalance across the hip is greatest in children with an L4 level lesion, yet these children have a lower rate of dislocation and a lower magnitude of flexion contracture than children with a thoracic level lesion and no power across the hips.[44] For this reason, Menelaus[44] warns against prophylactic surgery to correct muscle imbalance, because it will not necessarily prevent hip dislocation. The approach to treatment of hip disorders in this population should be founded on maximizing a patient's

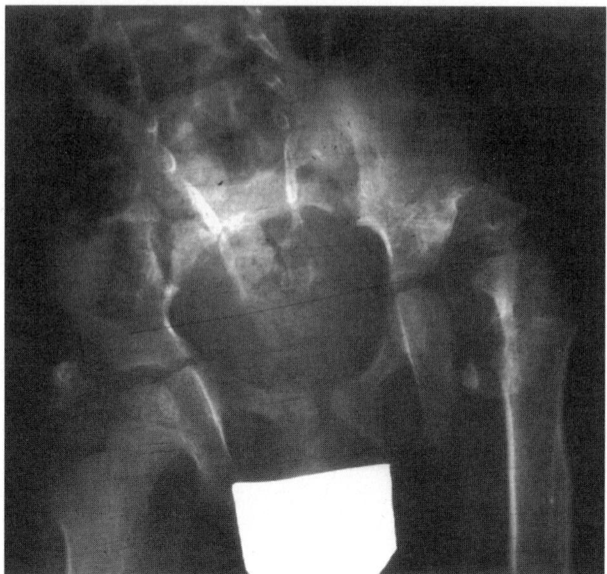

Figure 14-11 This radiograph demonstrates a high left hip dislocation with the formation of a pseudoacetabulum, or a new hip joint, on the iliac wing. Such unilateral dislocations lead to pelvic obliquity, which can create seating problems and pressure sores.

function through consideration of current and predicted ambulatory status.

Children with thoracic and high lumbar lesions have fixed flexion contractures and a relatively high rate of hip subluxation and dislocation. Although many of these patients are able to walk with extensive bracing and therapy, they can rarely do so after the age of 10. Nevertheless, some investigators believe that the psychological benefits of walking even temporarily can make the effort worthwhile.[45] Soft tissue releases can be beneficial to reduce hip flexion contractures and facilitate bracing and ambulation, but because the patients become wheelchair dependent at an early age, aggressive osteotomies are generally not recommended, and dislocated hips can generally be left unreduced. One indication for aggressive treatment of hip dislocation in this group is to treat skin ulcers that result from the hip deformity. There may be a theoretical benefit to standing and walking at a young age, in building denser bones and reducing the risk of fractures due to osteopenia in later life.

Lesions located at the L3 or L4 level are more difficult. The literature is littered with studies showing alternatively that hip dislocation or dysplasia does and does not affect ambulatory ability. For example, Lee and Carroll[46] reported twice as many community ambulators in children with stable hips, but Bazih and Gross[47] showed no difference in rates of walking between children with stable and unstable hips. Comparing such studies is challenging because often the neurologic level is not "pure" and can deteriorate with time. Some researchers recommend observing the hips of all children with spina bifida until the age of 3 or 4, years when the neurologic level can be more reliably ascertained.[48] Others support surgical treatment of hip subluxation in children with a functional quadriceps mechanism and a stable neurologic level early in life (18 to 36 months).[49] This latter philosophy requires close monitoring of a child's hips to identify hip subluxation before it deteriorates.

Treating hip problems that develop in first year of life is particularly challenging in children with meningomyelocele. Traditional bracing and surgical treatments are reported to have failure rates of 50%.[49,50]

In general, in the ambulatory patient with a unilateral dislocation and lesion at a low (L3 or lower) neurologic level, reduction is recommended to facilitate walking. This is accomplished by improving the pelvic obliquity and leg length discrepancy created by the hip dislocation. Also, hip instability has been shown to be significantly associated with scoliosis, although interestingly, there is no correlation between the side of instability and the direction of the curve.[51] Routine reduction of bilateral dislocations is not indicated. Menelaus recommends reduction only if surgery is required to release a flexion contracture.[48]

Severe flexion contractures or hip dislocation are rare in the child with lumbosacral lesion and should be treated aggressively. These children have strong legs and are typically community ambulators, so every effort should be made to preserve their function.

Spine

Not surprisingly, children with spinal dysraphism have a high incidence of scoliosis and kyphosis. The incidence has been reported to be as high as 90%,[52] but two excellent later studies put the number closer to 50%.[51,53] Although the majority of these curves are paralytic and occur in childhood, as many as 15% are congenital, resulting from abnormal development of vertebrae in utero.[52]

Scoliosis

The review by Trivedi and colleauges[51] has provided useful definitions and information on the incidence and prevalence of scoliosis in children with myelomeningocele. These investigators defined *scoliosis* in this population as any curve with a Cobb angle greater than 20 degrees, because smaller curves typically improved. In their series, 42% of all curves developed in children older than 9 years, some manifesting in children as old as 15 years. Many previous studies did not include adolescents and defined scoliosis with smaller Cobb angles. In children with a thoracic neurologic level or a last intact laminar arch (LILA) at the thoracic level, incidence of scoliosis is 90%, and in those with an LILA below L4, the incidence is closer to 10%. Additionally, incidence of scoliosis in community ambulators is about half that in nonambulators.

Scoliosis can affect sitting balance and lead to pressure sores and pulmonary compromise (Fig. 14-12). Balance problems can force a child to stabilize the body with the hands, which can then not be used for other tasks. Scoliosis can create pelvic obliquity that can lead to pressure sores, typically over the ischial tuberosity. In severe cases, deformity of the thorax can lead to a restrictive pulmonary insufficiency that could improve with surgery.[54,55]

Curves with a Cobb angle of less than 20 degrees can generally be observed, but progressive curves require treatment. Although brace treatment has been shown to be moderately effective with relatively few complications,[56] most surgeons shy away from conservative treatment of scoliosis.[57] Paralytic curves are notoriously resistant to brace therapy, and children with spina bifida can experience skin problems as a result of curves, including ulcers, which are challenging to heal. Therefore, in patients with documented progression of scoliosis, surgery is usually needed to balance the spine and prevent further progression.

Unfortunately, the complication rate of surgery is quite high. Banit and colleagues,[58] publishing their experience in 50 surgical cases, reported a complication rate of 48% with an average of nearly 1.5 procedures per patient. Rates of complications related to hardware, including loosening and pseudarthrosis, range from 15%[58,59] to 30%.[60,61] Deep wound infections are of particular concern, and achieving wound healing is enormously challenging in many cases (Fig. 14-13). An infection rate as high as 33%[62] has been described, although later studies have cited a rate closer to 8%.[58,63] Although lower, the rate is still an order of magnitude greater than the wound infection rate seen in children undergoing surgery for idiopathic scoliosis. The frequency of wound problems, which include superficial infection and wound breakdown, has lead many surgeons to recruit plastic surgeons to assist with mobilizing local flaps for the closure in children with spina bifida.

As previously mentioned, about 15% of children with myelomeningocele also have congenital abnormalities of the vertebrae separate from the posterior element defects.[52] The defect is one of formation, whereby the vertebra is incompletely developed and often wedge shaped, or one of segmentation, in which a bony bridge connects two or more consecutive vertebrae. Certain patterns of these deformities predictably lead to scoliosis and often require surgery for correction. However, it is important to realize that in these children, several factors may be in effect simultaneously, all of which must be explored before a course of treatment is chosen. Although a progressive curve must be arrested, it is essential to protect intact spinal levels to avoid worsening these patients' neurologic and functional status.[57]

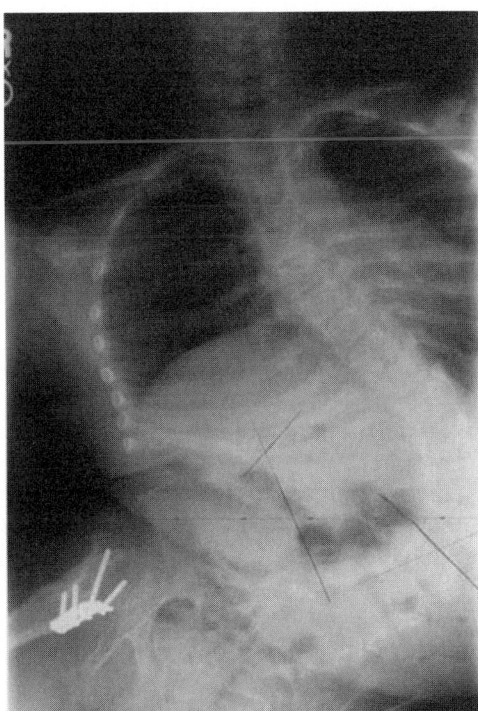

Figure 14-12 This seated anteroposterior spine radiograph shows a severe, 110-degree scoliosis in a girl with myelomeningocele. Note the severe pelvic obliquity and the hardware in the right hip from previous surgery for a dislocated hip.

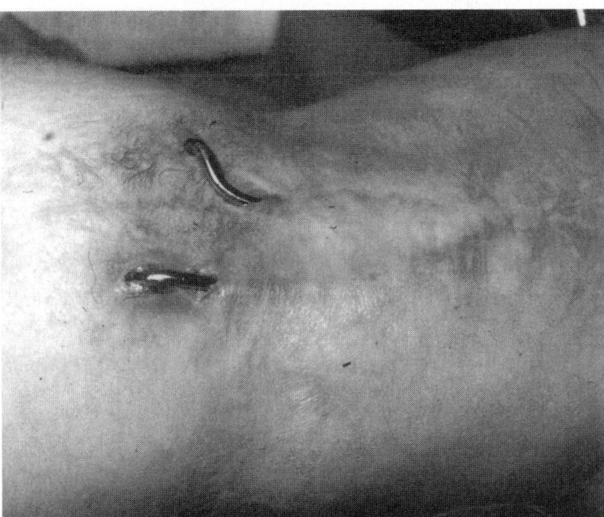

Figure 14-13 In this unfortunate girl patient who underwent spinal fusion for severe scoliosis, skin breakdown occurred over the surgical hardware. Obtaining adequate skin coverage for surgical procedures in children with myelomeningocele can be a major challenge, especially in the spine.

Finally, some cases of scoliosis are thought to result from syringomyelia, which is not uncommon in children with VP shunts and disturbances of CSF flow. The finding of a rapidly progressive curve or a curve that coincides with neurologic deterioration should raise the specter of syringomyelia, and magnetic resonance imaging should be considered.[64] In some cases, decompression of the syrinx has stabilized or improved the scoliosis.[65]

Kyphosis

In children with meningomyelocele, kyphosis has both congenital and paralytic causes. For example, Shurtleff and coworkers[66] reported that although 1 in 10 children with a thoracic lesion had kyphosis at birth, 1 in 3 demonstrated kyphosis by adolescence. The natural history of paralytic kyphosis is one of constant progression, making it difficult to treat. Gentle C-shaped curves tend to progress by about 3 degrees per year, whereas short, sharp curves are more malignant, progressing by 8 degrees per year (Fig. 14-14). This deformity is resistant to bracing for several reasons. Braces not only fail to control the deformity but also can actually cause problems on their own, own including skin ulceration and compression of the thoracic cage and abdominal wall.

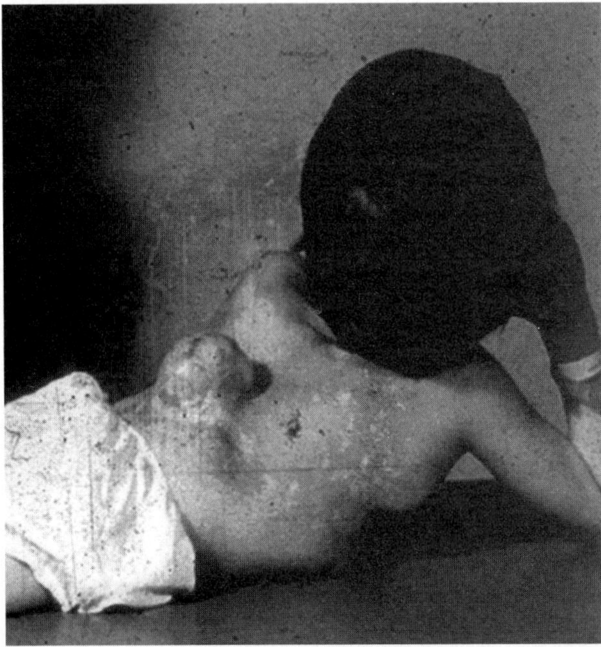

Figure 14-14 This older photograph shows a young boy with a severe, short kyphos that measured approximately 180 degrees on radiographs. Such lesions require surgical treatment, which often consists of excision of the vertebral bodies involved in the kyphos. The deformity acts as a pressure point, and persistent skin breakdown and osteomyelitis would occur without treatment. Seating is impossible with this level of deformity.

Untreated kyphosis leads to loss of truncal height, difficulty with sitting, and, in advanced cases, skin ulceration over the kyphos posteriorly and impingement of the ribs on the iliac crest. Increased abdominal pressure can cause respiratory compromise from loss of diaphragmatic breathing, and loss of access to the anterior abdominal wall can lead to problems caring for or creating urinary diversions or stomas.[67] The principal indication for surgery is to treat recurrent ulceration over the kyphos; however, the associated benefits are tremendous. In addition to improving the complications already mentioned, better truncal balance improves the child's ability to interact with the environment by freeing the arms, improving brace fitting, and enhancing seating. Unfortunately, there is a high complication rate; complications include infection, recurrence of deformity, hardware failure, and even sudden death,[68,69] making the decision to undertake surgery a very serious one.

Ambulation and Orthoses

As mentioned previously, orthotics are used to improve function. They are designed to replace muscles that are not working sufficiently to achieve this goal. However, it is important to remember that cannot actually correct a deformity. They are static devices capable of holding a limb or joint in a specific position, but each device must be shaped to the extremity, because a stiff limb will not contour to an orthotic. For example, a child with myelomeningocele and a severe equinus contracture must undergo posterior release of the ankle before a brace can be used to both hold the foot in a functional neutral position and help prevent the deformity from recurring.

Most orthotics are applied to the lower extremities, and they are often used to facilitate gait. Therefore, one must have a working knowledge of normal gait to understand how different braces help children with spina bifida. A simplified summary of one gait cycle, commonly called a stride, follows.

The two main phases of the gait cycle are stance and swing, each of which can be broken up into several components. The *stance phase* describes any time a foot is on the ground and the *swing phase*, any time a foot is off the ground. By convention, the gait cycle begins with stance phase, which is initiated by *heel strike*. In this phase, the ankle dorsiflexors (tibialis anterior muscle) are firing to hold the toes up to keep them from catching on the ground. After heel strike, the limb begins to accept the weight of the body during *loading response*, as the ankle slowly plantar-flexes to meet the ground. Next is *midstance*, in which the center of gravity of the body is directly over the ankle and the foot is flat on the ground. Stance is completed by *terminal stance* as the ankle progressively dorsiflexes again to tension the plantar flexors in preparation for *toe off*, which requires plantar-flexion of the ankle to propel the body forward.

The swing phase consists of *initial swing*, *midswing*, and *terminal swing*. Initial swing requires hip flexion, knee flexion, and ankle dorsiflexion to allow the foot to clear the ground as it is swung forward. During midswing and terminal swing the knee is extended as the foot is placed forward, and the swing phase ends once the heel contacts the ground, to begin yet another cycle.

Obviously, this basic mode of locomotion, repeated thousands of times a day by most normal children from the age of 1 year, requires tremendous coordination of several major muscle groups, and problems in any one area will lead to a disturbance in gait that may manifest as a limp, a fall, or an inability to walk at all. Orthotics help replace muscles that are not functioning normally and thus improve, if not normalize, gait. A detailed description of every type of orthotic is beyond the scope of this discussion. Nevertheless, a review of the basic types of orthoses is important for anyone involved in the care of children with myelomeningocele.

The ankle-foot orthosis is one of the most commonly used braces in orthopaedics (see Fig. 14-8). There are many different types, but all AFOs essentially hold the foot in a neutral position. In accomplishing this goal. The AFO restricts motion at both the ankle joint and the subtalar joint. However, an AFO helps the child with a weak tibialis anterior muscle child clear the foot during the swing phase of gait, so the child does not trip or have to compensate for a foot that does not dorsiflex. An AFO can also help children with weakness or absence of ankle plantar flexors by preventing the ankle from excessive dorsiflexion during the stance phase of gait, which could result in a crouch gait pattern.

Problems with the position of the subtalar joint, often from an imbalance between the tibialis posterior, tibialis anterior, and peroneal muscles, can be aided with a foot orthosis. The University of California Biomedics Laboratory (UCBL) shoe insert cups the heel and extends down to support the sole of the foot; this orthotic can help children with valgus ankles. Varus or valgus ankle can also be helped by placement of wedges in the shoe under half the ankle to make the foot roll into a more neutral position. For example, a heel in varus, if flexible, may be treated with a lateral heel wedge.

If the child has a neurologic level above L4 and certainly L3, the quadriceps muscle will be weak, and a knee-ankle-foot orthosis can be help compensate for inadequate knee extension (Fig. 14-15). As already described, the quadriceps muscle is very important; it helps extend the knee in swing phase and keeps the knee from bending and collapsing in midstance. The KAFO has a thigh cuff of variable design, a hinge at the level of the knee, and an anterior knee pad that provides posterior force on the knee to prevent unwanted flexion. Additionally, many devices are designed with a "drop-lock" at the knee hinge that will keep the brace, and hence the knee, from flexing

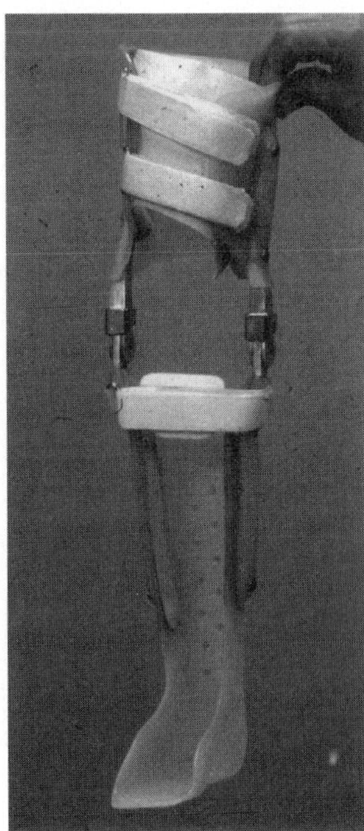

Figure 14-15 This knee-ankle-foot orthosis helps control both the knee and ankle joints. The knee hinges can be locked or unlocked, depending on the level of voluntary control of the knee.

The next stage of bracing is the hip-knee-ankle-foot orthosis (Fig. 14-16). Such orthotics serve several functions. For the child with a low lumbar lesion and severe internal torsion of the legs, the HKAFO can help position the legs properly for ambulation, specifically heel strike and weight acceptance. For the same patient, the HKAFO can facilitate ambulation in the absence of torsional problems if the patient has difficulty with quadriceps weakness and proper placement of the leg with each stride. Children with upper lumbar lesions (L3 and above) may also ambulate with an HKAFO, but more commonly, their weakness about the hip joint and their propensity for hip flexion contractures make the HKAFO less functional. In these children, the reciprocating-gait orthosis may be a better choice. The RGO has a mechanism that connects

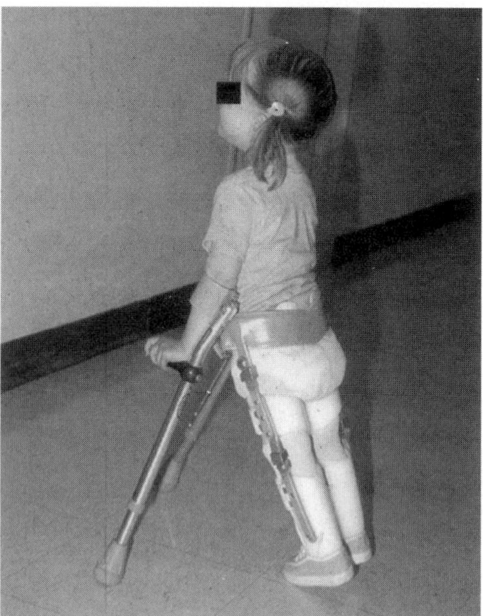

FIGURE 14-16 This hip-knee-ankle-foot orthosis helps control the entire lower extremity and can facilitate ambulation in children with high lumbar lesions.

the motion of the two legs so that one hip passively extends as the other is actively flexed (hence the term "reciprocal").

In a child in whom the neurologic level approaches the thoracic region, there is no volitional control of any of the muscles involved in ambulation, and the muscles of the thorax and upper extremity instead must be used to power gait if ambulation is to be achieved. The thoracic-hip-knee-ankle-foot orthosis (THKAFO) can be useful in this setting when combined with use of a walker or Lofstrand crutches. Other options for these children are the RGO or, for children in whom arm use is impaired, the swivel walker. The swivel walker converts side-to-side movements of the thorax into forward motion by means of swiveling bases.[17]

Pathologic Fractures

Wolff law states that bone forms in response to stress and, conversely, bone is resorbed when there is no stress. Therefore, the leg bones of paralyzed patients rapidly become thin and osteopenic when they are not loaded. The combination of sensory loss with osteopenic or outright osteoporotic bone is a setup for fracture in children with myelomeningocele. Barnett and Menelaus[70] report an overall incidence of about 20% for pathologic fractures, with a much higher incidence in children with thoracic lesions (69%), and no fractures in those with lesions at or below S2.

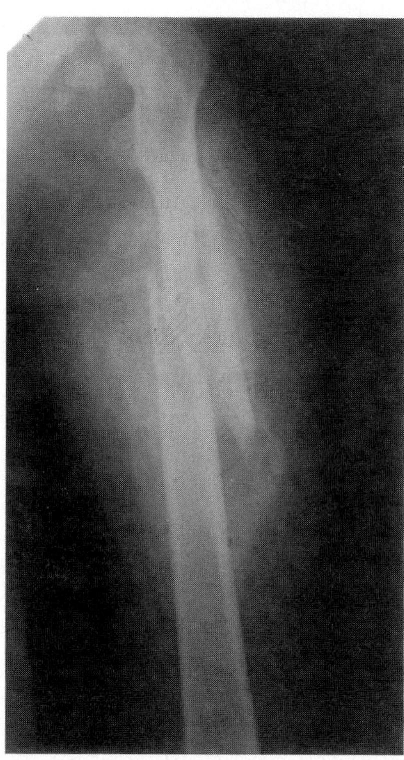

Figure 14-17 An anteroposterior radiograph of a left femur shows an old femur fracture with exuberant callus. Children with spina bifida have low bone density, especially those who do not walk, and are at risk for fracture. Such pathologic fractures, which can occur during transfers or physical therapy, often are unnoticed. The first sign may be redness and swelling over the fracture, which can be confused with infection. Keeping the possibility of pathologic fracture in mind and obtaining radiographs can prevent unnecessary delays in diagnosis.

The clinical presentation is similar to that of an infection, consisting of a swollen, red limb and, possibly, fever. Supracondylar femur fractures, the most common pathologic fracture in this population, often manifests a warm, red, swollen knee. The patient usually presents several days after the fracture, and there may be no history of trauma. Awareness of the frequency of pathologic fractures in children with spina bifida avoids unnecessary evaluation for infection. Treatment usually consists of brief brace or cast immobilization with a light compressive dressing to reduce edema. These fractures usually heal quickly with exuberant callus (Fig. 14-17). Prevention is best achieved by encouraging as much weight-bearing and activity as possible to stimulate the weight-bearing bones.

Of note, osteopenia and pathologic fractures in this population can rarely be secondary to metabolic problems such as renal osteodystrophy and even vitamin C deficiency.[71] Also, children with myelomeningocele can have physeal problems, including separation of the epiphysis from the metaphysis and spontaneous physeal arrest.

Charcot Arthropathy

Charcot arthropathy describes the breakdown of an insensate joint. The condition is typically heralded by swelling, erythema, and warmth of the joint. These signs are followed by joint instability, leading to subluxation and occasionally dislocation. With this instability, the joint surfaces fragment, creating osteochondral bodies. The first large study to examine the incidence and treatment of this condition in spina bifida was reported by Nagarkatti and colleagues in 2000.[72] In a review of 1600 patients from four major institutions, these researchers found 16 patients with a Charcot arthropathy, for an incidence of 1 per 100. We believe that this figure likely underrepresents the true incidence, because patients treated at children's hospitals are often lost to follow-up once they are older than 20 years.

Only community ambulators with a motor level of L4 or below and a sensory level of L4 or L5 have Charcot joints. The ankle was found by Nagarkatti and colleagues to be the joint most commonly involved, commonly followed by the knee and hip. Treatment consists of orthotic modification. Arthrodesis is to be avoided in this population because the results tend to be poor. Nagarkatti and colleagues concluded that the best results were achieved by brace modification in patients in whom the diagnosis was made early. Therefore, they recommended a high index of suspicion for Charcot arthropathy in community ambulators with a low lumbar neurologic level. In patients with myelomeningocele who present with red, swollen joints, the diagnosis of Charcot arthropathy should be considered (in addition to fracture) and ruled out.

FUTURE CHALLENGES

Since the mid-1970s, great strides have been made in the treatment of spina bifida, most notably with the successful prevention of many thousands of cases[12] and the promise of success for fetal surgery in this population.[25] However, all treatment is only a reaction to the symptoms of the disease. There is no cure for spina bifida, because we are unable as yet to repair spinal cord lesions or reconnect the spinal cord to the peripheral nervous system. This simple fact underlies the three-tiered approach to the future treatment of this disease recommended here.

First, the most effective "treatment" is to prevent it in the first place. The fact that adequate levels of maternal folic acid from the time of conception through the formation of the central nervous system can prevent neural tube defects such as spina bifida and anencephaly has been well established. That knowledge has been put to use, because maternal education and folic acid enrichment of grains have resulted in a significant drop in the incidence of neural tube defects in this country and around the world. Identification of other risk factors, if they exist, could similarly further reduce the incidence of the disorder.

Second, we need to better identify the best way to care for children born with spina bifida and to support their families. Our surgical indications are constantly evolving, and the establishment of the multidisciplinary clinic has improved both the quality and length of life for these children. Further clinical research with an emphasis on patient-based outcomes and quality of life issues will help all health care professionals optimize the care given to these patients.

Finally, the possibility of actually curing these children should be addressed. Some advances have been made toward repairing spinal cord tissue, greatly facilitated by the publicity given spinal cord injuries through the tragic accident of American actor Christopher Reeve. This research could potentially be applied to children with congenital spinal cord or neural tube defects, enabling us for the first time to actually treat the disease instead of just the symptoms.

SUMMARY

Spina bifida is a complex spectrum of diseases most typically affecting the caudal end of the spinal cord. Depending on the location of the lesion and other comorbidities, the clinical picture varies from that of an intellectually normal child who is a community ambulator and requires no assistive devices to the complete paraplegic with hydrocephaly, severe cognitive defects, and impaired use of the arms. We are currently unable to treat the underlying disease. But treating children with spina bifida in a multidisciplinary clinic achieves the best care for their problems, be they neurosurgical, urologic, or nursing related. Orthopaedic surgery is often required to realign the limbs or spine into a functional position, one that can often be held with the assistance of an orthotic. Great care must be taken with the insensate skin of such children, for whom decubitus ulcers are a major preventable source of morbidity.

MAJOR POINTS

There is strong evidence supporting the role of folic acid in reducing neural tube defects. Women considering pregnancy should be strongly encouraged to take supplements before they become pregnant.

The *neurologic level* of a child with spina bifida, or any spinal cord injury, is defined by the distal most nerve root functioning in a *clinically significant manner*.

Universal latex precautions should be observed for all children with spina bifida from the time of birth. This practice has been shown to greatly decrease the incidence of latex sensitivity in this group.

A multidisciplinary approach is vital for the appropriate care of these children, who have multiple physical and emotional needs.

Early intervention programs have been shown to possibly improve physical and cognitive function and should be encouraged.

Orthoses play an important role in the management of spina bifida. They improve function by maintaining joints in an advantageous position and even permitting ambulation in young children with high-level lesions.

Limbs cannot be forced into orthoses. Orthoses are not used to correct deformity; rather, they are static devices designed to maintain a position that is passively achievable.

Pressure sores are best treated with prevention, but when they occur, they require a multidisciplinary approach involving nurses, plastic surgeons, and orthopaedists.

Any time bony resection is contemplated for treatment of a pressure sore, consider a realignment procedure instead, which may provide longer-lasting and more predictable results.

Magnetic resonance imaging (MRI) evidence of spinal cord tethering alone is not an indication for neurosurgical release. Nearly all children with spina bifida have MRI evidence of tethering, but release is usually reserved for those with neurologic deterioration.

A swollen red limb or joint in a child with myelomeningocele is a fracture until proven otherwise.

Evidence now suggests that fetal surgery to close the neural tube may reduce the incidence of hydrocephalus and improve the child's neurologic level.

REFERENCES

1. Lary JM, Edmonds LD: Prevalence of spina bifida at birth—United States, 1983–1990: A comparison of two surveillance systems. Morbid Mortal Wkly Rep 45(SS-2):15-28, 1996.
2. Haddow J: Preventing neural tube defects: A major success story, with a chapter yet to be written. J Med Screen 6:169, 1999.
3. Blatter BM, Lafeber AB, Peters PW, et al: Heterogeneity of spina bifida. Teratology 55:224-230, 1997.
4. Seller MJ, Nevin NC: Periconceptional vitamin supplementation and the prevention of neural tube defects in south-east England and Northern Ireland. J Med Genet 21:325-330, 1984.
5. Riley MM, Halliday JL, Lumley JM: Congenital malformations in Victoria, Australia, 1983–95: An overview of infant characteristics. J Paediatr Child Health 34:233-240, 1998.
6. Carter CO, Evans K: Children of adult survivors with spina bifida cystica. Lancet 2(7835):924-926, 1973.
7. Laurence KM, Carter CO, David PA: Major central nervous system malformations in South Wales. II: Pregnancy factors, seasonal variation, and social class effects. Br J Prev Soc Med 22:212-222, 1968.
8. Pendleton HJ: Acute folic acid deficiency of pregnancy associated with oral ulceration and anencephaly. Proc R Soc Med 62:834, 1969.
9. Yates JR, Ferguson-Smith MA, Shenkin A, et al: Is disordered folate metabolism the basis for the genetic predisposition to neural tube defects? Clin Genet 31:279-287, 1987.
10. Folic acid for the prevention of neural tube defects. American Academy of Pediatrics. Committee on Genetics. Pediatrics 104:325-327, 1999.
11. Honein MA, Paulozzi LJ, Mathews TJ, et al: Impact of folic acid fortification of the US food supply on the occurrence of neural tube defects. JAMA 285:2981-2986, 2001.
12. Erickson JD: Folic acid and prevention of spina bifida and anencephaly: 10 years after the U.S. Public Health Service recommendation. MMWR Morbid Mortal Wkly Rep 51(RR-13):1-3, 2002.
13. Lindseth RE: Myelomeningocele. In Morrissy RT, Weinstein SL (eds): Lovell and Winter's Pediatric Orthopaedics, 5th ed. Philadelphia, Lippincott Williams & Wilkins, 2001, pp 601-632.
14. Lorber J: Selective treatment of myelomeningocele: To treat or not to treat? Pediatrics 53:307-308, 1974.
15. Hoeman SP: Primary care for children with spina bifida. Nurse Pract 22:60-62, 65-72, 1997.
16. Rudeberg A, Donati F, Kaiser G: Psychosocial aspects in the treatment of children with myelomeningocele: An assessment after a decade. Eur J Pediatr 154(Suppl 4):S85-S89, 1995.

17. Phillips D: Orthotics. In Broughton N, Menelaus M (eds): Menelaus' Orthopaedic Management of Spina Bifida Cystica. Philadelphia, WB Saunders, 1998, pp 67-76.

18. Madersbacher H: Neurogenic bladder dysfunction in patients with myelomeningocele. Curr Opin Urol 12: 469-472, 2002.

19. Urological management of spina bifida (including management of urinary tract infections). Aust Fam Physician 31:84-87, 2002.

20. Rintoul NE, Sutton LN, Hubbard AM, et al: A new look at myelomeningoceles: Functional level, vertebral level, shunting, and the implications for fetal intervention. Pediatrics 109:409-413, 2002.

21. Michejda M: Intrauterine treatment of spina bifida: Primate model. Z Kinderchir 39:259-261, 1984.

22. Brunelli G, Brunelli F: Experimental foetal microsurgery as related to myelomeningocele. Microsurgery 5:24-29, 1984.

23. Meuli M, Meuli-Simmen C, Yingling CD, et al: In utero repair of experimental myelomeningocele saves neurological function at birth. J Pediatr Surg 31:397-402, 1996.

24. Adzick NS, Sutton LN, Crombleholme TM, et al: Successful fetal surgery for spina bifida. Lancet 352(9141):1675-1676, 1998.

25. Bruner JP, Tulipan N, Paschall RL, et al: Fetal surgery for myelomeningocele and the incidence of shunt-dependent hydrocephalus. JAMA 282:1819-1825, 1999.

26. Alenius H, Palosuo T, Kelly K, et al: IgE reactivity to 14-kD and 27-kD natural rubber proteins in latex-allergic children with spina bifida and other congenital anomalies. Int Arch Allergy Immunol 102:61-66, 1993.

27. Degenhardt P, Golla S, Wahn F, et al: Latex allergy in pediatric surgery is dependent on repeated operations in the first year of life. J Pediatr Surg 36:1535-1539, 2001.

28. Nieto A, Mazon A, Pamies R, et al: Efficacy of latex avoidance for primary prevention of latex sensitization in children with spina bifida. J Pediatr 140:370-372, 2002.

29. Anderson TE, Drummond DS, Breed AL, et al: Malignant hyperthermia in myelomeningocele: A previously unreported association. J Pediatr Orthop 1:401-403, 1981.

30. Turner A: Hand function in children with myelomeningocele. J Bone Joint Surg Br 67:268-272, 1985.

31. Mazur JM, Menelaus MB, Hudson I, et al: Hand function in patients with spina bifida cystica. J Pediatr Orthop 6:442-447, 1986.

32. Abery CA, Galvin JL: Physiotherapy and occupational therapy. In Broughton N, Menelaus M (eds): Menelaus' Orthopaedic Management of Spina Bifida Cystica. Philadelphia, WB Saunders, 1998, pp 77-93.

33. Broughton NS, Graham G, Menelaus MB: The high incidence of foot deformity in patients with high-level spina bifida. J Bone Joint Surg Br 76:548-550, 1994.

34. Bliss DG, Menelaus MB: The results of transfer of the tibialis anterior to the heel in patients who have a myelomeningocele. J Bone Joint Surg Am 68:1258-1264, 1986.

35. Fraser RK, Hoffman EB: Calcaneus deformity in the ambulant patient with myelomeningocele. Bone Joint Surg Br 73:994-997, 1991.

36. Janda JP, Skinner SR, Barto PS: Posterior transfer of tibialis anterior in low-level myelodysplasia. Dev Med Child Neurol 26:100-103, 1984.

37. Drennan JC, Sharrard WJ: The pathological anatomy of convex pes valgus. J Bone Joint Surg Br 53:455-461, 1971.

38. Malhotra D, Puri R, Owen R: Valgus deformity of the ankle in children with spina bifida aperta. J Bone Joint Surg Br 66:381-385, 1984.

39. Fraser RK, Menelaus MB: The management of tibial torsion in patients with spina bifida. J Bone Joint Surg Br 75:495-497, 1993.

40. Williams JJ, Graham GP, Dunne KB, et al: Late knee problems in myelomeningocele. J Pediatr Orthop 13:701-703, 1993.

41. Greene WB: Treatment of hip and knee problems in myelomeningocele. Instr Course Lect 48:563-574, 1999.

42. Menelaus M: The knee. In Broughton N, Menelaus M (eds): Menelaus' Orthopaedic Management of Spina Bifida Cystica. Philadelphia, WB Saunders, 1998, pp 129-134.

43. Sandhu PS, Broughton NS, Menelaus MB: Tenotomy of the ligamentum patellae in spina bifida: Management of limited flexion range at the knee. J Bone Joint Surg Br 77:832-833, 1995.

44. Broughton NS, Menelaus MB, Cole WG, et al: The natural history of hip deformity in myelomeningocele. J Bone Joint Surg Br 75:760-763, 1993.

45. Mazur JM, Shurtleff D, Menelaus M, et al: Orthopaedic management of high-level spina bifida: Early walking compared with early use of a wheelchair. J Bone Joint Surg Am 71:56-61, 1989.

46. Lee EH, Carroll NC: Hip stability and ambulatory status in myelomeningocele. J Pediatr Orthop 5:522-527, 1985.

47. Bazih J, Gross RH: Hip surgery in the lumbar level myelomeningocele patient. J Pediatr Orthop 1:405-411, 1981.

48. Broughton N: The hip. In Broughton N, Menelaus M (eds): Menelaus' Orthopaedic Management of Spina Bifida Cystica. Philadelphia, WB Saunders, 1998, pp 135-144.

49. Tosi LL, Buck BD, Nason SS, et al: Dislocation of hip in myelomeningocele. The McKay hip stabilization. J Bone Joint Surg Am 78:664-673, 1996.

50. Breed AL, Healy PM: The midlumbar myelomeningocele hip: mechanism of dislocation and treatment. J Pediatr Orthop 2:15-24, 1982.

51. Trivedi J, Thomson JD, Slakey JB, et al: Clinical and radiographic predictors of scoliosis in patients with myelomeningocele. J Bone Joint Surg Am 84:1389-1394, 2002.

52. Samuelsson L, Eklof O: Scoliosis in myelomeningocele. Acta Orthop Scand 59:122-127, 1988.

53. Bowman RM, McLone DG, Grant JA, et al: Spina bifida outcome: A 25-year prospective. Pediatr Neurosurg 34: 114-120, 2001.

54. Banta JV, Park SM: Improvement in pulmonary function in patients having combined anterior and posterior spine fusion for myelomeningocele scoliosis. Spine 8:765-770, 1983.

55. Carstens C, Paul K, Niethard FU, et al: Effect of scoliosis surgery on pulmonary function in patients with myelomeningocele. J Pediatr Orthop 11:459-464, 1991.

56. Muller EB, Nordwall A: Brace treatment of scoliosis in children with myelomeningocele. Spine 19:151-155, 1994.

57. Banit DM, Iwinski HJ Jr, Talwalkar V, et al: Posterior spinal fusion in paralytic scoliosis and myelomeningocele. J Pediatr Orthop 21:117-125, 2001.

58. Stella G, Ascani E, Cervellati S, et al: Surgical treatment of scoliosis associated with myelomeningocele. Eur J Pediatr Surg 8(Suppl 1):22-25, 1998.

59. Geiger F, Parsch D, Carstens C: Complications of scoliosis surgery in children with myelomeningocele. Eur Spine J 8:22-26, 1999.

60. Parsch D, Geiger F, Brocai DR, et al: Surgical management of paralytic scoliosis in myelomeningocele. J Pediatr Orthop B 10:10-17, 2001.

61. Osebold WR, Mayfield JK, Winter RB, et al: Surgical treatment of paralytic scoliosis associated with myelomeningocele. J Bone Joint Surg Am 64:841-856, 1982.

62. Mazur J, Menelaus MB, Dickens DR, et al: Efficacy of surgical management for scoliosis in myelomeningocele: Correction of deformity and alteration of functional status. J Pediatr Orthop 6:568-575, 1986.

63. Torode I, Dickens D: The spine. In Broughton N, Menelaus M (eds): Menelaus' Orthopaedic Management of Spina Bifida Cystica. Philadelphia, WB Saunders, 1998, pp 145-167.

64. Samuelsson L, Bergstrom K, Thuomas KA, et al: MR imaging of syringohydromyelia and Chiari malformations in myelomeningocele patients with scoliosis. AJNR Am J Neuroradiol 8:539-546, 1987.

65. Hall PV, Campbell RL, Kalsbeck JE: Meningomyelocele and progressive hydromyelia: Progressive paresis in myelodysplasia. J Neurosurg 43:457-463, 1975.

66. Shurtleff DB, Goiney R, Gordon LH, et al: Myelodysplasia: The natural history of kyphosis and scoliosis: A preliminary report. Dev Med Child Neurol Suppl 37:126-133, 1976.

67. Eckstein HB, Vora RM: Spinal osteotomy for severe kyphosis in children with myelomeningocele. J Bone Joint Surg Br 54:328-333, 1972.

68. Houfani B, Meyer P, Merckx J, et al: Postoperative sudden death in two adolescents with myelomeningocele and unrecognized arrhythmogenic right ventricular dysplasia. Anesthesiology 95:257-259, 2001.

69. Winston K, Hall J, Johnson D, et al: Acute elevation of intracranial pressure following transection of nonfunctional spinal cord. Clin Orthop 128:41-44, 1977.

70. Barnett J, Menelaus M: Pressure sores and pathological fractures. In Broughton N, Menelaus M (eds): Menelaus' Orthopaedic Management of Spina Bifida Cystica. Philadelphia, WB Saunders, 1998, pp 51-65.

71. McKibbin B, Porter RW: The incidence of vitamin-C deficiency in meningomyelocele. Dev Med Child Neurol 9:338-344, 1967.

72. Nagarkatti DG, Banta JV, Thomson JD: Charcot arthropathy in spina bifida. J Pediatr Orthop 20:82-87, 2000.

Muscular Dystrophy and Arthrogryposis

RICHARD S. FINKEL
DENIS S. DRUMMOND

This chapter reviews inherited and acquired diseases of muscle that manifest in infancy and childhood, with an emphasis on general themes of presenting symptoms and signs, diagnostic issues, and common therapeutic concerns. We emphasize the impact of newer molecular genetic discoveries. Using Duchenne muscular dystrophy (MD) as the prototype, we offer a detailed discussion of its orthopedic management, with many of the points also applicable to other neuromuscular disorders.

WHEN TO SUSPECT A DISEASE OF MUSCLE

Identification of *hypotonia and weakness* in a patient should always prompt consideration of a neuromuscular disorder.[1] Multiple congenital contractures (arthrogryposis multiplex congenita) can be a result of a neuropathy or myopathy and warrants a neuromuscular evaluation.[3,5] Family history of a neuromuscular disorder may also prompt evaluation of a presymptomatic individual. Elevation of serum creatine kinase (CK) may be found incidentally; its presence suggests an underlying muscle disease, although modest elevations can also be seen in some neuropathic conditions.

EVALUATION OF THE CHILD WITH A SUSPECTED NEUROMUSCULAR DISORDER

The clinical examination should consist of a physical examination, a neurologic examination, and acquisition of the patient's history. The history should encompass the patient's developmental history and age at onset of symptoms, and should detail any related medical and functional impact (Box 15-1). The patient's biologic parents and siblings should be examined for any signs of weakness, handgrip or percussion myotonia, and ligamentous laxity; this procedure may yield a critical clue to the diagnosis of a genetically based disorder.

The *physical examination* should focus upon the *extent and distribution of hypotonia and weakness* in the trunk, limb, face, eye, and bulbar muscles. It is useful to consider neuromuscular disorders in two categories, genetically based and acquired. *Genetically based* neuromuscular disorders usually manifest in an indolent fashion with fixed weakness and delay in acquisition of motor skills (Table 15-1). *Acquired* neuromuscular disorders usually manifest as rapid or subacute progression of weakness and loss of motor function, often with significant muscle pain (Table 15-2).

Figure 15-1 illustrates the distribution of weakness in six of the more common muscular dystrophies.[6] It is important to search for related diaphragm weakness and

Box 15-1 Historical Points to Address in Patients with Suspected Neuromuscular Disorders

- Decreased fetal activity and risk factors of pregnancy or parturition (oligohydramnios, multiple fetus, breech)
- Age at onset of symptoms or when parents first had concerns
- Distribution of weakness
- Rate of progression versus a static process or one with slow improvement
- Presence of multiple joint contractures
- Early motor milestones
- Loss of skills?
- Decline in endurance?
- Muscle pain with simple ambulation or with extended exercise?
- Related musculoskeletal issues: scoliosis, contractures
- Dysphagia/aspiration and failure to thrive
- Potential cardiac involvement
- Possible ventilatory insufficiency and sleep apnea
- Family history

cardiomyopathy, though these disorders may be identified better on a chest radiograph and electrocardiogram (EKG) or echocardiogram. In children up to age 5 to 7 years, formal manual muscle testing of strength is often not reliable. Thus, the examination of the young infant focuses on functional indicators of weakness, such as the extent of head lag on traction from supine to sitting, "slip-through" at the shoulder girdle when the child is held vertically under the arms, and capacity to actively bear weight on extended legs. For the older infant and young child, the examiner considers sitting posture, ability to roll over and get to sit or pull to stand, gait, how the child rises from the supine to standing ("Gowers maneuver") (Fig. 15-2) or from a chair to standing, and stair-climbing (Fig. 15-3). Standard manual muscle testing on the 0 to 5 Medical Research Council scale (Table 15-3) and quantifiable measures of strength made with a handheld myometer can be used reliably in the school-aged child of normal intelligence. When used serially, quantified functional measures of endurance (e.g., time to walk or run 30 feet) can assess progression of disease and response to treatment.

When performing the physical examination, the clinician should keep in mind that some diseases (e.g., Duchenne MD, congenital myotonic dystrophy) are accompanied by cognitive delay or mental retardation. Muscle tenderness to palpation is a sign of acute inflammation (idiopathic or infectious myositis). In most pediatric neuromuscular disorders, deep tendon reflexes (DTRs) may be normal, reduced, or absent at the time of presentation and usually diminish as the disease progresses. Scoliosis is a common accompaniment of arthrogryposis, with a variable course depending on the underlying cause.[5]

Findings of the sensory examination are normal in a myopathy, dystrophy, pure motor neuropathy (spinal muscular atrophy), and neuromuscular junction disorder (myasthenia gravis).[1] However, they are abnormal in hereditary and acquired sensorimotor neuropathies.[7] The patient should be evaluated for mental status, occurrence of seizures, and other central nervous system (CNS) concerns. Table 15-4 summarizes *signs and*

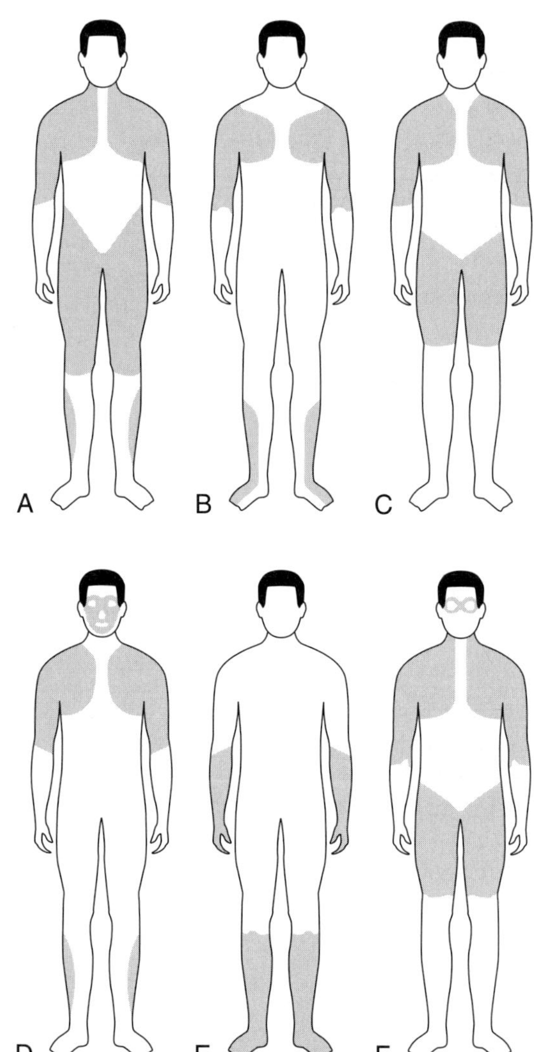

Figure 15-1 Distribution of prominent muscle weakness in different types of dystrophy, with shading indicating the affected areas: A, Duchenne and Becker; **B,** Emery-Dreifuss; **C,** limb-girdle; **D,** facioscapulohumeral; **E,** distal; **F,** oculopharyngeal. (From Emery AE: The muscular dystrophies (seminar). Lancet 359:687-695, 2002.)

Table 15-1 Selected Inherited Diseases of Muscle

Name	Mode of Inheritance	Age at Presentation (yrs)*	Rate of Progression†	Longevity
Muscular dystrophies (degenerative process) with progressive weakness				
Duchenne	XR	4	6 (100%)	20-30 yrs
Becker	XR	4 to 60	8 to variable	20 yrs to normal
Facioscapulohumeral	AD	3 to 44	Slow (20%)	Near normal
Limb-girdle category	AR>AD	2 to 30	5 to 60	Variable
Emery-Dreifuss	XR>AD	3 to adult	Slow	Variable
Congenital	AR	Birth to 2	Variable	0 to adult
Congenital myopathies (structurally abnormal muscle) with early onset weakness and static or slowly improving strength				
Myotubular	XR	Birth	Never walks	Weeks (years)
Centronuclear	AR/AD	Birth or infancy	Static to slow	Normal
Central core	AD	Birth or infancy	Static to slow	Normal
Nemaline	AD/AR	Birth to adult	Static to slow	Variable
Bethlem	AD	Infancy	Slow improvement	Normal
Myotonic disorders—mild weakness, stiffness and difficulty with muscle relaxation				
Myotonic dystrophy	AD	Teens onward	Slow (distal)	Risk of cardiac arrhythmia in adulthood
Congenital myotonic dystrophy	AD	Birth	Slow Improvement	25% early mortality
Myotonia congenita	AR>AD	Teens onward	Normal to mild	Normal
Periodic paralysis—episodic weakness				
Hypokalemic	AD>S	Childhood to 30	Attacks, hours to days	Normal
Hyperkalemic	AD	Childhood	Attacks ½–2 hours	Normal
Metabolic myopathies				
Glycogenoses				
Acid maltase deficiency (Pompe disease)	AR	Infant to adult	Rapid to slow	Infantile = fatal by age 2; adult = mildly weak
Myophosphorylase deficiency (McArdle disease)	AR	Teens	Slow	Normal
Lipid metabolism				
Carnitine palmityl transferase deficiency—exercise-induced muscle cramping, weakness, myoglobinuria	AR	Teens to adult	Slow	Normal
Mitochondrial myopathies—patterns of muscle weakness with CNS and systemic disease				
MELAS (mitochondrial myopathy, encephalopathy, lactic acidosis, and strokelike symptoms)	M>S	Infant-Adult	Variable	Variable
MERRF (myoclonic epilepsy with ragged red fibers)	S, M	Child-Adult	Variable	Variable
Kearns-Sayre syndrome (progressive ophthalmoparesis, ptosis, retinal degeneration, heart block, growth retardation)	S>M	Teen-Adult	Moderate	20–30 yrs

AD, autosomal dominant mode of inheritance; AR, autosomal recessive mode of inheritance; CNS, central nervous system; M, inherited through mother; S, sporadic mode of inheritance; XR, X-linked recessive mode of inheritance; >, more common than.

*Average age at time of diagnosis.

†Rate of progression = median years from diagnosis to nonambulatory state.

Adapted from Finkel RS: Muscular dystrophy and myopathy. In Maria BL (ed): Current Management in Child Neurology. Hamilton, Ontario, BC Decker, 2002.

symptoms of neuromuscular disorders and gives age at presentation.

Contractures may be evident at birth (Fig. 15-4) or may develop subsequently in the course of a neuromuscular disorder. Joint contractures are usually caused by weakness, an asymmetry of the muscle power at the joint, and gravitational forces. Thus, the presence of limitation in joint mobility on examination should always raise the suspicion of underlying weakness and imbalance of strength of the muscles at that joint. For example, with the equinus (plantar-flexion) contracture observed at the ankle, the calf muscles are noted to be

Table 15-2 Acquired Diseases of Muscle

Disease	Age at Presentation (years)*	Rate of Progression†
Idiopathic inflammatory myopathies		
Dermatomyositis	5-15 yrs>adults	Days to weeks
Polymyositis	Adults>children	Days to weeks
Infectious		
Viral		
Influenza	Children>adults	Acute, calf
Human immunodeficiency virus	Adults	Subacute, diffuse
Bacterial—usually tropical pyomyositis or in the immunocompromised host		
Staphylococcus aureus	All	Subacute, cramping
β-Hemolytic streptococci	All	Acute, sharp pain
Parasitic		
Cysticercosis (often asymptomatic)	All	Subacute
Trichinosis	All	Acute
Spirochetal		
Lyme disease *(Borrelia burgdorferi)*	All	Myalgias
Toxic		
Medication-induced		
Necrotizing (e.g., statins)	Adults	Subacute
Myalgias (e.g., ACE inhibitors, AZT, calcium-channel blockers)	Adults>children	Subacute
Glucocorticoid (iatrogenic)	2 yrs to adult	>4 wks
Critical illness myopathy—steroids + sepsis + nondepolarizing paralytic Rx	All ages	Acute
Endocrine—proximal weakness with myalgias, cramping, fatigue		
Hypothyroid	All	Chronic
Thyrotoxic	Adults>children	Subacute or chronic

ACE, angiotensin-converting enzyme; AD, autosomal dominant mode of inheritance; AR, autosomal recessive mode of inheritance; AZT, (azidothymidine), zidovudine; M, inherited through mother; S, sporadic inheritance; XR, X-linked recessive mode of inheritance; >, more common(ly) than.
*Average at time of diagnosis.
†Rate of progression = average years from diagnosis to nonambulatory state.
Adapted from Finkel RS: Muscular dystrophy and myopathy. In Maria BL (ed): Current Management in Child Neurology. Hamilton, Ontario, BC Decker, 2002.

functionally stronger than their antagonists, the dorsiflexors found in the anterior compartment of the leg. This difference results in an imbalance of strength with the foot gradually drawn plantar-grade and with tightness evolving in the Achilles tendon. Also, as children with an equinus contracture spend more time sitting and lying supine, gravity contributes to the plantarflexed position of the ankle, also contributing to the contracture.

The major causes of joint contracture are summarized in Table 15-5. Occasionally, contractures may result from a cramped environment in utero (e.g., a bifid uterus) or from an abnormality in type VI collagen.[5] Selected myopathies and dystrophies have distinguishing joint contractures relatively early in the course of weakness and can be an important clue in the diagnosis, as in Emery-Dreifuss MD (Fig. 15-5).

The history and physical examination enable a *differential diagnosis* to be made. It is useful to consider neuroanatomic localization, such as anterior horn cell, peripheral nerve, neuromuscular junction, muscle, and connective tissues when one is constructing a differential diagnosis for a patient with neuromuscular symptoms and signs. Table 15-6 gives examples of diseases for each category.

Features of hypotonia and weakness may also reflect CNS disorders and genetic syndromes.[8] In particular, newborns and infants presenting with hypotonia should be scrutinized for any related CNS disorder, dysmorphic features, and other organ system anomalies that would orient the focus of the evaluation toward a "central" etiology, metabolic disorder, or genetic syndrome rather than a "peripheral" neuromuscular one.[9] Limb weakness may mimic ataxia, and careful examination is needed to differentiate them. A focused diagnostic plan can then be pursued that establishes the specific diagnosis in the least invasive, most timely, and most cost-effective manner. The most commonly used diagnostic tests are summarized in the next section.

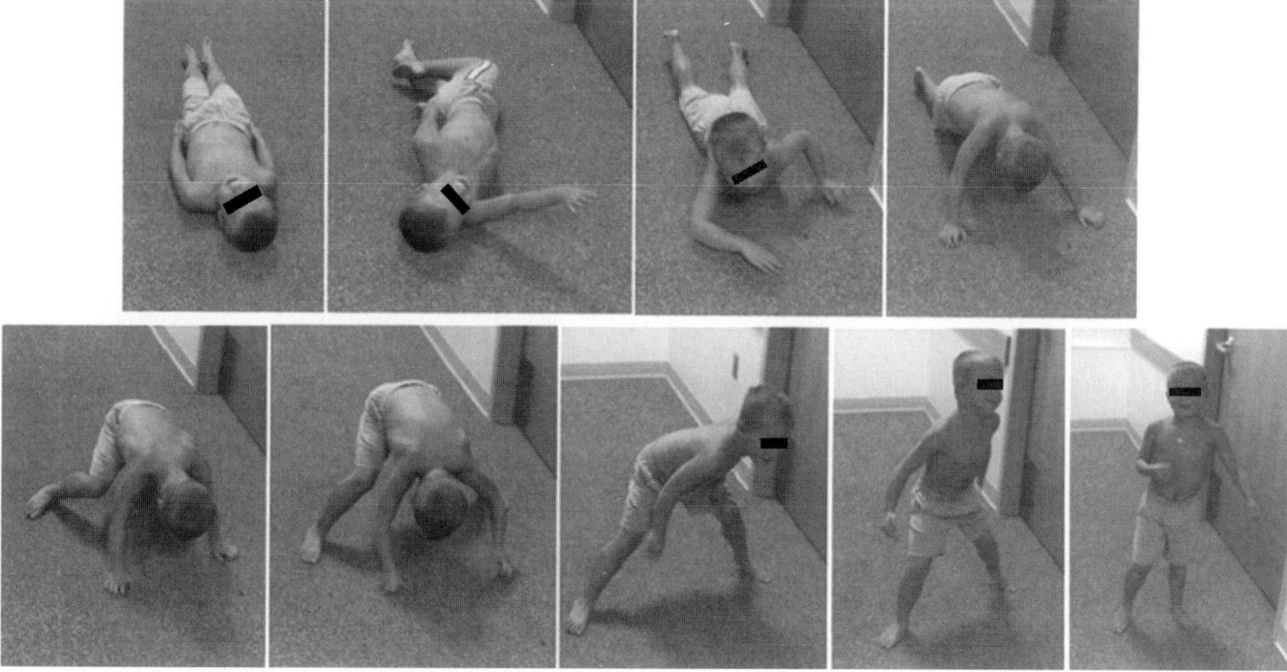

Figure 15-2 The Gowers maneuver demonstrates weakness of the pelvic-femoral musculature. The child lies supine and then is asked to stand up without assistance. In the fully positive response, the patient first rolls to the side, then prone, and elevates the trunk and buttocks by pushing up on the outstretched arms. Then the patient clasps the shins of the extended and widely spaced legs, and straightens the trunk into a vertical stance by "walking up" the legs with alternative hands and thrusting the upper torso and head backwards.

LABORATORY STUDIES AND DIAGNOSTIC TESTING

Serum creatine kinase determination is the most commonly obtained blood test to screen for a disease of muscle. The serum CK value is elevated in most myopathies and often 10- to 100-fold in some dystrophies. However, a normal CK value (≤250 IU) does not exclude a muscle disorder (e.g., some congenital myopathies and facioscapulohumeral dystrophy) or necessarily imply remission of myositis. Similarly, elevations to three times the upper limit of a normal CK range may represent a neurogenic disorder but can also be seen in otherwise healthy individuals (usually teenage boys with

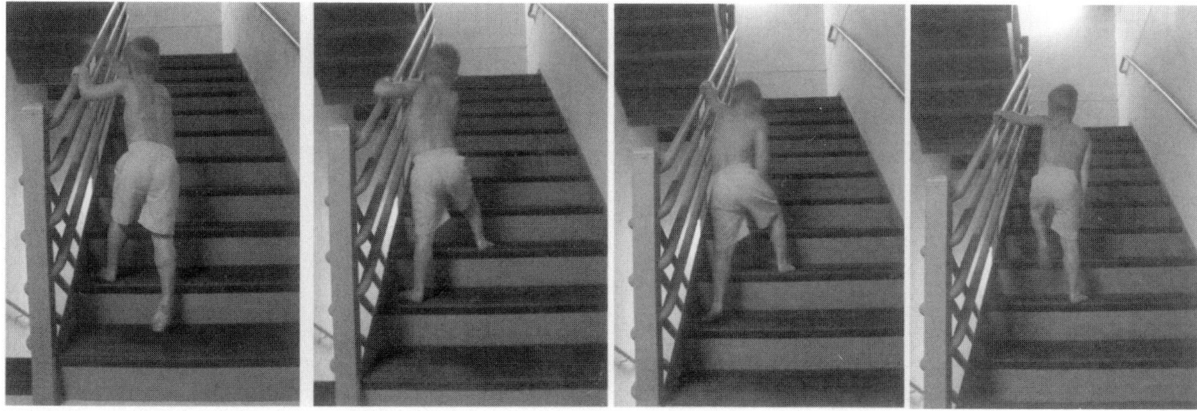

Figure 15-3 Six-year-old boy with Duchenne muscular dystrophy climbing stairs. Note the need to push off one knee and to pull up using the handrail to ascend one step at a time.

Table 15-3 The Medical Research Council Scale of Manual Muscle Testing

Grade	Description
0	No muscle contraction evident
1	Flicker or trace of muscle contraction
2	Active movement, with gravity eliminated
3	Active movement against gravity
4	Active movement against gravity and resistance
4–	Against slight resistance
4	Against moderate resistance
4+	Against strong resistance
5	Normal power

From Medical Research Council (UK): Aids to the Examination of the Peripheral Nervous System, 3rd ed. London, WB Saunders, 1986.

substantial muscle bulk). Vigorous exercise and contact sports may cause serum CK elevations, which should subside to normal after 2 to 3 days. Persistent elevation of the CK value above 1000 IU necessitates further evaluation for an underlying muscular disorder, even in the absence of specific symptoms or signs.

The serum *aldolase* value is often a more useful measure of disease activity in patients with myositis. *Blood lactate* and *pyruvate* and *carnitine* profiles are obtained when a mitochondrial disease of muscle is suspected. *Thyroid function studies* are important to consider, but hyperthyroidism is not often seen in children. When infectious causes are part of the differential diagnosis, complete blood count (CBC) with differential leukocyte count, erythrocyte sedimentation rate (ESR), cultures, and in some cases, specific antigen studies should be obtained. Toxic myopathies require special testing.

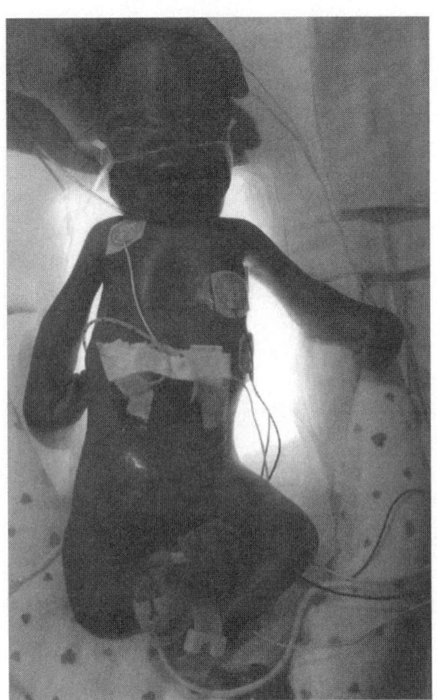

Figure 15-4 Arthrogryposis multiplex congenita. A premature boy (32 weeks gestation) with severe multiple congenital contractures and severe congenital neuropathy.

The impact of *molecular genetics* on the study of muscle diseases has been revolutionary. Since the cloning of the dystrophin gene for Duchenne and Becker MD in 1985, more than 50 genes for specific muscular dystrophies, myopathies, and ion channel disorders have been identified.[10] This development has radically changed the clinical approach to evaluation of a patient with a suspected muscle disorder, because specific diagnostic testing can, in many cases, establish a diagnosis

Table 15-4 Neuromuscular Symptoms and Signs by Age at Presentation[7]

Initial Finding	Newborn	Infancy	Childhood	Teen
Isolated hypotonia	C, G, L	C, G, L	C, G, L	L
Hypotonia and weakness	M, D, N, C, G	M, D, N, C, G	M, D, N, C, G	M, D, N
Contractures	M, D, N, C, G	M, D	M, D, N	M, D
Dysphagia-aspiration	M, D, N, C, G	M, D, N, C, G	M, N	D
Ventilatory insufficiency	M, D, N, C	M, D, N	M, D, N	M, D, N
Delay in motor milestones	N/A	M, D, N, C, L	M, D, N, C, G	N/A
Regression in motor skills	N/A	D, N	D, N, IM	D, N, IM
Loss of endurance-fatigue	N/A	M, D, N, L	M, D, N	M, D, N
Muscle pain or cramps	?	?	MM, D, IM	MM, D, IM
Elevation in CK enzyme*	D,	D, (N)	D, (N)	D
Presymptomatic identification	D, N	D, N		

C, central nervous system; G, genetic syndrome; IM, inflammatory or infectious myopathy; L, ligamentous laxity/connective tissue disorder; M, myopathy; MM, metabolic or mitochondrial myopathy; N, neuropathy (spinal muscular atrophy, peripheral nerve, neuromuscular junction); N/A = not applicable.
*Letters in parentheses represent variable findings.

Table 15-5 Joint Contractures

	Present at Birth	Evolves Later in Childhood
Single joint involvement	Idiopathic equinovarus (clubfoot) • Look for other joint involvement • Identify any underlying generalized weakness	Tethered spinal cord • Nerve root compromise leads to neurogenic atrophy • Often asymmetric
Multiple joint involvement	In utero constraint Brain dysgenesis Sacral dysgenesis and myelodysplasias Genetic syndromes (>150) Anterior horn cell disorders Hypomyelinating neuropathies Transient or congenital myasthenia gravis Congenital myopathies and muscular dystrophies Amyoplasia congenita	Genetically based: • Spinal muscular atrophy • Hereditary motor and sensory neuropathies • Myopathies • Dystrophies Acquired: • Idiopathic cerebral palsy (spastic diplegia) • Traumatic brain or spinal cord injury • Acute or chronic inflammatory demyelinating neuropathy • Dermatomyositis and polymyositis

without necessitating the traditional evaluation involving extensive laboratory testing, electromyography, and muscle biopsy. Traditional clinical nosologic entities have been redefined and new diseases discovered as new mutations are identified (e.g., the congenital muscular dystrophies and limb girdle muscular dystrophy [LGMD] categories).[11,12]

A single clinical entity may be caused by a mutation in one of a variety of genes resulting in a similar phenotype (e.g., nebulin, α-tropomyosin, and actin-α mutations in nemaline myopathy). Conversely, mutations within a single gene may result in different clinical phenotypes (e.g., ryanodine receptor gene mutations for central core myopathy and for malignant hyperthermia).

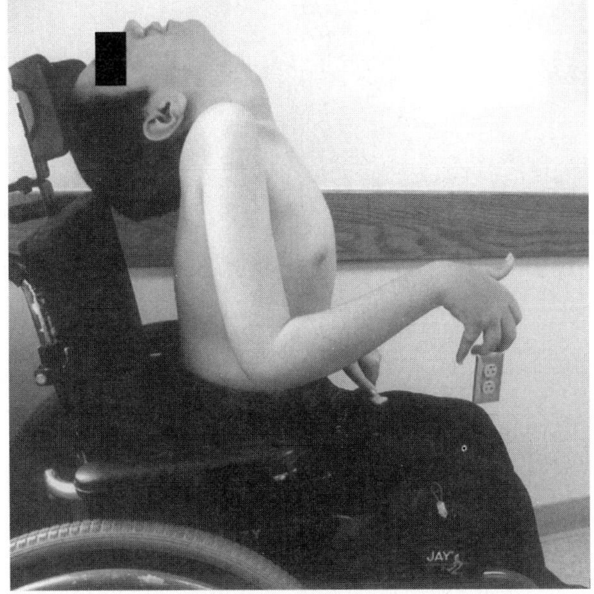

Figure 15-5 Emery-Dreifuss muscular dystrophy. Note the severe neck extension, elbow flexion, and wrist flexion contractures in this nonambulatory 19-year-old boy.

Genetic diagnostic testing for many neuromuscular disorders is now available from commercial and research laboratories.[10] This attempts to identify a specific mutation (deletion, duplication, point mutation, expansion of a triplet nucleotide repeat) within a gene from a peripheral blood sample or muscle tissue, or to identify an abnormal gene product. It is important to be aware of the limitations of these studies. For example, in Duchenne MD, a large-scale deletion in the dystrophin gene is identified in only 60% of patients through the use of standard polymerase chain reaction (PCR) primers. In deletion-negative cases, a muscle biopsy is then needed to obtain tissue that is examined for dystrophin protein on an immunostain and to measure protein quantity and size by Western blot analysis.

The role of *electromyography (EMG) and nerve conduction studies* has diminished since the advent of molecular DNA testing. They remain valuable, however, in differentiating an anterior horn cell neuropathy, peripheral neuropathy, or neuromuscular junction disorder from a primary disease of muscle.[1,7] Such testing is useful in defining electrical myotonia (in children older than 4 years) and may demonstrate characteristic features in certain myopathies and myositis.

The role of *muscle biopsy* has also evolved.[2] Evaluation by light microscopy remains important in confirming a suspected dystrophy or myopathy, particularly when clinical features and EMG findings are equivocal.[1] Certain congenital myopathies and myositis can

Table 15-6 Anatomical Approach to the Differential Diagnosis of Genetically Based and Acquired Disorders in Childhood*

Anatomic Localization	Hereditary Examples: Hallmark Features	Hereditary Examples: Typical Presentation	Acquired Examples
Anterior horn cell	Spinal muscular atrophy • Autosomal recessive • Hypotonia and proximal weakness in infants, limb-girdle weakness in teens • Tongue fasciculations • Areflexia • Normal intellect and sensation • Neurogenic electromyogram • Creatine kinase level normal to slightly increased • Deletion in Survival of Motor Neurons gene detected in about 98% of patients • Supportive treatment • Genetic counseling!	Type 1 (Werdnig-Hoffmann disease): • Diagnosis by 6 months • Never achieves sitting unsupported • Death usually by age 2 years from respiratory insufficiency Type 2 (intermediate form): • Diagnosis 6 months to 2 years • Sits but never stands unsupported • Variable course, often with long Plateau phases • Scoliosis Type 3 (Kugelberg-Welander disease): • Diagnosis 2 years to young adult • Walks but with proximal weakness • Static to slowly progressive course • May have long-term survival • Slowly progressive • Distal weakness and sensory loss • High arched feet and hammer toes • Foot orthotics and occasional surgery • Intrinsic hand wasting and contractures: OT, adaptive equipment, occasional tendon transfer surgery	Polio • Disease due to native virus is rare in immunized populations • Rare cases due to virulence from revertant mutation of attenuated oral live immunization virus • Can be due to other neurotropic viruses (enterovirus, West Nile virus) • Presents with gastrointestinal symptoms, followed by back pain and limb/respiratory/bulbar weakness; variable recovery. • Later decline in function ("post-polio syndrome") may occur decades later
Peripheral Nerve	Hereditary motor and sensory neuropathy (e.g., Charcot-Marie-Tooth disease) • Usually autosomal dominant, some recessive and X-linked • Demyelinating and axonal forms, characteristic nerve conduction findings • DNA testing available to confirm the diagnosis in the more common types		Acute inflammatory demyelinating polyradiculoneuropathy (Guillain-Barré syndrome): • Acute weakness, often ascending, may include respiratory failure and facial/bulbar weakness Chronic inflammatory demyelinating polyneuropathy (CIDP): • More indolent course, treated with immunosuppression
Neuromuscular junction	Myasthenia gravis • Usually autoimmune mediated • Congenital syndrome is rare • Fluctuating weakness and Muscle fatigue • May manifest as a medical emergency in respiratory failure	• Pure ocular, bulbar and limb forms versus generalized weakness • Characteristic repetitive nerve stimulation decremental response • Tensilon (edrophonium) test • Immune-suppression therapy • Thymectomy for generalized form	Botulism: • Neurotoxin from *Clostridium botulinum* • Infantile form is medical emergency with dysphagia, hypoventilation, generalized hypotonia, and weakness • Adult form from wound infection; may be less severe

Muscle	Refer to Table 15-1 Congenital myopathies: • Structural abnormality within the muscle fibers • May be weak at birth or "floppy baby" • Static or slow improvement usually • Many genes identified that encode for specific muscle cytoskeletal proteins Muscular dystrophies: • Degenerative process of muscle • Presents from birth to adult years, often with musculoskeletal complications and perhaps significant cardiac and pulmonary compromise • Detailed DNA and cellular protein analysis now available for most types of muscular dystrophy Myotonias: • Muscle stiffness or slow release of contracted muscle after sustained activity, usually with no or little weakness • Congenital form of myotonic dystrophy more severe Metabolic muscle diseases, variable presentation: • Hypotonia and weakness, cardiomyopathy, early demise (Pompe disease, early infantile form, acid maltase deficiency) • Hypotonia and hypoglycemia (glycogenosis, type 3) • Muscle cramping, weakness and myoglobinuria after exercise (McArdle disease, muscle phosphorylase deficiency; carnitine palmityl transferase deficiency type 2, a mitochondrial transport deficiency) Mitochondrial diseases and disorders of energy utilization: • Mitochondrial cytopathies may have diverse associated features, e.g., stroke (MELAS [mitochondrial encephalomyopathy–lactic acidosis–and strokelike symptoms] syndrome), myoclonic epilepsy (MERRF [myoclonus epilepsy with ragged red fibers] syndrome), ophthalmoparesis with retinitis pigmentosa (Kearns-Sayre syndrome), infantile hypotonia and encephalopathy (Leigh syndrome) • Lactic academia is a common feature	Refer to Table 15-2 Infectious, toxic, and idiopathic inflammatory myositis Endocrine-related myopathy
Collagen and connective tissue	Ligamentous laxity without weakness: benign hyperlaxity syndrome and Ehlers-Danlos and Marfan syndromes Ligamentous laxity with a related myopathy (Ullrich, Bethlem)	
Central nervous system	Congenital brain malformations Destructive processes: postinfectious, hypoxic-ischemic injury, posthemorrhagic Systemic metabolic disorders	
Genetic syndromes having prominent hypotonia	Trisomy 21 Prader-Willi syndrome Smith-Lemli-Opitz syndrome	

Adapted from Finkel RS: Muscular dystrophy and myopathy. In Maria BL (ed): Current Management in Child Neurology. Hamilton, Ontario, BC Decker, 2002.

also be diagnosed with the use of standard histochemical stains. Although specific diagnosis of some dystrophies and myopathies can be established solely by molecular genetic testing, muscle biopsy remains important for evaluating many metabolic disorders and should be performed at a center capable of obtaining and processing the specimen correctly to ensure satisfactory results.

Additionally, electron microscopy is occasionally useful in defining subcellular aspects of muscle disorders.

Sural nerve biopsy is occasionally needed to determine the nature of a peripheral neuropathy.[7] Also, the *ischemic forearm test* aids in the identification of a defect in glycogen metabolism in the evaluation of a patient with exercise-induced muscle cramping.

MANAGEMENT

Treatment of the child with a neuromuscular disorder is often best coordinated through a neuromuscular clinic with the combined help of the neurologist, orthopaedist, rehabilitation specialist, cardiologist, pulmonologist, and physical, occupational, and speech therapists. In selected cases, a gastroenterologist, nutritionist, geneticist, and social worker are needed as well.[15] The role of the primary care physician is critical in maintaining continuity and in coordinating the evaluation and treatment regimens. Once a specific diagnosis has been established, a long-term treatment algorithm can be formulated for the patient, one that is based on the knowledge of the natural history of the condition and notes the points at which particular issues are likely to arise. The treatment goals for patients with chronic neuromuscular disorders are summarized in Box 15-2.

Neuromuscular diseases give rise to a variety of symptoms that require specific treatments:

The treatment of *contractures* usually begins with passive range-of-motion stretching or serial casting. Surgical procedures may be needed to obtain optimal alignment and mobility.[13,16,17]

Cardiomyopathy and cardiac arrhythmia can occur in several muscle diseases and often warrants screening with ECG; if ECG findings are abnormal, echocardiography, Holter monitoring, cardiac consultation, or a combination of these measures is needed.

Restrictive lung disease resulting from weakness of the diaphragm and intercostal muscles may be a concern in an infant with a neuromuscular disorder or may arise insidiously in an older child several years after diagnosis. Respiratory complications may arise from a weak cough, preventing effective clearance of secretions and risking aspiration and atelectasis. Older children can be taught "air-stacking" breathing techniques, which, when used in conjunction with an abdominal thrust by a caregiver, can significantly increase the cough force.[14]

Box 15-2 Treatment Goals for Patients with a Chronic Neuromuscular Disorder

- *Maintain strength* via appropriate exercise, weight training, stretching and possibly the use of medication.
- *Promote safe ambulation* with orthotics, physical therapy, and orthopaedic management of scoliosis and contractures.
- *Maintain mobility* and independence, even when patient is not able to ambulate safely, with the use of a manual or power wheelchair or electric scooter.
- *Provide adaptive equipment to maintain independence in activities of daily living* at school and home, in recreation, and in employment settings.
- *Anticipate and prevent complications* (cardiac, respiratory, nutritional, musculoskeletal, and psychological) with regular physical evaluation, testing, therapy, medication, and surgery.
- *Ensure comfortable and functional* sitting.

Sleep apnea should be addressed in the history, searching for symptoms of noisy breathing or significant pauses in the breathing pattern when the child is asleep, headaches upon awakening, irritability, and excessive daytime somnolence. A sleep study and pulmonary consultation are then indicated.

Reliable pulmonary function tests can be performed by a trained technologist in a child older than 5 to 7 years who has no cognitive limitation. Measurements of maximal inspiratory-expiratory pressures, peak cough flow, spirometric parameters, and lung volumes can be made serially to monitor trends in a patient's disease and signal the need for a heightened level of concern.

Noninvasive assisted ventilation is often used when significant hypoventilation is present. Options are nasal continuous positive airway pressure (CPAP), Bi-PAP, In-Exsufflator, and occasionally a negative-pressure ventilator ("iron lung") or vest. An ethical dilemma may arise when intubation is considered and the prospects for future extubation are limited. Long-term tracheostomy and home ventilation are gaining acceptance in some settings; however, this measure requires enormous resources and commitment from the family. An annual influenza vaccination and the pneumococcal vaccination are recommended for all patients with chronic neuromuscular disorder and significant respiratory compromise. For infants, respiratory syncytial virus prophylaxis is often pursued in the winter months.

Adequate nutrition is essential to avoid muscle catabolism during times of illness and to promote optimal growth. Failure to thrive is a common concern in infants with dysphagia. A gastrostomy feeding tube, often with a fundoplication, is considered early for the infant whose oral intake is limited or when aspiration occurs.[15] For the child undergoing steroid treatment (e.g., some patients with Duchenne MD, those with dermatomyositis), it is important to address excessive weight gain and ensure adequate calcium intake.

DUCHENNE MUSCULAR DYSTROPHY

The dystrophic process of skeletal muscle associated with Duchenne MD is relentlessly progressive, leading to a breakdown of the muscle fibers and replacement of the muscle sarcoplasm with fibrofatty infiltrate. This process causes progressive weakness despite an incongruous increase in the bulk of the muscle mass, referred to as "pseudohypertrophy," that is a hallmark of this disease (Fig. 15-6). Typically, proximal muscles such as those around the shoulder and hip girdles are involved initially, followed by more distally placed muscles. The result is weakness and an inability to resist gravity, leading to frequent falls with difficulty in rising.

Contractures

In Duchenne MD and many other neuromuscular disorders, joint contractures evolve as weakness progresses beyond the grade 4 stage of muscle strength (less than active resistance; see Table 15-3). Contractures are especially common in nonambulatory patients.[16] Typically in patients with Duchenne MD, flexed, abducted, and externally rotated deformities of the hips develop, and the hips eventually become fixed in that position. Such patients experience flexion contractures of the knees approaching 90 degrees and stiff equinovarus contractures of both ankles. Often, one type of contracture influences body positioning and leads to the development of other contractures. For example, in a patient with flexion deformity of both the hips and knees who is lying supine in bed, hip abduction develops. The hip abductors shorten and the patient's hips become fixed in flexion and abduction—the so-called frog-leg position. This may make it difficult for the patient to sit comfortably in a wheelchair, the sides of which force adduction. Forcing the legs together in this manner results in discomfort in the area of origin of the hip abductors. Surgical release of the tight abductors may provide relief for some patients.

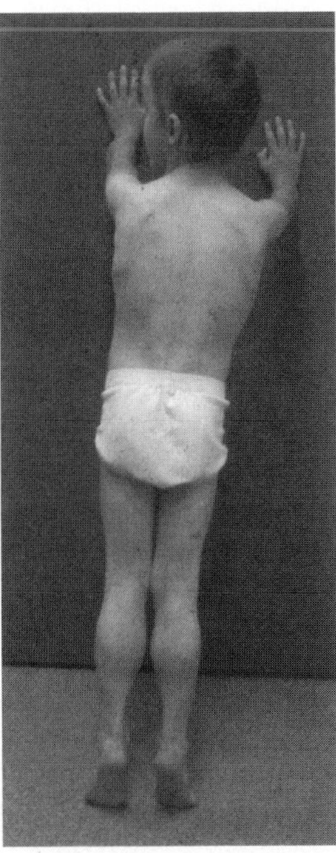

Figure 15-6 Boy with Duchenne muscular dystrophy. Note the marked calf hypertrophy and that the child is standing on his toes because of Achilles tendon contractures.

Gait and Posture

With progressive weakness around the hip girdle, walking becomes difficult, and falling with inability to rise becomes commonplace. The muscles responsible for standing upright, particularly the extensors of the hips and knees, become too weak to sustain an upright stance. The pelvis rotates forward, causing the knees to buckle into flexion, and the patient falls. Initially, most patients manage an upright stance with a compensatory posture marked by hyperlordosis of the spine (Fig. 15-7). This extreme lordotic posture shifts the patient's weight distribution so that the weight reaction line runs posterior to the center of rotation for the hips and anterior to the center of rotation for the knees (Fig. 15-8). This compensation is tenuous at best, as it is easily disturbed, leading to falls, a feeling of instability, and difficulty in rising.

Equinus of the ankles is helpful to the maintenance of the compensatory posture. It is not advisable to surgically correct the equinus in a patient at this stage of disease, because doing so would cause the patient to lean forward, leading to flexion of both hips and knees, failure of compensation, and falling. At this stage, a hindfoot release only allows standing with long-leg braces. Accordingly, heel cord lengthening or release is usually postponed to a later stage of disease.

Spinal Deformity

Spinal curvature results from progressive weakness of the paraspinal muscles and is a common component of many neuromuscular conditions (Fig. 15-9).[4,18,19,20] Scoliosis in boys with Duchenne MD is usually observed approximately 2 years after the patient becomes

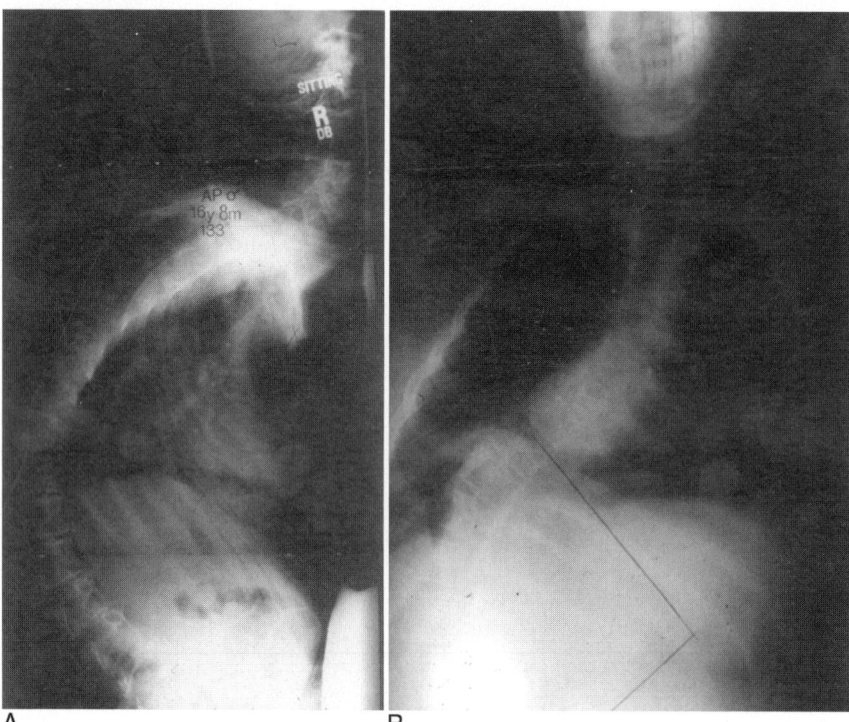

Figure 15-7 Lateral **(A)** and anteroposterior **(B)** radiographs demonstrating spinal deformity in Duchenne muscular dystrophy.

wheelchair dependent.[20] Initially, the curve is small and may be appreciated only on a radiograph; however, the deformity always progresses with time. Because there is some variability in the severity of the disease from patient to patient, and because the severity of the spinal deformity varies with the observed weakness, there are conflicting reports of the prevalence and natural history of scoliosis in this population.[13,20] These differences can be explained by the different time of follow-up reported in these studies. However, if observed long enough, virtually all children with Duchenne MD have a progressive spinal deformity, usually kyphotic scoliosis.[20] The annualized progression averages approximately 10 degrees. Invariably, the rate of progression accelerates with time, so that the annualized rate reaches 30 degrees or more. This phenomenon is frequently referred to as "spinal collapse." Spinal collapse reflects the state of the patient's weakness and course of disease. Over time, pulmonary and cardiac status deteriorate, and the spinal deformity becomes larger and more rigid.[13,20] Accordingly, surgical correction after the stage of spinal collapse is associated with a higher risk and greater difficulties than surgery performed before spinal collapse. Also, the reported blood loss with surgery in Duchenne MD after spinal collapse is higher than in most other types of neuromuscular scoliosis, although it varies with the stage of the disease at time of surgery.[20]

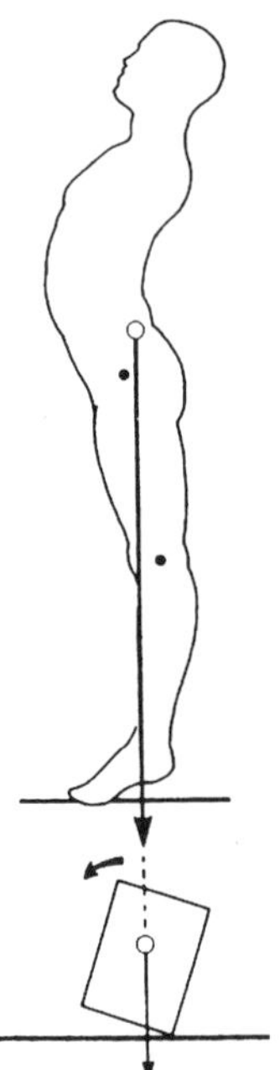

Figure 15-8 Axis of weight distribution in Duchenne muscular dystrophy. (From Siegel IM: Muscle and Its Diseases. Chicago, Year Book Medical, 1986.)

TREATMENT

The presence and evolution of scoliosis and joint contractures must be addressed with reference to functional limitation, medical complications, discomfort, and cosmetic issues.

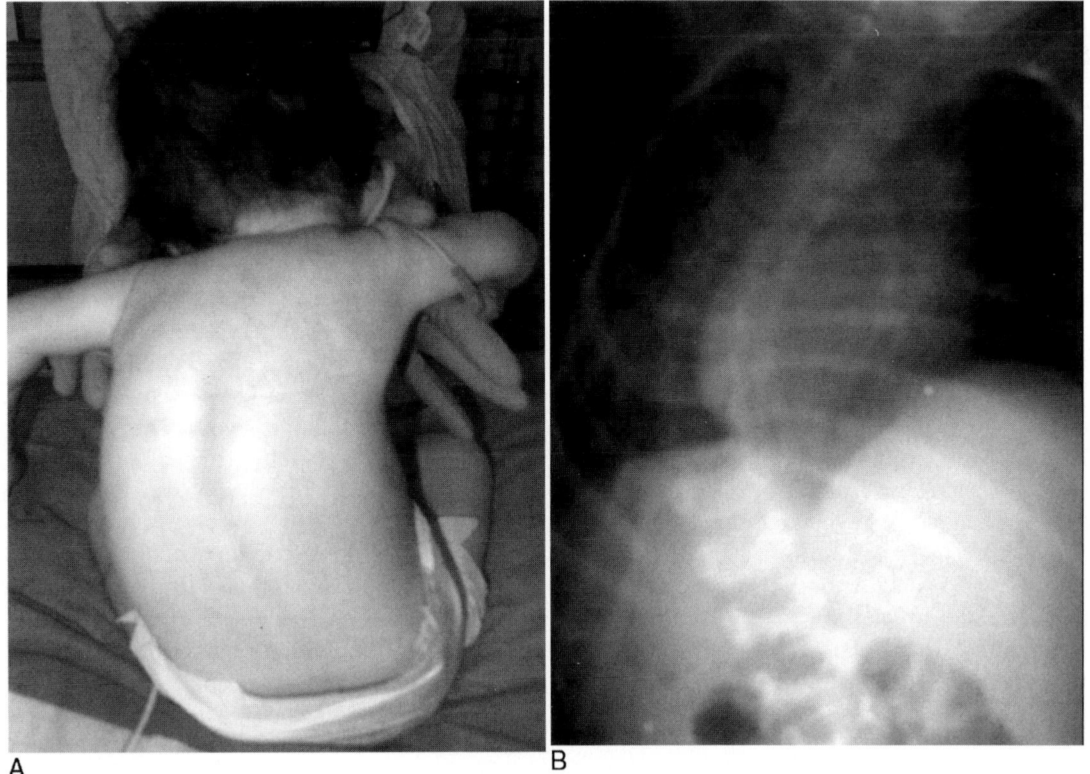

Figure 15-9 Neuromuscular scoliosis in a 9-month-old girl with spinal muscular atrophy type 1 (Werdnig-Hoffmann disease). A, Note the severe curvature of the spine when the patient is supported in a sitting posture. **B,** The corresponding chest radiograph.

Surgery

Limbs

The main goal of limb surgery is to prolong safe ambulation. The surgeon aims to correct the joint contractures so as to give the patient straight limbs, plantar-grade feet, and a stable stance.[16] Maintaining upright weight-bearing also preserves bone mineralization. However, there is controversy about the value of tendon release and transfer procedures in Duchenne MD, because after such procedures, locomotion requires added bracing, is frequently labored, and is still hazardous.[16] Shoulder girdle weakness prohibits the effective use of walking aids, and patients are unable to rise from a chair without help. Further, patients are often afraid of falling and may prefer the stability provided by a wheelchair. Weaker patients with more severe disease course seldom derive much benefit from aggressive surgery. Hence, limb surgery should be reserved for patients whose Duchenne MD has a less progressive course and for patients with Becker MD, who will derive more benefit from surgery.

Foot and Ankle

Some patients in wheelchairs find the equinovarus deformity of the foot and ankle bothersome; their feet get caught in the wheelchair platforms; they have difficulty with shoe wear; or they find the deformity cosmetically displeasing. Ankle and hind foot releases can be of value for such patients.

Frequently, severe contractures can be partially controlled by the use of prophylactic nighttime use of modified ankle-foot orthoses (MAFOs). These plastic braces help overcome the downward force of gravity. Although these devises do not eliminate the deformity, they can temporarily limit its severity.

A simple tenotomy of both Achilles tendons, performed early, can correct the ankle enough that the foot can be positioned flat or plantar-grade and can facilitate shoe wear. Later, a more aggressive approach is needed to correct severe equinovarus contracture, with release of all of the tight tissues in the posterior and medial aspects of the foot and ankle. Both of these situations require postoperative wearing of braces to prevent recurrence of contractures. However, in ambulatory patients with Duchenne MD, the equinus position of the ankle is helpful in maintaining balance with compensatory posture. Contracture release in these patients prohibits the compensatory mechanism, and patients are unable to achieve a balanced stance unless they are wearing braces that extend from the toes to the upper thighs. This issue is important in timing corrective surgery.

For ambulatory patients, particularly those with the Becker MD, the bilateral posteromedial release of the ankles is combined with a transfer of the tibialis posterior tendon from the medial side of the foot and ankle. The tibialis posterior tendon is rerouted through the interosseus membrane that runs between the tibia and fibula above the ankle, and attached to the midtarsus at the dorsum of the foot. This procedure achieves correction, a balanced foot, and some protection against recurrent deformity.

Hip and Knee

The release of contractures at the hip and knee are less commonly indicated because the contractures occur later in the disease course, once the goals for the patient have shifted from maintaining an upright stand to achieving and maintaining balanced sitting. However, patients who are unable to sit comfortably owing to contracted hip abductors may be treated with release of the tensor fascia lata and the anterior fibers of the gluteus medius. Generally, a simple bilateral release easily addresses this problem.

Scoliosis

The progressive nature of neuromuscular disorders leads to rigid and unbalanced spinal deformities, which eventually interferes with comfortable positioning in a wheelchair, reduces sitting tolerance to a few hours at a time and causes difficulty achieving comfortable positioning for sleep. Restrictive lung disease is accentuated on the concave side of the curve due to mechanical restriction in lung expansion. Surgical correction and stabilization with spinal instrumentation and arthrodesis, particularly if done before the curve becomes severe and the disease advanced, is the best way to handle this situation.

The use of a scoliosis brace is never definitive and does not avoid surgery, although it can slow progression of the curve and may gain some time to allow for somatic growth. Unfortunately, this is not a benefit in conditions like Duchenne MD, because the brace serves only to mask the problem while the disease continues to progress. If bracing is used, the seriousness of the situation becomes apparent later, when the patient has become weaker and the risks involved with surgery are greater. Further, brace wear is often uncomfortable for the child and not well tolerated.

It is essential for the spinal surgery procedure to occur *before spinal collapse*. Because the natural history of scoliosis in Duchenne MD is so predictable, optimal timing of treatment of the deformity can be achieved with radiographic evaluations every 6 months beginning approximately 2 years after the child begins full-time use of a wheelchair. It is wise to recommend spinal surgery as soon as the curve reaches 30 degrees. Delaying surgery risks spinal collapse, which further complicates Duchenne MD by causing numerous associated health problems.

Preoperative Preparation

The minimum preparation for spinal surgery in a patient with Duchenne MD is as follows:

- Cardiac consultation to ensure the presence or absence of cardiomyopathy and mitral valve prolapse and to assess the risk of cardiac failure. An echocardiogram and EKG should be included in this investigation.
- Pulmonary evaluation to determine the patient's pulmonary function, risk for pulmonary infection, and potential ventilation needs. This consists of a chest radiograph and pulmonary function tests, including measurements of pulmonary volumes and blood gases.
- Because of the tendency of children with Duchenne MD to bleed more than most other children, coagulopathy should be ruled out, and plenty of blood should be on hand for surgery.

Experienced anesthesiologists and critical care physicians are needed to help manage the patient during and after surgery. These children are at high risk for cardiac and pulmonary complications and should be treated only in tertiary care centers.

Surgical Procedure

The surgical approach for spinal correction is best made through a midline posterior exposure. A segmental spinal instrumentation, which attaches the vertebrae to two rods, is placed on either side of the midline of the spine. At the same time, a spinal arthrodesis or fusion is performed through the facet joints by addition of bone graft or graft substitute. Securing the purchase of the implants through multiple sites of attachment provides load sharing and stability. This maneuver ensures that there will be little postoperative loss of correction and enhances the chance of obtaining a solid arthrodesis. A brace is not required postoperatively with the biomechanical stability afforded by the segmental spinal instrumentation construct.

One topic of controversy for this procedure concerns whether the instrumentation should be extended to the sacrum and pelvis or stopped at L4. Champions of stopping the instrumentation short claim results in all but a few patients are similar to those reported by surgeons who extend the instrumentation. Additionally, shortened instrumentation saves about an hour of surgery and therefore reduces associated blood loss. Those who instrument the whole spine claim that doing so better ensures no further loss of correction of the scoliosis or the pelvic obliquity, thereby reducing the risk of associated unbalanced sitting. These surgeons also note that patients are generally at their healthiest at the time of the index surgery. Thus, taking the time to instrument the entire spine is necessary to ensure correction and avoid revision surgery at a later time—not a trivial undertaking. We subscribe to the belief that the initial correction should be extended to the sacrum and pelvis.

Equinus of the ankle plays an important role in maintaining the compensatory posture, helping to position the weight reaction line anterior to the knees. Disruption of the fragile compensatory posture causes the patient to fall. Physicians are cautioned to carefully consider all benefits and risks that a given procedure may incorporate. For example, an ill-advised release of the Achilles tendons to correct equinus disturbs this tenuous relationship of position and balance, resulting in a shift of the weight reaction line posterior to the knees. This causes the knees to flex and the patient to fall. The only way the patient can maintain an upright stance after heel cord release is by wearing a long leg brace, also known as a knee-ankle-foot orthosis (KAFO). Thus, if bracing is to be avoided at this time, it is wise to postpone hind foot release until the patient will accept the braces.

Nonoperative Management

Physical therapy with passive range of motion is particularly important for the patient with acute weakness and evolution of contractures, such as in severe dermatomyositis. For patients with slowly progressing weakness, the therapist can instruct caregivers in stretching techniques and can guide the family in appropriate activity modification (e.g., swimming, horseback riding, and adapted skiing). Fitting orthotics or braces and addressing mobility options (e.g., scooter, power chair) are also the specialized tasks of the physiatrist and physical therapist.

The role of *exercise and weight training* in patients with neuromuscular disorders is difficult to generalize because of the competing goals of augmenting strength in remaining healthy muscle tissue and minimizing accentuation of damage to vulnerable diseased fibers. The aims of such training are to increase strength and endurance, enhance aerobic capacity, maximize independent daily function, and promote inclusion of patients in sports and peer activities. Variables to consider in the design of an exercise regimen are (1) appropriate load for the level of weakness of the muscle being exercised, (2) intensity of the workout (i.e., number of repetitions and total work done), (3) rest periods between exercise sessions, (4) avoidance of overuse of the joints, and (5) stretching of contractures before exercising. Isotonic exercise with more concentric than eccentric activity is usually recommended. Isometric exercise (muscle contraction without joint movement) is helpful when there is related joint involvement, as in dermatomyositis, but should be curtailed during an active flare of disease activity. In general, the more sudden the evolution of the weakness, the more frequent and less intense the workout should be and the greater the emphasis put on stretching. Patients can also pursue aerobic exercise, but caution must be maintained for the patient with a cardiac or pulmonary condition. Low-resistance activity such as "spinning" on a stationary bicycle is often tolerated even when by patients with significant weakness. A supervised program with a trained therapist or experienced neuromuscular physiatrist is highly recommended to individualize the exercise regimen and to modify it as the course of disease evolves.

The *occupational therapist* addresses limitations in fine motor skills and related activities of daily living (dressing, bathing, toileting, food preparation, eating). Evaluation of the patient's home and school settings is often needed to ensure that proper adaptive equipment and safety devices are obtained.

The *speech therapist* evaluates oral-motor function related to feeding and speech limitation. In extreme cases in which speech is not possible, augmentative communication devices can facilitate communication.

Constipation is a common in patients with abdominal wall weakness and limited fluid intake. This complication must be treated vigorously with adequate fluid intake and the use of fruit juices, senna-based herbal tea or granules, mineral oil preparations, or an occasional suppository.

The *risk of malignant hyperthermia* in patients with certain muscle diseases when they undergo anesthesia must be recorded prominently in the patient's chart. The family should also be counseled about this issue.

The patient with a muscular dystrophy needs *psychosocial support* at home, at school, and in the community. The best resources are the clinic nurse and social worker, who can inquire about these issues when meeting with patients and identify local services. A representative of the Muscular Dystrophy Association (MDA) often attends MDA-sponsored neuromuscular clinics and offers additional resources. Several other focused support groups have evolved to provide current information on the diagnosis, treatment options, and research news for their particular issue (The Parent Project, for example, for Duchenne MD).

Medications

Corticosteroids have been demonstrated to slow the rate of progression of weakness in Duchenne MD and also transiently improve strength in some cases. The optimal dosage of prednisone is 0.75 mg/kg/day, although other regimens have also been proposed—1.5 mg/kg/ qod, 0.75 mg/kg on only the first 10 days of the month, and 10 mg/kg taken once a week.[21] Deflazacort, which is not available in the United States, is equally effective at 0.9 mg/kg/day and has fewer side effects. The decision to use long-term high-dose steroid therapy should not be taken lightly, and the parents should be counseled as to the short- and long-term side effects. A calcium supplement (1000 mg elemental calcium) and a multivitamin should be prescribed. The patient receiving such therapy should undergo screening for cataracts and bone density measurement annually and should be monitored closely for excessive weight gain, growth retardation, hypertension, glucose intolerance, gastrointestinal bleeding, and behavioral changes. Opinions vary as to the optimal time to initiate such treatment and whether to continue once the patient is nonambulatory. The role of steroids in preserving pulmonary and cardiac function has not been defined. The benefit of such agents to patients with severe Becker MD is probably similar, but for those with the milder form, the long-term side effects generally outweigh the benefits.

Oxandrolone, an anabolic steroid, may also slow the rate of progression of Duchenne MD. However, the use of steroids in other dystrophies is more empiric and occasionally beneficial. Prednisone is typically the first-line treatment for dermatomyositis and polymyositis. A low dosage, 10 mg/day, may be sufficient to achieve remission in a mild case, whereas in the patient with severe weakness and dysphagia, dosages of up to 2mg/kg/day divided bid are needed. Pulse intravenous methylprednisolone, 15 to 30 mg/kg every 2 to 4 weeks, may be needed in refractory cases, along with intravenous immunoglobulin (IVIG), azathioprine, methotrexate, cyclosporine, or cyclophosphamide. Albuterol has demonstrated limited benefit in fascioscapulohumeral muscular dystrophy.[4]

Supplementation with L-carnitine may be useful in patients selected mitochondrial myopathies, but use of this agent in other muscle diseases has not been demonstrated to be of benefit.

Creatine does increase muscle bulk and strength in exercising athletes but has not been shown to be of benefit in neuromuscularly weak patients. Glutamate, selenium, penicillamine with vitamin E, and allopurinol have all been used in variably controlled studies in Duchenne MD, without showing persuasive benefit. The use of such supplements in other neuromuscular disorders is empiric.

Figure 15-10 summarizes the principal clinical aspects of Duchenne MD and the related therapeutic interventions for each phase of the disease. The approach it describes can be adapted to other inherited and acquired muscular disorders, with adjustments for the age at onset, rate of progression, and extent of related musculoskeletal, respiratory, and cardiac issues. Specific orthopaedic management of the musculoskeletal issues is addressed in detail, and many of the principles apply to other neuromuscular disorders.[18]

FUTURE PROSPECTS FOR TREATMENT OF NEUROMUSCULAR DISORDERS

New hypotheses for the pathogenesis of a disease can be derived from an understanding of the role a particular gene plays in encoding for a specific structural protein or enzyme critical for normal muscle or nerve cell function. Specific adaptive mechanisms within the muscle or nerve cell can then be explored and possibly enhanced with the use of medication. The prospect of gene and stem cell therapies to correct the genetic defect and restore function is on the horizon; the first pilot human study using a viral vector in limb girdle MD was initiated in 1999. Understanding acquired muscle diseases continues to improve with current research (e.g., myositis-specific antigens in dermatomyositis). These newer tools allow for more accurate diagnosis and assessment of disease activity, thus enabling physicians to better counsel patients and their families about prognosis, genetic implications, and appropriate treatment options.

Typical Paradigm for Duchenne Muscular Dystrophy

Topic and *Intervention* — Time Frame in Years

Birth 2 4 6 8 10 12 16-20 20-30

1. Overview [pre-clinical] [diagnosis] [progression of disease.....................] [death..]

Genetic counseling: after the diagnosis has been established and when the parents are emotionally capable of addressing this topic.

2. Gross Motor Skills:
    Normal ....
    Slowly gaining ....
    Plateau phase ....
    Regression in gait ....
    Loss of ambulation ....
    Regression in upper limb function ....

Maintain mobility:
    Bracing ....
    Power chair ....

Adaptive equipment:
    Hydraulic lift for transfers, toileting ....
    Laptop computer ....

School adaptation:
School bus lift and classroom aide ....

3. Musculoskeletal:
    Scoliosis ....
    Joint Contractures
        heel cords ....
        tensor fascia lata ....
        hamstrings ....

Physiotherapy: ....
Bracing and/or tendon releases (variable) ....
Spinal fusion (variable) ....

4. Pulmonary:
    Restrictive lung disease ....
    Obstructive sleep apnea ....
Pulmonary function tests (and sleep study?) ....
Annual influenza vaccination ....
Pneumococcal immunization: at time of diagnosis
Non-invasive ventilatory support (variable) ....

5. Cardiomyopathy: ....
Annual ECG ....

6. Obesity: (variable) ....
Nutritional consultation ....

7. Learning Disability: (variable) ....
Psychoeducational evaluation, Individualized Educational Plan (IEP)

8. Depression: (variable) ....
Individualized and family counseling ....
Anti-depressant medication (SSRI) ....

9. Medication:
prednisone, deflazacort (?....................................)..(?.......................................)

Figure 15-10 Typical paradigm for Duchenne muscular dystrophy. See text for explanation. (Adapted with permission from Finkel RS "Muscular Dystrophy and Myopathy" in Current Management in Child Neurology, Maria BL [ed], 2002 BC Decker, Hamilton, Ontario.)

MAJOR POINTS

The hallmarks of a neuromuscular disorder (NMD) are hypotonia and weakness.

Musculoskeletal problems such as joint contractures and scoliosis are common features of many pediatric NMDs and may be an early or late component.

A focused history and physical exam can often suggest whether the neuromuscular features reflect a genetically based or acquired disorder. Duchenne MD serves as the prototype of a genetically based NMD and dermatomyositis for an acquired one.

The child with a NMD should always be evaluated for possible feeding, breathing and cardiac dysfunction. These issues are critical to address prior to any surgical procedure, to minimize the operative risk and ensure a favorable outcome.

The extent of functional motor impairment reflects a combination of weakness and musculoskeletal limitation and needs to be considered within the motor and developmental stage of the child.

Diagnosis of pediatric NMDs often requires detailed blood chemistry, molecular genetic, electromyography and/or muscle biopsy studies.

Treatment of pediatric NMDs should address maximizing motor function and promoting independence. This often requires the joint efforts of specialists in Neurology, Orthopaedics, Rehabilitation, Cardiology, Pulmonary and Genetics. Physical and occupational therapists are invaluable and a feeding program with a speech therapist critical for the child with dysphagia.

The optimal timing for initiating a medication or performing a surgical procedure is often handled by a team of physicians and therapists expert in Pediatric NMDs, such as through a Neuromuscular clinic.

With recent molecular genetic information defining the basis for many of the Pediatric NMDs comes the prospect of more targeted therapies, such as gene therapy. Meanwhile, prompt diagnosis and early management will provide effective genetic counseling and maximize the child's function.

REFERENCES

1. Finkel RS: Muscular dystrophy and myopathy. In Maria BL (ed): Current Management in Child Neurology. Hamilton, Ontario, BC Decker, 2002.
2. Anthony DC, De Girolami U, Shapiro F: Muscle Biopsy. In Jones, HR, De Vivo DC, Darras BT (eds): Neuromuscular Disorders of Infancy, Childhood, and Adolescence: A Clinician's Approach. Philadelphia, Butterworth/ Heinemann, 2003.
3. Hall J, Vincent A: Arthrogryposis: In Jones, HR, De Vivo DC, Darras BT (eds): Neuromuscular Disorders of Infancy, Childhood, and Adolescence: A Clinician's Approach. Philadelphia, Butterworth/Heinemann, 2003.
4. Shapiro F: Orthopedic Treatment: In Jones, HR, De Vivo DC, Darras BT (eds): Neuromuscular Disorders of Infancy, Childhood, and Adolescence: A Clinician's Approach. Philadelphia, Butterworth/Heinemann, 2003.
5. Hall JG: Arthrogryposis multiplex congenita: Etiology, genetics, classification, diagnostic approach, and general aspects. J Ped Ortho Part B 6:159-166, 1997.
6. Emery AEH: The muscular dystrophies [seminar]. Lancet 359:687-695, 2002.
7. Ouvier RA, McLeod JG, Pollard JD: Peripheral Neuropathy in Childhood, 2nd ed. London, Mac Keith Press, 1999.
8. Jones KL (ed): Smith's Recognizable Patterns of Human Malformation, 5th ed. Philadelphia, WB Saunders, 1997.
9. Darras BT: Neuromuscular disorders in the newborn. Clin Perinatol 24:827-844, 1997.
10. www.geneclinics.org. This website provides current reviews for many genetic conditions and lists where diagnostic testing can be obtained at commercial or research labs.
11. Mercuri E, Sewry C, Brown SC, et al: Congenital muscular dystrophies. Semin Pediatr Neurol 9:120-131, 2002.
12. Bonnemann CG, Finkel RS: Sarcolemmal proteins and the spectrum of limb-girdle muscular dystrophies. Semin Pediatr Neurol 9:81-99, 2002.
13. Birch JG: Orthopedic management of neuromuscular disorders in children. Semin Pediatr Neurol 5:78-91, 1998.
14. Bach JR, Zhitnikov S: The management of neuromuscular ventilatory failure. Semin Pediatr Neurol 5:92-105, 1998.
15. Tilton AH, Miller MD, Khoshoo V: Nutrition and swallowing in pediatric neuromuscular patients. Semin Pediatr Neurol 5:106-115, 1998.
16. Vignos PJ, Wagner MB, Karlinchak B, Katirji B: Evaluation of a program for long term treatment of Duchenne muscular dystrophy. J Bone Joint Surg 78-A:1844-1852, 1996.
17. McCluskey WP, Lovell WE, Cummings RJ: The cavovarus foot deformity: Etiology and management. Clin Ortho 247:27-37, 1989.
18. Merlini L, Granata C, Bonfiglioli S, et al: Scoliosis in spinal muscular atrophy: Natural history and management. Dev Med Ch Neurol 31:501-508, 1989.
19. Shapiro F, Specht L: The diagnosis and orthopaedic treatment of childhood spinal muscular atrophy, peripheral neuropathy, Friedrich ataxia and arthrogryposis. J Bone Joint Surg Am 75:1699-1714, 1993.
20. Oda T, Shimizu N, Yonenobu K, et al: Longitudinal study of spinal deformity in Duchenne muscular dystrophy. J Pediatr Orthop 13:478-488, 1993.
21. Wong BLY, Christopher C: Corticosteroids in Duchenne muscular dystrophy: a reappraisal. J Child Neurol 17: 183-190, 2002.

Index

Note: Page numbers followed by f indicate figures; those followed by t indicate tables; those followed by b indicate boxed material.

A

B

D

E

F

G

H

I

M

N

O

P

Q

R

S

T

U

V

W

X

Z